OTOLARYNGOLOGY

Volume 1
BASIC SCIENCES AND RELATED DISCIPLINES

Edited by

MICHAEL M. PAPARELLA, M.D.

Chairman, Department of Otolaryngology
The University of Minnesota

and

DONALD A. SHUMRICK, M.D.

Chairman, Department of Otolaryngology
and Maxillofacial Surgery
University of Cincinnati

W. B. SAUNDERS COMPANY – *Philadelphia* – *London* – *Toronto*

W. B. Saunders Company: West Washington Square
                          Philadelphia, Pa.   19105

                          1 St. Anne's Road
                          Eastbourne, East Sussex BN21 3UN, England

                          833 Oxford Street
                          Toronto, M8Z 5T9, Canada

Vol. 1 ISBN 0-7216-7058-X
Vol. 2 ISBN 0-7216-7059-8
Vol. 3 ISBN 0-7216-7060-1

Otolaryngology Volume 1

Print No.:   9   8   7   6   5

*This book is dedicated to the many American
otolaryngologists who, in the past few decades,
have made significant contributions to patient
care, research and teaching, thus helping to
establish otolaryngology as a regional specialty
with an ever-expanding scientific base.*

This book is dedicated to the many American otolaryngologists who, in the past few decades, have made significant contributions to patient care, research and teaching, thus helping to establish otolaryngology as a regional specialty with an ever-expanding scientific base.

CONTRIBUTORS

JOHN ADRIANI, M.D.

Professor of Surgery, Tulane University School of Medicine; Clinical Professor of Surgery and Pharmacology, Louisiana State University School of Medicine; Clinical Professor of Oral Surgery (Anesthesiology), Louisiana State University School of Dentistry; Director, Department of Anesthesiology, Charity Hospital, New Orleans, Louisiana

BARRY J. ANSON, Ph.D. (Med. Sc.)

Research Professor, The University of Iowa School of Medicine, Iowa City, Iowa; Robert Laughlin Rea Professor Emeritus of Anatomy Northwestern University Medical School; Honor List, Passavant Memorial Hospital, Chicago, Illinois

BERNARD S. ARON, M.D., D.M.R.T.

Associate Professor of Radiology, University of Cincinnati College of Medicine; Attending Physician in Radiation Therapy, Cincinnati General Hospital, Childrens Hospital, and Drake Hospital, Cincinnati; Consultant in Radiation Therapy, Veterans Administration Hospitals, Cincinnati and Dayton, Ohio

BYRON J. BAILEY, M.D.

Wiess Professor and Chairman, Department of Otolaryngology, University of Texas Medical Branch, Galveston, Texas

ABE B. BAKER, M.D., Ph.D.

Professor and Head of Department of Neurology, University of Minnesota Medical School, Minneapolis, Minnesota

JOHN D. BANOVETZ, M.D.

Clinical Assistant Professor, Department of Otolaryngology, University of Minnesota Medical School; Staff, Hennepin County General Hospital, Minneapolis, Minnesota

HUGH O. BARBER, M.D., F.R.C.S. (C)

Professor of Otolaryngology, University of Toronto; Head of Department of Otolaryngology, Sunnybrook Hospital, Toronto, Canada

ROGER BOLES, M.D.

Associate Professor of Otorhinolaryngology, University of Michigan School of Medicine, Ann Arbor; Active Staff, St. Joseph's Mercy Hospital, Ann Arbor; Consultant, Veterans Administration Hospital, Ann Arbor; Consultant, Wayne County General Hospital, Eloise, Michigan

PAUL B. BORGESEN, D.D.S., M.D.

St. Luke's Hospital and Medical Center, Phoenix, Arizona

JAMES F. BOSMA, M.D.

Chief, Oral and Pharyngeal Development Section, National Institute of Dental Research, National Institutes of Health, Bethesda, Maryland

K. GERHARD BRAND, M.D.

Professor, Department of Microbiology, University of Minnesota, Minneapolis, Minnesota

JACK BRUCHER, M.D.

Assistant Professor of Radiology, University of Cincinnati College of Medicine; Neuroradiologist, Department of Radiology, Bethesda Hospital, Cincinnati, Ohio

JOHN F. BRUGGE, Ph.D.

Associate Professor of Neurophysiology, University of Wisconsin Medical School, Madison, Wisconsin

HENRY BUCHWALD, M.D., Ph.D.

Associate Professor of Surgery, University of Minnesota Medical School; Attending Surgeon, University of Minnesota Hospitals, Minneapolis, Minnesota

RAYMOND CARHART, Ph.D.

Professor of Audiology and Otolaryngology, Northwestern University, Evanston, Illinois

v

ROBERT C. CODY, M.A.

Assistant Professor of Otolaryngology, University of Cincinnati Medical Center, Cincinnati, Ohio

JACK DAVIES, M.D.

Professor and Chairman of Anatomy, Vanderbilt University School of Medicine, Nashville, Tennessee

RONALD H. DIETZMAN, M.D., Ph.D.

Assistant Professor of Surgery, University of Minnesota Medical School, Minneapolis, Minnesota

JAMES A. DONALDSON, M.D.

Professor and Chairman, Department of Otolaryngology, University of Washington, Seattle; Attending Otolaryngologist, University Hospital, Harborview Medical Center, Children's Orthopedic Hospital, Seattle; Consultant, Madigan General Hospital, Tacoma, U.S.P.H.S. Hospital, Seattle, Washington

ARNDT JOHN DUVALL, III, M.D.

Professor, Department of Otolaryngology, University of Minnesota Medical School; Staff, University of Minnesota Hospitals, Consultant, Minneapolis Veterans Hospital, Minneapolis, Minnesota

GEORGE A. GATES, M.D.

Associate Professor and Head, Division of Otorhinolaryngology, University of Texas Medical School at San Antonio; Chief, Otorhinolaryngology Department, Bexar County Hospital; Staff, Santa Rosa Hospital; Consultant, Brooke Army Medical Center and Baptist Memorial Hospital, San Antonio, Texas

KENT K. GILLINGHAM, M.D.

Assistant Professor, University of Iowa College of Medicine, Iowa City, Iowa

ROBERT JAMES GORLIN, D.D.S., M.S.

Professor and Chairman, Division of Oral Pathology, University of Minnesota; Chief, Human Genetics Clinic, University of Minnesota Hospitals; Staff, University of Minnesota Hospitals, Mt. Sinai Hospital, Glenwood Hills Hospital, Hennepin County Hospital, Minneapolis, Minnesota

KENNETH N. HEHMAN, M.D.

Assistant Professor of Radiology, University of Cincinnati College of Medicine; Neuroradiologist, University of Cincinnati; Department of Radiology, Cincinnati General Hospital, Cincinnati, Ohio

WILLIAM B. HOFMANN, M.D.

Assistant Clinical Professor of Otolaryngology and Maxillofacial Surgery, University of Cincinnati; Assistant Attending Physician, The Christ Hospital; Staff, Bethesda Hospital, Our Lady of Mercy Hospital, Cincinnati, Ohio

RICHARD HONG, M.D.

Professor of Pediatrics, Department of Pediatrics, University of Wisconsin Medical Center, Madison, Wisconsin

DONALD B. HUNNINGHAKE, M.D.

Associate Professor, Departments of Medicine and Pharmacology, University of Minnesota, Minneapolis, Minnesota

THOMAS K. HUNT, M.D.

Associate Professor of Surgery, University of California School of Medicine, San Francisco, California

JOHN A. KIRCHNER, M.D., F.A.C.S.

Professor of Otolaryngology, Yale University School of Medicine; Chief of Section, Otolaryngology, Yale New Haven Hospital, New Haven, Connecticut

ICHIRO KIRIKAE, M.D.

Professor of Otolaryngology, Jichi University School of Medicine, Tochigi; Professor Emeritus, University of Tokyo; Staff, Jichi University Hospital, Tochigi, Japan

JAMES F. KOERNER, Ph.D.

Associate Professor, Department of Biochemistry, University of Minnesota Medical School, Minneapolis, Minnesota

FRANK M. LASSMAN, Ph.D.

Professor of Otolaryngology, Physical Medicine, and Communication Disorders, University of Minnesota Medical School; Director, Programs in Audiology and Speech Pathology, University of Minnesota Hospitals, Minneapolis, Minnesota

MERLE LAWRENCE, Ph.D.

Professor of Otorhinolaryngology and Director, Kresge Hearing Research Institute, University of Michigan Medical School, Ann Arbor, Michigan

RICHARD C. LILLEHEI, M.D., Ph.D.

Professor of Surgery, University of Minnesota Health Sciences Center, Minneapolis, Minnesota

DAVID J. LIM, M.D.

Associate Professor, Department of Otolaryngology, The Ohio State University College of Medicine; Director, Otological Research Laboratories, The Ohio State University College of Medicine, Columbus, Ohio

PAUL H. LOBER, M.D., Ph.D.

Professor of Pathology, University of Minnesota Medical School; Surgical Pathologist, University of Minnesota Hospitals, Minneapolis, Minnesota

RODERICK A. MALONE, M.D.

Assistant Professor of Anesthesia, University of Cincinnati School of Medicine; Attending Anesthesiologist, Cincinnati General Hospital, C. R. Holmes Hospital, and Shrine Hospital for Crippled Children, Cincinnati, Ohio

ROBERT L. MARESCA, M.D.

St. Luke's Hospital and Medical Center, Phoenix, Arizona

FRANK HENDERSON MAYFIELD, M.D.

Clinical Professor of Surgery (Neurosurgery), University of Cincinnati College of Medicine; Director of Neurosurgery, The Christ Hospital, Good Samaritan Hospital, Cincinnati, Ohio

BRIAN FRANCIS McCABE, M.D.

Professor and Head, Department of Otolaryngology and Maxillofacial Surgery, College of Medicine, The University of Iowa, Iowa City, Iowa

DONALD G. McQUARRIE, M.D., Ph.D.

Associate Professor of Surgery, University of Minnesota Medical School; Director, Surgical Research, and Chief, Head and Neck Surgery Section, Minneapolis Veterans Administration Hospital; Department of Surgery, University of Minnesota Hospitals, Minneapolis, Minnesota

JAY MELROSE, Ph.D.

Professor of Speech, Communication Disorders Area, University of Massachusetts, Amherst, Massachusetts

JOSEF M. MILLER, Ph.D.

Assistant Professor, Departments of Otolaryngology and Physiology, and Biophysics, University of Washington Medical School, Seattle, Washington

GEORGE J. MOTSAY, M.D.

Surgical Resident, University of Minnesota Hospital, Minneapolis, Minnesota

ARNOLD M. NOYEK, M.D., F.R.C.S. (C), F.A.C.S.

Assistant Professor of Otolaryngology, University of Toronto; Attending Otolaryngologist, New Mt. Sinai Hospital, Sunnybrook Hospital, Toronto; Consulting Otolaryngologist, Raycrest Hospital and Jewish Home for the Aged, Toronto, Canada

MICHAEL M. PAPARELLA, M.D.

Professor and Chairman, Department of Otolaryngology, University of Minnesota School of Medicine; Staff, University of Minnesota Hospitals, Minneapolis, Minnesota

G. O'NEIL PROUD, M.D.

Professor and Chairman, Department of Otolaryngology, University of Kansas School of Medicine, Kansas City, Kansas

CEDRIC A. QUICK, M.B., B.Ch. (Wales), L.R.C.P. (London), M.R.C.S. (Eng.), F.R.C.S. (Ed.)

Assistant Professor, Department of Otolaryngology, University of Minnesota School of Medicine; Staff, University of Minnesota Hospitals, Minneapolis, Minnesota

JOSEPH A. RESCH, M.D.

Professor, Department of Neurology, University of Minnesota Medical School, Minneapolis, Minnesota

FRANK N. RITTER, M.S. (OTOL.), M.D.

Clinical Associate Professor of Otorhinolaryngology, University of Michigan; Staff, University of Michigan Medical Center, St. Joseph's Mercy Hospital; Consultant, U.S. Veterans Hospital, Ann Arbor, and Wayne County General Hospital, Eloise, Michigan

KENNETH W. ROWE, Jr., M.D.

Associate Professor of Ophthalmology, University of Cincinnati College of Medicine; Chief Clinician, Ophthalmology, and Attending Ophthalmologist, Cincinnati General Hospital, Cincinnati, Ohio

WILLIAM HOWERTON SAUNDERS, M.D.

Professor and Chairman, Department of Otolaryngology at The Ohio State University College of Medicine; Staff, University Hospital, James Hospital, Ohio Penitentiary, Columbus, Ohio

LEE E. SCHACHT, Ph.D.

Supervisor, Human Genetics Unit, Minnesota Department of Health, Minneapolis, Minnesota

GILBERT M. SCHIFF, M.D.

Associate Professor, Internal Medicine, and Assistant Professor, Microbiology, University of Cincinnati College of Medicine; Director, Infectious Disease Division; Attending Physician, Cincinnati General Hospital, Cincinnati, Ohio

LEONARD S. SCHULTZ, M.D.

Medical Fellow, University of Minnesota Medical School; Staff, University of Minnesota Hospitals, Minneapolis, Minnesota

JAN SCHWARZ, M.D.

Associate Professor of Pathology; Associate Clinical Professor of Dermatology, University of Cincinnati College of Medicine; Associate Director, Clinical Laboratory, Jewish Hospital; Director, Laboratory of Mycology, Cincinnati General Hospital, Cincinnati, Ohio

DONALD A. SHUMRICK, M.D.

Professor and Director, Department of Otolaryngology and Maxillofacial Surgery, University of Cincinnati Medical Center, Cincinnati, Ohio

MELVIN E. SIGEL, M.D.

Clinical Associate Professor, Department of Otolaryngology, University of Minnesota Medical School; Chief, Department of Otolaryngology, Hennepin County General Hospital, Minneapolis, Minnesota

SOL RICHARD SILVERMAN, Ph.D., D.Litt., L.H.D., L.L.D.

Professor of Audiology, Washington University, St. Louis; Director, Central Institute for the Deaf, St. Louis, Missouri

JOHN McLELLAN TEW, Jr., M.D.

Instructor in Surgery (Neurosurgery), University of Cincinnati College of Medicine; Assistant Director of Neurosurgical Training Program, Good Samaritan Hospital, Cincinnati, Ohio

JUERGEN TONNDORF, M.D.

Professor of Otolaryngology, College of Physicians and Surgeons of Columbia University, New York, New York

GALDINO E. VALVASSORI, M.D.

Professor, Department of Radiology, University of Illinois School of Medicine, Chicago, Illinois

RICHARD L. VARCO, M.D., Ph.D.

Professor of Surgery, University of Minnesota Medical School; Attending Surgeon, University of Minnesota Hospitals, Minneapolis, Minnesota

JOHN J. WILL, M.D.

Professor, University of Cincinnati College of Medicine; Director of the Hematology Division of the Department of Medicine, Cincinnati General Hospital; Tumor Board, St. Elizabeth Hospital; Attending Physician, Cincinnati General Hospital, Cincinnati Veterans Administration Hospital, Drake Memorial Hospital, and C. R. Holmes Hospital, Cincinnati, Ohio

HENRY L. WILLIAMS, M.D., M.S.

Professor Emeritus, Otorhinology and Laryngology, Mayo Foundation Graduate School, University of Minnesota (Rochester); Professor, Otolaryngology, University of Minnesota Medical School; Consultant, Otolaryngology Service, Veterans Administration Hospital, Minneapolis, Minnesota

JEROME F. WIOT, M.D.

Professor of Radiology, University of Cincinnati College of Medicine; Director, Department of Radiology, Cincinnati General Hospital, Cincinnati, Ohio

RICHARD L. WITT, M.D.

Professor of Medicine, Director, Pulmonary Disease Division, Department of Medicine, University of Cincinnati College of Medicine, Cincinnati, Ohio

JUDAH ZIZMOR, M.D.

Director, Department of Radiology, Manhattan Eye, Ear and Throat Hospital; Attending Radiologist, New York Hospital, New York, New York

PREFACE

We, the editors, felt both honored and challenged when the Saunders Company invited us to prepare a new and definitive reference source in otolaryngology. The new book was to replace the classic Jackson work, *Diseases of the Nose, Throat and Ear,* which itself was one of the last in a proud line of tremendously influential books from the great Jackson Clinic (*Bronchoscopy and Esophagoscopy,* 1922; *Nose, Throat and Ear,* 1st edition, 1929; *Disease of Air and Food Passages of Foreign-Body Origin,* 1936; *The Larynx and Its Diseases,* 1937; *Cancer of the Larynx,* 1939; *Bronchoesophagology,* 1950).

The Jacksons typified a host of otolaryngologists who contributed in areas of clinical medicine, science and pedagogy. These productive and pioneering otolaryngologists, including our respective mentors, have broadened the scientific base of otolaryngology, thereby helping to establish the concept of regionalization for otolaryngology. Many of those to whom we are referring have written chapters for this work.

Otolaryngology is a regional specialty of medicine as well as of surgery. Indeed, the vast majority of new patients seen by an otolaryngologist are treated medically rather than surgically. Thus, the emphasis in this book is placed on the pathophysiology of head and neck diseases and related areas (excepting, of course, for intracranial and intraocular diseases) and on the principles of medicine and surgery.

These volumes are intended as a reference for graduate students—recognizing the physician to be a life-long student—and will, of course, be mainly of interest to residents and practitioners of otolaryngology. It is additionally of interest, however, that a study by the Minnesota Academy of General Practice, since replicated at the University of Florida and Johns Hopkins University, indicated that the commonest problems seen in the family physician's office are ear, nose and throat problems.* For this reason the work will also be an important source of information for medical students, who function as graduate students in most medical schools, and for primary physicians who wish a deeper understanding of the otolaryngologic problems with which they must deal frequently.

Our attempt to replace the Jackson and Jackson text, while maintaining an appropriately comprehensive scientific and clinical blend, resulted in the present three volume effort. Although each volume can stand alone, each is intended to be used best in conjunction with the other two. Volume I is subtitled *Basic Sciences and Related Disciplines.* Here the health sciences as they relate to otolaryngology are outlined in traditional manner, obviating the need, in most instances, for the reader to search for additional information in a basic science textbook. Following this, fundamental principles of surgery and of medicine are discussed. Other sections in the first volume include discussions of closely related disciplines such as Anesthesiology, Neurology and Ophthalmology. "Principles of Physical Diagnosis," "Audiology and Communication Disorders" and "Radiology and Radiotherapy" comprise the remaining sections of Volume I.

Volume II, *Ear,* is concerned with the medical and surgical aspects of otology. This volume is subdivided according to "Diseases of the External Ear," "Diseases of the Eustachian Tube, Mastoid and Labyrinthine Capsule," and "Diseases of the Inner Ear

---

*Reynolds, R. C.: Otolaryngology and family practice. Arch. Otolaryng. 94:289–293, 1971.

and Retrocochlear Region." Descriptions of surgical techniques are covered in the final chapter of each section, although we have attempted to prevent repetitive descriptions of the same operation (such as mastoidectomy) for different diseases.

Volume III covers the remaining areas of the discipline and is entitled *Head and Neck.* Sections of this volume include "Diseases of the Nose and Sinuses," "Dental Diseases," "Diseases of the Salivary Glands,"

"Maxillofacial Trauma and Cosmetic Surgery," "Diseases of the Trachea, Bronchi and Esophagus," and "Related Head and Neck Surgery and Reconstruction."

Because of the determination to establish a truly definitive "hunt book" of catholic scope, contributions by many experts were necessary. This made the task of coordination difficult, and we ask both the authors' and the readers' tolerance for some unevenness and for our first edition woes.

MICHAEL M. PAPARELLA, M.D.

DONALD A. SHUMRICK, M.D.

ACKNOWLEDGMENTS

We thank most sincerely the many contributors who made this effort possible. We are especially grateful to them for the excellence of their material and for their willingness to keep their chapters up to date. We are also indebted to our secretarial staffs and administrative assistants for their truly painstaking efforts. Finally we are most grateful to the W. B. Saunders Company, and especially Mr. Robert Rowan and Mr. John Hanley, for a very productive, pleasurable and friendly relationship.

CONTENTS

Section Three
BIOCHEMISTRY

Section Four
MICROBIOLOGY

Section Eight

MEDICAL PRINCIPLES OF OTOLARYNGOLOGY

Section Nine

OTOLARYNGOLOGY AND CLOSELY RELATED DISCIPLINES

Section Ten

PHYSICAL DIAGNOSIS (METHODS OF EXAMINATION)

Section One

EMBRYOLOGY
AND ANATOMY

Chapter 1

EMBRYOLOGY AND ANATOMY OF THE EAR

DEVELOPMENTAL ANATOMY OF THE EAR*

by

Barry J. Anson, Ph.D. (Med. Sc.)

PARTS OF THE EAR

The statoacoustic organ arose to present complexity in man from a humble beginning that is only partly predictive of its service in the human ear. In the structurally simple aquatic creature, the shark, the primordial element, the otocyst, never loses its original connection with the ectoderm from which it took origin (Fig. 1). Even after the auditory pit has be-

*Based upon studies carried out with the support of the Research Fund of the American Otological Society, Inc., and of the National Institutes of Health, U. S. Public Health Service (Grant No. NS 03855-08).

This chapter could not have been written without regular access to the monumental collection of serially sectioned temporal bones brought together by the late Professor Theodore H. Bast.

Following Doctor Bast's untimely death in April of 1959, the present author was encouraged to resume study of the series, thanks to the warm and long-term friendship of Dr. Otto A. Mortensen, Professor and Chairman of the Department of Anatomy at the University of Wisconsin. In this way a collaborative endeavor, begun more than 30 years ago, has been carried toward maturity.

Six graduate students in Doctor Mortensen's department have served in succession as Project Assistants in the course of this investigation: Doctors Shafik F. Richany, Gerald P. Stelter, Jerome R. Hanson, David G. Harper, Thomas R. Winch, and Michael J. Rensink.

Many of the sections in the series were prepared by Nicholas Quartuccio. The photomicrographs were taken by Homer Montegue, the drawings executed by George Buckley.

The author takes special pleasure in expressing his thanks to Mrs. Patricia Edberg for her judicious and meticulous secretarial supervision of all work on the manuscript and illustrations and for her indispensable aid in acting as conferee between the Production Department at W. B. Saunders Company and the writer.

come a vesicle, the contained fluid remains confluent with the circumambient water of the sea.

Differing from the condition in the aquatic creature, ectodermal continuity is lost in the human embryo; the contained fluid thereupon becomes the embryo's very own. Any change in its chemistry must henceforth depend upon processes that are shared with the general physiological economy of the whole body.

The otocyst is now a segregated epithelial sac. This simple vesicle must undergo profound change so that, when on the day of emergence from an "aquatic" habitation in the amnion, new connections will have been made to put its own fluid (the endolymph, not sea water) into physical (but indirect) relationship with the air of the postnatal terrestrial environment (Fig. 2). Thereby is initiated a series of remarkable modifications which depend mainly on salvage of structures already present. As a result of the refashioning, *air* is brought to act upon *fluid* through the intermediation of an *osseous chain*, parts of a branchial system useless on land: the first visceral (branchial) groove is converted into the external acoustic meatus; the first and second branchial arches into the auditory ossicles; and the first visceral pouch into the auditory tube, tympanic cavity, and related air spaces. A mechanism for aquatic respiration, by these changes, is altered to subserve the function of hearing.

This brief review of phylogenetic salvage suggests that familiarity with the teachings of embryology is nowhere more important than in

3

SHARK

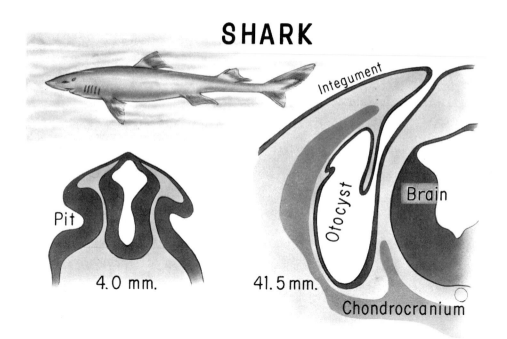

MAN

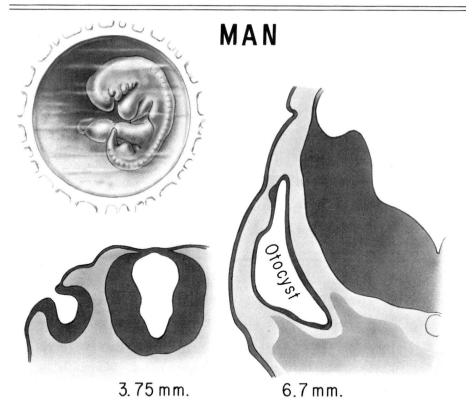

Figure 1. Comparative embryology of the otocyst in shark and man, especially in relation to environment. Sections from the Harvard Collection. (From B. J. Anson: Trans. Amer. Acad. Ophthal. & Otolaryng. *73*:17–38, 1969.)

Figure 2. Conversion of the parts of the branchial system and the related labyrinths to acoustic service in a terrestrial environment. Based upon a transverse section in an otological series from a fetus of nine weeks (40 mm. crown-rump length). Wisconsin Collection, series 168. × 16.

Air waves, conducted inward by the auricle and the external acoustic meatus (at 1) are transmitted to the labyrinthine fluids through the movement of the three bones of the ossicular chain (at 2) serving as "intermediaries" in the tympanic

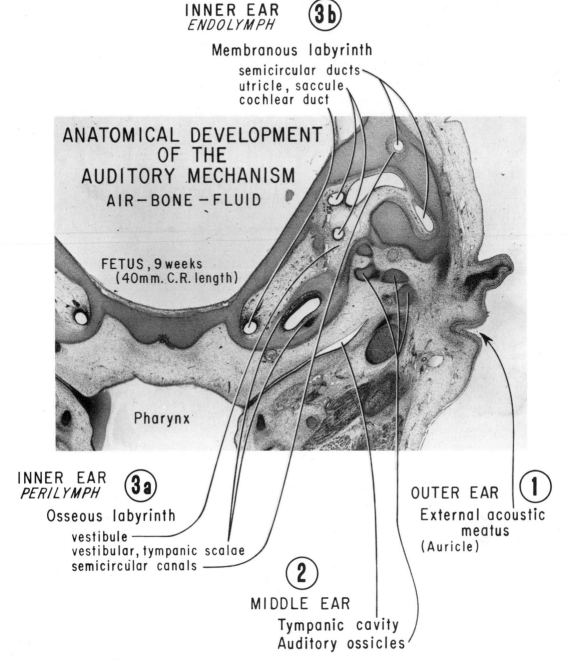

INNER EAR **3b**
ENDOLYMPH

Membranous labyrinth
semicircular ducts
utricle, saccule
cochlear duct

ANATOMICAL DEVELOPMENT
OF THE
AUDITORY MECHANISM
AIR — BONE — FLUID

FETUS, 9 weeks
(40mm. C.R. length)

Pharynx

INNER EAR **3a**
PERILYMPH

Osseous labyrinth
vestibule
vestibular, tympanic scalae
semicircular canals

OUTER EAR **1**
External acoustic
meatus
(Auricle)

MIDDLE EAR **2**
Tympanic cavity
Auditory ossicles

Figure 2. *Continued.*

cavity between the tympanic membrane and the vestibular fenestra (oval window) of the vestibule and the latter's contents (at 3 *a* and *b*).

The auricle, the external acoustic meatus and the outer (cuticular) layer of the tympanic membrane are derivatives of the ectoderm of the first pharyngeal groove. The auditory tube, the tympanic cavity and the inner (mucosal) layer of the tympanic membrane are derived from the entoderm of the first pharyngeal pouch, the latter prolonged toward the corresponding ectodermal groove from the wall of the pharynx. The auditory ossicles (malleus, incus and stapes) are refashioned, so to speak, from the cartilaginous branchial arches. Laterally, in the tympanic cavity, the manubrium of the malleus will become attached to the tympanic membrane; medially, the base (footplate) of the stapes will occupy the vestibular window in the lateral wall of the otic capsule. Within the capsule, perilymphatic spaces are forming in the reticulum whose source, like that of the capsule itself, is mesoderm (C).

The fundamental element, and the one first to appear, is the otocyst. Primordially a plaque on the ectoderm in the region of the hind brain, it becomes depressed below the surface as a pit. Next, losing continuity with the parental layer, it attains the form of an otocyst lodged in the mesenchyma (mesoderm). Finally, the originally simple ectodermal vesicle will undergo regional differentiation into the following: the cochlear duct (between the scalae of the perilymphatic system), the utricle and saccule (in the vestibule); the endolymphatic and associated ducts; and the semicircular ducts (in the canals).

5

the study of the anatomy of the ear and temporal bone. A comparison of the structure of the ear in two crucial stages (Figs. 3 and 4) will both establish these facts and prepare the way for presentation of adult anatomy.

In the nine-week fetus the *external ear* is represented by an elevation marginal to the first pharyngeal groove and by a sulcus anterior thereto (Fig. 3); the elevation will become the auricle, or pinna, while the sulcus will deepen to form the external acoustic meatus. The *middle ear* is a slitlike prolongation of the first pharyngeal pouch, which is beginning to invest the auditory ossicles. The *internal ear* is represented by the endolymphatic duct-system, lodged in mesenchymal tissue within which

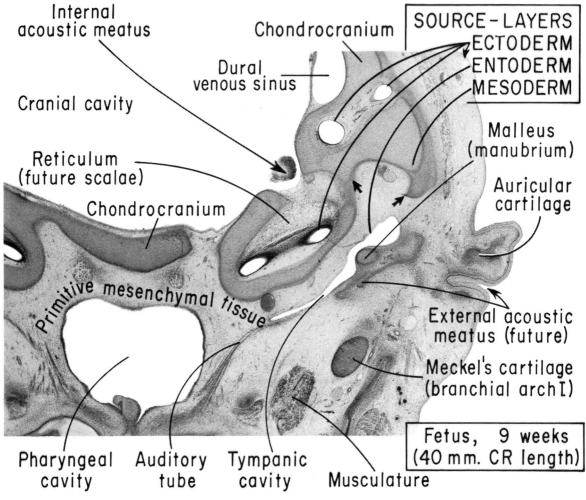

EAR AND RELATED ANATOMY

Internal acoustic meatus — Chondrocranium — SOURCE – LAYERS / ECTODERM / ENTODERM / MESODERM

Dural venous sinus

Cranial cavity

Malleus (manubrium)

Reticulum (future scalae)

Auricular cartilage

Chondrocranium

Primitive mesenchymal tissue

External acoustic meatus (future)

Meckel's cartilage (branchial arch I)

Fetus, 9 weeks (40 mm. CR length)

Pharyngeal cavity   Auditory tube   Tympanic cavity   Musculature

LABYRINTHS AND CARTILAGINOUS OTIC CAPSULE

Figure 3. Parts of the ear: Early developmental stage. Fetus of nine weeks (40 mm. crown-rump length). Transverse section. Wisconsin Collection, series 168. × 17.

The auricle appears as an elevation on the outer surface of the head, the external acoustic meatus as a sulcus (an inpushing of the primordial ectoderm). The tympanic cavity, continuous with the auditory tube, is an entodermal prolongation of the primitive pharynx.

The membranous labyrinth (derived from the ectodermal otocyst) consists, even at this early stage, of the following parts: cochlear and semicircular ducts; utricle and saccule; and the several intercommunicating channels (not sectioned at the level here illustrated).

The membranous labyrinth is lodged in mesenchyma within which the periotic tissue will give way to the spaces of the perilymphatic labyrinthine system. The surrounding cartilage will be transformed into bone.

Margins of the facial sulcus are indicated by the unlabeled arrows.

DIVISIONS OF THE OSSEOUS LABYRINTH

Cochlear Vestibular Canalicular

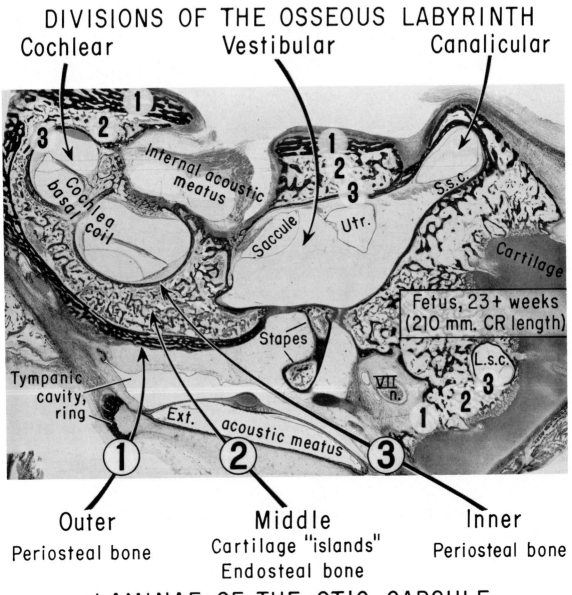

Figure 4. Parts of the ear: Later development stage. Fetus of 23+ weeks (210 mm.). Transverse section. Wisconsin Collection, series 47 A. ×8.

In the fetus at approximately the six-month stage, cartilage remains at the posterior part of an otic capsule that elsewhere consists of trilaminar bone. Retarded ossification in this canalicular division permits expansion of the canals and their contained ducts after the cochlear part of the capsule, formed in trilaminar bone, has attained adult dimensions (between the fourth and fifth month).

Periotic tissue, a remnant of the original reticulum, persists as anchorage in areas where portions of the membranous labyrinth are closely applied to the facing surface of the inner periosteal layer of the osseous capsule.

Abbreviations: *L. s. c.*, lateral semicircular canal; *S. s. c.*, superior semicircular canal; *utr*, utricle. The layers of bone are numbered.

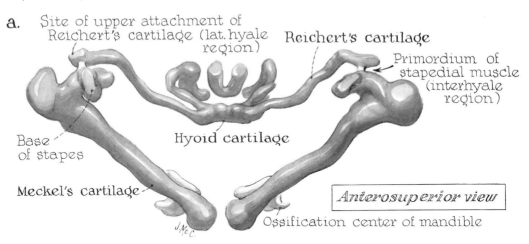

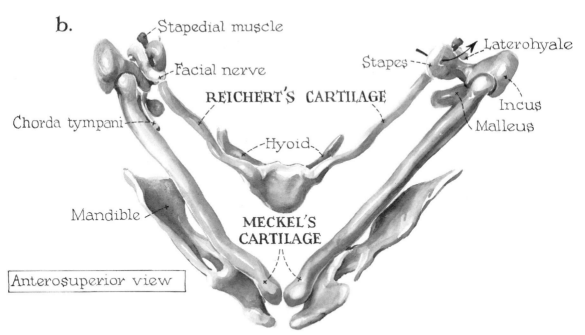

Figure 5.   First and second visceral (branchial) arches: Derivatives and related structures. Early developmental stages shown by reconstruction. Wisconsin Collection, series 10 and 174.

a, The mandibular and hyoid arches, respectively, have become true cartilage through the greater fraction of their length. The proximal extremity of each gives rise to the auditory ossicles. The primordium of the mandible is already formed in bone.

b, The stapes is changing from annular to stapedial form. The malleus and incus are less advanced. The osseous mandible is beginning to envelop the distal part of Meckel's cartilage. (Adapted from Hanson, Anson and Bast: Quarterly Bulletin, Northwestern University Medical School *33*:1–22, 1959.)

early vacuolization predicts the formation of the perilymphatic labyrinth. The otic capsule, formed in cartilage, invests the labyrinth.

Growth and differentiation proceed at such rapid rate that, in the fetus of approximately 23 weeks, the cochlea has attained full dimensions and the periotic spaces are well formed (Fig. 4). The inner periosteal layer of bone has encircled the labyrinth except in the territory of the fissula ante fenestram, where cartilage may persist even in the temporal bone of the adult. Ossification is retarded in the canalicular division of the otic capsule, where cartilage is rendered spongeous through the activity of invasive buds of vascular tissue; these enter through the subarcuate fossa, which at this stage is a relatively ample excavation. This process makes expansion possible in the arcs of the semicircular ducts. Concurrently the ossicles are undergoing initial ossification. Between the sixth and ninth months of fetal life ossification of the otic capsule advances slowly; it is accompanied by reorganization of bone of the wall of the vestibular aqueduct around the endolymphatic duct and sac (Fig. 28 a–c). In the latter process, the long axis of duct and sac changes from straight to curved and the sac enlarges.

Otherwise the internal (periosteal) layer remains a virtually unaltered shell for the perilymphatic and endolymphatic labyrinthine systems. The middle layer solidifies through application of endosteal bone on the cartilage islands, a process which is held in abeyance until birth. The outer (periosteal) layer increases rapidly in thickness through the successive external application of osseous laminae and the internal production of bone between adjacent layers. This, together with solidification of the middle layer, accounts for the density that is characteristic of the mature bone.

Many of the elements of the ear are derived from the branchial apparatus, which in aquatic and amphibious creatures serves a respiratory function (Fig. 5 a and b). In the process of conversion to new phylogenic use, the three germ layers contribute to the formation of the embryonic ear (Fig. 3).

The *ectoderm*, which lines the first branchial groove (between the mandibular and hyoid arches), contributes the cutaneous lining of the external acoustic meatus. The two arches which thus bound the groove give rise to the auricle through the production and subsequent fusion of nodular elevations on the facing margins. Deep in the depression the ectoderm contributes the outer, or cuticular, layer of the trilaminar tympanic membrane. Ectoderm is also the source layer of the membranous labyrinth. Beginning as a thickening situated dorsal to the first branchial groove, the placode becomes cup-shaped and then, successively, the following: a vesicle still attached by a stalk to the parent layer; an otocyst independent of the ectoderm; and, finally, by growth and differentiation into parts, the labyrinthine (endolymphatic) duct-system of the internal ear.

The *entoderm* of the primitive pharynx forms an entodermal pouch by pressing outward toward the ectoderm at the site of the corresponding branchial groove. The groove, situated between the first (mandibular) and second (hyoid) arches (and supported, respectively, by Meckel's and Reichert's cartilages), becomes the elongate auditory (eustachian) tube; the tympanic cavity; the latter's pneumatic extensions (namely, tympanic antrum and epitympanic recess); the air cells of the mastoid and petrous portions of the temporal bone, of the tympanic cavity and auditory tube; and the internal (mucosal) layer of the tympanic membrane.

From the third layer, the *mesoderm*, arise the remaining parts of the external, middle, and internal divisions of the ear. These are the following: the auricular cartilage and the intrinsic muscles of the external ear, the auditory ossicles with their associated muscles and ligaments, the submucosal tissue in which these structures are lodged, the middle (fibrous) layer of the tympanic membrane, the otic capsule, and the periotic tissue of the osseous labyrinth (enclosing the perilymphatic or periotic system of spaces).

The otic capsule develops in precartilage around the differentiating otocyst. Before the cartilage is converted into bone, reversal in development of the precartilage results in the production of a succession of channels between the capsule and the epithelial duct-system of the membranous labyrinth. Generally matching the former, but peripheral thereto and more capacious, these periotic spaces will be the scalae, the vestibule, and the semicircular canals of the osseous labyrinth of the adult ear.

The cartilage which thus encapsulates the perilymphatic system of intercommunicating spaces undergoes rapid ossification, attaining adult dimensions when the fetus has just reached the approximate middle of intrauterine life (Fig. 4). Thereupon is initiated the process of ossification, through the operation of which the primordial capsule, while retaining fetal di-

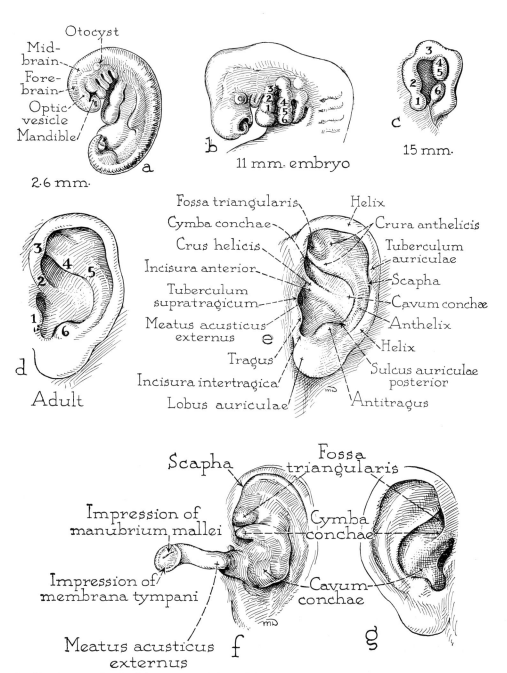

Figure 6. Developmental and adult anatomy of the auricle.

a, Primordial elevations on the first (mandibular) and second (hyoid) arches.

b to *d*, Progress of embryonic fusion of the hillocks and the adult configuration of the auricle (with corresponding numerals on the derived parts).

e, Adult form of the auricle with parts identified.

f and *g*, Fossae of the auricle and the external acoustic meatus, shown as a cast (in *f*) viewed from the medial side and the same foveate depression and bounding ridges from the lateral aspect (in *g*). (From Anson, B. J.: An Atlas of Human Anatomy. 2nd ed. Philadelphia, W. B. Saunders Co., 1963.)

mensions, becomes embedded in the *pars petrosa* of the temporal bone.

The inner periosteal and the middle layers of the trilaminar capsule remain histologically identifiable throughout the individual's lifetime. Retention of the original state is especially striking in the cochlea, where the architecture of these laminae in sections from an adult ear could be mistaken for that of an infant. Differing from this arrangement, the outer periosteal layer, in the course of its thickening, leaves no line of demarcation between its fetal and postnatal levels — that is to say, the initial boundary is, as it were, erased.

THE EXTERNAL EAR

Auricle

The auricle develops around the first branchial groove, the contributory tissue being furnished by both the first (mandibular) branchial arch and the second (hyoid) arch (Fig. 6 *a* and *b*). Six hillocks appear on these arches: three on the facing border of each (Fig. 6 *b* and *c*). They fuse to form the elevations, fossae, and sulci of the adult auricle (Fig. 6 *d* to *g*).

External Acoustic Meatus

The external acoustic meatus is a derivative of the first ectodermal branchial groove situated between the mandibular and hyoid arches (Fig. 7). The epithelium at the bottom of this groove is in contact with the entoderm of the first pharyngeal pouch. Connective tissue, derived from the mesoderm, intervenes between the epithelial layers to become the fibrous layer of the trilaminar tympanic membrane. The connective tissue around the margin of the membrane begins to ossify at about the third month. This tissue forms the tympanic ring, which serves as the circumferential skeletal support of the tympanic membrane (Figs. 8 and 9).

THE MIDDLE EAR

Tympanic Membrane

The three germ layers of the embryo take part in the formation of the tympanic membrane (Fig. 3). The ectoderm, carried inward as the wall of the external acoustic meatus, contributes the cutaneous layer; the entoderm,

prolonged from the primitive pharynx, forms the mucosal lamina; from the intervening mesoderm (mesenchyme) comes the fibrous layer (Fig. 7 *a* and *b*). With continuing development the last-named stratum becomes compressed into a thin sheet between the other two. As a consequence, the membrane in the fetus attains an adult appearance (Fig. 7 *c*).

Tympanic Ring

The tympanic ring does not begin as a cartilage "model"; it is formed from four minute ossification centers of membrane bone, the first of which appears precociously in the nine-week stage. Following fusion of the originally separate centers, growth proceeds rapidly with consequent increase in overall size (Fig. 8 *a* to *c*). In the 22-week specimen the ring is still independent of the otic capsule (Fig. 8 *d* and *e*). Fixation begins (in the posterior part) at the 34-week stage; progressing anteriorly, anchorage is complete in the newborn.

Considered as a separate skeletal element, the "ring" is never a finished annulus; in fact, at the time of fusion with related portions of the temporal bone it is still open along its cranial segment, the hiatus being the tympanic incisure (of Rivinus). Fixation results in the formation of temporary lines of suture with the squamous and petrous parts of the temporal bone (Fig. 9 *a*). Concurrently with fusion, two sets of changes are set in motion, viz., partitioning of the foramen enclosed by the ring, and growth of the ring itself along its sides and the floor. Subdivision of the original space is accomplished by ingrowth of two projections which ultimately meet and fuse (Fig. 9 *a* to *c*). The upper, lesser opening is the definitive external acoustic meatus; the lower opening is usually obliterated. In childhood it may persist as the foramen of Huschke (Fig. 9 *c* at unlabeled arrow). With further growth, that which arose as a partial ring, in addition to becoming the tympanic part of the temporal bone, contributes largely to the wall of the mandibular fossa and forms the sheath of the styloid process (Fig. 9 *d* and *e*). As a result of enlargement, it is as if the tympanic sulcus for attachment of the eardrum membrane were carried deeply into the internal acoustic meatus.

Tympanic Cavity

The cavity and the lining of the middle ear and of the auditory (eustachian) tube arise

(Text continued on page 18)

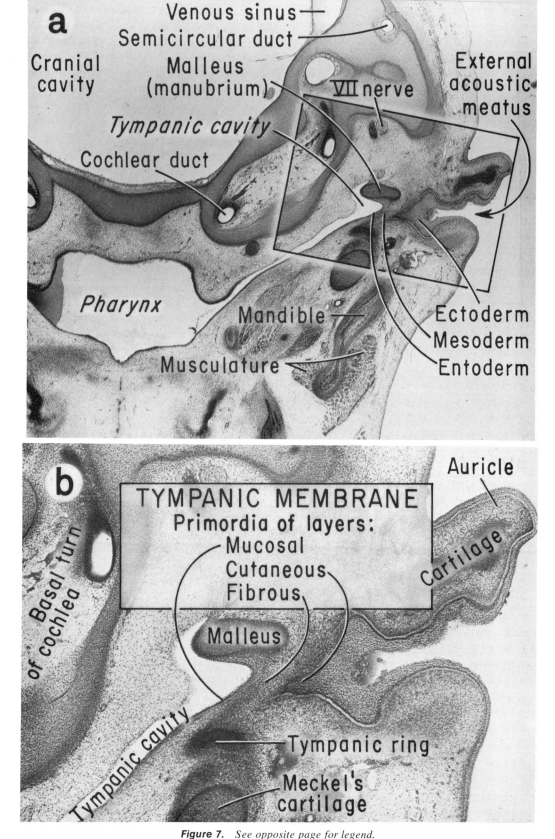

Figure 7. *See opposite page for legend.*

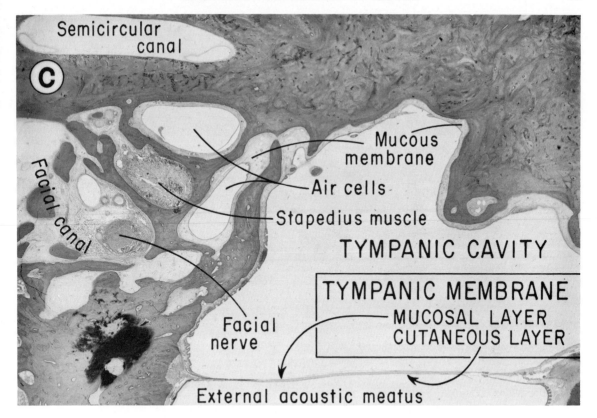

Figure 7. Tympanic cavity, external acoustic meatus and tympanic membrane: Developmental and adult anatomy. *a* and *b,* Fetus of 9 weeks (40 mm. CR length); *c,* child of 1 year, 10 months. Transverse sections. Wisconsin Collection, series 168 and 103. *a,* × 18; *b,* × 34; *c,* × 13.

a, The pharyngeal diverticulum from the first visceral pouch has grown as far as the primordial auditory ossicles, thereby forming the primitive auditory tube and the tympanic cavity. The integument of the corresponding visceral groove is continued inward as the epithelium of the external acoustic meatus and as the outer layer of the tympanic membrane. The area blocked in the rectangle is shown at higher magnification in the following figure (*b*).

b, This shows the primordial layers of the tympanic membrane in relation to the external acoustic meatus, the tympanic cavity and the intervening tissue. The outer (cutaneous) layer is derived from the ectoderm, the inner (mucosal) layer from the entoderm; the layer between them (the fibrous stratum) is contributed by the mesoderm.

c, In the fully differentiated condition, the membrane is excessively thin. The middle layer is not identifiable at low magnification.

The membrane is situated between the external acoustic meatus and the tympanic cavity. It is usually elliptical, but sometimes oval, in form. It is stretched out in the tympanic sulcus and the tympanic incisure (Rivini). In the newborn the incline of the membrane is such that it stands almost vertical. As a result of skeletal growth, the membrane in the adult ear faces medianward, backward and upward.

Far from being a smooth-walled space in the area of the tympanic membrane, the cavity of the middle ear regularly communicates with air cells that are associated with the facial canal. The largest and most constant air space is the tympanic sinus (see Fig. 10 *c*).

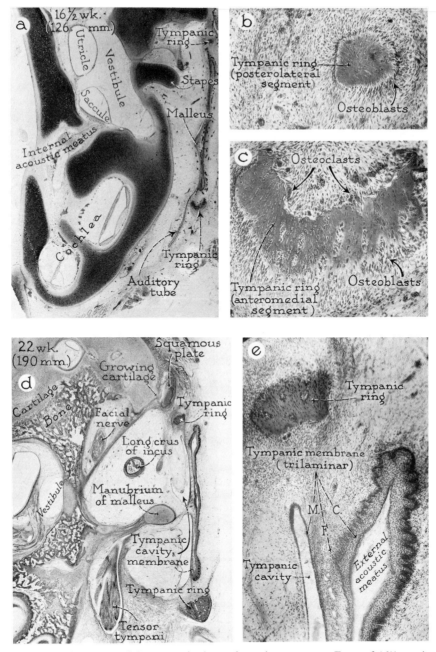

Figure 8.   Developmental anatomy of the tympanic ring and membrane. *a* to *c*, Fetus of 16½ weeks (126 mm. CR length); *d* and *e*, fetus of 22 weeks (190 mm.). Transverse sections. Wisconsin Collection, series 11 and 29 B. *a*, × 8; *b* and *c*, × 125; *d*, × 8; *e*, × 50.

a to *c*, In the four-month specimen, before the process of ossification of the otic capsule has begun, the tympanic ring is present in membrane bone. It is the site of intense cellular activity for growth; deposition is taking place on the convex (or outer) surface concurrently with resorption on the concave (inner) surface (*c*). The posterior limb is not yet sulcate (*b*), whereas the anterior limb has begun to assume characteristic form (*c*).

d and *e*, In a specimen approaching the six-month stage, ossification centers have appeared in the otic capsule and in the auditory ossicles. At this stage the posterior limb of the ring has begun to change configuration from a round column to one hollowed on its internal aspect. The primordial layers of the tympanic membrane are shown: cuticular (from ectoderm), mucosal (from entoderm) and fibrous (from mesoderm).

The hollow that is seen in the fetal specimen becomes the sulcus of the adult *pars tympanica* for attachment of the tympanic membrane. At each of the upper angles of the tympanic part, the sulcus runs out into a small pointed extremity, the greater and lesser tympanic spines. The space between the spines is not entirely filled up by attachment of the tympanic to the squamous part of the temporal bone; there remains an indentation termed the tympanic incisure (Rivini). (From Anson, B. J.: Quarterly Bulletin of Northwestern University Medical School *29*:21–36, 1955.)

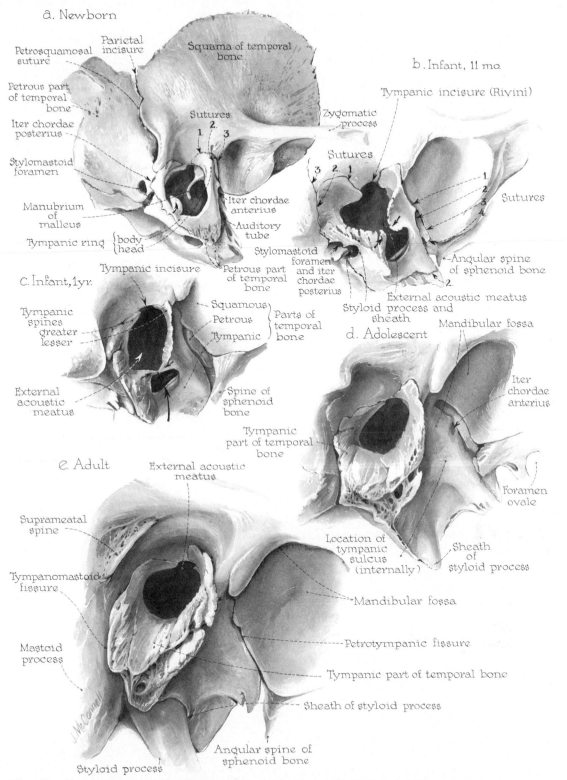

Figure 9. Developmental and adult anatomy of the tympanic ring. Skeletal preparations.

a, In the newborn, the tympanic ring has fused with the adjacent bone, the areas then persisting as suture lines: squamotympanic (at 1); petrotympanic (at 2); petrosquamous (at 3). A nodular projection appears on the posterior limb of the ring (at the unlabeled arrow).

b and *c*, With concurrent growth, a second nodule is formed on the anterior limb. These meet and fuse; thereby the annular space is subdivided into the meatus proper and an aperture which, when remaining unclosed, is termed the foramen of Huschke (unlabeled arrow in *c*). Sphenoid bone is in contact with the petrous part of temporal bone (at 4).

d and *e*, Superiorly, the notch (of Rivinus) remains as an adult feature. Inferiorly, continued growth accounts for the relatively great size of the tympanic part of the temporal bone. (From Anson, B. J.: Section X in Morris' Human anatomy. 12th ed. Used by permission of McGraw-Hill Book Company, New York.)

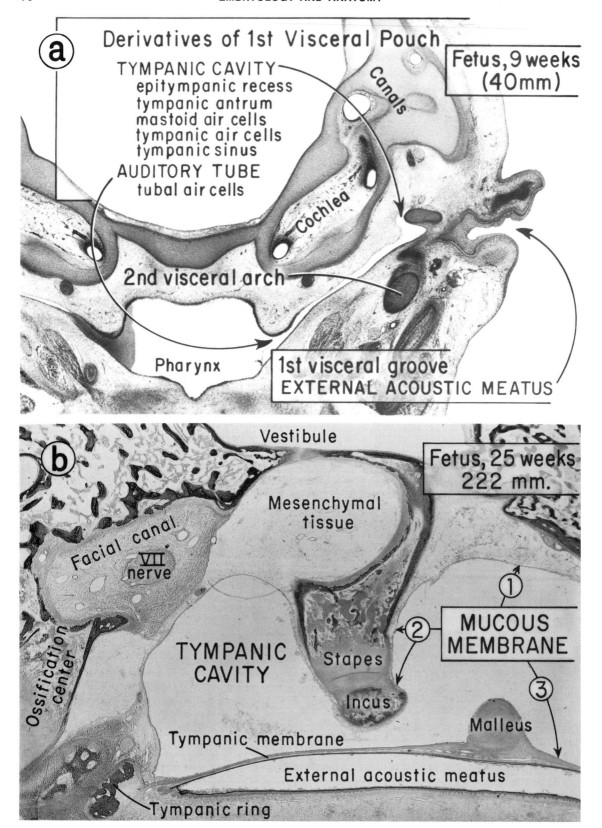

a Derivatives of 1st Visceral Pouch

Fetus, 9 weeks (40mm)

TYMPANIC CAVITY
epitympanic recess
tympanic antrum
mastoid air cells
tympanic air cells
tympanic sinus
AUDITORY TUBE
tubal air cells

Canals

Cochlea

2nd visceral arch

Pharynx

1st visceral groove
EXTERNAL ACOUSTIC MEATUS

b Vestibule

Fetus, 25 weeks
222 mm.

Facial canal
VII nerve

Mesenchymal
tissue

Ossification center

TYMPANIC
CAVITY

Stapes

Incus

① ②
MUCOUS
MEMBRANE

③

Malleus

Tympanic membrane

External acoustic meatus

Tympanic ring

Figure 10. See opposite page for legend.

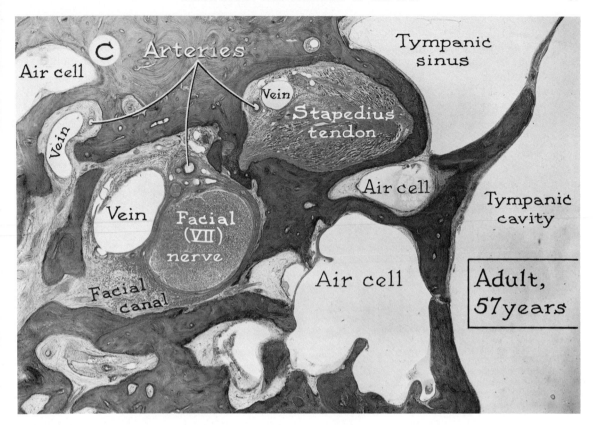

Figure 10. Development and adult form of tympanic cavity and related air cells. *a,* Fetus of 9 weeks (40 mm. CR length); *b,* fetus of 25 weeks (222 mm.); *c,* adult, 57 years of age. Transverse sections. Wisconsin Collection, series 168, 46 and 32, respectively. *a,* × 11; *b,* × 19; *c,* × 24.

a, The first visceral pouch, prolonged toward the ossicles, has formed the auditory tube and the proximal part of the tympanic cavity. Accessory spaces, to be formed later, are listed as derivatives.

b, In the six-month fetus, the mucous membrane has come to invest the lateral wall of the otic capsule (1); has contributed the mucosal layer of the tympanic cavity (3); and is spreading to invest the incus and stapes (2).

c, In addition to the general tympanic cavity and its recess and antrum, the mucous membrane replaces bone to produce a complex assemblage of air cells and a constant large cell above the ponticulus, the tympanic sinus. Further advance of mucous membrane into the otic capsule results in extensive, yet normal, pneumatization of the pyramid.

The ear drum, or tympanic cavity, is continuous behind and laterally with the mastoid air cells, formed by replacement of bone by mucous membrane. In front and medialward it opens into the pharynx by way of the auditory tube, the communication being retained from the embryonic stage of development. The lateral wall is in large part occupied by the tympanic membrane; the medial wall adjoins the labyrinth. (From B. J. Anson: Trans. Amer. Acad. Ophthal. & Otolaryng. *73:*17–38, 1969.)

from the expanding terminal end of the first (and possibly second) pharyngeal pouches (Figs. 10 and 11). The entodermal pharyngeal pouch appears early and is well formed in the embryo of three weeks; at the four-week stage, the tissue of the deep end is flattened dorso-ventrally against the facing layer of ectoderm of the infolding first branchial groove. Late in the second month the proximal part of the pharyngeal pouch becomes constricted to form the auditory tube; the distal end expands into a flattened sac, which is the early tympanic cavity (Fig. 10 *a*). In the fetus of 10 weeks the tip of this flattened tympanic cavity approaches the distal end of the first branchial groove, or future external acoustic meatus. The parietal layers of the two cavities are now separated from each other by cellular connective tissue which later condenses to form the fibrous layer of the thin trilaminar tympanic

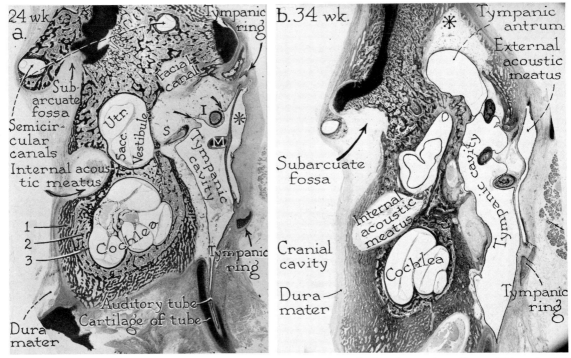

Figure 11. Tympanic cavity: Development, with accompanying change in the otic capsule. *a*, Fetus of 24 weeks (210 mm.); *b*, fetus, 34 weeks (310 mm.). Transverse sections. Wisconsin Collection, series 128 and 68, respectively.

a, This demonstrates a crucial stage in which the mucous membrane of the tympanic cavity (at *), advancing toward the canalicular part of the otic capsule, is being draped over the auditory ossicles (at unlabeled arrows). The middle layer of the capsule is still in a highly "cancellous" stage. Concurrently, on the opposite (medial) aspect of the capsule, bone is being formed to reduce the size of the subarcuate fossa (compare Figure 27 *a–c*). The capsule is composed of three laminae (see also Figure 23 *a–c*): 1, outer periosteal layer; 2, middle layer (intrachondral and endosteal bone); 3, inner periosteal layer. Abbreviations: I, incus; M, malleus; S, stapes.

b, Mucous membrane gradually replaces bone, mainly that of the middle layer of the capsule. Bone retreats ahead of the advancing membrane (at *). Replacement may take place to leave little more than thin trabeculae to support the semicircular canals and the cochlea.

Epithelium continues to take the place of bone, ultimately to produce a complex pneumatic pattern of spaces in the mastoid process of the temporal bone and in the wall of the antrum. Air cells arise in a similar way along the wall of the auditory tube; and, spreading from the middle ear, they may form around the carotid canal, above or below the cochlea and around the semicircular canals. Their number may be so great and their interconnections so wide that the supporting bone for the canals is reduced to a fragile trabecular framework.

In study of otological series in the Wisconsin Collection, it was learned that mastoid and antral air cells appear in the 34-week (310 mm., crown-rump length) fetus. Carotid air cells are first encountered in fetuses of 24 to 31 weeks (210 mm. to 280 mm.). Subtubal cells are present in the 27-week (240 mm.) stage.

From the same study it was concluded that there is no direct relation between air cells and bone marrow. Air cells do not invade marrow directly; rather, when air cells extend into diploic bone, the cells of bone marrow disappear. Most air cells are formed in young growing bone before the bone marrow is formed. When the production of air cells has been completed, the cells are separated from marrow either by plates of bone or by dense septa of connective tissue. (From Anson, B. J.: Section X in Morris' Human Anatomy. 12th ed. Used by permission of McGraw-Hill Book Company, New York.)

membrane of the adult ear (Fig. 7). The distal, expanded part of the auditory tube, which remains a slitlike flattened space up to the twentieth week of fetal life, soon begins to expand. In the fetus of 25 weeks, the loose mucoid connective tissue has given way to the expanding tympanic epithelium (Fig. 10 *b*). As the enlarging tympanum reaches the ossicles, its epithelium is wrapped around each of them, somewhat after the fashion in which peritoneal mesothelium envelopes the intestine.

Although pneumatization of the epitympanum lags somewhat behind that of the tympanum, pneumatization of both areas is virtually completed in the last month of fetal life. The antrum, a lateral extension of the epitympanum, begins to form at about the age of 22 weeks and is well advanced in the 34-week specimen. Formation of antral and mastoid air cells begins late in fetal life and progresses during infancy and childhood.

Petrous, or so-called apical, air cells occur in widely varying extent, number and position. They make their initial appearance soon after bone is laid down in the otic capsule; that is, at about the fetal age of 24 weeks (Fig. 11 *a* and *b*). Similar cells are concurrently formed in the wall of the tympanum and auditory tube. The largest of these is the tympanic sinus (Fig. 10 *c*).

Auditory Ossicles and Ossicular Muscles

General Development. The small ear bones, refashioned for the greater part from the tissue of the mandibular and hyoid arches (Meckel's and Reichert's cartilages), are first formed as cartilage "models." At the nine-week stage they have already attained the general configuration that characterizes their appearance in the adult (Fig. 12 *a*). Two portions have separate origins: the anterior process of the malleus, which forms independently and early in membrane bone; the vestibular portion of the base (footplate) of the stapes, which is primordially a part of the otic capsule. Branchial origin accounts for the broad continuity of the malleus with Meckel's cartilage, of which it is developmentally a part.

Growth of the ossicles is rapid; within a three-week period they have increased their overall dimensions by three times (Fig. 12 *b*). Just three months later, in the 15-week specimen, the ossicles have attained maximum size as chondral elements, with clear forecast of the adult morphology (Fig. 12 *c*).

Bone formation, initiated at the 16-week stage in the malleus and incus, begins somewhat later in the stapes (in one series at 19 weeks). In the latter stage (Fig. 12 *d*), periosteal bone is present in the head and in the proximal part of the manubrium of the malleus. On the incus the periosteal shell is spreading from the body to the short and long crura, while in the stapes ossification is taking place at the basal end of each crus. Endosteal bone is being formed beneath the periosteal lamina of the malleus and incus (its extent indicated by dark area in Figure 12 *d*). Meckel's cartilage currently undergoes conversion into a ligament, and the anterior process, hitherto free, becomes attached to the periosteal shell of bone of the head of the malleus. Ossification continues at such a rapid pace that the ossicles, except for permanently cartilaginous areas, are essentially adult skeletal elements in the 25-week fetus (Fig. 12 *e*).

The foregoing description accounts mainly for shape and size; it requires amplification in order to correlate these features with steps in the maturing histology of the three ossicles (Figs. 13 and 14).

Stapes. In the fetus of nine weeks the primitive "stapes" is a cartilaginous ring whose medial segment fuses with the wall of the otic capsule (Fig. 13 *a*). It is lodged in mesenchyma, the forerunner of the submucosal connective tissue.

In fetuses of approximately 16 weeks separation of the stapedial base (or footplate) is initiated (Fig. 13 *b*). The tissue in the oval-shaped zone thus produced will later differentiate into that of the annular ligament.

No sooner does each crus become a column of periosteal bone than resorption begins on the obturator surface, commencing in the crura. (Fig. 13 *c* and *d*). Endosteal bone, scattered as spicules through the primitive marrow, is quickly removed except at the capital and basal extremities of the ossicle, where it forms an osseous plate internal to the lamina of articular cartilage.

In the late fetus and in the newborn the stapes has almost attained mature histological structure (Fig. 13 *e*). As a result of the extensive removal of periosteal bone, the one-time marrow cavity of the head, crura, and base is open circumferentially toward the obturator foramen. Although mucous membrane is now draped over the internal surface of the periosteal shell, some of the primitive marrow persists.

The stapes of the adult is a fragile structure

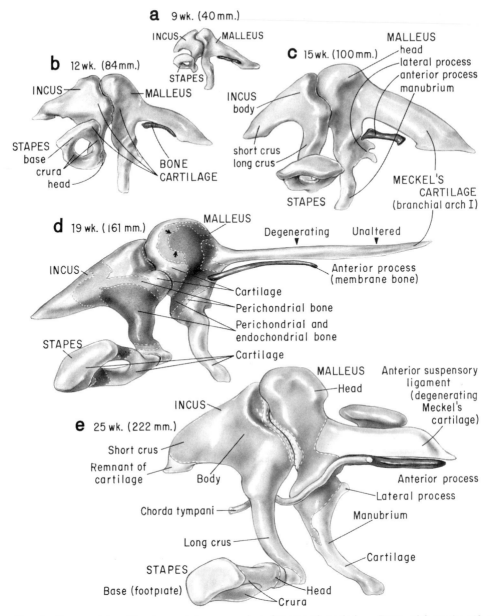

a 9 wk. (40 mm.)

INCUS — MALLEUS
STAPES

b 12 wk. (84 mm.)

INCUS — — MALLEUS

STAPES
base
crura
head
BONE
CARTILAGE

c 15 wk. (100 mm.)

MALLEUS
head
lateral process
anterior process
manubrium

INCUS
body

short crus
long crus

STAPES

MECKEL'S
CARTILAGE
(branchial arch I)

d 19 wk. (161 mm.)

MALLEUS

Degenerating   Unaltered

INCUS

STAPES

Anterior process
(membrane bone)

Cartilage
Perichondrial bone
Perichondrial and
endochondral bone
Cartilage

MALLEUS
Head

INCUS

Anterior suspensory
ligament
(degenerating
Meckel's
cartilage)

e 25 wk. (222 mm.)

Short crus
Remnant of
cartilage   Body

Chorda tympani

Long crus

Anterior process
Lateral process
Manubrium

Cartilage

STAPES
Base (footplate)   Head
Crura

Figure 12. Auditory ossicles: Developmental progress in a four-month period. *a,* Fetus of 9 weeks (40 mm. CR length); *b,* fetus of 12 weeks (84 mm.); *c,* fetus of 15 weeks (100 mm.); *d,* fetus of 19 weeks (161 mm.); *e,* fetus of 25 weeks (222 mm.). Wisconsin Collection, series 168, 162, 22, 13, and 46, respectively.

a to *c,* Cartilage "models," in assuming characteristic form, reach their maximum dimensions in cartilage at the four-month stage.

d, Bone formation, well under way in the five-month fetus, is both periosteal and endosteal (at darker areas at arrows). The anterior process of the malleus (formed in membrane bone) gains malleal attachment.

e, At approximately six months the ossicles are full size.

The following observations concerning the beginning of ossification will supplement the preceding accounts of ossicular development as demonstrated by the use of selected specimens.

In the embryo of approximately eight weeks (25 mm. crown-rump length), the ossicles and associated Meckel's bar (first branchial arch) are fully formed in true cartilage. The malleus is continuous with Meckel's cartilage, but the incus is separate from Reichert's cartilage (second branchial arch).

In the 14-week (100 mm.) fetus, the ossicles are still cartilaginous. A week later the first sign of impending ossification is seen in the malleus in the area of continuity with Meckel's cartilage. This change (in the 15-week, 111-mm. stage) takes the form of vacuolization of the cartilage — a process matched slightly later in the stapes and incus.

The first step in actual bone formation is taken by the incus; a thin periosteal shell appears on the long crus in the fetus of 16 weeks (117 mm.). A matching step is taken by the malleus in the 16½-week (126 mm.) specimen; a pellicle of bone

(Fig. 13 *f*). Its thin bilaminar base and deeply channeled crura differ strikingly from these portions of the robust cartilaginous "ossicle" of the four-month fetus (Fig. 13 *b*).

Stapedius muscle and facial canal. The stapedius muscle is a derivative of the second branchial arch. Even before ossification of the otic capsule begins, the future facial canal is identifiable as a sulcus on the tympanic wall of the canalicular division of the cartilaginous otic capsule (Fig. 13 *a* and *b*). The sulcus, still in preosseous stage, houses the stapedius muscle as well as the facial nerve and numerous blood vessels (Fig. 13 *b*). Closure is accomplished through the growth of periosteal bone (Fig. 13 *c* and *d*). In the newborn the mature condition has almost been attained (Fig. 13 *e*). In the newborn and in the child the service of the canal as a vascular conduit is clearly evident (Fig. 13 *e* and *f*). Vessels follow the stapedius tendon as it passes from the pyramidal eminence to the head of the stapes; other arteries and veins leave the canal through foramina in its walls to reach the mucous membrane. There, like the vessels around and within the tendon, they contribute to the tympanic plexus.

Vascularity is a striking feature of the anatomy of the facial canal in the temporal bone of the adult. In both the horizontal and the vertical segments, capacious veins in plexiform arrangement and smaller arteries surround the nerve (Fig. 13 *g* and *i*). They are prominently present in the compartment of the canal that transmits the stapedius muscle. Blood vessels of both compartments of the vertical segment of the canal communicate widely with those in the surrounding bone (Fig. 13 *h* and *i*).

Incus and malleus. The incus and malleus, like the stapes, arise in cartilage of the branchial arch system. But differing from the stapes, these two elements in the ossicular chain become relatively dense through continuing formation of endosteal bone in the course of fetal development. Unlike the stapes, and because deposition takes the place of erosion, both the malleus and incus thus retain the general form of the cartilage "model."

The malleus and incus in fetuses at approximately the four-month stage begin to change from cartilage to bone (Fig. 14 *a* and *b*).

In a fetus one month older the tissue in the area of the incudomalleal articulation serves to demonstrate two major steps in the progress of ossification: invasion of the short crus of the incus by vascular buds, preparatory to the formation of endosteal bone; and formation of such bone in the body of the malleus internal to the layer of periosteal bone (Fig. 14 *c*).

The relationship of the two laminae, periosteal and endosteal, is shown in the incus of a specimen somewhat younger but more advanced in histological change (Fig. 14 *d*). In the incus, cartilage is being resorbed beneath a still-thin periosteal plate, the latter rendered foraminous to permit the ingress of erosive vascular tissue; in the malleus, cartilage has been replaced by endosteal bone and primitive marrow.

In the seven-month fetus both layers are present (Fig. 14 *e*). Here two successive phases are demonstrated: whereas the endosteal bone in the long crus of the incus appears chiefly in the form of interconnected spicules, in the malleus it is a true lamina applied internally to the periosteal layer.

The structure of the malleus and incus in the adult ear is one of relative solidity (Fig. 14 *f*). The appearance bears some resemblance to that of a typical long bone in miniature, but one in which the marrow cavity of the "diaphysis" is replaced by vascularized endosteal bone.

It is generally accepted that the malleus and incus are derived from the first branchial arch (Meckel's cartilage). Actually the anterior process of the malleus develops independently in membrane bone (Fig. 12); and in addition to branchial source, the otic capsule contributes to the stapes the medial (vestibular) part of the base, termed lamina stapedis (Fig. 13).

Each of the branchial arches does much more than contribute ossicles: from the first (mandibular) arch are derived structures which begin proximally with the ossicles and terminate distally with the symphysis of the

(Text continued on page 34)

Figure 12. *Continued.*
is formed on the body of the ossicle near the area of articulation with the malleus. Not until the fetus has reached the age of 17+ weeks (146 mm.) does bone formation begin in the stapes. The single center appears on the obturator surface of the base, wherefrom it spreads along each crus, finally to involve the head. (Redrawn from Richany, Anson and Bast: Quarterly Bulletin of Northwestern University Medical School *28*:17–45, 1954.)

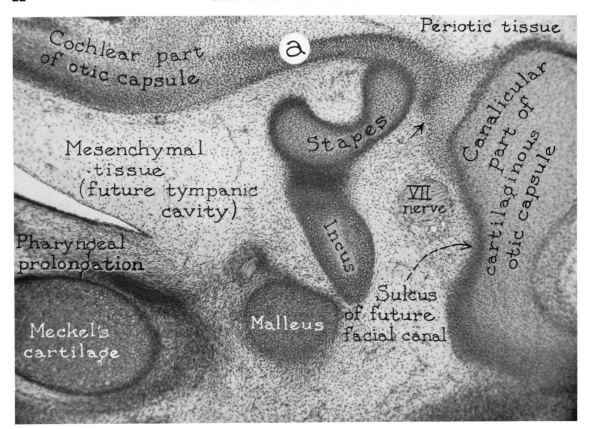

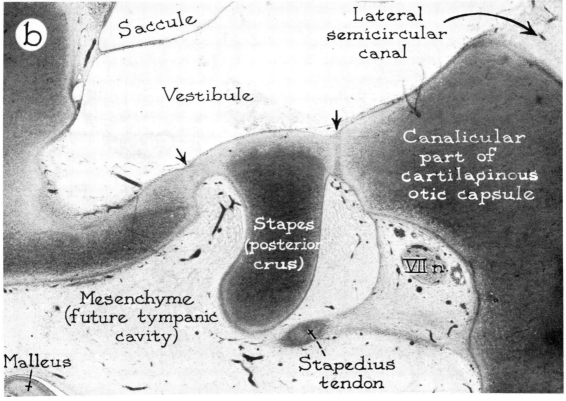

Figure 13. *See opposite page for legend.*

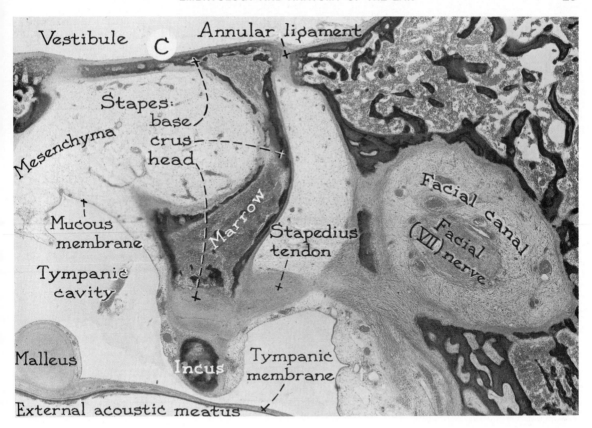

Figure 13. Stapes, stapedial muscle, facial canal and nerve: Developmental and adult anatomy. *a*, Fetus of 9 weeks (40 mm.); *b*, fetus, 16½ weeks (126 mm.); *c*, fetus, 26 weeks (230 mm.); *d*, fetus, 27 weeks (243 mm.); *e*, newborn (four-day premature); *f*, child, 6 years old. Transverse sections. Wisconsin Collection, series 168, 11, 64, 89, 124, and 81, respectively. *a*, × 62; *b*, × 30; *c*, × 22; *d*, × 24; *e*, × 30; *f*, × 16.

a, In the nine-week fetus, the stapes, like the malleus, incus and otic capsule, is composed of cartilage. The stirrup, still ring-shaped, impinges upon the capsular wall at the future site of the vestibular (oval) window (posterior margin indicated by the unlabelled arrow). Meckel's cartilage (second, or hyoid, visceral arch) is continuous with the malleus at other levels in the series of sections. The future facial canal is a sulcus on the wall of the canalicular division of the capsule.

b, At approximately eight weeks, the ossicles are formed in true cartilage; the first ossification center appears (in the stapes) as early as the 16-week stage in some specimens. During this period of two months, the ossicles increase rapidly in size and attain adult form.

In the specimen illustrated, differentiation of tissue is tardy; change is seen in the base of the stapes, where continuity with the capsule is being interrupted at the site of the future annular ligament (indicated by unlabeled arrows).

The facial "canal" is still a sulcus, its contents lodged in tissue that is histologically more advanced than the mesenchyma from which it is derived.

c, In the 26-week specimen, the ossicles have almost reached the midpoint in their approach to mature histological structure; they attained adult dimensions even earlier. Cartilage is retained on the articular surfaces of the three ossicles and in the manubrium of the malleus. Periosteal bone on the obturator surface of the crura is being removed; endosteal bone is deposited on the inner aspect of the head and base (footplate), converting each into a bilaminar plate. Mucous membrane of the expanding tympanic cavity is beginning to invest the stapes.

The periosteal layer of the otic capsule is complete on the deep surface of the facial canal, partial on the superficial (anterior) aspect.

Illustration continued on following page.

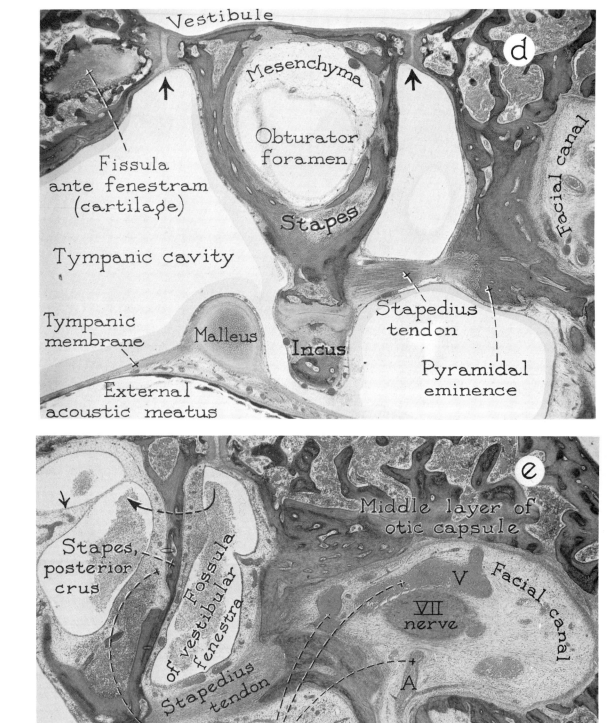

Figure 13. *Continued. See opposite page for legend.*

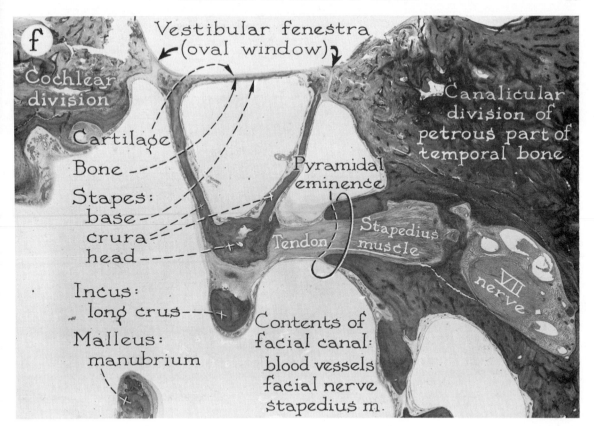

Figure 13. *Continued.*

d, The 27-week specimen is developmentally more advanced than the 26-week fetus (see *c*). The ossicles, almost adult in structure, are invested by mucous membrane. The cartilage of the stapedial base is discontinuous with that of the capsule—meaning that there is a true vestibular fenestra (oval window) and an annular ligament (at arrows).

e, Except for the persistence of some primitive marrow tissue in the submucosal layer, the stapes of the newborn infant is an adult ossicle. The schema of vascular supply is evident in the presence of blood vessels that are traceable from the facial canal, along the stapedius tendon to the crura, across the obturator foramen (at arrow) and, more prominently, in the occurrence of branches that leave the canal through vascular foramina near the pyramidal eminence. They contribute to the tympanic plexus.

f, Soon after birth the stapes, in every major respect, is an adult ossicle. Marrow tissue has been resorbed; "remodelling" has taken place at the extremities of the stapes to reduce the size of the channels for blood vessels at the circumference of the base and at the head.

It is evident that the developmental steps in formation of the auditory ossicles, of the vestibular window (with the annular ligament), and of the facial canal (with its highly vascular connective tissues) are both concurrent and structurally interrelated. In the earliest stage (nine-week) as here pictured, the base of the stapes is applied to the tympanic wall of the cartilaginous otic capsule where the fenestra will later appear. In the 16-week specimen, as histological difference between capsule and stapes becomes clear, blood vessels are traceable in the mesenchyma from the facial "canal" to the base (or footplate) of the stapes and from the same source vessels, with the stapedius tendon, to the head of the ossicle. As morphogenesis progresses, bone-formation in the 26-week fetus predicts closure of the sulcus to form a true facial canal, conversion of the stapes into an ossicle lacking a periosteal wall on its obturator aspect, and formation of a true fenestra and production of a vascular network around the stapedius tendon (late fetal and early infantile stages).

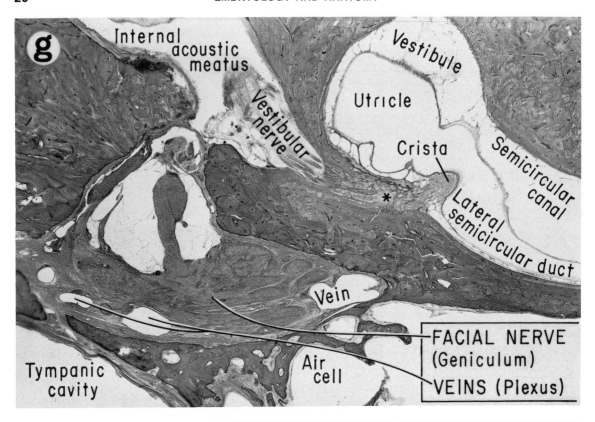

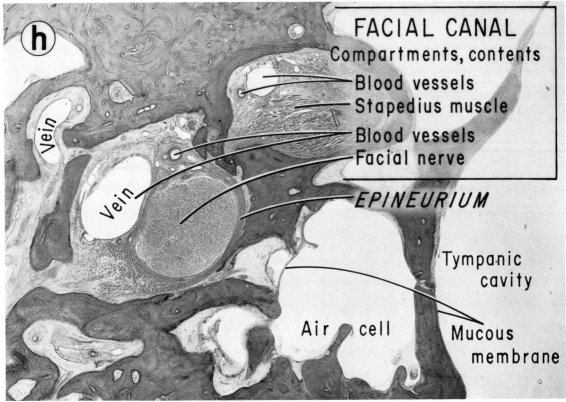

Figure 13. *Continued.   See opposite page for legend.*

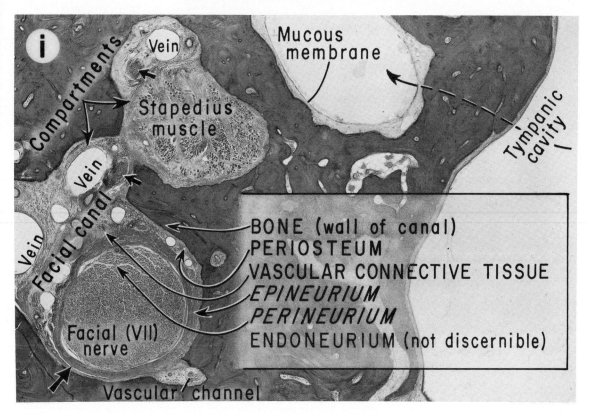

Figure 13. *Continued.*

Stapedial muscle, facial canal and nerve and related structures: Adult anatomy. Male, 57 years of age. Transverse sections. Right temporal bone. Wisconsin Collection, series 32. Selected levels in cranialcaudal order. g, × 15; h, × 26; i, × 30.

g, At the horizontal level of continuity of the utricle with the lateral semicircular duct, the facial (VIIth) nerve passes from the facial area of the fundus of the internal acoustic meatus into the geniculum of the facial canal. At the same level the vestibular division of the vestibulocochlear (VIIIth) nerve passes from the superior vestibular area of the fundus through foraminous bone (at *) to the superior cribrose macula on the wall of the elliptical recess of the vestibule. In the geniculum of the facial canal the similarly named part of the nerve begins its course backward, above the vestibular (oval) window and stapes. Here, and throughout the remainder of its course, the nerve is lodged in highly vascular tissue and is covered by a readily identifiable epineurium.

h. After turning in an even curve, the nerve begins its descent to the stylomastoid foramen. At or near the level of the pyramidal eminence, the canal is shared by the stapedius muscle. The muscle in its lower reaches is separated from the nerve by an osseous septum which divides the canal into two distinct channels, neural and muscular.

i, The stapedius muscle, like the facial nerve, is accompanied by capacious veins and less conspicuous, but numerous, arteries; those in the neural "semicanal" communicate freely with vessels in the surrounding bone. Most of the vessels lie in connective tissue external to the perineurium.

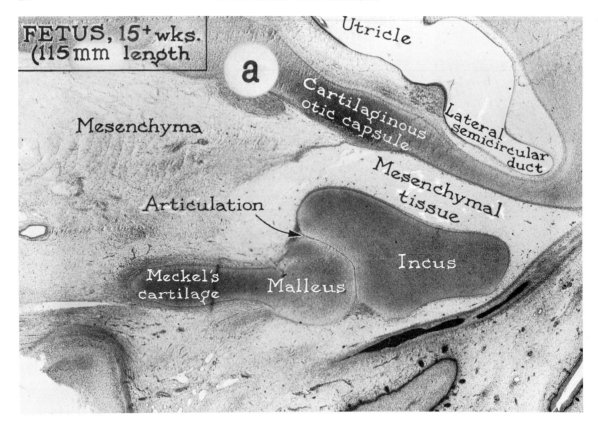

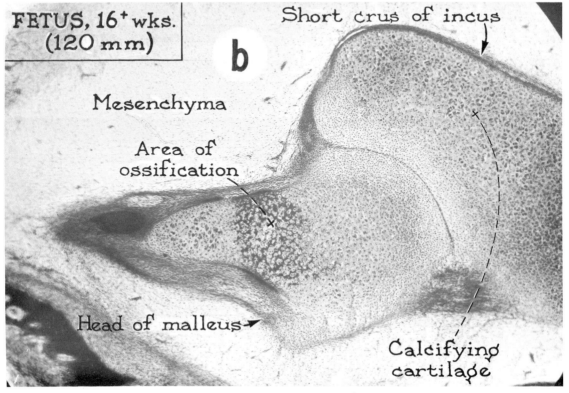

Figure 14.   *See opposite page for legend.*

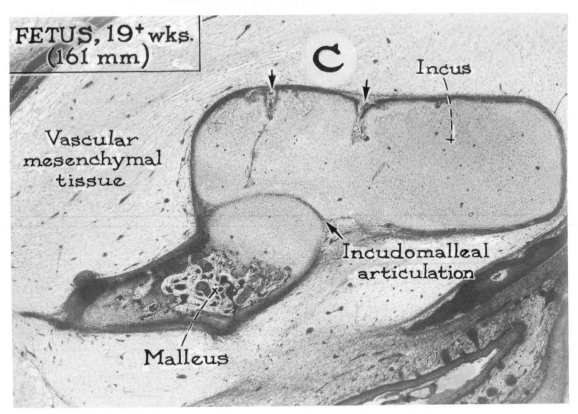

FETUS, 19⁺ wks. (161 mm)

Vascular mesenchymal tissue

C

Incus

Incudomalleal articulation

Malleus

Figure 14. Malleus and incus: Development. Level of the incudomalleal articulation. Six stages. *a*, Fetus of 15+ weeks (115 mm. CR length); *b*, fetus, 16+ weeks (120 mm.); fetus, 19+ weeks (161 mm.); *d*, fetus, 17+ weeks (146 mm.); *e*, fetus, 28+ weeks (255 mm.); *f*, adult, 19 years old. Transverse sections. Wisconsin Collection, series 54, 56, 13, 30, 111, and 29. respectively. *a*, × 22; *b*, × 47; *c*, × 31; *d*, × 57; *e*, × 36; *f*, × 31.

   a, In a specimen prior to the onset of ossification in the otic capsule, the auditory ossicles are, likewise, still wholly cartilaginous.

   b, Bone formation begins in specimens soon after the four-month stage.

   c, In the five-month specimen, buds of vascular tissue are invading the short crus of the incus. Periosteal and endosteal bone are present in the body of the malleus.

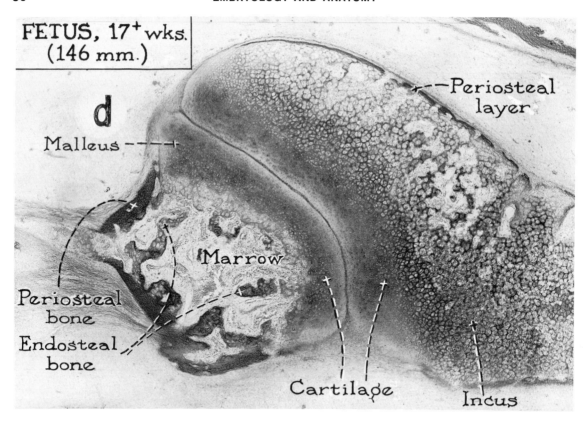

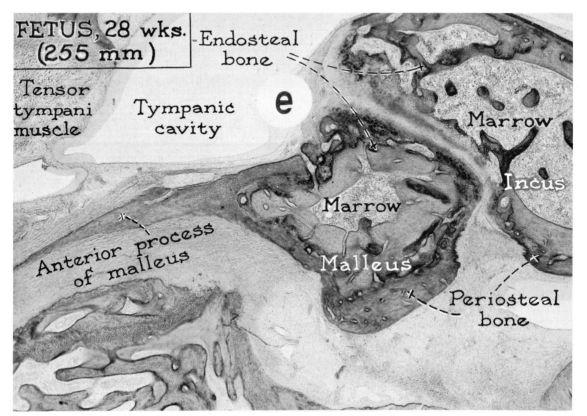

Figure 14. *Continued.   See opposite page for legend.*

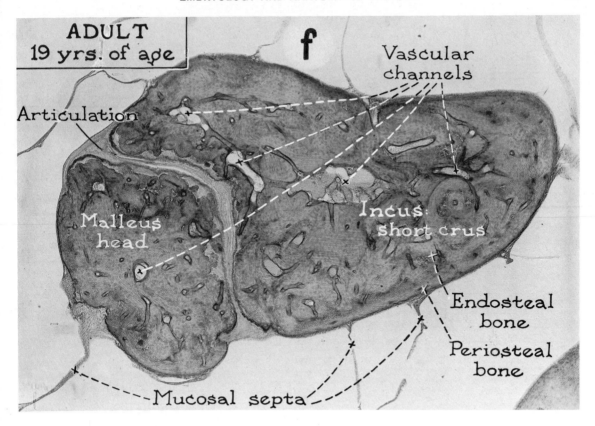

Figure 14. *Continued.*

d, A younger fetus, but of advanced development, demonstrates the formation of a periosteal layer and subjacent calcification in the incus, and production of spicules of endosteal bone in the malleus.

e, At seven months the nature of the mature ossicles is predicted in the bilaminar structure of the bone, and more especially in the rapid growth of the endosteal layer.

f, In the adult the result is seen in relative solidity of the bone. Space is limited to channels that transmit blood vessels.

As has already been shown (Fig. 13 *e*), the adult stapes occupies the part of the tympanic cavity that is bounded anteriorly by the cochlea and the semicanal of the tensor tympani muscle, posteriorly and superiorly by the facial canal. The space is named the fossula of the vestibular fenestra (stapes "niche" of otological terminology). The footplate, or base of the stapes, occupies and almost fills the vestibular (or oval) window. The opposite extremity, or head, articulates with the lenticular process of the long crus of the incus.

The short crus of the incus is directed horizontally backward; there its tip lies in the incudal fossa, attached to the wall by the posterior ligament.

The malleus, the largest of the three ear bones, lies farthest lateralward and forward. The upper part, or head, is situated in the epitympanic recess. This thick capital portion presents on its posterior and medial surfaces a saddle-shaped articular area for the body of the incus. The thin manubrium tapers to a tip where it ends like a spatula in an area of fixation to the tympanic membrane.

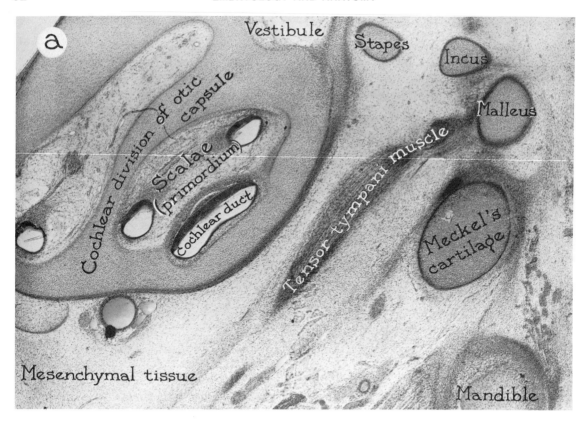

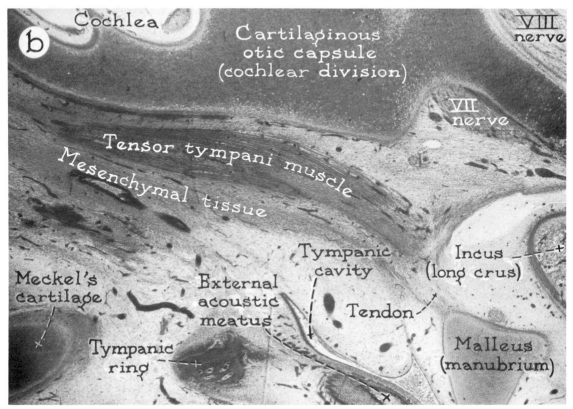

Figure 15.   See opposite page for legend.

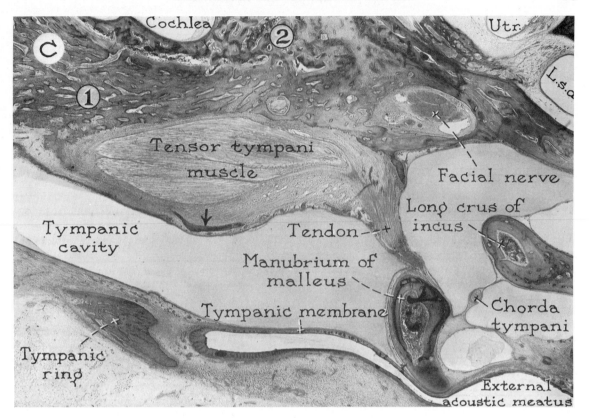

Figure 15. Ossicular muscles: Tensor tympani. Developmental stages. *a,* Fetus of 11+ weeks (62 mm.); *b,* fetus of 16½ weeks (126 mm.); *c,* fetus of 34+ weeks (310 mm.). Transverse sections. Wisconsin Collection, series 160, 11, and 68, respectively. *a,* × 31; *b,* × 31; *c,* × 14.

a, In the three-month fetus the primitive muscle courses through the mesenchyma which will become the submucosal connective tissue. It is inserted into the manubrium of the developing malleus, which, like the other ossicles and the otic capsule, is still cartilaginous.

b, Showing the form and relations of the muscle in the four-month specimen.

c, Accompanying ossification of the otic capsule, the tensor tympani becomes enclosed by bone of the semicanal. The wall (at arrow) is still incomplete as the fetus approaches term. For identification of the numbered layers of bone, see Figure 23.

The semicanal for the tensor tympani muscle is the upper and smaller part of the musculotubal canal, the lower and larger part being the canal for the auditory (Eustachian) tube.

The tensor muscle is spindle-shaped and bipennate. It arises from the wall of the semicanal (the bone of which is completed by tough connective tissue) and from the cartilaginous part of the auditory tube. The rounded tendon, upon emerging from the semicanal, turns at almost a right angle at the cochleariform process. It passes lateralward through the tympanic cavity, becoming invested by mucous membrane, to an attachment on the manubrium of the malleus near the neck of the ossicle.

mandible; from the second (hyoid) arch come structures which, again, start proximally with an ossicle and terminate distally (in the neck) with the hyoid bone (Fig. 5).

Like the stapes in the four-month stage (Fig. 13 *b*), the malleus and incus are still cartilage "models" of the future osseous hammer and anvil (Fig. 14 *a*). An outer layer of bone is soon formed. Concurrently the cartilage internal to this periosteal shell is replaced by marrow and by spicules of endosteal bone (Fig. 14 *b* to *d*). In the fetus of seven months endosteal bone has come to form a definite stratum. As a result, both ossicles are now bilaminar (Fig. 14 *e*). The process of ossification progresses until the time of birth approaches. Then the deposition of endosteal bone goes forward at such a rapid pace that the histological architecture of the malleus and incus in early postnatal specimens might be mistaken for that of an adult (Fig. 14 *f*). Both ossicles are solid except for the presence, regularly, of numerous vascular channels and for the occurrence, variably, of areas of secondary, sometimes tertiary, zones of resorption and new bone formation. The latter process seems to bear no relation to age.

Tensor tympani muscle. The tympanic tensor muscle is a derivative of the first branchial arch of the embryo. The stapedius muscle, as stated earlier, comes from the second arch.

In the specimen of approximately three months (prior to the onset of capsular ossification) the primordial tissue of the muscle lies in mesenchyma lateral to the cochlea (Fig. 15 *a*). The malleus, to which it will become attached, is, like the incus and stapes, a cartilage "model" of the mature ossicle.

One month later a histological difference between muscle and tendon is evident (Fig. 15 *b*). The latter is attached to the manubrium of the malleus.

In a late fetal stage periosteal bone is forming around the muscle to close the semicanal (Fig. 15 *c*).

Associated air chamber, cells. Formation of the antrum, a lateral extension of the epitympanum, begins about the twenty-second week of fetal life. At the age of 24 weeks the loose mesenchymal connective tissue of the primitive epitympanum tunnels lateralward toward the area which subsequently will be the antrum (Fig. 11 *a*). At the age of 34 weeks the fetal antrum is much larger; about one half of it is pneumatized (Fig. 11 *b*). It is undergoing expansion not only laterally in the direction of the future mastoid, but also medially, rostrally,

and posteriorly where, having destroyed the perichondral bone, the epithelium invades the endochondrial bone of the otic capsule. After the 34-week stage, pneumatization progresses very rapidly; enlargement of the antrum and the formation of antral and mastoid air cells, initiated in late fetal life, continue as developmental processes during infancy and early childhood.

Within the petrous portion of the temporal bone there usually occur additional pneumatic spaces, the air cells, derived as extensions of the tympanic cavity. They vary strikingly in size, number, and distribution, and from one individual to another. These spaces develop in a manner similar to that which produces the cavities of the tympanum, epitympanum, and antrum; bone, chiefly of the middle layer, retreats in advance of invading epithelium.

Auditory tube. In the embryo of six weeks, five pairs of pouches are identifiable in the primitive pharynx. Of these, only the first pair retains its embryonic relations in recognizable manner. During the eighth week each lengthens to form an auditory tube. By the ninth week the diverticulum is approaching the auditory ossicles (Fig. 3). The blind extremity of the outpocketing, further enlarged, becomes the tympanic cavity (Figs. 10 and 11). As already described, the tympanic epithelium, upon reaching the ossicles, wraps itself around them after the fashion of a miniature mesenteric investment.

THE INTERNAL EAR

Membranous Labyrinth

The membranous labyrinth is the fundamental part of the ear. It is the first to form, and even before any other part of the internal ear develops, the peripheral processes of the acoustic nerve reach its membranous wall. In these local areas the epithelium becomes modified into neuroepithelium for the end organs of hearing and equilibrium.

The primordium of the membranous labyrinth appears in the three-week embryo as a platelike thickening of the ectoderm situated on each side of the head dorsal to the first branchial groove in the region of the hind brain. This thickened plaque of epithelium, the otic placode, soon invaginates into the subjacent mesenchyma to form the otic pit. The invaginated portion then enlarges, and the

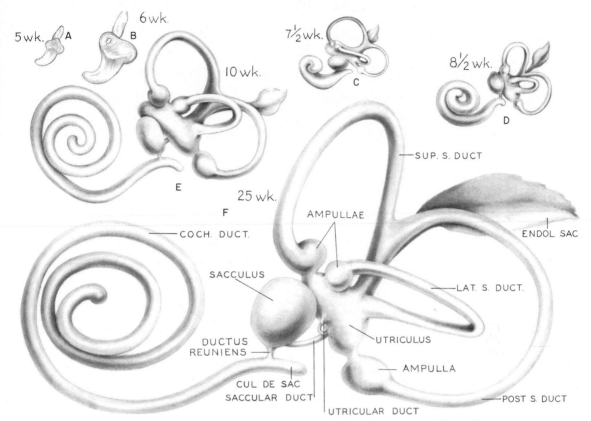

Figure 16. Membranous labyrinth: Development in a five-month period (5th to 25th week, approximate ages). Reconstructions prepared by the Born Method. A, embryo of 6.6 mm. (crown-rump length); B, embryo of 13 mm.; C, embryo of 20 mm.; D, fetus of 30 mm.; E, fetus of 50 mm.; F, fetus of 220 mm. Figures A to C, after Streeter. D, E, and F, Wisconsin Collection, series 92, 86, and 91, respectively. × 9. All drawn to scale.

In the vestibule the labyrinth is formed by two vesicles, the utricle and the saccule. The utricle communicates, by five openings, with three membranous semicircular ducts. The saccule is connected with the utricle, but only indirectly, through the endolymphatic duct as an intermediary. This arises as a very fine canal from the saccule and receives the utricular (utriculoendolymphatic) duct from the utricle. The cochlear part of the membranous labyrinth is formed by the cochlear duct which unites with the saccule by the *ductus reuniens*. The beginning of the cochlear duct is in the form of a blind extension, the vestibular caecum (or cul de sac). The duct describes two and three-quarters turns and terminates in the cupular caecum, the latter located in the cupular cavity of the apical turn. There it helps to form the helicotrema. (After Bast, T. H., and Anson, B. J.: The Temporal Bone and the Ear. Springfield, Ill., Charles C Thomas, 1949.)

mouth of the pit narrows by the growing together of the lips. When the margins meet and fuse, the otic pit is converted into a closed sac, the otocyst, or the otic vesicle.

The otic vesicle, now divorced from the parent layer, lengthens and changes form (Fig. 16 *A* and *B*). At first, the vesicle merely enlarges, lengthening faster than it widens. Next, the cranial part becomes marked off as the primordial endolymphatic duct and the caudal part as the forerunner of the cochlear duct (Fig. 16 *B*). The intermediate segment will become divided into utricle and saccule. The distal extremity of the endolymphatic appendage becomes the definitive endolymphatic sac (Fig. 16 *C*). When fully formed, at about midterm, the endolymphatic duct extends from the junction of the

saccular and utricular ducts through part of the vestibule just posteromedial and parallel to the common crus, then through the vestibular aqueduct of the otic capsule to terminate as an expanded intradural portion, the endolymphatic sac. In the mature form the sac occupies a foveate impression on the posterior surface of the petrous part of the temporal bone.

In embryos of approximately five weeks, three arciform outpocketings appear in the upper lateral or utricular part of the utriculosaccular portion of the otic vesicle (Fig. 16 *A*). A week later these ridges have become shelf-like bays of the utricular part of the differentiating otocyst (Fig. 16 *B*). At the center of each arched shelf, the opposing epithelial walls meet and fuse, with the result that the cavity is oblit-

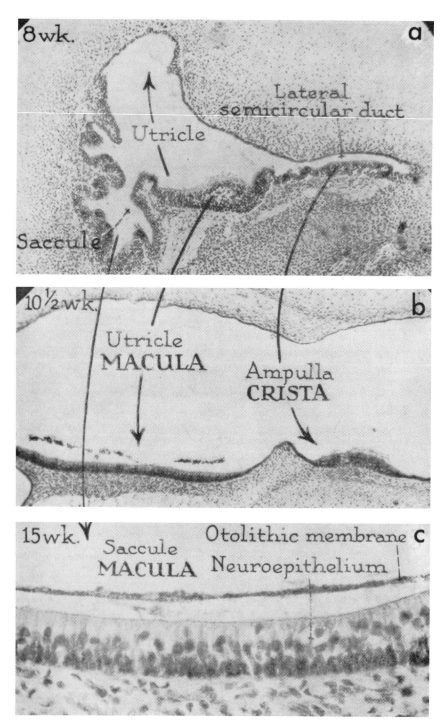

Figure 17. *See opposite page for legend.*

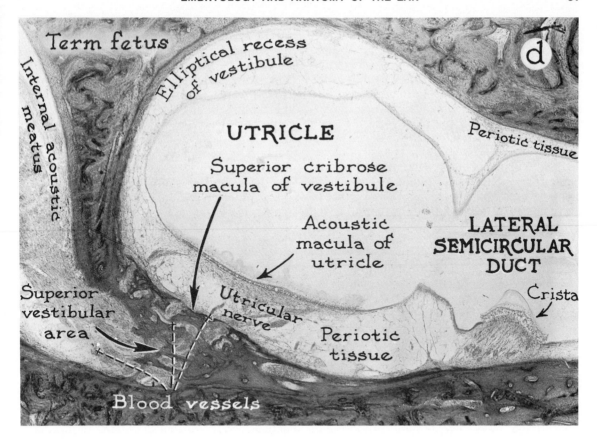

Figure 17. Crista and macula: Developmental and adult anatomy. *a,* Fetus of 8 weeks (25 mm.); *b,* embryo of 10½ weeks (50 mm.); *c,* fetus of 15+ weeks (115 mm.); *d,* fetus at term. Transverse sections. Wisconsin Collection, series 87, 86, 54, and 123, respectively. *a* and *b,* × 97; *c,* × 382; *d,* × 32.

a, Showing the early stage in differentiation of the acoustic macula of the utricle and of the crista of the lateral semicircular duct. The change from simple to neural epithelium occurs in those portions of the wall of the membranous labyrinth where the sensory nerves enter. Differentiation is initiated between the seventh and eighth week.

b, By the tenth to twelfth week, the typical cells are present: sensory cells which bear bristle-like hairs at their free margin, and supporting cells. Already the otolithic membrane is being formed. The ampullae of the semicircular ducts are widely continuous with the utricle and will remain so.

c, In fetuses of 15 weeks, the individual parts of the maculae and of the cristae are well differentiated. They appear to be similar to those seen in the adult. However, ossification has not yet been initiated; the surrounding otic capsule still consists of cartilage.

d, Demonstrating, in the fetus at term, the virtually mature form of the utricle and duct, and the structure of the surrounding system of perilymphatic spaces and investing osseous capsule (see Figures 20 *a–c*). Fibers of the upper terminal division of the vestibular nerve, accompanied by branches of the internal auditory blood vessels, are here shown as they pass from the superior vestibular area of the internal acoustic meatus to the acoustic macula of the utricle. Fibers of similar origin innervate the crista of the lateral membranous ampulla (following figure) and the crista of the superior ampulla (not sectioned at this level).

erated centrally. The area of epithelial fusion then disintegrates and is replaced by the surrounding mesenchymal tissue. The evaginations are thereby converted into semicircular ducts (Fig. 16 C). In the six-week embryo the superior ridge has already been converted into a semicircular duct; the other two protuberances are still ridgelike. They, too, are soon transformed into semicircular ducts, the posterior preceding the lateral in this phase of development. The ducts attain maximum size in the same order, final enlargement of their arcs being permitted by the spongeous structure of the canalicular part of the otic capsule (see subarcuate fossa).

The saccule undergoes considerable expansion in the embryonic and fetal stages (Fig. 16 C to F). Already in embryos of approximately five and six weeks, before the saccule is demarcated from the remainder of the vesicle, it sends out a single ventral evagination, the primordium of the cochlear duct (Fig. 16 B). This evagination grows in a medial direction and gradually bends to form a coil. At the eight-week stage it has formed one turn (Fig. 16 C); at 10 weeks, two turns (Fig. 16 E); at the 25-week stage, the cochlear duct has described almost two and one half turns and has virtually attained the form characteristic of the adult (Fig. 16 F). With the growth of the cochlear duct the communication of the latter with the saccule becomes constricted, as is already evident in the embryo of eight weeks. This segment, the ductus reuniens, while lengthening, continues to undergo relative narrowing. In the adult the duct is attenuated and the lumen so small that patency is sometimes questionable.

All the sensory end organs of the inner ear develop from epithelial areas of the otic labyrinth into which terminal nerve fibers from the vestibular and cochlear ganglia cells have grown. The cell processes, or nerve fibers, from both these ganglia make up the acoustic (vestibulocochlear, eighth cranial) nerve. The sensory epithelial areas are divided into two groups; viz., the vestibular end organ, which consists of the cristae and maculae (Figs. 17 and 18), and the cochlear end organ, or spiral organ of Corti (Fig. 19).

Maculae

The maculae develop from the epithelium which overlies the areas where the nerves enter the wall of the saccule and utricle (Fig. 17). In these zones the epithelium becomes modi-

fied into a complex pseudostratified layer (Fig. 17 a). Two types of cells are present, namely, the sensory cells, which bear bristlelike hairs at their free margin, and the supporting cells. The supporting cells secrete a gelatinous substance which forms a cushionlike membrane, the otolithic membrane (Fig. 17 b and c); the latter overlies the modified epithelium and bears superficial calcareous deposits, the otoconia. Differentiation begins between the seventh and eighth weeks of fetal life (Fig. 17 a). By the tenth to twelfth weeks the distinctive types of cells are apparent and the otolithic membrane is being formed (Fig. 17 b). In fetuses of 14 to 16 weeks, the individual parts of the maculae appear to be well formed and are similar to those seen in the adult (Fig. 17 c).

Cristae

The vestibular nerve sends a branch to each of the three ampullae of the semicircular ducts. The crista ampullaris is that modified and elevated portion of the epithelium of an ampulla into which the terminal fibers of an ampullary nerve extend. Here the epithelium is elevated into a ridgelike fold and its cells modified in a manner similar to that in which the macula is differentiated. The cristae are already distinguishable in a fetus of eight weeks as moundlike elevations (Fig. 18 a). Concurrently with the differentiation of the crista, the surrounding mesenchymal tissue of the fetus of 10 weeks (Fig. 18 b) becomes the cartilaginous labyrinthine wall and vacuolated periotic tissue of the 15-week stage (Fig. 18 c). When the crista attains virtually adult structure and size, in the fetus of 23 weeks, the capsular wall is formed in periosteal bone and the periotic labyrinth is well established.

Spiral Organ

The sensory end-organ in the cochlear duct develops from the epithelium along the posterior wall where the cochlear nerve fibers enter it (Fig. 19). Like the maculae and cristae, the spiral organ appears in early fetal life and attains adult proportions by midterm. Already in the placodal state, and also in the vesicle stage, the epithelium is stratified. This stratification is still a well defined feature in the eight-week fetus; in the anterior wall of the duct, however, it is much thinner than in the posterior and lateral walls. The other parts of the cochlea

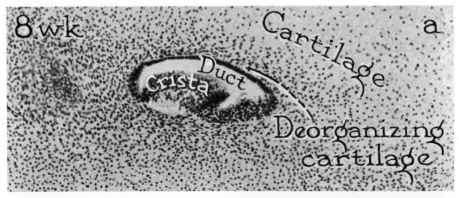

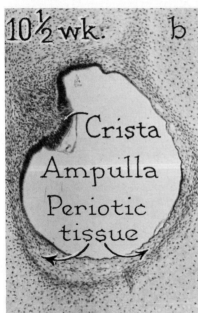 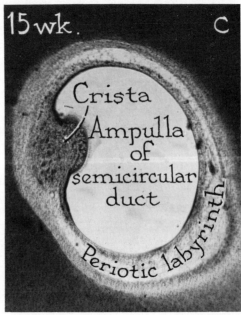

Figure 18. Crista of ampulla: Early development. *a,* Fetus of 8 weeks (25 mm.), lateral semicircular canal; *b,* fetus of 10½ weeks (50 mm. CR length), lateral canal; *c,* fetus of 15 weeks (100 mm.), posterior canal. Transverse sections. Wisconsin Collection, series 87, 86, and 22, respectively. *a,* × 127; *b,* × 82; *c,* × 38.

a, The crista of each membranous ampulla develops as a cushion-like elevation on the surface on the side of the ampullary wall where the sensory nerve enters. This corresponds to the convex side of the future semicircular canal (of the osseous labyrinth). At this stage the perilymphatic space of the bony labyrinth is represented by slight rarefaction of the cartilage in which the membranous ampulla is lodged.

b, As the ampulla enlarges, cartilage undergoes resorption, changing into a reticulum.

c, At the beginning of the fourth month the crista has attained sickle-shaped form. The primordial reticulum is giving way to space; this is the canalicular part of the perilymphatic labyrinthine system (or osseous labyrinth). In the five-month stage (not illustrated) the surrounding cartilage has changed to bone.

Each membranous semicircular duct lies eccentrically on the convex side of the osseous canal. The three ampullae are dilatations of the ducts; unlike the latter, they almost fill the corresponding expansion of the surrounding perilymphatic space. Each ampulla presents on the surface that corresponds to the convex side a transverse groove, the sulcus of the ampulla in which the nerve of supply enters, and the shelf-like ridge, or crista, which projects into the lumen.

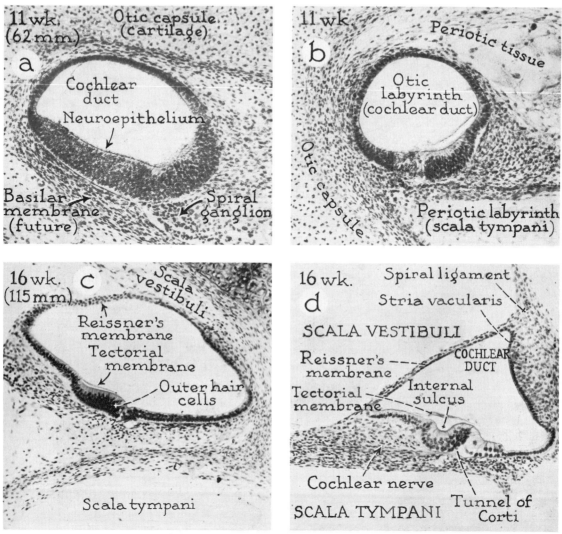

Figure 19. Regional development of the cochlear duct. Progress in a five-week period. *a,* Fetus of 11 weeks (62 mm. CR length) right ear, apical turn; *b,* same specimen, middle part of basal turn; *c;* fetus of approximately 16 weeks (115 mm.), left ear, apical turn; *d,* same specimen, middle part of basal turn. Transverse sections. Wisconsin Collection, *a* and *b,* series 160; *c* and *d,* series 54. *a,* × 130; *b,* × 134; *c,* × 125; *d,* × 128.

    a, In the apical turn of the cochlear duct of the 11-week fetus, the spiral organ (of Corti) is in a very early stage of development. The neuroepithelium is a simple stratified thickening of the primitive duct.

    b, In the basal turn of the same cochlea, elements of the future spiral organ are identifiable.

    c, In a specimen five weeks older, the apical turn of the cochlear duct is in a stage advanced beyond that of the corresponding segment in the younger fetus (*a*). The cochlear duct is set off from the scalae, the latter perilymphatic spaces being formed through resorption of the periotic reticulum (see Figure 21 *a*).

    d, In the basal turn of the same cochlea, all structures of the future duct are identifiable: internal sulcus, outer hair cells, vestibular (Reissner's) membrane, vascular stria, tunnel of Corti, and tectorial membrane. The cochlear nerve courses through tissue that will be contained in the osseous spiral lamina. (From Anson, B. J.: Section X in Morris' Human Anatomy. 12th ed. Used by permission of McGraw-Hill Book Company, New York.)

begin to differentiate at the beginning of the eighth week; these elements are the surrounding otic capsule, the centrally placed modiolus, and tympanic and vestibular scalae. The diameter of these scalae is greater than that of the cochlear duct. The interval is crossed by a spiral shelf (*lamina spiralis ossea*) which extends from the modiolus between the scalae to the posterior wall of the scala media. As the structures increase in size, the cross-sectional form of the cochlear duct changes from rounded (Fig. 19 *a* and *b*) to oval (Fig. 19 *b*), then finally to triangular. As a result, it comes to have three walls — anterior, posterior, and outer (Fig. 19 *d*). The anterior wall fuses with that of the scala vestibuli to form the vestibular membrane. The posterior wall merges with the wall of the scala tympani to form the basilar membrane; the outer wall rests on the spiral ligament; the inner angle of the cochlear duct is attached to the anterior surface of the osseous spiral lamina near the free margin of the latter.

With further growth of these structures, the epithelial duct becomes gradually modified. Along the anterior wall, in the area of the future vestibular membrane, it loses its stratification and becomes a simple columnar epithelium in the 11-week fetus. At 14 weeks this epithelium is cuboidal. Soon thereafter it flattens into a simple squamous type and continues so throughout life. The epithelium along the outer wall becomes modified in such a way as to resemble a glandular epithelium. The epithelial layer covers a vascular connective tissue, the *stria vascularis*, which in turn rests on the spiral ligament. The epithelium of the posterior wall (which is the basilar membrane) becomes highly modified into the spiral organ of Corti and the tectorial membrane.

The epithelium of the organ of Corti does not differentiate into its definitive parts in all cochlear turns until after midterm. Progress is most rapid in the basal turn, slowest in the apical turn. The epithelium of the apical turn in a fetus of 11 weeks is a thickened, pseudostratified layer (Fig. 19 *a*). But along the free surface of this epithelium in the lower turn there is an ill defined gelatinous membrane, the tectorial membrane (Fig. 19 *b*). In the lower turn the epithelium already shows a bulging and loosening of its cells in the region of the outer hair cells. In the 16-week fetus this condition in the lower turn is more marked, but in the apical turn differentiation has not yet taken place (Fig. 19 *c*). In the same stage the tunnel of Corti is beginning to appear in the basal turn

(Fig. 19 *d*), but not in the apical turn (Fig. 19 *c*). During the succeeding month the organ progressively completes its development toward its apical end, so that in a fetus of 21 weeks the tunnel of Corti is present in all turns. At about this age, or shortly thereafter, the internal ear attains its maximum size and becomes completely encased in its bony capsule. In the fetus of 25 weeks, the spiral organ closely resembles that of the adult.

Osseous Labyrinth

The perilymph-containing labyrinth consists of the tissue and the tissue-fluid spaces of mesodermal origin which surround most of the membranous labyrinth, thereby occupying the interval between the latter and the surrounding inner periosteal layer of the otic capsule.

Development of this labyrinthine system is rapid, being completed in approximately a four-month period, beginning near the second month of intrauterine life (Fig. 20). The process is similar in the three parts of the labyrinth — cochlear, vestibular, and canalicular (Fig. 21).

All parts of the perilymphatic labyrinthine system owe their formation to retrogressive alteration in which precartilage, halted in the course of its change into mature cartilage, is sacrificed to make way for fluid-containing, intracapsular space. This process may be very clearly demonstrated as it progresses in the canalicular division of the otic capsule (Figs. 20 *a* to *c*).

In the eight-week stage the tissue that immediately surrounds the semicircular duct begins to undergo resolution (Fig. 20 *a*). At 16 weeks cartilage has been replaced by a reticulum (Fig. 20 *b*). In the 24-week specimen the reticulum, in turn, has virtually disappeared (Fig. 20 *c*). This means that the change is accomplished in the space of four months, long before birth.

Formation of the perilymphatic spaces occurs first in the region which will become the vestibule. Next, similar spaces appear around the cochlear duct, those of the scala tympani before those destined to be the scala vestibuli. The appearance of the latter is, in turn, followed by the development of perilymphatic (periotic) spaces which, in surrounding the epithelial semicircular ducts, will be the corresponding semicircular canals.

Soon all these spaces fuse with one another

(*Text continued on page 46*)

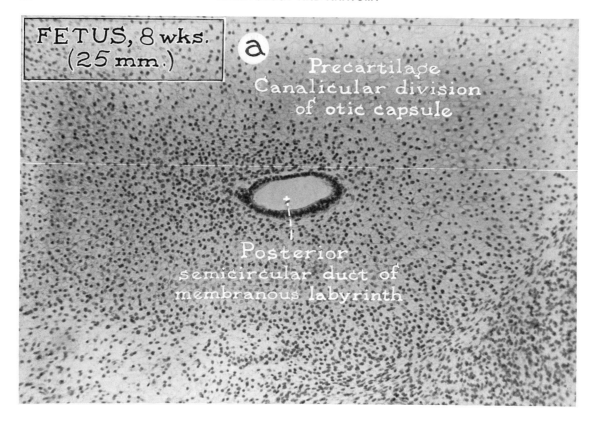

FETUS, 8 wks. (25 mm.)

a

Precartilage Canalicular division of otic capsule

Posterior semicircular duct of membranous labyrinth

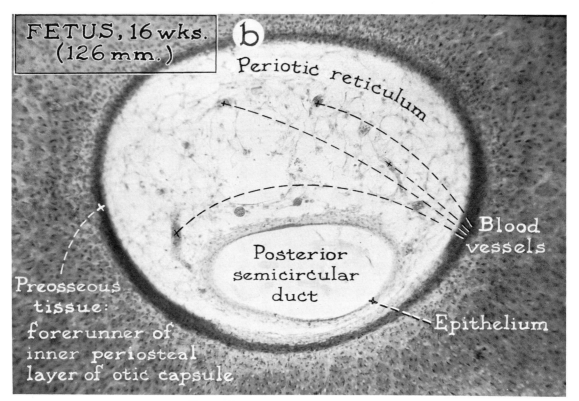

FETUS, 16 wks. (126 mm.)

b

Periotic reticulum

Blood vessels

Posterior semicircular duct

Epithelium

Preosseous tissue: forerunner of inner periosteal layer of otic capsule

Figure 20.   *See opposite page for legend.*

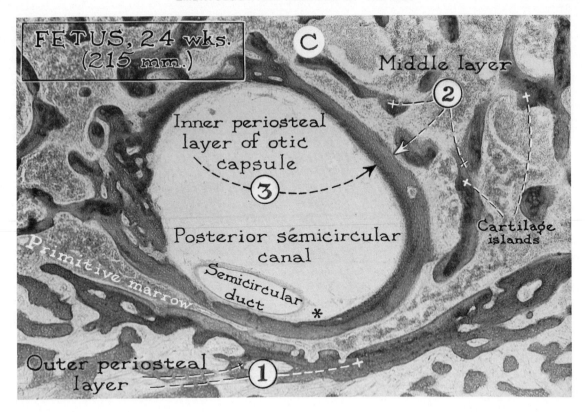

Figure 20. Perilymphatic space and surrounding capsule: Canalicular part. Developmental anatomy. Fetuses of two, four and six months. Transverse sections. Wisconsin Collection, series 87, 11, and 62, respectively. *a*, × 184; *b*, × 87; *c*, × 42.

a, In the two-month specimen, the precartilage around the epithelial duct system begins to undergo the kind of retrogressive change that will finally result in the formation of the space of the semicircular canals in this part of the otic capsule (the vestibule and scalae in the two other parts).

b, Precartilage is gradually replaced by a reticulum in which fibrils support small blood vessels. The latter have followed the route of the nerves from the internal acoustic meatus.

c, The delicate reticulum is largely lost, leaving virtually uninterrupted space between the epithelial duct and the periosteum that lines the semicircular canal. Where the duct is in contact with periosteum, periotic tissue remains chiefly as an anchorage (as at *). The surrounding otic capsule has undergone ossification; it consists of three distinctive layers of bone. (See Figure 4.)

The inner periosteal layer of the otic capsule (at 3), formed at midterm, remains apparently unaltered throughout life. The middle layer (at 2) at this stage is made up of cartilage islands or osseous globules. (See Figure 24.) These spicules of intrachondral bone are lodged in primitive marrow. They undergo little increase in bulk during the ensuing months of intrauterine life, until the time of birth approaches. Then the period of latency ends with onset of sweeping histological activity that soon converts the relatively solidified middle layer into part of the *pars petrosa*.

Differing from the middle layer, the outer periosteal layer undergoes, during the fetal months, steady increase in thickness and consistency. This is accomplished through deposition of bone (by osteoblasts) on the facing surfaces of the spicules. Although differing from the middle layer in developmental history and in histological appearance, it resembles, in gross appearance, the middle ear. The three layers are petrous in the adult temporal bone except where osseous tissue has been replaced by air cells. (From Anson, B. J.: Trans. Amer. Acad. Ophthal. & Otolaryng. *73*:17–38, 1969.

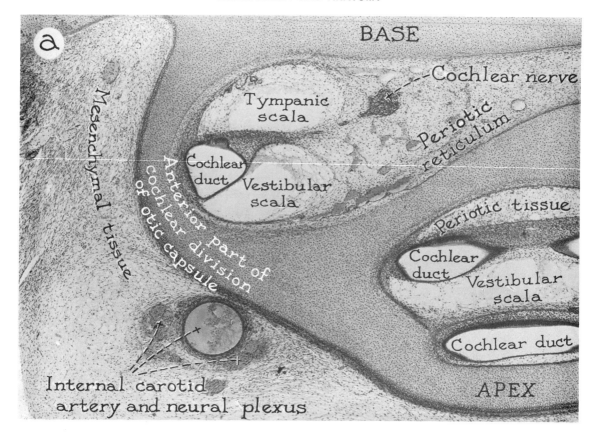

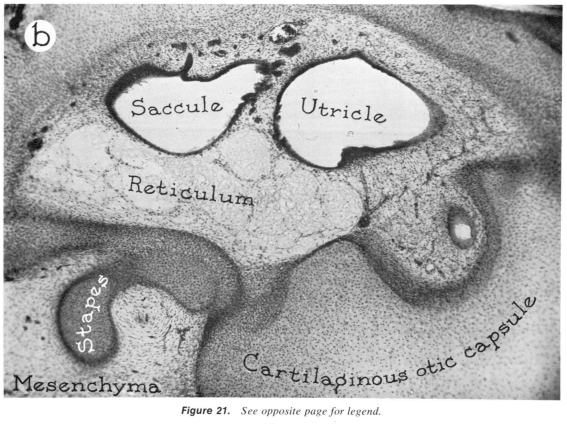

Figure 21. *See opposite page for legend.*

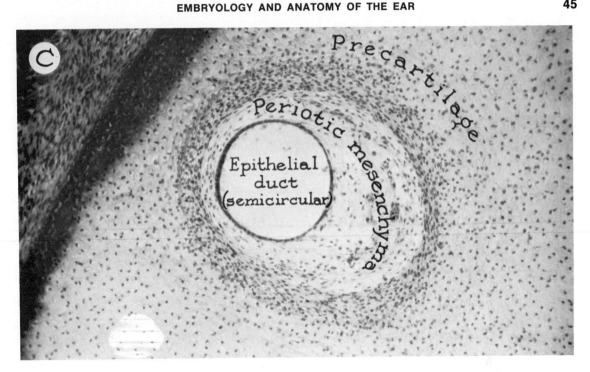

Figure 21. Perilymphatic space: Early development. *a*, Scalae of cochlea in a fetus of 12 weeks (84 mm.); *b*, vestibule in a fetus of 10 weeks (48 mm.); *c*, semicircular canal in a fetus of 10+ weeks (55 mm.). Transverse sections. Wisconsin Collection, series 162, 202, and 185, respectively. *a*, × 36; *b*, × 56; *c*, × 162.

a, In the three-month specimen, the reticulum that is closely related to the cochlear duct and to the developing spiral lamina is being resorbed. The small interfibrillar spaces that are thereby produced coalesce to form the scalae (here favorably demonstrated in the basal turn). The capsule is in the middle of its growth period as a wholly chondral element. After changing from precartilage in the second month, the first ossification center appears in the fourth month. (See Figure 26 *a*.)

b, In the vestibular part of the developing perilymphatic labyrinthine system, vacuole-formation is in a relatively advanced stage on the lateral aspect of the two membranous vesicles, the saccule and the utricle (this being the area in which such space first appears). On the opposite, or medial, aspect, the periotic tissue will undergo differentiation into supporting "ligaments" for the saccule and utricle and for the vessels and nerves of supply.

c, The periotic mesenchyma-like tissue is in a less advanced stage in the canalicular division of the otic capsule. The process of development of perilymphatic space, thereby slowed, is destined to go on for a longer time—until the fifth month, at which time the last of the fourteen ossification centers virtually completes envelopment of the semicircular canals.

The growth of the periotic labyrinth is virtually complete by the time the membranous labyrinth attains maximum size, at the middle of intrauterine life. Some strands of the periotic reticulum persist in the adult ear. Crossing the space between the endosteum of the osseous labyrinth and the membranous propria of the epithelial duct system (membranous labyrinth), they transmit small blood vessels to the latter.

to form a tortuous but uninterrupted, fluid-containing channel, the perilymphatic labyrinth.

In the early stage of development the histological structure of the perilymphatic reticulum is similar in the three portions of the labyrinth; they differ only in their relationship to the epithelial duct-system or membranous labyrinth. In the cochlea the two scalae are related to the cochlear duct (Fig. 21 a); in the canalicular division the canals surround the ducts (Fig. 21 c); the vestibule (between the cochlear and canalicular divisions) contains the utricle and saccule and portions of the communicating channels (Fig. 21 b).

Otic Capsule

The bony capsule develops rapidly from a cartilage model. It may, therefore, be classified as a cartilage bone, although in certain limited and special regions membrane bone takes part either in the initial process of ossification or in some phase of subsequent remodeling (in the modiolus, the tympanic wall of the lateral semicircular canal, the external ostium of the vestibular aqueduct, and the osseous spiral lamina).

During the early period of growth the internal ear is encased in a cartilaginous capsule. This cartilaginous forerunner of the osseous capsule goes on to the formation of bone in some areas and is deorganized in others in accommodation to increase in size of the labyrinthine system.

Here a comparison between a typical skeletal element and the petrous part of the temporal bone will serve to account for the exceptional developmental course and the retention of fetal structure of the otic capsule.

Like a typical long bone of the human skeleton, the capsule begins as a cartilage "model" (compare Fig. 22 a); but, differing therefrom, it grows with astonishing rapidity to attain adult dimension in the fifth month of intrauterine life (Fig. 22 d; compare Fig. 22 b). Even more striking in its deviation from the familiar pattern of development is its derivation from many (in fact, 14) ossification centers, each of which is trilaminar and without areas of epiphyseal growth (Fig. 23). The first center appears at the basal cochlear turn (Fig. 22 c), the last on the outermost part of the posterior semicircular canal.

The mesenchyme that surrounds the expanding otic vesicle changes into precartilage at about the seven-week stage. It will become true cartilage in embryos of eight weeks. Up to the sixteenth week of intrauterine life this capsule consists entirely of cartilage. Cartilage does not give way to bone until the underlying parts of the internal ear have attained their adult dimensions. In the canalicular region, where growth of the semicircular canals continues to about the twenty-first week, the capsule will remain cartilaginous until such growth is complete (Fig. 22 d). The earliest fusion takes place at the arch over the cochlear window; this occurs in the fetus of approximately 16 weeks, when the first three centers join. In a fetus of 19 weeks all but one of the centers (which appears at about the 20-week stage) has fused with one or more adjacent centers to form a unified skeletal element. The last center, the fourteenth, is present in the fetus of 21 weeks. At the 23-week stage, all centers have fused to form a complete bony capsule in which "suture lines" have been obliterated. There exists no histological mechanism to permit epiphyseal growth between centers.

Each constituent ossification center and, therefore, the otic capsule as a unit, is composed of three layers of bone; viz., the external periosteal, the intrachondral combined with the endochondral, and the internal periosteal. The outer periosteal stratum is formed from the cambium layer of the periosteum around the cartilaginous capsule. It is similar to the periosteal layer of long bones. The inner periosteal bone, immediately surrounding the labyrinthine spaces, is always thin and uniform in structure; it is derived from the inner periosteum. The middle layer is composed of combined intrachondral and endochondral bone. The intrachondral tissue of the middle layer consists of irregular areas of calcified hyaline cartilage, which contains true bone within the original cartilage lacunae. It forms the framework upon which endochondral bone is gradually deposited. Ultimately, through the increase of the latter, bone marrow is almost completely replaced; the originally capacious space is reduced to relatively small vascular channels.

Bone formation in the otic capsule is under way in the fifth fetal month, advancing more rapidly in the cochlear than in the canalicular division (Fig. 23 a and b). In the latter portion, cartilage is rendered spongeous to permit expansion of the semicircular ducts. Even in the six-month stage the canalicular capsule (area of the fourteenth center) has not yet changed

(Text continued on page 57)

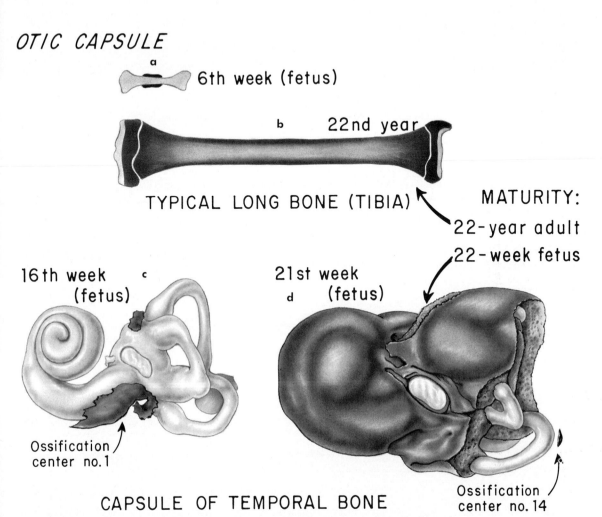

OTIC CAPSULE

a — 6th week (fetus)

b — 22nd year

TYPICAL LONG BONE (TIBIA)

MATURITY:
22-year adult
22-week fetus

16th week (fetus) — c

21st week (fetus) — d

Ossification center no.1

CAPSULE OF TEMPORAL BONE

Ossification center no.14

Figure 22. Development of the otic capsule in comparison with that of a typical long bone.

a, Cartilage "model" of a tibia in the six-week embryo. A collar of periosteal bone encircles the diaphyseal part of the future bone.

b, A typical long bone, with the epiphyseal centers of growth still present in the adult.

c, The beginning of bone formation in the otic capsule of man. The first ossification center appears along the basal turn of the cochlea in the area of the promontory. The perilymphatic space is shown in the reconstruction.

d, The last center appears at the 21-week stage in the canalicular part of the capsule, where spongeous cartilage (not shown) permits expansions of the arciform ducts.

In a typical long bone of the human skeleton, activity in a periosteal collar (a) accounts for diaphyseal growth, together with epiphyseal lengthening at proximal and distal areas of remnant cartilage. These processes may continue into the twenty-third year of adult life.

Bone formation in the otic capsule progresses on a wholly different pattern. Centers of ossification (c) fuse early, along contiguous surfaces without intervening zones of epiphyseal growth, to produce an osseous box for the labyrinth; one in which the constituent layers, three in number, continue to be histologically identifiable throughout life. (See Figure 23 *f.*) (From Anson, B. J.: Trans. Amer. Acad. Ophthal. & Otolaryng. *73:*17–38, 1969.)

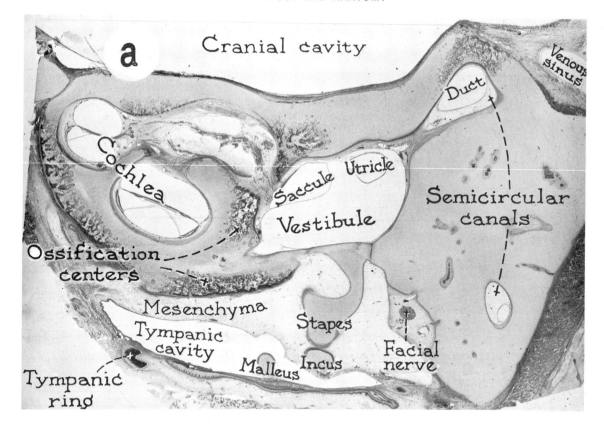

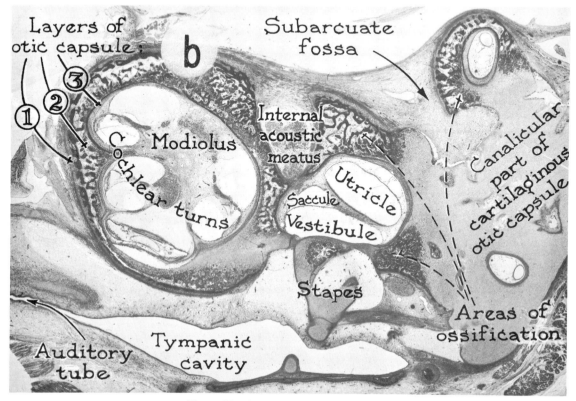

Figure 23.　*See opposite page for legend.*

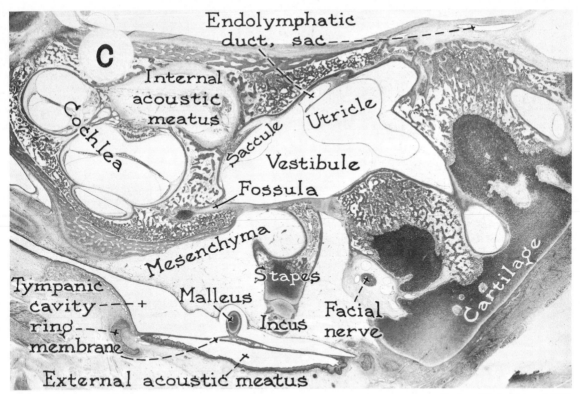

Figure 23. Otic capsule: Fetal and adult structure. *a*, Fetus of 20 weeks (167 mm. CR length); *b*, fetus of 19½ weeks (160 mm.); *c*, fetus of 23 weeks (202 mm.); *d* and *e*, newborn (4-day premature); *f*, adult, 19 years old. Transverse sections. Wisconsin Collection, series 105, 41, 70, 124, and 29, respectively. *a*, × 9; *b*, × 9; *c*, × 9; *d*, × 14; *e*, × 21; *f*, × 29.

a, In the fifth month of fetal life, ossification of the cartilaginous otic capsule has begun. Of the fourteen centers of bone formation, thirteen have appeared. Already it is evident that the change will progress more rapidly in the cochlear than in the canalicular division of the capsule. In the former part, vascular buds, having invaded the tissue around the semicircular canals, are beginning to render the cartilage spongeous.

b, In a specimen slightly younger, but more advanced than the preceding, the three typical layers of bone are present in much of the cochlea and vestibule: the outer periosteal (at 1); the middle (at 2), consisting of cartilage islands; the inner periosteal (at 3). Histogenesis in the canalicular part is characterized by extensive excavation. The blood vessels enter from the meningeal aspect, occupy the subarcuate fossa (Fig. 27 *a* and *b*); the fossa remains in the adult temporal bone in the form of an aperture of pinpoint size. Ossification is in progress in the ossicles.

c, In the sixth month of intrauterine life of the capsule, ossification centers, having fused peripherally to form a box-like case for the labyrinthine systems, remains cartilaginous in its posterior part and (in this specimen) in the *fissula ante fenestram*. The future facial canal is still a sulcus; the crura of the stapes are hollow columns of bone; mucous membrane of the tympanic cavity has enveloped the manubrium of the malleus; the tympanic ring is formed in membrane bone.

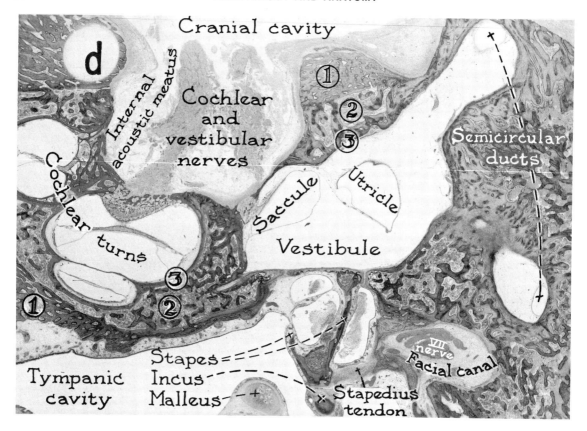

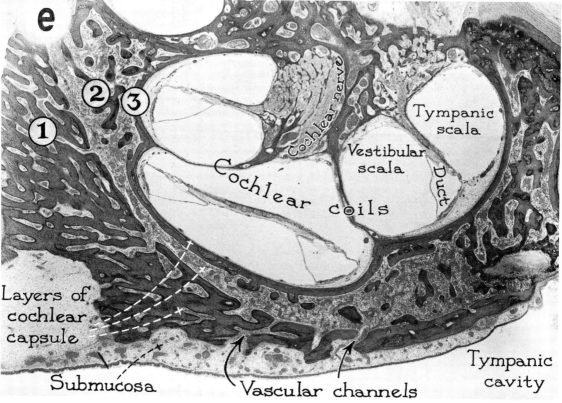

Figure 23. *Continued.   See opposite page for legend.*

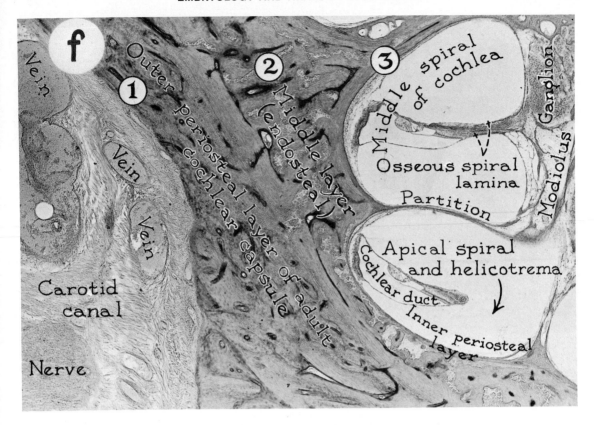

Figure 23. *Continued.*

d and *e,* In the late fetal stages and in the newborn, the following changes are evident: thickening of the outer layer in the cochlear division (1); endosteal bone formation in the middle layer of the canalicular part of the capsule (2). The inner periosteal layer (3) remains unaltered except insofar as it becomes connected with irregularly distributed islets of intrachondral bone (of the middle layer).

An area of the cochlea is shown in *e* (of a neighboring section) at higher magnification.

f, In the adult temporal bone, the middle layer (2) has become solidified, or petrous, in texture—matching that of the outer layer (1). Despite the deposition of endosteal bone on the cartilage islands, the latter areas remain throughout life as histologically diagnostic features of the middle layer. The capacious marrow spaces are reduced to small vascular canals.

It is clear from the photomicrographs herein described that the canalicular and cochlear divisions of the capsule are destined to attain similarly petrous fabric; except for a period of growth in cartilage, they pass through strikingly different series of morphogenetic steps.

The cartilaginous capsule arises as a unit from mesenchyma around the expanding otic vesicle. The mesenchymal tissue changes into precartilage at about the seven-week stage; precartilage becomes true cartilage in embryos of eight weeks. Between the second and fifth months the capsule grows in cartilage, keeping pace with enlargement of the contained membranous labyrinth. This means that the cartilage "model" of the capsule has attained maximum size before ossification begins.

With the very first step in bone formation, it is evident that the cochlear and canalicular divisions will go separate ways. Already in the five-month stage (Fig. 23 *a*), while ossification centers are forming in the cochlea, the cartilage around the semicircular canals is being invaded and resorbed by vascular buds from the internal auditory blood vessels through the arch of the superior semicircular canal; the channel thus formed is the subarcuate fossa. The vascular tissue reaches the height of its growth in the fetus of 21 weeks, at which stage the cochlear capsule is formed in trilaminar bone. Thereafter the vascular buds retreat and ossification of the canalicular capsule follows the pattern previously set in the cochlea (compare Figs. 23 *b* and 23 *c*). In the newborn, the divisions are similar in histological structure (Fig. 23 *d*).

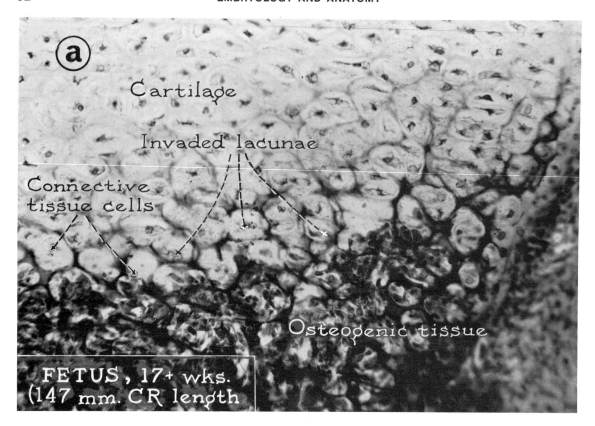

FETUS, 17+ wks.
(147 mm. CR length

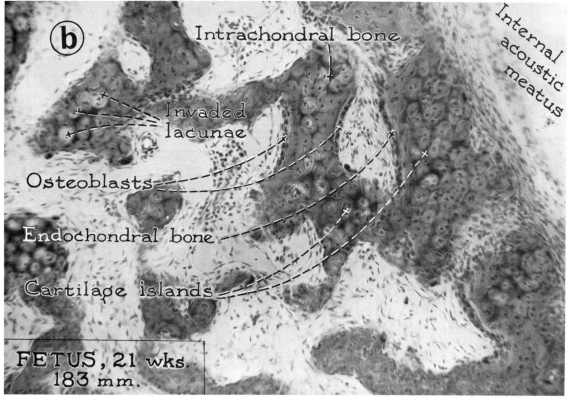

FETUS, 21 wks.
183 mm.

Figure 24.   *See opposite page for legend.*

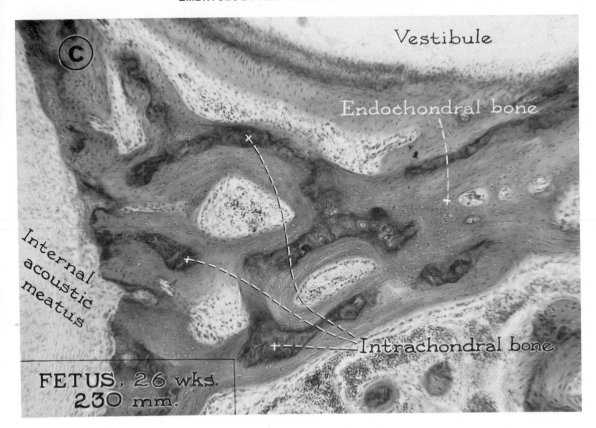

Figure 24. Otic capsule: Development of the middle layer. *a*, Fetus of 17+ weeks (147 mm. CR length); *b*, fetus of 21 weeks (183 mm.); *c*, fetus of 26 weeks (230 mm.). Transverse sections. Wisconsin Collection, series 38, 21 and 2. *a*, × 211; *b*, × 106; *c*, × 106.

a, The cartilaginous otic capsule, arising as a unit from mesenchyma around the membranous labyrinth, attains maximum growth before ossification is initiated (at approximately the beginning of the fifth month). In each of 14 centers of ossification, the process is similar: one in which the three constitutent layers follow different patterns of growth and differentiation and do so on independent timetables. Of the three laminae, the middle one is the most exceptional.

In the areas of growth, the cartilage cells enlarge, the matrix becomes calcified and the cells shrink and become atrophic. Osteogenic buds enter the lacunae of the calcified cartilage; in each excavated lacuna, the cartilage cell disappears and a nest of osteoblasts occupies the space.

b, The invading cells deposit an osseous lamina on the wall of the lacuna, without complete disappearance of the original cartilage. These islands, or bars, of separate derivation are termed "intrachondral bone." Osteoblasts deposit endochondral bone on the surface of the intrachondral bone. As a result, the middle layer of the capsule, as shown in the 21-week specimen, comes to consist of one type of bone imbedded within another.

c, Progressive deposition of endochondral bone widens the bars or spicules and reduces the size of the intervening marrow spaces to the dimensions of minute, sparsely distributed vascular channels (resembling Volkmann's canals). Just as the spicules fuse, so do the ossification centers which they comprise. Both the intrachondral and endochondral bone remain in their original form as primary bone; unlike skeletal elements generally, they are not re-excavated and rebuilt. Differing from all other bones that arise in cartilage, the otic capsule becomes an osseous box composed of a single skeletal element. The bone that comprises each center fuses, without epiphyseal interruption, with that of the adjacent centers of ossification.

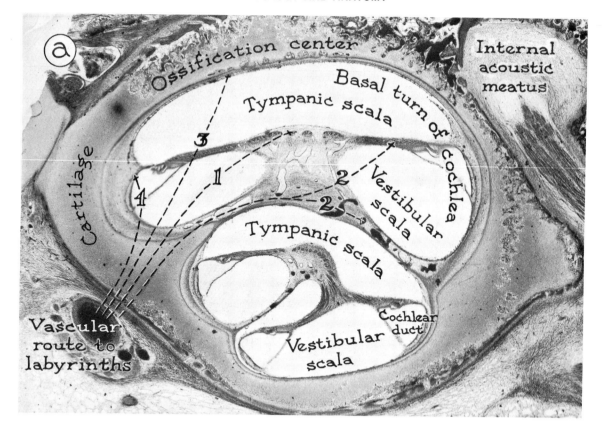

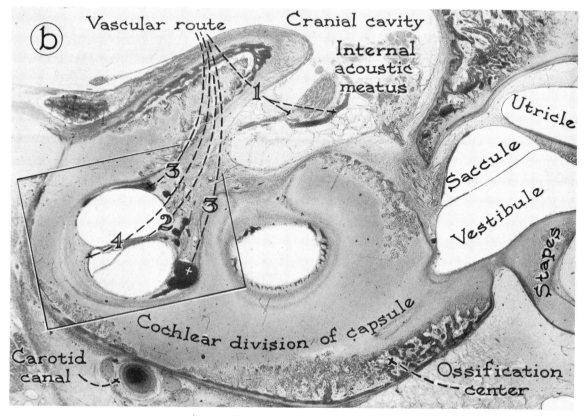

Figure 25. *See opposite page for legend.*

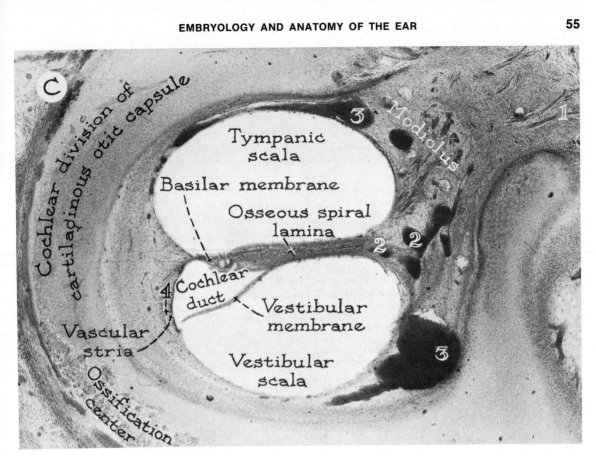

Figure 25.   Blood supply of the cochlea: Early development. Fetus of 19+ weeks (161 mm. crown-rump length). Transverse sections. Wisconsin Collection, series 13. *a*, × 18; *b*, × 16; *c*, × 44.

a, Demonstrating the pattern of branching and distribution of the internal auditory blood vessels from the internal acoustic meatus to the labyrinthine structures. They pass from the meatus to the modiolus of the cochlea (at 1), to the developing osseous spiral lamina and the partition between cochlear turns (at 2), to the walls of the scalae (at 3), and finally to the vascular stria of the cochlear duct (at 4).

b and *c*, Steps in the vascular route are traced from the internal acoustic meatus and modiolus (at 1), to the osseous spiral lamina (at 2), to the periotic tissue that lines the tympanic and vestibular scalae (at 3), finally to the *stria vascularis*. The rectangular area blocked in figure *b* is shown at higher magnification (with similar numbering) in figure *c*.

At this stage of bone formation in the cochlea, 12 of the 14 ossification centers are present in the otic capsule. Center No. 8 (cranially) has fused with Center No. 1 (caudally) to completely invest the labyrinth except in the area of the apical turn, where a seam of cartilage is still present. Each center is represented chiefly by an outer periosteal layer. Deep to this pellicle, cartilage is being invaded by vascular buds; conversion into islands of intrachondral tissue is, therefore, in progress. These islands of cartilage bone, once formed, will undergo exceedingly slow change in the remaining four months of fetal life. (See Figure 23.)

The cartilage that immediately invests the labyrinthine spaces of the cochlear capsule is a stratum in which blood vessels are wanting. But, within the scalae and around the cochlear duct, the vascular pattern is already established. Even after the cartilage has been replaced by bone of the middle and inner layers, the blood supply of the sensory elements of the membranous labyrinth continues to be independent of the supply to the capsule (*d*).

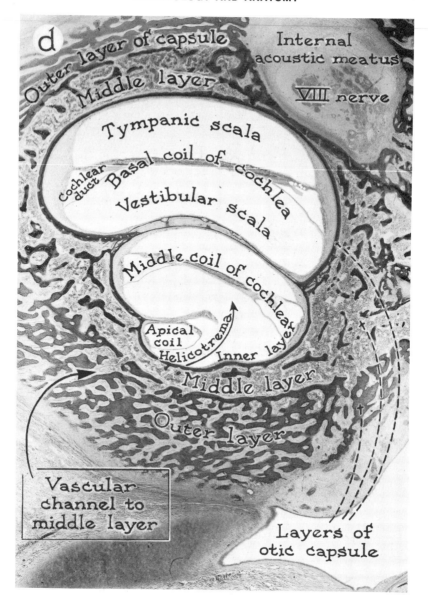

Figure 25. *Continued.*

d, Blood supply of the cochlea, later development. Fetus of 24 weeks (215 mm.). Transverse section. Wisconsin Collection, series 62. × 15.

Branches of the tympanic plexus of blood vessels, coursing through the submucosal tissue, pass inward by way of vascular channels in the outer periosteal layer of the capsule (as indicated by arrow at the lower left). They go as far as, but seem not to penetrate, the inner periosteal stratum. This means that the labyrinthine contents (vestibular and canalicular as well as cochlear) are supplied by the internal auditory artery and vein. The blood vessels follow the ramifications of the cochlear and vestibular divisions of the eighth nerve.

The vessels in the periotic tissue of the scalae (which is the peripheral remnant of the primitive reticulum) and in the developing osseous spiral lamina converge, so to speak, on the cochlear duct where they may be seen in the spiral ligament and in the vascular stria.

The schema here illustrated is substantially similar in the vestibular (for the utricle and saccule) and in the canalicular division of the otic capsule (for the semicircular ducts).

(Fig. 23 *c*). The middle layer of the entire capsule is still "cancellous" in structure. Solidification of this middle stratum is slow, being completed in early postnatal weeks (Fig. 23 *d* and *e*). Replacement of marrow by endosteal bone takes place with precipitate speed. The pattern then established is largely, sometimes totally, retained in the adult capsule (Fig. 23 *f*).

The dense, or stony, nature of the otic capsule is largely due to the compactness of the bone of the original centers of ossification.

Density is not, however, a characteristic of all portions of the "petrous" part of the temporal bone. The extracapsular part (composed of a late fetal and early postnatal extension of the outer periosteal layer) is not likely to remain petrous; rather it is usually pneumatic. The air cells, whose presence accounts for the "cancellous" nature of the bone, spread from the auditory tube and the tympanic cavity into the periosteal layer, and then into the endochondral bone (Fig. 11). It would appear that the innermost of the three layers normally remains unaltered throughout life.

The histogenesis of the middle layer calls for additional comment because it finds no counterpart in other bones of the human skeleton.

The cartilage of the primordial capsule begins to undergo change at the fetal stage of approximately 17 weeks. This initial step in ossification is marked by invasion of the chondral tissue by osteogenic buds of vascular connective tissue (Fig. 24 *a*). Some cartilage remains in the form of bars in which the lacunae, opened and invaded by osteoblasts, are converted into cartilage islands, or intrachondral bone (Fig. 24 *b*). Osteoblasts begin immediately to deposit endosteal bone on the outer surface of each such island. The intervening spaces that contain primitive marrow are thereby reduced to small vascular channels. As a result of these interrelated phases of development, the bone of the middle layer attains petrous character (Fig. 24 *c*).

The blood vessels in the vascular channels of supply to the otic capsule and to the immediately surrounding bone communicate mostly with arteries of the tympanic plexus located in the mucous membrane on the medial, or labyrinthine, wall of the tympanic cavity. Differing from the pattern of parietal supply, that of the sensory elements (within the cochlea, vestibule, and semicircular canals) comes through the internal acoustic meatus to the spiral organ, the acoustic maculae, and the cristae (Figs. 25 *a* to *d* and 26 *a* to *c*).

It is clear that the otic capsule is the most unusual skeletal element in the human body. The following developmental features are unique: origin, despite its small size, from 14 ossification centers, which appear within a period of six weeks, beginning with the fifteenth and ending with the twenty-first; fusion of the centers peripherally without intermediate zones of epiphyseal growth; trilaminar structure of each center and, consequently, of the total capsule; independent timetable of growth for each layer of every center; separate schema in attaining mature histological architecture. The outer periosteal layer grows by external application of lamellae and internal deposition of bone upon each such constituent; the inner periosteal layer seems never to change; the middle layer solidifies through increase in the endosteal bone, deposited upon islands of intrachondral bone. Fetal architecture, attained in these unusual ways, is kept throughout life in the total absence of those processes that elsewhere convert fetal into haversian bone.

Speed of growth is an equally arresting feature. A typical skeletal element (for example, the tibia), arising as a cartilage "model" (Fig. 22 *a*), attains adult dimensions in about 22 years (Fig. 22 *b*); the otic capsule in the fetus is as large as it will ever be (Fig. 22 *d*). A typical long bone arises from three centers: one diaphyseal, two epiphyseal. The otic capsule, about 1/150 as long, arises from 14, none of them epiphyseal (Fig. 22 *c* and *d*).

Capsular Channels

Considered as a space within an osseous box, the interior of the osseous labyrinth may be said to have eight channels of communication with the exterior: the internal acoustic meatus, subarcuate fossa and vestibular aqueduct on the medial surface; the cochlear aqueduct (or canaliculus) on the inferior surface; the two fenestrae, the fissula ante fenestram and fossula post fenestram on the lateral surface.

Internal Acoustic Meatus. The wall of the meatus is formed around the eighth nerve* and the internal auditory blood vessels. It is still a channel in cartilage in the four-month specimen (Fig. 26 *a*). Ossification centers are present at five months (Fig. 26 *b*). In the six-

---

*The stato-acoustic, later the vestibulocochlear, nerve of the *Nomina Anatomica*.

(Text continued on page 63)

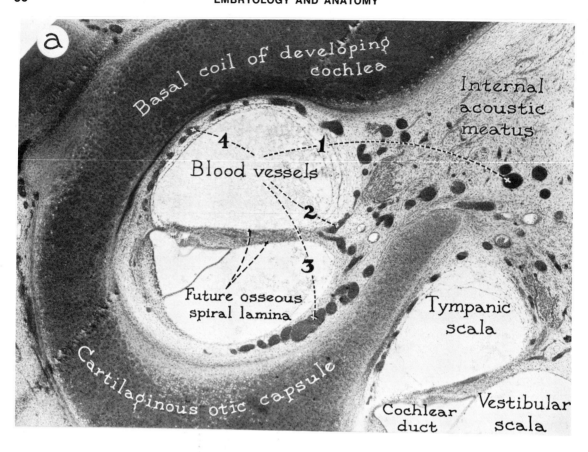

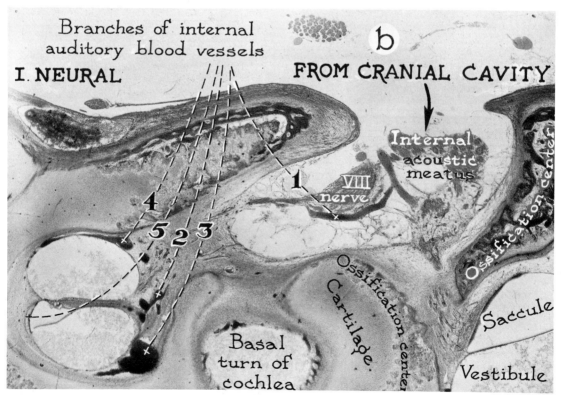

Figure 26.   *See opposite page for legend.*

month specimer
sule has become
spreading along
fetal dimensions
the adult (Fig. 2

Subarcuate Fc
tic meatus, the
temporal bone is
of blood vessels
the cerebellopo
However, in s
enough, and of s
course, as to l
proach to the ii
the similarity c
is a route for
render the carti
of the capsule
The resulting p
arcs of the semi
ceased in the ve
of the capsule (
fossa is reduced
life. It is usually
However, varia
striking (Fig. 2
anatomic "norn
quence where
approaches, or
ary site of the e
lar aqueduct (F
branches of the

Vestibular Aq
duct is formed a
and sac (Fig. 28
consists, in part
At this stage the
is undergoing a
the change in |
sac.

In the mature
pears typically a
rior surface of
considerable vai
tionships (Fig. 2

Cochlear Aqu
(or canaliculus)
the two-month f
precartilage on
turn of the cochl
ing cochlear (rot
from it runs thr
on the meninge
the pyramid. Its
the cochlear vei
29 b). Segregati
and 30).

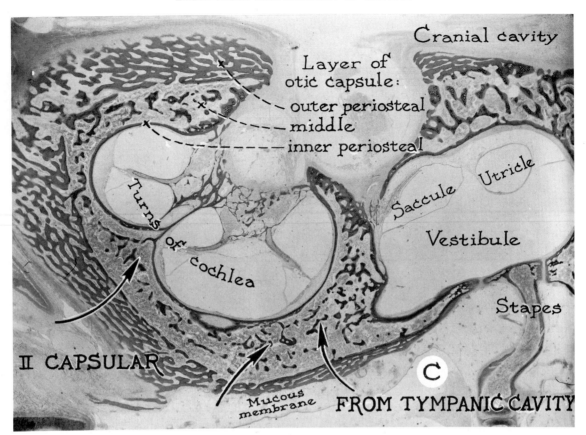

Figure 26. Development of the blood supply of the cochlear capsule and its contents. *a*, Fetus, 16 weeks (126 mm. CR length); *b*, fetus, 19½ weeks (161 mm.); *c*, fetus, 24+ weeks (215 mm.). Transverse sections. Wisconsin Collection, series 11, 13, and 62, respectively. *a*, × 43; *b*, × 17; *c*, × 13.

a, Showing the pattern of vascular supply to the membranous labyrinth in the four-month fetus (prior to the beginning of ossification of the otic capsule). Branches of the internal auditory vessels follow the rami of the vestibulocochlear (acoustic, or VIIIth) nerve. Here the cochlear vessels enter the internal acoustic meatus (1), to course in the osseous spiral lamina (2) along the wall of the scalae (3 and 4), finally reaching the spiral ligament and vascular stria.

b, Demonstrating the retention, in the five-month fetus, of the primordial scheme of blood supply. The branches pass from the internal acoustic meatus (1) to the turns of the cochlea (2). There, in each turn, the vessels course along the walls of the scalae (3 and 4) on their way to the *stria vascularis* (5). The pattern matches that of the neural ramification: the vessels come from sources in the cranial cavity that are primarily cerebrocerebellar.

c, Demonstrating that the vascular supply to the otic capsule differs from that of the contained sensory structures: the osseous shell receives tympanic vessels from the middle ear (anterior from the internal maxillary, superior from the middle meningeal, inferior from the ascending pharyngeal, and the posterior from the ascending pharyngeal).

On the promontory, the rami of the four arteries anastomose to form the tympanic plexus. The anterior tympanic artery (from the internal maxillary) enters the middle ear through the petrotympanic fissure (Glaseri). The superior tympanic (from the superficial branch of the internal maxillary) reaches the mucous membrane of the middle ear by passing through the tympanic canaliculus. The posterior tympanic artery (from the stylomastoid branch of the posterior auricular), coursing first through the facial canal, reaches the middle ear by way of the canaliculus for the chorda tympani, near the pyramidal eminence. The inferior tympanic (from the ascending pharyngeal artery) passes through the petrosal fossula and the tympanic canaliculus into the middle ear. (From Anson, B. J.: Trans. Amer. Acad. Ophthal. & Otolaryng. *73*:17–38, 1969.)

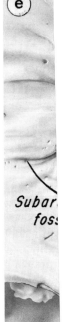

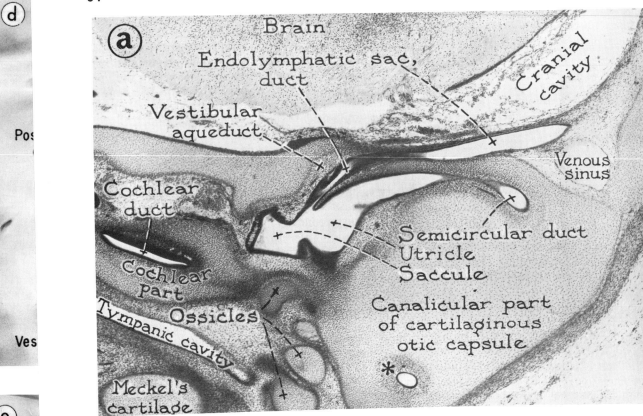

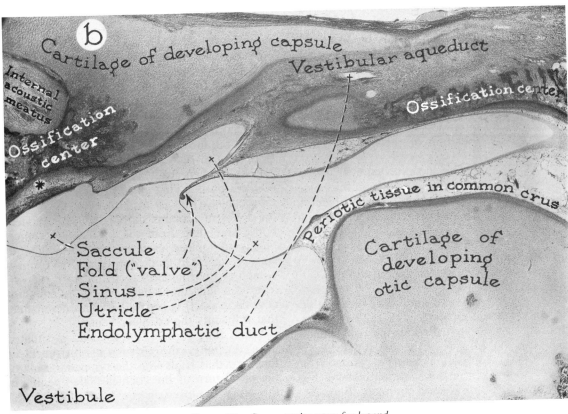

Figure 27.
d to *f.* Varia
d, The foss
The external
pyramid.
  e and *f,* Ap
petrosal sulcu

Figure 28.   *See opposite page for legend.*

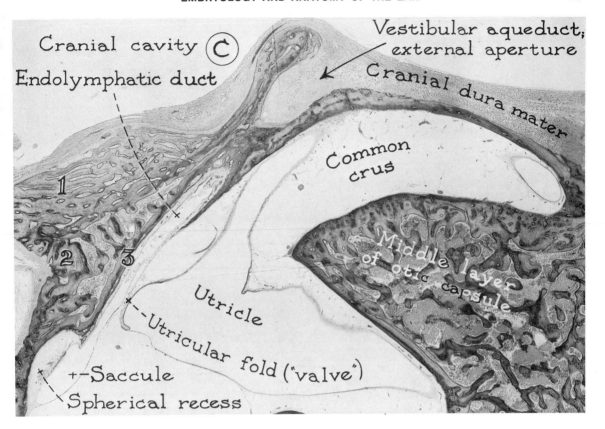

Figure 28. Vestibular aqueduct: Development. *a,* Fetus of 8½ weeks (28 mm.); *b,* fetus of 20 weeks (167 mm.); *c,* newborn (4-day premature). Transverse sections. Wisconsin Collection, series 158, 105, and 124, respectively. *a,* × 42; *b,* × 25; *c,* × 16.

a, In the fetus of two months, prior to the beginning of bone formation in the otic capsule, the cartilage immediately adjacent to the several divisions of the membranous labyrinth is undergoing retrogressive change; it is assuming the texture of a reticulum. This process accounts for the formation of the scalae, vestibule, cochlear aqueduct and semicircular canals (as at asterisk). The connective tissue thus produced contains numerous arterioles and venules, derived from the internal auditory blood vessels.

b, In the five-month fetus, in the early stage of capsular ossification, much of the periotic tissue has been resorbed, leaving perilymphatic spaces (in this section of the vestibule). The tissue of the aqueduct remains, later to assume the character of an adult connective tissue.

c, The aqueduct and its contents have assumed adult structure at birth. The internal aperture of the vestibular aqueduct opens on the wall of the elliptical recess of the vestibule. Traversing the bone of the pyramid, it terminates as an external aperture in the wall of the posterior cranial fossa. In the latter position, the sac occupies a foveate impression. (See gross specimens, Figure 29.) Proximally the duct communicates with the saccule and with the utricle. The opening is situated beneath a fold of valve-like form.

The surrounding capsule is trilaminar. It consists of an outer periosteal layer (at 1), a middle layer of intrachondral and endosteal bone (at 2) and an inner periosteal layer (at 3).

In the bone at the external aperture of the aqueduct further changes are destined to take place. In the 30-week stage, the middle layer is not only still left uncovered by periosteal bone, but apparently undergoes some resorption. At the time of birth new bone is deposited, with the result that the form of the aperture is changed. Here, the process of "remodelling" takes place in bone; whereas in the earlier modification of the canalicular part of the capsule, it is cartilage, not bone, that is involved in the remodelling.

The structure of the newly formed periosteal bone suggests that of membrane bone. Like much of the bone that lies peripheral to the area of the original otic capsule, it calls for further study. The gnarly character, lacking haversian pattern, places it in an uncatalogued position.

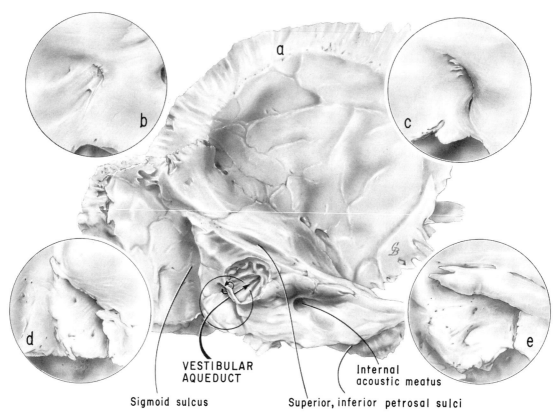

VESTIBULAR
AQUEDUCT

Internal
acoustic meatus

Sigmoid sulcus

Superior, inferior petrosal sulci

Figure 28A. Vestibular aqueduct: External aperture. Selected examples to demonstrate commonly encountered variations in size, form, and relationships. *a,* An example of a typical aperture and distal segment. *b* and *c,* Apertures of small and intermediate size. *d* and *e,* Apertures of large size lying close to vascular sulci in the "floor" of the fovea for the endolymphatic sac. (From Anson, B. J., Warpeha, R. L., and Rensink, M. J.: Ann. Otol. Rhinol. and Laryngol., *77:*583–607, 1968.)

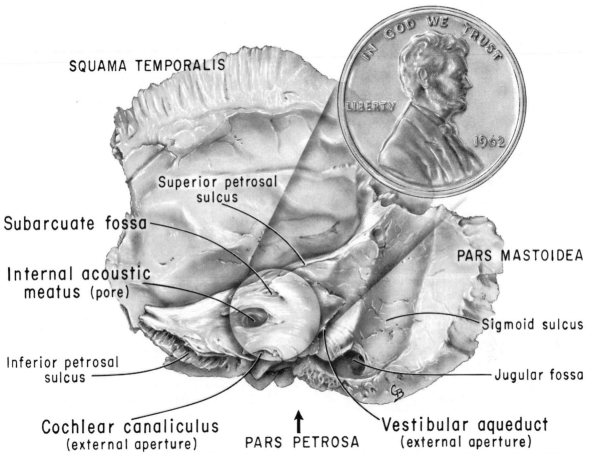

SQUAMA TEMPORALIS

Superior petrosal
sulcus

Subarcuate fossa

PARS MASTOIDEA

Internal acoustic
meatus (pore)

Sigmoid sulcus

Inferior petrosal
sulcus

Jugular fossa

Cochlear canaliculus
(external aperture)

PARS PETROSA

Vestibular aqueduct
(external aperture)

Figure 28B. Vestibular and cochlear aqueducts and related structures. The area is shown in comparison with the size of a copper cent outlined on the posterior surface of the petrous part of the temporal bone.

On this surface between the petrosal sulci are seen the external aperture of the vestibular aqueduct, the pore of the internal acoustic meatus, the opening of the subarcuate fossa, and notch marking the site of the external aperture of the cochlear aqueduct (or canaliculus) on the inferior surface of the bone.

(From Anson: Trans. Amer. Acad. Ophthal. Otolaryng. *73*:17–38, 1969.)

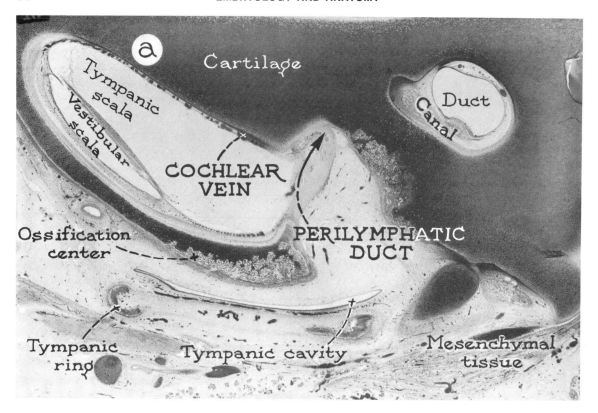

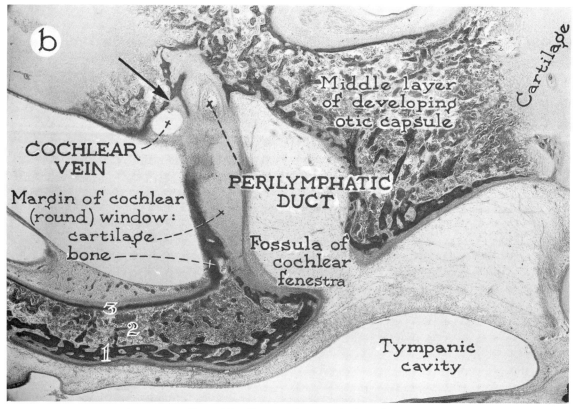

Figure 29.   *See opposite page for legend.*

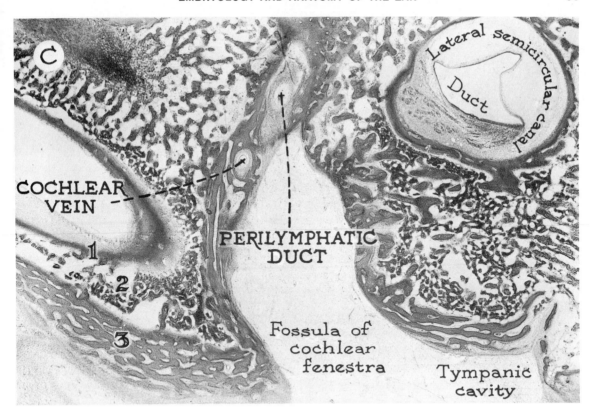

Figure 29. Cochlear aqueduct and perilymphatic "duct": Development. *a*, Fetus of 16½ weeks (126 mm. crown-rump length); *b*, fetus of 20 weeks (167 mm.); *c*, fetus of 21 weeks (183 mm.). Transverse sections. Wisconsin Collection, series 11, 105, and 21, respectively. *a*, × 15; *b*, × 20; *c*, × 21.

a, In the four-month specimen, at the beginning of ossification, the cochlear aqueduct (or canaliculus), containing the so-called perilymphatic (or periotic) "duct," is a stripe of retrogressively changing tissue in the cartilaginous otic capsule. (Compare Figure 27.) The internal aperture, shown here, is situated just inside of the developing cochlear window on the medial wall of the tympanic scala of the basal cochlear turn. It is already closely related to the cochlear vein.

b, In the five-month fetus, the otic capsule consists of three layers: an outer layer of periosteal bone (at 1), a middle layer composed of cartilage islands (at 2) and an inner lamina of periosteal bone (at 3). The outer layer is beginning to separate the cochlear aqueduct (with contained "duct") from a channel for the cochlear vein (see arrow).

c, In a slightly older specimen, the segregation is complete: each channel has an osseous wall.

The cochlear aqueduct (or canaliculus) in a skeletal preparation of an adult skull is observed to pass from the basal turn of the cochlea to the inferior surface of the pyramid between the jugular fossa and the external carotid foramen. In the fresh state its fibrous content is continuous at the internal aperture with the thin stratum of periotic connective tissue that lines the osseous labyrinth, and at the external aperture with the leptomeninges. The tissue within the aqueduct resembles that of the arachnoid; it is largely fibrillar. It is loosely meshed, the interfibrillar spaces outbulking the strands. Together the interstices make up the so-called perilymphatic (or periotic) "duct." Clinical observation points definitely to its service as a channel of communication between the perilymph of the osseous labyrinth and the cerebrospinal fluid in the subarachnoid space.

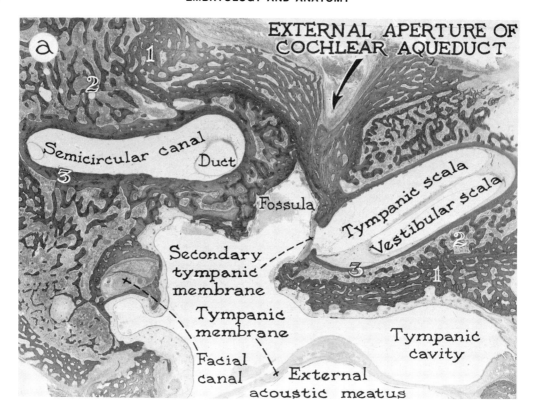

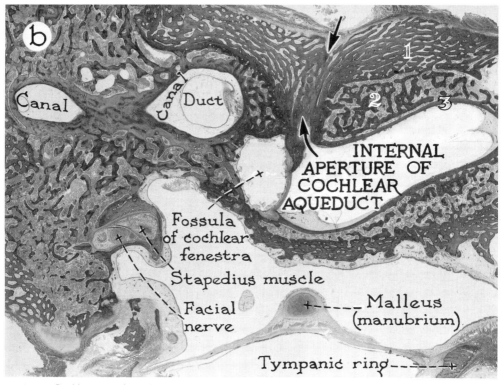

Figure 30. *a,* Cochlear aqueduct: Anatomy at the external aperture. The layers of capsular bone are numbered. (See Figure 23 *b, d, f.*) Newborn (four-day premature). Transverse sections. Wisconsin Collection, series 124. × 10.

b, Cochlear aqueduct, continued. Anatomy at the internal aperture. Same series. × 10.

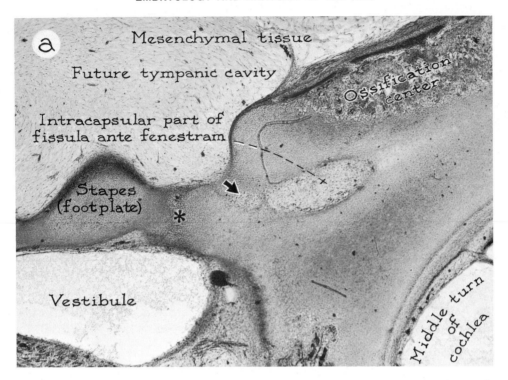

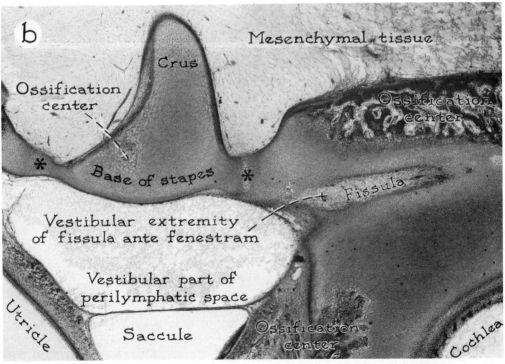

Figure 31. Fissula ante fenestram: Developmental stage. Fetus of 19 weeks (161 mm.). Transverse sections. Wisconsin Collection series 13. *a,* × 37; *b,* × 34.

a, The intraosseous portion, near the tympanic extremity (at arrow).

b, The vestibular extremity of the fissula. Here the tissue is continuous with that which lines the wall of the vestibule. In both figures the developing vestibular window is indicated by asterisks. Typically, as in this specimen, cartilage in the fissular tract undergoes retrograde change to become fibrous tissue. (Compare subarcuate fossa, Figure 27 *a* and *b.*) In some instances, the channel is occupied by cartilage or otosclerotic bone (Fig. 32 *a* to *c*).

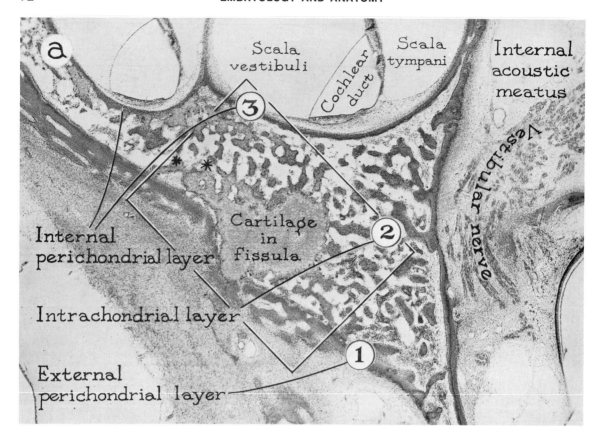

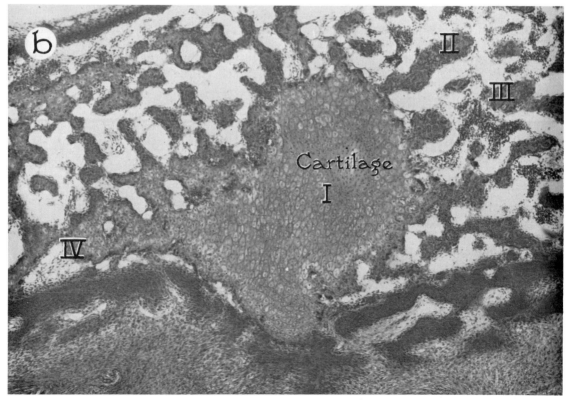

Figure 32. *See opposite page for legend.*

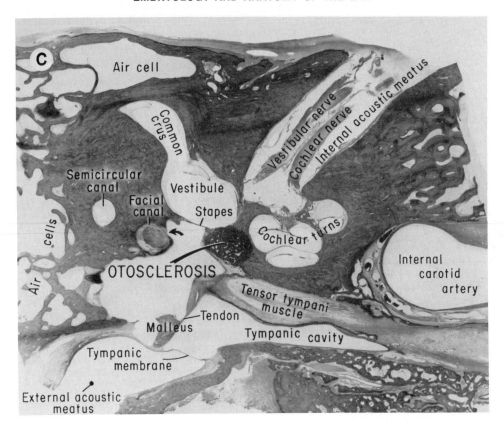

Figure 32. Fissula ante fenestram, continued: Aberrant and pathological tissue. *a* and *b*, Fetus of 21 weeks (183 mm.); *c*, adult, 54 years of age. Transverse sections. *a* and *b*, Wisconsin Collection, series 21. *c*, courtesy of Dr. C. M. Kos and Dr. J. A. Donaldson. *a*, × 34; *b*, × 71; *c*, × 4.

a, Showing an area of unresorbed cartilage in the customary location of the transcapsular tract of connective tissue termed the "fissula ante fenestram." The area blocked is shown at higher magnification in the following figure.

b, The histology of the middle layer (2), demonstrating stages in differentiation that lead to the formation of cartilaginous islands (*globuli interossei*). In the area shown, four stages in the change from cartilage to intrachondral bone are exhibited in the chondral nodule. The cartilage in the fissular area is unaltered tissue (I). As ossification proceeds, the cartilage lacunae are invaded by osteogenic buds (II) through whose activity cartilage is converted into intrachondral bone (III). Osteoblasts deposit layers of endosteal bone on the surface of these "islands" (IV).

c, Otosclerotic bone in the region of the fissula ante fenestram. (From Anson, B. J.: Trans. Amer. Acad. Ophthal. & Otolaryng. *73*:17–38, 1969.)

REFERENCES

References hereunder are limited to reports, in a collaborative program of otological research, upon which portions of the chapter are based.

Bast, T. H.: Early development of the bony capsule of the human ear. Laryngoscope 37:652, 1927.

Bast, T. H.: The utriculo-endolymphatic valve. Anat. Rec. 40:61–65, 1928.

Bast, T. H.: Ossification of the otic capsule in human fetuses. Carnegie Institution of Washington. Contrib. Embryol. 21:53–82, 1930.

Bast, T. H.: Blood supply of the otic capsule of a 150 mm. (C. R.) human fetus. Anat. Rec. 48:141–151, 1931.

Bast, T. H.: Development of the otic capsule. I. Resorption of the cartilage in the canal portion of the otic capsule in human fetuses and its relation to the growth of the semicircular canals. Arch. Otolaryng. 16:19–38, 1932.

Bast, T. H.: The utriculo-endolymphatic valve and duct and its relation to the endolymphatic and saccular ducts in man and guinea pig. Anat. Rec. 68:75–97, 1937.

Anson, B. J., Wilson, J. G., and Gaardsmoe, J. P.: Air cells of petrous portion of temporal bone in a child four and a half years old. A study based on wax-plate reconstructions. Arch. Otolaryng. 27:588–605, 1938.

Bast, T. H.: Development of the aquaeductus cochleae and its contained periotic duct and cochlear vein in human embryos. Ann. Otol. 55:278–297, 1946.

Anson, B. J., Cauldwell, E. W., and Bast, T. H.: The fissula ante fenestram of the human otic capsule. I. Developmental and normal adult structure. Ann. Otol. 56:957–985, 1947.

Anson, B. J., Cauldwell, E. W., and Bast, T. H.: The fissula ante fenestram of the human otic capsule. II. Aberrant form and contents. Ann. Otol. 57:103–128, 1948.

Anson, B. J., Bast, T. H., and Cauldwell, E. W.: The development of the auditory ossicles, the otic capsule and the extra-capsular tissues. Ann. Otol. 57:603–632, 1948.

Anson, B. J., and Bast, T. H.: The development of the otic capsule in the region of the vestibular aqueduct. Ann. Otol. 60:1072–1084, 1951.

Anson, B. J., and Bast, T. H.: The development of the otic capsule in the region of the cochlear fenestra. Ann. Otol. 62:1083–1116, 1953.

Richany, S. F., Bast, T. H., and Anson, B. J.: The developmental and adult structure of the malleus, incus and stapes. Ann. Otol. 63:394–434, 1954.

Anson, B. J., Bast, T. H., and Richany, S. F.: The fetal and early postnatal development of the tympanic ring and related structures in man. Ann. Otol. 64:802–823, 1955.

Strickland, E. M., Hanson, J. R., and Anson, B. J.: Branchial sources of the auditory ossicles in man. Part I. Literature. Arch. Otolaryng. 76:100–122, 1962.

Hanson, J. R., Anson, B. J., and Strickland, E. M.: Branchial sources of the auditory ossicles in man. Part II.

Observations on embryonic stages from 7 mm. to 28 mm. (CR length). Arch. Otolaryng. 76:200–215, 1962.

Anson, B. J., Harper, D. G., and Warpeha, R. L.: Surgical anatomy of the facial canal and facial nerve. Ann. Otol. 72:713–734, 1963.

Anson, B. J., Donaldson, J. A., Warpeha, R. L., and Winch, T. R.: A critical appraisal of the perilymphatic system in man. Laryngoscope 74:945–966, 1964.

Anson, B. J., Harper, D. G., and Winch, T. R.: Intraosseous blood supply of the auditory ossicles in man. Ann. Otol. 73:645–658, 1964.

Anson, B. J.: The endolymphatic and perilymphatic aqueducts of the human ear: Developmental and adult anatomy of their parietes and contents in relation to otological surgery. Acta Otolaryng. 59:140–151, 1965.

Anson, B. J., Donaldson, J. A., Warpeha, R. L., and Winch. T. R.: The vestibular and cochlear aqueducts: Their variational anatomy in the adult human ear. Laryngoscope 75:1203–1223, 1965.

Anson, B. J., Winch, T. R., Warpeha, R. L., and Donaldson, J. A.: The blood supply of the otic capsule of the human ear, with special reference to that of the cochlea. Ann. Otol. 75:921–944, 1966.

Anson, B. J., Harper, D. G., and Winch. T. R.: The vestibular system: Anatomic considerations. A.M.A. Arch. Otolaryng. 85:497–514, 1967.

Anson, B. J., Donaldson, J. A., Warpeha, R. L., and Winch, T. R.: The surgical anatomy of the ossicular muscles and the facial nerve. Laryngoscope 77:1269–1294, 1967.

Anson, B. J., Harper, D. G., and Winch, T. R.: The vestibular and cochlear aqueducts: Developmental and adult anatomy of their contents and parietes. Third Symposium on the Role of the Vestibular Organs in Space Exploration. NASA SP-152:125–146, 1968.

Anson, B. J., Harper, D. G., and Winch, T. R.: The vascular routes to the petrous part of the temporal bone: Developmental and adult anatomy. Third Symposium on the Role of the Vestibular Organs in Space Exploration. NASA SP-152:259–288, 1968.

Anson, B. J., Warpeha, R. L., Donaldson, J. A., and Rensink, M. J.: The developmental and adult anatomy of the membranous and osseous labyrinths and of the otic capsule. Otolaryng. Clin. N.A., October, 1968, pp. 273–304. (Also published as Meniere's Disease, Jack L. Pulec, ed.). Philadelphia, W. B. Saunders Company, 1968.

Anson, B. J., Warpeha, R. L., and Rensink, M. J.: The gross and macroscopic anatomy of the labyrinths. Ann. Otol. 77:583–607, 1968.

Anson, B. J.: Endolymphatic hydrops: Anatomic aspects. Arch. Otolaryng. 89:96–110, 1969.

Anson, B. J., The labyrinths and their capsule in health and disease. Trans. Amer. Acad. Ophthal. Otolaryng. 73:17–38, 1969. (Address of the Guest of Honor to the Joint Session, 1968.)

Litton, W. B., Krause, C. J., Anson, B. J., and Cohen, W. N.: The relationship of the facial canal to the annular sulcus. Laryngoscope, 79:1584–1604, 1969.

ANATOMY OF THE EAR

by

James A. Donaldson, M.D., and Josef M. Miller, Ph.D.

The peripheral auditory system functions to receive mechanical vibrations, to conduct these vibrations to the site of the primary receptor cells, and to transduce this energy into an encoded electrical form appropriate for conduction into and analysis by the central nervous system. The reception, conduction, and transduction processes are strictly determined by the structural characteristics of this special receptor. Corresponding in part to these functions, the ear can be divided into three regions, each of which has distinct structural and functional characteristics. The external ear, whose function is to receive sound waves, consists of the auricle and a short tube, the external acoustic meatus. The external meatus is closed medially by the tympanic membrane. The middle ear is an air-containing space in the petrous portion of the temporal bone containing the auditory ossicles. The main function of the middle ear is to conduct sound waves received by the external ear to the receptor cells with little energy loss. To do this the middle ear must act as an impedance matcher. The inner ear, consisting of the osseous and membranous labyrinths, serves a dual function as the primary receptor site for both hearing and balance.

EXTERNAL EAR

Auricle (Fig. 33). The auricle is a flexible appendage of thin elastic cartilage covered by skin. Anteriorly the skin is firmly attached, while posteriorly the skin is separated from the

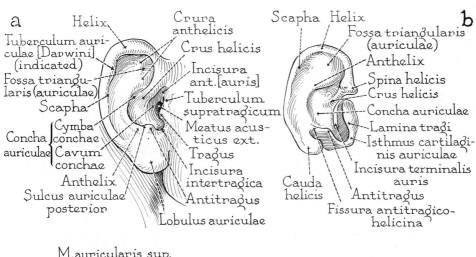

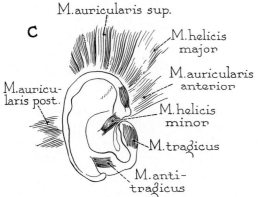

Figure 33. Auricle. *a*, Topographic anatomy of the auricle with skin intact. *b*, Supporting cartilaginous framework. *c*, Extrinsic and intrinsic auricular muscles. (From Section X, p. 1174, The Sense Organs. Morris' Human Anatomy. 12th ed. New York, Blakiston Division, McGraw-Hill Book Company, 1966.)

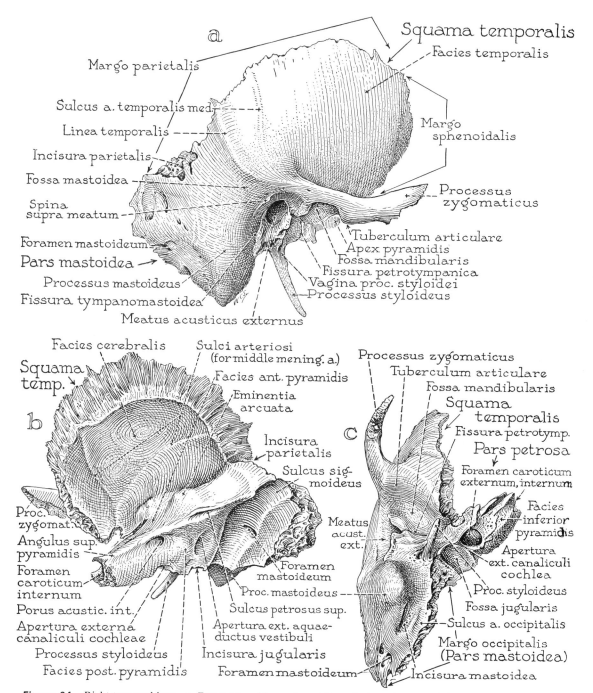

Figure 34. Right temporal bone. *a*, Dry temporal bone viewed from the lateral aspect. *b*, Same bone from the medial aspect. *c*, Inferior view. (From Anson, B. J.: An Atlas of Human Anatomy, 1950, p. 13.)

cartilaginous surface by a distinct subcutaneous layer. The tight adherence of the skin to the cartilage results in ridges and concavities of the auricle (Fig. 33 *a*) corresponding to the ridges and concavities of the auricular cartilage (Fig. 33 *b*). The absence of a subcutaneous layer between skin and cartilage anteriorly makes the auricle susceptible to frostbite despite a rich supply of superficial vessels. Other than a few small, downy hairs with associated sebaceous glands and scarce sweat glands, skin appendages are rare except in old age when stiff hairs may develop on the dorsal surface of the auricle and ear lobe.

The auricle is connected to the skull and scalp by three extrinsic muscles: the anterior, superior, and posterior auricular muscles. Development of the extrinsic muscles is quite variable in man; when well developed, they are capable of moving the ear. There are also a number of intrinsic muscles associated with the auricle; in man these muscles are indistinguishable grossly and have no functional significance.

Arterial supply to the auricle originates from the superficial temporal and posterior auricular arteries; venous drainage is supplied by the corresponding veins and the mastoid emissary vein. Lymphatic drainage is to the anterior, posterior, and inferior auricular nodes. The great auricular nerve innervates the medial side of the auricle; the upper portion is innervated by the lesser occipital nerve. The lateral side of the auricle is innervated by twigs of the great auricular nerve coursing over the helix and by the auriculotemporal nerve. Motor nerves to the extrinsic muscles extend from the temporal and posterior auricular branches of the facial nerve.

External Acoustic Meatus (Figs. 34 and 35). Between the auricle and the tympanic membrane, the external acoustic meatus assumes a medial and inferior "S" form. The shorter posterosuperior wall is 25 mm. long, while the longer antero-inferior wall is 31 mm. in length. The difference is caused by the oblique placement of the tympanic membrane. The size and shape of the canal vary. It is elliptical in cross-section, with the greater diameter of the ellipse being vertical at the auricular end and nearly horizontal at the tympanic end. Two prominences limit visibility of the tympanic membrane. The floor of the bony canal has an upward convexity at about its midpoint, while the anterior wall of the canal has a posterior convexity at its midpoint. Visibility of the drum membrane may be enhanced by pulling the auricle posteriorly, superiorly, and laterally. These irregularities in the external auditory meatus also predispose the canal to foreign body entrapment antero-inferiorly at the medial end of the bony canal. This region of the canal is known as the sulcus.

Slightly more than the medial half of the external acoustic meatus is bony, and the remaining lateral portion is a fibrocartilaginous tube open superiorly. The skin of the meatus is relatively thick in the cartilaginous portion, but gradually becomes very thin in the bony portion, especially anteriorly and inferiorly. It is firmly attached to perichondrium and periosteum, respectively. This skin of the cartilaginous meatus contains numerous fine hairs which continue only posteriorly and superiorly in the bony meatus. Sebaceous glands are exceptionally large in the cartilaginous portion, although present only on the posterosuperior wall of the bony meatus. Two horizontal clefts, the incisures of Santorini, are usually present in the anterior cartilaginous wall. While these allow increased flexibility of the meatus, they also allow extension of parotid abscesses into the meatus.

The blood supply to the external acoustic meatus is provided by the posterior auricular and superficial temporal arteries, as well as by the deep auricular artery which also supplies the tympanic membrane. Venous blood drains by way of the maxillary and external jugular veins and the pterygoid venous plexus. Lymphatic drainage is to the anterior, posterior, and inferior auricular nodes. Sensory innervation is supplied to the upper portion of the meatus and the tympanic membrane by the auricular branch (Arnold's) of the vagus nerve and by the auriculotemporal branch of the mandibular nerve.

Tympanic Membrane. The tympanic membrane is a membranous partition separating the external acoustic meatus from the tympanic cavity. It is semitransparent and elliptical — 9 to 10 mm. vertically and 8 to 9 mm. horizontally. Its external aspect is concave, the most depressed point being the umbo, which corresponds to the tip of the manubrium of the malleus. The manubrium itself extends from the umbo to the malleal prominence formed by the lateral process of the malleus (Fig. 36). From the malleal prominence, the anterior and posterior malleal folds extend to the edges of the tympanic notch (notch of Rivinus) and separate pars flaccida (Shrapnell's membrane) above from pars tensa below. The average thickness of the tympanic membrane is 0.074

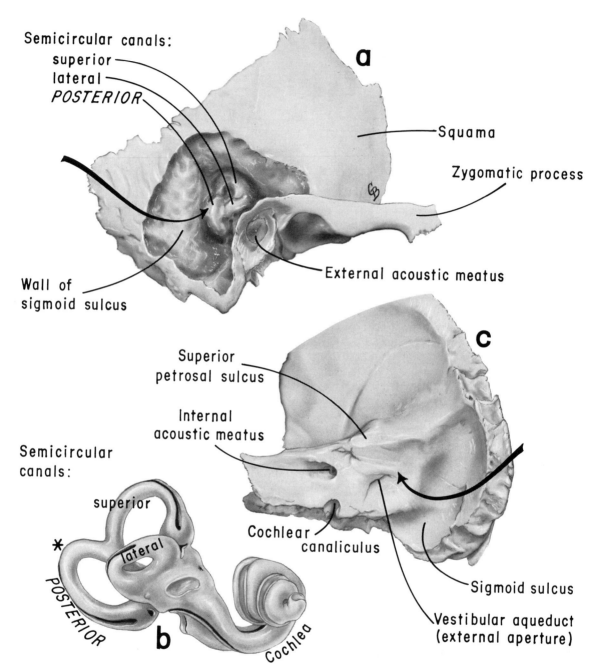

Figure 35. Right temporal bone.

a, The bone of the mastoid process has been removed, exposing to view the skeletonized semicircular canals.

b, Oriented in the same position as *a*, the entire skeletonized bony labyrinth is shown.

c, The posterior surface of the temporal bone is seen as if viewed through the posterior cranial fossa. The details of the posterior surface of the petrous portion are shown. (Anson, B. J.: Arch. Otolaryng. *89*:99, 1969.)

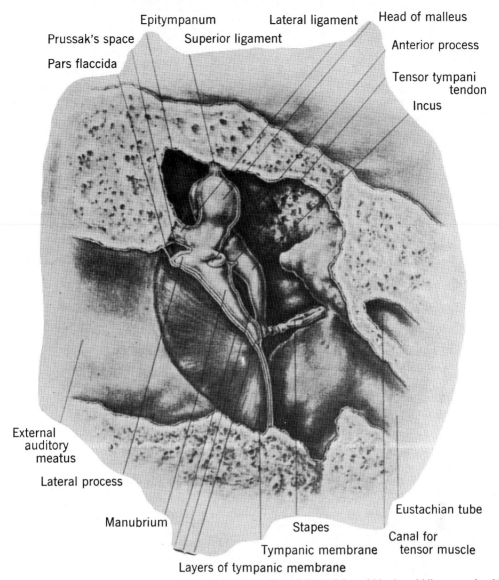

Epitympanum   Lateral ligament   Head of malleus

Prussak's space   Superior ligament   Anterior process

Pars flaccida   Tensor tympani tendon

Incus

External auditory meatus

Lateral process

Manubrium   Eustachian tube

Stapes   Canal for tensor muscle

Tympanic membrane

Layers of tympanic membrane

Figure 36. The middle ear. This view illustrates the suspension of the ossicles within the middle ear cavity. Note the attachment of the manubrium of the malleus to the tympanic membrane and the insertion of the stapes into the vestibular fenestra. (From Deaver, J. B.: Surgical Anatomy of the Human Body. Philadelphia, Blakiston Company, 1926.)

mm.; it is thickest (0.09 mm.) near the annulus inferiorly and antero-superiorly, and thinnest (0.055 mm.) in the middle of the posterosuperior quadrant.

The pars tensa of the tympanic membrane is composed of four layers. The lateral layer is continuous with the skin lining the external auditory meatus. It is 50 to 60 μ thick. Medial to this is a radiate fibrous layer with collagenous fibers passing from the umbo and manubrium to the peripheral fibrocartilaginous ring. More medial is the layer of nonradial fibers consisting of three types: circular, parabolic, and transverse. The parabolic fibers arise from the upper margin of the tympanic ring and partially cross the circular fibers. The transverse fibers are limited to the intermediate zone of the inferior quadrant where vibration amplitude is greatest. The inner layer of the tympanic membrane is a continuation of the mucosa of the tympanum and is 20 to 40 μ thick. Whereas the pars tensa contains all the above layers, the pars flaccida consists only of the lateral cutaneous layer and the mucosal layer. Epithelial migration of the tympanic membrane has been vividly demonstrated by Litton

(1963), who showed that it was centrifugal from the umbo at about 0.05 mm. per day.

The arterial supply laterally is from the tympanic branch of the deep auricular artery and medially from the anterior tympanic branch of the internal maxillary artery and the stylomastoid branch of the posterior auricular artery. The venous drainage corresponds to that of the external meatus and the tympanic cavity. Innervation is via the auricular branch of the vagus, the tympanic branch of the glossopharyngeus (of Jacobson), and the auriculo-temporal branch of the mandibular.

MIDDLE EAR

The tympanic cavity or middle ear is a mucous membrane-lined space between the tympanic membrane and the osseous labyrinth. The cavity is flattened, with vertical and antero-posterior diameters of 15 mm. and a mediolateral depth ranging from 6 mm. superiorly to 2 mm. at the umbo. The cavity can be divided into the tympanic cavity proper, medial to the tympanic membrane; the epitympanic recess, cephalad to the upper border of the tympanic membrane; the tympanic antrum with the mastoid air cells; and the hypotympanic recess, caudad to the tympanic membrane.

Acoustic Ossicles. The three acoustic auditory ossicles responsible for the conduction of sound waves from the external ear to the inner ear are suspended within the tympanic cavity (Fig. 36). The ossicles include the malleus, the incus, and the stapes. These bones are suspended as a chain which bridges the middle ear space from the tympanic membrane to the functional entrance of the inner ear, the vestibular fenestra, or oval window. As may be observed in Figure 37, the largest ossicle is the malleus. Its two major components are its head and manubrium. The length of this bone is from 8 to 9 mm. The incus consists of a body, a short process (5 mm.), and a long process (7 mm.). The stapes is the smallest bone of the body. Its overall height is approximately 3.3 mm.; its foot plate measures about 3 mm. by 1.4 mm.

Primary attachment of the malleus to the tympanic membrane is made via the manubrium, with the tip of the manubrium terminating at the umbo. The concave shape of the tympanic membrane is a result of the manner of suspension of the ossicles within the middle ear. The tip of the manubrium tends to retract the tympanic membrane into the middle ear cavity. Articular ligaments join the head of the

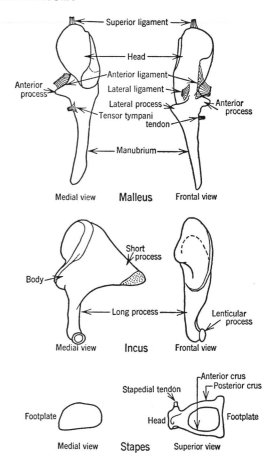

Figure 37. The auditory ossicles from the right ear, shown separately, five times natural size. (From Wever, E. G., and Lawrence, M.: Physiological Acoustics. 2nd ed. Princeton, New Jersey, Princeton University Press, 1954, p. 13.)

malleus to the body of the incus and the long process of the incus to the head of the stapes. The annular ligament holds the foot plate of the stapes in the vestibular fenestra. Aside from the annular ligament of the stapes and drum membrane attachment of the malleus, four other ligaments suspend this ossicular chain in the middle ear: the superior, anterior, and lateral ligaments of the malleus, and the posterior ligament of the incus. Additional support for the system is provided by two muscles, one attached to the malleus (the tensor tympani) and the other to the stapes (the stapedius). These muscles can restrain the movement of the system and play a role in the protection of the inner ear structure from intense sounds.

Walls of the Cavity. The tympanic cavity has six walls which are approximately paired. The roof or tegmen tympani separates the tympanic cavity from the middle cranial fossa. The floor of the hypotympanic recess is narrow transversely and is covered with tympanic cells. It is thin centrally and may be dehiscent, exposing the dome of the jugular bulb. This floor separates the hypotympanic recess from the internal carotid artery anteroinferiorly and the dome of the jugular bulb posteroinferiorly.

The posterior tympanic wall is open above (aditus ad antrum) and contains a recess (fossa incudis) for the short process of the incus. On this wall at the level of the stapes is a prominence, the pyramidal eminence (Fig. 38), through which the stapedius tendon travels from the stapedius muscle to the neck of the stapes. The general area lateral to the pyramidal eminence is the suprapyramidal recess, often referred to as the facial recess. Farther lateral is the aperture through which the chorda tympani enters the tympanum. Medial to the pyramidal eminence is a cavity, the sinus tympani, which usually extends medial to the stapedius muscle and which may extend medial to the vertical course of the facial nerve and/or even medial to its horizontal course. The anterior wall of the tympanum funnels into the tympanic orifice of the auditory tube, above which is the semicanal of the tensor tympani muscle, and posteroinferior to which is the internal carotid artery as it changes from its vertical to horizontal course through the temporal bone.

The lateral wall of the tympanic cavity proper is formed by the tympanic membrane, while that of the epitympanum is formed by the tympanic scutum (of Leidy), a portion of the squama closing the tympanic notch. The major feature of the medial wall (Fig. 39) is the promontory produced by the bulging basal turn of the cochlea. Coursing almost vertically over the promontory is a groove for the tympanic branch (Jacobson's) of the glossopharyngeal nerve. Posterior to the promontory the wall is divided into three depressions by two bony structures, the subiculum and the ponticulus. The subiculum is a ridge formed by the posterior prolongation of the cephalad border of the fossula of the cochlear fenestra. The ponticulus is a fine bony ridge passing from the area of the pyramidal eminence to the promontory. It is nearly parallel to the stapedius tendon. The lowest of these three depressions, caudad to the subiculum, is the fossula of the cochlear fenestra containing the secondary tympanic membrane. The central depression between the subiculum and the ponticulus is the anterior portion of the sinus tympani, and

above the ponticulus is the fossula of the vestibular fenestra containing the stapes.

The prominence of the facial canal (Fig. 40) is above the fossula of the vestibular fenestra. The anterior extent of the facial canal prominence is marked by the cochleariform process through which the tensor tympani changes its route and courses laterally to the malleus. The tensor is a relatively large muscle, 22 mm. long, forming part of the roof of the eustachian tube and part of the medial wall of the tympanum. It arises from the cartilaginous part of the tube, the great wing of the sphenoid, and the wall of its own semicanal, attaching to the manubrium of the malleus near its neck.

Tympanic Mucous Membrane. The tympanic cavity is lined with mucous membrane which covers its walls and all exposed contents. This lining is continuous anteriorly with the mucosa of the auditory tube (Fig. 41) and posteriorly with that of the tympanic antrum and mastoid cells. Recent studies have shown that part of the mucosa is covered with cilia which are supported in some areas by columnar pseudostratified cells and in other areas by low columnar epithelium. The cilia form distinct and consistent tracts over the anterior tympanic cavity, the hypotympanum, the epitympanum, and part of the promontory. These ciliary tracts appear related to the clearance function of the middle ear.

Tympanic Spaces. Prussak's pouch is a space which is triangular in vertical section. It is limited laterally by the pars flaccida, caudally by the short process of the malleus, and superiorly by the lateral mallear fold which passes from the neck of the malleus to the tympanic scutum. Attic retraction pockets and, frequently, cholesteatoma are found in Prussak's pouch.

The pouches of von Tröltsch include an anterior and a posterior pouch. These are adjacent to and limited by the handle of the malleus below the level of the short process. The anterior pouch is bounded posteriorly by the upper portion of the handle of the malleus, laterally by the pars tensa, and medially by the anterior mallear fold. The posterior pouch is bounded anteriorly by the upper portion of the handle of the malleus, laterally by the pars tensa, and medially by the posterior mallear fold.

Tympanic Antrum. The tympanic antrum is located posteriorly and slightly lateral to the upper half of the tympanic cavity. with which it communicates via the aditus ad antrum. The antrum is lined with mucous membrane which

(*Text continued on page 90*)

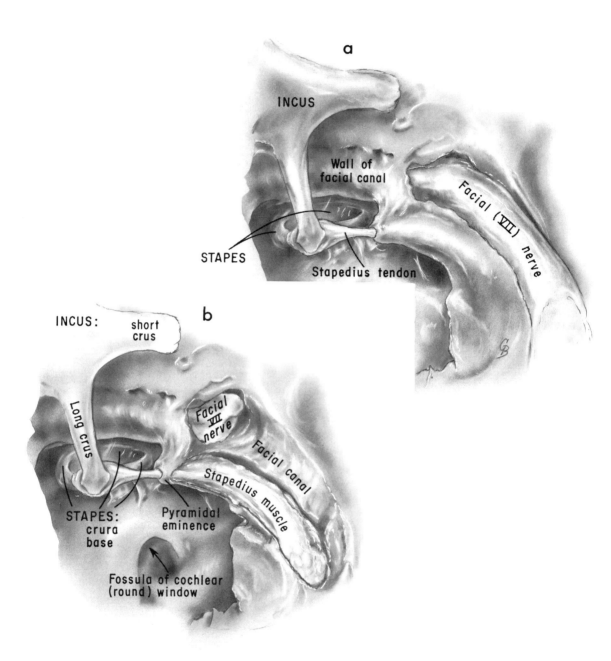

Figure 38.   Posterior tympanum. Dissected unembalmed temporal bone.

   a, The facial nerve has been uncovered as it finishes the horizontal course and curves gently toward its vertical course. The relationship of the intact facial nerve to the prominence of the stapedius muscle and its tendon can be seen.

   b, The facial nerve has been removed from the facial canal and the stapedius muscle uncovered. The compartment housing the stapedius muscle may be entirely separate from the facial canal, the two may communicate in part, or the two may be housed in a common compartment.

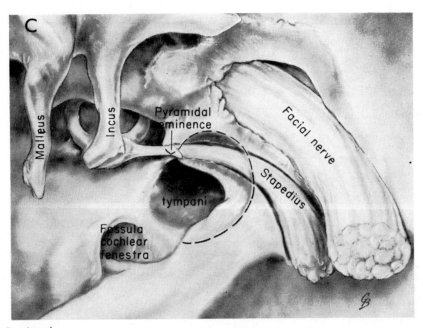

Figure 38. *Continued.*
c, In another specimen, the facial nerve and the stapedius muscle have been uncapped. The dotted line indicates the extent of the sinus tympani in this specimen. (*c* from Trans. Pacific Coast Oto-Ophthal. Soc., 1968, p. 101.)

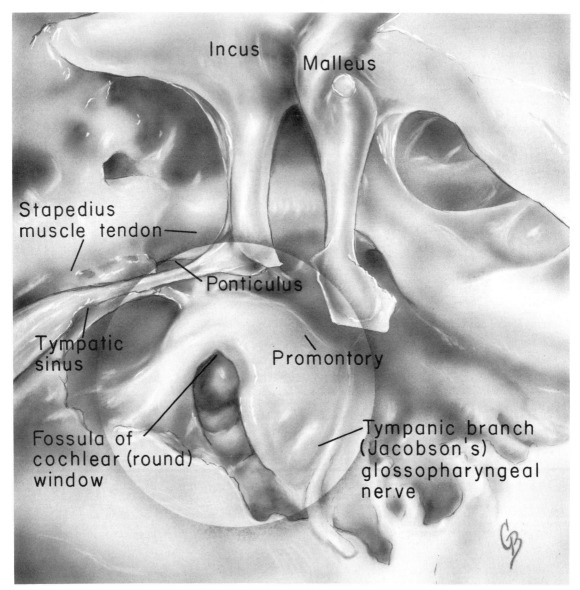

Figure 39. Anatomy of the medial wall of the tympanic cavity. Dissection of unembalmed specimen.

a, The tympanic membrane and external acoustic meatus have been removed, exposing the medial wall of the tympanum. The ossicles remain in situ. Note the ponticulus extending from the promontory to the pyramidal eminence. The encircled area contains the external aperture of the fossula of the cochlear fenestra.

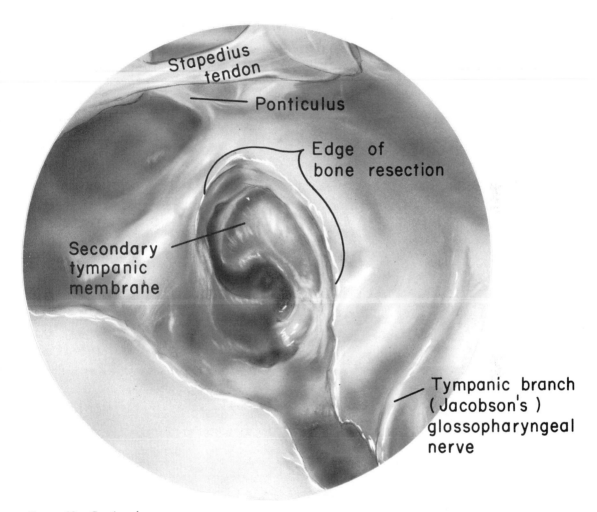

Figure 39. *Continued.*

b, The area encircled in *a* is shown after the anterior and posterior margins of the external aperture have been pared away, until the edge of the secondary tympanic membrane can be seen.

Figure 39. *Continued.*
 c, Horizontal section through the temporal bone, again showing the relationship of the orifice of the fossula to the secondary tympanic membrane. (Arch. Otolaryng. *88:*127, 1968.)

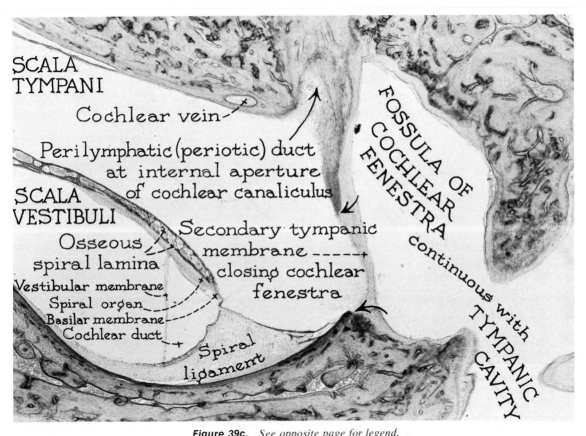

Figure 39c. *See opposite page for legend.*

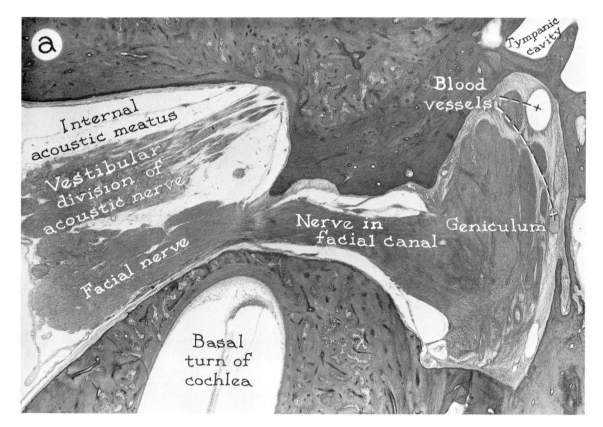

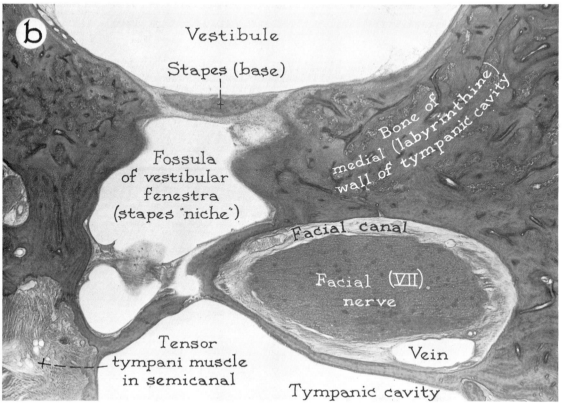

Figure 40. Facial canal—the contents, course, and related anatomy.

a, The nerve passes from the fundus of the internal acoustic meatus into the facial canal.

b, After bending sharply, the nerve passes posteriorly and laterally. The canal courses medial to the vestibular window. Note the prominent blood vessels within the canal.

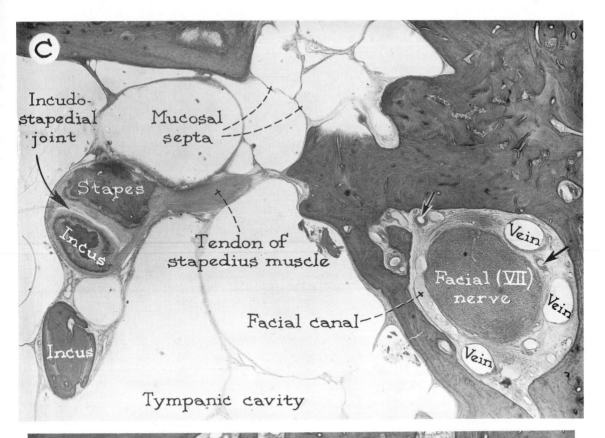

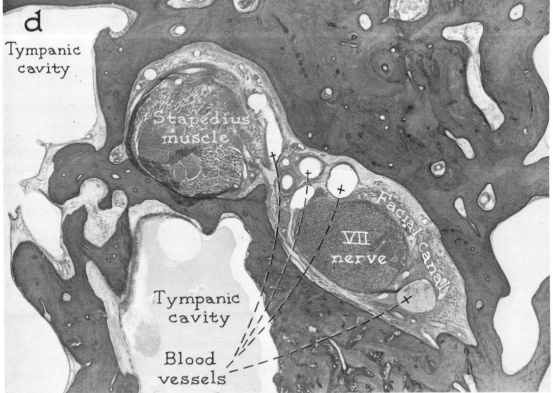

Figure 40. *Continued.*

c, Assuming its vertical course, the nerve descends to the stylomastoid foramen.

d, Near the lower limit of the stapedius muscle, the canal for the facial nerve and that for the stapedius muscle are continuous.

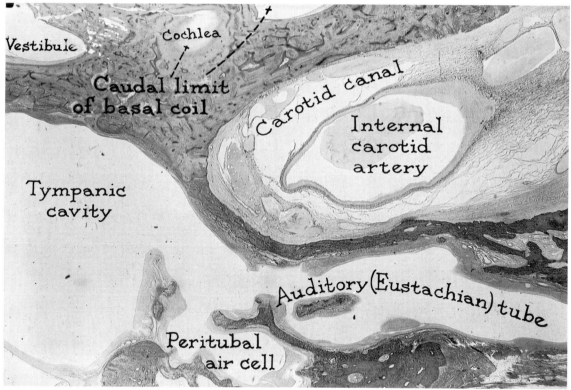

Figure 41. Horizontal section through the temporal bone at the level of the auditory tube. Note the peritubal air cell lateral to the auditory tube and the proximity of the internal carotid artery, in its canal, to the tube. (Anson, B. J., and Donaldson, J. A.: Surgical Anatomy of the Temporal Bone and Ear.)

continues from the epitympanum through the antrum to the numerous cells in the mastoid and petrous apex. Of particular interest to the surgeon is the relationship of the tympanic antrum to the surface landmarks of the temporal bone (Figs. 34 and 35). The major guide for the surgeon is Macewen's triangle. It is a triangle formed by the posterior prolongation of the upper border of the posterior root of the zygoma (the temporal line), the posterior wall of the external auditory meatus, and a line connecting the two which is perpendicular to the temporal line. The tympanic antrum is medial to the triangle.

Auditory Tube. The auditory tube descends downward medially and anteriorly from the anterior wall of the tympanum to the nasopharynx. It is about 37 mm. long and is shaped somewhat like an hourglass flattened anteroposteriorly, with the constriction at the junction of its lateral bony wall and medial cartilaginous portion. The size of the isthmus may be as small as 1.0 by 1.5 mm.

The cartilage of the tube is elastic except at the isthmus, where it becomes hyaline, losing its elastic fibers. In the bony part of the tube the mucous membrane of low columnar ciliated epithelium is firmly bound to periosteum. The lining of the cartilaginous tube, on the other hand, is of pseudostratified columnar cells, many of which are ciliated. Near the pharyngeal orifice are found goblet cells and tubulo-alveolar glands which secrete mucus into the tubal lumen. Surrounding the pharyngeal orifice is a ring of lymphoid tissue known as the tubal tonsil of Gerlach.

Vessels and Nerves. The arteries of the tympanic cavity derive mainly from the external carotid. The anterior tympanic artery branches from the internal maxillary artery and distributes to the anterior part of the cavity, including the tympanic membrane. The stylomastoid artery originates from the posterior auricular artery and proceeds to the posterior tympanic cavity and mastoid air cell region. The superficial petrosal artery extends from the middle meningeal artery; and the inferior tympanic artery, from the ascending pharyngeal. In addition, the caroticotympanic branch, from the internal carotid, supplies the anterior wall. The veins correspond roughly to the arteries and empty into the superior petrosal sinus and pterygoid plexus.

The lymphatics begin as a network in the mucous membrane and end chiefly in the retropharyngeal and parotid lymph nodes.

The nerves of the mucosa are principally represented by the tympanic plexus, formed by the tympanic branch of the glossopharyngeus (Jacobson's). Moreover, additional innervation is provided by the inferior and superior caroticotympanic nerves, from the internal carotid plexus of the sympathetic system, and from the small superficial petrosal nerve. The chorda tympani merely crosses through the tympanic cavity from the posterior to the anterior wall. The tensor tympani muscle is innervated by a branch of the mandibular nerve from the otic ganglion; the stapedius muscle is innervated by the facial nerve.

INNER EAR

Osseous Labyrinth. The osseous labyrinth housing the sense organs of hearing and balance is located in the petrous temporal bone (Figs. 42 and 43). It consists of several parts: the vestibule housing the saccule and utricle, the cochlea with its organ of Corti, the three semicircular canals, and the vestibular and cochlear aqueducts.

The vestibule is an irregular ovoid cavity approximately 4 mm. in diameter. It is located medial to the tympanic cavity with which it communicates through the fossula of the cochlear fenestra and the fossula of the vestibular fenestra. The three semicircular canals arise from recesses in the wall of the vestibule and return to it—each forming about two thirds of a circle. The ampullae of the superior and lateral semicircular canals are located at the anterosuperior aspect of the vestibule. The superior canal courses cranially, medially, and posteriorly and joins the returning posterior canal, forming the crus commune which then enters the posterior aspect of the vestibule. The course of the lateral semicircular canal, the shortest of the canals, is in a postero-inferior plane, returning to the posterior aspect of the vestibule. The lateral semicircular canal is intimately associated with the facial canal along its horizontal and vertical aspects. From the posterior portion of the vestibule the posterior semicircular canal courses in a posteromedial plane to join the superior canal, forming the crus commune.

Three recesses are formed in the posterior wall of the vestibule. The spherical recess, housing the saccule, is located antero-inferiorly. The elliptical recess, which contains the utricle, is located posterosuperiorly. The cochlear recess is located posteroinferiorly in the posterior wall of the vestibule. The cochlear recess contains the basal hook region of the cochlear duct. The vestibular crest separates the spherical recess from the elliptical recess and divides into two limbs which bound the cochlear recess. The opening of the vestibular aqueduct passes from the area of the elliptical recess to the posterior surface of the temporal bone. Through it the endolymphatic duct passes to the saccus endolymphaticus.

Antero-inferior to the vestibule is the bony cochlea, which is shaped like a flattened cone whose base is 9 mm. in diameter and whose height is 5 mm. The cochlea makes two and three fourths turns around a central axis known as the modiolus through which cochlear vessels and the cochlear division of the eighth cranial nerve pass to the cochlea. The canal of Cotunnius transmits the vein of the cochlear aqueduct to the posterior surface of the temporal bone.

Blood supply of the labyrinth. The labyrinth is supplied by the internal auditory artery which originates as a branch of either the basilar or antero-inferior cerebellar arteries (Fig. 44). The internal auditory artery subdivides into the vestibular artery, the cochlear artery proper, and the vestibulocochlear artery. The vestibular artery supplies parts of the saccule, utricle, and semicircular ducts. The cochlear artery supplies the apical two turns of the cochlea. The vestibulocochlear artery supplies two thirds of the basal coil of the cochlea, the greater part of the saccule, the body of the utricle, the posterior semicircular duct, and parts of the lateral and superior semicircular ducts. The labyrinthine venous drainage is via the internal auditory vein from the apical and middle cochlear turns; the vein of the cochlear aqueduct from the base of the cochlea, the saccule, and part of the utricle; and the vein of the vestibular aqueduct from the semicircular ducts and the remainder of the utricle.

Membranous Labyrinth. The membranous labyrinth (Figs. 43 and 45) is a system of epithelial-formed spaces and tubes containing endolymph. It is surrounded by the perilymph-filled periotic labyrinth which, in turn, is enclosed in the bony labyrinth of the otic capsule.

The membranous labyrinth consists of the

(Text continued on page 97)

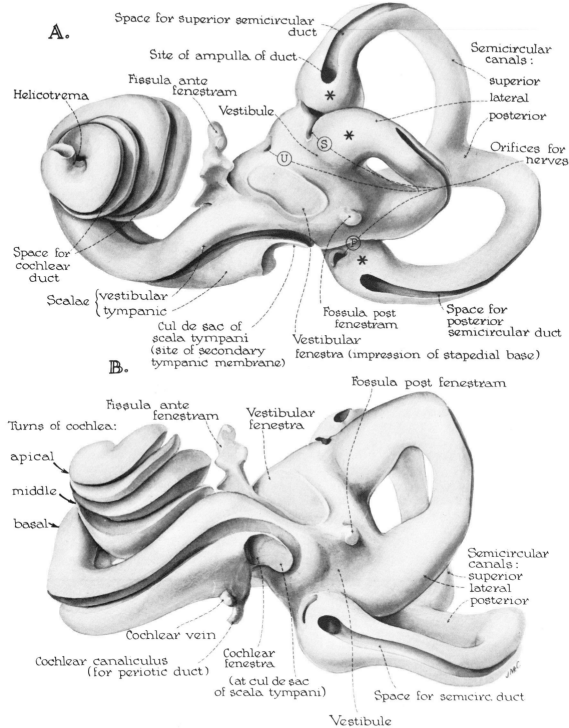

A.

Space for superior semicircular duct

Site of ampulla of duct

Fissula ante fenestram

Helicotrema

Vestibule

Semicircular canals :

superior

lateral

posterior

Orifices for nerves

(S)

(U)

(P)

Space for cochlear duct

Scalae {vestibular / tympanic

Cul de sac of scala tympani (site of secondary tympanic membrane)

Fossula post fenestram

Vestibular fenestra (impression of stapedial base)

Space for posterior semicircular duct

B.

Fissula ante fenestram

Turns of cochlea:

apical

middle

basal

Vestibular fenestra

Fossula post fenestram

Semicircular canals :

superior

lateral

posterior

Cochlear vein

Cochlear canaliculus (for periotic duct)

Cochlear fenestra (at cul de sac of scala tympani)

Space for semicirc. duct

Vestibule

Figure 42. Reconstruction of osseous labyrinth, demonstrating form of perilymphatic space proper and its continuity with fossula ante fenestram, fossula post fenestram, and cochlear canaliculus (310 mm. fetus).

a, Anterior-lateral view. Note form of labyrinthine system for perilymph comprising scali, vestibule, semicircular canals, and perilymphatic appendages; spaces (represented by sulci) of cochlear and semicircular ducts; points of entry of the utricular part of the acoustic nerve at *u*, of saccular part at *s*, and of nerve to ampulla on lateral semicircular duct at *p*; extension of tympanic scala as a cul de sac related in fresh state to a corresponding prolongation (cecum) of the cochlear duct. Asterisk indicates ampulla.

b, Inferior-lateral view with reconstruction rotated on its long axis through approximately one eighth of a turn, demonstrating to advantage: relation of two windows (vestibular and cochlear fenestrae) to each other, and their relation, in turn, to perilymphatic appendages; proximity of cochlear canaliculus to channel for cochlear vein; form of saucer-shaped cul de sac of tympanic scala (produced by shape of secondary tympanic membrane); relatively great capacity of osseous labyrinth, compared with that of a membranous labyrinth.

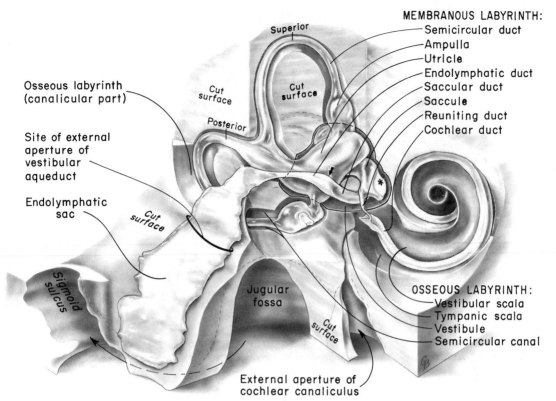

MEMBRANOUS LABYRINTH:
- Semicircular duct
- Ampulla
- Utricle
- Endolymphatic duct
- Saccular duct
- Saccule
- Reuniting duct
- Cochlear duct

Superior

Cut surface

Cut surface

Osseous labyrinth (canalicular part)

Posterior

Site of external aperture of vestibular aqueduct

Endolymphatic sac

Cut surface

Sigmoid sulcus

Jugular fossa

Cut surface

OSSEOUS LABYRINTH:
- Vestibular scala
- Tympanic scala
- Vestibule
- Semicircular canal

External aperture of cochlear canaliculus

Figure 43. Membranous and osseous labyrinth. Reconstruction prepared by the Born method. Adult, 69 years of age. (Wisconsin Collection.) This demonstrates especially the relations between the membranous and bony labyrinths, but in particular, the form, size, and relations of the endolymphatic sac. The saccus extends for a considerable distance beyond the external aperture of the vestibular aqueduct into the posterior cranial fossa. In the latter position it occupies a foveate impression on the posterior surface of the petrous pyramid where it may be prolonged inferiorly to the level of the sulcus for the sigmoid venus sinus. The unlabeled arrow points to the utriculo-endolymphatic duct; the asterisk is on the saccule.

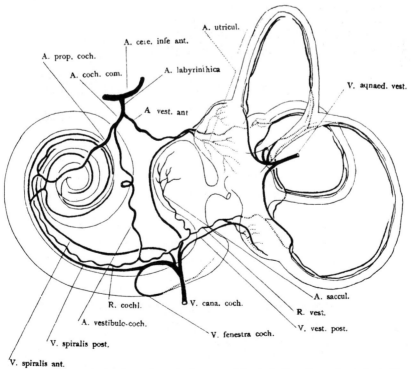

A. utricul.

A. cere. infe ant.

A. prop. coch.

A. coch. com.

A. labyrinthica

A vest. ant

V. aqnaed. vest.

A. saccul.

R. vest.

R. cochl.

V. cana. coch.

A. vestibule-coch.

V. vest. post.

V. fenestra coch.

V. spiralis post.

V. spiralis ant.

Figure 44. Schematic drawing of blood supply to the inner ear labyrinth. See discussion in text. (From Axelsson, A.: Acta Otolaryng. (Suppl.) *243*:8, 1968.)

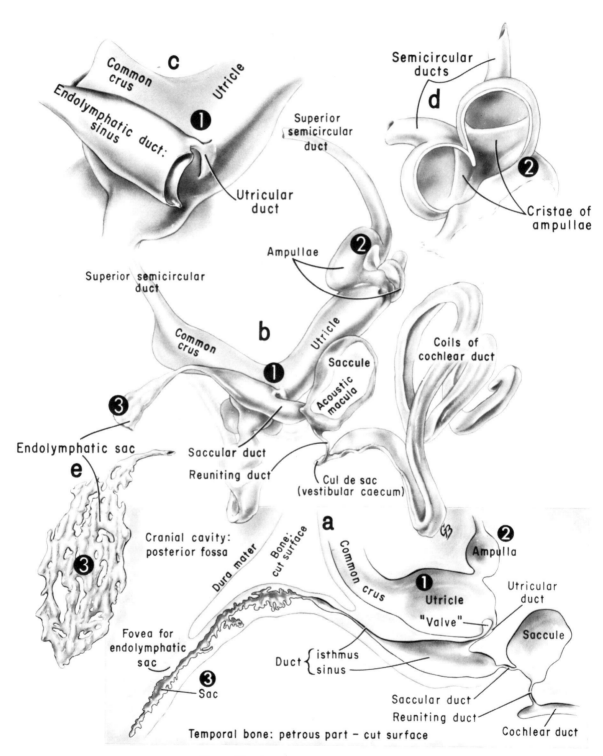

Figure 45. *See opposite page for legend.*

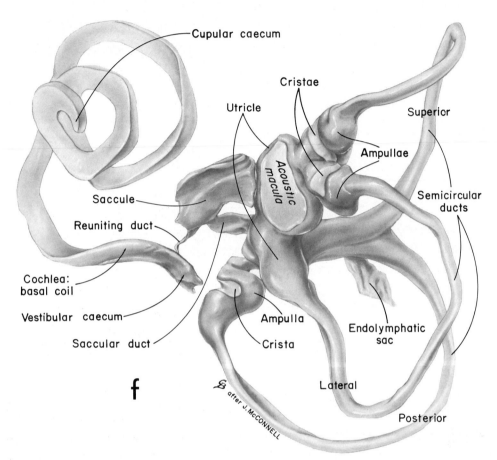

Cupular caecum

Cristae

Utricle

Superior

Ampullae

Acoustic macula

Saccule

Semicircular ducts

Reuniting duct

Cochlea: basal coil

Ampulla

Endolymphatic sac

Vestibular caecum

Saccular duct

Crista

Lateral

f

after J. McCONNELL

Posterior

Figure 45. Membranous labyrinth. Based upon a reconstruction by David G. Harper, M.D. Infant of 6 months. (Wisconsin Collection, series 121.)

a, This shows schematically the form of the labyrinth in the area of the endolymphatic duct, the utricle, and the interconnecting utricular (or utriculo-endolymphatic) duct. The numeral designations correspond throughout the succeeding figures. The utricle (at *1*) communicates widely with the common crus and with the semicircular ducts (at *2*). Differing from this relationship, the utricle opens into the endolymphatic duct beneath a valvelike form, formed by their epithelial walls and the intervening connective tissue. The endolymphatic duct expands proximally, where it communicates with the utricle. The sinuslike enlargement continues into a narrowed segment, the isthmus. While wide at the sinus, the endolymphatic duct narrows at the isthmus to widen again in the plicated sac.

b, The utricle (at one end) and the common crus together form a V-shaped common chamber. The utricle communicates widely with the ampullae (at *2*).

c and *d,* Toward the cochlear side (in *c*) the connection of the utricle with the sinuslike expansion of the endolymphatic duct is through an aperture which has a spatulate form (compare valve in *a*). It is to be likened to a chink. Comparably, the space at the free surface of the cupula of each crista is also narrow (less than at *2* in *c*, shrinkage having resulted in widening of the opening).

e, The termination expansion of the endolymphatic duct is characterized by multiple folds (*3*). As this "cast" of the lumen demonstrates, the facing epithelial surfaces meet, dividing the entire space into intercommunicating chambers.

f, Reconstruction of the entire membranous labyrinth as viewed from the lateral aspect to bring into perspective all the details depicted in *a* through *e*.

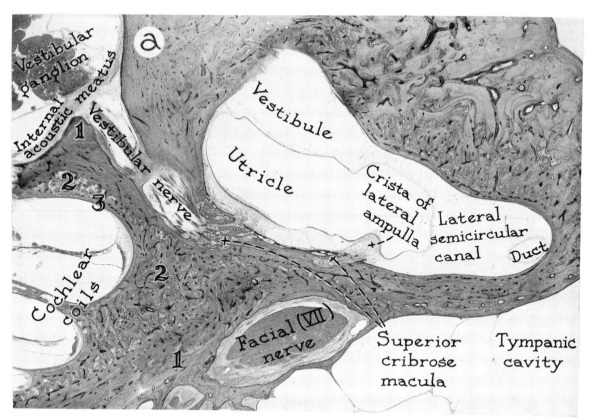

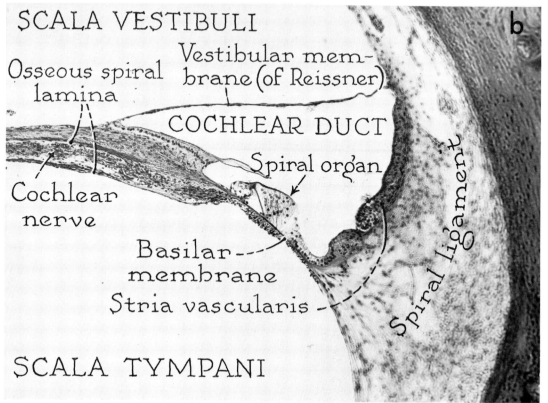

Figure 46. *See opposite page for legend.*

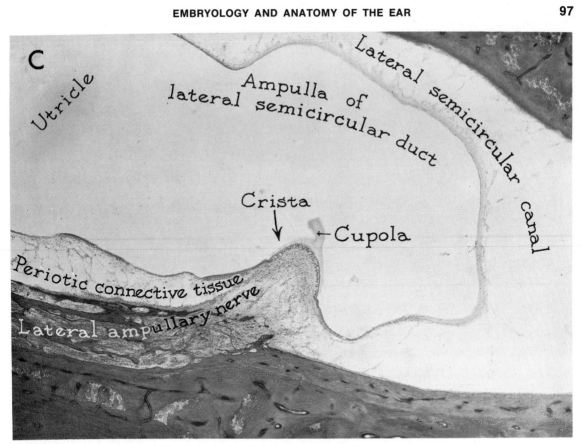

Figure 46. Sense organs of the inner ear: cochlear duct, saccule, utricle, and semicircular ducts. Transverse sections. (Wisconsin Collection.)

a, This shows the interrelationships between the sense organs of hearing and equilibrium, at the horizontal level of the utricle.

b, The cochlear duct (scala media) is in large part triangular in cross-section. The outer wall unites with the periosteum of the inner surface of the cochlear canal. The second wall, the one parallel to the base of the cochlea, runs in the direction of the osseous spiral lamina and extends from the latter's free margin to the spiral ligament of the cochlea—a ridgelike projection of the periosteum of the outer surface of the cochlear canal. This wall consists of a fibrous plate of connective tissue, the basal lamina, and supports the spiral organ (of Corti), the epithelial sensory structure which receives the terminal fibers of the cochlear nerve. The third wall, the vestibular membrane of Reissner, is exceedingly thin. Arising from the osseous spiral lamina near its free margin it passes at an angle of approximately 45 degrees.

c, Ampulla of lateral semicircular canal. Cross-section shows the crista with the cupula arising from it and its innervation via the ampullary nerve.

endolymphatic duct and sac, the saccule, the utricle, the semicircular canals, and the cochlear duct (Fig. 46). These are interconnected by small canals: the utricular duct, the saccular duct, and the ductus reuniens (Fig. 45 *f*).

Endolymphatic Duct and Sac. The endolymphatic sac usually lies partly within the vestibular aqueduct and partly on the posterior surface of the petrous portion of the temporal bone between the layers of the cranial dura mater. There is, however, much variation in size, shape, and position of the external aperture of the vestibular aqueduct (Fig. 47), as well as in the amount of expansion of the aqueduct immediately inside the external aperture. The location of the sac and the proportion of it within or outside the temporal bone is correspondingly variable. The sac itself varies considerably in size, shape, and position. Its lumen is frequently quite rugose. Its outer wall is surrounded by vascular connective tissue.

The endolymphatic sac can usually be reached through the temporal bone by removing the cells between the posterior semicircular canal and sigmoid portion of the transverse sinus. In this location its cephalad border is most frequently found at or below a line through the lateral semicircular canal.

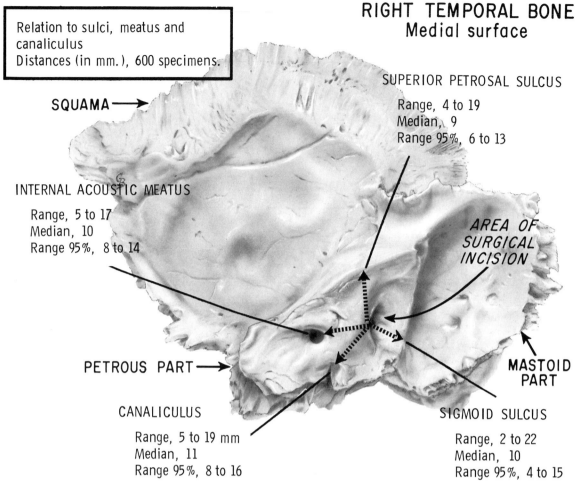

RIGHT TEMPORAL BONE
Medial surface

Relation to sulci, meatus and canaliculus
Distances (in mm.), 600 specimens.

SQUAMA ➤

SUPERIOR PETROSAL SULCUS

Range, 4 to 19
Median, 9
Range 95%, 6 to 13

INTERNAL ACOUSTIC MEATUS

Range, 5 to 17
Median, 10
Range 95%, 8 to 14

AREA OF SURGICAL INCISION

PETROUS PART ➤

MASTOID PART

CANALICULUS

Range, 5 to 19 mm
Median, 11
Range 95%, 8 to 16

SIGMOID SULCUS

Range, 2 to 22
Median, 10
Range 95%, 4 to 15

Figure 47. Right temporal bone, medial surface. The relation of the external aperture of the vestibular aqueduct to known landmarks is shown. The variability of this relation in 600 specimens is indicated.

The Utricle and Saccule. The utricle is an oblong, slightly flattened sac with a rounded end (Fig. 48). It occupies the elliptical recess in the posterosuperior portion of the vestibule. The saccule is a spherical organ, smaller than the utricle, located in the antero-inferior portion of the vestibule in the spherical recess. The sensory receptors and supporting structures responsive to positional changes of the body form the maculae of the utricle and saccule. The macula acoustica utriculi is a spade-shaped, thickened area situated anteriorly and laterally within the utricle. The macula of the saccule is a 2 by 3 mm. sensory structure located on the medial wall of the saccule. The macula of the saccule lies in approximately a vertical plane, perpendicular to the utricular macula. These maculae are innervated by the utricular and saccular branches of the vestibular nerve.

Both maculae are structured similarly. The primary receptor cells are hair cells. These hair cells are of two types (Fig 49): Type I tends to have an expanded base (flasklike) and is surrounded by chalice-type afferent nerve endings. The Type II cells are more tubular in shape and are supplied by smaller afferent and efferent nerve endings. The upper surface of these cells is cuticular, in which nonmotile stereocilia are embedded. A kinocilium is located in one region of the upper surface of each cell. Each of the hair cells is surrounded and held firmly by a matrix of supporting cells. The kinocilia and stereocilia hairs of these cells project into an otolithic membrane which lies atop each macula (Fig. 50). Many crystals of calcium carbonate, the otoconia, are found within the otolithic membrane. The increase in mass of this membrane provided by the presence of the otoconia plays a major role in

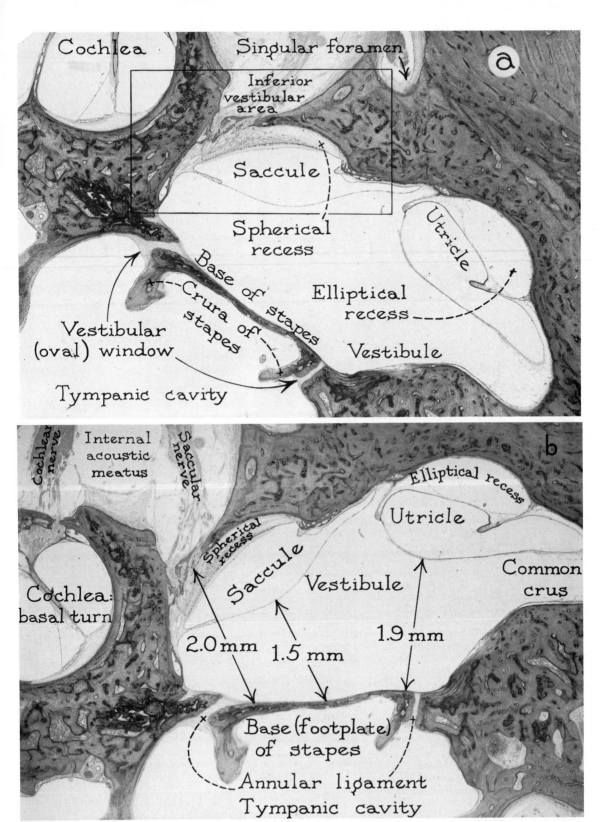

Figure 48. Vestibule, contents, and related anatomy. Ten week old infant. Transverse section. (Wisconsin Collection, series 83.)

The saccule and utricle occupy recesses (spherical and elliptical, respectively) on the wall of the vestibule. At the level of the midpoint of the stapes foot plate, the interdistance between the stapes and saccule is 1.5 mm., between the ossicle and utricle, approximately 2.0 mm. The latter distance is matched by that between the stapes and foramenous wall, where nerve fibers pass from the cribromacula of the bone to the acoustic macula of the saccule. It should be noted that these distances would be lessened either by dilation of the membranous labyrinth or by thickening of the footplate of the stapes.

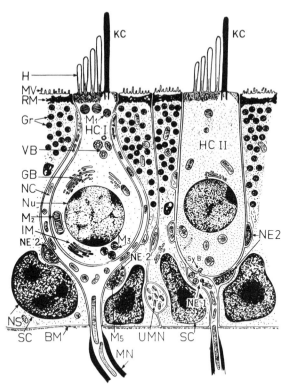

Figure 49. Diagrammatic representation of Types I and II vestibular hair cells. The flask-shaped Type I cell (*HC I*) is surrounded by a nerve calyx (*NC*), which makes contact on its outer surface with granulated (presumably efferent) nerve endings (*NE 2*). Unmyelinated fibers (*UMN*) are extensions of myelinated fibers (*MN*) which lose their myelin sheaths as they pass through basement membrane. Type II sensory cell (*HC II*) is roughly cylindrical and is supplied by two types of nerve endings (*NE 1* and *NE 2*) which can be seen at its basal end. Several groups of mitochondria (M_1-M_5) are found in the sensory cells and neural elements. Two kinds of hairs project from the surfaces of sensory cells, stereocilia (*H*) and kinocilium (*KC*), single kinocilium always being the longest on each cell. Supporting cells are easily distinguished from sensory cells by virtue of their numerous population of rather uniformly distributed granules (*Gr*). (From Ades, H. W., and Engstrom, H.: Form and enervation of the vestibular epithelia. *In* Graybiel, A.: The Role of the Vestibular Organs in Space. Washington, D.C., National Aeronautics and Space Administration, 1965. NASA Publication No. SP-77.)

Figure 50. *a,* View of the guinea pig macula of the saccule from above. Otoconia, compressing white surface, show "snowdrift" distribution. "Snowdrift" line is a common feature of this structure and corresponds to polarization line of sensory epithelium. Polarization of stereocilia and kinocilium is directed away from "snowdrift" line. (From Ades, H. W., and Engstrom, H.: Form and enervation of the vestibular epithelia. *In* Graybiel, A.: The Role of the Vestibular Organs in the Exploration of Space. Washington, D.C., National Aeronautics and Space Administration, 1965. NASA Publication No. SP-77.)

b, Diagrammatic drawing of sensory receptors and supporting structure of macula. (From Wersall, J., and Lundquist, P-G.: Morphological polarization of the mechanoreceptors of the vestibular and acoustic systems. *In* Graybiel, A.: Second Symposium on the Role of the Vestibular Organs in Space Exploration. Washington, D.C., National Aeronautics and Space Administration, 1966. NASA Publication No. SP-115.)

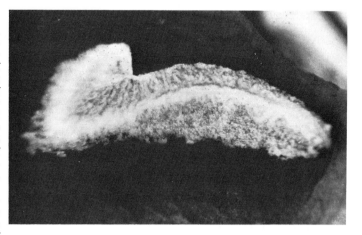

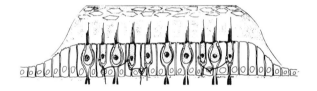

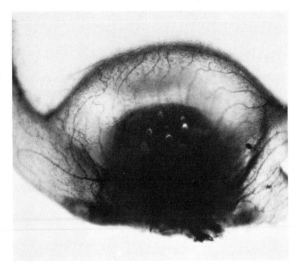

Figure 51. Macula of semicircular duct as seen through wall of ampulla. Note the rich network of blood vessels along the wall of the membranous labyrinth of the ampulla and in the ampullar crest. (From Ades, H. W., and Engstrom, H.: Form and enervation of the vestibular epithelia. *In* Graybiel, A.: The Role of the Vestibular Organs in the Exploration of Space. Washington, D.C., National Aeronautics and Space Administration, 1965. NASA Publication No. SP-77.)

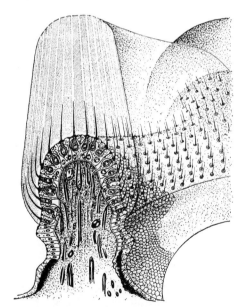

Figure 52. Diagrammatic representation of section through ridge of crista ampullaris. The organization of hair cells along the surface of the crista may be seen. Moreover, the insertion of the cilia into the cupula is shown. (From Wersall, J., and Lundquist, P-G.: Morphological polarization of the mechanoreceptors of the vestibular and acoustic systems. *In* Graybiel, A.: Second Symposium on the Role of the Vestibular Organs in Space Exploration. Washington, D.C., National Aeronautics and Space Administration, 1966. NASA Publication No. SP-115.)

determining the adequate stimulus for excitation of these hair cells.

Examination of the pattern of orientation of the stereocilia and kinocilia of the cells of the maculae reveals a systematic spatial organization. Observations suggest that this organization is of some functional significance. Thus, bending of the hairs in the direction of the kinocilium results in a depolarization and excitation of the cells, whereas bending the hairs in the opposite direction results in a hyperpolarization of the cell.

The utricle connects posteriorly with the semicircular canals and anteriorly via the utricular duct with the endolymphatic and saccular ducts. Communication between the utricle and the utricular duct may be limited by the utricular fold or valve (of Bast). The saccule communicates inferiorly via the ductus reuniens with the cochlear duct. It is at the junction of the utricular and saccular ducts that the endolymphatic duct arises.

Semicircular Ducts.   The membranous labyrinth of the semicircular canals is tubular in form. At one end of each canal is an enlargement: the ampulla. These ducts occupy only about one quarter of the diameter of the respective bony canals and open into the utricle through five orifices. Each canal opens directly at its ampullar end, but the posterior and superior ducts open through a common crus at their posterior end. The ampulla of each canal is an expanded area containing a transverse ridge of sensorineuroepithelium and supporting structures, the crista ampullaris (Figs. 51, 52, and 53). Although grossly of a different form, microscopically the crista ampullaris is very similar to the maculae of the saccule and utricle. Type I and Type II hair cells are found in this structure. The outer surface of each hair cell is cuticular, with about 50 stereocilia. The surface of each cell contains a cuticular-free region and one kinocilium.

The hairs of these cells insert into a gelatinous cupula which caps this ridge of sensorineuroepithelium. The cupula ampullaris extends from the surface of the crista to the roof of the ampulla. Movement of the endolymphatic fluid within the semicircular duct moves the cupula relative to the surface of the crista, thus providing the adequate stimulus for bending these hairs and concomitant excitation of the hair cells. The posterior, superior, and lateral ampullaris nerves of the vestibular portion of the eighth cranial nerve provide the afferent innervation for these sensory receptors.

Cochlear Duct.   This portion of the mem-

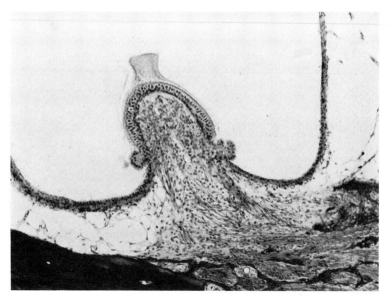

Figure 53. Photomicrograph of crista ampullaris of the squirrel monkey, showing the entrance of nerve fibers into the base of the crista. (From Paparella, M. M. (ed.): Biomechanical Mechanisms in Hearing and Deafness. Springfield, Ill., Charles C Thomas, 1970.)

branous labyrinth (Fig. 46) follows the spiral canal of the bony cochlea throughout its two and one half to two and three fourths turn length. The duct extends from the cochlear recess of the vestibule to end as a blind pouch, the cupular cecum, at the level of the apex of the cochlea. At its basal extent the small ductus reuniens allows communication of the endolymph of the cochlear duct with that of the saccular membranous labyrinth.

In transverse section the cochlear duct is somewhat triangular in form. The floor of the duct is formed principally by the rigid basilar membrane which inserts laterally along the tough spiral ligament. Overlying the spiral ligament, and forming the lateral wall of the cochlear duct, is the highly vascular stria vascularis. At the upper limit of the stria, the thin bicellular-layered vestibular membrane (Reissner's) extends from the spiral ligament to the limbus overlying the osseous spiral lamina, thus forming the third wall of the cochlear duct.

The basilar and Reissner's membranes divide the cochlear labyrinth into three canals: The closed central canal is, of course, the endolymph-filled cochlear duct, or scala media. Adjacent to Reissner's membrane is the scala vestibuli. Adjacent to the basilar membrane is the scala tympani. Both the scalae vestibuli and tympani are perilymph-filled. The fluid of these two scalae is in communication beyond the

apical closed end of the cochlear duct through the helicotrema.

The organ of Corti. The sensory receptors and supporting structures responsive to acoustic energy are located on the basilar membrane. These structures, forming the organ of Corti, are best examined from two views—a transverse view and a horizontal view. In the former case the midmodiolar sections of decalcified tissue illustrate the relations of the organ of Corti to the other structures of the membranous and periotic labyrinths (Figs. 46 and 54). In the horizontal view, obtained by examining from above strips of dissected basilar membrane and organ of Corti, the relationship of the various organ of Corti structures is well shown (Fig. 55). Indeed, from this view the basis for the radial development of this structure becomes abundantly clear. By combining these approaches, the cytoarchitecture of this complex three-dimensional structure can best be appreciated.

The spiral length of the basilar membrane is approximately 32 mm. Its width increases from 80 μ at the base to approximately 500 μ one half turn from the apex. In transverse section one of the most prominent features of the organ of Corti is the tunnel of Corti formed by the two pillar cells. The basilar membrane has been divided into two sections: the zona arcuata, which extends from the tympanic lip of the osseous spiral lamina to the base of the

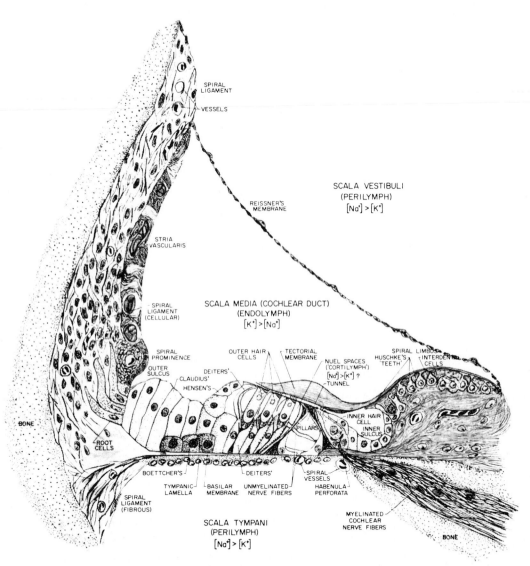

Figure 54. Diagram of transverse (mid-modiolar view of cochlear duct). See text. (From Hawkins, J. E., Jr.: Hearing: Anatomy and acoustics. *In* Best, C. H., and Taylor, N. B. (eds.): The Physiological Basis of Medical Practice. 8th ed. Baltimore, The Williams & Wilkins Company, 1966, Chapter 17.)

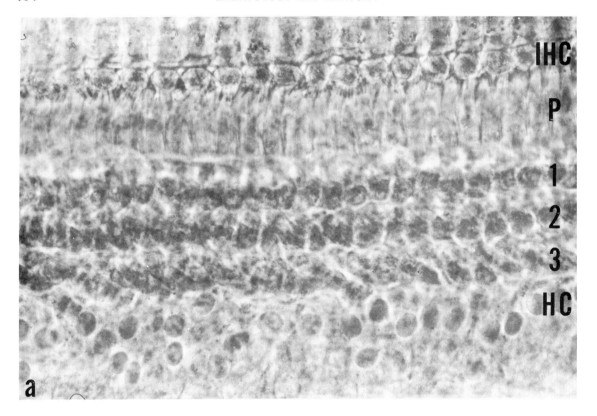

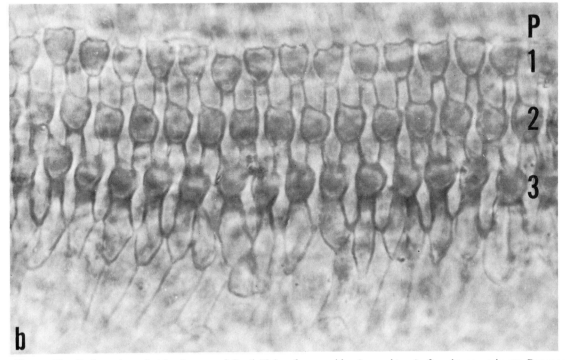

Figure 55.   Surface view of strip of organ of Corti. Taken from cochlea (second turn) of nonhuman primate. Because of the curvature of organ of Corti different structures are shown by focusing at different levels.

a, Focus on surface of inner hair cells (*IHC*). Hairs of inner hair cells are visible. *P*, pillar cells forming tunnel of Corti. *1*, *2*, and *3*, first, second, and third rows of outer hair cells. Nuclei of outer hair cells are visible. *H*, Henson's cells.

b, Focus, superficial to that of *a*, on surface of outer hair cells. Reticular lamina is clearly shown.

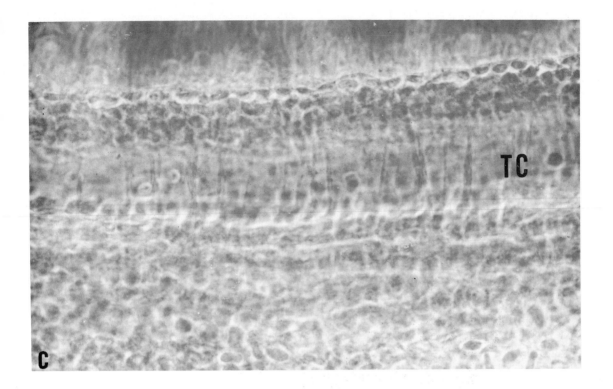

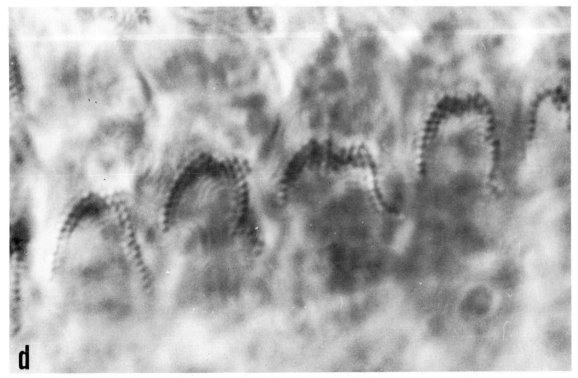

Figure 55. *Continued.*
c, Focus, deep to that of a, on nerve fibers crossing tunnel of Corti (TC).
d, High magnification photomicrograph of hair pattern of stereocilia on outer hair cells.

outer pillars; and the zona pectinata, which extends from the lateral pillar to the spiral ligament.

Following the radial organizations of the organ of Corti so well illustrated in the surface preparation view (Fig 55 *a*), a single row of inner hair cells just medial to the tunnel of Corti may be seen. Lateral to the tunnel three rows of outer hair cells are evident (Fig. 55 *a* and *b*). This pattern of hair cell representation is followed throughout the length of the organ of Corti. Near the apical extent, however, fourth and even fifth row outer hair cells may be found. These hair cells are the primary receptors sensitive to acoustic energy; other structures of the organ of Corti serve as supporting elements, determining to a great extent the range of mechanical stimuli capable of eliciting a response from the hair cells.

The single row of inner hair cells includes approximately 3500 cells. Observations have suggested that there are over 20,000 outer hair cells in the organ of Corti. Figure 56 *a* and *b* illustrates diagrammatically the major characteristics of these hair cells. Inner hair cells are flasklike in shape as opposed to the more "test-tubular" shape of the outer hair cells. The upper surface of the hair cells is formed by a thickened cuticular plate. It is in this cuticular plate that the stereocilia hairs of these cells are embedded. Two straight rows of approximately 50 nonmotile stereocilia are found on the inner hair cell. On the outer hair cell the stereocilia are arranged in three rows, forming a "W" pattern (Fig. 55 *d*). The angle formed by the legs of the "W" extends from approximately 70 degrees on apical-placed hair cells to approximately 120 to 130 degrees on basal turn hair cells.

A cuticular-free region is found on the surface of each hair cell lateral to the stereocilia. In this region the basal body of a kinocilium may be observed. As noted in electron microscopic studies of the hair cells, a high concentration of Golgi apparatus and mitochondria are formed beneath this cuticular-free region. Based upon such observations, it has been suggested that this high metabolic region of the hair cell may be primarily involved in the transduction process by which mechanical energy is converted into an electrical form.

Each inner hair cell rests in a cuplike phalangeal cell (Fig. 54). These cells send their phalangeal processes up to the level of the cuticular plates of the hair cells. Outer hair cells rest similarly on supporting Deiters' cells. Similar to the supporting cells at the base of the inner hair cells, Deiters' cells send phalangeal processes to the surface of the organ of Corti, forming a rigid contact with the cuticular plates of the outer hair cells.

From the surface view, a characteristic reticulated pattern is seen at the upper surface of the organ of Corti (Fig. 55 *b*). This reticular lamina is formed by the phalangeal processes of the cells surrounding the inner and outer hair cells, by the cuticular plate of the inner and outer hair cells, and by the expanded heads of the inner and outer pillar cells forming the tunnel of Corti. Medially each inner hair cell is surrounded and interdigitated with the process of the phalangeal cell. Laterally the head of the inner pillar cells extends adjacent to the inner hair cell. Similarly lateral to the tunnel of Corti, the first structure forming the reticular lamina is the extended process of the head of the outer pillar cell. This is then followed by the first row of outer hair cells. Beyond this the reticular lamina is formed by an interdigitation of phalangeal processes of the Deiters' cells, followed by one row of outer hair cells. It is to be noted that the phalangeal processes of the Deiters' cells extend to and join the reticular lamina at a level three or four hair cells further toward the apex than the hair cell which the Deiters' cell supports. Thus, this system forms a cross-structure of supporting elements of great structural rigidity that surrounds the hair cells.

The cells of Hensen are located beyond the most laterally placed phalangeal process (Fig. 54). These cells extend from the lateral border of the organ of Corti down to the tall columnar epithelial cells, the cells of Claudius, which rest upon the basilar membrane and extend laterally to the spiral ligament and stria vascularis.

As noted in Figure 54 (the transverse section of the cochlea), medial to the supporting cells of the inner hair cells may be found a series of cuboidal inner sulcus cells extending from the inner hair cells to the fibrous spiral limbus which rests upon the osseous spiral lamina. It is from the superior surface of the spiral limbus that the tectorial membrane takes its origin. This ribbonlike membrane extends over the organ of Corti throughout the spiral extent of the cochlear duct. The stereocilia extending from the hair cells are embedded in this structure.

The cross-sectional view of the cochlear duct shows that beneath the tectorial membrane and within the organ of Corti exist a number of fluid-filled spaces. The major ones are the inner sulcus and the tunnel of Corti. In addition to this, adjacent to the hair cells are the small spaces of Nuel. These regions are filled with cortilymph, a material considered to be similar in its ionic constituents to that of perilymph.

Evaluation of the mechanics of the organ of Corti suggests that major support for the hair cells is provided at the superior surface, that is, at their attachment to the reticular lamina. The rigid reticular lamina has been found to be stiffly attached to the basilar membrane via the pillar cells. Thus, the hair cells are provided with a rigid attachment to the basilar membrane. On the other hand, the tectorial membrane, in which the hairs of the hair cells are embedded, forms a loose attachment with the basilar membrane via the spiral limbus. As a result of this arrangement, it may be seen

that movement of the basilar membrane will differentially influence the cell bodies of the hair cells and the tectorial membrane. It may be seen, then, how a differential response on these structures through movement of the basilar membrane may result in a bending of the stereocilia of the hair cells and thus initiate the transduction response of these sensory receptors.

Innervation. Beneath each hair cell two types of nerve endings have been observed through electron microscopic study. The primary endings are agranular, dendritic terminations of the afferent eighth nerve fibers. These endings extend as unmyelinated fibers through the tunnel of Corti and enter the osseous spiral lamina via the habenula perforata. It is at this point that these fibers acquire a myelin sheath and proceed through Rosenthal's canal into the modiolus to join the main body of the afferent eighth nerve fibers destined for the brain stem

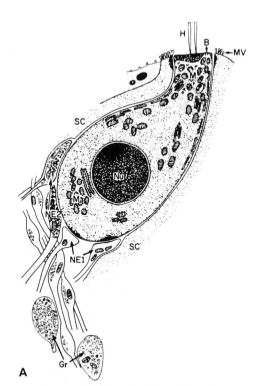

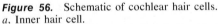

A   **B**

Figure 56.   Schematic of cochlear hair cells.
a, Inner hair cell.
b, Outer hair cell. *H,* stereocilia; *B,* basal body of kinocilium; *MV,* microvilli on supporting cell; *NE₁,* afferent nerve ending (agranulated); *NE₂,* efferent nerve ending (granulated); *M,* mitochondrion; *Ph,* phalangeal process. (From Hawkins, J. E., Jr.: Hearing: Anatomy and acoustics. *In* Best, C. H., and Taylor, N. B. (eds.): The Physiological Basis of Medical Practice. 8th ed. Baltimore, The Williams & Wilkins Company, 1966.)

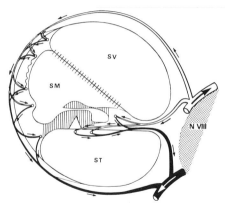

Figure 57. Diagrammatic drawing of cross-section of one turn of the cochlea. Shows major division of blood supply to the membranous labyrinth of the cochlea. One major group of vessels forms the spiral vessels under the basilar membrane. A second group forms a series of capillary networks in the lateral wall of the labyrinth. (From Axelsson, A.: Acta Otolaryng. Suppl. *243*:107, 1968.)

cochlear nuclei. In addition to these afferent fibers with their agranular endings, a number of granulated endings have been observed to make contact with both the hair cells and the terminal endings of the afferent fibers. These granulated endings are efferent fibers originating from the brain stem in Rasmussen's olivo-cochlear bundle. The major influence of the efferent nerve fibers on cochlear function appears to be one of inhibition.

Blood supply. The blood supply to the organ of Corti and other structures of the cochlear duct is provided by the vessels within the stria vascularis and the spiral vessels underlying the basilar membrane. The arterial supply to the cochlea enters through the modiolus along with the eighth nerve fibers. Arterioles divide at the level of the spiral lamina, with one group of vessels proceeding to a position underlying the basilar membrane. The second

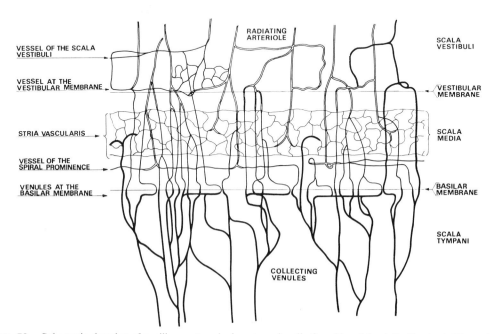

Figure 58. Schematic drawing of capillary networks in external wall of cochlear labyrinth. See text. (From Axelsson, A.: Acta Otolaryng. Suppl. *243*:62, 1968.)

arteriole system travels within the periosteal lining across the wall of the scala vestibuli to the region of the spiral ligament (Fig. 57). At this point the arterioles break up to form four capillary networks along the lateral wall of the periotic labyrinth (Fig. 58). The first group of vessels supplies the region of the spiral ligament about the insertion of Reissner's membrane. The second group of vessels forms the highly anastomosed capillary bed of the stria vascularis. The third set of capillaries supplies the vessels of the spiral prominence, and the final set supplies the lower portion of the spiral ligament. These vessels, including the spiral vessels underlying the basilar membrane, drain into venules which form the posterior spiral vein and, finally, into the internal auditory vein.

It may be noted that neither the structures of the organ of Corti nor the cortilymphatic space includes the presence of blood vessels. The neuroepithelium of the organ of Corti must thus receive oxygen and nutrients indirectly from either the vessels of the lateral wall of the cochlear duct or the spiral vessels underlying the basilar membrane.

The cooperation of Dr. Barry J. Anson in providing previously unpublished illustrations is gratefully acknowledged. Support of this work was derived from PHS Research Grant NB 08181 and from a Deafness Research Foundation Grant.

REFERENCES

Ades, H. W., and Engstrom, H.: Form and enervation of the vestibular epithelia. *In* The Role of the Vestibular Organs in the Exploration of Space, A. Graybiel, General Chairman. NASA Publication No. SP-77. Washington, D.C., National Aeronautics and Space Administration, 1965.

Amjad, A. H., Starke, J. J., and Scheer, A. A.: Tympanofacial recess in the human ear. Arch. Otolaryng. *88*:131–137, 1968.

Amjad, A. H., Scheer, A. A., and Rosenthal, J.: Human auditory canal. Arch. Otolaryng. *89*:709–714, 1969.

Anson, B. J. (ed). Morris' Human Anatomy. 12th ed. New York, Blakiston Division, McGraw-Hill Book Company, 1966.

Anson, B. J., and Donaldson, J. A.: The Surgical Anatomy of the Temporal Bone and Ear. Philadelphia, W. B. Saunders Company, 1967.

Anson, B. J.: Endolymphatic hydrops. Anatomic aspects. Arch. Otolaryng. *89*:70–84, 1969.

Axelsson, A.: The vascular anatomy of the cochlea in the guinea pig and in man. Acta Otolaryng. Suppl. 243, 1968.

Bast, T. H., and Anson, B. J.: The Temporal Bone and the Ear. Springfield, Ill., Charles C Thomas, 1948.

Bloom, W., and Fawcett, D. W.: A Textbook of Histology. 8th ed. Philadelphia, W. B. Saunders Company, 1966.

Bredberg, G.: Cellular pattern and nerve supply of the human organ of Corti. Acta Otolaryng. Suppl. 236, 1968.

Donaldson, J. A.: The fossula of the cochlear fenestra. Arch. Otolaryng. *88*:124–130, 1968.

Donaldson, J. A., Anson, B. J., Warpeha, R. L., and Rensink, M. J.: The surgical anatomy of the sinus tympani. Arch. Otolaryng. *91*:219–227, 1970.

Duvall, A. J.: The ultrastructure of the external sulcus in the guinea pig cochlear duct. *Laryngoscope 79*:1–29, 1969.

Engstrom, H., Ades, H. W., and Anderson, A.: Structural Pattern of the Organ of Corti. Stockholm, Almqvist and Wiksells, 1966.

Engstrom, H., Ades, H. W., and Hawkins, J. E., Jr.: Cellular pattern, nerve structures, and fluid spaces of the organ of Corti. *In* Neff, W. D. (ed): Contributions to Sensory Physiology. Vol. 1, New York, The Academic Press, Inc., 1965.

Flock, A.: Transducing mechanisms in the lateral line canal organ receptors. *In* Cold Spring Harbor Symposia on Quantitative Biology, Vol. 30. Frisch, L. (ed.): Sensory Receptors. Cold Spring Harbor, New York, Cold Spring Harbor Laboratory of Quantitative Biology, 1965.

Hawkins, J. E., Jr.: Cytoarchitectural basis of the cochlear transducer. *In* Cold Spring Harbor Symposia on Quantitative Biology, Vol. 30. Frisch, L. (ed.): Sensory Receptors. Cold Spring Harbor, New York, Cold Spring Harbor Laboratory of Quantitative Biology, 1965.

Hawkins, J. E., Jr.: Hearing: Anatomy and Acoustics. *In* Best, C. H., and Taylor, N. B. (eds.): The Physiological Basis of Medical Practice. 8th ed. Baltimore, The Williams & Wilkins Company, 1966.

Hollingshead, W.: Anatomy for Surgeons. 2nd ed. Vol. 1, The Head and Neck. New York, Hoeber Medical Division, Harper and Row, 1968.

Igarashi, M.: Dimensional study of the vestibular end organ apparatus. *In* Second Symposium on the Role of the Vestibular Organs in Space Exploration, A. Graybiel, General Chairman. NASA Publication No. SP-115. Washington, D.C., National Aeronautics and Space Administration, 1966.

Iurato, S.: The Submicroscopic Structure of the Inner Ear. London, Pergammon Press, 1967.

Kirikae, I.: The Structure and Function of the Middle Ear. Tokyo, The University of Tokyo Press, 1960.

Litton, W. B.: Epithelial migration over tympanic membrane and external canal. Arch. Otolaryng. *77*:254–257, 1963.

Neff, W. D. (ed.): Contributions to Sensory Physiology. Vols. 1 and 2. New York, The Academic Press, Inc., 1965.

Nomura, Y., and Hiraide, F.: Cochlear blood vessel. Arch. Otolaryng. *88*:231–241, 1968.

Proctor, B.: Surgical anatomy of the posterior tympanum. Ann. Otol. *78*:1026–1040, 1969.

Ruch, T. C., and Patton, H. D. (eds.): Physiology and Biophysics. 19th ed. Philadelphia, W. B. Saunders Company, 1965.

Smith, C. A.: Capillary areas of the membranous labyrinth. Ann. Otol. *63*:435–447, 1954.

Smith, C. A.: Structure of the stria vascularis and the spiral prominence. Trans. Amer. Otol. Soc. *45*:50–65, 1967.

Spoendlin, H.: The Organization of the Cochlear Receptor. New York, S. Karger and Sons, 1966.

Van Bergeijk, W. W.: Evolution of vertebrate hearing. *In* Neff, W. D. (ed.): Contributions to Sensory Physiology. Vol. 1. New York, The Academic Press, Inc., 1965.

Wersall, J., Flock, A., and Lundquist, P-G.: Structural basis for directional sensitivity in cochlear and vestibular sensory receptors. *In* Cold Spring Harbor Symposia on Quantitative Biology. Vol. 30. Frisch, L. (ed.): Sensory Receptors. Cold Spring Harbor, New York, Cold Spring Harbor Laboratory of Quantitative Biology, 1965.

Wersall, J., and Lundquist, P-G.: Morphological polariza-tion of the mechanoreceptors of the vestibular and acoustic systems. *In* Second Symposium on the Role of the Vestibular Organs in Space Exploration. A. Graybiel, General Chairman. NASA Publication No. SP-115. Washington, D.C., National Aeronautics and Space Administration, 1966.

Williams, H. L.: Developmental variations of the temporal bone that influence the evolution of chronic suppurative otitis media and mastoiditis and the medical and surgical treatment of this syndrome. Ann. Otol. 79:827–859, 1969.

Chapter 2

EMBRYOLOGY AND ANATOMY OF THE HEAD AND NECK

by Jack Davies, M.D.

BASIC EMBRYOLOGY

Formation of the Foregut

The human embryo is developed at the interface between two sacs, a dorsal amniotic sac and a ventral yolk sac. It consists, therefore, of a dorsal plate of ectoderm and a ventral plate of endoderm. The ectoderm is thickened caudally to form a linear mass of cells, the primitive streak, which recedes caudally as growth in length of the embryonic disc occurs, and in so doing leaves behind a linear rod of cells subjacent to the midline ectoderm; this is the head process and is later converted into the notochord (Fig. 1 *A*). Under the influence of the head process the overlying midline ectoderm is induced to thicken first into a neural plate and later into a neural groove, from which the central nervous system is formed by a process of fusion. The intra-embryonic mesoderm spreads out from the primitive streak and the head process to all parts of the embryonic disc except in two areas: the buccopharyngeal area anteriorly and the cloacal membrane posteriorly. In these two sites the ectoderm and endoderm remain in firm contact and later break down to permit continuity between the amniotic sac and the yolk sac at the mouth and at the anus, respectively. Anterior to the buccopharyngeal area the mesoderm spreads across the midline, forming the primitive diaphragm or septum transversum in which the pericardium, the heart, and the associated great vessels are formed. Caudal to the cloacal mem-

brane the mesoderm is continuous with the mesoderm investing the amnion dorsally and the yolk sac ventrally on the one hand, and on the other with the body stalk through which vascular connections between the embryo and the placental structures are developed; the latter is subsequently converted into the umbilical cord.

The next important step in the development of the embryo by which its definitive internal and external form is established is the formation of the head and tail folds (Fig. 1 *B*). The ectodermal surface of the embryo and the rapidly elongating neural tube grow more rapidly than does the yolk sac, with the result that the embryo as a whole begins to arch dorsally into the amniotic sac around an arbitrary axis marked anteriorly by the attachment of the amnion to the septum transversum and posteriorly by the attachment of the amnion to the cloacal membrane and body stalk. In this manner the anterior and posterior ends of the embryonic disc begin to overhang the yolk sac, forming the head and tail folds, and at the same time the upper part of the yolk sac is incorporated bodily into the C-shaped embryonic body to form the gut cavity. The septum transversum containing the heart and pericardium is likewise carried caudally under the overhanging head of the embryo into its definitive position in relation to the diaphragm; the cloacal membrane and body stalk are carried cranially under the tail of the embryo.

Progressive closure of the connection (vitello-intestinal isthmus) between the intra-embryonic part of the yolk sac (gut) and the extra-

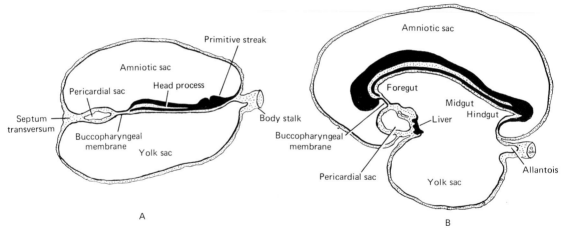

Figure 1. Longitudinal sections of the embryonic disc before (A) and after (B) the formation of the head and tail folds ("reversal of the pericardium and septum transversum"). As a result, the dorsal part of the yolk sac is incorporated into the embryo, forming the foregut anteriorly, the hindgut posteriorly, and the midgut which communicates through a "vitello-intestinal isthmus" with the extra-embryonic part of the yolk sac.

embryonic part then takes place and the connection is ultimately obliterated. The peripheral part of the yolk sac takes no further part in development but becomes atrophic. Connections may persist between the yolk sac and the gut, in which case they form varieties of the so-called Meckel's diverticulum, usually found in the small intestine about 1 m. proximal to the ileocecal valve. That part of the yolk sac incorporated anteriorly into the head fold forms the foregut; it ends caudally at an arbitrary point dorsal to the septum transversum and immediately caudal to the liver outgrowth or hepatic diverticulum (Fig. 1 *B*). The hindgut is formed from that portion of the yolk sac incorporated caudally into the tail fold. The intermediate portion of the intra-embryonic yolk sac forms the midgut. We shall be concerned in this chapter exclusively with the further development of the foregut. Its salient relationships are illustrated in detail in Figure 2.

The foregut is related dorsally to the central nervous system caudal to about the level of the hindbrain. The notochord lies between the roof of the foregut and the nervous system in a bed of mesoderm and has important relationships anteriorly, where it ends immediately caudal to the dorsal attachment of the buccopharyngeal membrane. Rathke's pouch, the primordium of the anterior pituitary, lies immediately anterior to the buccopharyngeal membrane, arising as an upgrowth of the dorsal ectoderm of the mouth or stomodeum. Thus, the notochord in the adult may be considered to terminate anteriorly in the body of the basisphenoid immediately posterior to the sella turcica. Here tumors

of the notochord (chordomas) may be found in relation to the base of the skull and the roof of the pharynx. Here also tumors of the anterior pituitary (craniopharyngiomas) or benign rests and adenomas of the pituitary may be found.

The foregut is related ventrally to the roof of the pericardium and more caudally to the septum transversum (Fig. 2). Two outgrowths of the foregut into these mesodermal beds dorsal to the foregut are observed: the laryngotracheal groove (primordium of the tracheal and pulmonary diverticula) and the hepatic diverticulum (primordium of the liver and gallbladder). Laterally the foregut is limited by a thick wall of mesoderm in which the branchial or pharyngeal arches are developed. These arches are five in number and superficially resemble the gill arches of a fish. (See Figure 4 *A*). The arches are separated by external grooves also reminiscent of the gill slits of the fish. The external grooves do not, however, communicate at any stage with the cavity of the foregut as in the fish. The external branchial or pharyngeal arches correspond on the inside of the foregut to a set of internal arches also separated by internal pharyngeal grooves (Fig. 15). A transverse section of the foregut at the level of the primitive pharynx is shown in Figure 3. The section passes through a pharyngeal arch on the right side and through an external and internal groove on the left side. The plate of apposed ectoderm and endoderm in the depth of the internal and external grooves is the closing membrane. A typical branchial or pharyngeal arch artery and nerve are shown on the right of the figure.

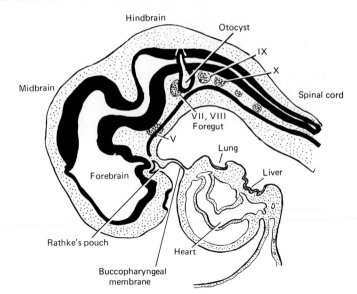

Figure 2. Longitudinal section of the anterior part of the embryo showing details of the brain, foregut, and adjacent parts of the pericardium and septum transversum. The primordia of the sensory ganglia of the fifth (V), seventh (VII), eighth (VIII), ninth (IX), and tenth (X) cranial nerves are stippled.

Further Development of the Foregut and the Evolution of the Pharyngeal (Branchial) Arches

The primitive foregut is converted by subsequent elongation and growth into the pharynx, esophagus, stomach, and proximal part of the small intestines as far caudally as the origin of the bile duct. All these parts of the foregut are surrounded by mesoderm and are also related ventrally either to the mesoderm in the roof of the pericardium or of the septum transversum. The pulmonary outgrowths arise from the ventral wall of the caudal pharynx (hypopharynx), as will be described in Chapter 2.

The pharyngeal arches, as stated previously, are five in number and are counted cranial to caudal, beginning with the first or mandibular arch immediately caudal to the mouth or stomodeum (Fig. 4 *A*). The fifth arch does not appear on the surface but lies buried around the site or origin of the laryngotracheal outgrowth. It is conventionally called the sixth arch for reasons of evolution and comparative anatomy, which cannot be discussed here. The arches are thus described as follows: first (mandibular) arch; second (hyoid) arch, third arch, fourth arch, sixth arch. Since the arches consist of mesoderm, they are capable of differentiating into a variety of tissues, e.g., connec-

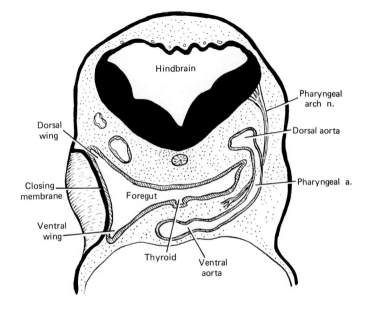

Figure 3. Transverse section of the embryo through the hindbrain and foregut. The section passes through a pharyngeal (branchial) cleft and pouch on the left side, and through the intervening pharyngeal arch on the right side. The arch contains a nerve and a pharyngeal arch artery.

tive tissue, cartilage, bone, blood vessels, and muscle. Nerves from the overlying ectodermal nervous system grow into the arches but are not differentiated from them. An understanding of the development of the pharyngeal arch cartilages, arteries, and nerves forms an excellent basis for an understanding of the adult anatomy of the head and neck and for a rational approach to the developmental abnormalities frequently found in this region.

SKELETAL DERIVATIVES OF THE PHARYNGEAL ARCHES

Cartilaginous bars are differentiated in each of the pharyngeal arches (Fig. 4 *A*). Two stages in their subsequent differentiation into the adult structures of the head and neck are shown in Figure 4 *B* and *C*. The fate of each of the arch cartilages is as follows:

First (Mandibular) Arch. The cartilage of this arch is known as Meckel's cartilage. It extends dorsally to make contact with another cartilaginous mass surrounding the otocyst or primordium of the inner ear, the otic capsule. It extends ventrally to fuse with the opposite cartilage in the floor of the pharynx. Meckel's cartilage becomes enveloped by membrane bone, which forms the body of the mandible and disappears without trace from the level of the lingula (at the entrance to the dental foramen) to the mental tubercles. Dorsal to the lingula, Meckel's cartilage becomes converted into the sphenomandibular ligament (Meckel's ligament), the anterior ligament and process of the malleus, the malleus, and the incus.

Second (Hyoid) Arch. The cartilage of this arch, much slenderer than that of the first, is like it in that it also reaches the otic capsule dorsally and meets its fellow in the midline ventrally. It becomes converted into the upper part of the body of the hyoid bone, the lesser cornu of the hyoid bone, the stylohyoid ligament, the styloid process, and possibly the

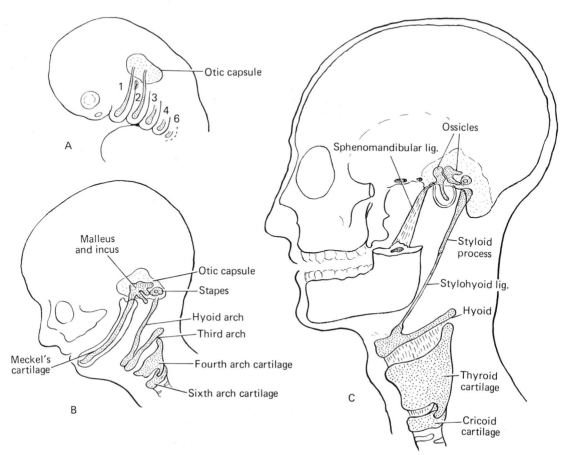

Figure 4. Three stages in the differentiation of the skeletal derivatives of the pharyngeal arches. The adult derivatives of the cartilage are stippled in C.

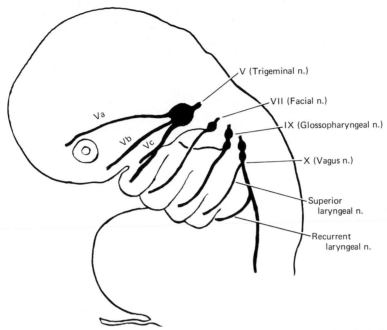

Figure 5. Scheme of the nerves of the pharyngeal arches: first arch, trigeminal; second arch, facial; third arch, glossopharyngeal; fourth arch, superior laryngeal branch of the vagus; sixth arch, recurrent (inferior) laryngeal branch of the vagus nerve.

stapes. There is evidence in lower forms that the stapedial homolog is not developed from the second arch but independently from the otic capsule.

Third Arch. This cartilage meets with the opposite arch in the floor of the pharynx but falls short of the otic capsule dorsally. It is converted into the lower part of the body and the greater cornu of the hyoid bone.

Fourth Arch. This arch cartilage is also limited to the ventral mesoderm of the pharynx and becomes converted into the thyroid cartilage and associated ligamentous structures.

Sixth Arch. This cartilage is small in extent and is transformed into the cricoid cartilage, the arytenoid cartilages, and the small accessory cartilages of the larynx. (See Chapter 4.)

Thus, the phylogenetically ancient suspensory and respiratory cartilages of the pharynx undergo a remarkable evolution in mammals in which their identity is maintained but their function is entirely altered. The skeletal structures of the cranial vault, the face, and the jaws are formed by phylogenetically new bone, called dermal bone since it is formed "in membrane," i.e., in mesoderm surrounding the brain, the eyes, the nose and the face. The old branchial cartilages become superseded in this supportive function and either disappear or are transformed into new structures of peculiar impor-

tance and function in terrestrial mammals. Thus, the Meckelian and hyoid cartilages become transformed into the ossicles of the middle ear. The rest of the hyoid cartilage and the third arch cartilage take on important functions in relation to the hyoid suspensory apparatus and swallowing. The fourth and sixth cartilages form the supporting and functional cartilages of the larynx.

NERVES OF THE PHARYNGEAL ARCHES

In addition to the cartilaginous structures developed within the arches, there are also vascular and neural structures. The arches become penetrated at an early stage by nerve fibers of the cranial nerves, which establish functional connections with the muscles and other structures within the arches, including the overlying skin. These connections are probably prerequisites for the full functional differentiation of these structures. The cranial nerves of the five arches and the muscles which they innervate are as follows (Fig. 5).

First Arch. The nerve of the first arch is the trigeminal or fifth cranial nerve. The proper nerve of the arch is its third or mandibular division. The first and second divisions of the nerve do not enter the arch but pass in front of the eye and mouth, respectively, as the ophthalmic and maxillary nerves. The ganglion of the fifth nerve is large (Gasserian ganglion). The motor branches of the nerve are distributed only through the mandibular division. The muscles innervated by this division, and so developmentally derived from the first arch mesoderm, are the muscles of mastication (masseter, temporalis, medial and lateral pterygoids), the anterior belly of the digastric and mylohyoid, the tensor tympani, and the tensor veli palatini (tensor palati).

Second Arch. The nerve of this arch is the facial or seventh cranial nerve. Its ganglion (geniculate) is small and lies in relation to the otic capsule. A small branch of the facial nerve, the chorda tympani, passes into the first arch and joins the mandibular branch of the fifth nerve. It is called a "pretrematic nerve" (in front of the gill slit) since it passes into the arch next anterior to its proper arch; it is described in connection with the development of the middle ear (Chapter 3). The muscles innervated by the facial nerve, and so of second arch origin, are the platysma and the muscles of facial expression—the stylohyoid, the posterior belly of the digastric, and the stapedius.

Third Arch. The third arch nerve is the glossopharyngeal or ninth cranial nerve. It has two small sensory ganglia. It also has a small "pretrematic" branch, the lesser superficial petrosal nerve, which will be described in connection with the middle ear. The muscles supplied by the ninth nerve are the stylopharyngeus and the upper (superior and middle) constrictor muscles of the pharynx.

Fourth Arch. The nerve of the fourth arch is the superior laryngeal branch of the vagus (tenth cranial nerve). This nerve has a sensory component (internal branch), supplying the mucosa of the laryngopharynx and larynx as far down as the true vocal cords, and a motor branch (external branch), which supplies the cricothyroid muscle.

Sixth Arch. The nerve of the last arch is the inferior (recurrent) laryngeal branch of the vagus nerve. It supplies all the intrinsic muscles of the larynx, the inferior constrictor muscle (wholly or in part), the upper fibers of the esophagus, as well as the mucous membrane of the larynx below the vocal cords and that of the lower pharynx and upper esophagus.

The position of the pharyngeal arch nerves in the adult is fixed in relationship with the skeletal derivatives of the arch cartilages (Fig. 6). Thus, the mandibular branch, with its two terminal divisions (lingual and inferior alveolar or dental), lies internal to the saphenomandibular ligament within the pterygoid region. The facial nerve (of the second arch) lies immediately lateral to the base of the styloid process after emerging from the stylomastoid foramen. The glossopharyngeal nerve (of the third arch) lies deep and posterior to the stylopharyngeus muscle and then enters the tongue in the angle between the stylohyoid ligament and the greater cornu of the hyoid bone. The internal branch of the superior laryngeal nerve (of the fourth arch) lies on the thyrohyoid membrane in the interval between the greater cornu of the hyoid bone and the upper margin of the thyroid cartilage. The inferior or recurrent laryngeal nerve (of the sixth arch) lies in the groove between the esophagus and the trachea and enters the larynx posterior to the cricothyroid joint under cover of the thyroid cartilage. The reason for the devious course of this nerve will be explained in a subsequent paragraph.

ARTERIAL DERIVATIVES OF THE PHARYNGEAL ARCHES

Following the basic plan of the pharyngeal arch system, five arteries are developed within the mesoderm of the arches (Fig. 7). The vessels arise by the confluence of small vascular islands within the mesoderm (angioblastic islands) and are formed one after the other in cranial to caudal sequence. All five vessels are probably not found at any one stage, as shown in Figure 7, since the first and second arterial arches degenerate before the third and subsequent arteries are formed. The arteries arise from the ventral aorta in the roof of the pericardium and pass dorsally through the arch to unite with the dorsal aorta on either side (Figs. 3 and 7). The dorsal aortae pass cranially to supply the rapidly developing forebrain and midbrain. They unite at a level caudal to the arch field to form a single dorsal aorta from which the arteries to the foregut (celiac axis), to the midgut (superior mesenteric), and to the hindgut (inferior mesenteric) arise in sequence. Small intersegmental arteries are given off from the dorsal aortae along the length of the embryo, passing between the segmental mesodermal blocks (somites) which later take part in the formation of the vertebrae; they supply the spinal cord and postvertebral skin and musculature. The arrangement of the pharyngeal arch (branchial aortic) arteries is strikingly similar to that in a primitive vertebrate such as the dogfish.

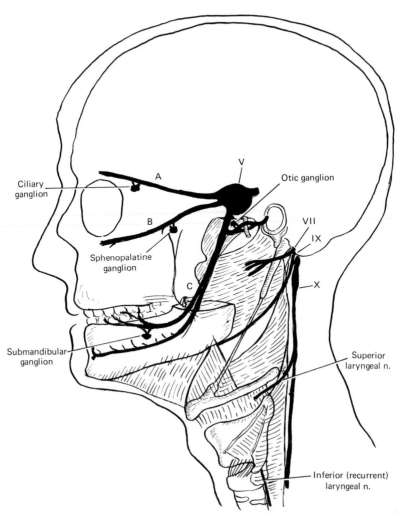

Figure 6. Muscles of the floor of the mouth and of the pharyngeal wall and their relationship to the pharyngeal arch nerves. Parasympathetic ganglia are related to the three divisions of the trigeminal nerve: ciliary ganglion to the ophthalmic branch, sphenopalatine ganglion to the maxillary branch, otic and submandibular ganglia to the mandibular branch.

The flow of blood in the pharyngeal arch arteries is dorsally from the heart into the dorsal aortae. The fused dorsal aortae give rise caudally to two umbilical arteries through which the deoxygenated blood is carried to the placenta. It is returned as oxygenated blood to the heart by the umbilical veins.

Note that in every instance but one the pharyngeal arch nerves come to lie *anterior* to their respective arch arteries. The exception is the nerve of the sixth arch (inferior or recurrent laryngeal), which lies *posterior* to its respective arch artery (Fig. 7). This exceptional circumstance has important consequences in relation to the adult course of this nerve.

The adult derivatives of the pharyngeal arch arteries on each side will now be described.

The arrangement of the arteries in relation to the nerves in Figure 8 is shown from the left side.

The first and second arteries become atrophic and disappear, probably before the third and more caudally placed arch arteries are fully formed. The dorsal segment of the second arch artery persists for a time during fetal life as the "stapedial artery," passing through the crura of the stapes which are ossified around the vessel. This artery may rarely persist in the adult and may cause bleeding during operations on the middle ear and during mobilization of the stapes. In some animals the vessel persists normally and takes part in the blood supply of the intracranial structures. The third arch artery becomes the proximal part of the

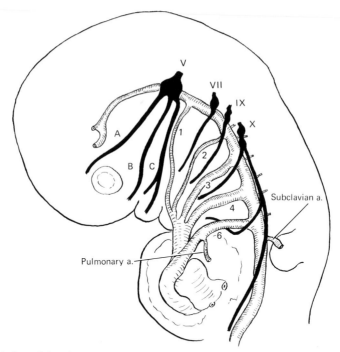

Figure 7. Left lateral view of the pharyngeal arch arteries and nerves. All the arch nerves lie cranial to their respective arch arteries with the exception of the nerve of the sixth arch (recurrent laryngeal nerve), which lies caudal to its arch artery. The subclavian is derived from the seventh intersegmental artery.

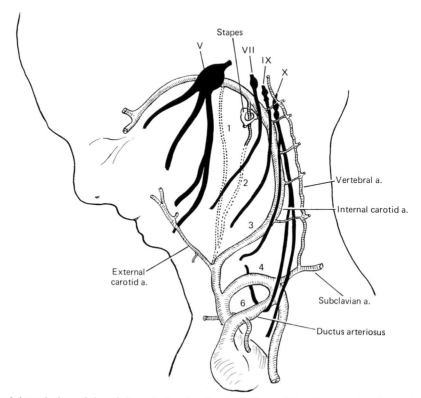

Figure 8. Left lateral view of the adult neck showing the derivatives of the pharyngeal arch arteries and their relationship to the nerves. Due to persistence of the connection of the sixth arch artery with the dorsal aorta (ductus arteriosus), the recurrent laryngeal nerve turns around it caudally.

internal carotid artery. The dorsal aorta cranial to the third arch artery forms the remaining part of the internal carotid artery, including its intracranial portion. The external carotid artery develops late as a small offshoot of the ventral part of the third arch artery and passes cranially to supply the face and jaws. The short segment of the third arch artery proximal to the origin of the external carotid artery becomes elongated and becomes the common carotid artery. Note that the trigeminal, facial, and glossopharyngeal nerves pass into their respective arch structures *lateral* to the dorsal aorta, and so lateral to the internal carotid artery; these cranial nerves are found in this relationship to the great vessel in the adult.

The fourth arch artery (Figure 8, at the left) is transformed into the arch of the aorta. The dorsal aorta connecting this vessel to the third arch artery disappears. The left subclavian artery is developed from a persisting seventh intersegmental artery arising from the dorsal aorta and passing into the primordium of the forelimb. The vertebral artery is formed as a longitudinal anastomotic connection between the seventh intersegmental artery (subclavian) caudally and the individual intersegmental arteries cranial to this. That portion of the vertebral artery curving posteriorly and medially around the lateral mass of the atlas to enter the foramen magnum lateral to the medulla oblongata represents a persisting first or perhaps second intersegmental artery. Note that the internal branch of the superior laryngeal nerve (fourth arch nerve) also descends lateral to the internal carotid artery and enters the larynx through the thyrohyoid membrane. (See also Figure 6.)

The sixth arch artery on the left forms a large and important vessel in fetal life (Fig. 8). Soon after the appearance of the lung diverticulum from the floor of the pharynx, a small pulmonary artery is given off from the caudal face of the sixth arch artery. Distal to this point, the sixth arch artery persists in fetal life as the ductus arteriosus. This important shunt provides a "by-pass" for the deoxygenated blood from the right ventricle, returning it quickly to the placenta without passing through the lungs, which are not functional. The flow of blood in this vessel is reversed at birth following inflation of the lungs and expansion of the pulmonary vascular bed. The ductus arteriosus remains open during the postnatal period of adjustment to fluctuating right and left ventricular pressures and then undergoes an endarteritis which obliterates its lumen. In about 1 per cent of newborns the ductus remains patent as late as the end of the first year. In abnormal cases it may remain widely patent in the adult, giving a characteristic "machinery murmur" on auscultation. Right ventricular decompensation and congestive heart failure supervene in later adult life unless the vessel is closed surgically.

Note that the inferior or recurrent laryngeal nerve (nerve of the sixth arch) is found caudal to its proper artery, as described on p. 116. Since the sixth arch artery persists as the ductus arteriosus, the recurrent laryngeal nerve curves around this vessel on its caudal or inferior surface before assuming its final position in the groove between the esophagus and the trachea. Its final entry into the larynx (Fig. 6) is through the cricothyroid interval, that is, between the derivatives of the fourth and sixth arch cartilages. The ductus arteriosus becomes converted in the adult into the ligamentum arteriosum, which connects the left pulmonary artery to the undersurface of the aortic arch. The recurrent laryngeal nerve is properly described as curving around the ligamentum arteriosum rather than the arch of the aorta.

The final disposition of the arch arteries on the right side is shown in Figure 9. The first and second arch arteries disappear, as on the left side, with the possible exception of the persisting "stapedial artery." The third arch artery is converted into the internal carotid artery. The right fourth arch artery forms the proximal segment of the subclavian artery up to its point of union with the dorsal aorta. Beyond this point, the right subclavian artery is developed from the seventh intersegmental artery, which passes into the limb bud. Thus, on the left side the subclavian artery is formed only from the seventh intersegmental artery; on the right side it is formed from the fourth arch artery and also from the seventh intersegmental artery. The sixth arch artery gives off a small pulmonary artery, as on the left side. Dorsal to this point, however, the sixth arch artery disappears, so that there is no ductus arteriosus on this side. The effect of this on the position of the right recurrent laryngeal nerve is to cause it to curve around the next most cranial persisting arch vessel (the fourth), in this case the subclavian artery. The external carotid and vertebral arteries are developed as on the left side.

The primitive arrangement of the arch arteries in relation to the foregut is shown in Figure 10 *A* as viewed from the front. Note that the vessels arise from the ventral aorta *ventral* to the pharynx; they join dorsally on either

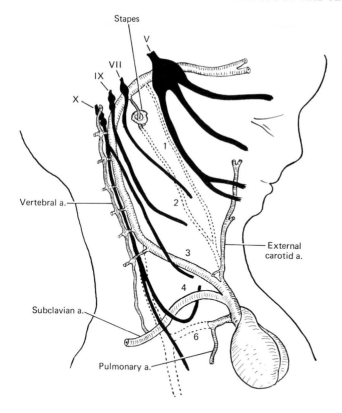

Figure 9. Right lateral view of the adult neck showing the derivatives of the pharyngeal arch arteries and their relationship to the nerves. On this side the connection of the sixth arch artery with the dorsal aorta disappears, thus causing the recurrent laryngeal nerve to turn around the next most cranial artery, in this case the right subclavian artery. The subclavian artery on the right is formed from the fourth arch artery and the seventh intersegmental artery.

side to form the dorsal aortae, which fuse caudally *dorsal* to the esophagus. In a real sense, therefore, the persisting arch vessels (internal carotid, aorta, ductus arteriosus, right subclavian) embrace the lateral surfaces of the esophagus. The final disposition of the vessels and the normal course of the recurrent laryngeal nerves on the left and the right are shown in Figure 10 *B* from the front.

Nonrecurrence of the Right Inferior Laryngeal Nerve

This not infrequent anomaly is accidentally discovered during thyroidectomy and is *invariably* associated with a retroesophageal right subclavian artery. This anomalous vessel arises distally from the aorta beyond the attachment of the ligamentum arteriosum. The anomaly arises as a persistence of the right dorsal aorta distal to the origin of the seventh intersegmental artery (right subclavian). The sixth arch artery on this side disappears distal to the point of origin of the pulmonary artery (Fig. 11). Thus, the recurrent laryngeal nerve on this side is now shifted cranially and curves anteriorly around the next most cranial, persisting

arch artery, in this case the right internal carotid artery. The nerve accordingly descends almost vertically in relation to the internal carotid artery and enters the larynx through the cricothyroid interval. A necessary corollary of this variation is the existence of a right subclavian artery which arises from the dorsal aorta

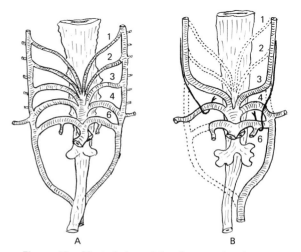

Figure 10. Ventral view of the pharyngeal arch arteries (A) and their derivatives (B).

Anomalies of the azygos and hemiazygos veins are legion and are usually unimportant.

Development of the Pharyngeal Pouch System

A striking feature of the development of the pharynx is the origin of the principal endocrine glands of the head and neck (thyroid, parathyroid) and of the large lymphatic organs such as the tonsil and thymus in relation to endodermal diverticula. It must be presumed that in the early evolution of these glandular structures in vertebrates, they developed as endodermal diverticula of the foregut. It will be recalled (Fig. 3) that the lumen of the primitive pharynx conforms to the external and internal configuration of the mesodermal pharyngeal arches. Thus, the pharynx is relatively narrow from side to side at the level of the arches and is extended laterally in the form of recesses or pouches in the grooves between the arches. The appearance of these pharyngeal pouches as seen from the ventral surface and also in relation to the persisting third, fourth, and sixth arch arteries is shown in Figure 13.

The pharynx is seen to be wide anteriorly in relation to the arches and pouches, and to nar-

row poste[r]
the pulm[o]
pouches, [
caudal. A
pendage [
dependent
lumen. Th
passes do[
pouches, [
third and [
artery bet[
appendage
hypophar[
shown ari[
floor of t[
derivative

In later
pouches b[
pharynx, [
ryngeal lu[
gated pha
The first [
the tubo[
middle ea[
tiated, as [
3. The ve
pouch do[
tubotymp[
pocket ar[

beyond the left subclavian artery and passes to the right behind the esophagus (Fig. 11). These two variations must coexist, and one without the other is embryologically impossible. Aortograms in cases of nonrecurrence of the left inferior laryngeal nerve will always reveal a retroesophageal right subclavian artery. The latter may be symptomless or may cause dysphagia. The abnormal course of the left inferior laryngeal nerve also predisposes it to possible damage during thyroidectomy.

In situs inversus the thoracic and abdominal viscera are reversed in position, and in these instances there is a persistence of the right dorsal aorta rather than the left. The ductus arteriosus is then found on the right side. The inferior laryngeal nerve on the right turns around the abnormal ductus, and the nerve on the left side turns around the subclavian artery.

Evolution of the Great Veins of the Head and Neck and Thorax

The rather simple pattern of veins in the early human embryo at about the fifth week

of development is shown in Figure 12 *A* as seen from the front. A bilaterally symmetrical system of venous channels, the cardinal system, empties into the caudal chamber of the heart or sinus venosus within the septum transversum. Anterior cardinal veins on either side drain caudally from the head region. Posterior cardinal veins from the caudal parts of the embryo join with the anterior cardinal veins to form a large venous channel on either side, the common cardinal veins or ducts of Cuvier, which enter the lateral horns of the sinus venosus. Also emptying caudally into the sinus venosus are two bilaterally symmetrical systems of veins, the umbilical (right and left) and the vitelline (right and left). The former are the placental veins which convey oxygenated blood from the placenta to the heart; the latter are the veins of the yolk sac.

At a later stage the pattern of veins is modified (Fig. 12 *B*). The right anterior and common cardinal veins become enlarged, while the left common cardinal system is reduced. This relative preponderance of the right over the left cardinal system is associated with the development of a massive venous shunt between the anterior cardinal veins anterior to the trachea (Fig. 12 *B*). This is the left innominate (left brachiocephalic) shunt which becomes the adult vein of the same name. At the same time the posterior cardinal veins become reduced in size on both sides, and their former function of receiving the intersegmental venous drainage of the body wall (Fig. 12 *A*) is taken over by a new and more dorsally placed system of veins, the supracardinal or perisympathetic veins.

Complex changes also occur in the veins entering the sinus venosus from the body wall and yolk sac. The four veins (two umbilical and two vitelline) (Fig. 12 *A*), which formerly entered the sinus venosus, no longer do so; instead, a single vein, usually considered to be the terminal portion of the right vitelline vein (Fig. 12 *B*), is the only one to enter the chamber at this level. This short vessel forms the terminal segment of the inferior vena cava. The development of this great vessel more caudally is of no concern in relation to this chapter, and details may be sought in standard embryology books. The right umbilical vein disappears and the left umbilical vein enlarges to become the single definitive placental vein.

The final disposition of the great veins is shown in Figure 12 *C*. The right anterior cardinal vein as low as the right seventh intersegmental vein (subclavian) forms the right in-

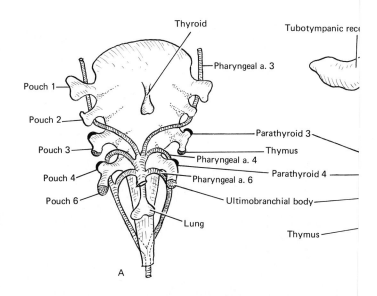

Figure 13. Thyroid, Tubotympanic rec[ess], Pharyngeal a. 3, Pouch 1, Pouch 2, Pouch 3, Parathyroid 3, Thymus, Pharyngeal a. 4, Pouch 4, Parathyroid 4, Pharyngeal a. 6, Pouch 6, Ultimobranchial body, Lung, Thymus, A

Figure 13.   Ventral views of the derivatives of the pharyngeal pouches A) become incorporated into the tubotympanic recess (middle ear and eus[tachian tube] in black. The thymus arises from the ventral wing of the third pouch and

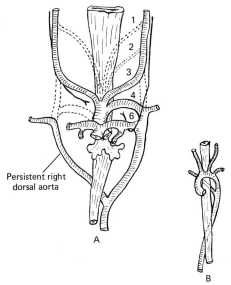

Persistent right dorsal aorta, A, B

Figure 11.   Scheme showing the genesis of retroesophageal right subclavian artery. The fourth arch artery, which normally forms the proximal segment of the right subclavian artery, disappears and the distal part of the fourth arch artery and its connection with the dorsal aorta persists. The right recurrent laryngeal nerve, as a consequence, turns around the next most cranial arch artery (the third) and so descends almost vertically to the larynx in proximity to the internal and common carotid arteries. A retroesophageal right subclavian artery is always found in association with nonrecurrence of the right recurrent laryngeal nerve.

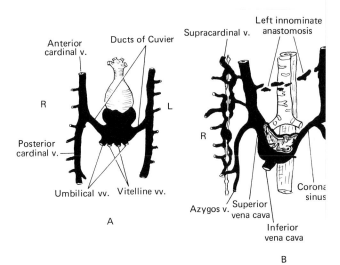

A

B

Figure 12. Three stages in the development of the great veins jugular systems and that of the azygos and hemiazygos systems. the left superior intercostal vein in C which represents the forme vena cava.

ternal jugular vein. The right anterior cardinal vein caudal to the subclavian vein forms the right innominate (brachiocephalic) vein. The left anterior cardinal likewise forms the left internal jugular vein as low as the left seventh intersegmental vein (subclavian); these two veins fuse to form the left innominate (brachiocephalic) vein. The latter passes across the midline anterior to the trachea and unites with the right innominate vein to form the superior vena cava. The right posterior cardinal vein persists as that part of the azygos vein which arches over the root of the right lung. The distal portion of the azygos vein, which receives the intersegmental drainage (intercostal) of the body wall, is developed from the supracardinal or perisympathetic plexus of veins (Fig. 12 *B*). The right superior intercostal vein, a vessel of considerable radiological importance, is also of supracardinal origin and drains into the azygos vein above the root of the lung. It is of interest that in rare cases the lung, in its growth into the thoracic wall, may encounter the azygos vein, and a portion of the upper lobe may be entrapped medial to this vessel, forming an azygos lobe. (See Chapter 3.) This is usually an incidental finding on radiological study and is without symptoms. The right common cardinal vein forms the terminal segment of the superior vena cava, which passes into the pericardium and enters the right atrium.

On the left side the common cardinal vein

forr
cor
veir
still
hon
liga
is
inno
ante
sup
peri
syst
A
and
lary
ven
abs
inno
dov
righ
sinu
sym
cult
moi
dotl
the
abn
left
ven
sub
abe
that
"lef

gregate, forming the palatine tonsil. The ventral remnant of the second pouch is represented in the adult by the intratonsillar fossa.

The third, fourth, and sixth pouches give rise to important glandular structures by a process of epithelial (endodermal) proliferation and differentiation. The dorsal wing of the third pouch gives rise to the parathyroid-3, so called because of its origin. The dorsal wing of the fourth pouch gives rise to parathyroid-4. The ventral wing of the third pouch proliferates to form the thymus. The thymus becomes greatly elongated (Fig. 13 *B*) and extends into the superior and anterior mediastinum of the thorax. In this later growth and caudal displacement the parathyroid associated with it (parathyroid-3) is also displaced caudally. Thus, the parathyroid derived from the third pouch becomes the inferior parathyroid of the adult, though it is developmentally the more cranial of the two parathyroids. Parathyroid-4 remains at a more cranial level and is the superior parathyroid of the adult. Rarely a rudimentary thymus may develop from the ventral wing of the fourth pouch, forming an accessory thymus in relation to the superior parathyroid.

The sixth pouch, observed previously as an appendage of the fourth pouch, gives rise to the ultimobranchial body. This conspicuous spherical body differentiates into glandular tissue which resembles fetal thyroid tissue. Its subsequent fate is unknown. In the pig it is conspicuous at birth and resembles embryonic thyroid tissue. It seems possible that the ultimobranchial body in man may become absorbed into the lateral lobe of the thyroid gland

without trace or may possibly be implicated in the formation of the so-called solitary nodules.

Development of the Cervical Sinus

Closely bound up with the development of the pharyngeal pouches, which are of endodermal origin, is that of the cervical sinus (cervical sinus of His), which is derived from the ectoderm. At first (Fig. 14 *A*) the external pharyngeal arches from the first to the fourth are visible; the sixth is buried beneath the surface. At a slightly later stage (Fig. 14 *B*) there is a relative caudal growth and enlargement of the first and second arches in such a way that the third and fourth arches become submerged in a shallow ectodermal pit, the cervical sinus. The depth of this pit is further enhanced by the appearance of a V-shaped swelling caudal to the arch field, the epipericardial ridge. The V lies on its side with the point facing caudally and the arms of the V embracing the caudal arches anteriorly. The epipericardial ridge is raised up by the proliferation of the underlying mesoderm, in which the musculature caudal to the arch field is differentiated (sternomastoid-trapezius complex), the infrahyoid muscles, and the muscles of the floor of the mouth and tongue (Fig. 14 *C*). Contained within this mesodermal ridge are the spinal branch of the accessory (eleventh) and the hypoglossal (twelfth) cranial nerves. These nerves are not properly cranial nerves but belong to the cranial group of spinal nerves which are presumed to have been incorporated into the skull in the

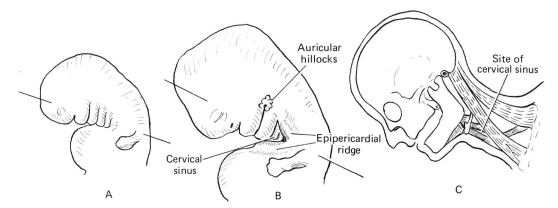

A   B   C

Figure 14. Left lateral views of the pharynx and of the adult neck showing the origin of the cervical sinus of His. In B the arches caudal to the second are becoming submerged by the elevation of the mesodermal epipericardial ridge. The adult muscles derived from the epipericardial ridge (C) are the trapezius, sternomastoid, infrahyoid muscles, and muscles of the tongue, which form the caudal and posterior boundaries of the pharyngeal arch field. Remnants of the cervical sinus lie cranial to these boundaries.

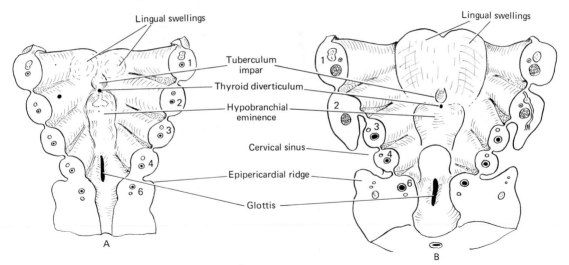

Figure 15. Floor of the embryonic pharynx at two stages showing the formation of the tongue and epiglottis and the origin of the thyroid diverticulum. The development of the cervical sinus is shown in B; the third and fourth arches become submerged by the overlapping mass of the second arch anteriorly and that of the epipericardial ridge posteriorly.

process of the evolution of mammals. The caudal growth of the second or hyoid arch, which is innervated by the seventh cranial nerve, resembles the growth of the so-called operculum in the bony fish which overhangs and partially occludes the underlying gill slits. Thus, the earlier stage (Fig. 14 *A*) resembles the cartilaginous fish or "sharklike" stage of human ontogenesis; the later stage (Fig. 14 *B*) resembles the bony fish stage.

The approximate area of the cervical sinus in the angle between the limbs of the epipericardial ridge is illustrated in the adult neck in Figure 14 *C*. The upper and caudal limb of the V is represented by the trapezius and sternomastoid muscles. The inferior limb of the V is represented by the infrahyoid muscles, the muscles of the floor of the mouth, and the intrinsic muscles of the tongue. The arch field, represented in the adult by the mandibular structures, the hyoid bone, and the thyroid and cricoid cartilages, is contained within the angle made by the two muscular limbs of the epipericardial ridge. The arching course of the hypoglossal nerve lateral to the internal and external carotid results from the differentiation of the epipericardial ridge caudal to the arch field (see Figure 16); the nerve subsequently migrates cranially until it is arrested by the lower sternomastoid branch of the occipital artery. The loop of the ansa hypoglossi, containing fibers of the first, second, and third cervical nerves, is also determined by the ridge. The patterns of fibers from the platysma muscle,

innervated by the facial nerve, which overlie the arch field and sweep down onto the anterior part of the upper thorax, result from the growth and migration of second arch mesoderm lateral to the arch field. It is evident from a consideration of the above developmental facts that any persisting connection between the surface and the cervical sinus, or between the latter and the deeper endodermal pouches of the pharynx, must lie deep to the platysma muscle and also must lie anterior to the derivatives of the epipericardial ridge and the hypoglossal loop.

In order to illustrate more carefully these important relationships, two sections have been illustrated in Figure 15 *A* and *B* along the planes indicated in Figure 14 *A* and *B*, respectively. The floor of the pharynx, flanked laterally by the arches, is shown as viewed from the top, the roof of the pharynx having been removed. The arches are seen (Fig. 15 *A*) passing down into the floor of the pharynx like the ribs of a ship meeting in a keel-like mass of midline structures to be described later. The endodermal pouches lie laterally between the arches and are in immediate contact with the ectoderm at the closing membranes. The arch arteries and nerves are also shown within the arches. The formation of the cervical sinus by the caudal extension of the second arch and the raising of the epipericardial ridge caudally is shown in Figure 15 *B*. The effect of this is to close off from the surface an ectodermally lined pit in the floor of which are the third and fourth arches and the related closing membranes. The hypoglossal nerve and branches of the spinal accessory and upper cervical nerves are contained within the epipericardial ridge and so lie caudal to the arch field. The cervical sinus is eventually cut off from the surface by the closure of the external orifice; the sinus itself is obliterated and normally no trace of it remains.

PERSISTENCE OF THE CERVICAL SINUS

Lateral Cysts of the Neck. The cervical sinus may persist, clinically recognized as a lateral cyst of the neck. The cyst is of ectodermal origin and so is lined by epidermal epithelium which, by desquamation, may produce a cholesteatoma. The cyst is also prone to repeated infection and to malignant change, giving rise to an epidermoid carcinoma. Its complete removal is, therefore, imperative. The cyst differs from the midline cysts of the neck (usually of thyroglossal cyst origin) in that it does not move on swallowing. Fistulous connections between the cyst and the surface may exist, in which case they may exude cholesterol-like material, pus, or infected material. The orifice lies at some point along the anterior surface of the sternomastoid, as would be expected from the manner of its development. The cyst itself lies deep to the platysma, since the latter is a second arch derivative. It also lies in close relationship to the carotid sheath.

The persistence of fistulous connections between the cervical sinus cyst and the deep pharyngeal pouches is easily explained on the basis of their development. The anatomical relationships of these tracts are of importance and give a vital clue to the precise endodermal pouch involved. Connections with the second endodermal pouch are the commonest. Connections with the third pouch are probably rare but possible. Connections with the fourth pouch must be very rare, if they occur at all.

Connection of Cervical Sinus Cyst with Second Pouch. The cyst and its fistulous connection with the pharynx are shown in Figure 16. The tract ascends from the cyst along the carotid sheath until it reaches the hypoglossal nerve above the hyoid bone lateral to the internal and external carotid arteries and the loop of the lingual artery. Note that the hypoglossal nerve is tethered by the small but important lower sternomastoid branch of the occipital artery. This vessel, considered to be a persisting intersegmental artery, may be absent, in which case the hypoglossal nerve descends almost vertically from the base of the skull. The fistulous tract loops over the hypoglossal nerve since the nerve belongs to the epipericardial ridge and not the arches. It then pierces the

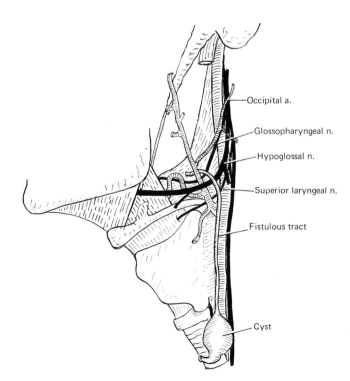

— Occipital a.

— Glossopharyngeal n.

— Hypoglossal n.

— Superior laryngeal n.

— Fistulous tract

— Cyst

Figure 16. Left lateral view of the adult pharynx showing the relationships of a fistulous tract between a persistent cervical sinus and the remains of the second pharyngeal pouch. The tract loops around the hypoglossal nerve and pierces the middle constrictor after passing through the "fork" of the two carotid arteries.

pharyngeal wall at the level of the middle constrictor muscle and opens into the intratonsillar fossa, which is the remnant of the ventral wing of the second pharyngeal pouch (see p. 124). Note that the tract must necessarily pass anterior to the internal carotid artery (third arch artery) and so between the fork of the internal and external carotid arteries (Fig. 15). It must also pass cranial to the third arch nerve, in this case the ninth (glossopharyngeal) nerve. Damage to this nerve must be avoided.

Connection of Cervical Sinus Cyst with Third Pouch. The course of the cyst and of the fistulous tract over the loop of the hypoglossal nerve (Fig. 17) is as in the previous case. However, the tract in this case passes posterior to the internal carotid artery (artery of the third arch). It then descends in close relation to the pharyngeal wall caudal to the glossopharyngeal nerve. It pierces the thyrohyoid membrane between the hyoid bone (third arch) and the thyroid cartilage (fourth arch) to enter the pharynx in the region of the pyriform sinus, generally held to be the approximate site of the third endodermal pouch. The tract pierces the thyrohyoid membrane cranial to the internal branch of the superior laryngeal nerve (nerve of the fourth arch).

Theoretical Connections Between the Cervical Sinus and the Fourth or Sixth Pouches. Connections between the cervical sinus and the caudal pouches are theoretically possible but are not described in the literature. The characteristic loop of the tract over the hypoglossal nerve could scarcely survive the extensive caudal displacement of the arteries of the fourth and sixth arches. However, remnants of the tract or of the endodermal pouches may possibly persist, in which case they would be found caudal to the fourth or sixth arch derivatives in the root of the neck or upper mediastinum. Cysts in relation to the subclavian artery, the arch of the aorta, or the pulmonary arteries could conceivably be of cervical sinus or endodermal pouch origin. In the former case the lining of the cyst is ectodermal in origin and could be expected to give rise to epidermoid carcinoma. In the latter case, the cyst is lined by noncornified squamous epithelium of pharyngeal or esophageal type or a columnar epithelium of intestinal type. Resulting malignant change could, therefore, give rise to epidermoid carcinoma or adenocarcinoma. Some of the so-called dermoid cysts in the upper mediastinum could also be of cervical sinus origin.

Development of the Tongue

The tongue arises as a composite structure in the floor of the pharynx (Fig. 15). Its cover-

Figure 17. Left lateral view of the adult pharynx showing the connection of a persistent cervical sinus and fistulous tract with the remains of the third pharyngeal pouch. The tract loops around the hypoglossal nerve and descends to the larynx by passing posterior to the internal carotid artery. It enters the pyriform sinus by piercing the thyrohyoid membrane cranial to the superior laryngeal nerve.

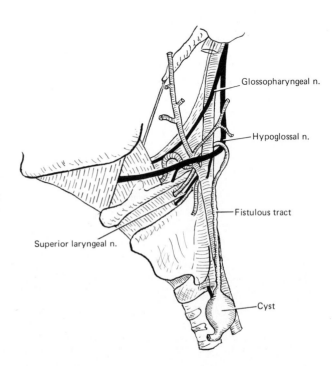

Glossopharyngeal n.

Hypoglossal n.

Fistulous tract

Superior laryngeal n.

Cyst

ing epithelium is endodermal. It arises ante- riorly as two symmetrical swellings (lingual swellings) at the ventral ends of the two first pharyngeal arches. An unpaired swelling pos- terior to the lingual swellings is the tuberculum impar. Posterior to the tuberculum impar is an extensive linear swelling, the hypobranchial eminence, with which the ventral ends of the third and fourth arches merge. The thyroid gland arises as an outgrowth of the floor of the pharynx between the tuberculum impar and the hypobranchial eminence (Fig. 15 *A*).

At a later stage (Fig. 15 *B*) the lingual swell- ings are enlarged and soon fuse to form the anterior two thirds of the tongue. This part of the tongue, therefore, is bilateral in origin, a fact which accounts for the area of low vascu- larity in the midline of the tongue. The tuber- culum impar is now small and becoming sub- merged by the piling up of the hypobranchial eminence posterior to it to form the posterior third of the tongue. At the same time there is a general migration of the third arch mesoderm into the posterior third of the tongue, merging with the hypobranchial eminence. The hypo- branchial eminence also develops a horizontal groove dividing it into an anterior component, which assists in the formation of the posterior third of the tongue, and a posterior component, which forms the epiglottis.

Thus, the adult tongue (Fig 18 *A*) consists of several parts. The anterior two thirds is of first

or mandibular arch origin, and so is supplied by the mandibular (lingual) branch of the tri- geminal nerve. The posterior third is derived in part from the hypobranchial eminence and in part from third arch mesoderm, and so re- ceives its sensory innervation from the supe- rior laryngeal nerve (supplying the hypobran- chial eminence anterior to the epiglottis) and from the glossopharyngeal nerve (third arch). Special sensation (taste) to the anterior two thirds of the tongue is mediated by the chorda tympani branch of the facial. This nerve was previously observed within the first arch as the pretrematic branch of the facial nerve (p. 116). Taste is carried to the posterior third through lingual branches of the glossopharyngeal and the internal branch of the superior laryngeal nerves.

The division between the anterior two thirds and posterior third of the adult tongue corre- sponds approximately with the V-shaped line of the circumvallate papillae (Fig. 18). The pala- tine tonsil, as has been described (p. 124), is formed by the aggregation of lymphoid tissue around the ventral wing of the second pouch (intratonsillar fossa). The site of the third pouch is probably high up in the floor of the pyriform sinus. The site of the fourth and sixth pouches is also unknown but may reasonably be expected to be in the lower part of the pyriform sinus caudal to the internal branch of the superior laryngeal nerve. The vallecula

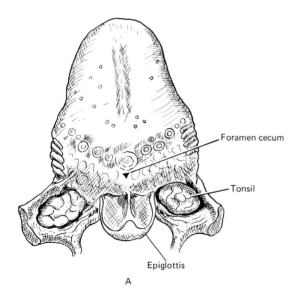

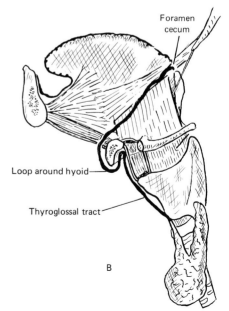

Figure 18.   The adult tongue (A) showing the foramen cecum which indicates the former site of origin of the thyro- glossal duct. In B the course of a persistent thyroglossal duct is shown.

corresponds to the groove between the anterior (lingual) and posterior (epiglottal) parts of the hypobranchial eminence, and so has no relationship to any pharyngeal pouch.

The anterior and posterior pillars of the fauces correspond approximately with the second and third internal arches, respectively, and the second pouch or intratonsillar fossa lies between them. The pharyngoepiglottic fold may correspond with the fourth arch. The aryepiglottic folds mark the site of evagination of the laryngotracheal diverticulum to be described in Chapter 6. Identification of these adult structures with the primitive arches has little validity, however, and serves little practical purpose.

Development of the Thyroid Gland; Thyroglossal Cysts

The thyroid gland develops as the earliest of the endocrine derivatives of the pharynx as a single midline evagination of the endoderm in the floor of the pharynx (Figs. 3 and 15 *A*). The site of the thyroid outgrowth later lies between the tuberculum impar and the hypobranchial eminence (Fig. 15 *A*). The thyroid diverticulum then grows caudally in a loose subpharyngeal plane of mesoderm and also proliferates at its tip into two lateral lobes (Fig. 15 *B*). The thyroid lobes come early into anterior relationship with the third arch artery as it emerges from the ventral aorta (Fig. 15 *A*) and so is related intimately in the adult to the internal carotid artery (Fig. 15 *B*). The connecting (thyroglossal) duct between the thyroid and the floor of the pharynx becomes attenuated and normally disappears. The pyramidal lobe indicates its former site of attachment to the thyroid gland.

Persistence of the thyroglossal duct may occur and may give rise to cystic masses at any point along its path, from the floor of the pharynx to the pyramidal lobe of the gland. When the tract persists throughout its length, its course is characteristic (Fig. 18 *B*). The tract ascends from the pyramidal lobe, which lies, as a rule, to the left of the midline. It necessarily passes anterior to the pharyngeal arch derivatives and so ascends anterior to the thyroid cartilage and the body of the hyoid bone. It then pierces the floor of the mouth between the two mylohyoid muscles and penetrates the base of the tongue, finally opening into the foramen cecum. The foramen cecum represents the site of origin of the original thyroid diverticulum and lies at the junction of the anterior two thirds and the posterior third of the tongue (Fig. 18 *A*).

The relationship of the thyroglossal tract to the body of the hyoid bone is important. Note that the attachment of the thyrohyoid membrane is to the upper and posterior rim of the body of the hyoid bone. The thyroglossal tract ascends on the anterior surface of the membrane, then curves caudally in intimate apposition to the posterior surface of the hyoid (Fig. 18 *B*). It then ascends once more anterior to the body of the hyoid bone, usually slightly to the left of the midline, and passes through the floor of the mouth. In removing the tract it is essential to eliminate it throughout its length from the foramen cecum to the pyramidal lobe. In order to remove completely the hyoid portion of the tract, it is usual to remove the middle segment of the body of the hyoid bone with bone shears. Failure to remove all the tract may result in recurrence. Unlike the lateral cysts of the neck, which are of cervical sinus origin (ectodermal), the thyroglossal or midline cysts of the neck move on swallowing since they are firmly attached to the thyroid cartilage and hyoid bone. Since they are of endodermal origin, they may give rise to adenocarcinoma.

RELEVANT CONCEPTUAL ANATOMY OF THE HEAD AND NECK

The anatomy of the adult head and neck is built around the pharynx and its associated branchial derivatives which together form a "median visceral column" attached above to the base of the skull. Flanking the pharyngeal arch field posteriorly and anteriorly is the V-shaped muscle mass, differentiated within the epipericardial ridge, containing the sternomastoid trapezius complex and the infrahyoid and suprahyoid muscles and the muscles of the tongue. Lateral to the median visceral column is a fascial space or compartment, the laterovisceral space, which contains the vascular structures and the components of the pharyngeal arch nerves. This space has important relationships and anatomical continuities with other potential spaces, which are of the greatest importance in determining the spread of infectious and neoplastic processes.

Anatomy of the Median Visceral Column

The pharynx is a musculomembranous tube supported by overlapping constrictor muscles of striped muscle and other muscles arising from the base of the skull and styloid process (Fig. 19).

The superior constrictor muscle of the pharynx arises by a continuous origin from the lower half of the medial pterygoid plate, the pterygoid hamulus, the pterygomandibular ligament, and the bone immediately adjacent to the attachment of the ligament to the mandible. Since the pterygomandibular ligament is oblique, extending from the pterygoid hamulus medially to the mandible laterally, those fibers of the superior constrictor taking origin from it are in the same oblique plane as the ligament (Fig. 20). Moreover, since the buccinator muscle arises from the anterior surface of the pterygomandibular ligament, this muscle and the superior constrictor must also be in the same plane. Thus, an anatomical structure which descends from the pterygoid region (infratemporal fossa) above the level of the pterygomandibular ligament is automatically carried into the soft tissues of the cheek, e.g., the

buccal branch of the mandibular nerve. Likewise, any infectious process related to the upper fibers of the superior constrictor muscle tends to pass into the cheek.

The superior constrictor muscle has an arching, free, lower border below the level of the pterygomandibular ligament (Fig. 19). Below this edge the fibers of the muscle sweep forward into the tongue in the vertical plane of the pharyngeal wall. A triangular gap between the pterygomandibular and lingual fibers of the superior constrictor muscle and the lingual constitute the "gateway" to the tongue (Fig. 20). Through this space pass the styloglossus muscle, the lingual artery, and lingual nerve, and the glossopharyngeal nerve.

The upper fibers of the superior constrictor also have a free border. The fibers arising from the medial pterygoid plate are often described as constituting a sphincteric mechanism at the junction of the naso- and oropharynx (nasopharyngeal or Passavant's sphincter). The arching upper fibers of the superior constrictor are at-

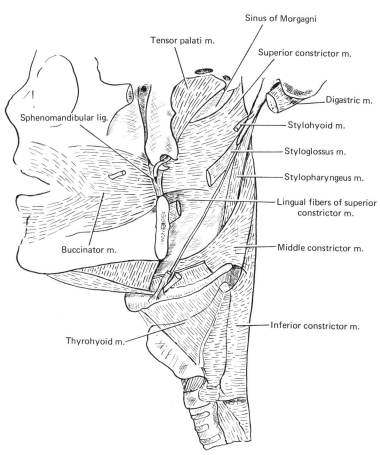

Figure 19.   Details of the constrictor muscles of the adult pharynx and of the muscles arising in relationship to the styloid process.

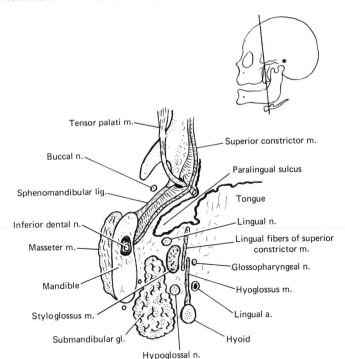

Figure 20. Coronal section through the adult mandible and adjacent parts of the face in the plane indicated in the small diagram. The tendon of the tensor palati is shown piercing the pharyngeal wall and curving around the pterygoid hamulus. The structures beneath the paralingual sulcus, in the "gateway" to the tongue, are also shown.

Tensor palati m.

Superior constrictor m.

Buccal n.

Paralingual sulcus

Sphenomandibular lig.

Tongue

Inferior dental n.

Lingual n.

Masseter m.

Lingual fibers of superior constrictor m.

Glossopharyngeal n.

Mandible

Hyoglossus m.

Styloglossus m.

Lingual a.

Submandibular gl.

Hyoid

Hypoglossal n.

tached to the midline pharyngeal tubercle (Fig. 21) of the basisphenoid.

The middle constrictor muscle of the pharynx arises from the lower part of the stylohyoid ligament, the lesser cornu of the hyoid bone, and from the entire length of the greater cornu of the hyoid bone (Fig. 19). The muscle also has free upper and lower borders. Posteriorly the muscle overlaps the superior constrictor and is also inserted by a pointed tendon into the pharyngeal tubercle.

The inferior constrictor muscle of the pharynx arises from the oblique line of the thyroid cartilage, from a fibrous arch over the cricothyroid muscle, and from the side of the cricoid cartilage. The muscle also has a free upper margin; its lower fibers merge with the circular fibers of the esophagus (Fig. 19).

There are nonmuscular areas in the muscular wall of the pharynx: (1) between the base of the skull and the upper fibers of the superior constrictor (sinus of Morgagni), (2) between the superior constrictor and the middle constrictor muscles, and (3) between the middle and inferior constrictor muscles. The first area (sinus of Morgagni) is occupied by a "eustachian complex" containing the pharyngotympanic tube, the tensor veli palatini (tensor palati) muscle and the levator palati muscle (Fig. 19). The second area contains the lingual fibers of the superior constrictor passing into the tongue, also the stylohyoid ligament, the lin-

gual artery and nerve, and the glossopharyngeal nerve. This area (Fig. 19) lies opposite the palatine tonsil so that the aforementioned structures form important lateral relationships of the tonsil. Here also the external maxillary (facial) artery may make a conspicuous high loop in immediate lateral relationship to the tonsil which it supplies. This vessel, as well as the internal carotid artery itself, may be injured during tonsillectomy. The third nonmuscular area between the middle and inferior constrictors lies close to the posterior margin of the thyrohyoid membrane (Fig. 19). Here it is crossed by the internal branch of the superior laryngeal nerve and is related deeply to the pyriform sinus. A less conspicuous nonmuscular area lies between the inferior constrictor and the upper circular fibers of the esophagus (Fig. 19) The latter are exposed at this point since the longitudinal fibers pass forward and insert by a pointed tendon into the back of the cricoid cartilage. This and, to a lesser extent, the second and third nonmuscular areas constitute zones of relative weakness in the pharyngeal wall through which pulsion diverticula may develop.

The Styloid Muscles

The styloid process and the stylohyoid ligament are parts of the second or hyoid arch cartilage. The stylohyoid is the proper muscle of this arch and is accordingly supplied by the facial nerve. The facial nerve turns laterally around the base of the styloid process and then passes forward to enter the parotid gland. The two other muscles attached to the styloid process, the styloglossus, supplied by the hypoglossal nerve, and the stylopharyngeus, supplied by the glossopharyngeal nerve, become secondarily attached to the bony process during the development of the pharyngeal region. These three muscles form part of the suspensory apparatus of the tongue, the hyoid bone, and the thyroid cartilage, and assist in swallowing.

The stylohyoid is the most superficial of the three styloid muscles. It arises by a slender tendon near the tip of the process and inserts onto the hyoid bone lateral to the lesser cornu. Here it splits to allow passage of the intermediate tendon of the digastric muscle; the tendon itself is anchored to the bone by a fascial sling containing a bursa. The styloglossus is intermediate in depth and arises from the anterior surface of the lower part of the styloid process and the upper part of the stylohyoid ligaments; it inserts into the side of the tongue after passing under the arching free margin of the pterygomandibular fibers of the superior constrictor (Figs. 19 and 20). The muscle pulls the tongue posteriorly during the first phase of swallowing. The stylopharyngeus is the deepest of the styloid muscles. It arises from the inner side of the base of the process, descends almost vertically, then passes deep to the upper fibers of the middle constrictor and is attached to the posterior margin of the thyroid cartilage. The glossopharyngeal nerve makes a characteristic turn around the muscle near its origin, passing to its lateral side. The muscle elevates the thyroid cartilage during the later phases of swallowing.

The "Eustachian Apparatus"

The pharyngotympanic (eustachian) tube is developmentally an outgrowth of the pharynx (see Chapter 4), and its cartilaginous component lies within the upper part of the pharyngeal wall. This part of the tube lies in the petrosphenoidal fissure (Fig. 21) and so is obliquely placed. The cartilaginous tube is continuous with the bony portion in the petrosphenoid angle and (at its pharyngeal end) rests on a small spine on the posterior margin of the medial pterygoid plate. The tensor veli palatini (tensor palati) muscle arises immediately lateral to the cartilaginous tube from the edge of

the greater wing of the sphenoid adjoining the petrosphenoidal fissure, and also from the lateral wall of the tube itself. The muscle is triangular and narrows into a slender tendon which winds around the lateral surface of the pterygoid hamulus, which serves as a pulley for it (Figs. 19 and 20). A bursa is found at this point. The tendon then pierces the pharyngeal wall and expands into the palatal aponeurosis within the soft palate. The aponeuroses of the two sides are fused in the midline so that simultaneous action of the two muscles tenses and flattens the soft palate during swallowing. The tensor palati also opens the cartilaginous portion of the tube during swallowing as a result of its attachment to the lateral surface of the tube. It is supplied by the mandibular division of the fifth nerve through small branches arising near the foramen ovale. The levator palati arises medial to the cartilaginous tube from the inferior surface of the apex of the petrous temporal bone (Fig. 21). It then descends almost vertically to be attached to the upper and posterior surface of the palatal aponeurosis. Its action is to raise the soft palate during swallowing. It is supplied by nerves of the pharyngeal plexus containing fibers of the cranial accessory (eleventh) nerve. The muscle also has some fibers of origin from the wall of the tube itself, and so assists in opening the tube.

The cartilaginous tube and its associated muscles form a functional group of structures conveniently grouped as the eustachian apparatus. Since they occupy the sinus of Morgagni between the upper fibers of the superior constrictor and the base of the skull (Figs. 19 and 22), they are an integral part of the wall of the pharynx in this area.

Composition of the Pharyngeal Wall

The composition of the pharyngeal wall in vertical section is shown schematically in Figure 22. From above down, it comprises the eustachian apparatus: the superior, the middle, and the inferior constrictor muscles. The lateral surface of the pharyngeal wall is covered by a thin layer of connective tissue, the buccopharyngeal fascia. This fascia is carried into the cheek by the common attachment of the fibers of the superior constrictor and of the buccinator to the pterygomandibular ligament. Below this level it fades out in the floor of the mouth in relation to the styloglossus and the side of the tongue. The internal surface of the constrictor muscles is lined by a strong elastic fas-

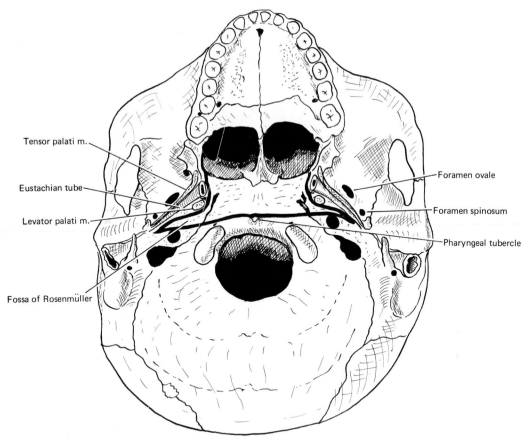

Tensor palati m.

Eustachian tube

Levator palati m.

Fossa of Rosenmüller

Foramen ovale

Foramen spinosum

Pharyngeal tubercle

Figure 21. Base of the skull with the attachment of the pharynx (heavy, black line) projected onto it. The pharyngeal attachment is rhomboidal, the lateral angles lying opposite the sphenoidal spine. The posterior attachment sweeps horizontally across the base of the skull anterior to the carotid canals and the foramen magnum, meeting in the midline at the pharyngeal tubercle.

cial layer, the pharyngobasilar fascia. It is attached above to the skull medial to the eustachian apparatus; below it merges with the muscularis mucosae of the esophagus. Internal to the pharyngobasilar fascia is the mucous membrane of the pharynx. Opposite the gaps between the constrictors and between the last of these and the esophagus, as described previously, the pharyngeal wall consists only of the buccopharyngeal and pharyngobasilar fasciae and the underlying mucous membrane.

The Lateropharyngeal and Laterovisceral Spaces

The medial visceral column of structures, comprising the pharynx above and the esophagus and trachea below, is related throughout its length to a laterovisceral space of great clinical importance. This space will be termed the "lateropharyngeal space" as low as the sixth cer-

vical vertebra where the pharynx joins the esophagus; below this level, it will be termed the "laterovisceral space."

THE LATEROPHARYNGEAL SPACE

The lateropharyngeal space is illustrated at three levels from above down in Figures 23 to 26. At the highest level (Fig. 23) the lateropharyngeal space is the same as the pterygoid region (infratemporal fossa, deep parotid space). The attachment of the pharynx to the base of the skull in the region of the eustachian apparatus is oblique, as a result of the obliquity of the petrosphenoidal fissure and the tube which lies in it. Thus, the attachment of the pharynx, when both sides are visualized (Fig. 21), is rhomboidal. The most lateral point of attachment on either side is the petrosphenoid angle, between the spine of the sphenoid and the petrous temporal bone. The obliquity of

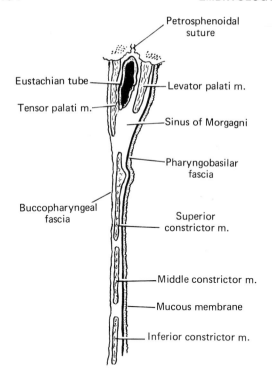

Petrosphenoidal suture

Eustachian tube

Levator palati m.

Tensor palati m.

Sinus of Morgagni

Pharyngobasilar fascia

Buccopharyngeal fascia

Superior constrictor m.

Middle constrictor m.

Mucous membrane

Inferior constrictor m.

Figure 22. Vertical section through the pharyngeal wall. The eustachian apparatus (tube, levator palati, tensor palati) occupies the sinus of Morgagni. The buccopharyngeal fascia invests the constrictors laterally and the pharyngobasilar fascia invests them internally.

this attachment results in the formation of the lateral recess of the pharynx or fossa of Rosenmüller (Fig. 23). It is possible to palpate the entire inner surface of the cartilaginous portion of the eustachian tube in the wall of the lateral recess. Advantage is taken of the recess to cannulate the tube. The tip of the cannula is introduced into the recess posterior to the pharyngeal opening of the tube and gradually drawn forward; the tip then slides into the tube without difficulty. The lateropharyngeal space at the level of the lateral recess lies anterolaterally because of the obliquity of the pharyngeal wall at this level (Fig. 23). Immediate contents of the space are the two pterygoid muscles (medial and lateral), the mandibular branch of the trigeminal nerve emerging from the foramen ovale, and the internal maxillary artery, especially its middle meningeal branch, which enters the skull through the foramen spinosum.

The auriculotemporal nerve arises from the mandibular nerve immediately below the skull and encircles the middle meningeal artery, splitting into two branches which reunite beyond the artery. The nerve then passes laterally posterior to and in close contact with the capsule of the temporomandibular joint. It then passes upward over the root of the zygoma and supplies the skin on the side of the head and the upper part of auricle. It sends branches into the capsule of the temporomandibular joint and also into the bony auditory meatus to supply its mucosal lining and the external surface of the tympanic membrane. The latter branches enter the meatus through the squamotympanic fissure with branches of the posterior auricular artery. The nerve is an important source of referred pain from the teeth to the joint and the external ear.

The otic ganglion lies medial to the mandibular branch of the trigeminal nerve, between it and the tensor palati and close to the foramen ovale. Here it receives the lesser superficial petrosal nerve (Fig. 23), a parasympathetic nerve arising from the glossopharyngeal nerve and conveying secretomotor fibers to the parotid gland (see p. 145) via the auriculotemporal nerve. The chorda tympani nerve, described previously as the pretrematic branch of the facial nerve, emerges from the middle ear through the petrotympanic fissure (Fig. 23), grooves the spine of the sphenoid (groove of Lucas) and then descends lateral to the tensor palati muscle deep to the mandibular division of the fifth nerve. It joins the lingual branch of this nerve and carries secretomotor fibers to the submandibular and sublingual glands and taste fibers from the anterior two thirds of the tongue (see p. 128). Deep infections of the lateropharyngeal space at this level may arise from the maxillary molars and are very chronic, deep-seated, and painful.

Other important anatomical relationships of the lateral recess of the pharynx are the great vessels (Fig. 23), the internal carotid artery, and the internal jugular vein. An aneurysm of the internal carotid artery at this point may bulge into the lateral recess of the pharynx and resemble a retropharyngeal or peritonsillar abscess. Pulsation of the swelling should be detected and may deter incision. The retropharyngeal space at this level lies between the constrictor muscle and its covering of buccopharyngeal fascia on the one hand and the atlas and axis vertebrae with their investing prevertebral muscles and prevertebral fascia on the other. This space, which contains no important structures except for lymph nodes, may also be the site of an abscess.

The lateropharyngeal space at a lower level (Fig. 24) shows important relationships to the parotid gland. For this reason it is referred to as the deep parotid space. Also evident at this

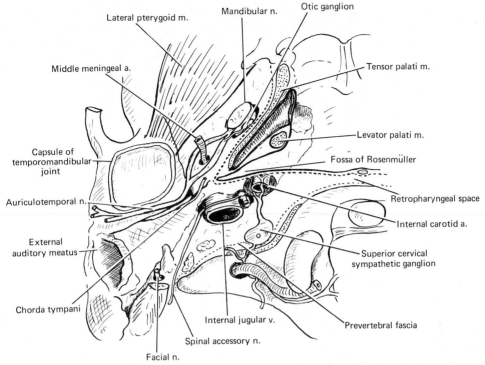

Lateral pterygoid m.

Mandibular n.

Otic ganglion

Middle meningeal a.

Tensor palati m.

Levator palati m.

Fossa of Rosenmüller

Capsule of
temporomandibular
joint

Retropharyngeal space

Auriculotemporal n.

Internal carotid a.

External
auditory meatus

Superior cervical
sympathetic ganglion

Chorda tympani

Internal jugular v.

Prevertebral fascia

Spinal accessory n.

Facial n.

Figure 23. Relationships of the upper attachment of the pharynx (interrupted lines) at the base of the skull. The contents of the infratemporal fossa (pterygoid region) lie anterolaterally. Posterior to the lateral angle (fossa of Rosenmüller) are the internal jugular vein, the internal carotid artery, and the ninth, tenth, and eleventh cranial nerves.

Figure 24. Transverse section through the parotid gland showing the superficial and deep parts of the gland and its connecting isthmus. The prestyloid and poststyloid compartments of the lateropharyngeal space with their contents are separated by a strong stylopharyngeal aponeurosis.

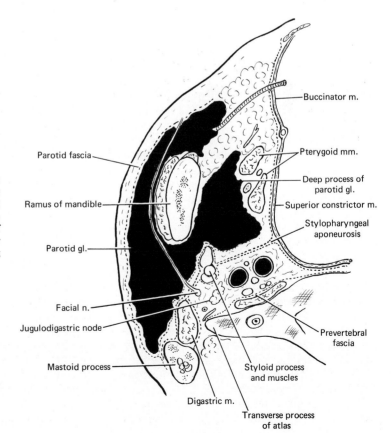

Parotid fascia

Buccinator m.

Pterygoid mm.

Deep process of
parotid gl.

Ramus of mandible

Superior constrictor m.

Stylopharyngeal
aponeurosis

Parotid gl.

Facial n.

Jugulodigastric node

Prevertebral
fascia

Mastoid process

Styloid process
and muscles

Digastric m.

Transverse process
of atlas

level is a strong aponeurotic sheet extending from the pharyngeal wall to the styloid process and its muscles (Fig. 24).

A similar but less dense fascial sheet extends from the styloid process and its muscles to the mastoid process and posterior belly of the digastric muscle. These two fascial sheets constitute a strong "styloid diaphragm," which effectively separates the parotid space anteriorly from the space enclosing the great vessels posteriorly. Anterior to the styloid diaphragm (prestyloid region) are the two pterygoid muscles and the deep (pterygoid) process of the parotid gland. The deep process of the gland is continuous with the superficial lobe through a narrow isthmus of glandular tissue between the ramus of the mandible and the sternomastoid muscle; it fills all the available space in the prestyloid region. It also has an anterior extension which fills the angle between the medial and lateral pterygoids, and a deep or pharyngeal extension which reaches to the pharyngeal wall. Extension of the parotid into the vascular or retrostyloid space is prevented by the styloid diaphragm. Similarly, malignant extension of the gland is prevented by the styloid diaphragm and rarely involves the retrostyloid space and the great vessels.

Contained within the retrostyloid space are the internal carotid artery, the internal jugular vein, the seventh, ninth, tenth, eleventh, and twelfth cranial nerves, and the superior sympathetic ganglion of the cervical chain. One of these in particular, the jugulodigastric gland, lies lateral to the internal jugular vein and between it and the posterior belly of the digastric and receives afferent lymphatics from the pharynx and tonsil. It may become infected and present as a painful swelling below the mastoid, causing a diagnostic problem. The transverse process of the atlas projects laterally and may be palpated in the narrow gap between the ramus of the mandible and the tip of the mastoid process. It is overlaid by the posterior belly of the digastric muscles and is also crossed by the occipital artery and the spinal accessory nerve. The nerve may be irritated or caught up in an inflammatory process involving the jugulodigastric lymph node and give rise to considerable pain. The facial nerve (Fig. 23) has only a brief course through the retrostyloid space after leaving the skull by the stylomastoid foramen. It pierces the lateral portion of the styloid diaphragm and enters the superficial lobe of the parotid gland.

The lateropharyngeal space at the level of the body of the mandible is shown schematically in Figure 25. The styloid diaphragm is still present. In addition, however, there is a strong band of fascia, a thickening of the deep cervical fascia, the stylomandibular "ligament," extending from the styloid process to the angle of the mandible. It separates the superficial lobe of the parotid gland from the submandibular gland. The lateropharyngeal space (Fig. 23) is continuous at this level with a fascial space occupied by the submandibular gland. The submandibular gland consists of two parts, a superficial and larger part, and a deep part. The two parts are continuous around the posterior free margin of the mylohyoid muscle (Fig. 25). The superficial part lies in the floor of the mouth inferior and lateral to the oral diaphragm (mylohyoid and anterior belly of the digastric). The deep part, from which Wharton's duct arises, lies in the forward extension of the lateropharyngeal space, which fades out anteriorly in relation to the side of the tongue. Here the gland lies lateral to the styloglossus and hypoglossus muscles and is related superiorly to the mucous membrane in the floor of the mouth (paralingual sulcus). The lingual fibers of the superior constrictor also enter the submandibular space and the buccopharyngeal fascia investing, then fade out in relation to the areolar tissue of the region (Fig. 25). The retrostyloid compartment at this level is limited anteriorly by the styloid diaphragm and contains the great vessels, the cranial nerves (9-12), the sympathetic chain, and the deep cervical lymph nodes. It is readily infected by lymphatics from the tonsil. The lateropharyngeal space becomes descriptively the laterovisceral space at the lower margin of the pharynx where it joins the esophagus. The styloid diaphragm disappears near the tip of the styloid process, merging anteriorly with the parotid fascia and the stylomandibular ligament, and inferiorly with the deep cervical fascia covering the anterior triangle of the neck.

LATEROVISCERAL SPACE

The laterovisceral space lies lateral to a median visceral column made up of the esophagus and trachea (Fig. 26).

Integral with it, but separated from it by an independent, thin, fascial sheath, is the thyroid gland. The parathyroid glands may lie within the fascial sheath of the thyroid gland, embedded in its substance, or outside the sheath. The superior parathyroid is usually more constant in position than the inferior parathyroid.

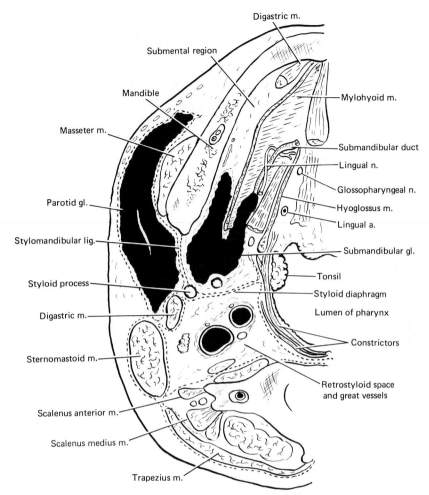

Figure 25. Transverse section of the neck at the level of the body of the mandible. The lower pole of the parotid glands is separated from the submandibular gland by the stylomandibular ligament. The lateropharyngeal space is divided, as at a higher level, into prestyloid and poststyloid compartments.

The infrahyoid, or "strap," muscles lie anterior to the median visceral column (Fig. 26). They are surrounded by a thin fascial sheath, independent of that enveloping the median visceral column, and continuous laterally with the fascia of the omohyoid and sternomastoid muscles. This fascia is part of the enveloping deep fascia of the neck and is continued posteriorly across the posterior triangle, enclosing the trapezius and finally reaching the cervical spinous processes.

A layer of fascia covering the prevertebral muscles is the prevertebral fascia (Fig. 26). Between it and the fascia of the median visceral column is a potential space of considerable importance, the retroesophageal space, continuous above with the retropharyngeal space (Fig. 26). The prevertebral fascia extends laterally across the scalenus anterior muscle which

arises from the anterior tubercles of the transverse processes of the cervical vertebrae. The prevertebral fascia passes laterally in relation to the scalenus anterior (scalene fascia) and forms the anterior wall of the axillary sheath. Here it meets with the deep cervical fascia covering the posterior triangle, forming a tubular fascial sheath around the trunks of the brachial plexus and, at a lower level, around the axillary artery and vein (Fig. 26).

The phrenic nerve, arising from the anterior rami of the third and fourth cervical nerves, lies deep to the scalene fascia on the anterior surface of the scalenus anterior, passing obliquely across the muscle from above down and from lateral to medial. It can be preserved intact in operations on the deep neck as long as this fascial layer is undamaged. The scalenus medius and the scalenus posterior muscles

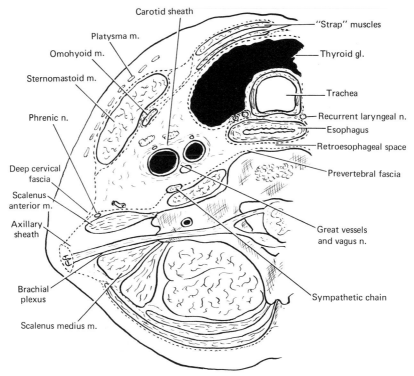

Figure 26. Transverse section through the laterovisceral space at the level of the thyroid gland. The poststyloid compartment, containing the great vessels, is continuous with the laterovisceral space at this level. Note the continuity of the prevertebral fascia with the scalene fascia. The latter, together with the fascia of the posterior triangle, constitutes the axillary sheath.

arise from the posterior tubercles of the cervical transverse process, and so lie posterior to the emerging roots of the brachial plexus (C5, 6, 7, 8 and T1).

The laterovisceral space in the neck lies in the more or less triangular region (as seen in cross-sections of the neck, Fig. 26), bounded medially by the median visceral column, anterolaterally by the sternomastoid and inferior belly of the omohyoid, and posteriorly by the prevertebral muscles and the scalenus anterior. It is traversed throughout its length from the thoracic inlet to the pharynx by the common carotid artery and the internal jugular vein. The loose areolar tissue within the laterovisceral space allows distension of these great vessels, as in extreme exertion. Added space is gained by the contraction of the omohyoid and its fascia. It is slightly condensed around the vessels forming the carotid sheath, which is exaggerated by formalin fixation and is much less real in life than in the dissecting room. Within the posterior wall of the sheath is the tenth cranial (vagus) nerve. In the anterior wall of the sheath is the ansa hypoglossi, a loop of nerve fibers made up of the descendens hypo-

glossi (containing fibers of C1) and the descendens cervicalis (containing fibers of C2 and 3). The ansa hypoglossi gives off branches to the infrahyoid muscles (sternohyoid, sternothyroid, omohyoid): its characteristic curving course reflects, as does that of the hypoglossal nerve, the development of the epipericardial ridge (p. 124) caudal to the arch field. There are also lymph nodes of the deep cervical chain within the areolar tissue of the laterovisceral space. They drain the floor of the mouth, the tonsillar area, the larynx and lower pharynx, as well as the median visceral column of structures below the level of the pharynx. The cervical sympathetic chain lies closely adherent to the prevertebral fascia in the posterior wall of the laterovisceral space (Fig. 26): it will be described in more detail later.

The extensions of the laterovisceral space and the retroesophageal space into the thorax are of great clinical importance (Fig. 26). The median visceral column is continued into the superior mediastinum and remains invested with a thin fascial sheath. The retroesophageal space also continues into the posterior mediastinum and comes to an end at the level of the diaphragm. Infections of this space, arising in the vertebral bodies or by lymphatic or direct extension from the pharynx, may thus extend into the posterior mediastinum throughout its length.

The laterovisceral space also continues into the upper thorax lateral to the median visceral column (Fig. 27). The space, filled with loose areolar tissue, here contains the roots of the great arteries arising from the arch of the aorta (left subclavian, left common carotid, innominate [brachiocephalic] arteries). The apex of the lung and its pleura occupy each side of the thoracic inlet and close off the laterovisceral space laterally. There are unimportant extensions into a retropleural space in relation to the neck of the first rib and also into the extrapleural space. The dome of the pleura is thickened superiorly by a tentlike extension of fascia stretching from the transverse process of the seventh cervical vertebra to the inner surface of the first rib (Sibson's fascia). Crossing the dome of the pleura at the thoracic inlet are the subclavian artery and vein. The sharp tendon of the scalenus anterior attached to the first rib

at the scalene (Lisfranc's) tubercle separates the two vessels. The artery may be partially occluded by the tendon, especially when the neck is rotated. There may also be pressure on the lower trunk and cords of the brachial plexus, giving pain or paresthesia along the dermatomes of C8 and T1. These findings (scalenus anterior syndrome) are relieved by tenotomy of the scalenus anterior. A differential diagnosis must be made between it and the effects of a cervical rib. Branches of the subclavian artery and vein also arch across the dome of the pleura: the internal thoracic (mammary) vessels anteriorly, and costocervical trunk posteriorly. The latter divides at the level of the neck of the first rib (Fig. 27) into the superior intercostal artery and the deep cervical artery. It lies with the inferior ganglion of the cervical sympathetic chain in a retropleural fossa. The first thoracic nerve is closely related to this fossa. It emerges between the first and second thoracic vertebrae, passes laterally, first inferior to the neck of the first rib, and then superior to the shaft of the first rib where it joins the eighth cervical nerve.

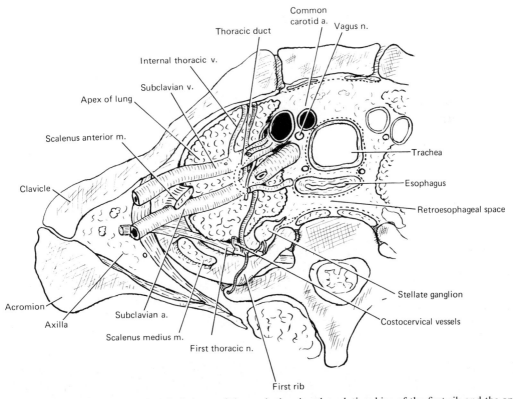

Figure 27. Transverse section through the root of the neck showing the relationships of the first rib and the apex of the lung. Note the stellate ganglion and branches of the costocervical trunk lying in a "retropleural fossa" opposite the neck of the first rib. The apex of the axilla is formed by the "cervicoaxillary canal" bounded by the first rib, the clavicle, and the upper border of the scapula.

The median visceral column of structures sinks deeper into the neck as it approaches the thoracic inlet. Thus, a space is opened up between it and the posterior surface of the manubrium sterni and the attachment of the infrahyoid ("strap") muscles to the sternum and first rib (Fig. 27). This pretracheal or retrosternal fascial space is occupied by loose areolar tissue and may permit infectious processes or tumors to expand widely before producing pressure symptoms on the trachea or great veins. In the fetus, the newborn, and the child up to about the age of puberty, the retrosternal space contains the upper part of the thymus gland, which may also produce pressure symptoms. The retrosternal space is entered during tracheostomy. In young children the thymus with large superior thymic veins may be encountered. A large artery to the thyroid, the arteria thyroidea ima, may also be encountered anterior to the trachea. The innominate (brachiocephalic) artery may also lie in the retrosternal space behind the right sternoclavicular joint and may be injured. Techniques have been developed in recent years for performing biopsies of the hilar lymph nodes or of masses in this area by passing a needle into the mediastinum through the retrosternal space.

GENERAL NEUROANATOMY OF THE HEAD AND NECK

The neuroanatomy of the head and neck of importance to otolaryngologists includes: (1) the nerve supply of the special sense organs (eye, ear, and nose), (2) the nerve supply of the extrinsic muscles of the eye (third, fourth, and sixth cranial), (3) the nerve supply of the pharyngeal or branchial arch derivatives (fifth, seventh, ninth, and superior and inferior laryngeal branches of the tenth), (4) the nerve supply of the supporting muscles of the head (trapezius, sternomastoid), the infrahyoid muscles, and the muscles of the tongue (eleventh, twelfth, upper cervical), and (5) the autonomic nerve supply of the smooth muscle and glandular tissue of the head and neck (sympathetic and parasympathetic).

Nerve Supply of the Special Sense Organs

The sense organs (eye, inner ear, and nose) are of ectodermal origin, as will be described in Chapter 3, where the detailed innervation of these structures, insofar as it concerns the otolaryngologist, will also be described.

NERVE SUPPLY OF THE EXTRINSIC OCULAR MUSCLE

These muscles are of somitic origin, that is, they are derived from condensations of mesoderm lateral to the neural tube. They are striated and so are innervated by motor axons growing out from the ventral (basal) part of the neural tube. The nerves involved are: the oculomotor or third nerve which supplies the superior rectus, the medial rectus, the inferior rectus, and the inferior oblique muscles; the trochlear or fourth nerve which supplies the superior oblique muscle; and the abducens or sixth nerve which supplies the lateral rectus. They are of importance in that they may be irritated or paralyzed by infections or neoplastic processes invading the orbit. Irritative lesions cause spasm of the muscles supplied by the nerves. Paralysis of the nerves permits the eye to be pulled by unopposed antagonistic muscles into abnormal positions (strabismus) with double vision or inability to direct the gaze. Paralysis of the oculomotor nerve in all its branches results in a squint in which the eye is pulled laterally by the lateral rectus and also downward by the superior oblique. There is also mydriasis (dilated pupil) due to the paralysis of the sphincter pupillae, loss of accommodation due to paralysis of the ciliary muscle, and drooping of the eyelid (ptosis) from paralysis of the levator palpebrae superioris muscle. Paralysis of the sixth nerve results in double vision when attempts are made to gaze laterally. Such a lesion may be accompanied by deep orbital pain arising from an infectious process at the apex of the petrous temporal bone (Gradenigo's syndome). Paralysis of the fourth nerve results in double vision when the gaze is directed downward and outward. These patients characteristically see double when going downstairs. Thrombosis of the cavernous sinus may also result in damage to these cranial nerves.

NERVE SUPPLY OF THE PHARYNGEAL OR BRANCHIAL DERIVATIVES

These have been studied in detail (p. 115 to 116) and will be reviewed only briefly. The first arch derivatives are supplied by the trigeminal (fifth) nerve. The nerve supplies the forehead and face, the side of the head, and the lateral surface of the auricle and drum, the mucosa of the oral cavity, the teeth, and the mucosa of the nasal cavity. Motor fibers are distributed by the mandibular division to the muscles of mastication (masseter, temporalis, pterygoids) and the muscles of the floor of the mouth (anterior belly of the digastric, mylohyoid). The tensor veli palatini and the tensor tympani are also supplied by this nerve (See Chapter 3.) The second arch derivatives are supplied by the facial or seventh nerve. It has no cutaneous supply. It supplies taste to the anterior two thirds of the tongue and to adjacent parts of the hard and soft palate. It distributes motor fibers to the stylohyoid, the posterior belly of the digastric, the platysma, the muscles of facial expression, and the stapedius muscle. Parasympathetic fibers are distributed to the lacrimal gland, the submandibular and sublingual glands, and to all the mucous and serous glands of the nose and palate (see later). The third arch derivatives are supplied by the glossopharyngeal or ninth nerve. The nerve has no cutaneous distribution. It supplies the posterior third of the tongue (taste and ordinary sensation), the adjoining vallecula, epiglottis and tonsillar area, and the nasopharynx in the region of the eustachian tube and the fossa of Rosenmüller. It also takes part in the pharyngeal plexus on the surface of the middle constrictor, and may share in the supply of this muscle and of the superior constrictor. The only muscle definitely known to be supplied by the glossopharyngeal nerve is the stylopharyngeus, which is involved in swallowing. The derivatives of the fourth arch are supplied by the superior laryngeal branch of the vagus nerve. It supplies by its internal branch the mucous membrane of the larynx above the level of the vocal cords and the adjoining areas of the pharynx, including the pyriform sinus and epiglottis. It supplies by its external branch the cricothyroid muscle, which is a tensor of the vocal cords. The sixth arch derivatives are supplied by the inferior or recurrent laryngeal branch of the vagus nerve. It supplies the intrinsic muscles of the larynx and the mucous membrane of the larynx below the vocal cords, also the mucosa of the cervical and upper thoracic portion of the trachea and esophagus.

**NERVE SUPPLY OF THE DERIVATIVES
OF THE EPIPERICARDIAL RIDGE**

There are only ten cranial nerves in vertebrates below the birds and reptiles. In higher vertebrates there are twelve, the additional nerves being the eleventh or accessory and the twelfth or hypoglossal nerves. These nerves are supposed to have been incorporated into the skull during evolution and represent upper cervical spinal nerves. These nerves enter the pharyngeal region within a V-shaped mesodermal bed or epipericardial ridge caudal to the arch area (p. 124). The sternomastoid, the trapezius, the infrahyoid, and the intrinsic muscles of the tongue are differentiated within this mesodermal mass. The nerves supplying these muscles are the accessory, the hypoglossal, and the upper three spinal nerves. The accessory nerve has a cranial and a spinal component. The cranial component is really a part of the vagus and is often included with it as the "vago-accessory complex." Its precise distribution is uncertain. It is considered to be responsible for the supply of the branchial musculature developed within the fourth and sixth arches, and so properly belongs with the branchial group of cranial nerves. It is distributed to the lower constrictor fibers of the pharynx, the extrinsic and intrinsic muscles of the pharynx, and the striated fibers of the upper and middle esophagus. The nerve may also be distributed to the lungs and great vessels, including the heart, these fibers being both sensory and motor.

The spinal accessory nerve arises from the lateral cells of the anterior gray matter in the upper four or five segments of the cervical spinal cord. It ascends immediately anterior to the denticulate ligament of the spinal cord within the subarachnoid space and enters the foramen magnum. It leaves the skull with the vagus and cranial root of the accessory, with which it is fused, through the jugular foramen and then parts company with the cranial root. It then passes laterally either to the outside (Fig. 23) or the inside of the internal jugular vein, crosses laterally to the transverse process of the atlas vertebra deep to the posterior belly of the digastric, and enters the sternomastoid muscle just below the mastoid process. It supplies this muscle and then crosses the posterior triangle, where it is rather superficially situated within the deep cervical fascia. It is readily injured in this part of its course, especially when caught up in the inflammatory processes involving the deep cervical lymph nodes at this level. The nerve enters the trapezius about halfway down its anterior border and is reinforced by branches of the third and fourth cervical nerves, which form with it a "subtrapezial plexus."

The hypoglossal nerve enters the tongue immediately above the greater cornu of the hyoid bone (Fig. 16), deep to the mylohyoid and superficial to the hyoglossus. It supplies the intrinsic muscles of the tongue and also the styloglossus. The hypoglossal nerve carries fibers of the first cervical nerve which leave it near the tip of the greater cornu of the hyoid bone as the nerve to the thyrohyoid. Other fibers of the first cervical nerve leave the hypoglossal as the descendens hypoglossi; this joins the descendens cervicalis, which contains fibers of the second and third cervical nerves, to form a loop on the anterior wall of the carotid sheath (ansa hypoglossi). From this loop motor fibers are distributed to the two bellies of the omohyoid, the sternohyoid, and the sternothyroid.

Autonomic Nervous System of the Head and Neck

General Principles. The autonomic nervous system of the body is subdivided into two components: the thoracolumbar outflow comprising the sympathetic nerves, and the craniosacral outflow comprising the parasympathetic nerves. These nerves are concerned with the supply of smooth muscle and glandular tissue and are grouped together as general visceral efferent fibers (see Fig. 31).

SYMPATHETIC

The thoracolumbar outflow arises in the intermediolateral column of small neurons within the spinal cord from the first thoracic to the second lumbar levels (Figs. 28 and 29).

A typical cross-section of a spinal cord segment (Fig. 28) illustrates the arrangement of the sympathetic outflow. Axons arise in the intermediolateral column, leave the spinal cord by the ventral (motor) root, and enter the spinal nerve. They leave the spinal nerve as a white ramus communicans, so-called since it has a well developed myelin sheath. Such a nerve fiber is preganglionic since it has not yet had a synapse. It enters one of the sympathetic ganglia lying ventrolateral to the vertebral column (paravertebral ganglia) and may take one of the following courses: (1) It may have an immediate synapse with a second order neuron within the ganglion and then return to the spinal nerve as a gray ramus communicans, so-called because it lacks a well developed myelin sheath. The gray ramus communicans is distributed with the spinal nerve to the blood vessels (vasomotor fibers), sweat glands (sudomo-

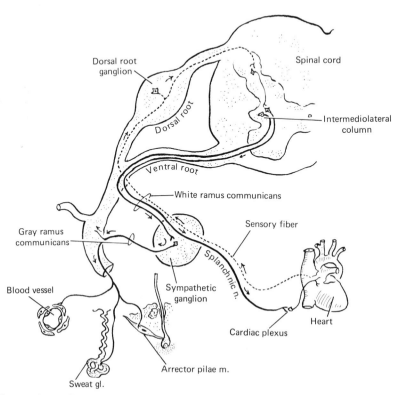

Figure 28. Scheme of a typical spinal nerve and cord segment. The sympathetic components, both sensory and motor, are shown in relation to the nerve roots and their peripheral distribution.

tor fibers), and the pilo-erector muscles (pilo-motor fibers). (2) It may ascend or descend in the sympathetic chain and have a synapse at any level with a second order neuron within a ganglion distant from its level of exit from the spinal cord. It may then leave the ganglion as a gray ramus communicans to enter a spinal nerve and be distributed as in (1). (3) The white ramus communicans may pass through a ganglion at any level without synapse and continue as an elongated splanchnic nerve to a distant collection of second order neurons within one or another of the visceral cavities, e.g., the cardiac and pulmonary plexuses in the thorax, the celiac and superior mesenteric plexuses in the abdomen, or the pelvic plexuses. Postganglionic fibers arise here and are distributed to the smooth muscle and glandular tissue of the viscera and to that of the blood vessels. (4) Second order neurons in the sympathetic ganglia may also pass directly into the visceral cavities to supply the viscera. Fibers which have not had a synapse, e.g., splanchnic nerves, are called preganglionic. Those which have had a synapse, e.g., gray rami communicantes, are called postganglionic.

The chemical mediator release at the synaptic terminal of preganglionic sympathetic fiber is acetylcholine, and such fibers are termed cholinergic. The chemical mediator of postganglionic fibers to smooth muscle and pilo-erector muscles is adrenaline or noradrenaline, and such fibers are called adrenergic fibers. The postganglionic fibers to the sweat gland are cholinergic. Cholinergic fibers are blocked at the synapse by atropine and anticholinergic drugs such as methantheline bromide (Banthine), propantheline bromide (Pro-Banthine) and methscopolamine bromide (Pamine). They are stimulated by cholinergic drugs such as acetylcholine and pilocarpine. The drug physostigmine (Eserine) mimics the action of acetylcholine by inhibiting the enzyme cholinesterase that normally hydrolyzes acetylcholine at the synapse. Pilocarpine is used to promote sweating. Postganglionic sympathetic fibers to the viscera are adrenergic, but the response of the smooth muscle depends on the type of receptors. Thus, sympathetic stimulation of the bronchial and coronary musculature causes dilation; stimulation of the smooth muscle of the vessels usually causes constriction. Postganglionic adrenergic fibers may be blocked by drugs such as Dibenamine. They are stimulated or mimicked by adrenaline or noradrenaline.

The spatial limits of the sympathetic preganglion outflow (thoracolumbar outflow) are determined by the location of the cells of the intermediolateral column, which is found only between the first thoracic and the second lumbar levels of the spinal cord (Fig. 29). Thus, white rami communicantes are found only between T1 and L2, whereas gray rami communicantes are found at all levels (see (2)).

Afferent or sensory fibers also enter the spinal cord with the sympathetic system (Fig. 28). Sensory fibers arising in the viscera or great vessels ascend to the sympathetic ganglia along the splanchnic nerves. They enter the dorsal root (Fig. 28) with somatic sensory fibers, and their cell bodies lie within the dorsal root ganglion. Central processes of the cell body enter the cord and gray matter where they set up simple reflex arcs with motor neurons of the intermediolateral column (Fig. 28). Pain fibers from the heart, for example, ascend to the sympathetic chain of the neck via the cervical and upper thoracic splanchnic nerves. The pain is often referred to the somatic nerves arising from the cord at the same level as the incoming sympathetic fibers, in this case the cervical and upper thoracic nerves. The pain may accordingly be felt in the angle of the jaw (great auricular nerve), the shoulder, and along the inner side of the arm, forearm, and hand (dermatomes of C8 and T1).

The manner in which the head and neck are supplied by sympathetic nerves is illustrated in Figure 29. The cells of origin lie in the intermediolateral column of the upper two or three thoracic segments of the cord. Preganglionic fibers leave the cord via the ventral roots of the upper thoracic nerves. They then ascend within the upper thoracic and cervical chain and enter into synapse with second order neurons at any level up to the superior cervical ganglion at the base of the skull; this is the highest point at which a synapse takes place. Postganglionic fibers then leave the cervical chain: (1) gray rami communicantes which join the nerves of the cervical plexus and are distributed to the blood vessels, sweat glands, and pilo-erector muscles of the neck and face; (2) reinforcing twigs to plexuses on the walls of the branches of the external carotid and vertebral arteries; and (3) the carotid plexus on the wall of the internal carotid artery. The plexuses on the vertebral and carotid arteries are distributed with their terminal branches to the face, the skull, and the contents of the cranial cavity, including the brain.

The postganglionic fibers along the internal carotid artery (carotid plexus) are of particular

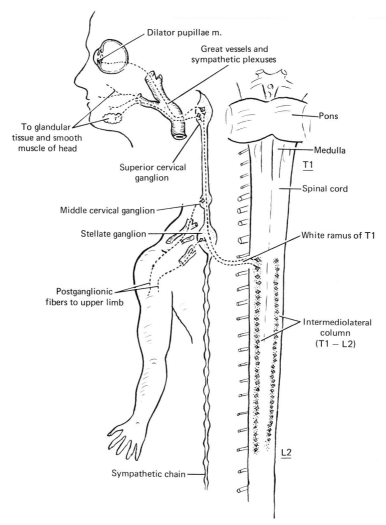

Figure 29. Scheme of the sympathetic innervation of the upper extremity and head and neck. The highest level at which neurons of the sympathetic (thoracolumbar) outflow extend is T1.

importance. They enter the skull with the artery and are distributed with the anterior and middle cerebral arteries and the ophthalmic artery. The ophthalmic plexus carries fibers (postganglionic) to the dilator pupillae, the smooth muscle in the floor of the orbit (Horner's muscle), the smooth muscle in the upper eyelid, and the blood vessels of the orbit and eye. Paralysis of the postganglionic fibers along the ophthalmic artery results in pupil constriction (miosis), drooping of the upper eyelid, and enophthalmos, in which the eye is sunken into the orbit. These ocular findings are part of Horner's syndrome (see later). Postganglionic fibers of the carotid plexus are also distributed to the sphenopalatine ganglion via the deep petrosal nerve and are distributed to the lacrimal and nasopalatine glands and to the blood vessels of the nose and palate (Chapter 2).

There are three cervical sympathetic ganglia: inferior, middle, and superior. The inferior ganglion is often fused with the first thoracic ganglion, forming the stellate ganglion (Fig. 27). It lies on the neck of the first rib in a retropleural fossa where it is closely related to the first thoracic nerve, the superior intercostal artery and vein, and the dome of the pleura. It is connected to the first thoracic nerve by white and gray rami communicantes, and to the eighth cervical nerve by gray rami; some variation is observed, however. It is important to note that the inferior cervical sympathetic ganglion (or the stellate ganglion) is the highest point at which preganglionic fibers enter the cervical chain, since the intermediolateral column of cells does not lie above T1 (occasionally as high as C8). Removal of this ganglion, therefore, interrupts completely the entire preganglionic supply of sympathetic fibers to the head and neck. Horner's syndrome results from interruption of this preganglionic outflow. It consists of: loss of sweating, vasodilation of the affected side, and ocular signs as described previously (pupillo constriction, enophthalmos, ptosis). Pain in the cervical region may also be encountered. The syndrome may result from surgical interference or from pressure of a tumor at the level of the neck of the first rib (superior sulcus [Pancoast] tumor). It may be avoided in a thoracic sympathectomy by careful separation of the stellate ganglion into an upper (inferior cervical) component and a lower (first thoracic) component, the upper part being left intact. The paralysis of the sudomotor fibers may be demonstrated by painting the skin with starch and iodine powder and then injecting the sudorific drug pilocarpine; areas of skin which sweat normally turn blue.

The sympathetic (postganglionic) nerve supply of the upper extremity enters the limb via the middle cervical and stellate ganglia and the gray rami connecting these with the brachial plexus (Fig. 29). Thus, the sympathetic nerve supply to the upper limb may be cut by removing the middle and inferior cervical ganglia and the intervening chain. In practice it is necessary to remove also the upper thoracic chain ganglia, owing to variations in the sympathetic outflow. In this operation the second order neurons are removed, so that the operation is a "postganglionic sympathectomy." Under these circumstances the loss of the trophic unit comprising the second order neuron and the effector organ (sweat gland or smooth muscle of a blood vessel) becomes hypersensitive to adrenaline (Loewi's effect). The results of the operation are accordingly apt to be disappointing since the patient's limb vessels go into spasm during emotional stress. Removal of the lumbar sympathetic chain for peripheral vascular disease of the lower extremity does not remove at the same time the second order neurons of the pelvic sympathetic chain. The operation is thus a "postganglionic sympathectomy," and sensitization of the leg vessels to adrenaline does not occur.

Details of the sympathetic innervation of the nose, pharynx, ear, and larynx will be given in Chapter 3 in connection with the description of these areas.

PARASYMPATHETIC

The parasympathetic system of the body, unlike the sympathetic system, is subdivided into two outflow components: the cranial and the sacral. The cranial outflow arises in nuclei within the brain stem (Fig. 30) and emerges through the third (oculomotor), the seventh (facial), the ninth (glossopharyngeal), and the tenth (vagus) nerves. The sacral outflow emerges from the lateral gray matter of the spinal cord at the level of the third and fourth sacral nerves; it forms the so-called nervi erigentes, which supply the pelvic viscera, the distal colon, and the external genitalia. The cranial outflow supplies the head and neck as well as the derivatives of the foregut and midgut: pharynx, larynx, esophagus, lungs, stomach, small intestine, liver, pancreas, and intrinsic glands of the gut, and the colon as far distally as the splenic flexure where the superior and inferior mesenteric arterial territories overlap. The sacral outflow supplies the hindgut and cloacal derivatives (descending colon, sigmoid and rectum, pelvic viscera, and external genitalia).

The cranial outflow only will be considered here. (See Chapter 3 for details.) The outflow of the third (oculomotor) nerve arises in the neurons of the Edinger-Westphal nucleus, a collection of small cells associated with the motor nucleus of the third nerve in the midbrain at the level of the superior colliculus. The preganglionic fibers leave the inferior branch of the oculomotor nerve within the orbit and enter the ciliary ganglion, a small collection of second order parasympathetic neurons lateral to the optic nerve (Fig. 30). Here the fibers synapse, and postganglionic fibers are distributed to the eye through the long and short ciliary nerves. They supply the sphincter pupillae and the ciliary muscle. Paralysis of the third nerve, in addition to the loss of function of the levator palpebrae superioris and the extrinsic muscles of the eye (except the superior oblique and the lateral rectus), results in a dilated pupil (mydriasis) and loss of accommodation. Since both preganglionic and postganglionic synapses of the parasympathetic system are cholinergic, they are stimulated by cholinergic drugs (acetylcholine, physostigmine, pilocarpine) and blocked by anticholinergic drugs (atropine, Banthine, Pamine). Atropine-like compounds are used to dilate the pupils. Since they also paralyze the ciliary muscle, they are likely to impede the removal of aqueous humor at the iris-mesh angle and so may precipitate glaucoma in a susceptible patient.

The parasympathetic outflow through the facial or seventh nerve arises in the hypothetical

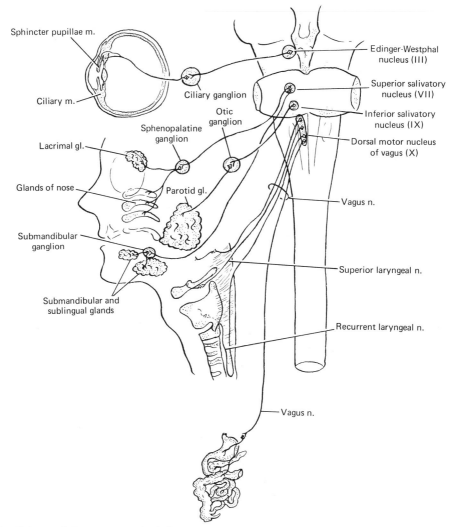

Figure 30. Scheme of the parasympathetic innervation of the head and neck. Central nuclei of the visceral efferent column are indicated in the brain stem.

"superior salivatory nucleus," supposed to lie in the midpons. Preganglionic fibers leave the brain in the pars intermedia (nerve of Wrisberg) between the motor branch of the facial and eighth nerve in the cerebellopontine angle. The pars intermedia is both motor and sensory. It contains preganglionic parasympathetic (secretomotor) fibers as well as taste fibers from the anterior two thirds of the tongue. It may be involved with the facial and the eighth nerve in cerebellopontine angle tumors, usually acoustic neuromas. The preganglionic fibers of the pars intermedia enter the internal auditory meatus with the facial and eighth nerves and fuse with the facial nerve proximal to the geniculate ganglion. They leave the facial nerve at the level of the ganglion as the greater superfi-

cial petrosal nerve which supplies preganglionic fibers to the sphenopalatine ganglion. (See Chapter 3.) Postganglionic fibers leave the sphenopalatine ganglion and are distributed to the lacrimal gland and the serous and mucous glands of the nose, paranasal sinuses, palate, and nasopharynx. Preganglionic fibers also leave the facial nerve as the chorda tympani about 5 mm. above the stylomastoid foramen. (See Chapter 3.) They cross the inner surface of the tympanic membrane, emerge from the skull through the petrotympanic fissure (Fig. 23), descend through the infratemporal fossa lateral to the tensor veli palatini, and join the lingual branch of the mandibular division of the trigeminal nerve. They are distributed through the lingual nerve to the submandibular ganglion where the second order neurons lie and the postganglionic fibers to the submandibular and sublingual glands arise. Sensory fibers (taste) from the anterior two thirds of the tongue are also distributed through the chorda tympani and enter the brain stem through the pars intermedia.

The parasympathetic outflow of the ninth or glossopharyngeal nerve arises in neurons of a hypothetical "inferior salivatory nucleus" within the pons. They leave the skull with the glossopharyngeal nerve. Immediately below the jugular foramen these fibers leave the glossopharyngeal nerve as the tympanic branch (Jacobson's nerve). It pierces the floor of the middle ear through a small foramen in the bony ridge between the carotid canal and the jugular foramen and forms a plexus on the promontory of the middle ear (Chapter 3). It then leaves the middle ear as the lesser superficial petrosal nerve, which emerges from the anterior surface of the petrous temporal bone in the middle cranial fossa and leaves the skull either through the foramen ovale or through a small accessory foramen (foramen Vesalius). It enters the otic ganglion (Fig. 23), which lies on the tensor veli palatini muscle, between it and the mandibular branch of the trigeminal nerve. Postganglionic fibers arise from the second order neurons of the otic ganglion and are distributed to the auriculotemporal nerve by which they are carried to the parotid gland.

The parasympathetic outflow of the vagus and of the cranial root of the accessory nerves (vago-accessory complex) arises in the dorsal motor nucleus of the vagus in the floor of the fourth ventricle at the level of the medulla. They are distributed to the wall of the pharynx and larynx as well as to the derivatives of the foregut and midgut distal to these. The second order neurons, unlike those of the sympathetic, lie in the walls of the structures supplied (Fig. 30), e.g., the submucosal and myenteric plexuses of the gut. Postganglionic fibers are supplied from these "mural ganglia" to glandular tissue and smooth muscle. Stimulation of the cholinergic fibers of the vago-accessory complex by acetylcholine, physostigmine, and pilocarpine produces hypermotility of the visceral muscle and promotes a secretion rich in water and enzymes. Blockade of the system by atropine or drugs such as Banthine causes reduction of motility as well as reduction in secretion, especially of hydrochloric acid by the oxyntic cells of the stomach. Dryness of the mouth (xerostoma) is also an unpleasant side effect.

Central Connections of the Cranial Nerves

Though the cranial nerves, with some exceptions (e.g., olfactory, optic, acoustic, oculomotor, and trochlear), are mixed, having sensory, motor and, often, autonomic components, the central connections of the nerves within the brain are much simpler (Fig. 31). The fibers are regrouped within the brain in relation to function and without regard to the complex composition of the individual cranial nerves. Six major nuclear columns (collections of neurons) are recognized in the brain stem. Three of these (1 to 3) lie in the upper half (alar plate) of the neural tube, which is sensory in function; three of them (4 to 6) are in the lower half of the neural tube (basal plate), which is motor in function. The primary cell bodies of the incoming fibers to the sensory columns are outside the brain or spinal cord in the sensory ganglia of the cranial nerves, e.g., the trigeminal ganglion, the geniculate ganglion, the superior and inferior ganglia of the ninth and tenth nerves, or the dorsal root ganglia of the spinal nerves. The cell columns related to these incoming sensory fibers are, therefore, second order neurons and send their axons to other parts of the brain stem or to the cortex. The first three sensory columns in sequence from dorsal areas to ventral are as follows (Fig. 31):

Special Somatic Afferent Column. This column is associated with the special sense organs (nose, eye, ear) which are of ectodermal origin and so are "somatic" in origin. (See Chapter 3.) The olfactory neurons of the second order within the olfactory bulb, though situated in the cerebral hemisphere, must be considered to belong to this group. The lateral geniculate bodies, containing late order neurons of the primary visual pathway, represent the special somatic afferent nucleus of the optic nerve. The medial geniculate bodies likewise represent the tertiary end-station of the auditory pathway. The vestibular and cochlear nuclei in the pons represent the second order neurons of the auditory and vestibular pathways. They are also representative of the special somatic afferent column.

General Somatic Afferent Column. This column lies ventral to the special somatic afferent column and contains sensory fibers mediating sensations of pain, temperature, touch, vibration, and proprioception from the skin, joints, and tendons. It receives incoming cutaneous fibers of the trigeminal (fifth) nerve from the face and from the muscles of mastication and the temporomandibular joint. The main sen-

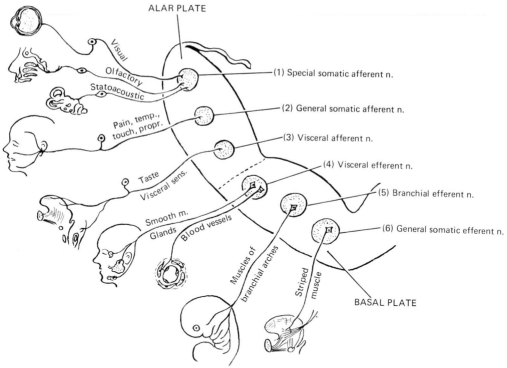

ALAR PLATE

(1) Special somatic afferent n.

(2) General somatic afferent n.

(3) Visceral afferent n.

(4) Visceral efferent n.

(5) Branchial efferent n.

(6) General somatic efferent n.

BASAL PLATE

Figure 31.   Scheme of the principal nuclear groups of the brain stem. Sensory neurons lie in the "alar plate" dorsal to the sulcus limitans (dotted line) and motor nuclei in the "basal plate."

sory nucleus of the fifth nerve (midpons) is believed to receive mostly tactile impulses. The long nucleus of the spinal tract of the fifth nerve, which extends from the midpontine level to the upper cervical region of the cord, is believed to receive predominantly pain stimuli. The ophthalmic, maxillary, and mandibular areas of the trigeminal territory are represented upside down in the spinal tract and nucleus (i.e., the forehead at the bottom, the jaw at the top). Proprioceptive impulses from the muscles of mastication are believed to enter the mesencephalic nucleus of the trigeminal nerve which lies lateral to the lower part of the midbrain aqueduct. This nucleus is unique in that the primary sensory neurons lie within the neural tube and not outside as do other primary sensory neurons. Also included in this column is the posterior horn of the gray matter, in which first order sensory neurons mediating pain, temperature, touch, and some proprioception have their synapse.

Visceral Afferent Column.   This column lies dorsal to the sulcus limitans, delimiting the basal from the alar plate (Fig. 30). It receives sensory impulses from the foregut and midgut derivatives, mainly taste sensation (conscious or unconscious) from the viscera. It also re-

ceives afferent stimuli from the walls of the great vessels (for example, the carotid sinus via Hering's nerve) which enter into important vascular reflexes affecting blood pressure and cardiac output. Sensory impulses from the viscera, not necessarily at the conscious level, entering the visceral afferent column, mediate important visceral reflexes such as coughing, swallowing, and vomiting. The nucleus of the tractus solitarius which lies in the medulla oblongata medial to the spinal tract and nucleus of the spinal tract of the trigeminal nerve forms the visceral afferent column and receives afferent fibers of the facial nerve (e.g., tympani, chorda tympani, greater superficial petrosal nerve), of the glossopharyngeal nerve (from carotid sinus, tongue, and pharynx), and of the vago-accessory complex (from larynx, pharynx, great vessels of thorax, esophagus, stomach, and small and large intestine as far distally as the splenic flexure). The nucleus is linked by a poorly defined "solitariospinal" tract with the spinal cord and mediates reflexes involving the diaphragm (phrenic C3 and 4) and the intercostal and abdominal muscles. Thus, in swallowing, the reflex is initiated by the contact of food with the posterior wall of the pharynx (ninth nerve); in sneezing, the afferent side of the reflex is the maxillary branch of the trigeminal nerve; in coughing, the afferent impulses reach the solitary tract and its nucleus through the vagus or cranial accessory nerve; and in vomiting, the afferent side of the reflex passes from the mucous membrane of the stomach to the solitary tract and nucleus through the vagus nerve. The efferent or motor side of these reflexes is mediated by connections between the solitary tract and the motor neurons of the medulla (respiration, etc.) and the spinal cord (diaphragm, intercostal and abdominal muscles).

Visceral Efferent Column. This group of cells, located ventral to the sulcus limitans (Fig. 30), is the site or origin of the preganglionic fibers of the parasympathetic cranial outflow (see p. 145). The neurons of this column supply smooth muscle and glandular tissue through the facial, the glossopharyngeal and the vago-accessory complex. The nuclei of this column are the "superior salivatory nucleus" (high pons), the "inferior salivatory nucleus" (midpons), and the motor nucleus of the vagus (medulla and floor of fourth ventricle). This column is connected by short, connecting or internuncial neurons with the visceral afferent column (previously discussed) and is concerned in reflexes such as coughing and vomiting. Reflex contraction of smooth muscle, salivation, and gastric hypersecretion, for example, are parts of the vomiting reflex.

Branchial Efferent (Special Visceral Efferent) Column. This column comprises those nuclei concerned in the innervation of the musculature of the pharyngeal or branchial arches. It is, therefore, uniquely based on the embryological origin of these muscles (see p. 115 to 116). The nuclei from above down are the motor nucleus of the trigeminal nerve (high pons), the motor nucleus of the facial nerve (midpons), and the nucleus ambiguus (low pons and medulla). The motor nucleus of the trigeminal nerve supplies motor fibers to the muscles of the first arch (the muscles of mastication—tensor veli palatini, tensor tympani, mylohyoid, anterior belly of the digastric). The motor nucleus of the facial nerve supplies fibers to the muscles of the second arch (stapedius, platysma, stylohyoid and posterior belly of the

digastric—the muscles of facial expression). The nucleus ambiguus supplies motor fibers to the muscles of the third, fourth, and sixth arches through the glossopharyngeal, superior laryngeal, and recurrent laryngeal branches of the vagus, respectively. Thus it supplies constrictors of the pharynx, the stylopharyngeus, the levator veli palatini, the intrinsic and extrinsic muscles of the larynx, and the striped musculature of the upper esophagus. The branchial efferent column is thus involved in swallowing and phonation. The nucleus ambiguus may be damaged by bulbar poliomyelitis or ascending paralysis of the brain stem, in which case the soft palate and the constrictor mechanism of the pharynx may fail. An ominous sign is regurgitation of fluid down the nose, indicating failure of the palatopharyngeal reflex. Phonation may also be defective following strokes which interrupt the corticobulbar fibers from the motor cortex to the nucleus ambiguus.

General Somatic Efferent Column. This column, which is the most ventral of the six columns, is made up of large neurons of motor type with prominent Nissl substance. The neurons supply fibers to the striated muscle of the head and neck that is derived from the somites (see p. 115 to 116). These include the extrinsic muscles of the eye, the muscles of the epipericardial ridge (sternomastoid, trapezius, and infrahyoid), and the intrinsic muscles of the tongue and the styloglossus. The cranial nerves and nuclei of this column are: the nucleus of the oculomotor nerve (superior colliculus of midbrain), the trochlear nerve (inferior colliculus of midbrain), the hypoglossal nucleus (low medulla), and the lateral group of anterior horn cells of the upper five cervical segments of the spinal cord, which give rise to the spinal root of the accessory nerve. The general somatic efferent column also receives "upper motor neuron fibers" from the motor cortex of the opposite side and so is involved in strokes and injuries to the brain stem. Paralysis of the ocular muscles may occur (see p. 140). Paralysis of the muscles of the tongue and the styloglossus causes the protruded tongue to deviate to the affected side. Paralysis of the sternomastoid and trapezius is easily recognized.

Chapter 3

EMBRYOLOGY AND ANATOMY OF THE FACE, PALATE, NOSE AND PARANASAL SINUSES

by Jack Davies, M.D.

BASIC EMBRYOLOGY

Development of the Face

The face is developed in the mesodermal tissues ventral to the overhanging forebrain (Fig. 2, Chapter 2). The presumptive facial area is covered externally by ectoderm which also lines the slitlike mouth cavity or stomodeum. The junction between the ectoderm of the stomodeum and the endoderm of the foregut is the buccopharyngeal membrane (Fig. 2, Chapter 2), which disappears in the early somite stage. The position of this membrane, marking the junction of ectoderm and endoderm, is shown in the adult in Figure 13 and will be referred to later. Following the development of the pharyngeal arches, the stomodeum is flanked caudally by the first or mandibular arch, cranially and laterally by the maxillary extensions of the arch, and by the area of mesoderm and ectoderm in the midline which cover the overhanging forebrain (Fig. 1). Rathke's pouch may be seen in the roof of the stomodeum; it lies immediately anterior to the upper attachment of the buccopharyngeal membrane and so marks the posterior limit of the ectoderm in the roof of the mouth. Rathke's pouch gives rise to the anterior and middle lobes of the pituitary gland. Its position in the roof of the embryonic mouth is a useful point of reference during the rapid develop-

mental changes that result in the formation of the nasal cavities and nasopharynx.

The face of an embryo of about 5 mm. (28 days) is shown in Figure 1 *A*. The most significant early event in the formation of the face is the development of the nasal pits. These arise bilaterally as placodes or thickenings of the surface ectoderm, indicated by dotted lines in Figure 1 *A*. The nasal placodes then sink in to form bilateral nasal pits (Fig. 1 *B*). The area between the nasal pits is the frontonasal area ("process"). Note that the frontonasal area is not in any sense a "process" since it is formed inevitably by the sinking in of the nasal pits on either side; it is formed by the mesoderm and its covering ectoderm between the deepening pits. The external openings of the nasal pits are flanked by flairing edges or nasal fins which merge imperceptibly ventrally with the tissues anterior to the mouth. At this stage (Fig. 1 *B*), from an embryo of about 10 mm. (33 days), the region of the future upper lip is thickened by the formation of swellings indicating proliferative changes within the underlying mesoderm. A lateral swelling, which merges with the mandibular area at the angle of the mouth, is the maxillary growth area ("process"). A prominence in the midline between the nasal pits is the frontonasal swelling. There is a shallow groove between the maxillary and frontonasal swellings on either side. Note at this point in the description that there is at no stage a cleft between the frontonasal swellings and the max-

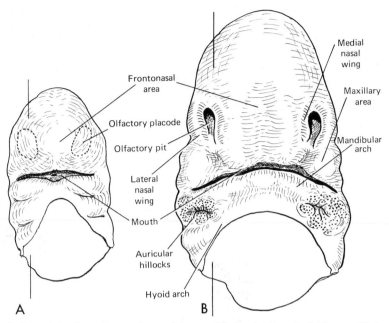

Figure 1.   Ventral view of the face of an embryo of 5 mm. (28 days) (*A*) and of 10 mm. (33 days). (After Streeter, Developmental Horizons in Human Embryos, 1948.)

illary swellings; in fact, a "hare-lip" does not exist at any stage in normal development. The external ear or pinna is already foreshadowed at the 10 mm. stage (Fig. 1 *B*) by growth centers around the upper end of the second external pharyngeal groove. These growth centers are also reflected as surface swellings, the six auricular swellings or "auricular hillocks" of His. Note that the cranial three of the swell-

ings properly belong to the mandibular arch, and so are eventually supplied by the mandibular division of the trigeminal nerve, while the caudal three swellings lie in the second arch and so are eventually supplied by the seventh or facial nerve.

The face is shown at a later stage (15 mm.; 37 days) in Figure 2. The changes in the surface contours of the components of the face

Figure 2.   Ventral view of the face of an embryo of 15 mm. (37 days). (After Streeter, Developmental Horizons in Human Embryos, 1948.)

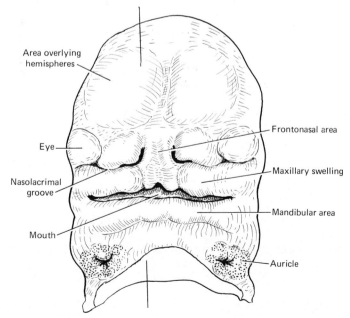

are evident. The nasal pits are smaller relative to the face, and the lateral nasal flange or wing is rounded and more prominent. The groove between the maxillary swellings laterally and the somewhat depressed frontonasal area in the midline is deeper. There is another groove extending from the inner side of the eye to the lateral edge of the nasal pits (external nares) which marks the future site of the nasolacrimal duct. The duct is formed somewhat later by the deepening of the groove and the closure of its ectodermal edges to form a duct: a secondary opening into the inferior meatus of the nose is then formed. Apart from these specific changes in the relative proportions and details of the face, there are two other notable changes. One of them is the prominence of the cerebral hemispheres which now impress themselves upon the overlying ectoderm and mesoderm, forming a definite forehead region. The prominence of the hemispheres is a specifically human feature at this early stage of development. The second change is the progressive displacement of the eyes from the lateral to the anterior surface of the head. This displacement is brought about by the pressures of the rapidly growing mesoderm behind the eyes, that is, in the regions destined to form the parietal bones, the squamous temporal bones, and the greater wings of the sphenoid. This shift in position of the eyes is a necessary prerequisite for binocular vision and involves an overlapping of the visual fields. In the absence of the pressures from the temporal and parietal area of mesoderm, as from some unexplained growth failure, the eyes and ears tend to remain abnormally placed on the side of the head. Other changes in the conformation of the face at this stage (Fig. 2) are the narrowing of the mouth by proliferations of maxillary and mandibular mesoderm at the angles, and a relative increase in prominence of the auricular hillocks. Note that these hillocks are situated far caudally with respect to the angle of the mouth. This is their primitive position and tends to be retained in certain genetic defects often associated with mental retardation and extensive mesodermal defects involving dermal bones of the skull. Its persistence in the adult should alert the clinician to associated genetic defects.

In the final evolution of the face, the salient features are the development of a prominent nasal bridge resulting from delayed growth in the frontonasal area between the medial nasal wings, and smoothing out of the grooves between the various growth centers ("processes") of the face.

Facial Growth Centers ("Processes") and the Genesis of Harelip

For many years, since the classic descriptions of His, it has been customary to describe the components of the embryonic face as consisting of "processes." The early mode s of His show such processes, which clearly have free extremities coated externally by ectoderm. It was commonly supposed that the upper lip, for example, was completed by fusion of the frontonasal process and the maxillary processes, in which the abutting ectoderm first fused and then was absorbed (Fig. 3 A). Harelip was supposed to be a persistence of the embryonic condition resulting from failure of the processes to fuse.

Streeter, in his classic "Developmental Horizons in Human Embryos," first pointed out the error of this concept. He observed that processes, in the sense that they were free at some point and had overlying ectoderm, never exist at any stage in the development of the human face. He writes: "In reality they (the processes) are not prolongations having free ends which meet in the nasal region; nor is the ectoderm absorbed over the abutting surfaces. . . . It is more precise to speak of these structures as swellings or ridges which correspond to centers of growth in the underlying mesenchyme. The furrows that lie between them on the surface are smoothed out as the proliferations and fusion of the growth centers fill in beneath. Under these circumstances no ectoderm requires absorption; it is simply flattened out in adaptation to the changed surface." An attempt to compare the classic concept of "processes" with the revised version of Streeter is shown in Fig. 3 A and B. Streeter's version is certainly correct, since a study of embryos at critical periods fails to reveal any processes in the sense of His, nor is any trace of absorbing ectoderm between the so-called recesses to be found. The genesis of harelip must be re-evaluated in the light of Streeter's concept.

Development of the Upper Lip and the Genesis of Harelip

According to Streeter's concept, the upper lip is completed by the fusion of growth centers in the maxillary and frontonasal areas beneath the overlying ectoderm, the intervening shallow grooves being simply "ironed out" and brought to the general level of the surrounding tissues (Fig. 3 B). The defect resulting in harelip must then be considered in the light of a

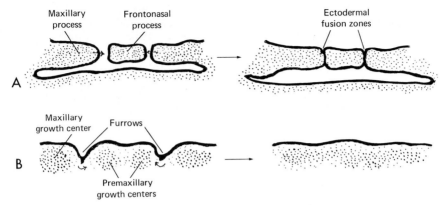

Figure 3. Schematic horizontal sections through the area of the upper lip showing two concepts of how the upper lip is developed. *A* is the classic concept of "processes" which fuse and the overlying ectoderm at the areas of contact is secondarily absorbed. *B* is the concept of subectodermal "growth centers" in the maxillary and premaxillary mesoderm which fuse and in so doing "iron out" the intervening groove; no absorption of abutting ectoderm is involved.

growth failure in the mesoderm involved rather than a failure of free processes to fuse. Thus, if the maxillary or frontonasal mesoderm should be delayed in its proliferation, the intervening groove, so far from being smoothed out, might rather be deepened. The cause of such a mesodermal growth failure is, of course, unknown. It could be a nutritional failure or could result from some genetic failure in the growth and differentiation of the mesoderm.

The subsequent development of a frank defect or cleft in the upper lip, either passing through into the vestibule of the mouth or, in more severe cases, extending deeper into the palate lateral to the premaxilla on one or both sides, also requires further explanation. In the genesis of these defects a further phenomenon may also be involved. This is the formation of the primary dental lamina and its subsequent division into the dental lamina and the labiodental lamina. It occurs much later than the events already described in the formation of the face and begins in embryos of about 18 mm. (38 to 40 days). There is an ingrowth of ectoderm in the roof and floor of the mouth near its external opening, in a curving manner following the contour of the future vestibule of the mouth and the line of the teeth. The primary dental lamina then becomes subdivided into an anterior labiodental lamina and a posterior dental lamina (Fig. 4 *A*). Cavitation of these anterior or labiodental laminae results in the formation of the vestibule of the mouth, between the lips and the teeth. The cavitation is incomplete anteriorly, forming the frenulum. More extensive failure of cavitation results in various degrees of "tongue-tie." The teeth are developed from the dental lamina.

It is evident from the foregoing description that soon after the definitive form of the face is laid down there appears on the deep surface of the future upper and lower lip a linear tract of ectoderm, the labiodental lamina, later the labiodental sulcus or vestibule of the mouth.

Figure 4. Sagittal schematic sections through the upper jaw showing the formation of an ectodermal ingrowth in *A* which becomes subdivided in *B* into an anterior lamina and a posterior dental lamina. The former cavitates to form the vestibule of the mouth; the teeth are developed from the latter. *C* and *D* show sections through the vestibule before and after cavitation.

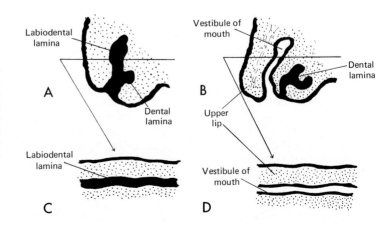

From this point its relationship to the genesis of harelip becomes conjectural. It is conceivable, however, that the coexistence of a deep furrow between the maxillary and frontonasal growth centers, resulting from a delayed growth of one or the other of these centers, associated with the formation of the labiodental sulcus, may result in fusion of the ectoderm of the upper lip with that of the labiodental sulcus. Under these circumstances, which probably occur about the 20 mm. stage (end of the 6th week), the possibility of restitution of the upper lip by fusion of the maxillary and frontonasal growth centers is gone forever, and subsequent breakdown of the intervening ectoderm results in a simple harelip. The cases of harelip which also involve the hard palate are to be explained on a similar basis, but will be described after the description of the formation of the hard palate.

Developmental Abnormalities of the Face

In addition to harelip there are many abnormalities in the development of the face, based largely on its origin from several discrete growth centers in the mesoderm. Microstomia and macrostomia, in which the mouth cleft is respectively narrowed or widened, result from excessive or defective proliferations at the angles of the mouth. Macrostomia may be so severe that the angle of the mouth extends far posteriorly, cutting the ramus of the mandible off from developing its normal articulation with the base of the skull. In this case there is frequently persistence of Meckel's cartilage (mandibular or first arch cartilage [see Chapter 2]), which may be ossified and constitute the only connection between the mandible and the skull on the affected side. There is frequently an associated defective development or failure of the malleus and incus and of the external auditory meatus. In such cases the stapes and the inner ear are always normal, so that the surgeon may reconstitute the ossicular chain with confidence of restoring hearing.

Microstomia is often associated with and probably results from failure of growth of the mandibular arch. The mandibular arch normally shows a delay in development compared with the more cranial components of the face and skull. This relative delay may result, in its less severe manifestations, in a simple undershooting of the lower jar, common in new babies and a cause of faulty bite in older children. In more severe cases in which the mandibular arch

is partially or almost completely suppressed there results micrognathia or agnathia. The mouth is usually minute, the mandible vestigial, and there may be fusion of the middle ear cavities in the midline caudal to the mouth. The external ear, which depends on the growth pressure of the mandibular arch in reaching its normal position, retains its primitive position low down in the neck and close to the midline (Fig. 2). In severe micrognathia or agnathia the auricles are fused in the midline caudal to the mouth.

Clefts of the face may also exist and may, in some cases, be related to the boundaries between the developmental regions of the face. Macrostomia is a persistence of the normal wide cleft of the mouth. An oblique cleft may run from the medial angle of the eye to the upper lip and may be associated with a harelip. Such a cleft is a persistence of the normal nasolacrimal groove between the maxillary swelling and the lateral nasal wing (Fig. 2). In such cases the lacrimal groove is laid open and discharges tears onto the surface of the face. Other clefts of the face may run in almost any direction, but do not conform to any normal geographic boundaries of the face and so are not easily explained.

Development of the Auricle or Pinna

The auricle or pinna develops as six swellings or "hillocks" surrounding the upper end of the second external pharyngeal groove (Figs. 1, 2, and 5 A). The auricle becomes established by the growth and fusion of these disparate growth centers (Fig. 5 B). The first hillock (most anterior on the mandibular arch) becomes the tragus; the second, the crus helicis; the third, the helix. The fourth hillock (most posterior on the second or hyoid arch) becomes the antihelix; the fifth, the antitragus; and the sixth (most anterior on the hyoid arch), the lobule.

Abnormalities or genetically determined variations in the pattern of fusion of the auricular hillocks account for the frequent abnormalities of the auricle and for the striking familial resemblances between people with respect to the ear. Accessory nodules, usually anterior to the tragus, arise from accessory or additional hillocks. They are of little consequence except cosmetically. Their removal, however, is often accompanied by considerable hemorrhage. Grossly deformed auricles, as described, especially when associated with a low position of

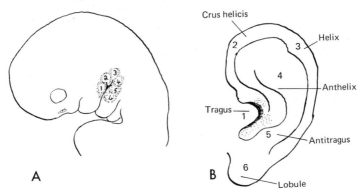

Figure 5. Development of the external ear or auricle. The sixth "auricular hillocks" surrounding the dorsal end of the first external pharyngeal groove are stippled in *A*. The parts of the auricle derived from the six auricular hillocks are shown in *B*.

the ear on the side of the head, should alert the clinician to accompanying mesodermal and neural defects.

Developmental Territories of the Face in Relation to Nerve Supply

The broad developmental regions of the face, namely, the frontonasal, the maxillary and the mandibular areas, are reflected in their pattern of sensory supply from the fifth or trigeminal nerve (Fig. 6).

The first or ophthalmic division of the tri-geminal nerve (VA) supplies the frontonasal area. The maxillary division (VB) supplies the area derived from the maxillary swellings (Fig. 2). The mandibular division (VC) supplies the mandibular arch, including the lateral and upper half of the auricle, but excluding the angle of the jaw.

The nerve of the frontonasal "process" is generally held to be the anterior ethmoidal nerve, a branch of the nasociliary arising within the orbit. It leaves the medial wall of the orbit through the anterior ethmoidal canal between the frontal bone and the lamina papyracea of the ethmoid and enters the anterior cra-

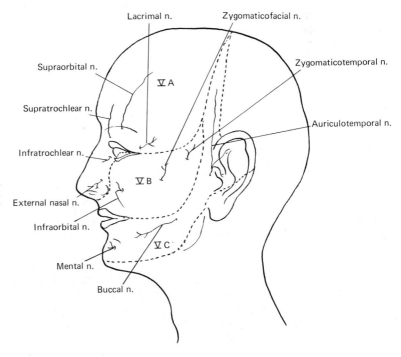

Figure 6. Parts of the face derived from the three developmental areas of the face: frontonasal area (ophthalmic nerve), maxillary area (maxillary nerve), and mandibular area (mandibular nerve).

nial fossa of the skull on top of the cribriform plate of the ethmoid. It then pierces the anterior cranial fossa lateral to the crista galli and descends into the nasal cavity deep to the nasal bone, lying in a groove in the bone. It reaches the skin between the lower edge of the nasal bone and the nasal cartilage of the ala and, as the lateral nasal nerve, supplies the skin of the lateral surface of the nose. The curious course of this nerve is explained as follows: The nerve originally has a simple course, descending into the frontonasal region of the face. It is later trapped between the cartilaginous nasal capsule (later forming the ethmoid) and the orbital plate of the frontal and the nasal bones, both of which are "dermal bones," i.e., developed "in membrane" in the superficial mesoderm. Thus, the nerve lies in its definitive position before the bones are formed. The bones are then laid down around them and so determine their complex anatomical course in the adult skull. The remaining ophthalmic territory of the face (Fig. 6) includes the forehead (via the supraorbital and supratrochlear nerves), the upper eyelid, including the conjunctiva and upper half of the cornea (via the lacrimal and supratrochlear nerves), and the side of the nose (via the infratrochlear and external nasal nerves).

The maxillary territory of the face includes the area below the palpebral fissure (lower eyelid, including the lower half of the cornea) and the upper lip (via the infraorbital nerve), the zygomatic region and the side of the temple (via the zygomaticofacial and zygomaticotemporal nerves) (Fig. 6).

The mandibular territory includes the area below the mouth (via the mental nerve), the cheek (via the buccal nerve), and the side of the temple, including the upper part of the auricle (via the auriculotemporal nerve). Note that the palpebral fissure and the angle of the mark delineate the territories of the three divisions of the trigeminal nerve on the face (Fig. 6). The angle of the jaw is supplied by the cervical plexus through the great auricular nerve (C2 and C3) and so is excluded from the mandibular territory. The lower part of the auricle is supplied by the great auricular nerve and the lesser occipital nerve (C2 and C3), and so is also excluded from the trigeminal territory.

The trigeminal nerve is notorious for mediating referred pain, often making exact diagnosis difficult. Pain arising in the teeth (via the superior and inferior dental nerves) is also referred through the auriculotemporal nerve to the external ear and parotid region, thus imitating the pain of external otitis or an impacted foreign body. Pain may also be referred from the teeth to the temporomandibular joint or in the reverse direction. Note the close anatomical relationship between the auriculotemporal nerve and the posterior surface of the capsule of this point (Fig. 23, Chap. 2). Areas of the trigeminal sensory territory may also be "trigger areas" for pain in trigeminal neuralgia or tic douloureux.

The large size of the trigeminal nerve and its sensory representation are reflected in its extensive sensory connections in the brain. The nuclei connected with the incoming fibers belong to the "general somatic afferent column" (Fig. 31, Chap. 2) and mediate pain, temperature, touch and conscious proprioception. The fibers for pain and temperature descend in the spinal tract of the trigeminal nerve through the lateral part of the lower pons and medulla as low as the second or third cervical segment of the spinal cord, where they are continuous with the dorsolateral fasciculus (Lissauer's tract). The pain-temperature fibers then enter into synaptic contact with the adjacent cells of the nucleus of the spinal tract of the trigeminal, beginning at the lower border of the pons. The ophthalmic fibers lie anteriorly in the part of the spinal tract of the trigeminal, the mandibular nerves dorsally and the maxillary fibers intermediate in position. The ophthalmic fibers descend into the upper cervical cord; the maxillary fibers descend only to the lower border of the medulla; the mandibular fibers descend only as far as the middle of the medulla. Neurons of the second order arising in the nucleus of the spinal tract of the trigeminal nerve cross the midline and ascend in at least two ascending secondary tracts to reach the posterior part of the ventral nucleus of the thalamus where they have a second synapse. Fibers of the third order then pass through the internal capsule to project onto the posterocentral or somesthetic cortex. Here the body is depicted upside down. The face, however, is represented on a disproportionately large area of the sensory cortex, low down near the sylvian fissure. The large area for the thumb is represented close beside the face area of the cortex. This approximation of sensory projections for the face and thumb perhaps reflects the evolutionary importance of sucking and feeding actions in the development of the brain.

The pain-temperature fibers of the ophthalmic nerve can be surgically interrupted by an incision into the posterolateral surface of the medulla at the lower border of the pons. Here the spinal tract becomes superficial in an area known as the tuberculum cinereum, immediately dorsal to the olive and ventral to the restiform body. To render the maxillary and mandibular nerves analgesic, it is necessary to sever the tract higher in the medulla. Severance of the tract for intractable trigeminal neuralgia or pain from carcinoma of the face results in loss of pain and temperature sensation from the same side of the face in one or all of the three divisions, depending on the level of section. In all instances in which the sensory territory of the trigeminal nerve is denervated in relation to the ophthalmic or maxillary territories, either by resection of the trigeminal (gasserian) ganglion or by medullary tractotomy, the loss of innervation of the cornea and conjunctiva is of great significance. Loss of pain sensation in these areas may result in corneal ulceration.

Fibers of the trigeminal nerve mediating touch enter the main sensory nucleus of the fifth nerve at the level of the midpons and also enter the upper part of the spinal tract. Proprioceptive fibers from the muscles of mastication enter the mesencephalic nucleus of the fifth nerve, a small linear group of neurons extending from the level of the main sensory nucleus into the midbrain lateral to the aqueduct of Sylvius. These neurons are unusual in that the primary cell bodies do not lie in the gasserian ganglion but lie within the mesencephalic nucleus, that is, within the brain stem.

Development of the Palate

The development of the premaxillary portion of the palate (primordial palate), i.e., that part which carries the incisor teeth, differs fundamentally from that of the rest of the palate both in manner and in the time at which it is formed.

The formation of the premaxillary portion of the palate occurs early (from the 33rd to the 37th day) in conjunction with the development of the face (see Figs. 1 and 2) and as an inevitable consequence of the development of the bilateral nasal pits. As the nasal pits sink into the paraxial mesoderm of the face and deepen, there is left between them a midline mass of mesoderm which constitutes the nasal septum. Ventral to the nasal pits there is a block of mesoderm which constitutes the upper lip and is necessarily continuous above with the primitive nasal septum (Figs. 7 A and B, and 9 A). At a slightly later stage the nasal pits approach

the ectoderm in the roof of the mouth just anterior to the point of origin of Rathke's pouch (Fig. 7 B). Fusion between the ectoderm of the nasal pits and that of the roof of the mouth results for a time in a thick bucconasal septum, which then becomes attenuated, forming the bucconasal membrane. The bucconasal membrane then breaks down (Fig. 7 C), establishing a posterior opening into the roof of the mouth from the nasal pits, the primitive posterior nares. It is now possible to speak of nasal cavities on either side, separated by a thick nasal septum, opening anteriorly through the anterior nares and posteriorly through the primitive posterior nares. The roof of the nasal cavity, which is in close relationship to the overlying forebrain, becomes differentiated into the olfactory epithelium, a primary sensory receptor for smell. Sensory cells from this area send out processes, comparable to axons, toward the overlying olfactory bulbs and establish primary synaptic connections with the cells of the bulbs (Fig. 7 C and D). The differentiation of the olfactory epithelium goes hand in hand with that of the olfactory bulb, and the interaction between the two is an example of primary induction. In the absence of the olfactory bulbs, the olfactory epithelium fails to develop, resulting in congenital anosmia.

It is necessary to re-emphasize that the primordial palate is merely a block of mesoderm lying transversely ventral to the nasal pits. It represents that part of the mesoderm of the face anterior to the mouth not involved in the formation of the nasal pits which, from the manner of its formation, must necessarily be continuous above with the nasal septum between the two pits. The primordial palate presents onto the surface of the face as a depressed area between the maxillary swellings, continuous with the frontonasal area (Fig. 2). As noted elsewhere, at no stage is there a condition resembling harelip; the ectoderm of the tissues anterior to the mouth forms an unbroken stretch from side to side. The primordial palate cannot in any sense be considered a "process."

The subsequent growth of the head results in a progressive increase in the anteroposterior and lateral extent of the mouth and pharynx. This process is illustrated insofar as it affects the nasal septum in Figure 8. The posterior nares become progressively enlarged posteriorly (in the directions of the small arrows) as the nasopharynx deepens and, as a consequence, the nasal septum also becomes elon-

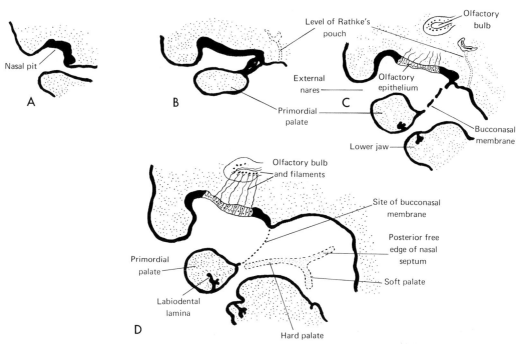

Figure 7. Series of sagittal sections through the nasal area in the planes indicated in Figures 1 and 2 showing the deepening of the nasal pit (*A* and *B*), the breakdown of the bucconasal membrane (*C*) and the opening into the roof of the mouth to form the posterior nares. Increase in the anteroposterior extent of the pharyngeal cavity posterior to the primordial palate is followed by horizontal partitioning of the nasal cavity from the mouth cavity by the maxillary shelves (hard palate, *D*).

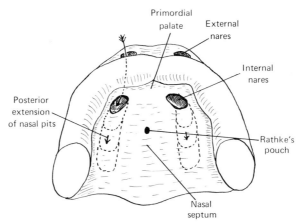

Figure 8. Roof of the mouth showing the backward extension of the posterior nasal aperture and the concomitant lengthening of the nasal septum. The latter is necessarily continuous anteriorly with the primordial palate. The opening of Rathke's pouch is presumably carried on to the free edge of the nasal septum.

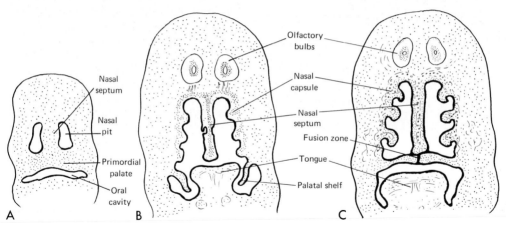

Figure 9. Frontal schematic sections through the nose at the level of the primordial palate in an early stage (*A*), and at later stages through the maxillary shelves before (*B*) and after (*C*) fusion with the nasal septum. (After Streeter, Developmental Horizons in Human Embryology, 1948.)

gated. It now presents into the roof of the mouth as a broad extensive area between the posterior nares. In this process of extension of the posterior nares, the point of origin of Rathke's pouch must be assumed to be taken up into the area involved in the new part of the nasal septum (Fig. 8). At this stage, beginning about the 9th week, the maxillary and palatal portions of the hard palate are developed and fill in most of the roof of the mouth posterior to the primordial palate (Fig. 7 *D*).

Development of the Palate Posterior to the Premaxilla

The large orifices of the posterior nares resulting from their posterior extension and the increased depth of the nasopharynx and base of the skull (Fig. 8) are now partially closed off by the development of maxillary shelves on either side. The maxillary shelves appear about the 35th day (in embryos of 12 mm.) and are true processes in that they have free extremities and are covered on all sides except where they are continuous with the maxillary mesoderm (Fig. 9 *B*). The shelves grow in from the lateral wall of the oronasal cavity and at first lie freely within the paralingual sulcus. They are prevented for a considerable time from making contact with the undersurface of the nasal septum by the tongue, which is pressed hard against it. The tongue is withdrawn from contact with the nasal septum about the 9th week, thus allowing the free edges of the palatal

shelves to fuse with the nasal septum (Fig. 9 *C*). Fusion then occurs rapidly along approximately the anterior three fourths of the free surface of the nasal septum. The palatal shelves fall short of the nasal septum posteriorly and constitute the soft palate (Fig. 7 *D*). That part of the nasal septum posteriorly which fails to fuse with the palatal shelves forms the definitive posterior edge of the nasal septum. The posterior nares of the adult are not finally established until the process of palatal fusion is complete, by about the 12th week.

The pattern of fusion of the palatal shelves with the nasal septum and the primordial palate is shown in Figure 10. The fissure observed in complete cleft palate also follows this pattern. It may be unilateral or bilateral.

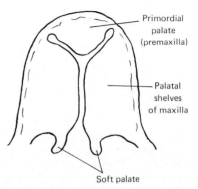

Figure 10. Pattern of fusion of the maxillary shelves with the primordial palate and nasal septum.

Genesis of Cleft Palate

Understanding of the genesis of cleft palate must take into consideration the normal facts of development. Failure of the palatal shelves to fuse with the undersurface of the nasal septum is clearly the immediate cause of cleft palate. This failure may be partial, complete, unilateral or bilateral. The soft palate may be divided since it is developmentally a bilateral structure. The cleft, whether unilateral or bilateral, passes laterally around the primordial palate anteriorly and so passes between the lateral incisor teeth and the canine teeth. The possible factors involved in the formation of harelip have already been considered. Harelip is often associated with cleft palate, though not necessarily. It is obvious from the close clinical association between these two defects that there must be certain common developmental causes. If the primary defect is considered to be a failure of or delay in mesodermal growth centers, notably those of the maxillae, it is reasonable to suppose that not only will a harelip be produced but that also there will be a predisposition for maldevelopment of the palatal shelves. Mechanical factors in the failure of the palatal shelves to fuse with the nasal septum have also been considered. The continued apposition of the tongue to the nasal septum precludes fusion of the palatal shelves, and it is supposed that the withdrawal of the tongue is a definitive factor in determining the success or failure of this fusion. That the mandibular region is relatively delayed in its growth has been observed. It is conceivable that the growth of the mandible finally results in the withdrawal of the tongue from the nasal septum. Extensor movements of the neck of the fetus have also been considered as factors influencing the withdrawal of the tongue. Many teratogenic agents, notably cortisone in susceptible strains of rats, cause cleft palate. It seems reasonable to suppose that such agents affect mesodermal growth or differentiation and that mechanical factors are here relatively less important. The enormous number of chemical and hormonal agents that may result in cleft palate in susceptible strains suggests that (1) genetic factors are involved, (2) there is no specific inducer of cleft palate, but rather the maxillary mesoderm and its palatal shelves are for some reason highly susceptible, and (3) the delayed pattern of fusion of the palatal shelves with nasal septum and possibly the influence of mechanical factors also render the process highly susceptible.

Further Development of the Nasal Cavities and Paranasal Sinuses

The olfactory organs are phylogenetically ancient structures and, like the inner ear, are enclosed within the equally ancient chondroskeleton of the skull. The nasal cavities become surrounded by a condensation of mesenchyme which then chondrifies, forming the nasal capsule (Figs. 9 *B* and *C*). The chondrification spreads down into the nasal septum and also into the lateral wall. Processes of the lateral walls give rise to the superior, middle and inferior conchae (turbinates), which provide added mucosal surface for the warming of the incoming air. The olfactory epithelium, on the upper surface of the nasal septum, the adjacent roof and the lateral wall of the nasal cavity, lies in a cul-de-sac relatively secluded from the main flow of air. This arrangement avoids excessive drying and also permits the odorous materials in the air to remain in contact with the olfactory epithelium. The sensory fibers arising from specialized receptor cells in the olfactory epithelium pass through the roof of the nasal capsule (future cribriform plate of the ethmoid) to reach the olfactory bulbs. They are surrounded for a part of their length distal to the olfactory bulbs with extensions of the meninges which resemble central tracts in that they do not regenerate after section, so that the anosmia resulting from trauma is permanent. The olfactory filaments are also important in that they are able to transmit certain agents such as viruses from the nose to the primary olfactory centers of the brain. This pathway is suggested for rabies, thus accounting for the presence of the inclusion bodies (Negri bodies) in the primary cortical receptor, the hippocampus. They may also be involved in the transmission of other viruses including poliomyelitis virus. Associated with the olfactory epithelium are serous glands which lubricate the area and keep it moist. They receive their secretomotor supply from the facial nerve via the sphenopalatine ganglion and the nerve of the pterygoid canal (vidian nerve) (see Fig. 24).

The paranasal sinuses are developed as outgrowths from the lateral wall of the nasal cavities, that is, from the meatuses bounded by the three conchae and the adjacent roof and floor. The maxillary sinus appears as an outpouching of the nasal mucosa in the third month of fetal life. The frontal sinus develops as an upgrowth of one of the anterior groups of ethmoidal air cells. It does not penetrate the frontal bone, as a rule, until after birth. It invades the bone in the first and second years after birth, undergoes a growth spurt about the ninth year, and reaches its full size at about age 20. The ethmoidal air cells, growing from the superior and inferior meatuses, are present at birth, grow slowly after birth, and reach their full development at about puberty. The sphenoidal air sinuses are not enclosed by bone at birth. They increase rapidly about the third year and show additional growth at puberty. The maxillary sinuses are small cavities at birth in the shallow maxillae. They extend laterally as far as the infraorbital nerve by the end of the first year and grow steadily thereafter until about the tenth year. Their subsequent growth occurs in association with the eruption of the permanent teeth. The posteroinferior angle of the sinus is added last in connection with the eruption of the last molar teeth.

Development of the Lacrimal Apparatus

As described earlier, the lacrimal duct is developed along the line of the nasolacrimal furrow between the lateral nasal wing and the maxillary swelling (Fig. 2). The ectoderm in the floor of the furrow deepens and the margins then close over to form the duct, which loses its connection with the surface. The duct then acquires a secondary opening into the inferior meatus of the nasal cavity. At its upper end the duct bifurcates and establishes connections with the conjunctival sac at the inner canthus of the eye (lacrimal canaliculi). The lacrimal gland develops as an ectodermal proliferation of the conjunctival sac at the upper and outer angle of the eye. It receives its secretomotor supply from the sphenopalatine ganglion and the facial nerve via the zygomaticotemporal nerve. Note that the gland is an ectodermal structure and quite superficial. It lies external to the orbital septum and its removal does not involve invasion of the orbit itself.

Development of the Salivary Glands

The parotid gland is ectodermal in origin and arises as a proliferation at the angle of the mouth in embryos of about 12 mm. The opening of the duct (Stensen's duct) then shifts posteriorly and comes to open into the vestibule of the mouth at the level of the second upper molar tooth. The submandibular gland develops as a groove in the endoderm in the floor of the mouth in the paralingual sulcus.

The edges of the groove then close over except anteriorly at the external opening of the duct (Wharton's duct). Since the duct arises from the epithelium in the floor of the mouth, the lingual nerve must lie inferior to it. This accounts for the characteristic curving course of the lingual nerve, at first lateral, then under and, finally, medial to the submandibular duct (see Fig. 20, Chap. 2). The sublingual glands arise as multiple proliferations of the endoderm in the floor of the mouth.

ANATOMY OF THE NASAL CAVITY AND NASOPHARYNX

Nasal Cavities and Nasopharynx

The general features of the nasal cavities and nasopharynx (Fig. 11) are familiar and require only superficial comment. Prominent features of the lateral wall of the nasal cavity are the three scroll-like conchae or turbinate bones. The mucosa overlying these, as over the nasal septum and in the sinuses, is a typical mucoperiosteum or, where cartilage is present, a mucoperichondrium. The epithelium is pseudostratified columnar and ciliated. It rests on a basement lamina which is attached firmly to the underlying bone or cartilage by dense but highly vascular connective tissue. Submucous resection is carried out by separating the mucosa with the periosteum or perichondrium, which together form a structural and functional unit. In certain areas, notably the conchae, the submucosal connective tissue contains large venous channels which are capable of engorgement. They serve to warm the incoming air but may give rise to obstruction when engorged from inflammation. Most of the serous glands which moisten the nasal mucosa (serous glands of Bowman) lie in the upper reaches of the cavity in relation to the olfactory epithelium. There are numerous mucous glands or goblet cells scattered throughout the nasal mucosa. These, like the serous glands, are supplied from the sphenopalatine ganglion and the facial nerve.

The conchae form the boundaries of three horizontal passages or meatuses (superior, middle, and inferior). The spheno-ethmoidal recess (Fig. 11) lies above the superior concha and receives the opening of the sphenoidal sinus. The superior meatus (between the superior and middle conchae) receives the openings of the superior, and possibly a few of the middle, ethmoidal sinuses. The middle meatus

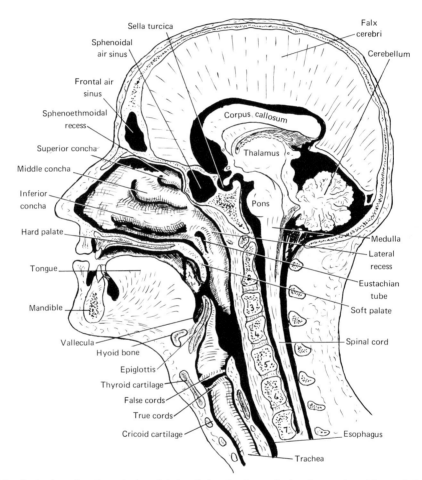

Figure 11.   Sagittal section through the adult head showing in particular the nasal cavities and the pharynx.

lies between the middle and inferior conchae and receives the openings of the anterior and some of the middle ethmoidal sinuses, the opening of the maxillary sinus and, anteriorly, the opening of the frontal sinus. These will be described in detail later. The inferior meatus between the floor of the nasal cavity and the inferior concha receives the opening of the nasolacrimal duct. Note that the superior and middle conchae are parts of the ethmoid bone, whereas the inferior concha is a bone in its own right.

The roof of the nasal cavity is formed by the cribriform plate of the ethmoid (which transmits the olfactory filaments), by the undersurface of the sphenoid bone and by the nasal area of the frontal and nasal bones. The nasal septum is made up of vomer and the perpendicular plate of the ethmoid (Fig. 12). The perpendicular plate of the ethmoid rests below on the vomer and projects far forward to carry the nasal bones. The vomer articulates above with the undersurface of the base of the sphenoid, and inferiorly makes contact with the whole length of the hard palate, made up of the horizontal plate of the maxilla anteriorly and the horizontal plate of the palatine posteriorly. The vomer is marked by a groove in which lies the nasopalatine (long sphenopalatine) nerve on its way to the incisive canal. The nasal septum is completed anteriorly by cartilage (Fig. 12). Posteriorly the nasal cavities open into the nasopharynx through the posterior nares, which are bounded in the midline by the vomer, superiorly by the articulation of the vomer with the vaginal process of the medial pterygoid plate (Fig. 16), laterally by the vertical plate of the palatine, and below by the horizontal (palatal) process of the palate bone.

The nasopharynx (Fig. 11) is a cavity which, unlike the rest of the pharynx, has rigid walls except inferiorly where it is bounded by the soft palate, and so is never obliterated under normal conditions. In transverse section the nasopharynx (Fig. 23, Chap. 2) is rhomboidal. It narrows anteriorly where it joins the posterior nares. Its lateral angles are prolonged out as far as the spine of the sphenoid, forming the lateral recesses of fossae of Rosenmüller (Fig. 23, Chap. 4). The lateral recesses owe their existence to the oblique attachment of the pharynx to the base of the skull along the line of the petrosphenoidal suture. Here the wall is formed by the "eustachian apparatus," comprising the pharyngotympanic tube, the tensor and levator veli palatini muscles and associated fascial layers (Fig. 22, Chap. 2). The lateral recess has important relationships in addition to those structures comprising the eustachian apparatus. It is related posterolaterally to the internal carotid artery and the venous and neural components of the retrostyloid space. Posteriorly it is related to the retropharyngeal space (Fig. 24, Chap. 2). An abscess in the retropharyngeal space may bulge or point into the lateral recess of Rosenmüller. Likewise an aneurysm of the internal carotid artery may bulge into the space and result in fatal hemorrhage if accidentally incised in mistake for an abcess. The recess is a useful factor in cannulating the eustachian tube. The instrument is placed first in the recess and slowly drawn forward so that it will traverse the whole inner surface of the cartilaginous tube until it enters the orifice.

The orifice itself (Fig. 11) lies about 1 cm. behind and a little below the posterior end of the inferior concha. It is thickened above and

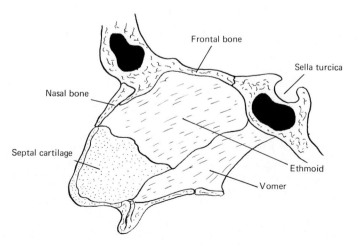

Figure 12. Composition of the nasal septum in the adult.

Frontal bone

Sella turcica

Nasal bone

Septal cartilage

Ethmoid

Vomer

behind by lymphoid tissue, forming the tubal tonsil of Gerlach. The roof and posterior wall of the nasopharynx are continuous and sloping. They are formed by the inferior surface of the body of the sphenoid, the basi-occipital, and anterior atlanto-occipital membrane, the anterior arch of the atlas, and the body of the second or axis vertebra (Fig. 11). Inferiorly the nasopharynx opens into the oropharynx. The opening is closed off during deglutition by the soft palate and by the contraction of the sphincteric fibers of the superior constrictor (Passavant's sphincter). These fibers may raise up a definite ridge on contraction over which the epithelium is stratified squamous and which comes into contact with the soft palate during swallowing. The sphincter may also make examination of the nasopharynx by a mirror difficult.

The oropharynx is the intermediate portion of the pharynx (Fig. 11) and stretches from the level of the soft palate to the level of the upper border of the epiglottis. Its lateral walls are shown in Figure 19, Chapter 2. They include the superior constrictor, the middle constrictor muscles, the gap between these muscles containing the stylohyoid ligament and the styloglossus, and also the curve of the glossopharyngeal nerve and the external maxillary artery. The oropharynx communicates with the mouth anteriorly through the oropharyngeal isthmus. The isthmus is guarded laterally by the palatine tonsils, which lie in the tonsillar fossa between the anterior and posterior pillars of the fauces. The former is produced by the palatoglossus muscle and the latter by the palatopharyngeus muscle. The posterior wall of the oropharynx is formed by the body of the second and possibly part of the third cervical vertebrae (Fig. 11); like the rest of the pharynx it is here related to the important retropharyngeal space.

The laryngopharynx extends from the upper level of the epiglottis to the lower border of the cricoid cartilage where it is continuous with the esophagus (level of the upper part of the sixth cervical vertebra). It is described in connection with the larynx.

Lymphoid Tissue of the Pharynx and Waldeyer's Ring

The lymphoid tissue that surrounds the oropharyngeal isthmus and the opening of the nasopharynx into the oropharynx defensive is referred to as Waldeyer's ring (Fig. 13). It is formed superiorly by the midline pharyngeal tonsil or "adenoids." It is continuous laterally on either side with the tubal tonsil. Lower

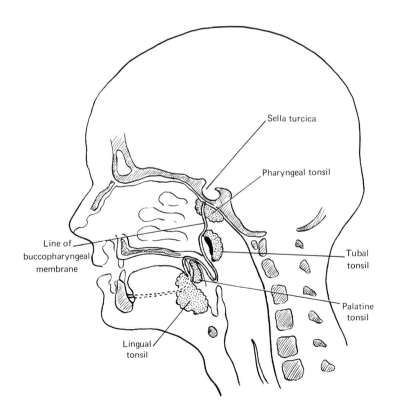

Figure 13. Schematic sagittal section through the head showing the approximate position of the former buccopharyngeal membrane (junction of ectoderm anteriorly and endoderm posteriorly). The lymphoid tissue at the oropharyngeal isthmus (Waldeyer's ring) is also shown.

down on either side are the palatine tonsils. The ring is completed inferiorly by the lymphoid tissue in the posterior third of the tongue (lingual tonsil). In the newborn child and infant the craniocaudal extent of the pharynx is much less than in the adult, so that the normal hypertrophy of the lymphoid tissue of Waldeyer's ring readily occludes the posterior nares and the opening from the nasopharynx into the oropharynx, especially when inflammation is present. Nasal obstruction and mouth breathing, accordingly, are very common and may require surgical correction.

Nerve Supply of Nasal Cavity and Pharynx

The nasal cavity receives its sensory nerve supply from the maxillary and the ophthalmic nerves. Sensory fibers reach the sphenopalatine ganglion via the nasopalatine (from nasal septum and anterior part of the palate), greater palatine (posterior part of the palate), lesser palatine nerves (soft palate), by branches from the sphenoidal sinus and ethmoidal sinuses, and by branches from the maxillary sinus via the superior dental nerves. Blocking the sphenopalatine ganglion, therefore, provides satisfactory anesthesia for most parts of the nasal region, including the sinuses. The ethmoidal nerves, branches of the nasociliary branch of the ophthalmic nerve, are exceptions. The anterior ethmoidal nerve supplies the anterior group of ethmoidal cells and the anterior part of the nasal septum. The posterior ethmoidal nerve, which may be absent, supplies the posterior ethmoidal cells and the sphenoidal air sinus.

The parasympathetic fibers to the glandular tissue of the nasal cavities and sinuses, including the lacrimal gland, are derived from the sphenopalatine ganglion. They reach the ganglion through the nerve of the pterygoid canal (vidian nerve), formed by the union of the greater superficial petrosal nerve and the deep petrosal nerve (Figs. 24 and 30, Chap. 2). The greater superficial petrosal nerve arises from the facial nerve at the level of the geniculate ganglion and emerges through the anterior surface of the petrous temporal bone in the midline cranial fossa. Here it lies deep to the dura, forming the floor of Meckel's cave in which is lodged the gasserian ganglion. Traction on the nerve at this point in trigeminal ganglionectomy may pull on the facial nerve and give a transient or permanent facial paralysis. The nerve then joins with a sympathetic branch

(deep petrosal) from the caroticotympanic plexus on the internal carotid artery, which together form the nerve of the pterygoid canal (vidian nerve). The vidian nerve traverses a canal in the sphenoid at the root of the pterygoid process (Fig. 16) and emerges in the pterygopalatine fossa where it enters the sphenopalatine ganglion. The parasympathetic fibers have a synapse here, and the postganglionic fibers pass via the branches of the ganglion to the glandular tissue of the nose and sinuses. The sympathetic fibers do not relay, having had their last synapse in the superior cervical sympathetic ganglion, and are distributed to glandular tissue and blood vessels of the nose and sinuses. The branches of the sphenopalatine ganglion described previously are generally accompanied by arteries derived from the internal maxillary artery.

Destruction of the sphenopalatine ganglion, a common operation at one time for hay fever and allergic conditions, is followed by catastrophic atrophy of the glandular tissue of the nose, palate, and sinuses. This results in loss of smell and a chronic malodorous inflammatory condition (ozena) of the nasal passages. The ganglion may be approached for temporary blocking by two routes. One is through the nose, the needle being directed through the mucous membrane at the posterior end of the inferior meatus. The second route is laterally through the cheek, the needle being directed through the infratemporal region until it passes into the pterygopalatine fossa between the pterygoid plates and the maxilla. The sensory supply of the nasopharynx is via the pharyngeal nerve. This small branch of the sphenopalatine ganglion lies in a groove completed by the articulation of the vaginal process of the medial pterygoid plate and the sphenoidal process of the palatine bone (Fig. 16). It passes backward and innervates the area round the eustachian tube and the lateral pharyngeal recess.

Sensory impulses are transmitted from this nerve to the maxillary branch of the trigeminal; sympathetic and parasympathetic fibers are transmitted by the vidian nerve. The oropharynx derives its sensory fibers from the pharyngeal plexuses on the lateral surface of the middle constrictor muscle. These fibers pass up to the brain in the glossopharyngeal nerve but also in the pharyngeal branches of the vagus and the superior and inferior laryngeal branches of the vagus. Secretomotor branches are distributed to the pharynx via the pharyngeal plexus comprising fibers of the ninth, tenth, and possibly eleventh cranial nerves.

Sympathetic fibers enter the pharyngeal plexus through the sympathetic branches of the superior and middle cervical sympathetic ganglia. The sensory territories of the glossopharyngeal nerve may act as trigger zones for paroxysmal attacks of pain analogous to trigeminal neuralgia. All the afferent fibers from the pharynx on reaching the brain enter the tractus solitarius (general visceral afferent column) (Fig. 31, Chap. 2). They relay in the nucleus of the tractus solitarius and make internuncial or short intermediary connections with other nuclei of the medulla and also connect with the spinal cord through the solitariospinal tract.

The motor fibers to the constrictors of the pharynx belong to the group of special visceral (branchial) efferent neurons. They arise in the nucleus ambiguus in the medulla and pass to the pharynx through the glossopharyngeal, vagus, and possibly the cranial component of the eleventh or accessory nerve. These connections of the tractus solitarius and nucleus ambiguus are important in reflexes such as coughing, sneezing, swallowing, gagging, vomiting, and so forth.

The Mechanism of Deglutition

Following mastication of the food, the process of swallowing is initiated by the contraction of the tongue and the muscles in the floor of the mouth. The bolus of food is passed through the oropharyngeal isthmus and enters the oropharynx. The mouth is then closed. The opening between the nasopharynx and the oropharynx is then closed by the elevation of the soft palate by the tensor and levator veli palatini muscles and by the contraction of Passavant's sphincter. There is approximation of the palatoglossal and palatopharyngeal arches (anterior and posterior pillars of the fauces) to the back of the tongue. The pharynx is thus converted into a closed box. The larynx and pharynx are then elevated by contraction of the stylopharyngeus and thyrohyoid muscles so that the floor of the pharyngeal compartment rises. The larynx then descends, carrying with it the lower pharynx (hypopharynx), producing a pistonlike effect on the closed upper pharynx. The bolus of food is sucked toward the esophagus with great speed, perhaps assisted momentarily by contraction of the middle and inferior constrictors. Most if not all of this phase of swallowing, however, is too rapid to be primarily peristaltic in character. It is so rapid that when corrosive liquids are

swallowed, the area of damage may be in the hypopharynx or in the esophagus. That pressure differences are fundamental in the act of swallowing is shown when regurgitation takes place due to failure of closure of the nasopharyngeal "pinchcock." Under these circumstances fluids are projected through the nose with considerable violence. This may happen inadvertently but may be an ominous sign in a patient with bulbar paralysis, indicating involvement of the nucleus ambiguus, the first sign that the process has ascended to the level of the medulla.

The importance of a proper mechanism for closure of the nasopharynx in normal speech is also recognized.

Limits of Ectodermal and Endodermal Territories in the Adult Nose, Mouth and Pharynx

The approximate site of the buccopharyngeal membrane which marks the posterior limit of the ectoderm and the anterior limit of the foregut endoderm is indicated by the double line in Figure 13. The line begins superiorly near the pharyngeal tonsil, at the approximate site of origin of Rathke's pouch. It then passes down the lateral wall of the nasopharynx anterior to the eustachian orifice, which is of endodermal origin. It then passes into the floor of the mouth anterior to the palatoglossal fold (anterior pillar of the fauces) and inside the line of the teeth. It finally reaches the symphysis menti to join the line of the opposite side. All structures posterior to this line are endodermal in origin and are supplied by nerves caudal to the fifth (seventh, ninth, tenth, eleventh, and twelfth).

ANATOMY OF THE PARANASAL SINUSES

The paranasal air sinuses comprise the maxillary, the ethmoidal, the frontal, and the sphenoidal sinuses. They are developed as diverticula of the nasal mucosa and, like it, are lined by a mucoperiosteum. The mucoperiosteum consists of a pseudostratified ciliated columnar epithelium, with scattered mucus-secreting goblet cells, firmly attached to the periosteum. The cilia beat toward the nasal cavities, though drainage is often hampered by the small size of the opening from the sinus to the nose and by the absence of mechanical and gravitational effects. The sinuses are poorly developed or absent at birth, reach more or less adult size by puberty but may continue to extend (pneumatization) until 20 or more years of age.

Maxillary and Ethmoidal Sinuses

The maxillary sinus occupies the pyramidal body of the maxilla and lies in relation to the canine, premolar and molar teeth. The apex of the sinus lies at the root of the zygomatic process of the maxilla. The base faces toward the lateral surface of the nasal cavity. The roof of the sinus is separated by a thin plate of bone from the orbital cavity and its contents. The anterolateral wall is related to the face in the somewhat concave region of bone lateral to the incisive fossa. The posterior wall of the sinus is related to the infratemporal fossa or pterygoid region, where it is in contact with the buccal pad of fat and the posterior superior dental nerves. The infraorbital branch of the maxillary nerve traverses the roof of the sinus in a thin-walled or partly dehiscent canal. The nerve gives off the middle and anterior superior dental nerves within the roof of the sinus

which then descend along its anterolateral wall, supply the mucoperiostium of the sinus, and innervate the upper teeth. The maxillary nerve emerges from the anterior wall of the sinus as the infraorbital nerve (Fig. 6). The lower part of the anterolateral wall of the sinus is covered by the mucous membrane of the vestibule of the mouth, through which it may be drained, as in the Caldwell-Luc procedure.

The base of the maxillary sinus, which faces into the nasal cavity, is the most complex and also the most important surgically. When the isolated maxilla is examined (Fig. 14 *A*), the opening or ostium of the maxillary sinus is seen to be large and involves almost all the nasal surface of the bone. This large opening is filled in by a series of bones which, along with the overlying mucous membrane, reduce the definitive opening to a small hole. The lacrimal occludes it anteriorly and articulates inferiorly with the inferior concha. The inferior concha, which is a bone in its own right, fills in the lower part of the sinus. Its articulation with the lacrimal bone completes a bony canal through which the nasolacrimal duct discharges into the inferior meatus of the nose. The vertical

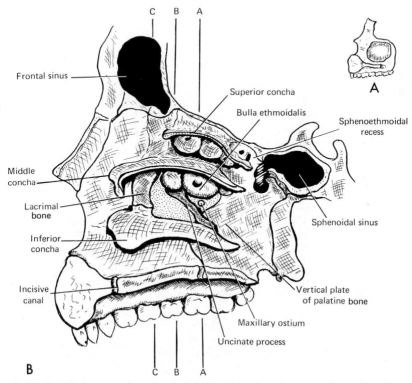

Figure 14. Lateral wall of the nasal cavity of the adult. The three conchae or turbinates have been removed to show the bony structures which form the lateral wall and almost completely occlude the large ostium in the maxilla. The very extensive ostium of the dry maxilla (*A*) is filled in by the bones illustrated in *B*.

plate of the palatine bone occludes the ostium posteriorly. It articulates anteriorly with the inferior concha and above with the ethmoid and the base of the sphenoid. The ethmoid bone occludes the upper part of the maxillary ostium and is hollowed out by air cells. A slender uncinate process springs from the anterior part of the ethmoidal labyrinth and articulates inferiorly and posteriorly with the inferior concha. These relationships are shown in Figure 14 *B*, in which the nasal wall of the sinus has been exposed by removal of the conchae. A prominent middle ethmoidal sinus, the bulla ethmoidalis, bulges into the middle meatus above the uncinate process. The entire nasal surface of the sinus with its accompanying bones is overlaid with mucous membrane except for a small hole, the definitive maxillary ostium, which lies immediately below the bulla and above the uncinate process (Fig. 14 *B*). The curving space between the uncinate process and the bulla is the hiatus semilunaris, into which the definitive maxillary ostium opens. The frontal sinus opens anteriorly into the hiatus semilunaris under cover of the anterior group of ethmoidal cells. The ethmoidal air cells are variable in number and disposition but

are generally disposed of in three overlapping groups: an anterior, middle, and posterior group. The anterior group open into the hiatus semilunaris separately or with the frontal air sinus. The middle group, of which the bulla ethmoidalis is one, open into the middle meatus above the uncinate process. The posterior group open into the superior meatus between the superior and middle conchae (Fig. 14 *B*) or, rarely, into the spheno-ethmoidal recess.

A series of sections through the maxillary sinus and adjacent parts of the nose along the planes A, B, and C (Fig. 14 *B*) may clarify the complex anatomical interrelationships of the air sinuses. In Figure 15 *A* the section passes through the maxillary ostium. The mucosa is shown in dotted lines. Note that as the mucosa of the middle meatus is traced into the sinus, it passes over the uncinate process and forms a recess of sulcus on the lateral side of the process before ascending again to enter the sinus. This recess or cul-de-sac is the floor of the hiatus semilunaris which appears from the medial surface of the nasal cavity as a curving slit between the uncinate process and the bulla ethmoidalis (Fig. 14 *B*). In order to enlarge the maxillary ostium surgically it is necessary to

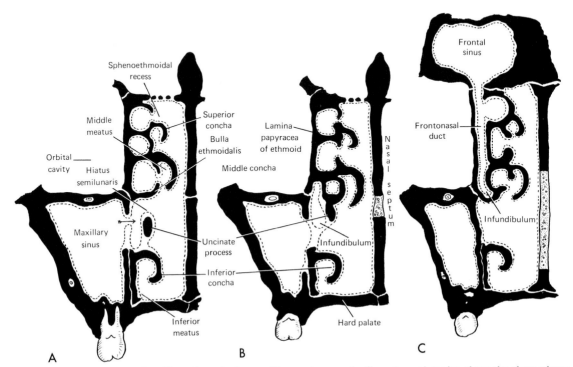

Figure 15.   Three coronal sections through the maxillary antrum and adjacent nasal cavity along the three planes indicated in Figure 14 *B*. The arrow in *A* indicates the maxillary ostium opening into the hiatus semilunaris. The infundibulum (*B*) receives the frontonasal duct in *C*.

break the uncinate process of the ethmoid and also to enlarge the ostium, which is purely mucosal, lateral to the uncinate process. In this way adequate drainage can be established.

In the second section (Fig. 15 *B*) anterior to the first (see Figure 14 *B* for plane of sections A, B, and C), the uncinate process is fused anteriorly with the bulk of the ethmoid. This fusion, plus the disappearance of the maxillary ostium at this level, converts the mucosal recess or cul-de-sac into a channel, the infundibulum. In the third section (Fig. 15 *C*), anterior to B, the infundibulum is shown receiving the frontonasal duct or duct of the frontal air sinus. In about 50 per cent of the population the frontal air sinus opens directly into an infundibulum. In the remaining 50 per cent it opens into the anterior ethmoidal cells before opening into the hiatus semilunaris.

The premolar, molar, and sometimes the canine teeth lie in the floor of the maxillary sinus. The roots of the teeth may be covered by an extremely thin shell of bone, and infection of the sinus from infected roots is not uncommon. Infection originating in the sinus may extend through the thin roof, setting up serious intraorbital infection. Spread of infection from the sinus backward into the infratemporal fossa, though rare, is possible and is one way in which the lateropharyngeal deep space may become infected, as well as from an infected last molar tooth.

Frontal Sinuses

The drainage of this sinus and its relationship to the other paranasal sinuses has been described (Fig. 15). The sinus is usually asymmetrical, extending for considerable distances into the orbital plates, as well as superiorly and laterally into the diploë of the frontal bones. It is frequently loculated. The important relationships of the sinus are anteriorly the skin of the forehead, inferiorly the orbit and roof of the nasal cavity, and posteriorly the anterior cranial fossa with its contents (frontal lobe, olfactory tracts, meninges). Also posteriorly are the falx cerebri and the superior and inferior sagittal sinuses contained within its attached and free borders, respectively. These sinuses receive venous tributaries from the diploë and from the bone around the frontal sinus, constituting pathways of infection. Direct infection of the sinus is most common following a crushing injury of the forehead, and there may be extension to the frontal lobe and the meninges.

Sphenoidal Sinuses

The sphenoidal sinuses are deeply situated. Their relationships are complicated and can occasion important clinical signs when the sinuses are infected. The two sinuses open anteriorly into the spheno-ethmoidal recess above the superior concha (Fig. 14 *B*). The large opening of the sinus in the base of the sphenoid on either side is partially enveloped by a scroll-like bone, the sphenoidal concha or turbinate (bones of Bertin). The bone resembles a small trumpet with its long axis lying anteroposteriorly. The opening of the trumpet is anterior and opens into the spheno-ethmoidal recess.

The anatomical relationships of the sinuses are considered in sections at two levels of the skull in Figures 16 and 17.

The first section is at the level of the superior orbital fissure and optical foramen (Fig. 16). Immediately lateral to the sinus on either side, separated from them by bone of variable thickness, are the optic foramina containing the optic nerve and the ophthalmic artery, also the superior orbtal fissure and its contents. The medial part of the fissure contains the superior ophthalmic vein and four components of the cranial nerves: the superior branch of the oculomotor nerve, the nasociliary nerve, and inferior branch of the oculomotor nerve, and the abducens or sixth cranial nerve. These nerves, the vein, and the contents of the optic foramen are encircled by a fibrous ligament, the annulus tendineus or annulus of Zinn. This gives origin to the extrinsic ocular muscles, which thus arise in the form of a cone at the apex of the orbit. These structures enter the orbit within the cone of muscles. More laterally placed structures which enter the orbit outside the muscle cone are the lacrimal nerve, the frontal nerve, and the trochlear or fourth nerve. Lateral spread of infection from the sinus may involve the optic nerve and its coverings or meninges. It may involve the superior ophthalmic vein, possibly leading to retrograde thrombosis of the cavernous sinus. It may cause irritation of the nerves within the medial end of the superior orbital fissure. Irritation of the abducens nerve leads to spasm of the lateral rectus muscle. Irritation of the superior and inferior branches of the oculomotor causes spasm of the muscles supplied (superior rectus, levator palpebrae superioris, medial rectus, inferior rectus, inferior oblique). Retro-orbital pain and pain in the eye may be caused by irritation of the nasociliary nerve. Autonomic

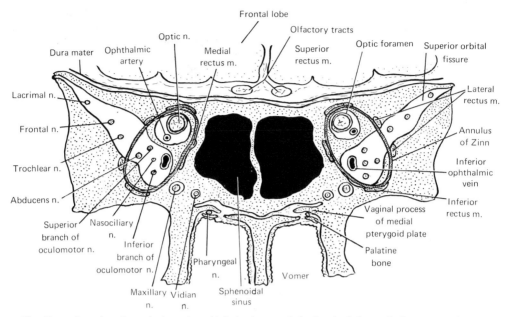

Figure 16. Frontal section through the sphenoidal air sinus and the level of the optic foramen and superior orbital fissure.

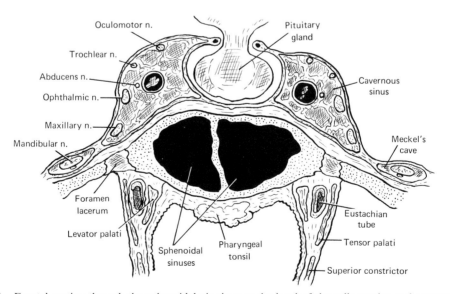

Figure 17. Frontal section through the sphenoidal air sinus at the level of the sella turcica and cavernous sinus.

effects may also ensue since this nerve carries parasympathetic fibers through the ciliary ganglion to the sphincter pupillae and ciliary muscle.

The sphenoidal sinuses are related above to the anterior cranial fossa in the region of the jugum sphenoidale. Here they are related to the orbital surfaces of the frontal bones and the olfactory tracts. Inferiorly the sphenoidal sinuses are related to the roof of the nasal cavities and to the nasopharynx behind them. The small pharyngeal nerve, a branch of the sphenopalatine ganglion, lies below the sinus in a small canal formed by the apposition of the vaginal process of the medial pterygoid plate and the sphenoidal process of the palatine bone (Fig. 16). The nerve carries secretomotor fibers from the vidian nerve to the region around the eustachian tube and lateral recess of the nasopharynx. It also carries sensory fibers to the maxillary nerve via the sphenopalatine ganglion. It may serve as a trigger for trigeminal neuralgia. Inferolateral to the sinus is the canal for the maxillary nerve and inferiorly is the pterygoid or vidian canal.

On a more posterior plane the sphenoidal sinuses have important relationships to the cavernous sinus and adjacent parts of the middle cranial fossa (Fig. 17). The sinuses are separated above on either side by a thin plate of bone from the sella turcica containing the dura mater and the pituitary gland. At one time the pituitary was approached surgically through the roof of the nasopharynx by a trans-sphenoidal route. Above and laterally the sinuses are related to the cavernous sinuses. The cavernous sinuses are traversed by the internal carotid arteries. The abducens nerve on either side lies lateral to the internal carotid artery within the cavernous sinus. In the lateral wall of the cavernous sinus, from above down, are: the oculomotor nerve, the trochlear nerve, the ophthalmic nerve, and the maxillary nerve. The mandibular nerves are situated more laterally and are not in immediate relationship with the cavernous sinus or the sphenoidal air sinus.

The sphenoidal sinuses are related inferiorly to the roof of the nasopharynx and the pharyngeal tonsils. The section (Fig. 17) passes through the lateral recess of the pharynx or fossa of Rosenmüller and shows the attachment of the eustachian apparatus at the base of the skull. The eustachian tube lies immediately below the foramen lacerum at the level of this section; further laterally the tube lies obliquely in the petrosphenoidal suture.

THE ANATOMY OF THE EAR

The ear is a complex sensory organ of triple origin. The phylogenetically most ancient part of it is the stato-acoustic organ within the cartilaginous otic capsule. The cochlea and ossicular apparatus are phylogenetically more recent and are evolved as modifications of the first and second branchial arch cartilages. The cochlea is also recent and shows a parallel evolution with that of the middle ear and ossicular chain. The middle ear is developmentally an air sinus and develops as an outgrowth of the pharynx. The ossicular chain is developed from the upper ends of the first (mandibular) and second (hyoid) cartilages. The original function of the mandibular cartilage in the support of the lower jaw is taken over during evolution by a new dermal bone, the mandible. The external ear is a modification of the surface ectoderm by which the skin is brought into functional relationship with the ossicles at the drum, and the external canal is modified for protection and for the reception and concentration of sound.

Development of the Ear

The arrangement of the pharyngeal (branchial) arches in the floor of the mouth in young embryos of about 4 mm. is shown in Figure 15, Chapter 2. At a somewhat later stage (Fig. 18) the tubotympanic recess is demarcated from the midline structures by the lateral expansion of the pharyngeal lumen opposite the first, second, and third arches. The tubotympanic recess is partially constricted medially by the forward migration of the third arch into the base of the tongue (see arrows in Figure 18).

The tubotympanic recess forms an expanded cavity which contains the lateral extensions of the first, second, and third arches as well as the intervening endodermal pouches (first and second). The lateral part of the tubotympanic recess becomes the middle ear and the connecting passage between it and the midline structures of the pharynx becomes the pharyngotympanic or eustachian tube. Since the third arch bounds the eustachian tube posteriorly, the artery of this arch (the internal carotid) comes to lie posterior to the tube in the adult. The artery then passes forward above the tube as the forward continuation of the dorsal aorta (see Fig. 8, Chap. 2).

The external auditory meatus develops as

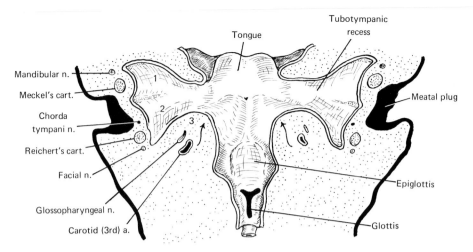

Figure 18. Floor of the pharynx of an embryo showing the formation of the tubotympanic recess. The recess arises as a lateral expansion of the pharyngeal lumen at the level of the first three internal pharyngeal grooves and pouches. The external auditory meatus is shown as a solid "meatal plug" of ectoderm growing deeply into the mesoderm from the upper end of the first external pharyngeal groove to make contact with the tubotympanic recess, the "drum" being formed at the area of contact.

a thickening of the ectoderm at the upper end of the second external pharyngeal cleft (see Fig. 5). The floor of the groove sinks into the underlying mesoderm as a cylindrical meatal plug (Fig. 18) which becomes applied to the lateral wall and floor of the expanded end of the tubotympanic recess. Contact with the tubotympanic recess is made in such a way that when the drum is formed at the interface between the ectodermal and endodermal surfaces it lies obliquely, and such that the roof and anterior wall of the external auditory canal are shorter than the floor and posterior wall. The ectodermal meatal plug then hollows out to form a canal in which hair follicles and ceruminous glands develop. The "drum area" or tympanic membrane is the circular area of contact between the meatal plug and the endoderm of the tubotympanic recess.

Further Development of the Tubotympanic Recess, Otic Capsule and Cartilages of the First Two Arches

The otic capsule is the cartilaginous mass which encloses the inner ear and which later forms the petrous temporal bone. It lies above the lateral extremity of the tubotympanic recess, as shown in Figure 19 *A*. The cartilage of the first arch (Meckel's cartilage) lies anterior to the tubotympanic recess; the cartilage of the second arch (Reichert's cartilage) lies behind it. The two cartilages soon become joined by fibrous, later cartilaginous, condensations or roof processes above the tubotympanic recess, between it and the overlying otic capsule (Fig. 19 *A*). The roof processes differentiate into the body of the malleus and incus. Later processes of the two ossicles form the long and short process of the incus and also the anterior and inferior process (handle) of the malleus. The handle of the malleus projects downward lateral to the tubotympanic recess and is later trapped between it and the meatal plug (Fig. 18).

The tegmen tympani is formed as a flange growing out from the otic capsule and passing above and anterior to the tubotympanic recess (Fig. 19 *B*). It forms the roof and anterior bony wall of the tubotympanic recess. The mandibular cartilage escapes under the free edge of the tegmen tympani (Fig. 19 *B*) to enter the lower jaw. In a later stage (Fig. 19 *C*) the otic capsule and the tegmen tympani become overlaid laterally by a sheet of membrane or dermal bone, the squamous temporal bone. The squamous temporal bone eventually overgrows the petrous temporal bone except for the mastoid process and free edge of the tegmen tympani in relation to the floor of the temporomandibular fossa (Fig. 19 *C* and *D*). The upper part of Meckel's cartilage, as mentioned, forms the malleus and the incus with their various bony processes. The rest of Meckel's cartilage becomes transformed into the anterior ligament of the malleus and the sphenomandibular ligament (Figs. 19 *D* and 20).

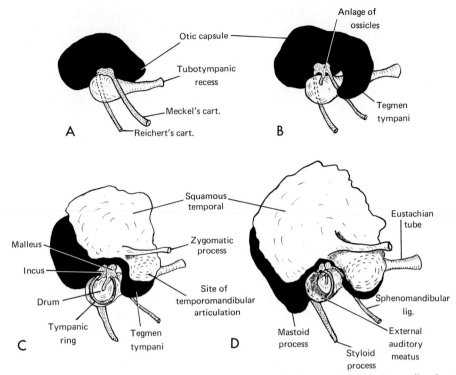

Figure 19. Four stages in the development of the middle ear. In *A* the otic capsule (in black) overlies the tubotympanic recess. In *B* the tegmen tympani is formed anterior to the recess as a flange. In *C* the squamous temporal bone is formed in membrane and overlaps the otic capsule and middle ear laterally and inferiorly; the temporomandibular joint is formed in relation to it. In *D* the external bony meatus is formed as a lateral extension of the tympanic ring.

The tympanic ring is formed in membrane around the drum where the meatal plug and the tubotympanic recess are in contact. At birth (Fig. 19 *C*) the ring is present but has not as yet become elongated into a definite bony meatus. As a result, the drum is very superficial in a baby and is easily injured by forceps or instrumental examination. The mastoid process is also absent at birth so that the facial nerve emerging from the stylomastoid canal is superficial and easily injured by the use of obstetrical forceps. The tympanic ring extends after birth by further intramembranous ossification. The new bone is added laterally so that a bony meatus is developed, the drum being at its medial or deep end (Fig. 19 *D*). As the bony

Figure 20. Section through the adult middle ear showing the structures developed from the otic capsule (petrous temporal bone, in black), the membranous bones (tympanic ring, squamous temporal), and the derivatives of Meckel's cartilage (sphenomandibular ligament), and of Reichert's cartilage (styloid process).

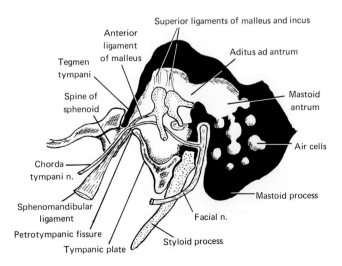

external auditory meatus is established, the formation of the temporomandibular fossa and its complex fissures is also complete (Fig. 20). The fissure (glaserian fissure) which lies in the floor of the temporomandibular fossa is compound. Laterally it lies between the squamous temporal and the tympanic bone (squamotympanic fissure). Medially the squamotympanic fissure is subdivided by the interpolation of the free edge of the tegmen tympani (now a portion of the petrous temporal bone, shown in black in Figure 19). The fissure thus becomes the petrosquamous fissure anteriorly and the petrotympanic fissure posteriorly. From the fact of the development of the tegmen tympani, it can be seen that any structure escaping from the middle ear (e.g., Meckel's cartilage, chorda tympani nerve) must leave under cover of the tegmen tympani, that is through the petrotympanic fissure (Fig. 21). The capsule of the temporomandibular joint is attached along the glaserian fissure. The fossa posterior to this is occupied by a process of the parotid gland and also contains the auriculotemporal nerve in close apposition to the capsule of the joint (Fig. 23, Chap. 2).

The second arch cartilage (Reichert's) gives rise to the styloid process, the stylohyoid ligament, the lesser cornu bone and the upper part of the body of the hyoid bone (Fig. 19). The stapes may be derived from the condensation at the upper end of Reichert's cartilage. There is evidence that the stapes ossifies in connection with the otic capsule. The form of the stapes is determined by the passage of the stapedial artery through the preosseous condensation of the ossicle. This vessel may represent the upper end of the second pharyngeal arch artery (Fig. 8, Chap. 2). It may persist and cause hemorrhage in operations on the middle ear.

Development of the Drum

The tympanic membrane or drum develops at the area of contact between the ectodermal meatal plug and the endodermal tubotympanic recess (Figs. 18 and 22 A). The contact is oblique so that the drum lies obliquely with respect to the axis of the external meatus. The chorda tympani nerve, the handle of the stapes, and a layer of mesoderm are trapped between the meatal plug and the tubotympanic recess (Fig. 22 A). Thus, the drum consists of three layers: an outer ectodermal layer continuous with the skin of the external auditory meatus, an intermediate mesodermal layer containing the handle of the malleus and the chorda tympani nerve, and an inner endodermal layer continuous with the mucous membrane of the middle ear. The nerve supply of the drum reflects its origin. The ectodermal (outer) surface is supplied by the auriculotemporal branch of the trigeminal nerve and by the auricular branch of the vagus (Arnold's) nerve posteriorly. The last nerve is of interest in that it is the only somatic afferent branch of the vagus nerve. It may represent the last remnant of a once extensive system in lower vertebrates, including the lateral line system of fish. The same nerves that supply the drum also supply the external auditory meatus. Irritation of the auricular branch of the vagus nerve may cause reflex coughing or vomiting (hence its former name, the "alderman's nerve"). Foreign bodies in the ear may, therefore, simulate thoracic conditions, and syringing of the external ear in old patients may cause fatal syncope. The afferent connections of the auricular branch of the vagus are uncertain; there is evidence that they pass to the nucleus of the spinal tract of the trigeminal nerve.

Postnatal Developments in the Ear

At birth the ear is essentially as depicted in Figure 19 C. The four elements of the temporal bone are easily distinguished: the petrous (including the tegmen tympani), the squamous

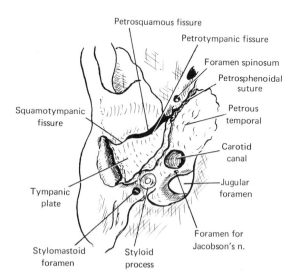

Figure 21. Base of the adult skull in the region of the temporomandibular fossa. The tegmen tympani interpolates itself between the squamous temporal bone and the tympanic plate (ring), forming the petrosquamous fissure anteriorly and the petrotympanic fissure posteriorly.

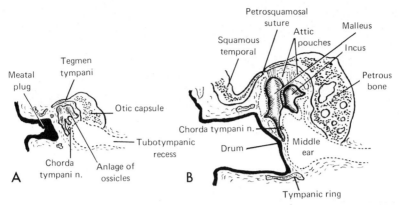

Figure 22. Two longitudinal sections of the external and middle ear showing the progressive dorsal extension of the mesenchyme ("epitympanic tissue") by which the attic recesses are formed and the ossicles become surrounded by mucous membrane.

temporal bone, the tympanic ring, and the styloid process. The mastoid antrum is present as a posterior extension of the middle ear, but there is no mastoid process. The mastoid process does not form a definite prominence until the end of the second year, and the mastoid air cells follow soon after. The tympanic ring extends laterally after birth, forming the bony canal. The temporomandibular fossa is small and faces more laterally at birth; thereafter it becomes deeper and faces more ventrally. Ossification of the petrous temporal is complex and from multiple centers. Being phylogenetically ancient, the petrous bone (otic capsule) rarely shows developmental abnormalities. At birth the middle ear cavity does not extend beyond about the origin of the handle of the malleus from the body (Fig. 19 A). Above this level the epitympanic recess or attic is occupied by gelatinous mesenchymatous material or epitympanic tissue. This tissue is very susceptible to infection and may also impede the movement of the ossicles at first. There is a progressive extension of the middle ear cavity during the first year at the expense of this epitympanic tissue (Fig. 19 B). This extension takes place by a process of cavitation and differentiation so that the cavity extends dorsally to envelop the ossicles completely. When this extension is complete, the attic region forms a complicated labyrinth of mucosal spaces and recesses (e.g., pouches of Tröltsch, pouch of Prussak). The ossicles develop outside the tympanic cavity. They are extramucosal but are secondarily incorporated into the tympanic cavity by the formation of the attic recesses. The superior ligaments of the malleus and the incus are the remnants of the original epitympanic tissue in which the ossicles were once embedded. The secondary mucosal extension also takes place around the stapes,

the tendons of the stapedius and of the tensor tympani muscles and all other intratympanic structures so that these also are extramucosal, though technically they are within the middle ear cavity.

Development of the Inner Ear

The inner ear is developed as a thickening or placode of the ectoderm on the lateral surface of the head at the level of the fourth ventricle in embryos of 4 mm. (Fig. 23 A). The placode then sinks in, forming first a pit, then a vesicle cut off from the surface (Fig. 23 B and C). The vesicle or otocyst then gives off a diverticulum from its dorsal surface, the endolymphatic duct in embryos of 6 mm. (Fig. 23 C and D). The semicircular canals appear in embryos of 15 mm. and 37 days (Fig. 23 D) as flanges sticking out from the surface of the otocyst. The walls of the flanges then come into contact centrally where they break down, giving rise to canals which are well developed by the 30 mm. stage (Fig. 23 E). The cochlea appears in the 15 mm. stage (Fig. 23 D) as a diverticulum at the lower pole of the otocyst. It coils progressively, finally attaining two and three quarter turns by the end of the embryonic period (end of third month). The otocyst becomes constricted at its middle between the part bearing the semicircular canals and that bearing the cochlea, forming the utricle and the saccule (Fig. 23 F). The endolymphatic duct becomes shifted down by differential growth onto the connection between the utricle and the saccule, so that it is ultimately attached to the utriculosaccular duct.

Statoreceptors (maculae) are developed by differentiation of the ectodermal epithelium lining the utricle and saccule. Similar receptors

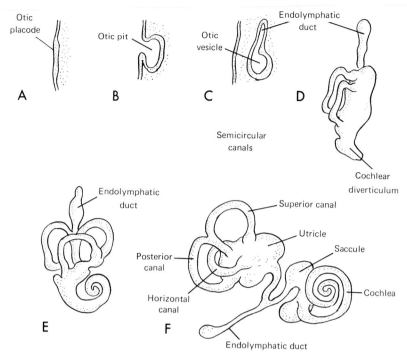

Figure 23. Stages in the development of the otocyst: *A* as an ectodermal placode; *B* as a pit; *C* as an elongated vesicle isolated from the surface ectoderm. From *D* to *F* are illustrated the events leading to the formation of the membranous labyrinth. (Modified from Streeter.)

(cristae) are developed in the ampullae of the semicircular canals and respond to motion. The organ of Corti differentiates in the wall of the cochlear duct throughout its length. The neurons of the vestibular and cochlear ganglia develop by proliferation from the walls of the otocyst and its subdivisions. The manner of origin of these neurons resembles the origin of the dorsal root ganglion cells from the neural crest. For this reason the ectoderm which gives rise to the otocyst is referred to as the presumptive neural crest. The vestibular ganglion cells remain close to the saccule and utricle, and peripheral fibers grow into the ampullae and into the maculae of the utricle and saccule to make synaptic contact with the sensory receptors there. The ganglion cells of the cochlear system (spiral ganglion) become arranged along the length of the cochlear spiral. Peripheral processes of the cells enter into synaptic contact with the sensory cells of Corti's organ.

Central Connections of the Vestibular and Cochlear Ganglia

Central fibers of the vestibular and cochlear ganglia grow toward the brain stem and enter it at the lower border of the pons, later the cerebellopontine angle. There are four vestibular nuclei: superior, lateral (Deiter's), medial, and inferior, which is continuous with the spinal vestibular nucleus. Connections of the vestibular nuclei are with the cerebellum, especially the flocculonodular lobe and with the anterior horn cells of the spinal cord through the vestibulospinal tract. A longitudinal system of fibers on either side of the midline throughout the brain stem, the medial longitudinal fasciculus, receives many secondary vestibular fibers from the same and the opposite side. The function of the medial longitudinal fasciculus is to unite the nuclei of the cranial nerves supplying the muscles of the eye (third, fourth, and sixth) with the vestibular nuclei, and lower down with the anterior horn cells of the upper part of the spinal cord. Complicated reflexes involving eye, ear, neck, and trunk functions are thus coordinated. Examples are the so-called neck and body righting reflexes of Magnus and Levi. When a cat is dropped upside down, the eyes are first leveled, then the head, followed by the neck and the trunk, so that the animal lands on all fours. Destruction of the optic pathways and of the vestibular pathways impairs these reflexes, leaving only proprioceptive impulses from the neck and trunk to allow the animal to orient itself in space.

The central cochlear fibers make synaptic contact with the dorsal and ventral cochlear nuclei, above and below the inferior cerebellar peduncle (restiform body), respectively. The secondary fibers of the ventral cochlear nucleus pass to the opposite side, forming an ovoid mass of fibers or trapezoid body. They then turn cranially as the lateral lemniscus, which is the central auditory pathway in the brain stem. The dorsal cochlear fibers sweep across the floor of the fourth ventricle as the striae acousticae and sink into the gray matter to join the lateral lemniscus of the opposite side. The lateral lemniscus enters the inferior colliculus in the midbrain and has secondary synaptic connections there. The third order fibers pass to the medial geniculate body via the inferior quadrigeminal brachium and have another synapse in this body. Fibers of the fourth order then pass through the sublenticular part of the internal capsule to reach the auditory projection area on the temporal lobe of the brain (margin of the superior temporal gyrus and floor of the sylvian fissure).

Nerve Supply of the Ear

The nerve supply of the ear and related parts is illustrated in the fetus in Figure 24. The trigeminal ganglion and its three branches lie anterior to the otic capsule (petrous temporal). Associated with each branch are parasympathetic ganglia: the ciliary, the sphenopalatine, the otic, and the submandibular. The facial nerve is caught up in the chondrification of the otic capsule and so lies in a canal within its substance. The nerve has a sharp bend immediately dorsal to the middle ear at the level of the geniculate ganglion. This ganglion is analogous to a dorsal root ganglion and contains the cell bodies of all the visceral afferents in the facial nerve. From the ganglion at this level emerges the greater superficial petrosal nerve, a parasympathetic secretomotor nerve arising in the visceral efferent column of the brain stem (superior salivatory nucleus). Its fibers pass through a canal in the otic capsule and emerge on its anterior surface deep to the mandibular branch of the trigeminal nerve. They then enter the upper part of the foramen lacerum, without actually traversing it, and are joined by sym-

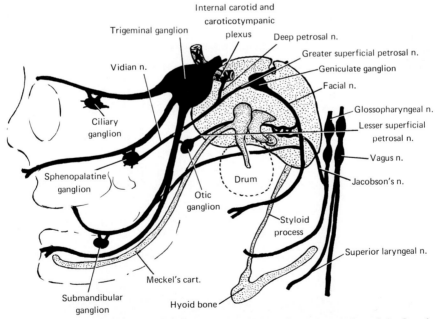

Figure 24. Diagram of the cranial nerves in immediate relationship to the otic capsule and the first three branchial arch derivatives. Parasympathetic ganglia are associated with each of the branches of the trigeminal nerve: ciliary with the ophthalmic, sphenopalatine with the maxillary, otic and submandibular with the mandibular branch. Note also the greater superficial petrosal joining with the deep petrosal to form the vidian nerve, and also the chorda tympani and the lesser superficial petrosal nerves.

pathetic filaments (deep petrosal nerve) from the caroticosympathetic plexus on the internal carotid artery. The two groups of fibers constitute the nerve of the pterygoid canal (vidian nerve) which passes forward to the sphenopalatine ganglion (Fig. 24). The subsequent distribution of this nerve has been described.

The chorda tympani nerve arises from the facial nerve in the stylomastoid canal about half a centimeter before its exit (Fig. 21). The nerve is visceral. It carries sensory fibers of taste from the anterior two thirds of the tongue and also secretomotor fibers to the submandibular and sublingual glands. The latter arise in the visceral efferent column (superior salivatory nucleus) of the brain stem. The nerve crosses the tympanic membrane lying between the mucous membrane of the middle ear and the handle of the malleus. It leaves the middle ear under cover of the free edge of the tegmen tympani through the petrotympanic fissure (Fig. 21). It then grooves the spine of the sphenoid and descends with the sphenomandibular ligament. It joins the lingual nerve and is distributed by it to the tongue and the submandibular and sublingual glands.

The glossopharyngeal and vagus nerves lie behind the otic capsule in the jugular foramen.

Each has two sensory ganglia. The tympanic branch of the glossopharyngeal (Jacobson's) nerve arises from the ninth nerve soon after its exit from the jugular foramen and immediately re-enters the skull through a small canaliculus on the bony ridge between the carotid canal and the jugular foramen (Fig. 20). It enters the middle ear and forms a plexus on the promontory (tympanic plexus). Here it receives fibers from the facial nerve and passes forward as the lesser superficial petrosal nerve (Fig. 24). It emerges on the anterior wall of the petrous temporal bone and leaves the skull either through the foramen ovale or through a small hole behind it (canaliculus innominatus). It then enters the otic ganglion where synaptic connections are made. Postganglionic fibers are distributed to the parotid via the auriculotemporal nerve. The tympanic branch of the glossopharyngeal is the main sensory nerve to the middle ear and outer part of the eustachian tube and also supplies parasympathetic fibers to the mucous membrane.

The nerve supply of the external ear has been described; it is somatic since the external meatus is of ectodermal origin.

Further amplification of the embryology and anatomy of the ear is found in Chapter 1.

Chapter 4

EMBRYOLOGY AND ANATOMY OF THE LARYNX, RESPIRATORY APPARATUS, DIAPHRAGM AND ESOPHAGUS

by Jack Davies, M.D.

As shown in Chapter 2, the embryonic fore-gut is derived from the anterior part of the yolk sac. It extends anteriorly from the buccopharyngeal membrane and caudally as far as the origin of the liver, the future site of the common bile duct (Fig. 1). The respiratory apparatus (larynx, trachea, lungs) arise as an outgrowth of the ventral wall of the foregut. The rest of the foregut caudal to the pulmonary outgrowth differentiates into the esophagus, the stomach, and the duodenum as far caudally as the common bile duct.

DEVELOPMENT OF THE PULMONARY DIVERTICULUM

The pulmonary diverticulum arises in embryos of about 3 mm. (26 days) as a groove (laryngotracheal groove) in the midventral wall of the foregut immediately caudal to the last of the pharyngeal arches (Fig. 1 *A*). At this stage the groove occupies a large area of the anterior wall of the foregut. There is only a short length of foregut between the pulmonary outgrowth and the origin of the liver. The pulmonary outgrowth then grows caudally as an independent tube (trachea). It is uncertain how the tracheal tube becomes independent of the esophagus. There are two theories: One theory attributes the separation of the trachea from the esophagus to the formation of a tracheo-esophageal

septum. The other theory is that the growth and separation of the trachea is by simple growth and elongation at its distal, blind extremity. There is no proof for one or the other theory. However, the two theories must be considered in attempts to explain the development of tracheo-esophageal fistulas.

The appearance of the laryngotracheal groove and its early growth caudally as an independent tube is shown in two transverse sections, one at the point of separation and another just caudal to it (Fig. 1 *B*). It is impossible to determine by a study of serial sections whether the separation is effected by the formation of lateral folds which then fuse to form a horizontal partition, or whether the diverticulum simply grows caudally as an independent tube. However the separation is brought about, the tracheal tube soon appears as an independent blind passage opening anteriorly into the pharynx and ending caudally in the mesodermal tissues dorsal to the pericardium.

DEVELOPMENT OF THE LUNGS

The blind end of the tracheal tube divides into the main-stem bronchi (Fig. 2 *A* and *B*). Between the 7 mm. stage (28th day) and the 16 mm. stage (37th day) the secondary and tertiary bronchi are differentiated (Fig. 2 *C*, *D* and *E*). The mesoderm surrounding each sub-

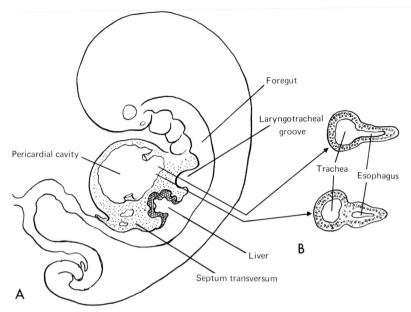

Figure 1. Schematic sagittal section of embryo of 3 mm. (26 days) showing the origin of the pulmonary outgrowth from the foregut into the mesoderm of the septum transversum dorsal to the pericardial sac (*A*). Transverse sections at two levels through the pulmonary diverticulum are shown in *B* above and below the area of separation from the foregut. (After Streeter, Developmental Horizons in Human Embryos, 1942.)

division of the bronchial tree condenses and differentiates into the supporting and vascular structures of the lung. The bronchopulmonary segments are formed by progressive division of the bronchi followed by differentiation of the mesoderm around them.

The pulmonary arteries arise as endothelial outgrowths from the caudal surface of the sixth

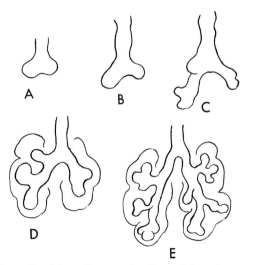

Figure 2. Schematic reconstructions of the pulmonary outgrowth up to about the 16 mm. stage (37 days, *E*). Condensations of mesenchyme around the subdivisions of the bronchial tree form the vascular and supporting framework of the lung. (After Streeter, Developmental Horizons in Human Embryos, 1948.)

pharyngeal arch arteries. They grow caudally into the lung and form the vascular plexuses within it. The pulmonary veins arise as a simple endothelial outgrowth from the posterior surface of the left atrium and join the capillary plexuses within the substance of the lungs. The single orifice of the pulmonary vein is later absorbed into the wall of the left atrium so that four pulmonary veins eventually open into this chamber.

DEVELOPMENT OF THE LARYNX

The larynx develops as a differentiation of the mesoderm surrounding the upper end of the pulmonary diverticulum. This opening, or primitive glottis (Fig. 18, Chap. 3), lies immediately caudal to the floor of the pharynx between the last (sixth) pharyngeal arches and immediately caudal to the hypobranchial eminence (Figs. 3 *A*; 15, Chap. 2; 18, Chap. 3). The primitive glottis is at first slitlike, with its axis disposed anteroposteriorly. The medial ends of the sixth arches then enlarge, forming the bilateral arytenoid swellings which encroach on the glottis, converting it into the T-shaped opening (Figs. 3 *B* and 18, Chap. 3). The horizontal component of the T-shaped glottis is bounded anteriorly by the hypobranchial eminence. This part of the hypobranchial eminence differentiates into the epiglottis (Fig.

3 *B* and *C*). Some claim that the epiglottis is formed from the medial extremities of the fourth pharyngeal arches. There is a deep cleft between the arytenoid swellings extending as far caudally as the cartilage of the sixth arch (cricoid) (Fig. 3 *C*).

The differentiation of the larynx at a slightly later stage (8 mm., 28 days) is shown in Fig. 3 *C*). The epiglottis is clearly defined. The margins of the arytenoid swellings adjoining the glottis show two additional swellings corresponding to underlying growth centers in the mesoderm; they are the cuneiform and corniculate swellings in which small cartilages are formed. The interarytenoid cleft is conspicuous at this stage. Immediately lateral to the arytenoid swellings which bound the entrance to the larynx, a depression in the pharyngeal

wall forms the pyriform sinus. It is reasonable to suppose that the ventral ends of the fourth and sixth arches here merge with the tissues around the glottis. Any remnants of the connections between the third and fourth pouches (pharyngobranchial ducts) may also be expected to open into the upper and lower regions of the pyriform sinus, respectively (Fig. 3 *C*).

In the later differentiation of the larynx there is a marked epithelial proliferation around the glottis by which the entrance is almost or completely obliterated for a short time. A small slitlike canal persists in the region of the interarytenoid cleft and communicates with the lumen of the larynx. The definitive shape of the laryngeal entrance emerges following recanalization of the epithelial fusion zone and oblit-

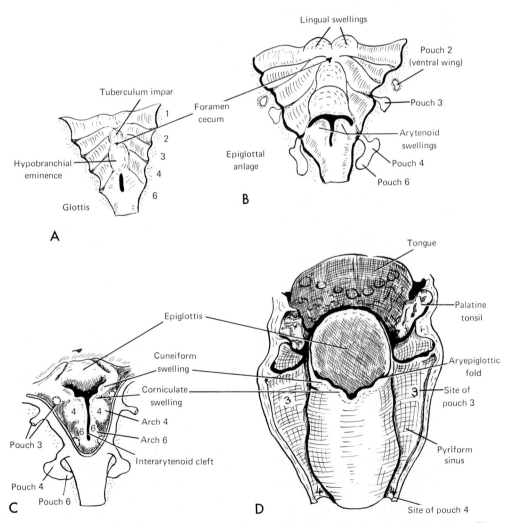

Figure 3. Developmental changes in the floor of the pharynx leading to the formation of the larynx. The numbers in (*C*) and (*D*) indicate the presumptive sites of the internal openings of the pharyngobranchial ducts.

eration of the interarytenoid cleft. The aryepiglottic folds differentiate in the margins of the arytenoid swellings and enclose the cuneiform and corniculate cartilages. The vocal cords appear as differentiations in the lateral wall of the larynx in embryos of about 20 mm. (40 days). The ventricle appears a little later as a solid epithelial bud which acquires an independent lumen by the third month. It is not a remnant of a pharyngeal pouch since it lies within the laryngotracheal diverticulum and is caudal to the arch area.

The larynx is relatively small in the fetus and only acquires its proper dimensions after birth. It is also much higher in the fetus and newborn relative to the cervical spine than in the adult. In the fifth month of fetal life the epiglottis rests upon the dorsal surface of the soft palate, a normal condition in most mammals. Descent of the pharynx is incomplete at birth and the level of the glottis is at about the disc between the second and third cervical vertebrae. In the adult the glottis lies opposite the body of the fifth cervical vertebra. The high larynx and the relative shallowness of the nasopharynx in the infant renders it peculiarly susceptible to obstruction of the nasal and laryngeal passages.

Developmental Summary of the Larynx and Congenital Abnormalities

The larynx of man is a complex organ developmentally. Its skeletal framework is derived in evolution and in individual ontogeny by modification of the pharyngeal or branchial arch cartilages now released from their former role in supporting the gill structures. The hyoid bone is derived from the second and third arch cartilages. The thyroid cartilage, to which the vocal cords become attached, is derived from the fourth arch cartilage. The cricoid cartilage is derived from the sixth arch cartilage and surrounds the upper end of the tracheal tube. The arytenoid cartilages are developed within the arytenoid swellings which are thought to be derivatives of the sixth arch. The epiglottis is developed in the posterior mesoderm of the pharyngeal floor behind the root of the tongue and contains derivatives of the hypobranchial eminence and possibly also the ventral ends of the fourth arches. The true and false vocal cords, as well as the ventricle, develop from the mucous membrane in the lateral wall of the laryngeal cavity and are not of significance in relation to the arches or the pouches. The pyriform sinus lateral to the laryngeal inlet and the

aryepiglottic folds occupies the region of the ventral ends of the fourth and sixth arches (Fig. 3 C and D). Any remnants of the third and fourth endodermal pouches must be sought in the area of the pyriform sinus and not within the larynx itself.

The interarytenoid cleft (Fig. 3 B and C) may fail to undergo secondary closure. This would account for an epithelial cleft between the arytenoid cartilages extending caudally as far as the cricoid cartilage. The epithelial fusion of the laryngeal inlet is a normal feature of the development of the larynx toward the end of the sixth week. Failure to recanalize may result in atresia of the laryngeal inlet. Congenital cysts of many kinds are also described in the larynx and may give rise to obstruction and stridor at birth. Cysts may arise within the larynx, from the ventricle or saccule, or from any part of the mucosa above and below the true vocal cords. The explanation of these is without satisfactory embryological basis. Cysts or tumors in the base of the tongue (lymphangioma, lingual thyroids, and so forth) may also overlie the larynx and give rise to obstruction at birth. Examination of the larynx by laryngoscopy can be lifesaving in cases of congenital stridor.

Nerve Supply of the Larynx

The nerve supply of the larynx is best understood in terms of the development of the larynx. The epiglottis, vallecula, and adjacent parts of the laryngopharynx are supplied by the glossopharyngeal nerve (nerve of the third arch) and by the superior laryngeal nerve (nerve of the fourth arch). These nerves subserve both common sensation and taste. The internal branch of the superior laryngeal nerve (a branch of the vagus) enters the larynx between the derivatives of the third and fourth arch, i.e., through the thyrohyoid interval (Fig. 6, Chap. 2). It then lies deep to the mucous membrane of the pyriform sinus and supplies the mucosa of the sinus and the mucous membrane of the larynx above the level of the true vocal cords. Injury to this nerve, as by invasive carcinoma, is early and painful. It may be necessary to section the nerve bilaterally at the posterior part of the thyrohyoid interval. Loss of sensation to the laryngeal inlet may lead to aspiration pneumonia. The inferior or recurrent laryngeal branch of the vagus nerve enters the larynx under cover of the fourth arch cartilage (thyroid cartilage) and supplies the mucous membrane below the vocal cords, as well as all the intrinsic muscles of the larynx. It will be recalled that the inferior laryngeal nerve turns around the ligamentum arteriosum (sixth arch) on the left and around the subclavian artery on the right (fourth left aortic arch). The fibers which supply the abductor muscles of the vocal cord (crico-arytenoideus posterior) are so placed in the nerve at this level that the abductor fibers are most susceptible to damage, i.e., are more vulnerable than the adductor fibers (Semon's law). In bilateral section of the recurrent laryngeal nerve the vocal cords lie in the "cadaveric position," totally relaxed and abducted. The inferior laryngeal nerves enter the larynx posterior to the cricothyroid joint. Here they may be involved in arthritis of the joint, giving rise to pain and spasm of the vocal cords. The cricothyroid muscle, which is a tensor of the vocal cords, is supplied by the small external branch of the superior laryngeal nerve. This nerve descends in close proximity to the superior thyroid artery and may be cut during thyroidectomy. Reference was made in Chapter 2 to the nonrecurrence of the inferior laryngeal nerve associated with a retro-esophageal right subclavian artery.

DEVELOPMENT OF THE PLEURAL CAVITIES AND DIAPHRAGM

As described in Chapter 2, the pericardioperitoneal canals develop as cleavage spaces within the intra-embryonic mesoderm and are connected anteriorly with the pericardium and posteriorly with the peritoneal cavity. Following the formation of the head and tail folds, the canals lie lateral to the foregut (Fig. 4 *A*) and dorsal to the pericardium from which they arise. More posteriorly the canals lie dorsal to the septum transversum before opening out into the general peritoneal cavity. The septum transversum forms a primitive diaphragm in which lie the sinus venosus and the confluence of the great veins (ducts of Cuvier), and the phrenic nerves on either side lie in the body wall lateral to the pericardioperitoneal canals (Fig. 4 *A*) on their way to the septum transversum.

The pleural cavities are formed by extension of the pericardioperitoneal canals into the body wall. This extension, which takes place by a process of cavitation of the mesoderm, occurs in a plane *lateral* to the ducts of Cuvier and the phrenic nerves. The two pleural cavities approach each other anteriorly but do not fuse (Fig. 4 *B*). An important result of the excavation of the body wall by the pleural cavities is the formation of an inner sheet or lamina of mesoderm, the pleuropericardial membrane, enclosing the ducts of Cuvier and the phrenic nerves. It forms the fibrous pericardium of the adult which, accordingly, contains the phrenic nerves and the derivatives of the ducts of Cuvier on either side. On the right side the duct of Cuvier is transformed into the superior vena cava and on the left side into the coronary sinus, the oblique vein of the left atrium and

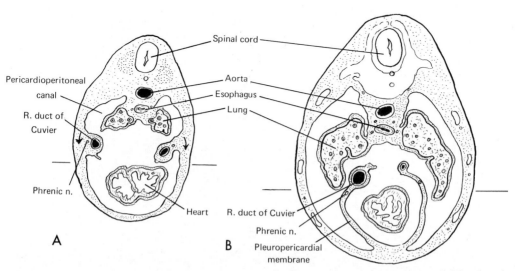

Figure 4. Two schematic transverse sections of the embryonic thorax showing the development of the pleural spaces and the formation of the definitive chest wall and fibrous pericardium. The latter, representing the mesodermal partition between the pleural spaces and the pericardial sac, contains the derivatives of the ducts of Cuvier (superior vena cava on the left) and the phrenic nerves.

the vestigial ligamentum venae cavae sinistrae. The opening from the pleural cavities to the pericardial cavity lies immediately dorsal to these structures, between them and the root of the lung (Fig. 4). The serous pericardium differentiates from the original pericardial sac formed by mesodermal cavitation in the early embryo (Chapter 2). It is made up of a mesothelial layer resting on a thin layer of mesoderm. The inner or visceral layer of the serous pericardium differentiates in relation to the surface of the heart as the epicardium; the outer or parietal layer lines the fibrous pericardium.

Following the penetration of the pleural cavities into the body wall the lungs grow into the preformed cavities (Fig. 4 *B*). In so doing they carry with them their original serous covering of visceral pleura but remain free within the pleural cavities, separated from the parietal pleura by a thin layer of fluid. The parietal and visceral pleural layers are continuous with each other at the root of the lung. Since the parietal pleura is formed by splitting of the body wall, it is a somatic structure and so is supplied by somatic (intercostal) nerves. The visceral layer applied to the lung is supplied by autonomic nerves since it is a visceral structure (splanchnopleure). The pericardial pleura differentiates from the surface of the pleuropericardial membrane; and since it is also a so-

matic structure, being once part of the body wall, it is supplied by the phrenic nerve.

A further result of the excavation of the pleural cavities on either side into the body wall is the formation between them of a septum of mesoderm containing the pericardium and heart, the median visceral column of the esophagus and trachea, and the great vessels. This septum or partition is the mediastinum of adult anatomy. The openings between the pericardium and the pleural cavities are closed at an early date by fusion of the tissues between the ducts of Cuvier and the roots of the lungs.

Development of the Diaphragm

The consequences of pleural development and the concomitant growth in width and depth of the chest itself are shown in coronal sections at two stages (Fig. 5 *A* and *B*). The ventral wall of the pericardial sac and thoracic wall is removed in each case and the embryos are viewed from the front. In *A* the pleural cavities have not yet begun to excavate the thoracic wall. The lungs lie dorsal to the ducts of Cuvier and the slitlike openings between the pericardial sac and the pleural cavities. The septum transversum or primitive diaphragm is a horizontal block of mesoderm between the pericardial sac and the peritoneal cavity. It contains the sinus venosus and also the liver.

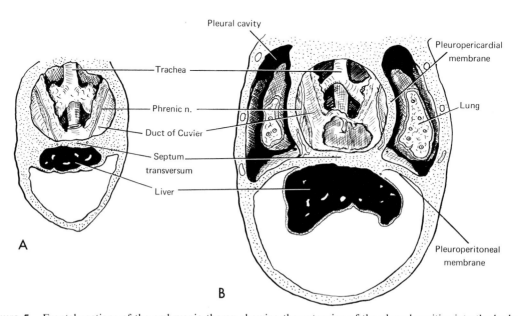

Figure 5.   Frontal sections of the embryonic thorax showing the extension of the pleural cavities into the body wall and septum transversum. The extension into the septum transversum results in the formation of a lamina of mesoderm (pleuroperitoneal membrane, *B*), which contributes to the sternocostal part of the diaphragm in the adult.

The small openings from the pleural cavities to the peritoneal cavity lie dorsally close to the vertebral column and the large adrenals. In *B* the effects of extension of the pleural cavities and the increased width of the thorax are shown. A second sheet or lamina of mesoderm, the pleuroperitoneal membrane, is delaminated from the thoracic wall and applied to the upper surface of the liver. It is attached centrally to the septum transversum. The pleuroperitoneal membrane forms the lateral or muscular leaflet of the diaphragm in the adult. Muscle differentiates within it, and it is supplied by the phrenic nerve.

The adult diaphragm is of multiple origin. The central tendon represents the septum transversum on which rests the pericardium. The lateral muscular leaflet (sternocostal part) of the diaphragm is formed from the pleuroperitoneal membranes. The crura of the diaphragm are formed by the extension of muscle into the dorsal mesentery of the foregut.

Congenital Defects of the Diaphragm

Rarely the small opening from the pleural cavity to the peritoneal cavity may persist. The opening is almost always on the left since it is thought that the pressure of the large right lobe of the liver and the adrenal may predispose the right side to early closure. The opening must be sought far posteriorly near the spinal column, between the crura and the sternocostal part of the diaphragm.

Large defects of the diaphragm may involve the sternocostal portion and must be attributed to failure of the pleuroperitoneal membrane. Abdominal contents may be herniated into the pleural cavity, again almost invariably on the left side.

A "congenitally short esophagus" may predispose to the development of hiatal hernia. The sliding hernial sac lies in relation to the esophageal hiatus and has no apparent developmental relationship to the primitive pleuroperitoneal openings or to failure of the pleuroperitoneal membrane. There is no indication that adult hiatal hernias are congenital in origin or are related to congenital shortness of the esophagus, though there may be a congenital weakness in the muscle around the esophageal hiatus.

Rare diaphragmatic defects in the region of the central tendon must be attributed to secondary breakdown of the mesoderm of the septum transversum. In this case the pericardial sac is deficient caudally and the abdominal contents are herniated into the pericardium. This condition may be associated with other extensive mesodermal defects of the anterior abdominal wall such as omphalocele.

DEVELOPMENT OF THE ESOPHAGUS

The esophagus is formed by elongation and differentiations of the foregut caudal to the pulmonary diverticulum. This part of the esophagus is very short at first and the pulmonary diverticulum or laryngotracheal groove occupies an extensive area in the ventral wall of the foregut cranial to the esophagus (Fig. 1 *A*). Elongation of the esophageal part of the foregut takes place as the trachea elongates. The manner of growth of the esophagus and the separation of the trachea from the foregut are implicated in the development of fistulous connections between the esophageal and tracheobronchial passages. The commonest type of fistula is one in which the esophagus communicates by a small hole with the lower end of the trachea close to the bifurcation (H-type of tracheo-esophageal fistula). More severe forms include those in which the esophagus is atretic distal to the bifurcation while the proximal segment of the esophagus opens into the trachea.

The genesis of these forms of tracheo-esophageal fistulas is unknown. If the separation of the trachea from the foregut involves the formation of a horizontal tracheo-esophageal septum (Fig. 1), the fistula may represent a failure of complete fusion of this septum. If, however, the trachea separates as an independent tube without the formation of a septum, the fistulous connection must be regarded as a secondary opening rather than the persistence of an existent connection. The atresia of the esophagus distal to the bifurcation may be explained on the basis of the normal epithelial hyperplasia characteristic of the esophagus shortly after the separation of the trachea. The epithelial lining completely obliterates the esophageal lumen for a time, and the lumen is slowly established by recanalization. Atresia may result from inadequate or complete failure of recanalization of the esophagus.

Chapter 5

NEUROANATOMY FOR THE OTOLARYNGOLOGIST

by Roger Boles, M.D.

CEREBROSPINAL FLUID AND ITS CIRCULATION

Cerebrospinal fluid is produced largely by the choroid plexuses. These are capillaries arranged in tufts from the tela choroidea. They are covered by a fine layer of ependymal cells. The choroid plexuses are located in each of the ventricles. Most of the cerebrospinal fluid is produced in the lateral ventricles and passes through the interventricular foramina of Monroe into the third ventricle, then via the aqueduct of Sylvius into the fourth ventricle. The fluid from the fourth ventricle can then escape into the subarachnoid space by (1) *the foramen of Magendie*, in the roof of the ventricle, to the cisterna magna, or (2) the *foramina of Luschka* into the pontine cistern. The fluid in the subarachnoid space flows upward over the cerebellum, pons, and cerebral hemispheres. It finally reaches the arachnoid villi where it is reabsorbed into the venous dural sinuses, especially the superior sagittal sinus.

BLOOD SUPPLY AND VENOUS DRAINAGE OF THE CENTRAL NERVOUS SYSTEM

Arterial Blood Supply

Brain

The main arterial blood supply to the brain is through the internal carotid arteries anteriorly and the vertebral arteries posteriorly. The *internal carotid arteries* enter the skull via the carotid canals. They cross the foramen lacerum and pass into the middle cranial fossa, ascending in the carotid grooves on either side of the sphenoid bone. The carotid is encased between dural layers in this tortuous ascension along the sphenoid bone and is also enveloped by the cavernous sinus. In this segment it gives off small branches to the hypophysis, semilunar ganglion, and the cavernous and petrosal sinuses. Occasionally it gives off an anterior meningeal branch here. Just as the internal carotid artery emerges from the cavernous sinus, it gives off the ophthalmic artery. At the level of the lateral cerebral fissure, the internal carotid divides into several branches: the anterior cerebral arteries, the middle cerebral arteries, the posterior communicating arteries, and the anterior choroidal arteries.

Anterior Cerebral Arteries. The anterior cerebral arteries course rostrally and medially to the beginning of the longitudinal fissure over the optic tract. Here, the vessels of the two sides lie close together and are joined by the important anastomotic *anterior communicating artery*. Each anterior cerebral artery then arches upward and backward in the longitudinal fissure, following the dorsum of the corpus callosum and anastomosing posteriorly with branches of the posterior cerebral artery. In its course it gives off branches to the medial aspects of the frontal and parietal lobes, the anterior perforated substance, and the corpus callosum.

Middle Cerebral Arteries. These arteries are the largest branches of the internal carotid arteries. They course laterally in the lateral cerebral fissure and then arch upward and backward over the lateral portions of the hemispheres. The medial and lateral striate arteries are given off near the origin of the middle cerebral and these penetrate the anterior perforated substance to supply the basal ganglia and internal capsule.

Posterior Communicating Arteries. The posterior communicating arteries run backward to join the cerebral branches of the vertebral-basilar system. They supply the internal capsule and thalamus.

Anterior Choroidal Arteries. These arise just below the main divisions of the internal carotid artery and pass backward to supply the choroid plexus of the lateral ventricle. In their posterior course they supply the optic tract, the hippocampus, the basal ganglia and internal capsule, the cerebral peduncle, and the lateral geniculate body.

The *vertebral arteries* enter the skull through the foramen magnum and ascend along the lateral ventral side of the medulla. They join at the rostral end of the medulla to form the *basilar artery*. Intracranially the vertebral

arteries give off the *anterior and posterior spinal arteries* and the *postero-inferior cerebellar artery*. The anterior spinal arteries join to form a single vessel which runs ventrally along the medulla and spinal cord. The posterior spinal arteries descend onto the cord along the dorsal roots of the spinal nerves. The postero-inferior cerebellar artery usually arises from the vertebrals just before they join to form the basilar artery, although they, occasionally, arise as branches of the basilar artery (Fig. 1).

The basilar artery ascends in the midline on the ventral surface of the pons and ends by dividing into the *posterior cerebral* arteries. It gives off several pontine branches, internal auditory arteries, and the antero-inferior and superior cerebellar arteries. The latter, in addition to supplying the cerebellum, also supply the superior and inferior colliculi, the pineal body, and the choroid plexus of the third ventricle. The *posterior cerebral arteries* pass laterally, and after receiving the posterior communicating artery from the internal carotid, they curve posteriorly to supply the under- and me-

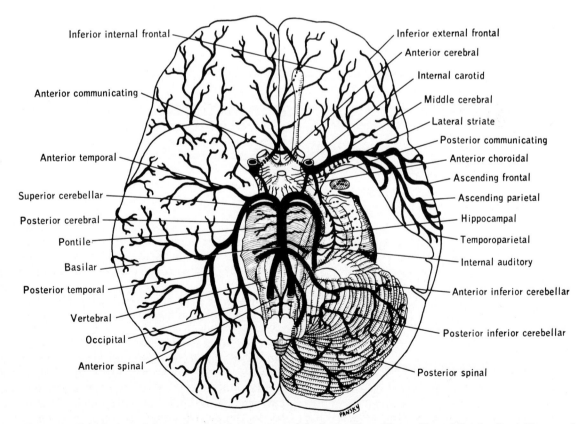

Inferior internal frontal
Anterior communicating
Anterior temporal
Superior cerebellar
Posterior cerebral
Pontile
Basilar
Posterior temporal
Vertebral
Occipital
Anterior spinal

Inferior external frontal
Anterior cerebral
Internal carotid
Middle cerebral
Lateral striate
Posterior communicating
Anterior choroidal
Ascending frontal
Ascending parietal
Hippocampal
Temporoparietal
Internal auditory
Anterior inferior cerebellar
Posterior inferior cerebellar
Posterior spinal

Figure 1. Principal arterial vessels on the basal aspect of the brain. (From House, E., and Pansky, B.: A Functional Approach to Neuroanatomy. 2nd ed. New York, McGraw Hill Book Company, Inc., 1967.)

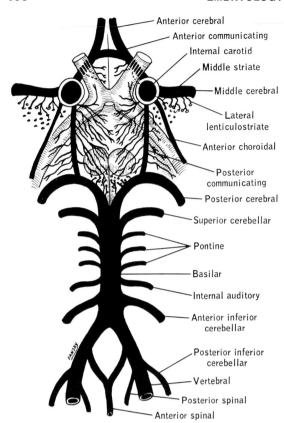

Anterior cerebral
Anterior communicating
Internal carotid
Middle striate
Middle cerebral
Lateral lenticulostriate
Anterior choroidal
Posterior communicating
Posterior cerebral
Superior cerebellar
Pontine
Basilar
Internal auditory
Anterior inferior cerebellar
Posterior inferior cerebellar
Vertebral
Posterior spinal
Anterior spinal

Figure 2. Enlargement of the central portion of Figure 1, showing some of the smaller branches in greater detail. (From House, E., and Pansky, B.: A Functional Approach to Neuroanatomy. 2nd ed. New York, McGraw-Hill Book Company., Inc., 1967.)

dial surfaces of the occipital and temporal lobes. They also give off branches to the choroid plexus (Fig. 2).

The circle of Willis is formed by the circular anastomotic pattern of internal carotid and vertebral systems. This rich anastomosis allows for excellent collateral circulation in the brain when one of the vertebrals or carotids becomes occluded.

Spinal Cord

The spinal cord is supplied by the anterior and posterior spinal arteries which, as they descend, richly anastomose with smaller spinal branches of the vertebral, intercostal, lumbar, and sacral arteries.

Meningeal Arteries

Cranial

The meninges of the posterior fossa are supplied by meningeal branches of the ascend-

ing pharyngeal, occipital, and vertebral arteries. Meninges in the middle fossa receive their blood supply from the middle and accessory meningeal arteries, both of which are branches of the internal maxillary artery. The meninges of the anterior fossa are supplied by the ethmoidal arteries from the ophthalmic branches of the internal carotid arteries.

Spinal

The same arteries which supply the cord also supply the spinal meninges.

Venous Drainage

Venous blood from both the brain and the meninges drains into the venous dural sinuses.

Superior Sagittal Sinus. This sinus begins anteriorly at the foramen cecum where it receives a branch from the nasal cavity. It courses dorsally and posteriorly in the upper border of the falx cerebri, which is attached to the roof of the cranium in the midline. Most of the time the sagittal sinus turns to the right side posteriorly at the occipital protuberance to become confluent with the transverse sinus of the right side. The sagittal sinus receives drainage from the superior cerebral veins and also from the meningeal veins. It also receives cerebrospinal fluid from the arachnoid villi and the venous lacunae.

Inferior Sagittal Sinus. The inferior sagittal sinus occupies most of the posterior portion of the inferior free margin of the falx cerebri. It ends posteriorly in the straight sinus. It receives veins from the medial surfaces of the cerebrum.

Straight Sinus. The straight sinus runs in the dural fold at the junction of the falx cerebri and the tentorium cerebelli. Posteriorly, at the occipital protuberance, it turns laterally into the transverse sinus, usually on the left side. Anteriorly it receives the great cerebral vein (of Galen). It also receives superior cerebellar veins.

Transverse or Lateral Sinuses. These run laterally from the internal occipital protuberance in the fold of tentorium cerebelli attached to the occipital bone. At the base of the temporal bone they turn downward and forward as the *sigmoid sinuses* to reach the jugular bulb at the jugular foramen. At the top part of the sigmoid sinus the jugular bulb receives the superior petrosal sinus. The jugular bulb at the lower end of the sigmoid sinus

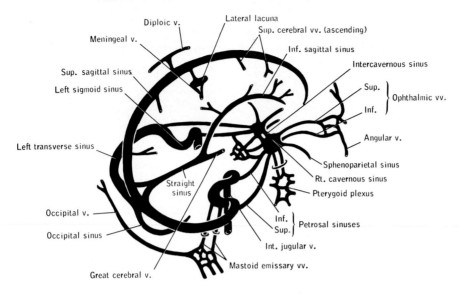

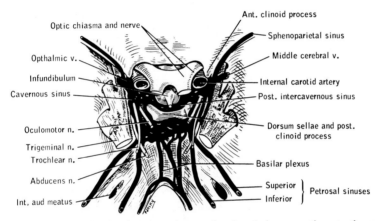

Figure 3. Upper figure, Diagram of the dural venous sinuses showing their connections to the extracranial venous system. Lower figure, Detailed diagram of the cavernous sinus showing its relations to the pituitary gland, the internal carotid artery, and cranial nerves II, III, IV, V, and VI. (From House, E., and Pansky, B.: A Functional Approach to Neuroanatomy. 2nd ed. New York, McGraw-Hill Book Company, Inc., 1967.)

receives the inferior petrosal sinus. The transverse and sigmoid sinuses also receive the inferior cerebral and cerebellar veins, the mastoid and condyloid emissary veins, and the diploic veins.

Occipital Sinus. The occipital sinus is the smallest of the sinuses and begins at the foramen magnum by the convergence of small veins and runs posteriorly and superiorly in the attached margin of the falx cerebelli. It empties into the confluence of sinuses at the internal occipital protuberance, known as the *torcular Herophili,* where the superior sagittal, straight, transverse, and occipital sinuses join. The occipital sinus receives the inferior cerebellar veins.

Cavernous Sinus. The cavernous sinus is irregular in shape and fills in the space between the body of the sphenoid bone and the dura, forming the medial boundary of the middle fossa from the superior orbital fissure to the petrous portion of the temporal bone (Fig. 3). It is broken up by trabeculae into many venous cavernous spaces; thus its name, the cavernous sinus. Within its lateral wall are incorporated the third, fourth, and first and second divisions of the fifth nerves. The sixth nerve and internal carotid artery are suspended more centrally in the sinus. The chief afferent vessels are the superior, and sometimes inferior, ophthalmic veins and some cerebral veins. The efferent channels are the superior and inferior

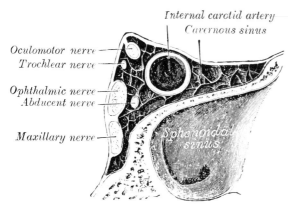

Internal carotid artery
Cavernous sinus
Oculomotor nerve
Trochlear nerve
Ophthalmic nerve
Abducent nerve
Maxillary nerve
Sphenoidal sinus

Figure 4. Oblique section through the right cavernous sinus. (From Goss, C. M. (ed.): Gray's Anatomy. 28th ed. Philadelphia, Lea & Febiger, 1967.)

petrosal sinuses and the intercavernous sinuses. The intercavernous sinus connects the two cavernous sinuses across the midline. It communicates with the pterygoid plexus by several emissary veins in the base of the skull. It consists of an anterior limb which passes in front of the hypophysis and a posterior limb behind the hypophysis (Fig. 4). Along with the two cavernous sinuses, the intercavernous sinuses form a venous circle around the hypophysis known as the *circular sinus*.

Superior Petrosal Sinuses. These leave the cavernous sinus and run posteriorly along the petrous ridge of the temporal bone in the tentorium cerebelli. They empty into the transverse sinuses as they turn downward as the sigmoid sinuses on the inner surface of the mastoid portion of the temporal bone. The superior petrosal sinus receives cerebellar and inferior cerebral veins, and also veins from the tympanic cavity.

Inferior Petrosal Sinuses. These sinuses begin in the cavernous sinuses and course caudally along the inferior petrosal sulcus formed by the junction of the petrous part of the temporal bone and the basilar part of the occipital. They end in the anterior part of the jugular bulb. They receive the internal auditory veins and also veins from the medulla, pons, and cerebellum.

Basilar Plexus. The basilar plexus consists of several interlacing channels in the dura over the clivus which interconnect the inferior petrosal sinuses and also communicate with the anterior vertebral venous plexus.

Diploic Veins

The diploic veins form venous plexuses in the diploë between the inner and outer tables of the skull and communicate intracranially with the meningeal veins and the venous dural sinuses and extracranially with the veins of the pericranium. They are drained by four main trunks on each side: frontal, anterior temporal, posterior temporal, and occipital.

Frontal. The frontal vein connects the supraorbital vein with the superior sagittal sinus.

Anterior Temporal. The anterior temporal vein anastomoses with the sphenoparietal sinus and one of the deep temporal veins through an aperture in the greater wing of the sphenoid bone.

Posterior Temporal. The posterior temporal vein ends in the transverse sinus through an aperture in the mastoid angle of the parietal bone or through the mastoid foramen.

Occipital. The occipital vein is the largest of the four and opens either externally into the occipital vein or internally into the transverse sinus or the confluence of sinuses.

Emissary Veins

Emissary veins connect the intracranial venous dural sinuses with extracranial veins through various foramina and openings in the skull. Blood can flow in either direction in these veins and they therefore constitute a major pathway for the intracranial extension of extracranial infection. The principal veins are the main emissary, the parietal emissary, the foramen ovale and foramen lacerum emissary, the internal carotid plexus, and the foramen cecum emissary.

Mastoid Emissary Vein. This vein runs through the mastoid foramen, connecting the transverse sinus with the posterior auricular or occipital veins.

Parietal Emissary Vein. The parietal emissary vein passes through the parietal foramen, connecting the veins of the scalp with the superior sagittal sinus.

Foramen Ovale and Foramen Lacerum Emissary Veins. These connect the cavernous sinus with the pterygoid plexus.

Internal Carotid Plexus of Emissary Veins. This accompanies the carotid artery in the carotid canal, connecting the cavernous sinus with the internal jugular vein.

Foramen Cecum Emissary Vein. This vein connects the superior sagittal sinus with the veins in the nose.

Other Anastomoses. There are other important anastomoses between the dural venous sinuses and extracranial veins which are not classed in the strict sense as emissary veins.

These include the superior ophthalmic and basilar plexus.

The superior ophthalmic vein. This vein connects the facial and angular veins with the cavernous sinus.

Basilar plexus. The basilar plexus connects the inferior petrosal sinuses with the vertebral veins.

Clinical Considerations of Cerebral Circulation

Intracranial Hemorrhages

Extradural or Epidural Bleeding. This type of bleeding occurs between the dura and the skull and is almost always arterial. It is usually the result of traumatic disruption of the middle meningeal artery.

Subdural Bleeding. Subdural bleeding occurs between the dura and the arachnoid, a noncommunicating space, and is predominantly venous. It is frequently caused by trauma.

Subarachnoid Hemorrhage. Subarachnoid hemorrhage occurs between the arachnoid and pia and directly contaminates the cerebrospinal fluid. It is usually arterial, involving the cerebral vessels. It may be traumatic or spontaneous, frequently from rupture of a cerebral arterial aneurysm.

Cerebral Hemorrhage. Cerebral hemorrhage is arterial bleeding within the brain substance and is usually spontaneous.

Hydrocephalus

Two general types occur.

Communicating Hydrocephalus. In this the ventricular system and subarachnoid communication are open, but the arachnoid villi and perivascular spaces become obstructed by blood, serum, or an inflammatory process and impede the resorption of cerebrospinal fluid.

Noncommunicating Hydrocephalus. In this form of hydrocephalus various portions of the ventricular system may become blocked by tumors, strictures, or other processes. The flow of cerebrospinal fluid rostral to the obstruction is impeded or totally blocked, resulting in retrograde distention of ventricular systems.

PERIPHERAL NERVOUS SYSTEM

The peripheral nervous system carries impulses between the central nervous system and the other structures of the body. It is composed of nerve fibers, ganglia, and end organs. Because of the many different functions the peripheral nervous system subserves and the many different structures it supplies, it is subdivided into the afferents and efferents of both the somatic and visceral systems of fibers. For descriptive purposes, the peripheral nerves may be further subdivided into (1) the cranial nerves (Fig. 5), (2) the spinal nerves, and (3) the autonomic nervous system.

Cranial Nerves

Olfactory Nerve

The olfactory nerve is entirely afferent and subserves exclusively the sense of smell. It consists of a number of bundles of nerve fibers which are situated in the olfactory groove of the nasal cavity and are the central processes of special neuroepithelial cells in the mucous membrane of the upper reaches of the nose. The *olfactory cells* are bipolar cells which are scattered throughout the other nonspecialized, columnar, supporting epithelium. The peripheral process of these bipolar cells extends to the surface of the epithelial membrane where it sends out a tuft of fine *olfactory hairs* beyond the surface (Fig. 6). The central process extends through the basement membrane and joins the neighboring process to create a submucosal unmyelinated plexus. These finally unite into about 20 nerves which pass through the opening in the cribriform plate as the *fila olfactoria*. These central processes terminate in the glomeruli of the olfactory bulb, synapsing here with the mitral and tufted cells. The mitral and tufted cells send their axons into the olfactory tract and end in the central olfactory areas previously described under the rhinencephalon.

Optic Nerve

This nerve of sight consists mainly of the axons of the cells in the ganglionic layer of the retina. These converge toward the optic disc where they then gather into bundles and pierce the choroid and scleral coats through the multiple openings in the lamina cribrosa of the sclera. From this point centrally they are jointly known as the optic nerve. The nerve passes through the posterior portion of the orbit for a distance of 2 to 3 cm., and throughout this

Nerves	Components	Function	Central Connection	Cell Bodies	Peripheral Distribution
I. Olfactory	Afferent Special visceral	Smell	Olfactory bulb and tract	Olfactory epithelial cells	Olfactory nerves
II. Optic	Afferent Special somatic	Vision	Optic nerve and tract	Ganglion cells of retina	Rods and cones of retina
III. Oculomotor	Efferent Somatic	Ocular movement	Nucleus III	Nucleus III	Branches to Levator palpebrae, Rectus superior, medius, inferior, Obliquus inferior
	Efferent General visceral	Contraction of pupil and accommodation	Nucleus of Edinger-Westphal	Nucleus of Edinger-Westphal	Ciliary ganglion; Ciliaris and Sphincter pupillae
	Afferent Proprioceptive	Muscular sensibility	Nucleus mesencephalicus V	Nucleus mesencephalicus V	Sensory endings in ocular muscles
IV. Trochlear	Efferent Somatic	Ocular movement	Nucleus IV	Nucleus IV	Branches to Obliquus superior
	Afferent Proprioceptive	Muscular sensibility	Nucleus mesencephalicus V	Nucleus mesencephalicus V	Sensory endings in Obliquus superior
V. Trigeminal	Afferent General somatic	General sensibility	Trigeminal sensory nucleus	Trigeminal ganglion (Gasserian)	Sensory branches of ophthalmic maxillary and mandibular nerves to skin and mucous membranes of face and head
	Efferent Special visceral	Mastication	Motor V nucleus	Motor V nucleus	Branches to Temporalis, Masseter, Pterygoidei, Mylohyoideus, Digastricus, Tensores tympani and palatini
	Afferent Proprioceptive	Muscular sensibility	Nucleus mesencephalicus V	Nucleus mesencephalicus V	Sensory endings in muscles of mastication
VI. Abducent	Efferent Somatic	Ocular movement	Nucleus VI	Nucleus VI	Branches to Rectus lateralis
	Afferent Proprioceptive	Muscular sensibility	Nucleus mesencephalicus V	Nucleus mesencephalicus V	Sensory endings in Rectus lateralis
VII. Facial	Efferent Special visceral	Facial expression	Motor VII nucleus	Motor VII nucleus	Branches to facial muscles, Stapedius, Stylohyoideus, Digastricus
	Efferent General visceral	Glandular secretion	Nucleus salivatorius	Nucleus salivatorius	Greater petrosal nerve, pterygopalatine ganglion, with branches of maxillary V to glands of nasal mucosa. Chorda tympani, lingual nerve, submandibular ganglion, submandibular ganglion, and sublingual glands
	Afferent Special visceral	Taste	Nucleus tractus solitarius	Geniculate ganglion	Chorda tympani, lingual nerve, taste buds, anterior tongue
	Afferent General visceral	Visceral sensibility	Nucleus tractus solitarius	Geniculate ganglion	Great petrosal, chorda tympani and branches
	Afferent General somatic	Cutaneous sensibility	Nucleus spinal tract of V	Geniculate ganglion	With auricular branch of vagus to external ear and mastoid region
VIII. Acoustic	Afferent Special somatic	Hearing	Cochlear nuclei	Spiral ganglion	Organ of Corti in cochlea
	Afferent Proprioceptive	Sense of equilibrium	Vestibular nuclei	Vestibular ganglion	Semicircular canals, saccule, and utricle
IX. Glosso-pharyngeal	Afferent Special visceral	Taste	Nucleus tractus solitarius	Inferior ganglion IX	Lingual branches, taste buds, posterior tongue
	Afferent General visceral	Visceral sensibility	Nucleus tractus solitarius	Inferior ganglion IX	Tympanic nerve to middle ear, branches to pharynx and tongue, carotid sinus nerve
	Efferent General visceral	Glandular secretion	Nucleus salivatorius	Nucleus salivatorius	Tympanic, lesser petrosal nerves, otic ganglion, with auriculotemporal V to parotid gland
	Efferent Special visceral	Swallowing	Nucleus ambiguus	Nucleus ambiguus	Branch to Stylopharyngeus
X. Vagus	Efferent General visceral	Involuntary muscle and gland control	Dorsal motor nucleus X	Dorsal motor nucleus X	Cardiac nerves and plexus; ganglia on heart. Pulmonary plexus; ganglia, respiratory tract. Esophageal, gastric, celiac plexuses; myenteric and submucous plexuses, muscle and glands of digestive tract down to transverse colon
	Efferent Special visceral	Swallowing and phonation	Nucleus ambiguus	Nucleus ambiguus	Pharyngeal branches, superior and inferior laryngeal nerves
	Afferent General visceral	Visceral sensibility	Nucleus tractus solitarius	Inferior ganglion X	Fibers in all cervical, thoracic, and abdominal branches; carotid and aortic bodies
	Afferent Special visceral	Taste	Nucleus tractus solitarius	Inferior ganglion X	Branches to region of epiglottis and taste buds
	Afferent General somatic	Cutaneous sensibility	Nucleus spinal tract V	Superior ganglion X	Auricular branch to external ear and meatus
XI. Accessory	Efferent Special visceral	Swallowing and phonation	Nucleus ambiguus	Nucleus ambiguus	Bulbar portion, communication with vagus, in vagus branches to muscles of pharynx and larynx
	Efferent Special somatic	Movements of shoulder and head	Lateral column of upper cervical spinal cord	Lateral column of upper cervical spinal cord	Spinal portion, branches to Sternocleidomastoideus and Trapezius
XII. Hypoglossal	Efferent General somatic	Movements of tongue	Nucleus XII	Nucleus XII	Branches to extrinsic and intrinsic muscles of tongue

Figure 5. Outline of the cranial nerves. (From Goss, C. M. (ed.): Gray's Anatomy. 28th ed. Philadelphia, Lea & Febiger, 1967.)

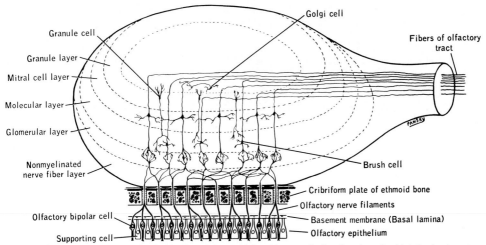

Figure 6. Section through the olfactory epithelium and the olfactory bulb, showing the histologic structure of each. (From House, E., and Pansky, B.: A Functional Approach to Neuroanatomy. 2nd ed. New York, McGraw-Hill Book Company, Inc., 1967.)

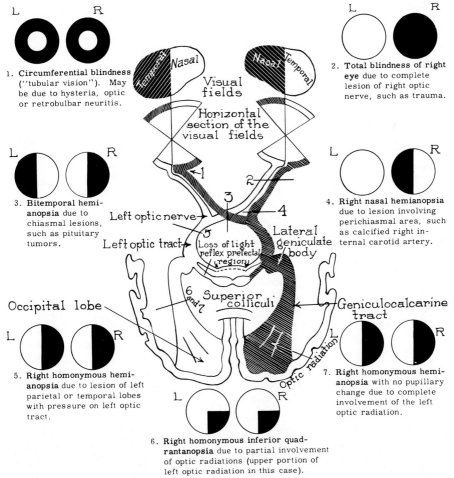

Figure 7. Visual field defects associated with lesions of the visual system. (From Chusid, J. G., and McDonald, J. J.: Correlative Neuroanatomy and Functional Neurology. Los Altos, Calif., Lange Medical Publications, 1970.)

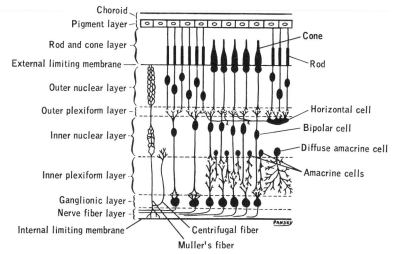

Figure 8. Structure of the retina. (From House, E., and Pansky, B.: A Functional Approach to Neuroanatomy. 2nd ed. New York, McGraw-Hill Book Company, Inc., 1967.)

length it is covered by dura, arachnoid, and pia. It exits from the orbit through the optic foramen and then curves toward the midline to converge with the nerve of the opposite side as the optic *chiasma*. The optic chiasma resembles an "X," with the optic nerves in front and the optic tracts behind. It rests upon the tuberculum sellae of the sphenoid bone and on the diaphragm sellae of the dura. Just posterior to it is the stalk of the hypophysis. Just lateral to it on each side are the internal carotid arteries. Within the optic chiasma some of the fibers of the optic nerves cross and some remain uncrossed. Those fibers in the medial aspect of the nerve, which arise in the nasal half of the retina, cross at the chiasma; whereas the fibers in the lateral aspect of the nerve, which arise from the temporal half of the retina, remain uncrossed and continue on in the tract of the same side (Fig. 7).

Because of its embryonic origin and structure, the optic nerve corresponds more to a central tract of brain fibers than to a peripheral cranial nerve. Embryologically it develops from the lateral aspect of the forebrain. It is supported by neuroglia instead of Schwann cells and has meningeal coverings like those of the brain. Further, the optic nerve is actually a third order neuron to the brain from the actual receptors in the retina (Fig. 8), the rods, and the cones. Beyond the chiasma the fibers continue in the diverging *optic tracts*. Most of the fibers of the optic tract end in the lateral geniculate body and are then relayed to the visual cortex and other lower nuclei which mediate reflex responses to ocular stimuli.

The ganglion cells of the optic nerve are actually not the primary receptor cells of the retina but rather are connected through the layers of the retina with the actual receptor cells, the *rods* and *cones,* by numerous bipolar cells.

Oculomotor Nerve

The oculomotor nerve is primarily a somatic motor nerve (Fig. 9). It also carries parasympathetic fibers to the ciliary ganglion and some afferent proprioceptor fibers from the ocular muscles. It supplies the levator palpebrae superioris muscle, all the extrinsic ocular muscles except the superior oblique and lateral rectus, and all the intrinsic muscles except the dilatator pupillae.

The somatic motor fibers arise in the oculomotor nucleus in the midbrain just ventral to the cerebral aqueduct and are both crossed and uncrossed. The fibers pass ventrally to emerge from the oculomotor sulcus medial to the cerebral peduncle in the posterior fossa. The nerve then passes forward to pierce the dura of the lateral wall of the cavernous sinus. After traversing the lateral wall of the cavernous sinus, it passes forward into the superior orb tal fissure and divides into *superior* and *inferior divisions.* The superior division passes medialward, sending branches to the *superior rectus* and the *levator palpebrae superioris muscles.* The inferior division supplies the *medial* and *inferior recti muscles* and the *inferior oblique muscle.* It also sends a *root* to the ciliary ganglion.

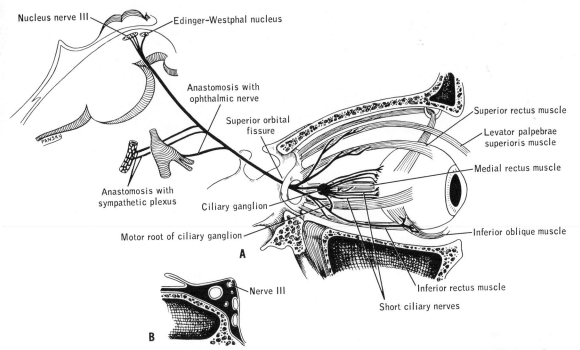

Figure 9. Oculomotor nerve (III). *A*, Its course, distribution within the orbit, and relations. *B*, The relations of nerve III to other nerves and vessels within the cavernous sinus. (From House, E., and Pansky, B.: A Functional Approach to Neuroanatomy. 2nd ed. New York, McGraw-Hill Book Company, Inc., 1967.)

The parasympathetic fibers arise in the *autonomic nucleus of the oculomotor nerve,* which is just rostral and dorsal to the somatic motor nucleus and is known as the *Edinger-Westphal nucleus* (Fig. 10). Its fibers remain uncrossed and join the inferior division in the superior orbital fissure and enter the ciliary ganglion as its preganglionic fibers. The vast majority of these fibers are for the innervation of the ciliary muscle of the iris while only a few are for the pupillary sphincter muscles.

The *ciliary ganglion* is a small parasympathetic ganglion which lies in the orbit about 1 cm. anterior to the optic foramen near the lateral aspect of the optic nerve. Its preganglionic fibers enter the *root* of the ciliary ganglion from the inferior division of the oculomotor nerve; its postganglionic fibers pass out through the *short ciliary nerves* to innervate the ciliary muscle of the iris and the pupillary sphincter muscle. The ciliary ganglion receives two important *communications:* (1) one from the *nasociliary nerve* carrying sensory fibers from the fifth nerve to the cornea, iris, and ciliary body; and (2) one with the *sympathetics* from the cavernous plexus which innervate the pupillary dilator muscle and the blood vessels of the globe. These communications pass directly through the ganglion without synapsing

with the ganglion cells and join the *short ciliary nerves* to the globe.

The branches of the ciliary ganglion are eight to ten short *ciliary nerves* which pass forward into the globe along with the long ciliary nerves from the nasociliary.

The proprioceptor fibers in the oculomotor nerve are probably from the mesencephalic nucleus of the fifth nerve.

The cortical fibers controlling eye movements end mostly in the nuclei of the reticular substance of the midbrain where conjugate movements of the eyes are integrated. Internuncial neurons then carry these cortical impulses to the nuclei of the eye muscles. The eye muscle nuclei also receive connections through the medial longitudinal fasciculus from the vestibular nuclei (crossed and uncrossed), from various other nuclei of the reticular formation, from interconnections between eye muscle nuclei and nuclei controlling head and neck movements, from proprioceptors in the cervical cord, and from the superior colliculi.

The superior colliculus is the center for coordination of eye movements. It receives fibers from (1) the optic tract; (2) sensory fibers from the spinal cord through the spinotectal tract; (3) sensory fibers from the trigeminal nerve; (4) auditory fibers from the lateral lem-

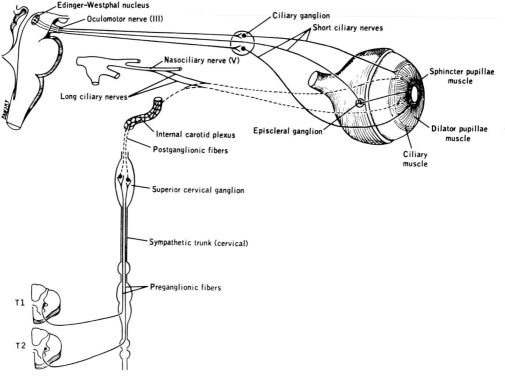

Figure 10. Autonomic connections of the cillary and episcleral ganglia through the oculomotor nerve (III) and the superior cervical ganglion. Dotted lines—postganglion fibers of the thoracolumbar outflow. (From House, E., and Pansky, B.: A Functional Approach to Neuroanatomy. 2nd ed. New York, McGraw-Hill Book Company, Inc., 1967.)

niscus for reflex movements of the eyes in response to sound; (5) fibers from the visual cortex through corticotectal tracts; and (6) fibers from the thalamic nuclei for primary and cortical olfactory associations. The descending efferent fibers of the superior colliculus cross mostly in the *fountain decussation of Meynert* in the dorsal portion of the tegmentum and continue caudally as the tectobulbar and tectospinal tracts. The tectobulbar tracts give off connections to the eye muscle nuclei and to the nucleus of the facial nerve. The tectospinal tracts connect with the ventral horn cells of the spinal cord, especially the cervical cord, to coordinate head and neck movements with eye movements.

Trochlear Nerve

The trochlear nerve is a somatic motor nerve which innervates the *superior oblique muscle* of the eye. It arises in the midbrain from the trochlear nucleus which is just ventral to the cerebral aqueduct, adjacent to the midline, and at the level of the inferior colliculus. The fibers curve dorsalward and cross to the opposite side in the roof of the cerebral aqueduct as it becomes the fourth ventricle. It then emerges just lateral to this dorsal decussation and just posterior to the inferior colliculus. It runs forward and pierces the dura along the lateral border of the cavernous sinus. It continues forward through the cavernous sinus and enters the orbit through the superior orbital fissure. It then courses medially and enters the superior oblique muscle.

In the wall of the cavernous sinus the trochlear nerve forms connections with the cavernous plexus of sympathetics and with the ophthalmic division of the fifth nerve.

Trigeminal Nerve

The trigeminal nerve is the largest of all the cranial nerves. It is the great sensory nerve for the skin of the face and the mucous membranes and other internal structures of the head; it is also the motor nerve for the muscles of mastication. It contains proprioceptive fibers.

The sensory nucleus of the fifth nerve is quite extensive. It has a large rostral head, the *main sensory nucleus,* and a tapering caudal portion, the *spinal tract,* which is continuous with the substantia gelatinosa (of Rolando) of the spinal cord. The main sensory nucleus is primarily for discriminative sense, whereas the spinal tract is primarily a sensory nucleus for pain and temperature.

The main sensory nucleus receives its afferents from the semilunar ganglion, called the sensory root, through the lateral part of the ventral surface of the pons (Fig. 11). Its axons then cross to the opposite side and ascend to the thalamic nuclei where they are then relayed to the postcentral cerebral cortex. The descending sensory root fibers from the semilunar ganglion course through the pons and

medulla in the spinal tract of the fifth nerve and end in nuclei of this tract as far down as the second cervical segment. The axons of these spinal tract nuclei cross to the opposite side and ascend to the thalamic nuclei in the spinothalamic tract and are from there relayed to the cerebral cortex. The sensory trigeminal nuclei also have many connections with the motor nuclei of the pons and medulla. In addition to receiving the sensory fibers of the trigeminal nerve, the descending tract probably also receives the somatic sensory fibers of the vagus, glossopharyngeal, and facial nerves.

The proprioceptor fibers of the trigeminal nerve arise in the muscles of mastication and

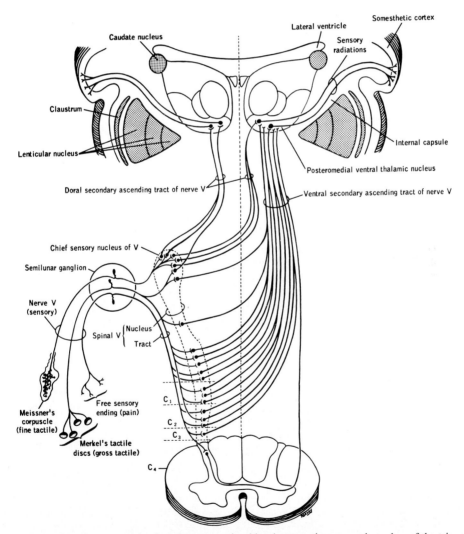

Figure 11. Projection of exteroceptive impulses transmitted by the somatic sensory branches of the trigeminal nerve. Note: the chief sensory nucleus transmits only impulses of gross and fine tactile stimuli; pain is transmitted only via the caudal part of the spinal nucleus. Gross tactile impulses are transmitted throughout all parts of the nuclear complex. (*Modified after Crosby, Humphrey, and Lauer,* 1962.) (From House, E., and Pansky, B.: A Functional Approach to Neuroanatomy. 2nd ed. New York, McGraw-Hill Book Company, Inc., 1967.)

probably also in the extraocular muscles. They terminate in the *mesencephalic root of the fifth nerve*. These mesencephalic root cells form collaterals with the motor nuclei of the nerve.

The *motor nucleus* lies near the lateral angle of the fourth ventricle in the rostral part of the pons. It receives cortical fibers for voluntary motor control from the pyramidal tracts, mostly crossed, but some uncrossed. It also receives reflex input from the sensory nucleus and the mesencephalic root of the fifth nerve. The axons emerge from the lateral aspect of the pons as the *motor root* just anterior to the sensory root and pass anterior with the sensory root to the semilunar ganglion.

TRIGEMINAL GANGLION (SEMILUNAR GANGLION; GASSERIAN GANGLION)

It is the great sensory ganglion of the fifth nerve that contains the cell bodies of the sensory fibers of the three main divisions of the trigeminal nerve. The ganglion lies within folds of dura, known as Meckel's cave, and sits in the trigeminal impression in the petrous apex. Anteriorly it receives the three large sensory divisions: ophthalmic, maxillary, and mandibular. The central sensory root fibers leave the posterior aspect of the ganglion to pass to their insertion into the pons. The motor root fibers pass beneath the ganglion, between it and the petrous bone, and join the sensory mandibular division as it exits from the skull through the foramen ovale. The ganglion also receives sympathetic filaments from the carotid plexus and gives out small branches to the dura.

Accessory ganglia of the trigeminal nerve consist of several small parasympathetic ganglia and are anatomically, but not functionally, associated with the trigeminal nerve. They are: (1) the ciliary ganglion with the ophthalmic nerve, which actually receives its preganglionic fibers from the oculomotor nerve; (2) the pterygopalatine (sphenopalatine) with the maxillary nerve, which receives its fibers from the facial nerve; and (3) the otic and submandibular ganglia with the mandibular nerve, which receive their fibers from the glossopharyngeal and facial nerves, respectively.

Ophthalmic Nerve. The ophthalmic nerve courses anteriorly from the gasserian ganglion in the dura of the lateral wall of the cavernous sinus. It receives sympathetic filaments from the cavernous plexus and also communicating branches from the third, fourth, and fifth nerves. Just before it exits from the skull in the

superior orbital fissure, it gives off a branch to the dura and then divides into three branches: frontal, lacrimal, and nasociliary.

Frontal nerve. The frontal nerve is the largest branch of the ophthalmic. It courses between the levator palpebrae superioris and the periorbita, and about halfway through the orbit it divides into a large supraorbital and a small supratrochlear branch.

SUPRAORBITAL NERVE. The supraorbital nerve leaves the orbit through the supraorbtal notch or foramen. It sends branches to the upper lid and then turns upward over the forehead beneath the frontalis muscle, dividing into medial and lateral branches. These nerves supply the scalp as far back as the lambdoidal suture.

SUPRATROCHLEAR NERVE. The supratrochlear nerve passes medially in the orbit, gives off branches to the conjunctiva and upper lid, and then exits from the orbit deep to the frontalis and corrugator muscles to supply the skin of the lower and medial part of the forehead.

BRANCH TO THE FRONTAL SINUS. This nerve pierces the floor of the frontal sinus in the supraorbital notch and supplies the mucous membrane of the frontal sinus.

Lacrimal nerve. The lacrimal nerve passes through the lateral, narrow portion of the superior orbital fissure and courses between the rectus lateralis and the periorbita to the lacrimal gland. It gives off branches to the gland and to the conjunctiva before piercing the orbital fascia to supply the skin of the upper lid.

In the orbit the lacrimal nerve receives a communication from the zygomatic branch of the maxillary nerve which carries postganglionic parasympathetic secretory fibers from the sphenopalatine ganglion to the lacrimal gland. The preganglionic fibers for lacrimation reach the sphenopalatine ganglion via the greater petrosal and vidian nerves from the seventh nerve.

Nasociliary nerve. The nasociliary nerve, after entering the orbit through the superior orbital fissure, passes to the medial wall of the orbit. Here it passes through the anterior ethmoid foramen as the *anterior ethmoidal nerve,* entering the intracranial cavity just above the cribriform plate. It then runs forward along the cribriform plate and finally drops down into the nasal cavity through a slit alongside the crista galli. Here, along with its intranasal branches, it supplies the mucous membrane of the upper and anterior part of the nasal septum, the lateral wall of the nose, and the frontal and anterior ethmoidal sinuses. It then slips downward between the nasal bone and the upper lateral cartilage to emerge as the *external nasal branch,* which supplies the skin of the ala and nasal tip.

As the nasociliary nerve enters the orbit, it gives off a *communicating branch to the ciliary ganglion,* which carries sensory fibers right through the ganglion to the globe without synapsing. It supplies sensation to the cornea, iris, and ciliary body.

The *long ciliary nerves* are two or three in number and are also given off by the nasociliary nerve toward the back of the orbit. They course with the short ciliary nerves from the ciliary ganglion to the back of the globe where they pierce the sclera and pass forward to the iris and cornea, giving sensation to these parts. Also, from the cavernous plexus they carry sympathetic filaments which innervate the pupillary dilator muscle.

Prior to entering the anterior ethmoidal foramen, two more branches are given off, the *posterior ethmoidal nerve* and the *infratrochlear nerve.* The posterior ethmoidal passes through the posterior ethmoidal foramen and supplies the posterior ethmoidal and sphenoid sinuses. The infratrochlear nerve passes forward to the medial angle of the eye to supply the skin of the lids and the side of the nose, the conjunctiva, and the lacrimal sac.

The Maxillary Nerve. The maxillary division of the trigeminal nerve, like the ophthalmic, is also entirely sensory. It supplies the mid third of the face and the mucous membranes of the upper portions of the mouth and pharynx, the maxillary sinus, as well as the upper teeth. As it leaves the semilunar ganglion anteriorly, it passes forward in the dura of the lower lateral wall of the cavernous sinus, then forward under the dura to reach the foramen rotundum, through which it exits from the cranial cavity. It then crosses the pterygopalatine fossa to enter the inferior orbital fissure where it becomes the *infraorbital nerve.* In the posterior part of the orbit, it lies in the infraorbital groove, but anteriorly it enters the infraorbital canal. It emerges on the face of the maxilla from the infraorbital foramen and divides into several branches which supply the skin of the cheek, nose, lower eyelid, and upper lip.

Prior to entering the foramen rotundum, a dural branch is given off, called the *middle meningeal nerve,* which accompanies the middle meningeal artery. In the pterygopalatine fossa, three major branches are given off:

zygomatic nerve, pterygopalatine (sphenopalatine) nerves, and *posterior superior alveolar nerves.*

Zygomatic nerve. The zygomatic nerve enters the orbit through the inferior orbital fissure and divides into the *zygomaticotemporal* and *zygomaticofacial* branches. The zygomaticotemporal branch runs along the lateral wall of the orbit. Here it gives off a communication to the lacrimal nerve which carries postganglionic parasympathetic fibers from the sphenopalatine ganglion for lacrimation. It then leaves the orbit through a small foramen to enter the temporal fossa, where it finally pierces the temporal fascia an inch above the zygomatic arch to innervate the skin of the side of the forehead. The zygomaticofacial branch courses more inferiorly in the orbit and then traverses the zygomatic bone to emerge on the cheek, where it supplies the skin of that area.

Pterygopalatine (sphenopalatine) nerves. These are two short trunks which unite the *sphenopalatine ganglion* with the maxillary division of the trigeminal nerve (Fig. 12). They transmit mostly afferent sensory fibers of the maxillary nerve from the nose, palate, and pharynx which pass through but do not synapse in the ganglion. They also carry important postganglionic parasympathetic secretory fibers from the ganglion to the maxillary nerve where they pass in a retrograde fashion for a short distance to the zygomatic nerve, out which they flow to the lacrimal nerve and lacrimal gland. The preganglionic fibers are derived from the seventh nerve via the greater petrosal and vidian nerves. In addition to giving off secretory fibers to the lacrimal gland, the sphenopalatine ganglion also sends postganglionic secretory fibers to the glands of the nasal cavity, pharynx, and palate through other branches of the pterygopalatine nerves. Sympathetic fibers also pass through the ganglion without synapsing and are derived from the carotid plexus and pass to the ganglion via the deep petrosal and vidian nerves. They pass on to the nose and palate through branches of the pterygopalatine nerves.

BRANCHES OF THE SPHENOPALATINE NERVES

Orbital

1. Filaments to the periosteum of orbit through the inferior orbital fissure.

2. Sphenoethmoidal fibers which supply the mucous membrane of the posterior ethmoidal and sphenoid sinuses.

Greater Palatine Nerve. The greater pala-

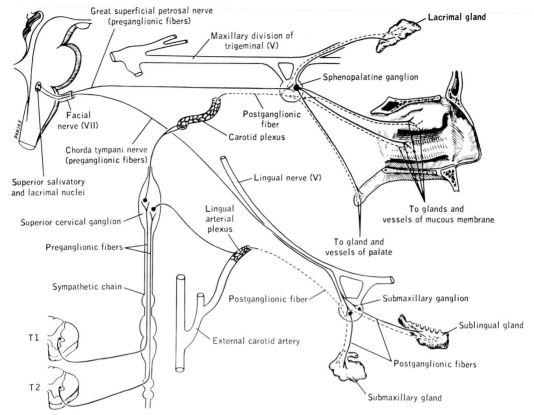

Figure 12. Autonomic connections of the sphenopalatine ganglion, mainly from nerve VII and the superior cervical ganglion. Dotted lines—postganglionic fibers of the thoracolumbar outflow. (From House, E., and Pansky, B.: A Functional Approach to Neuroanatomy. 2nd ed. New York, McGraw-Hill Book Company, Inc., 1967.)

tine nerve descends through the pterygopalatine canal and emerges upon the posterior aspect of the hard palate through the greater palatine foramen. It divides into several branches and passes forward to supply the mucosa of the hard palate. In its descending portion in the pterygopalatine canal it usually gives off *posterior inferior nasal branches* which supply the posterior aspects of the inferior turbinate and middle and inferior meati. It also gives off lesser *palatine nerves* which emerge from the lesser palatine foramen and disburse over the soft palate, uvula, and tonsil.

Posterior Superior Nasal Branches. These enter the posterior part of the nasal cavity through the sphenopalatine foramen and supply the mucous membrane of the superior and middle turbinates, the posterior ethmoid sinuses, and the posterior part of the nasal septum.

Pharyngeal Branch. The pharyngeal branch passes through the pharyngeal canal to the nasopharynx posterior to the eustachian tube.

Posterior superior alveolar nerves. These are usually two in number and supply the mucosa and gums of the posterior cheek and alveolar ridge. They enter the posterior alveolar canals and send twigs to each molar tooth.

In the infraorbital canal two additional alveolar branches are given off, the *middle* and *anterior superior alveolar nerves*. The middle superior nerve supplies the two premolar teeth and the anterior superior nerve supplies the incisor and canine teeth. It also gives off a nasal branch which supplies the inferior meatus and the floor of nose anteriorly. The nerves descend from the infraorbital canal in the wall of the maxillary antrum. All the alveolar nerves form a superior dental plexus.

Mandibular Nerve. The mandibular nerve is the third division of the trigeminal nerve and the largest of the three divisions. It has mixed motor and sensory fibers. The motor fibers innervate the following muscles: (1) muscles of mastication, (2) mylohyoid, (3) anterior belly of the digastric, (4) tensor tympani, and (5) tensor veli palatine.

The sensory fibers supply the skin of the lower one third of the face and the temporal region, the anterior ear, and the external auditory canal; the mastoid air cells; the mucous membranes of the cheek, tongue, and floor of mouth; the lower gums and teeth; the mandible and temporomandibular joint; and part of the dura and skull.

Just below the foramen ovale the *otic ganglion* lies close to the medial surface of the nerve and is connected by several communications with branches of the mandibular nerve.

The branches of the main trunk of the mandibular nerve are: (1) recurrent meningeal, (2) medial pterygoid, (3) masseteric, (4) deep temporal, (5) lateral pterygoid, (6) buccal, (7) auriculotemporal, (8) lingual, and (9) inferior alveolar.

Recurrent meningeal branch. This supplies the dura and enters the skull through the foramen spinosum with the artery.

Medial pterygoid nerve. This nerve supplies the medial pterygoid muscle after passing through the otic ganglion without synapsing. It also gives off branches to the *tensor veli palatini muscle* and the *tensor tympani muscle,* which also pass without synapsing through the otic ganglion.

Masseteric nerve. The masseteric nerve passes through the mandibular notch to innervate the masseter muscle. It also sends a twig to the temporomandibular joint.

Deep temporal nerves. These are usually two in number, the anterior and posterior, and supply the temporalis muscle.

Lateral pterygoid nerve. This nerve supplies the lateral pterygoid muscle.

Buccal nerve. The buccal nerve passes between the two heads of the lateral pterygoid muscle and beneath the anterior border of the masseter muscle. It divides into upper temporal and lower buccinator branches, which are entirely sensory to the skin of the cheek and the mucous membranes of the mouth and gums.

Auriculotemporal nerve. The auriculotemporal nerve usually begins as two roots which encircle the middle meningeal artery near the base of the skull. It then runs as a single trunk posteriorly and laterally to the medial aspect of the neck of the mandible and emerges superficially between the ear and the condyle of the mandible deep to the parotid gland. It continues superiorly with the superficial temporal artery over the root of the zygomatic arch and divides into superficial temporal branches. The auriculotemporal nerve has

important communications and branches from the standpoint of the otolaryngologist:

Communications with the facial nerve in the parotid gland accompany the facial fibers to supply the skin over the facial muscles.

Communications with the otic ganglion join the roots of the auriculotemporal nerve near the base of the skull and contain postganglionic parasympathetic fibers carrying secretory impulses to the parotid gland. The preganglionic fibers to the otic ganglion are supplied by the ninth nerve through the lesser petrosal nerve.

Anterior auricular branches supply the helix and tragus of the ear.

External auditory meatus branches enter the canal through the bony-cartilaginous junction and supply the skin of the canal and part of the tympanic membrane.

Articular branches supply the temporomandibular joint.

Parotid branches carry the postganglionic secretory fibers to the parotid gland.

Lingual nerve. The lingual nerve runs parallel with the inferior alveolar nerve and is joined by the chorda tympani nerve near the internal maxillary artery. It courses forward and medially between the hyoglossus muscle and the deep portion of the submandibular gland alongside the tongue. As it passes forward beneath the floor of the mouth, it crosses over the submandibular duct to run lateral to it immediately beneath the mucous membrane. Here it is vulnerable to injury in dissections of the duct, either from within the mouth or through an external approach. The most important communications of the lingual nerve are with the chorda tympani nerve and the submandibular ganglion. The chorda tympani nerve carries preganglionic parasympathetic secretory fibers destined for the submandibular and sublingual glands via the submandibular ganglion. The chorda tympani also carries special sensory fibers supplying taste to the anterior two thirds of the tongue. The communications of the lingual nerve with the submandibular ganglion are several short roots which carry pre- and postganglionic secretory fibers for the submandibular and sublingual glands. The ganglion lies in close proximity to the submandibular gland. Besides secretory and taste fibers which the lingual nerve carries from the chorda tympani nerve, it supplies its own important sensory fibers to the mucous membranes of the anterior two thirds of the tongue, the floor of mouth, and the gums.

Inferior alveolar nerve. The inferior alveolar nerve accompanies the inferior alveolar artery into the mandibular foramen on the medial aspect of the ascending ramus of the mandible. It continues in the mandible through the mandibular canal to the mental foramen, where it divides into terminal branches.

BRANCHES OF THE INFERIOR ALVEOLAR NERVE

Mylohyoid Nerve. The mylohyoid nerve leaves the inferior alveolar just before the latter enters the mandibular foramen. It then passes downward and forward in a deep groove on the medial surface of the mandible to reach the mylohyoid muscle. It supplies motor fibers to the mylohyoid muscle and also to the anterior belly of the digastric muscle.

Dental Branches. The dental branches arise from the intracanalicular portion of the nerve and supply the molar and premolar teeth.

Incisive Branch. This is one of the terminal branches at the mental foramen which continues anteriorly within the bone to supply the canine and incisor teeth.

Mental Nerve. The mental nerve is the other terminal branch which exits through the mental foramen to supply the lower lip and chin.

Abducent Nerve

The abducent nerve supplies motor innervation to the lateral rectus muscle of the eye. It also probably contains proprioceptive fibers to the mesencephalic nucleus of the fifth nerve. Its main motor nucleus lies close to the floor of the fourth ventricle. The motor fibers pass ventrolaterally to emerge in the furrow between the inferior border of the pons and the superior end of the pyramid of the medulla. It passes forward to pierce the dura at the dorsum sellae of the sphenoid bone. It then passes below the posterior clinoid process to enter and traverse the cavernous sinus and finally enter the orbit through the superior orbital fissure. It enters the medial aspect of the lateral rectus muscle after passing through the two heads of the muscle.

The abducent nucleus receives voluntary impulses via the corticobulbar tracts and has rich reflex connections with the medial longitudinal fasciculus and other tracts and nuclei of the brain stem and spinal cord similar to the oculomotor and trochlear nuclei.

Facial Nerve

The facial nerve has two roots, the larger being the main motor root which supplies the facial muscles; and the smaller being the *nervus intermedius* (nerve of Wrisberg) which contains special sensory fibers of taste from the tongue, and parasympathetic secretomotor fibers to the submaxillary and sublingual salivary glands, the nasal and palatine glands, and the lacrimal gland (Fig. 13). In addition, the seventh nerve carries a few general somatic and visceral afferent fibers. The somatic afferents join the auricular branch of the vagus to supply sensation to the external acoustic meatus. The cell bodies of these fibers are in the geniculate ganglion and centrally they probably end in the spinal tract of the fifth nerve. The visceral afferents probably innervate the mucous membranes of the nose, palate, and pharynx through the greater petrosal nerve. They also have their cell bodies in the geniculate ganglion and connect centrally with the tractus solitarius.

The main motor nucleus of the seventh nerve lies deep in the reticular formation of the pons just rostral to the nucleus ambiguus of the tenth nerve. Its axons pass dorsally and continue dorsomedially to the floor of the fourth ventricle where they turn sharply to run for a short distance in a rostral direction dorsal to the medial longitudinal fasciculus and medial to the abducent nucleus. The fibers then make an abrupt turn laterally to arch over the abducent nucleus, producing an elevation in the floor of the fourth ventricle called the facial colliculus. This part of the facial nerve which arches abruptly over the sixth nerve nucleus is known as the internal genu of the nerve. From this genu the axons pass ventrolaterally and also slightly caudalward to emerge from the brain stem at the caudal border of the pons in a recess between the olive and inferior cerebellar peduncle.

The primary central connections of the motor cells of the facial nucleus are with the corticobulbar fibers of the aberrant pyramidal tracts. The corticobulbar fibers reaching the motor nuclei of the lower part of the face are entirely crossed, whereas those connecting with the cells of the upper part of the face are both crossed and uncrossed. This difference in the corticobulbar fibers supplying the upper and lower facial muscles accounts for the sparing of the forehead movements in supranuclear lesions of the seventh nerve. The main motor nucleus also has many reflex connections with other cranial nerve nuclei, namely the fifth and eighth, and with other nuclei of the reticular formation of the pons and medulla. Emotional facial expression is largely

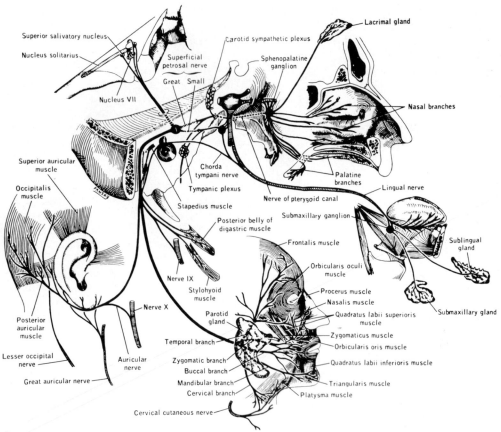

Figure 13. Complete distribution, course, and relations of the facial nerve (VII). (From House, E., and Pansky, B.: A Functional Approach to Neuroanatomy. 2nd ed. New York, McGraw-Hill Book Company, Inc., 1967.)

mediated through these latter reticular reflex connections.

The parasympathetic secretory fibers of the nervus intermedius arise from cell bodies in the superior salivatory nucleus, which is dorsomedial to the facial nucleus. These fibers are preganglionic and are distributed to the submandibular ganglion via the chordatympani nerve for innervation of the submandibular and sublingual glands, and to the sphenopalatine ganglion via the greater petrosal nerve for innervation of the lacrimal, nasal, and palatine glands.

Taste fibers from the anterior two thirds of the tongue reach their cell bodies in the geniculate ganglion via the chorda tympani nerve and connect centrally with the nucleus of the tractus solitarius. This nucleus has reflex connections with the salivary nucleus, the nucleus ambiguus and dorsal nucleus of the vagus, and the hypoglossal nucleus and with spinal cord nuclei through the reticulospinal tract.

Both the motor and intermediate roots exit from the brain stem at the posterior border of the pons and pass lateralward with the acoustic nerve into the internal acoustic meatus, the motor root of the facial being more medial; the acoustic, lateral; and the intermedius, in between the two. At the lateral extremity of the internal auditory canal, the facial and intermediate nerves separate from the acoustic nerve and enter the bony facial canal (fallopian canal). The nerve continues lateralward in the first part of the fallopian canal between the cochlea and semicircular canals to reach the anterosuperior part of the medial wall of the tympanic cavity. Here it turns sharply posterior to run horizontally along the medial wall of the middle ear just above the oval window. As the nerve makes its sharp bend posteriorly at the upper anterior aspect of the medial wall of the middle ear, the nerve becomes swollen as incorporates the geniculate ganglion. T sharp posterior bend is sometimes called *geniculum.*

Just posterior to the oval window a neath the overhanging horizontal semi canal, the facial nerve again makes a tinct turn, this time in a downward direction. It then courses downward in a vertical direction just posterior to the posterior bony tympanic annulus and exits through the stylomastoid foramen just medial to the mastoid tip and posterior to the styloid process. As the nerve emerges from the stylomastoid foramen, it passes lateral to the root of the styloid process in an anterior direction to enter the parotid gland. Within the gland it shortly divides into its two primary divisions, the upper temporofacial division and the lower cervicofacial division. Each of these divisions breaks up into several terminal branches which interconnect with each other in a plexiform arrangement, usually within the substance of the parotid gland but sometimes anterior to the gland. These terminal facial branches innervate the various facial and scalp muscles.

COMMUNICATIONS OF THE FACIAL NERVE

In the internal auditory canal
    With the acoustic nerve.
At the geniculate ganglion
    With the otic ganglion via filaments which join the lesser petrosal nerve.
    With the sympathetics of the middle meningeal artery via the external petrosal nerve.
In the facial canal
    With the auricular branch of the vagus near the stylomastoid foramen.
Extracranially
    With the glossopharyngeal nerve.
    With the vagus nerve.
    With the great auricular and lesser occipital nerves of the cervical plexus.
    With the auriculotemporal nerves and other branches of the fifth nerve.

BRANCHES OF THE FACIAL NERVE

From the Geniculate Ganglion
Greater petrosal nerve (greater superficial petrosal nerve). This branch leaves the geniculate ganglion anteriorly, passing for a short distance in the anterior part of the petrous before emerging through the hiatus of the facial canal into the middle cranial fossa. It passes beneath the dura in a groove on the anterior surface of the petrous apex and runs rostrally to the foramen lacerum where it joins with the deep petrosal nerve to form the *nerve of the pterygoid canal* or the *vidian nerve*. The vidian

nerve traverses the pterygoid canal a exiting, crosses the pterygopalatine foss. enter the sphenopalatine ganglion.

The greater petrosal nerve is a mixed nerve, containing sensory and parasympathetic fibers. The parasympathetics are preganglionic secretomotor fibers from the nervus intermedius which pass through the geniculate ganglion without synapsing. They connect with postganglionic fibers in the sphenopalatine ganglion which ultimately innervate the lacrimal, nasal, palatine, and pharyngeal glands. The bulk of the greater petrosal nerve consists of sensory fibers which take origin from cell bodies within the geniculate ganglion and are distributed to the soft palate through the lesser palatine nerves. A few sensory filaments are given off to the eustachian tube.

Branches Within the Fallopian Canal
Nerve to the stapedius muscle. This nerve arises from the facial nerve as it begins its vertical course in the posterior aspect of the middle ear. The stapedial branch reaches the muscle through a small opening in the base of the pyramid.

Chorda tympani nerve. The chorda tympani nerve arises from the vertical portion of the facial nerve in the mastoid, just before it exits from the stylomastoid foramen. As the chorda arises about 6 mm. from the stylomastoid foramen, it passes cranialward in the opposite direction of the facial nerve, paralleling the facial nerve for a distance in the posterior wall of the middle ear and then diverging to emerge through a small aperture (*iter chordae posterius*) between the base of the pyramid and the bony tympanic annulus. It then courses anteriorly across the lateral aspect of the tympanic membrane, crossing the neck of the malleus, and exits anteriorly through the *iter chordae anterius*. It traverses the *canal of Huguier* in the petrotympanic fissure and emerges from the skull on the medial surface of the spine of the sphenoid bone. It then joins the lingual nerve between the internal and external pterygoid muscles. The majority of the fibers of the chorda tympani nerve are special afferents for taste which have their cell bodies in the geniculate ganglion and which are distributed to the anterior two thirds of the tongue. The chorda also contains preganglionic parasympathetic secretory fibers which end by synapsing in the submandibular ganglion and which carry impulses destined for the submandibular and sublingual salivary glands as well as other minor salivary glands and mucous glands in the floor of the mouth.

SUBMANDIBULAR GANGLION. This is a 3 to 4 mm. ganglion lying just above the deep lobe of the submandibular gland on the hyoglossus muscle near the posterior border of the mylohyoid muscle. It is suspended from the lingual nerve by two 0.5 cm. nerve filaments. These connecting filaments carry both parasympathetic and sympathetic fibers to and from the ganglion. The proximal communicating filament consists mainly of preganglionic secretory parasympathetics which join the lingual nerve from the nervus intermedius via the chorda tympani. In the submandibular ganglion these preganglionic fibers synapse with cell bodies whose postganglionic fibers pass directly into the submandibular gland. Some pass back to the lingual nerve through the distal communicating filament and are distributed along with the peripheral branches of the lingual nerve to the sublingual glands and other minor salivary glands in the floor of the mouth.

The submandibular ganglion also receives some sympathetic communications from the sympathetic plexus accompanying the facial artery, but these pass through the ganglion without synapsing.

A few visceral afferent fibers also pass through the ganglion en route to their cell bodies in the geniculate ganglion via the lingual and chorda tympani nerves. They have no synapses in the submandibular ganglion.

Branches of the Facial Nerve in the Face and Neck

Posterior auricular nerve. This supplies the posterior auricular muscle, the muscles of the posterior aspect of the pinna, and the occipital muscle. It leaves the facial nerve just outside the stylomastoid foramen and runs upward between the external auditory meatus and the mastoid tip and, thence, to its muscles of distribution.

Digastric branch. The digastric branch also arises close to the stylomastoid foramen and supplies the posterior belly of the digastric muscle.

Stylohyoid branch. The stylohyoid branch innervates the stylohyoid muscle and arises near, or in conjunction with, the digastric branch.

Parotid Plexus. The most peripheral part of the facial nerve becomes a plexiform branching of the nerve within the substance of the parotid gland, the ultimate terminals of which supply somatic motor innervation to the facial muscles. The main trunk of the facial nerve divides into *temporofacial* and *cervicofacial divisions* which, in turn, subdivide into the specific branches which innervate the various facial muscles. Five main such subdivisions are usually identifiable.

Temporal branches. The temporal branches are the uppermost branches which cross the zygomatic arch and supply the anterior and the superior auricular muscles, the frontalis, the orbicularis oculi and the corrugator.

Zygomatic branches. Zygomatic branches also arise from the temporofacial division and run parallel to the zygomatic arch to innervate the orbicularis oculi. The lower branches often join with the buccal branches to form an infraorbital plexus which innervates the muscles of the midface.

Buccal branches. The main buccal branch may arise from either the temporofacial division or the cervicofacial division. Its branches usually communicate freely with the zygomatic branches above and the mandibular branches below, innervating the muscles of the midface, including the procerus, orbicularis oculi, zygomaticus, levator anguli oris, levator labii superioris, buccinator, orbicularis oris, nasalis, and depressor septi.

Mandibular branch. This branch usually dips inferior to the horizontal ramus of the mandible and deep to the platysma as it runs forward to innervate the depressor anguli oris, orbicularis oris, depressor labii inferioris, and mentalis and risorius.

Cervical branch. The cervical branch is the lowest branch from the cervicofacial division and runs deep to the platysma muscle, which it innervates.

Acoustic (Eighth) Nerve

The acoustic nerve consists of two distinct sets of fibers, the cochlear and the vestibular. The peripheral portions of the cochlear and vestibular nerves join to form the common acoustic nerve at the lateral portion of the internal auditory canal, where they are also joined by the facial nerve in the internal auditory canal.

COCHLEAR NERVE

Ascending Auditory Pathways. This pathway is also referred to as the classical or projective system or the afferent acoustic pathway. It transmits impulses from the organ of Corti to the auditory cortex.

The receptor cells are the hair cells which lie along the entire length of the organ of Corti in the cochlear duct. Unmyelinated nerve fibers pass from the hair cells to the bony modiolus of the cochlea where the fibers become myelinated. After a short course in the modiolus, the peripheral process joins its cell body located in the *spiral ganglion*. This is the first of four neurons between the cochlea and the cerebrum. From the ganglion cells the central fibers of these bipolar neurons enter the internal acoustic meatus to be joined by the fibers from the vestibular division of the eighth nerve. They traverse the auditory canal and meatus and enter the posterior cranial fossa where they immediately enter the brain stem in the cerebellopontine angle.

After entering the brain stem, the cochlear fibers divide into two main bundles. One group passes lateral and dorsal to the restiform body to terminate in the dorsal cochlear nucleus. The other group remains slightly ventral and medial to the restiform body and ends in the ventral cochlear nucleus. It has been found that the fibers coming from the basal coils of the cochlea terminate in the dorsal part of the dorsal cochlear nucleus. Those fibers arising in the apical coils end in the ventral part of the dorsal cochlear nucleus and in the ventral nucleus. However, some fibers pass to higher order neurons farther along the pathway before they synapse.

The cell bodies of the second order neurons lie in the dorsal and ventral cochlear nuclei. The axons from these cells follow two alternate pathways, the direct route and the indirect relay circuit (Fig. 14). By the direct route, fibers from the ventral cochlear nucleus, and perhaps most of the fibers from the dorsal cochlear nucleus that cross through the dorsal and intermediate trapezoid bodies, bend rostrally and continue in the lateral lemniscus of the other side. They do not terminate in the superior olivary nucleus but continue on directly to the medial geniculate body of the thalamus, bypassing the inferior colliculus. It is believed that the uncrossed fibers from the dorsal nucleus which pass in the ipsilateral lateral lemniscus also go directly to the medial geniculate body.

The indirect relay circuit begins in the ventral cochlear nucleus, the axons passing medially in the ventral trapezoid body, with some of them terminating in the nucleus of that body where a third order neuron arises. The superior olive is an important relay station,

receiving fibers from both of the cochlear nuclei and from the nucleus of the trapezoid body. From the olives, fibers ascend in the lateral lemniscus, some synapsing in its nucleus while others continue on to the inferior colliculus. Some of these fibers probably reach the medial geniculate body without synapsing in the inferior colliculus. From the inferior colliculus, the fibers eventually terminate in the medial geniculate nucleus of the thalamus. This nucleus is divided into a small ventral and a large dorsal portion. It is the latter that receives most of the auditory impulses directed toward conscious levels.

The cell bodies of the fourth order neurons are located in the dorsal parts of the medial geniculate body. Their axons, called auditory radiations or the geniculotemporal tract, pass laterally to terminate in the transverse temporal gyri of the cerebral hemispheres. Tones of different frequencies have specific reception areas in the auditory cortex.

The ascending auditory pathways make numerous connections with nuclei throughout the central nervous system as part of a complex auditory reflex system (Fig. 15).

Descending Auditory Pathways. Besides the conscious and reflex afferent auditory pathways, there are also descending efferent auditory pathways. The descending pathways, in general, have an inhibiting effect upon the ascending fibers and thereby tend to provide some degree of self-regulation to the auditory system. Each relay station of the auditory pathway has been considered to be dually innervated, thus providing a way for incoming impulses to be internally influenced, negated, or modified.

THE VESTIBULAR NERVE

The vestibular nerve arises from bipolar cells in the vestibular ganglion (Scarpa's ganglion) situated in the upper part of the lateral end of the internal auditory meatus. The peripheral fibers divide into three branches:

1. The *superior branch* supplies the macula of the utricle and the cristae in the ampullae of the superior and lateral semicircular ducts.

2. The *inferior branch* supplies the macula of the saccule.

3. The *posterior branch* traverses the foramen singulare and supplies the crista in the ampulla of the posterior semicircular duct.

Medially the vestibular fibers join the com-

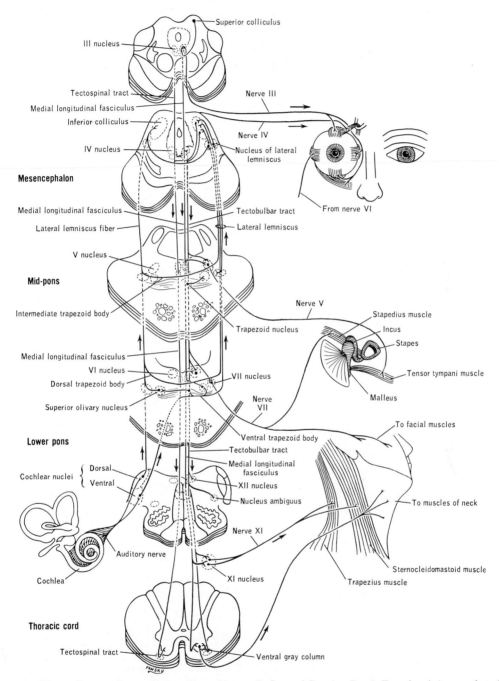

Figure 14. The auditory reflex pathway. (From House, E. L., and Pansky, B.: A Functional Approach to Neuro-anatomy. 2nd ed. New York, McGraw-Hill Book Co., Inc., 1967.)

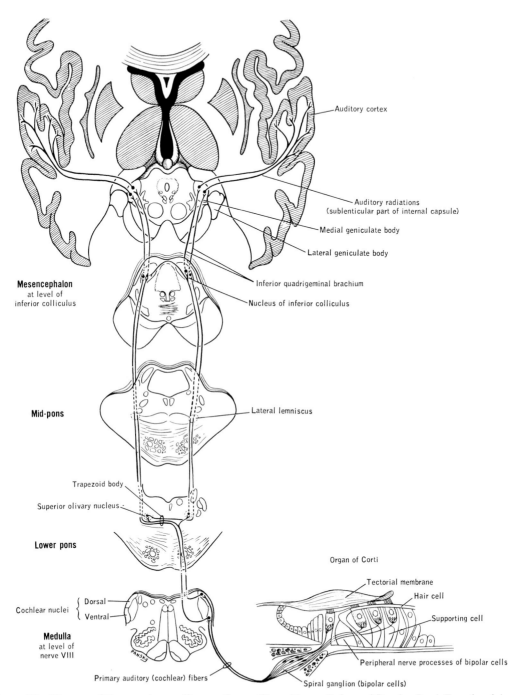

Figure 15. Diagram of the conscious auditory pathway. (From House, E. L., and Pansky, B.: A Functional Approach to Neuroanatomy. 2nd ed. New York, McGraw-Hill Book Co., Inc., 1967.)

mon acoustic nerve and traverse the internal auditory canal and posterior fossa to enter the medulla, where they divide into ascending and descending branches. The ascending branches pass to the medial, lateral, and superior vestibular nuclei, to the fastigial nuclei, and to the vermis of the cerebellum. The descending branches form the spinal root of the vestibular nerve and terminate in the inferior (spinal) vestibular nucleus. The connections of the second order vestibular neurons are diffuse and participate in a complex reflex system for maintaining the position of the eyes and body in relation to changes in orientation of the head. The second order neurons from the medial vestibular nucleus make widespread connections throughout the medulla and pons to the nuclei of the reticular formation and to motor nuclei of the cranial nerves and autonomic centers. They also contribute many ascending and descending fibers to the medial longitudinal fasciculi. Connections from the superior vestibular nucleus are particularly associated with the cerebellum. The lateral nucleus sends second order neurons via the reticular formation into the important direct vestibulospinal tract, which is probably the chief antigravity mechanism of the central nervous system. The lateral nucleus also contributes fibers to the medial longitudinal fasciculus. The inferior (spinal) nucleus has widespread connections with the nuclei of the reticular formation of the medulla and pons. It contributes fibers to the medial longitudinal fasciculus and some of its fibers also form the crossed vestibulospinal spinal tract (Fig. 16).

There are important descending association connections between the cerebellum and the vestibular nuclei through which the cerebellum exerts its coordinating influence directly upon the vestibular nuclei.

The conscious vestibular pathways are apparently not well understood nor uniformly agreed upon. Some feel the ascending vestibular pathways to consciousness follow those of the auditory pathways.

Glossopharyngeal Nerve

The ninth nerve is a mixed sensory and motor nerve (Fig. 17). The sensory components consist of somatic afferents supplying sensation to the mucous membranes of the pharynx, tonsillar region, and back of the tongue; special visceral afferents which supply taste to the posterior part of the tongue; and general visceral afferents which supply the blood pressure receptors of the carotid sinus and carotid body. The motor components of the glossopharyngeal nerve include the motor innervation of the stylopharyngeus muscle and the secretomotor innervation of the parotid gland and other minor salivary and mucous glands of the posterior tongue and adjacent pharynx.

The special visceral afferent fibers for taste of the ninth nerve have their cell bodies in the *inferior (petrosal) ganglion* at the base of the skull and terminate centrally in the nucleus solitarius via the tractus solitarius in the medulla (Fig. 18). The motor fibers to the stylopharyngeus arise in the cephalic end of the nucleus ambiguus. Somatic afferents have their cell bodies in the *inferior (petrosal) ganglion.* The central processes pass into the tractus solitarius, where they become widely distributed. Many synapse in the nucleus of the tractus solitarius. The special visceral afferents from the carotid body and sinus join the main tunk of the nerve and end with the rest of the visceral afferents in the tractus solitarius. From here they are distributed to the dorsal motor nucleus of the vagus and to the vasomotor and respiratory centers in the brain stem. The secretomotor fibers to the salivary and mucous glands arising in the inferior salivatory nucleus reach their glandular destinations via relays in the otic ganglion. The salivatory nucleus has many connections with other central pathways and nuclei, particularly with the nucleus and tractus solitarius.

The superficial origin of the glossopharyngeal nerve from the brain stem is by three or four rootlets in the groove between the olive and inferior peduncle. It passes laterally along the lower border of the petrous bone and exits from the skull through the jugular foramen. It then runs anteriorly between the internal carotid artery and the internal jugular vein following the posterior border of the stylopharyngeus muscle for a few centimeters before crossing over the stylopharyngeus to penetrate deelpy into the pharyngeal terminations at the posterior border of the hyoglossus muscle. As the glossopharyngeal nerve exits through the jugular foramen, it has a pair of ganglionic swellings, the superior (jugular) ganglion and the inferior (petrosal) ganglion. The superior is very small and inconstant. The ganglia contain the cell bodies for the sensory fibers of the nerve. The ninth nerve communicates with the

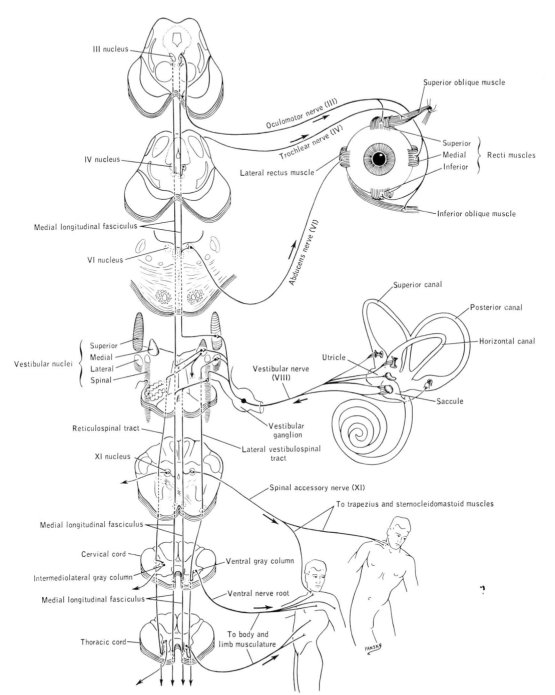

Figure 16. Simple vestibular reflex pathways. (From House, E. L., and Pansky, B.: A Functional Approach to Neuro-anatomy. 2nd ed. New York, McGraw-Hill Book Co., Inc., 1967.)

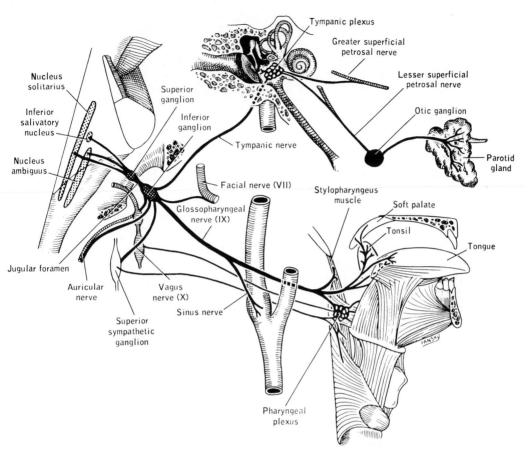

Figure 17. Course, distribution, and relations of the glossopharyngeal nerve (IX). (From House, E., and Pansky, B.: A Functional Approach to Neuroanatomy. 2nd ed. New York, McGraw-Hill Book Company, Inc., 1967.)

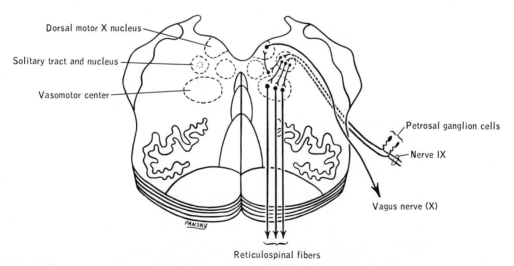

Figure 18. Open part of the medulla with the vasomotor center enlarged. (From House, E., and Pansky, B.: A Functional Approach to Neuroanatomy. 2nd ed. New York, McGraw-Hill Book Company, Inc., 1967.)

vagus nerve, the superior sympathetic ganglion, and the facial nerve.

BRANCHES OF THE GLOSSOPHARYNGEAL NERVE

Tympanic (Jacobson's) Nerve. The tympanic nerve has both sensory and secretory fibers. It supplies sensory fibers to the middle ear and parasympathetic secretory fibers to the parotid gland via the otic ganglion. It arises from the main trunk of the petrosal ganglion and penetrates into the floor of the middle ear through a small foramen in the base of the petrous between the carotid canal and the jugular fossa. It continues upward in a groove on the promontory where it enters into the tympanic plexus. It re-enters a small bony canal near the cochleariform process, passes medial to the semicanal for the tensor tympani muscle, and continues on as the lesser petrosal nerve.

The *tympanic plexus* lies in grooves on the promontory of the middle ear and is made up of tympanic branches of the ninth nerve and the caroticotympanic nerves from the sympathetic plexus surrounding the carotid artery. The tympanic plexus communicates with the greater petrosal nerve.

SENSORY BRANCHES. These branches are given off to the epithelium of the middle ear and its accessory chambers.

LESSER PETROSAL NERVE. The lesser petrosal nerve is the continuation of the tympanic branch of the ninth nerve beyond the tympanic plexus as it courses medial to the semicanal for the tensor tympani and re-enters the cranial cavity on the superior surface of the petrous, just lateral to the hiatus of the facial canal. It then leaves the cranial cavity again after a short anterior course, exiting through a small opening in the region of the suture line between the petrous and the greater wing of the sphenoid. Here it communicates with the geniculate ganglion of the seventh nerve by a small

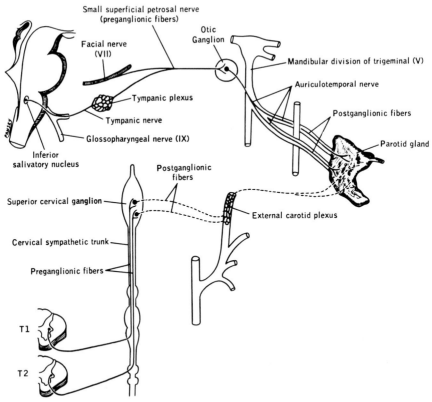

Figure 19. Cranial autonomic nerves, with special emphasis on the connections of the otic ganglion, chiefly through nerve IX and the superior cervical sympathetic ganglion. Dotted lines—postganglionic fibers of the thoracolumbar outflow. (From House, E., and Pansky, B.: A Functional Approach to Neuroanatomy. 2nd ed. New York, McGraw-Hill Book Company, Inc., 1967.)

filament. Just outside the skull it joins the otic ganglion.

Otic ganglion. The otic ganglion measures 2 to 4 mm. in diameter and closely approximates the medial surface of the mandibular division of the fifth nerve just below the foramen ovale (Fig. 19). The motor root of the otic ganglion is made up of the preganglionic parasympathetic fibers of the lesser petrosal nerve. The postganglionic parasympathetic fibers arising from the cell bodies in the otic ganglion are distributed mainly to the parotid gland via communications with the auriculotemporal nerve and its branches. Some postganglionics pass via the other nerves to the mucous and minor salivary glands in the mouth and pharynx. Other branches of communication with the otic ganglion are: *sympathetic,* from the middle meningeal plexus; the *medial pterygoid nerve* via trigeminal motor fibers which pass on through the ganglion as the motor fibers to the tensor tympani and tensor velli palatini muscles; the *mandibular nerve* via trigeminal sensory branches; the *sphenoidal branch* from the vidian nerve; and the chorda tympani communication. All these communicating branches pass without synapsing through the otic ganglion.

The *carotid sinus nerve* arises from the main trunk of the glossopharyngeal nerve just beyond the jugular foramen. It runs down the internal carotid artery to the carotid bifurcation where it terminates in the blood pressure receptors in the walls of the carotid sinus. It sends a branch to the intercarotid plexus, which is made up largely of vagal and sympathetic fibers. This intercarotid plexus terminates in the chemoreceptors of the carotid body.

Pharyngeal Branches. Pharyngeal branches are several in number and join vagal and sympathetic fibers at the level of the middle pharyngeal constrictor muscle to form the *pharyngeal plexus.* This plexus supplies the muscles and mucous membranes of the pharynx.

Branch to the Stylopharyngeus Muscle. This is the only muscular branch of the glossopharyngeal nerve.

Tonsillar Branches. The tonsillar branches supply sensory fibers to the faucial tonsils and their surrounding palatal and pillar membranes.

Lingual Branches. These supply afferent fibers for taste and general sensation to the posterior aspect of the tongue and secretomotor fibers to the mucous glands of the posterior tongue.

Vagus Nerve

The vagus nerve is the longest of the cranial nerves and has the widest distribution. It contains both somatic and visceral afferents and both general and special visceral efferent fibers. The somatic sensory fibers supply the external auditory canal and the posterior aspect of the pinna. The visceral afferent fibers supply the mucous membranes of the pharynx, larynx, bronchi and lungs, and the heart, esophagus, intestines, stomach and kidneys. The general visceral efferents are parasympathetics and go to the heart and nonstriated muscle and glands of the esophagus, stomach, trachea, bronchi, biliary tract, and most of the intestine. Special visceral efferents supply the striated muscles of the larynx, pharynx, and palate.

The afferent fibers in general have their cell bodies in the jugular and nodose ganglia of the vagus nerve at the base of the skull. Their central connections vary with the different types of afferents. The somatic sensory fibers from the external ear probably join the spinal tract of the fifth nerve and have connections with the thalamus, sensory cortex, and medullary and spinal nuclei. The visceral afferent fibers join the tractus solitarius and end in its nucleus. These, in turn, make associations with other centers in the reticular formation, much as did those of the glossopharyngeal nerve; namely, with the respiratory (Fig. 20), vasomotor, cardiac, vomiting, and swallowing centers (Fig. 21). These are then relayed to medullary and spinal nuclei as well as to the dorsal motor nucleus of the vagus. A few special visceral afferent taste fibers of the vagus, from a few receptors on the epiglottis and in the larynx, end in the tractus and nucleus solitarius.

The special visceral efferent fibers of the vagus which innervate the striated muscle of the pharynx and larynx arise in the nucleus ambiguus in the medulla, then turn ventrally and laterally to join the sensory fibers in a common emergence from the brain stem. The nucleus ambiguus connects with corticobulbar fibers from the same and opposite sides as well as with other central tracts from the trigeminal, glossopharyngeal, vagus, and spinal nerves. It is this crossed as well as uncrossed cortical representation in the nucleus ambiguus that probably accounts for the rarity of vocal paralysis on the basis of isolated central nervous system lesions.

The general vsiceral efferents of the vagus are preganglionic parasympathetics for smooth

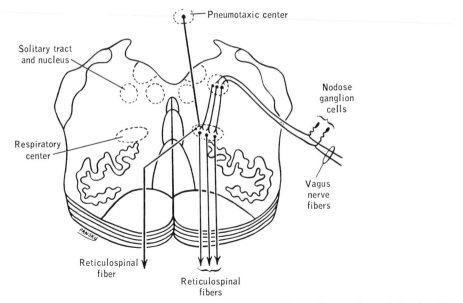

Figure 20. Open part of medulla with the respiratory center enlarged. (From House, E., and Pansky, B.: A Functional Approach to Neuroanatomy. 2nd ed. New York, McGraw-Hill Book Company, Inc., 1967.)

muscle and glands of the gastrointestinal tract and lungs as well as inhibitory fibers to the heart. They arise in the *dorsal nucleus of the vagus.* The nucleus has extensive connections with other central nuclei and tracts, particularly those of the reticular formation.

The common superficial origin of the combined sensory and motor fibers of the vagus nerve is by eight to ten rootlets from the dorsolateral aspect of the medulla in the same groove between the olive and the inferior peduncle shared more rostrally by the glossopharyngeal nerve and more caudally by the spinal accessory nerve. The rootlets merge and pass laterally to exit from the skull through the jugular foramen in a common dural sheath with the spinal accessory nerve. In the jugular fossa, the vagus has two ganglionic swellings, which are the sensory ganglia of the nerve.

The superior (jugular) ganglion is in the jugular foramen and is less than 0.5 cm. in diameter. Most of the peripheral sensory fibers of the cells of this ganglion make up the auricular branch of the vagus, with a few going to the pharyngeal branches. *The inferior (nodose) ganglion* is much bigger, measuring 2.5 cm. in length, and lies about 1 cm. distal to the superior ganglion. The peripheral processes of the inferior ganglion supply the larynx, esophagus, trachea and bronchi, and other thoracic and abdominal organs.

COMMUNICATIONS OF THE TENTH NERVE

At the superior ganglion the tenth nerve connects with the accessory nerve (cranial portion), the inferior ganglion of the glossopharyngeal nerve, the facial nerve, and the superior cervical sympathetic ganglion.

The cranial portion of the accessory nerve joins the vagus just proximal to the inferior ganglion and constitutes the greater portion of the motor fibers to the pharynx and larynx.

At the inferior ganglion the tenth nerve joins the hypoglossal nerve, the superior cervical sympathetic ganglion, and the first and second cervical spinal nerves.

COURSE OF THE VAGUS NERVES

The upper main trunk of each vagus nerve passes downward in the neck within the carotid sheath between the internal jugular vein and the carotid arteries (Fig. 22). Below the root of the neck the course of the nerve differs on the two sides.

The *right vagus* passes anterior to the first part of the subclavian artery and continues downward alongside the trachea to the root of the lung. Here it breaks up into the posterior pulmonary plexus. Below this plexus it further

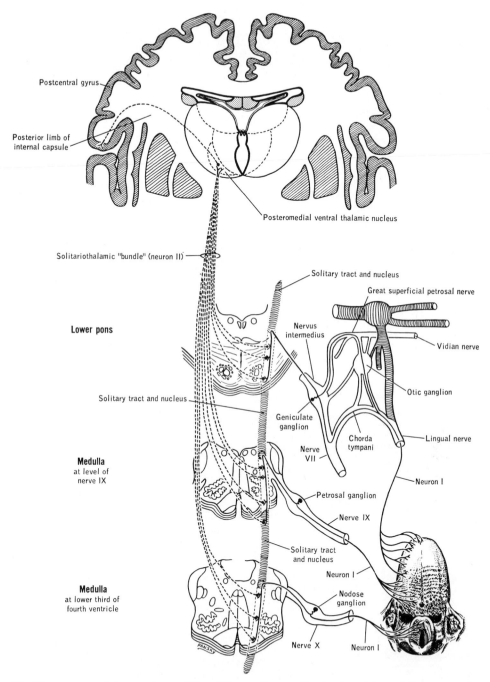

Figure 21. Conscious gustatory pathway. (From House, E., and Pansky, B.: A Functional Approach to Neuroanatomy. 2nd ed. New York, McGraw-Hill Book Company, Inc., 1967.)

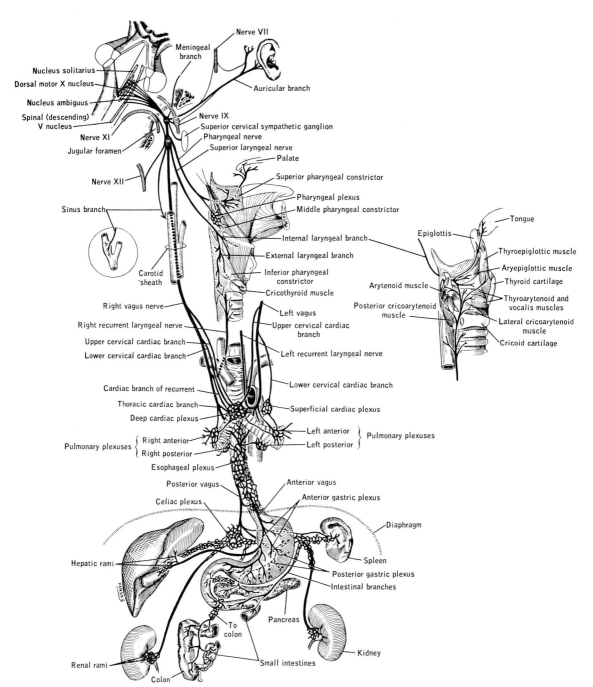

Figure 22. Course, relations, and complete distribution of the vagus nerve (X). (From House, E., and Pansky, B.: A Functional Approach to Neuroanatomy. 2nd ed. New York, McGraw-Hill Book Company, Inc., 1967.)

forms the dorsal esophageal plexus. Here it communicates with the left vagus, and then all the plexiform fibers join into one trunk, the posterior vagus nerve, which passes through the diaphragm on the posterior aspect of the esophagus. The posterior vagus then continues along the lesser curvature of the stomach and divides into celiac and gastric branches.

The *left vagus* runs between the left carotid and subclavian arteries as it enters the chest. It crosses the left side of the arch of the aorta and finally also divides up into a posterior pulmonary plexus behind the root of the left lung. It then forms the ventral esophageal plexus and finally re-forms into a single ventral trunk which pierces the diaphragm on the ventral aspect of the esophagus. In the abdomen the anterior vagus nerve divides into hepatic and gastric branches on the anterior aspect of the stomach.

BRANCHES OF THE VAGUS NERVE

In the Jugular Fossa
Meningeal branch. The meningeal branch arises at the superior ganglion and re-enters the cranium through the jugular foramen to supply the dura of the posterior fossa.

Auricular branch. The auricular branch arises from the superior ganglion and enters the mastoid canaliculus in the lateral aspect of the jugular fossa. It exits again through the tympanomastoid suture to reach the surface, where it supplies sensation to the posterior aspect of the pinna and to the posterior part of the external auditory meatus. It communicates with the seventh and ninth cranial nerves.

Branches in the Neck
Pharyngeal branches. The pharyngeal branches arise from the inferior ganglion and contain both sensory and motor fibers, the latter contributed by the accessory nerve. They join the *pharyngeal plexus,* made up of branches from the glossopharyngeal, vagus, and sympathetic nerves. Branches of the plexus are distributed to the muscles and mucous membranes of the pharynx and palate, except for the tensor palatini. Vagal filaments from the pharyngeal plexus also join glossopharyngeal and sympathetic fibers to form the *intercarotid plexus* at the carotid bifurcation. The vagal fibers are visceral afferents which end in the carotid body and mediate impulses set up by the chemoreceptors in that body which are sensitive to changes of carbon dioxide and possibly oxygen tensions in the blood.

Superior laryngeal nerve. This nerve arises from the inferior ganglion and passes downward and medially, deep to the internal carotid artery, to the lateral aspect of the thyrohyoid membrane where it divides into internal and external branches.

INTERNAL BRANCH. The internal branch pierces the thyrohyoid membrane with the superior laryngeal artery and veins and supplies sensory fibers to the mucous membranes and parasympathetic secretory fibers to the glands of the epiglottis, base of the tongue, aryepiglottic folds, and intrinsic parts of the larynx as far down as the vocal cords. It communicates with the recurrent nerve inferiorly.

EXTERNAL BRANCH. The external branch extends caudally outside the larynx to give motor innervation to the cricothyroid muscle and inferior constrictor muscle of the pharynx. It communicates with the pharyngeal plexus and the cervical sympathetics.

Superior cardiac branches. These arise from the vagus both high and low in the neck and are two or three in number. They follow the course of the carotid artery downward to join the cardiac plexuses in the thorax.

Recurrent laryngeal nerve. The recurrent laryngeal nerve arises in the root of the neck, curves around the great vessels in the root of the neck or upper thorax and then ascends again to its ultimate termination, the larynx. The origin and course of the nerve are different on the two sides. On the right side the recurrent nerve arises in the root of the neck as the vagus crosses the first part of the subclavian artery. The recurrent branch loops under the subclavian artery and passes deep to the common carotid artery to follow along the tracheoesophageal groove beneath the lateral lobe of the thyroid gland. On the left side the recurrent nerve actually arises in the cervical thorax as the vagus crosses the left side of the arch of the aorta. The recurrent branch loops around the aorta just distal to the ligamentum arteriosum and then, like its fellow on the right side, follows the tracheoesophageal groove upward to the larynx. Both left and right nerves come into close but variable relationships with the inferior thyroid artery. They finally dip under the inferior border of the inferior pharyngeal constrictor muscle and enter the larynx through the cricothyroid membrane. This entry is usually just posterior to the articulation of the inferior cornu of the thyroid cartilage with the cricoid cartilage. Either just before or just after entry into the larynx, the recurrent nerve breaks up into muscular branches and supplies all the intrinsic muscles of the larynx (except the cricothyroideus).

BRANCHES OF THE RECURRENT LARYNGEAL NERVE

Cardiac Branches. These are given off as the nerve loops around the subclavian artery and aorta and contribute to the cardiac plexuses.

Tracheal and Esophageal Branches. These arise all along the nerve and supply both muscular and sensory fibers to the mucous membranes and muscular coats of these structures and the subglottic region of the larynx.

Pharyngeal Branches. Pharyngeal branches are motor fibers to the inferior pharyngeal constrictor muscle.

Inferior Laryngeal Nerves. These are the terminal muscular branches to the intrinsic laryngeal muscles (excluding the cricothyroid muscle).

Esophageal branches. The esophageal branches arise superiorly from the recurrent nerves in the midthorax from the main trunks of the vagus; inferiorly they arise from the esophageal plexus. The motor efferents from the recurrent nerve end for the most part directly in the striated muscle of the upper one third of the esophagus. The efferents from the esophageal plexus in the lower one third of the esophagus are almost exclusively preganglionic parasympathetics which synapse with groups of ganglion cells in the Auerbach-Meissner plexus in the wall of the esophagus. The postganglionics of the plexus innervate the muscle and mucous glands of the esophagus. The middle one third of the esophagus, which has an admixture of striated and nonstriated muscle, is innervated by both general somatic efferent fibers and parasympathetics. The visceral afferents of these branches and plexus have their cell bodies in the inferior ganglion of the vagus.

The *esophageal plexus* is formed by the left vagus posteriorly and the right vagus anteriorly, as both main trunks tend to break up into multiple strands below the bifurcation of the trachea. The plexus also includes sympathetics in its makeup. Just above the diaphragm the plexuses gather into one or two main strands to form the anterior and posterior vagus nerves which then penetrate the diaphragm along with the esophagus.

Spinal Accessory (Eleventh) Nerve

The accessory nerve is entirely motor and derives from both cranial and spinal origins (Fig. 23).

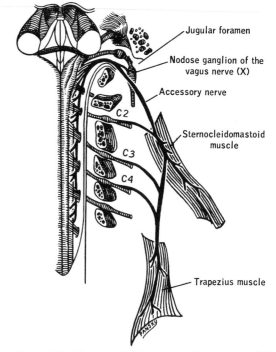

Figure 23. Course, distribution, and relations of the spinal accessory nerve (XI). (From House, E., and Pansky, B.: A Functional Approach to Neuroanatomy. 2nd ed. New York, McGraw-Hill Book Company, Inc., 1967.)

CRANIAL ORIGIN

The cranial part of the eleventh nerve is indeed accessory to the vagus nerve. It has an origin in the nucleus ambiguus like the vagus; it joins the vagus immediately upon leaving the cranium; and its fibers are distributed with the branches of the vagus. The cells of origin in the caudal part of the nucleus ambiguus appear to be cranial extensions of the anterior horn cells of origin of the spinal part of the nerve. The nucleus ambiguus makes central connections with crossed pyramidal fibers and also with other sensory cranial nuclei. The axons of the cranial portion pass ventral to the spinal tract of the fifth nerve and emerge in the posterior lateral sulcus of the medulla as a series of rootlets, in series with the emergence of the vagal fibers more rostrally. They then pass laterally to the jugular foramen where they are joined by the fibers from the spinal origin. The two joined portions then exit from the cranium through the jugular foramen in a common dural sheath with the vagus. At the level of the nodose ganglion, the spinal and cranial portions again divide from each other. The cranial fibers join the vagus and are distributed to the muscles of the pharynx, larynx, and esophagus.

SPINAL ORIGIN

The spinal part of the accessory nerve arises from the lateral cell groups in the anterior horn of the first five or six cervical segments of the spinal cord. These anterior horn cells connect with pyramidal fibers. They also connect with fibers from the medial longitudinal fasciculus, rubrospinal, and vestibulospinal tracts for the coordination of head and eye movements. They also connect with spinal and cranial sensory muscles and tracts. The spinal fibers emerge from the lateral funiculus of the cord and join each other as they pass cranialward alongside the cord and enter the posterior cranial fossa through the foramen magnum. They join the cranial portion at the jugular foramen, but again separate after exiting from the skull through the jugular foramen.

It pierces the anterior border of the cranial portion of the sternocleidomastoid muscle, courses through the upper one third of the muscle and emerges from the posterior border in its midportion. It then courses obliquely downward across the posterior triangle of the neck just beneath the superficial layer of the deep cervical fascia. It is in this area that the nerve is particularly vulnerable to injury from relatively minor surgical procedures or lacerations. The nerve then enters the anterior border of the trapezius muscle. It continues on the deep surface of the trapezius almost to its caudal border and forms a plexiform arrangement with communications from the second, third, and fourth cervical nerves. The branches of the spinal portion are the sternomastoid and trapezius, which innervate the respective muscles.

Hypoglossal (Twelfth) Nerve

The twelfth nerve is the motor nerve of the tongue (Fig. 24). The hypoglossal nucleus lies near the central canal in the caudal closed part of the medulla. The axons of the nucleus pass ventrally through the reticular substance, medial to the inferior olive, and emerge from the

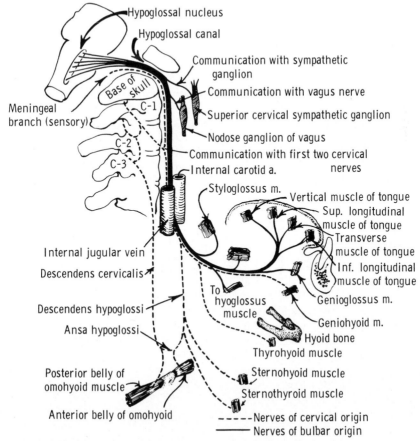

Figure 24. The hypoglossal nerve. (From Chusid, J. G., and McDonald, J. J.: Correlative Neuroanatomy and Functional Neurology. 14th ed. Los Altos, Calif., Lange Medical Publications, 1970.)

medulla as multiple rootlets in the ventral lateral sulcus between the inferior olive and the pyramid. The nucleus of each side communicates with the other across the midline via their dendrites. They also have rich central connections with crossed and uncrossed pyramidal fibers and with secondary sensory pathways from the trigeminal, facial, glossopharyngeal, and vagus nerves.

The rootlets from the brain stem merge into a main trunk which exits from the skull through the hypoglossal canal. The main trunk of the nerve passes downward along the carotid sheath to the level of the occipital artery where it hooks beneath this artery and passes sharply forward superficial to the internal and external carotid arteries. It turns slightly cranialward just above the hyoid bone and passes deep to the tendon of the digastric muscle and forward between the mylohyoid and hyoglossus muscles into the intrinsic muscles of the tongue which it innervates. The true fibers of the hypoglossal nerve also innervate the styloglossus, hyoglossus, and genioglossus muscles.

COMMUNICATIONS OF TWELFTH NERVE

The twelfth nerve connects with the vagus near the base of the skull, the pharyngeal plexus, the sympathetics from the superior cervical ganglion, the lingual nerve, and a loop connecting the anterior primary divisions of the first, second and third cervical nerves. This communication is important because it contains cervical motor fibers destined for the strap muscles, including the geniohyoideus. This communication also provides sensory fibers from the cranialmost cervical dorsal root ganglia.

BRANCHES OF TWELFTH NERVE

Dural branches. Dural branches to the posterior cranial fossa are given off in the hypoglossal canal and are probably contributed by the cervical sensory communications.

Descending hypoglossal branch. This is derived from fibers from the first cervical nerve, leaves the hypoglossal nerve as it loops around the occipital artery, and descends in the lateral neck to form the loop, the *ansa hypoglossi (ansa cervicalis),* with the lateral arm of the loop from the second and third cervical segments, the descending cervical nerve. The branches from this loop supply the inferior strap muscles.

Thyrohyoid and geniohyoid branches. These are muscular branches and are also made up of fibers from the first cervical nerve. They leave the hypoglossal nerve near the posterior border of the hyoglossus muscle.

Muscular branches. Muscular branches are the true hypoglossal fibers which terminate in the styloglossus, hyoglossus, and genioglossus muscles as well as the intrinsic muscles of the tongue. These branches also contain proprioceptor fibers, probably contributed by the cervical root communications.

Spinal Nerves

The spinal nerves arise from the spinal cord within the spinal canal and exit through the intervertebral foramina (Fig. 25). There are 31 pairs and they are grouped as follows: eight cervical, 12 thoracic, five lumbar, five sacral, and one coccygeal. Each spinal nerve attaches to the spinal cord by two roots, a ventral or motor root and a dorsal or sensory root. Both roots unite immediately beyond the spinal ganglion to form the spinal nerve, which exits through the intervertebral foramen.

The *spinal (dorsal root) ganglion* is a collection of nerve cells on the dorsal root of the spinal nerves and constitutes the cell bodies for the peripheral sensory nerves.

The *gray (postganglionic) rami communicantes* contain the postganglionic fibers from the adjacent sympathetic ganglia received by the spinal nerves just distal to the junction of the dorsal and ventral roots. These are sympathetic visceral efferents which reach their destinations in the periphery via the spinal nerves and their branches (Fig. 26). In the cervical region the first four cervical nerves receive their rami from the superior cervical sympathetic ganglion, the fifth and sixth from the middle cervical ganglion, and the seventh and eighth from the inferior cervical ganglion. In the thoracic region there is one ganglion for every spinal nerve, but in the lumbosacral region the ganglia again become more variable and less segmentally arranged with the spinal nerves.

The *white (preganglionic) ramus communicans* is the branch of the spinal nerve through which the preganglionic fibers from the spinal cord reach the sympathetic chain of ganglia. They leave the ventral primary divisions of the spinal nerve just after it has left the intervertebral foramen. The white rami occur on the 12 thoracic and first two lumbar nerves only. The sympathetic ganglia in the chain above and below these segments receive their pregan-

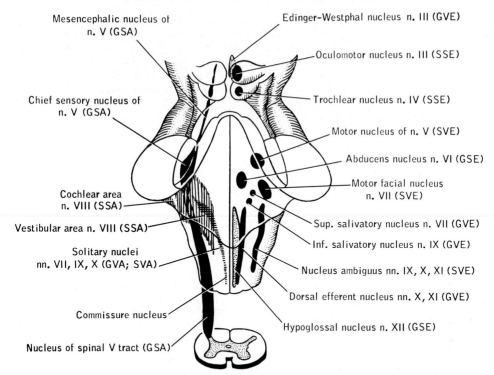

Mesencephalic nucleus of n. V (GSA)

Edinger-Westphal nucleus n. III (GVE)

Oculomotor nucleus n. III (SSE)

Trochlear nucleus n. IV (SSE)

Chief sensory nucleus of n. V (GSA)

Motor nucleus of n. V (SVE)

Abducens nucleus n. VI (GSE)

Motor facial nucleus n. VII (SVE)

Cochlear area n. VIII (SSA)

Vestibular area n. VIII (SSA)

Sup. salivatory nucleus n. VII (GVE)

Inf. salivatory nucleus n. IX (GVE)

Solitary nuclei nn. VII, IX, X (GVA; SVA)

Nucleus ambiguus nn. IX, X, XI (SVE)

Dorsal efferent nucleus nn. X, XI (GVE)

Commissure nucleus

Hypoglossal nucleus n. XII (GSE)

Nucleus of spinal V tract (GSA)

Figure 25. Outline of the brain stem with a projection of the cranial nerve nuclei and their components. Afferents are shown on the left, efferents on the right. (From House, E., and Pansky, B.: A Functional Approach to Neuroanatomy. 2nd ed. New York, McGraw-Hill Book Company, Inc., 1967.)

glionic fibers through these same white rami, with the preganglionic fibers passing vertically up and down the chain to reach the more remote ganglia.

A recurrent *meningeal branch* is given off from each spinal nerve as soon as it emerges from the intervertebral foramen.

Primary Divisions of the Spinal Nerves

The spinal nerve divides into two primary divisions, ventral and dorsal, almost as soon as the two roots have joined to form a single spinal nerve. Each primary division receives fibers from both roots.

DORSAL PRIMARY DIVISIONS OF THE SPINAL NERVES

With only a few exceptions, the dorsal primary divisions supply the muscles and skin of the dorsal part of the neck and trunk.

Cervical Nerves. The dorsal primary division of the first cervical (suboccipital) nerve is usually entirely motor, supplying deep muscles in the suboccipital triangle.

The dorsal division of the second cervical nerve is the largest of the cervical dorsal divisions and is both motor and sensory. It emerges between the atlas and axis and divides into a large medial branch, the *greater occipital nerve,* and a smaller *lateral branch.* The greater occipital nerve gives off a few muscular fibers and then becomes subcutaneous near the nuchal line to supply sensation to the scalp posteriorly and superiorly. The smaller lateral branch gives off muscular fibers.

The dorsal division of the third cervical nerve is also mixed motor and sensory and supplies sensation to the scalp over the lower occipital region. The dorsal divisions intercommunicate rather freely, forming what is sometimes called the *posterior cervical plexus.* The dorsal primary divisions of the fourth through eighth cervical nerves are all mixed, supplying the deep paraspinous muscles and the skin over the back of the neck.

Thoracic Nerves. The dorsal primary divisions of all the thoracic nerves are mixed motor and sensory and supply the large deep muscles of the back and the skin over the back as far down as the buttocks.

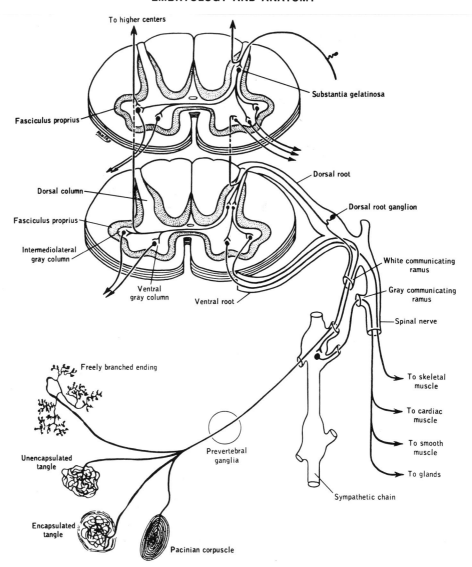

Figure 26. General visceral afferent reflex pathway for impulses entering the CNS through spinal nerves. (From House, E., and Pansky, B.: A Functional Approach to Neuroanatomy. 2nd ed. New York, McGraw-Hill Book Company, Inc., 1967.)

VENTRAL PRIMARY DIVISIONS OF THE SPINAL NERVES

The ventral primary divisions of the spinal nerves supply the ventral and lateral parts of the trunk and all the extremities. In the cervical, lumbar, and sacral regions they unite to form plexuses.

Cervical Nerves. The ventral primary divisions of the first four cervical nerves form the cervical plexus, while the last four cervical nerves together with the first thoracic form the brachial plexus.

Cervical plexus. The cervical plexus originates high in the neck opposite the upper four

vertebral bodies (Fig. 27). It emerges anterior to the deep prevertebral muscles but deep and posterior to the sternocleidomastoid muscle.

SUPERFICIAL OR CUTANEOUS BRANCHES
Smaller Occipital Nerve. This ascends along the posterior aspect of the upper part of the sternomastoid muscle and supplies the skin of the side of the head behind the ear.

Great Auricular Nerve. The great auricular nerve winds around the posterior border of the sternomastoid muscle in its midportion and ascends on the surface of the muscle, dividing into anterior and posterior branches.

The *anterior (facial) branch* is distributed to the skin over the parotid gland.

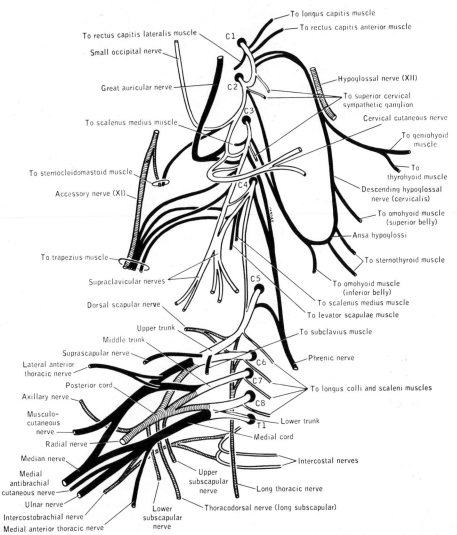

Figure 27. Diagram of the formation and distribution of the cervical and brachial plexuses. In the brachial plexus, black denotes the anterior branches, striped fibers represent the posterior branches. (From House, E., and Pansky, B.: A Functional Approach to Neuroanatomy. 2nd ed. New York, McGraw-Hill Book Company, Inc., 1967.)

The *posterior (mastoid) branch* supplies the skin over the mastoid process and the back of the ear.

Anterior (Cervical) Cutaneous Nerve. This bends around the posterior border of the sternomastoid muscle at its midportion and passes forward on the surface of the muscle, dividing into ascending and descending branches. The ascending branches supply the skin of the submandibular region and the anterior and lateral parts of the upper neck. The descending branches supply the skin of the lateral and anterior aspects of the lower part of the neck as far down as the sternum.

Supraclavicular Nerves. These nerves emerge from beneath the posterior border of the sternomastoid muscle at about its midportion and descend across the posterior triangle under the superficial layer of the deep cervical fascia. Near the clavicle they pierce the fascia in three groups of supraclavicular nerves: *medial (anterior), intermediate,* and *lateral (posterior);* these supply the skin over the upper anterior chest and shoulder.

DEEP OR MUSCULAR BRANCHES. These include numerous branches which go to two large groups of muscles, the deep prevertebral muscles in the lateral neck and the strap muscles, including the geniohyoideus. The communications of these nerves with the hypoglossal nerve in supplying the strap muscles and forming the ansa cervicalis (ansa hypoglossi) have already been described under the discussion of hypoglossal nerve.

The *phrenic nerve* is an important deep branch of the cervical plexus and carries some sensory as well as motor fibers. It is the main motor nerve to the diaphragm, although the diaphragm is also innervated by the lower thoracic nerves. The phrenic nerve originates mainly from the fourth cervical but also receives fibers from the third and fifth nerves. It courses downward and medially on the anterior surface of the anterior scalene muscle into the chest. It passes ventral to the root of the lung and then along the lateral aspect of the pericardium until it reaches the diaphragm. It receives a communication with the sympathetics at the root of the neck.

Brachial plexus. The brachial plexus supplies the nerves, both motor and sensory, to the upper limb (Fig. 25). It is formed by the ventral primary divisions of the fifth through the eighth cervical nerves and by the first thoracic. It courses across the lower lateral neck deep to the prevertebral fascia, emerging from beneath the lateral border of the anterior scalene muscle and running beneath the clavicle into the axilla.

The Autonomic Nervous (Visceral Efferent) System

The autonomic nervous system is the motor system which regulates the organs (viscera) of the body, including the smooth (involuntary) muscles, cardiac muscles, and glands. The basic morphological difference between this visceral motor system and the somatic motor system is that two neurons (preganglionic and postganglionic) are required to transmit an impulse from the central nervous system (CNS) to the active effector organ in the viscera, whereas only a single neuron is required to carry impulses from the CNS to skeletal muscle. The autonomic nervous system is composed of two divisions or systems, the *sympathetic (thoracolumbar)* and *parasympathetic (craniosacral),* which differ morphologically and which are for the most part physiologically antagonistic to each other. The sympathetic system is connected with the CNS through the thoracic and upper lumbar segments of the spinal cord, and its ganglia tend to be more centrally situated near the spinal column. The parasympathetic system is connected with the CNS

through certain cranial nerves and through the middle three sacral segments of the spinal cord; its ganglia tend to be more peripherally located near the organs innervated. The sympathetic and parasympathetic systems both innervate many of the same organs, both systems usually being antagonistic to each other physiologically in the respective organs. The two systems frequently travel together, particularly in the thorax, abdomen, and pelvis, where they form great autonomic plexuses.

Sympathetic Systems

The cells of origin of this system lie in the lateral gray column of the thoracic and lumbar segments of the spinal cord. The axons of these cells leave the cord through the ventral roots of the spinal nerves and reach the paraspinal sympathetic chain by traversing the white rami communicantes. They either terminate in the ganglia of this chain or may pass on through to terminate in the collateral ganglia of the prevertebral plexuses. These are preganglionic fibers and are mostly myelinated. The postganglionic fibers are usually unmyelinated and are distributed to the viscera via communications with other cerebrospinal nerves and various plexuses and by some of their own visceral branches.

SYMPATHETIC TRUNK

This consists of a chain of ganglia connected by intervening cords and extending along the lateral aspect of the vertebral column from the base of the skull to the coccyx. The trunk is also generally considered to include the preganglionic and postganglionic fibers as well. Both types of fibers may run up and down the trunk for a few or many segments. The ganglia of the trunk (chain ganglia) measure in length anywhere from 1 to 10 mm. in diameter and may fuse with one another as in the cervical ganglia (Fig. 28). The roots of the ganglia are the white rami communicantes, so named because of the preponderance of myelinated fibers in their makeup. Many of the preganglionic fibers in the lower thoracic and upper lumbar levels pass out of the trunk through the splanchnic nerves to synapse in the celiac and related collateral ganglia (Fig. 29).

Branches of the Sympathetic Trunk. Branches of distribution of the sympathetic trunk may be made up of either postganglionic fibers (gray rami) or preganglionic fibers which

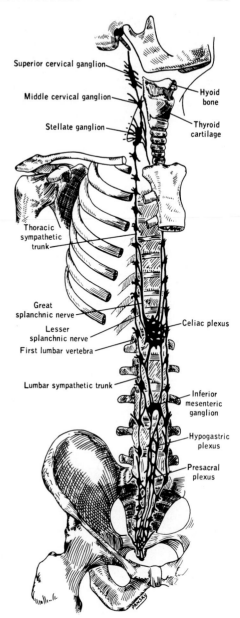

Superior cervical ganglion

Middle cervical ganglion

Stellate ganglion

Hyoid bone

Thyroid cartilage

Thoracic sympathetic trunk

Great splanchnic nerve

Lesser splanchnic nerve

First lumbar vertebra

Lumbar sympathetic trunk

Celiac plexus

Inferior mesenteric ganglion

Hypogastric plexus

Presacral plexus

Figure 28. Sympathetic ganglionated chain, the communicating rami, and the splanchnic nerves of the human adult. (From House, E., and Pansky, B.: A Functional Approach to Neuroanatomy. 2nd ed. New York, McGraw-Hill Book Company, Inc., 1967.)

have passed through without synapses on their way to collateral ganglia in the abdomen. These branches may be distributed in a number of ways by (1) spinal nerves, (2) cranial nerves, (3) arteries, (4) separate branches to individual organs, and (5) great autonomic plexuses.

Cephalic Portions of the Sympathetic System. This part of the sympathetic system contains no ganglia of its own but is essentially a direct extension of the superior cervical ganglion through the internal and external carotid plexus fibers as well as by fibers along the vertebral arteries. Within the cranial cavity the inter-

nal carotid plexus gives off branches which form the cavernous plexus.

Branches of the internal carotid plexus

1. Communication to the trigeminal nerve.

2. Communication to the abducent nerve.

3. *Deep petrosal nerve* leaves the carotid plexus at the foramen lacerum and joins the greater petrosal nerve to form the vidian nerve.

4. *Caroticotympanic nerves* join the tympanic plexus on the promontory of the middle ear.

Branches of the cavernous plexus

1. Communication with the oculomotor nerve.

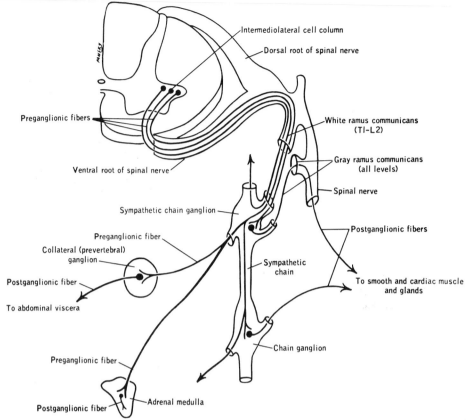

Figure 29. Diagram of a section of the spinal cord, two sympathetic chain ganglia, a collateral ganglion, a terminal ganglion, and the connecting nerves to show the distribution of pre- and postganglionic fibers. (From House, E., and Pansky, B.: A Functional Approach to Neuroanatomy. 2nd ed. New York, McGraw-Hill Book Company, Inc., 1967.)

2. Communication with the trochlear nerve.

3. Communication with the ophthalmic division of the trigeminal nerve.

4. Nerve fibers to the *dilator pupillae muscle* pass to the iris of the eye via the communication with the ophthalmic nerve which joins the nasociliary nerve and the long ciliary nerves to the posterior part of the bulb where they pierce the sclera and pass forward to the iris.

5. Communication with the *ciliary ganglion* via the nasociliary nerve or via a branch of its own through the superior orbital fissure.

6. Fibers to the pituitary gland.

7. Terminal filaments along anterior and middle cerebral arteries and ophthalmic arteries.

Branches of the external carotid plexus. The external carotid filaments follow along the many branches of this artery to their terminations in the erector pilae muscles and sweat glands of the skin as well as in the smooth muscle in the arterial walls themselves. They give off several distinct communications with facial ganglia.

1. filaments to the *submandibular ganglion* from the facial artery.

2. filaments to the *otic ganglion* from the middle meningeal artery.

3. Communication with the *geniculate ganglion* via the *external superficial petrosal nerve.*

Cervical Portion of the Sympathetic System. This portion of the sympathetic system consists of three cervical ganglia: *superior, middle,* and *inferior (stellate ganglion),* connected by intervening cords of sympathetic fibers (Fig. 30). This cervical chain lies posterior to the carotid artery between it and the transverse processes of the cervical vertebrae. They receive no white rami communicantes from the cervical spinal nerves; all their preganglionic fibers arise from the upper five thoracic spinal segments and nerves and ascend in the sympathetic trunk to the cervical ganglia.

Superior cervical ganglion. This ganglion

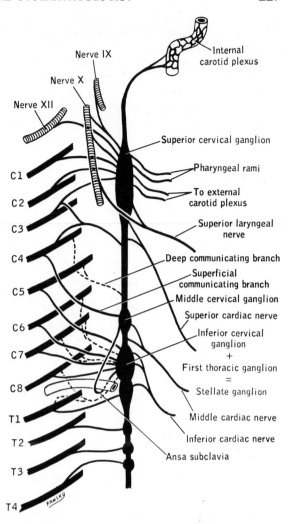

Figure 30. The cervical sympathetic trunk and its ganglia. (Adapted from Woerdeman: Atlas of Human Anatomy. New York, Blakiston Division, McGraw-Hill Book Company, Inc., 1950.)

is much larger than the other two and is usually the largest of all the trunk ganglia. It is fusiform, measuring 28 mm. long and 8 mm. wide, and lies over the longus capitus muscle at the level of the second cervical vertebra.

BRANCHES OF THE SUPERIOR CERVICAL GANGLION

1. Internal carotid plexus.

2. Communications with cranial nerves nine, ten and twelve.

3. Gray rami communicantes to the first three or four cervical spinal nerves.

4. Pharyngeal branches via the vagus and glossopharyngeal nerves to the pharyngeal plexus.

5. Nerves to the *external carotid artery plexus.*

6. Branch to the *intercarotid plexus* which supplies the carotid sinus and carotid body.

7. *Superior cardiac nerve* leaves the superior ganglion and runs down the neck in the posterior fascia of the carotid sheath. On the left side it crosses the subclavian artery and follows the innominate artery to the deep part of the cardiac plexus in the chest. On the right side the superior cardiac nerve follows the common carotid artery into the chest where it crosses the arch of the aorta to reach the superficial part of the cardiac plexus.

Middle cervical ganglion. This ganglion is the smallest of the three cervical ganglia and is sometimes entirely absent. It varies in both position and size. Like the other cervical ganglia it has no white rami communicantes but receives its preganglionic fibers through the sympathetic trunk from the second and third thoracic nerves.

BRANCHES OF THE MIDDLE CERVICAL GANGLION

1. *Gray rami communicantes* to the fifth and sixth cervical nerves.

2. *Middle cardiac nerve* is the largest of the

three cardiac nerves in the neck. It follows the carotid artery into the thorax where it joins the deep cardiac plexus.

3. *Thyroid nerves* form a plexus on the inferior thyroid artery and communicate with the superior and inferior laryngeal nerves.

The trunk between the middle and inferior ganglia is always double, encircling the subclavian artery and supplying the artery with branches. This encirclement of the subclavian is known as the *ansa subclavia*.

Inferior cervical ganglion. The inferior ganglion is usually fused with the first thoracic ganglion, in which case it is known as the *stellate ganglion.* The inferior ganglion lies between the base of the transverse process of the seventh cervical vertebra and the neck of the first rib on the medial side of the costocervical artery. It has no white ramus but receives its preganglionic fibers through the trunk from the upper thoracic nerves. When it is fused with the first thoracic ganglion as the stellate ganglion, it receives the white ramus communicans of the first thoracic nerve.

BRANCHES OF THE INFERIOR CERVICAL GANGLION

1. *Gray rami communicantes* to the sixth, seventh and eighth cervical nerves, and also to the first thoracic in the case of a stellate ganglion. Most of the sympathetics to the upper extremities are provided by the stellate ganglion through the eighth cervical and first thoracic nerves.

2. *Inferior cardiac nerve* may arise from the inferior ganglion, the first thoracic ganglion, the stellate ganglion, or the ansa subclavia. It runs down the anterior surface of the trachea to the deep cardiac plexus.

3. *Vertebral nerves* accompany the vertebral artery through the vertebral foramina and into the cranial cavity on the basilar, posterior cerebral, and cerebellar arteries.

Oculomotor nerve. The oculomotor nerve contains visceral efferents for the nonstriated muscle of the ciliary and pupillary sphincter muscles of the eye. The preganglionic fibers arise in the Edinger-Westphal nucleus in the anterior part of the oculomotor nucleus in the midbrain. They course through the inferior division of the third nerve to the ciliary ganglion. The postganglionics pass in the short ciliary nerves to the eyeball.

Facial nerve. The facial nerve contains parasympathetic efferents to the lacrimal, submandibular, and sublingual glands and to the many mucous and minor salivary glands of the nose, palate, and tongue. The preganglionic fibers arise in the superior salivatory nucleus in the reticular formation of the pons and pass out of the brain stem in the nervus intermedius.

SPHENOPALATINE GANGLION. Those preganglionics of the nervus intermedius which leave the facial nerve at the geniculate ganglion via the greater petrosal nerve pass via the vidian nerve to terminate in the sphenopalatine ganglion. Postganglionics then pass to the lacrimal gland via the maxillary, zygomatic, and lacrimal nerves, while others accompany branches of the maxillary nerve to the glands of the nose, nasopharynx, palate, and tonsils.

SUBMANDIBULAR GANGLION. The preganglionic fibers leaving the facial nerve via the chorda tympani nerve join the lingual nerve to terminate in the submandibular ganglion. The postganglionics pass to the submandibular and sublingual glands.

Glossopharyngeal nerve. The ninth nerve contains efferent parasympathetics to the parotid gland and also to mucous and minor salivary glands in the buccal mucosa, tongue, and floor of mouth. The preganglionic fibers arise in the inferior salivatory nucleus in the medulla, leave the glossopharyngeal in the tympanic nerve, and traverse the lesser petrosal nerve to terminate in the otic ganglion. Most of the postganglionic fibers join the auriculotemporal nerve and are distributed to the parotid gland. Other branches reach the smaller glands of the oral and lingual mucous membranes via the branches of the mandibular nerve.

Vagus nerve. The tenth nerve contains efferents to the nonstriated muscle and glands of the tracheobronchial tree, the alimentary tract as far as the transverse colon, the gallbladder, bile ducts and pancreas, and the inhibitory fibers to the heart. The preganglionic fibers arise from cells in the dorsal motor nucleus of the vagus in the medulla and course in the vagus nerve and its branches to ganglia in or near the organs innervated.

BASIC STRUCTURE OF THE NERVOUS SYSTEM

Neurons

The neuron is the basic unit of structure and function of the nervous system and is composed of a cell body and one or more processes called axons and dendrites. Functionally speaking, axons carry impulses away from the cell body; dendrites conduct impulses toward the cell body.

Neurons can be classified according to the number of processes they have.

Unipolar. These cells have a single process which splits into two branches a short distance from the cell. Neurons of this type are predominantly sensory and are found almost exclusively in the peripheral nervous system.

Bipolar. These cells are fusiform and have an axon attached at one end and a dendrite at the other. They are found in the retina, in cochlear and vestibular ganglia, and in certain places in the central nervous system.

Multipolar. These comprise the majority of central nervous system neurons and are also typical of the peripheral autonomic nervous system. The cell has several poles to which usually attach several dendrites but only one axon.

Cell Body

This the portion of neuron which contains the nucleus. The nucleus is surrounded by the *cytoplasm* of the cell body. The cytoplasm is composed of several components: *neurofibrils,* fine fibrils which extend throughout the cell body and out into all processes; *neuroplasm,* a semiliquid substance surrounding neurofibrils. The neuroplasm of axons is known as *axoplasm.*

Nissl Substance. Also known as *nissl bodies,* this is clumped or particulate matter, usually scattered among the neurofibrils. It extends into the dendrites but not into the axons. It is thought to be responsible for the production of new cytoplasm which flows continuously down the axon (axoplasmic flow).

Pigments

Golgi Net and Mitochondria. These are scattered between the neurofibrils and nissl bodies and probably function, as in other cells, in protein synthesis, respiration, and production of secretions.

Supporting Elements in the Central Nervous System

Ependyma. The ependyma constitutes the epithelium lining the ventricles of the brain and the central canal of the spinal cord.

Neuroglia

Astrocytes. Astrocytes are found throughout the central nervous system in both the gray and white matter.

Oligodendroglia. Oligodendroglia are also found throughout the gray and white matter of the CNS and appear to be the counterpart of the Schwann cells of the peripheral nervous system; that is, they are responsible for the formation of myelin in the white matter.

Microglia. Microglia are the smallest of all the neuroglia. They are highly mobile and

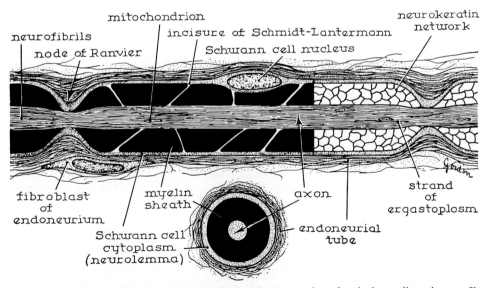

Figure 31. Semidiagrammatic drawing of a longitudinal and cross section of a single myelinated nerve fiber and its endoneurial sheath. The left side of the upper drawing reveals what would be seen after fixation in osmium tetroxide, while the right side of the drawing represents what is seen after the fatty component of myelin has been dissolved away, as occurs with ordinary technics. (From Ham, A. W.: Histology. 6th ed. Philadelphia, J. B. Lippincott Co., 1969.)

move about as macrophages, especially in response to pathological conditions.

Myelin — Insulating Substance of the Nervous System. Myelin is a lipid substance which probably exists in the nervous system as a lipid-protein complex. It is present in the white substance of the CNS and around the axis cylinders of most peripheral nerves. (Fig. 31). It seems to enhance the conduction of nerve impulses which lead to delicate and precise movements.

Components of a Peripheral Nerve (Fig. 32)

Axis Cylinder. The axis cylinder consists of bundles of neurofibrils set in axoplasm.

Myelin. This surrounds the axis cylinders of most peripheral nerves. The notable exceptions which are unmyelinated are the postganglionic fibers of the autonomic nervous system which have their cells of origin in ganglia. The myelin sheaths are interrupted at intervals by constrictions known as *nodes of Ranvier.*

Neurilemma. The neurilemma is a fine membrane of Schwann cells, also known as the *sheath of Schwann,* which surrounds all peripheral nerves, myelinated and unmyelinated. On myelinated nerves there is one Schwann cell between each node of Ranvier. Neurilemma plays both a supporting and metabolic role for the axon. It is apparently responsible for the production of myelin in myelinated nerve fibers.

Endoneurium. Endoneurium consists of fine strands of connective tissue which infiltrates between the individual nerve fibers.

Perineurium. This is a connective tissue sheath which surrounds groups of nerve fibers, dividing the entire nerve into bundles and fascicles.

Epineurium. Epineurium is a rather dense connective tissue which surrounds the entire nerve trunk.

Degeneration and Regeneration of Neurons in Peripheral Nerves

When a peripheral nerve is injured, two types of degeneration occur, *retrograde* and *wallerian.*

Retrograde degeneration constitutes a breakdown of both myelin and the axis cylinder for a few millimeters from the site of injury back along the proximal nerve trunk toward the cell body. The Schwann cells, however, remain alive and may actually proliferate.

Wallerian degeneration refers to the disintegration and disappearance of the myelin and axis cylinders distal to the site of injury in a peripheral nerve.

Schwann cells remain alive in this peripheral portion of the injured nerve and even proliferate to form a longitudinally oriented syncyt-

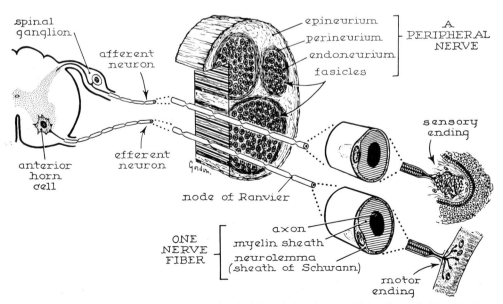

Figure 32. Diagram showing the various parts of a sizable peripheral nerve. (From Ham, A. W.: Histology. 6th ed. Philadelphia, J. B. Lippincott Co., 1969.)

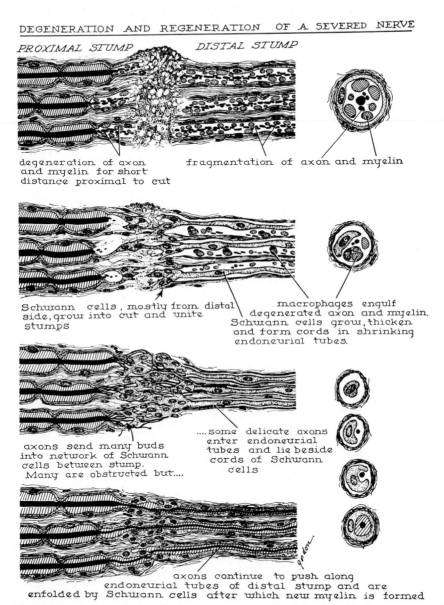

DEGENERATION AND REGENERATION OF A SEVERED NERVE

PROXIMAL STUMP   DISTAL STUMP

degeneration of axon
and myelin for short
distance proximal to cut

fragmentation of axon and myelin

Schwann cells, mostly from distal
side, grow into cut and unite
stumps

macrophages engulf
degenerated axon and myelin.
Schwann cells grow, thicken
and form cords in shrinking
endoneurial tubes.

axons send many buds
into network of Schwann
cells between stump.
Many are obstructed but....

....some delicate axons
enter endoneurial
tubes and lie beside
cords of Schwann
cells

axons continue to push along
endoneurial tubes of distal stump and are
enfolded by Schwann cells after which new myelin is formed

Figure 33.   Diagram showing the changes that occur in a nerve when it is severed and regenerates. (From Ham, A. W.: Histology. 6th ed. Philadelphia, J. B. Lippincott Co., 1969.)

ium along which axoplasm may flow in the regenerative process. Under favorable conditions, axoplasm is said to flow along the distal degenerated segment of nerve at the rate of 1 to 2 mm. per day. It is produced by the viable cell bodies of the nerve proximal to the injury (Fig. 33).

REFERENCES

Bailey, F. R., and Copenhaver, W. M.: Textbook of Histology. 15th ed. Baltimore, The Williams & Wilkins Co., 1964.

Crosby, E. C., Humphrey, T., and Lauer, E. W.: Correlative Anatomy of the Nervous System. New York, The Macmillan Co., 1962.

Gray, H., and Goss, C. M.: Anatomy of the Human Body. 28th ed. Philadelphia, Lea & Febiger, 1969.

Ham, A. W.: Histology. 6th ed. Philadelphia, J. B. Lippincott Co., 1969.

House, E. L., and Pansky, B.: A Functional Approach to Neuroanatomy. 2nd ed., New York, McGraw-Hill Book Co., 1967.

Mcdonald, J. J., and Chusid, J. G.: Correlative Neuroanatomy and Functional Neurology. 12th ed. Las Altos, California, Lange Medical Publications, 1964.

Chapter 6

EMBRYOLOGY AND ANATOMY OF THE SALIVARY GLANDS

by George A. Gates, M.D.

The salivary glands may be divided into two groups: the paired major salivary glands—parotids, submandibulars, and sublinguals, and the minor salivary glands. The major salivary glands are located outside the oral cavity proper and are connected to it by a complex ductal system. The minor salivary glands are situated beneath the mucosa of the oral cavity and empty their secretions directly through short rudimentary ducts. Structurally the major salivary glands are compound tubulo-alveolar in type; the minor salivary glands are simple tubular and tubulo-alveolar. The parotid gland is the largest of the salivary glands and occupies the space immediately in front of and beneath the external ear. The submandibular gland is next largest in size and largely fills the submandibular triangle. The smallest of the major salivary glands is the sublingual gland, which is located under the anterior portion of the floor of the mouth. The minor salivary glands are composed of collections of secretory acini scattered throughout the lining of the buccal cavity, palate, and tongue and are also found, to a lesser extent, in the nasopharynx, nasal cavity, and paranasal sinuses.

EMBRYOLOGY

The major salivary glands and many of the minor salivary glands are derived from stomodeal ectoderm, although those minor glands of the nasopharynx and base of the tongue which arise from pharyngeal entoderm show no histological differences in the adult which would indicate a difference in origin (Patton, 1968).

Each of the major salivary glands develops in a generally similar fashion by the ingrowth of oral epithelium into the underlying mesenchyme. The bud of epithelial cells proliferates to form a cylindrical mass which, with continued growth, extends away from the oral cavity toward its eventual destination. As this cord of cells elongates, budding and branching of the distal segments occur, resulting in the formation of primordial ducts and acini. As the outer ductal cells differentiate into a secretory epithelium, the ductal lumen is formed by degeneration of the central cells. Serous and mucous acini develop from the terminal buds. The myoepithelial cells probably arise here as well. While epithelial growth and differentiation is taking place, the connective tissue stroma of the glands forms by condensation of the regional mesenchyme. Fibrous septa appear between the branching ductal and acinar structures while the investing fascial capsule, which delineates the gland from adjacent structures, is formed. The minor variations shown by each of the major salivary glands from this general developmental pattern are discussed later.

Parotid Gland

The parotid gland primordium can be recognized in the six-week embyro at a point in the cheek where the duct orifice is eventually located. It grows outward and backward across the lateral aspect of the masseter muscle, ending its course against the developing ear canal structures. Simultaneously the facial nerve migrates anteriorly through the developing gland and becomes surrounded by it. The growing glandular parenchyma insinuates itself into the many spaces related to the mandible, temporal bone, and adjacent muscles, forming the many irregularly shaped processes that characterize the adult parotid gland. The ductal system branches distally in an arboreal fashion, increasing in number and decreasing in caliber. The fascial septa within the gland are relatively prominent and adherent to the investing capsule. Only serous cells develop in parotid acini.

Submandibular Gland

Arising near the midline in the floor of the oral cavity, the submandibular primordium is seen late in the sixth week of fetal life. The point of origin is marked in the adult by the orifice of the submandibular duct. The duct elongates posteriorly nearly to the angle of the mandible, where it turns inferiorly and begins to branch in the same manner as the parotid. The intralobular and interlobular fascial septa are less dense than in the parotid gland. The cells in the terminal alveoli differentiate into both serous- and mucus-secreting types.

Sublingual Gland

The sublinguals are the last of the major salivary glands to appear. They can be seen by the end of the seventh week and develop, not as a single anlage, but rather as several closely related groups of cell buds. While these groups merge into a single gross structure which is surrounded by a common fascial envelope, the multicentricity of origin is evidenced in the adult by the presence of multiple ducts which open directly into the floor of the mouth into the submandibular duct. The sublingual gland is the smallest of the major salivary glands and its acini are composed of mucus-secreting and serous-secreting cells, with a predominance of the former.

Minor Salivary Glands

The development of the minor salivary glands is presumed to follow the same general pattern as that of the major salivary glands. The acinar cell types may be mucus-secreting, serous-secreting, or mixed.

ANATOMY

Parotid Gland

The parotid gland varies in weight from 14 to 28 gm. (Gray, 1966) and averages 5.8 cm. in height and 3.4 cm. in width in the adult male (Davis et al., 1956). The gland lies immediately in front of and beneath the external ear on the lateral side of the face. Its lateral surface is convex and smoothly lobulated where it is limited by the superficial layer of deep cervical fascia. The deep surface of the gland is characterized by several irregular processes which project into the intervals between the bony, cartilaginous, muscular, and fascial structures that comprise the medial boundary of the parotid space. The lateral surface of the gland is roughly triangular or ovoid in shape, being wider above where it extends toward the zygomatic arch, than below where it narrows to form the so-called tail which may be elongated and overlap the sternocleidomastoid muscle and mastoid tip. Inferiorly the gland is grooved by the superior surface of the posterior belly of the digastric muscle. Anteriorly the gland overlaps the mandible and its associated muscles both superficially and deeply. The anterior margin of the superficial part of the gland may extend forward for some distance over the masseter muscle as the so-called accessory lobe. In many instances, however, this accessory lobe is separated from the main body of the gland and empties directly into the main parotid duct. Posteriorly the gland is intimately applied to the cartilaginous and bony segments of the external auditory canal and the anteroinferior surface of the temporal bone.

As the gland passes into the space between the mandible in front and temporal bone behind, it is narrowed somewhat and enlarges medially to form the deep or retromandibular portion of the gland. The gland is in medial relation below to the styloid process, the styloid muscles, the internal carotid artery, and the internal jugular vein; above to the thin stylomandibular membrane which separates the gland from the parapharyngeal space; and anteriorly to the internal pterygoid muscle. The stylomandibular process of the gland invaginates the stylomandibular fascia just above the stylomandibular ligament and, on occasions, forms a distinct tunnel (Patey and Thackray, 1957). The inferior process of the retromandibular portion, when present, passes beneath the stylomandibular ligament and enters the parapharyngeal space area (Work and Habel, 1963) (Fig. 1). Above, the glenoid process of the gland extends deeply toward the glenoid fossa. The parotid duct emerges from the undersurface of the anterior portion of the gland and, lying on the masseter muscle, passes forward about 1 cm. below the zygomatic arch accompanied by a buccal branch of the facial nerve. It turns medially at the anterior border of the masseter muscle and pierces the buccal fat pad and buccinator muscle to enter the mouth opposite the second upper molar tooth. The duct is 4 to 6 cm. in length and 0.5 mm. in diameter (Woodburne, 1965). The small accessory portion of the parotid gland, when present, lies above the duct and drains directly into it. Intraorally the duct orifice is seen at the tip of a small papilla and will usually admit a No. 0 or No. 1 probe without difficulty.

The superficial layer of deep cervical fascia divides to completely encase the parotid gland and is known as the parotid fascia. The dense fibrous septa which compartmentalize the gland are fused with the parotid fascia, thereby preventing the ready development of a surgical plane between the gland and the fascia. This fascia is continuous with the fascia of the sternocleidomastoid and digastric muscles posteriorly and the masseter muscle anteriorly. It is attached to the mastoid tip behind and the zygoma above. The fascia covering the medial surface of the gland is thinner and is continuous with the fascia of the styloid muscles and attaches to the styloid process.

The facial nerve enters the parotid gland posteriorly and deeply immediately after giving off the motor branches to the auricular and posterior digastric muscles. The major division of the nerve, the pes anserinus, usually occurs within 1.3 cm. of where the main trunk leaves the stylomastoid foramen (Dargent and Duroux, 1946). At the pes the nerve branches to form the temporofacial division above and the cervicofacial division below. The nerve continues to branch within the parotid gland as the fibers pass obliquely through its substance and exits the gland anteriorly to innervate the muscles of facial expression. Vertical anastomotic branches are commonly seen between the branches of the temporofacial division; are occasionally seen between a buccal branch of the cervicofacial division and one or more branches of the temporofacial division; are rarely seen between the mandibular branch and other branches; and are unknown between the branches of the cervicofacial division (Davis et al., 1956). Occasionally the nerve has a plexiform arrangement within the gland but a system of discrete branches is the rule.

Sharp disagreement exists as to whether the parotid gland is bilobed in character, with the facial nerve branches passing around a connecting isthmus in a discrete fascial space, or whether the nerve passes through the sub-

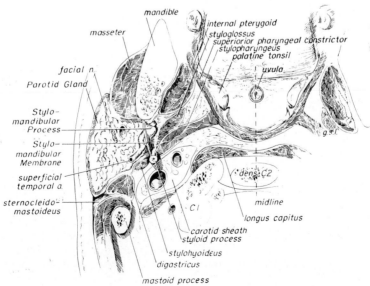

Figure 1. Horizontal section at the level of C1 demonstrating the deep relationships of the parotid gland. (Work, W. P., and Habel, D. W.: Ann. Otol. *72:*842, 1963.)

stance of a unilobar gland, being separated from it only by the perineural sheath. From a surgical point of view the division of the gland into lobes is an iatrogenic rather than an anatomical circumstance. Normally the main trunk of the facial nerve occupies, as it enters the gland, a constant relationship to the superior border of the posterior digastric muscle insertion, the posterolateral border of the styloid process, and the groove formed by the junction of the tympanic bone and mastoid process. In addition, the sharply pointed inferior edge of the cartilaginous ear canal serves as a superficial guide to the general area of the stylomastoid foramen (Gaughran, 1961). The styloid process is frequently absent or only rudimentarily developed in many cases. Anteriorly a buccal branch of the temporofacial division maintains a nearly constant relationship to the superior border of the main parotid duct. Inferiorly the mandibular branch is seen crossing the lateral surface of the posterior facial vein. The vein is occasionally doubled or duplicated, with the nerve passing in between.

The greater auricular nerve which lies deep to the platysma on the superficial layer of deep cervical fascia usually divides below the external ear. The anterior branch sends sensory fibers to the skin and fascia overlying the parotid gland. The auriculotemporal branch of the mandibular division of the fifth cranial nerve passes on or in the superior deep portion of the gland as it leaves the infratemporal fossa to innervate the scalp. It sends several branches to the parotid gland which carry, in addition to sensory fibers, the postganglionic parasympathetic fibers from the otic ganglion which are secretomotor to the parotid gland. The preganglionic fibers arise in the inferior salivatory nucleus, leave the medulla in the ninth cranial nerve, and take a circuitous route across the promontory of the middle ear and pass to the otic ganglion via the lesser superficial petrosal nerve. Postganglionic sympathetic nerves arise in the superior cervical ganglion and pass to the parotid gland with its arterial supply.

The vascular relationships of the parotid gland are principally with branches of the external carotid artery, although the internal carotid artery may occasionally lie in close proximity to the retromandibular portion of the gland. The external carotid artery enters the gland deeply and divides within its substance into the internal maxillary and superficial temporal arteries. The latter gives rise to the transverse facial artery, which passes laterally to cross the mandible and exits the parotid gland near its superior border. Branches of these vessels, as well as those of the posterior auricular artery, provide a rich arterial supply to the gland. The venous relationships are quite variable but, in general, the posterior facial vein arises within the gland from the junction of the internal maxillary and superficial temporal veins. It exits the gland inferiorly, often dividing into an anterior branch which unites with the anterior facial vein to form the common facial vein and a posterior branch which, with the posterior auricular vein, forms the external jugular vein. The veins lie superficial to the arteries and deep to the facial nerve.

The parotid gland is richly invested with lymph nodes which are located immediately under the parotid fascia and within the substance of the gland. These nodes carry lymph from the parotid gland and serve as the principal collecting system for the frontotemporal region of the scalp, the upper face, the lacrimal gland, and the pinna. The nodes vary in number from three to 20. There are a few nodes in relation to the deep surface of the gland whose afferent channels drain the palate, nasopharynx, auditory tube, and middle ear. The efferent channels communicate with both the superficial and deep lymphatic systems of the neck.

Submandibular Gland

The submandibular gland is the second largest of the major salivary glands. Its external surface is finely lobulated in appearance and rounded in shape. It occupies the bulk of the submandibular triangle whose superior border is the body of the mandible and whose sides are formed by the anterior and posterior bellies of the digastric muscle. Superficially the gland is covered by skin, subcutaneous tissue, platysma muscle, and the superficial layer of deep cervical fascia. This fascia, which is attached below to the hyoid bone and above to the mandible, stretches across the submandibular triangle and is readily separable from the capsule of the gland. The gland is in medial relationship to the hyoglossus muscle posteriorly and genioglossus muscle anteriorly and to the lingual and hypoglossal nerves. Anteriorly the gland is indented by the mylohyoid muscle and overlaps it superficially to a considerable extent when large, and underlaps it deeply where the gland and duct pass forward under its cover. Posteriorly the gland rests against the posterior digastric and stylohyoid muscles and against the parotid gland, from which it is separated by the quadrangular fascia.

The duct emerges from the hilum of the gland on its deep surface and passes forward and medialward to open into the anterior floor of the mouth through a constricted orifice located in the sublingual papilla. The duct is 5 cm. in length and thin walled. It is crossed twice by the lingual nerve; first, laterally, as the nerve enters the submandibular triangle from above and behind, and again, anteriorly, as the nerve passes medial to the duct, sending its terminal branches upward to supply sensory endings in the tongue and mouth. The duct can readily be seen in the mouth as a ridge passing obliquely posterolateral from the papilla. The duct orifice is small and will admit a 3-0 or 4-0 probe and can be dilated in most cases to admit a No. 1 or 2 probe.

Postganglionic parasympathetic fibers to the submandibular gland arise in the submandibular ganglion and from scattered ganglion cells located within the hilum of the gland (Langley's ganglion). The submandibular ganglion lies on the hypoglossus muscle at the posterior border of the mylohyoid and is attached to the gland by a short stalk and to the lingual nerve from which it is suspended by two nerve rootlets. The posterior rootlet carries preganglionic fibers to both the submandibular and Langley's ganglion. The anterior rootlet carries postganglionic fibers to the sublingual gland and the minor salivary glands in the oral cavity. The preganglionic fibers arise in the superior salivatory nucleus, leave the pons in the nervus intermedius, and are carried across the middle ear by the chorda tympani nerve which joins the lingual nerve deep in the infratemporal fossa. Postganglionic sympathetic fibers from the superior cervical ganglion enter the gland with its arterial supply.

The facial artery is the principal nutrient vessel of the gland. It enters the submandibular triangle deep to the posterior digastric and stylohyoid muscles and lies in a groove on the deep surface of the gland as it courses upward. At the superior margin of the gland the artery turns upward and passes over the body of the mandible in a notch located at the anterior border of the masseter muscle. The gland receives many small arterial branches from the facial artery and from the submental artery. The submental artery leaves the facial artery at the superior border of the gland and passes forward on the mylohyoid muscle. Venous drainage is via the anterior facial vein, which lies on the superficial layer of cervical fascia.

Several lymph nodes lie on the gland under the cervical fascia. There are no lymph nodes in the substance of the gland. The nodes drain to the deep cervical lymphatic system.

Sublingual Gland

The sublingual gland is the smallest of the three major salivary glands. It is located deep to the mucus membrane of the floor of the mouth and is covered inferiorly by the mylohyoid muscle and laterally by the mandible. It lies on the genioglossus muscle, from which it is separated by the lingual nerve and submandibular duct. Posteriorly it abuts the deep anterior projection of the submandibular gland. It empties its secretions into the mouth through 10 to 12 small caliber ducts, some of which empty into the submandibular duct. Its arterial supply is via the submental branch of the facial artery and the sublingual branch of the lingual artery. Secretomotor innervation is from the postganglionic fibers carried from the submandibular ganglion by the lingual nerve. Lymphatic drainage is to the submandibular nodes.

Minor Salivary Glands

The oral cavity receives the secretions of multiple small collections of salivary gland tissue located in the submucosa of the lips, cheeks, hard and soft palates, and the tonsillar pillars. In addition, numerous glands are found in the muscle of the base of the tongue posterior to the vallate papillae and along the underside of the lateral edges of the tongue. These glands are serous, mucous, and mixed in type. Each gland opens directly into the oral cavity through small separate ducts. The vascular and lymphatic relationships are the same as the area of mucosa under which they are situated. The parasympathetic innervation is via the lingual nerve, except for the glands of the palate whose secretomotor fibers are distributed from the sphenopalatine ganglion through the palatine nerves.

REFERENCES

Dargent, M., and Duroux, P. E.: Données anatomiques concernant la morphologie et certains rapports du facial intra-parotidien. Press Méd. *54*:523–524, 1946.

Davis, R. A., Anson, B. J., Budinger, J. M., and Kurth, L. E.: Surgical anatomy of the facial nerve and parotid gland based upon a study of 350 cervico-facial halves. Surg. Gynec. Obstet. *102*:385–412, 1956.

Gaughran, G. R.: The parotid compartment. Ann. Otol. *70*:31–51, 1961.

Gray, H.: Anatomy of the Human Body. 28th ed. Philadelphia, Lea & Febiger, 1966.

Patey, D. H., and Thackray, A. C.: The pathological anatomy and treatment of parotid tumors with retropharyngeal extension. Brit. J. Surg. *44*:352–358, 1957.

Patton, G. M.: Human Embryology. 3rd ed. New York, McGraw-Hill Book Co., 1968.

Woodburne, R.: Essentials of Human Anatomy. 3rd ed. New York, Oxford University Press, 1965.

Work, W. P., and Habel, D. W.: Mixed tumors of the parotid gland with extension to the lateral pharyngeal space. Ann. Otol. *72*:842–860, 1963.

Section Two

PHYSIOLOGY

Chapter 7

PHYSICS OF SOUND

by Juergen Tonndorf, M.D.

The following account is written for people whose background is not in physics and who therefore have little if any training in mathematics. Mathematics will be used with respect to only one point (*impedance*), but it will be very elementary, not going beyond simple calculus. Those desiring a more formal treatment are referred to other textbooks such as are listed in the bibliography.

Sound is a form of physical energy. The ear as well as the larynx are mechanical devices (receiver of sound and generator, respectively); in this respect they must both obey the appropriate laws of physics, i.e., of *acoustics,* as the particular subfield is called that deals with sound.

A good case can be made for the fact that the larynx operates like certain types of wind instruments. However, to simply compare the action of the ear to that of a microphone is quite misleading. Microphones are so designed that they only measure, but do not disturb, an existing sound field, and especially so that they do not draw acoustic power from it. By contrast, the ear does consume acoustic power, although admittedly in quite small quantities.

It has been customary for a long time to describe sound in terms of tones (or mixtures of such) of very long durations, mainly because of certain powerful mathematical descriptions that can be applied to such cases. However, sounds in our everyday experience are usually not of the latter type. More typically, they are short, in the order of 0.1 sec. and often much shorter; for example, speech sounds in running speech. Therefore, we must also consider short-lasting, so-called *transient,* sounds. In counterdistinction, the long duration sounds are then referred to as *steady-state* events.

It may be noted in this connection that the information carrying capacity of steady-state sounds is essentially nil. It takes sound signals that change rapidly with time and have little predictability to transmit information.

THE DECIBEL (dB)

Before entering the discussion of acoustics proper, we must define the *decibel* (dB), a measure that has found widespread acceptance not only in acoustics, but also in electrical engineering, optics, and many other fields. As will be pointed out in detail later, sound signals may vary in intensity from low to high, corresponding to variations in loudness from soft to loud. Intensity is a physical measure and is defined as the average rate of energy flow through a unit area (1 cm.^{2}) at a given point in a specified direction. Its unit is the watt/cm.^{2}. Since power = energy per sec., it may also be considered a measure of "power density."

In acoustics one is frequently interested in mere relative changes, i.e., how much more intense one given sound is as compared to another. Moreover, more often than not, effects such as the attenuation afforded by a wall are independent of the actual level. (Note that the term "level" refers to absolute power values in watts/cm.^{2}; there are also energy levels, sound pressure levels, and so forth.) Typically, such a wall may attenuate sound to one tenth its original value. If the original value is L_0 and the attenuated one L_a we may have

$$L_0 \quad 10, 100, 1000\ldots\ldots \atop L_a \quad 1 \quad 10 \quad 100\ldots\ldots \qquad (I)$$

In all three cases the result is a *ratio of 10*. We can rewrite the values of (I) as

$$
\begin{array}{llll}
L_0 & 10^1 & 10^2 & 10^3 \ldots \ldots \\
L_a & 10^0 & 10^1 & 10^2 \ldots \ldots
\end{array}
\qquad \text{(II)}
$$

We see then that the ratio, being 10^1, can be conveniently expressed by its exponent, 1 in the present example. These exponents, as is well known, are *logarithms to the base of ten*. This is the basis of the decibel notation which also contains a scaling factor of 10:

$$
N_{dB} = 10 \log \frac{I'}{I''}
\qquad \text{(1)}
$$

The result is a number (*N*), since the ratio between two values (*I*-intensity) that have the same dimension (e.g., watts/cm.^{2}) is dimensionless.

In actual practice, sound is more conveniently measured in terms of pressure than in terms of intensity. Sound pressure (p) is given as dyne/cm.^{2} (i.e., force per area), and is related to sound intensity (I) as in

$$
p^2 \sim I
\qquad \text{(2)}
$$

Therefore

$$
N_{dB} = 10 \log \left(\frac{p'}{p''}\right)^2 = 20 \log \frac{p'}{p''}
\qquad \text{(3)}
$$

Hence, a ratio of 10 in terms of intensity equals 10 dB, whereas the same ratio in terms of sound pressure equals 20 dB; doubling an intensity value means an increment of 3 dB, whereas doubling a pressure value means an increment of 6 dB. The 5 dB step of a clinical audiometer is thus seen to represent almost a doubling of the sound pressure value. The short table (III) gives a few representative values.

The acceptance of the decibel was aided by another fact. Communication engineers had found out quite early that the range of intensities between the hearing threshold (the level at which one barely hears a sound) and those sounds painful to the ear is quite large. In the middle frequency range (1000 Hz to 3000 Hz) in which a normal ear is most sensitive (for an exact definition of frequency see later), this range is close to 1:10,000,000. Moreover, it

was commonly believed until recently that the response of the ear varies as a logarithm of the signal magnitude, the so-called *Weber-Fechner* law. (We know now that this law is only an approximation, and that the responses of *all* senses vary as power functions of signal magnitude whereby the exponent of such functions is a characteristic of each particular sense – the power law of Stevens and of Plateau.) Engineers had already found it convenient at the time when radios were first introduced to use volume controls that were logarithmically rather than linearly tapered. (Such controls are nothing but variable resistors.) In this manner the user has the impression that he is actually controlling "loudness" in a linear manner.

If one wishes to express the results of a given measurement, of a noise level for example, in absolute terms, but still use the dB, one simply has to form the dB ratio between the power (or sound pressure) level in watts/cm.^{2} or dynes/cm.^{2}, respectively, to a given *standard reference level*. For many years the values of these reference levels have been set at 10^{-10} watts/cm.^{2} or 0.0002 dynes/cm.^{2}, respectively. The arbitrariness of such reference levels is reflected by the fact that in underwater acoustics a level of 1 dyne/cm.^{2} is used as a reference. Still other values are used in audiometry, where the zero reference level is determined as a sort of an average threshold for healthy young ears. It varies with frequency to account for the frequency dependence of human hearing. The 1951-ASA (American Standards Association, now ANSI (American National Standards Institute) levels have in 1969 been replaced by the 1964 ISO (International Standards Organization) levels, which differ slightly, but consistently, from the former.

SIMPLE HARMONIC MOTION

Sound is usually produced by structures that are set into vibration by mechanical, electromagnetic, or a host of other means.

The simplest sustained tone that can be produced, for example by a tuning fork, is based upon very uniform, pendulumlike motions of its tines. If we plot such to and fro motions against time, we obtain a *time course*, a section of which is shown in Figure 1. This is called a *simple harmonic* motion (for a reason that will become obvious presently) or, because of its derivation from *sine* (or *cosine*) functions, a

dB	10	20	30	40	
Sound intensity ratios	10	100	1000	10,000	(III)
Sound pressure ratios	3.162	10	31.62	100	

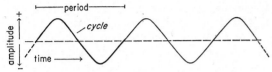

Figure 1. Time pattern of a sine wave. The first cycle is drawn slightly heavier. Its duration is called a period. The dashed continuations at both ends indicate that this pattern is a mere fraction of an event which, at least theoretically, lasts infinitely long. (From Glorig, A. (ed.): Audiometry Principles and Practice. Baltimore, The Williams & Wilkins Co., 1965, Chapter II.)

sinusoidal waveform. In a true sinusoidal wave the time duration of one cycle, the *period,* is rigidly maintained. One cycle may be counted from any given starting point until the waveform has returned to the same point having the same tendency of motion. For example, starting at the zero line on the left of Figure 1, the trace goes upward to the positive maximum, downward again to zero, passes the negative maximum, and returns to zero. Such count could be started at any other point. The number of cycles per second is a measure of the frequency (unit: 1 Hertz [Hz]). The closest psychophysical equivalent to frequency is pitch.

The excursions of the tracing from zero in either direction represent the *displacements* of the vibrating structure from its resting position. The height is called amplitude. Starting from the zero line at any point in time, this may be the *instantaneous* amplitude, and it may be either positive or negative; at the point of maximum displacement it is known as the *peak* amplitude; that from a positive peak to a negative one, the *peak-to-peak* amplitude.

One other important measure is the so-called *root-mean square* (RMS) amplitude. It represents a statistical average and is registered by many measuring instruments. For sinusoidal events it is equal to the peak amplitude divided by $\sqrt{2}$, i.e., approximately to 0.707 times the value of the peak amplitude. The importance of RMS values lies in *power* considerations. A unidirectional (dc) current of electricity passing through a wire dissipates energy in the form of heat. It is clear that an alternating (ac) current that changes direction, reducing even to zero at regular intervals (like the tracing of Figure 1), will heat the wire to a lesser extent. The RMS value then designates the magnitude of a dc current that has the same heating capacity as an ac current of a given peak value. Since power considerations are principally alike in electrical, mechanical, and other phys-

ical processes, the RMS concept has universal validity. The nearest psychophysical equivalent to the displacement amplitude of a sound generator (at least for a given frequency) is *loudness.*

SUPERPOSITION OF SINE-WAVE EVENTS

A given structure may be subjected to more than one sinusoidal event at the same time. Obviously the structure cannot execute two different vibrations at the same time, but will follow their *resultant* from instant to instant. We will limit consideration to two such events applied simultaneously and will start out with a special case in which both are of the same frequency.

Phase. In order to determine the resultant, we must know in what part of its cycle one event happens to be with respect to the other. Because of their derivation from sine functions (see previous discussion), the tracing of a full "cycle" may be said to represent the circumference of a circle of a radius equal to the peak amplitude. Thus, each point along the cycle, or its projection upon the time axis, may be expressed in terms of an angle between zero and 360 degrees, starting at any point—a zero-crossing, for example. Such an angle, which then determines uniquely the relative state of the vibratory event, is called a *phase angle.* Since the circumference of a circle may also be expressed in *radians,* one can also employ multiples or fractions of π to quantify a phase angle (2π radians $=360°$).

Figure 2 gives two pairs of events that have different phase relationships. It is seen that for either pair the phase relation determined at any one point in time holds for any other point. (This arises from the fact that we had assumed that both events have the same frequency. In such a case it takes exactly the same time for either event to complete one cycle or any fraction thereof.) In tracing (A) of Figure 2, the phase relation is 90° $(1/2\pi)$, with event A *leading* event B, or event B *lagging* behind event A. In tracing (B) of Figure 2, the phase relation is exactly 180° (1π); lead or lag cannot be determined in this case. The latter situation is often referred to as *phase opposition.* If there is no phase difference, the events are said to be *in phase* (0° phase angle).

Once the phase angle is determined, the resultant waveform of the two events can be determined by adding their instantaneous am-

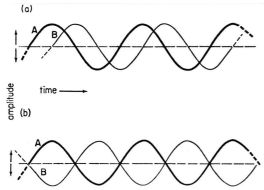

Figure 2. Phase relationships between two sinusoidal events. (*a*) The two events are 90 degrees apart in phase with event A leading event B; (*b*) both events are now in opposite phase relation. (From Glorig, A. (ed.): Audiometry Principles and Practice. Baltimore, The Williams & Wilkins Co., 1965, Chapter II.)

plitudes, so-called *linear superposition,* with proper regard to their signs in the manner of Figure 3. Of special interest are cases (a) and (b). In both of them, amplitudes of the primary events are equal. When the phase angle is 0° (case a), the resultant R has twice the amplitude of each single event since amplitude is simply doubled at all times (*reinforcement*). When the phase angle is 180° (case b), the resultant R is a straight line, amplitudes of the primary events being equal and of opposite signs at all times (*cancellation*). In all other cases (for example, case c), that is, when phase angles are neither 0° nor 180° and/or amplitudes of the primaries are not equal to each other, there is partial reinforcement or partial cancellation. For the case of equal amplitude of the two primary signals, the limiting phase angle is 120°. If the latter is smaller than

this value, there will be partial reinforcement; if it is larger, partial cancellation.

It is noted that all resultants, with the exception of the case of complete cancellation, are also sine waves having the same frequency as the primary events.

Beats. If we now allow the two events to have different frequencies, although such differences should be small (500 Hz and 510 Hz, for example), an interesting phenomenon will develop. In contrast to the cases just discussed, the phase relation between the two events does not stay put, but alters continuously. Inspection of Figure 4, line C, indicates that whenever a period of time is elapsed that is the reciprocal of the difference of the two signal frequencies (10 Hz = 1/0.1 sec. in the present example) a given phase relation will repeat itself, only to change once more at the next instant. The superposition of two such events must lead to a waveform such as given in line D of Figure 4. Its amplitude no longer stays uniform; it fluctuates in a sinusoidal manner at a rate once more equal to the difference between the signal frequencies. Furthermore, as can be seen from Figure 4, the waveform of the resultant has a period different from that of either of the two signal frequencies. It is equivalent to their average (1/2[500 + 510] = 505 Hz in the present example).

When the amplitudes of the two primaries are equal, there is one instant of complete cancellation followed by a later one at which amplitude is exactly twice that of each primary (see line D of Figure 4). This had to be expected from the results of Figure 3, that is, from the principle of linear superposition.

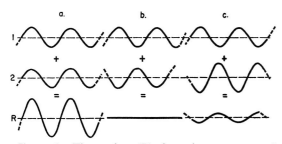

Figure 3. The resultant (R) of two sine-wave events (1 and 2) when combined in different phase relationships. Column *a* (in-phase relation, equal amplitudes) shows amplitude doubling; column *b* (phase opposition, equal amplitudes) shows complete cancellation; column *c* (phase opposition, amplitude not equal) shows partial cancellation. (From Glorig, A. (ed.): Audiometry Principles and Practice. Baltimore, The Williams & Wilkins Co., 1965, Chapter II.)

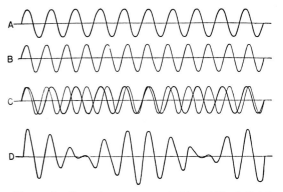

Figure 4. Two sine-wave events (A and B) of slightly different frequencies when superimposed upon each other (C) result in a beat pattern. (D). For the sake of illustration, a frequency ratio of 5:6 between primaries has been chosen. (From Glorig, A. (ed.): Audiometry Principles and Practice. Baltimore, The Williams & Wilkins Co., 1965, Chapter II.)

Since beats are heard especially well under this latter condition, they are known as "best beats." When the amplitudes of the primaries are not equal, neither cancellations nor reinforcements are complete. Moreover there are slight variations of frequency in addition to those of amplitude. However, the resultant beats sound less distinct to the ear.

The example of Figure 4 concerned two primaries that were only slightly apart in frequency. Musicians who tune their instruments while listening to the disappearance of beats call this type an *imperfect unison*. Physicists refer to them as *simple beats*.

Beats may also appear between primaries that are not quite in *harmonic relationship* (see later), that is, when their frequency ratio is not quite an integral number such as 1:2; 1:3; 2:3; etc. For example, the combination of 500 Hz and 1010 Hz leads also to a 10 Hz beat. (The correct harmonic relationship would be 500 Hz and 1000 Hz [1:2].) This is then known either as a *mistuned consonance* or as *complex beats* in musical or physical terminology, respectively.

Complex Harmonic Motion. Finally, we must examine the waveforms resulting from superposition of events having frequencies that are related to one another by exact integral numbers, e.g., 500 Hz and 1000 Hz (1:2); 500 Hz and 1500 Hz (1:3); 500 Hz and 750 Hz (2:3); 750 Hz and 1000 Hz (3:4); etc. Beats, obviously, cannot occur in such cases. Although in the case of 1:2 relationship, for example, one primary waveform will complete two cycles at the same time the other one completes only one, this relationship is strictly maintained at all times, and there is no gradual shift in phase. Figure 5 shows the waveform resulting from such a combination for two different phase relationships between the primaries. In contrast to the simple sinusoidal waveform of Figure 1, those of Figure 5 are known as *complex* waveforms. To be sure, Figure 5 still appears relatively "simple," but when several frequencies are superpositioned, the resultant waveform will soon become quite complex, especially since its shape does not only depend upon the number of the components but also upon their relative strength and their phase relationships (Figs. 5 and 6).

In music such whole number relationships play a special role. For example, the 1:2 ratio represents an octave, the 2:3 ratio a fifth, the 3:4 ratio a fourth, and so forth. For this reason the term *harmonic relationship* has been in use for a long time. In a given harmonic series one

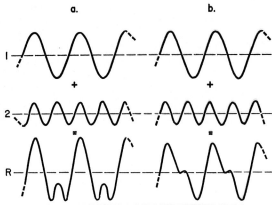

Figure 5. Combined effect (R) resulting from the combination of two sine-wave events (1 and 2); event 2 has twice the frequency of event 1. Right and left columns differ with respect to the phase relationship between primaries. Note the difference in resultant waveforms. (From Glorig, A. (ed.): Audiometry Principles and Practice. Baltimore, The Williams & Wilkins Co., 1965, Chapter II.)

refers to the lowest common divisor (e.g., 100 Hz of the series 100, 200, 300, 400, ... Hz) as the *fundamental* or the *first partial*. The 200 Hz component would be the first overtone or the second partial, and so forth. The terms "fundamental" and "overtones" are most commonly used in musical terminology, whereas "partials" are employed more commonly in physical terminology. (The term "basic frequency" is occasionally employed for the first partial.) We realize now that the relationship between beating primaries is an *inharmonic* one.

Fourier Analysis. Actually, the *synthesis* of complex waveforms as described in the foregoing has become possible only relatively recently after suitable devices had become available. The knowledge that complex waveforms show a *periodicity*, that is, the periodic repetition of a characteristic waveform, however complex, is somewhat older. This important discovery is credited to the French mathematician Fourier. *Fourier analysis* is a powerful mathematical tool and is used today in many different fields, not only in acoustics. Fourier first described his theorem for the problem of heat transfer in 1811. Its application to acoustics, and particularly to the performance of the ear, was first suggested by G. S. Ohm in 1843. This is known as *Ohm's law of acoustics*, in contrast to his better known *electrical law*.

The point must be stressed that for any given waveform there is only one solution in terms of the contained frequencies and their amplitude and phase relationships. It is then possible to record this information in the form

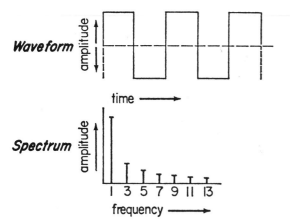

Figure 6. Spectroanalysis of a complex waveform. Chosen for this purpose is a so-called square wave having infinitely steep slopes and flat tops and bottoms. This type of wave is used extensively in instrumental testing. Its spectrum, a discrete line spectrum, is infinitely wide, although the relative amplitude of the higher harmonics is decreasing rapidly with rank order. (From Glorig, A. (ed.): Audiometry Principles and Practice. Baltimore, The Williams & Wilkins Co., 1965, Chapter II.)

of a *spectrum*, i.e., relative amplitude *vs.* frequency (including phase information). In such a plot each frequency appears as a line of a given height. (For an example, see Figure 6.) All complex sounds, including inharmonic sounds, have *discrete line spectra*. It is a curious fact, however, that as one gains information about the frequency composition of a given complex sound one loses sight of its waveform. There is no denying that by experience one learns to some degree to associate some of the waveforms of lesser complexity with their spectra, but that is an *acquired* faculty, not one that is inherent.

Either notation, waveform or spectrum, is complete and unique. When information is being stored for future playback (phonograph records, recording tape) it is more convenient to record waveforms. For purposes of analyzing the performance (potential or real) of electro-acoustic systems, Fourier transformation is an indispensable and powerful tool. G. S. Ohm, as just mentioned, had postulated that the ear performs a Fourier analysis upon incoming sound. This hypothesis was based upon the observation that the ear can differentiate complex tones to some degree, a faculty that can be improved by training. Moreover, the ear distinguishes musical instruments and voices partly by recognizing their characteristic *timber* or *quality*. (The word timbre is used in musical terminology and the word quality in physical terminology.) Instruments do not produce pure tones (*i.e.,* simple sinusoidal sounds); their timbre depends upon the number and distribution of the higher harmonics they invariably contain. This is so not only for given types of instruments, but also for instruments of the same kind, making it possible, for example, to distinguish high-quality violins from those of lesser quality. The same difference in timbre applies to human voices, i.e., to typical sopranos, altos, tenors, and bassos.

GENERATION OF SINUSOIDAL VIBRATIONS

We may now raise the question of the factors that let a tuning fork or a similar instrument execute its vibrations. As everyone knows, one has only to strike a tuning fork once in order to activate it. It will then vibrate for quite a while, say one to two minutes, at slowly diminishing amplitudes. (The latter point will be ignored for the time being.)

Events in mechanical systems are governed by their physical properties and by forces that are either external or inherent. When the tines of a tuning fork have been displaced by an external force (e.g., after having been struck by a rubber mallet), a force is evoked that tends to restore the fork to its previous equilibrial state. In most instances such *restoring forces* are given by the *elastic* properties of the material, their magnitude being governed by Hooke's Law, i.e., that the resultant stress equals the strain. (This law holds only for relatively small displacements. Beyond certain limits, things get more complicated, as we will see later.) Under the effect of the elastic, restoring force the tines return to their resting position. However, in doing so they pick up velocity. Because of their inherent mass, this means an increase in their *momentum* (mass × velocity = momentum). The momentum is highest, but the restoring force lowest, just when the tines reach their resting position. Therefore, the movement is carried right through that point, initiating a displacement of opposite sign. In turn, the growing displacement evokes a restoring force, also of opposite sign, slowing down the motion which eventually, at some maximal amplitude, comes to a standstill. Now the elastic force takes over, tending again to bring the tines back to their equilibrial position. Once more the momentum increases and the whole event repeats itself, only running in the opposite direction.

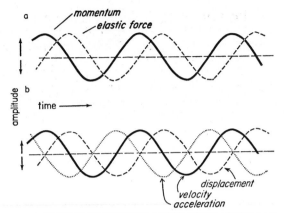

Figure 7. *a*, Phase relationship between the momentum of and the elastic force underlying a sinusoidal event. The momentum leads the elastic force by a phase angle of 90 degrees. *b*, Phase relationship between the displacement, velocity and acceleration of a sinusoidal event. The displacement lags behind the velocity by 90 degrees and is in phase opposition to the acceleration. Comparison of sections *a* and *b* indicates that the displacement is proportional to the elastic force, the velocity to the momentum, and the acceleration to the inertial properties of the system. All these events have sinusoidal waveforms (provided the displacement is sinusoidal), but are not necessarily of equal amplitude as shown in this schematic example. (From Glorig, A. (ed.): Audiometry Principles and Practice. Baltimore, The Williams & Wilkins Co., 1965, Chapter II.)

It is clear then that the vibration is maintained by alternate effects of the elastic restoring force and the momentum. If the event is sinusoidal, both vary sinusoidally with time. The elastic force reaches its maximum at the point of maximal displacement, and its minimum (it actually becomes zero) in the resting position. The momentum, on the other hand, is zero at the point of reversal, that is, the position of maximal displacement, and maximal when the tines pass through their resting position. Inspection of Figure 7 indicates that such a condition is fulfilled when and only when the phase relationship between the displacement or the restoring force on the one hand and the velocity or the momentum on the other is 90 degrees, with the velocity leading the displacement.

The rate of velocity is not uniform. In other words, acceleration and deceleration alternate with each other. Both are highest when the tines come to their standstill at the point of maximal displacement and then get going again in the opposite direction. This means that displacement and acceleration reach their respective maxima at the same time, but are in phase opposition. The phase relationship between the displacement, the velocity, and the acceleration of a sinusoidal vibratory event is depicted

in Figure 7. It may be mentioned here that all three entities have "amplitudes." Thus, to avoid confusion one should always refer to an amplitude of displacement, of velocity, or of acceleration.

Tuning forks are known to maintain their frequency very precisely. In fact, some modern chronometers employ small tuning forks as time-keeping devices. Thus, the frequency is a built-in feature of these forks; it is known as their *natural* frequency. The latter does not depend upon the amplitude vibration or the force with which the tuning fork is struck. It depends upon (1) the elastic coefficient of the material (the stiffer, the higher the natural frequency) and (2) its mass (the heavier, the lower the natural frequency). Obviously, then, the natural frequency is related to the two factors that maintain the vibrations, the elastic restoring force, and the inertia. (f_0 = natural frequency; E = elasticity; M = mass).

$$f_0 = \tfrac{1}{2}\,\pi\sqrt{\frac{E}{M}}$$

Instruments like tuning forks start their vibrations very easily, "resonating" with another nearby fork of the same frequency. Therefore, their natural frequency is also known as the *resonance frequency.*

Damping. Earlier in the discussion we disregarded the fact that tuning forks do not actually maintain their vibratory amplitude but show a gradual decrement with time. This decrement results from the effect of *friction,* both external (e.g., air resistance) and internal (e.g., friction within the crystal lattice of the material). Any form of movement, one directional (dc) or alternating (ac), is opposed by friction, its magnitude being proportional to the velocity of such movement. Thus, it leads the displacement by 90 degrees in phase (Figure 7). Its effect on vibratory events is known as *damping.*

Since the velocity of sinusoidal vibrations is always in some proportion to their displacement amplitudes (see previous discussion), it is clear that the absolute magnitude of the effect of damping decreases proportionally as the displacement amplitude is diminished. Expressed differently, in a given event the effect of damping is always at a fixed ratio to the displacement amplitude. (It is only at the start or at the end of such an event that it becomes appreciably higher as a result of the effect of *static* friction.) This fact will make the assessment of damping a relatively simple task. All one has to do is to measure the amplitude ratio of any

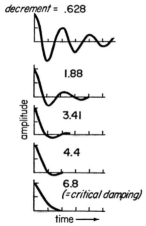

decrement = .628

1.88

3.41

4.4

6.8
(=critical damping)

amplitude

time ⟶

Figure 8. Decremental wave pattern for various damping factors. Note that the decrement becomes steeper with increasing damping and that, finally, at critical damping the event has become aperiodic. (From Glorig, A. (ed.): Audiometry Principles and Practice. Baltimore, The Williams & Wilkins Co., 1965, Chapter II.)

two successive periods (A_n/A_{n+1}). This ratio is called the *decrement* and defines damping uniquely. In practice the logarithmic decrement is usually used, that is, the natural logarithm of the above ratio ($\delta = \log_e A_n/A_{n+1}$). The higher the damping the less the number of cycles a vibratory event will go through before coming to a complete stop. Figure 8 shows the effect of such variation in damping. It covers a range of slightly more than one order of magnitude.

It is evident that the damping of tuning forks is very much less than that of any of the examples shown, for its decrement is much slower. The value of $\delta = 6.8$ is of special interest. It is exactly at this damping value that a structure, after having been displaced, is unable to execute even a single vibratory cycle. Instead it is returning asymptotically to its resting position. This damping value is known as *critical damping*. If damping is even higher (overdamping), the return to the resting position is executed in a creeping manner, making its duration longer and longer than that of a half cycle of the corresponding vibratory event. This retarding effect of damping makes itself already felt at a level below critical damping. It is for that reason that the natural frequency of a given system goes down slightly with increased damping as we shall see later (Fig. 10).

Free Vibrations, Maintained Vibrations, Forced Vibrations. As was just mentioned, tuning forks struck once vibrate for a long time. Thus, by definition, their damping must be very low. Since they receive but one initial

impulse and none thereafter, their vibrations are an example of so called *free vibrations*. The latter, as we know from the example of tuning forks, occur always at the natural frequency of the system in question. There are also ways of driving tuning forks continuously, for example, by having one tine of a steel fork act as the arm of electromagnetic interrupter. Forks of this or of similar construction were used extensively as generators of steady tones before the advent of electronic instruments, since they can be made to maintain their amplitude at any desired level. Such vibrations are known as *maintained vibrations*. Finally, an earphone or a loudspeaker can be driven at many different frequencies, not only at their natural frequencies. Otherwise, they could not reproduce speech signals or music, which changes rapidly in frequency with time. Such vibrations are known as *forced vibrations*. When the driving force is withdrawn, there is usually a very brief period of free vibrations before the system comes to rest.

Laryngeal Voice Production. One generator that is of special interest to otolaryngologists is the larynx. Simultaneously, it may serve as an example of how vibrations are generated by a unidirectional force. During expiration, when voice production usually takes place, the air current flowing through the organ is unidirectional, but the vocal cords vibrate in an alternating mode. The underlying process is as follows: The laryngeal muscles must first position the vocal cords, preferably in the midline position, and put them under proper longitudinal tension. This tension provides the "tuning" of the cords. A chest contraction will now increase the air pressure in the subglottic space. This pressure, finally, overcomes the muscular opposition and forces the glottic chink open. At this moment an air current gets under way, and the subglottic pressure decreases accordingly. Owing to the latter change, the vocal cords approximate each other once more. This latter event is aided by the fact that an air current flowing through a narrow channel (where current velocity and channel width are reciprocally related) exerts a negative pressure upon the channel walls, sucking them into the channel (so-called Bernouilli effect). After the glottis is closed once more, the subglottic pressure rises again, and the next cycle is started. The restoring force in this case is partially given by muscular tension and partially by the Bernouilli effect. The momentum is that of the moving air. Both factors are again seen to be 90 degrees out of phase with each other. Varying the muscular tension of the vocal cords will vary the frequency produced.

Actually it is not necessary that the vocal cords be tightly approximated. Even when the glottis is open, but the vocal cords are tensed and the rate of the expiratory air current is increased, the vocal cords are set into motion by the air current flowing through the glottic chink. This is another application of the Bernouilli effect leading once more to an oscillatory motion. In this latter case, a voiceless "whispered" sound is produced, whereas the output in the first case is of the voiced type.

The resultant waveform of the vocal cords in either case is not sinusoidal, although for a voiced output it is periodic when sustained sounds are produced. In the first case (closed glottis = voiced output), there are brief pulses corresponding to the opening phases separated from another by longer lasting quiescent intervals corresponding to glottic closure.

It is clear then from waveform considerations that the output of the larynx is not a pure tone but a complex tone. In the case of an unvoiced output it is essentially a noise, which we will define later. We have yet to describe the role of the respiratory tract in voice production (see the section on filters).

It may be noted that the present brief account of laryngeal voice production follows the so-called *aerodynamic* concept. The so-called *neuromuscular theory* that was briefly in vogue in the early 1950's is untenable from the acoustic standpoint. The aerodynamic function of the larynx has great similarity to the working mechanism of brass musical instruments—bugles, trumpets, and the like. The role of the vocal cord is then played by the lips of the player.

Another way of converting a dc motion into ac vibrations is shown by the action of a bow upon a violin string. The horsehair of the bow is covered with resin to make it sticky. When the bow is drawn over the strings with some force, the friction resulting from the sticky resin will take the string along for a short distance. After a while the elastic restoring force must overcome the driving force and the string returns fast to its resting position and usually beyond it. The resulting waveform is of the so-called *sawtooth* type, that is, the first slope (that corresponding to the forced motion) is more gradual than the second one (that corresponding to the return motion). Thus, in this case the output is not sinusoidal. In general, generators of this kind are known as *relaxation oscillators*.

ACOUSTIC TRANSIENTS

With the exception of the larynx in its unvoiced mode, all generators described so far produce simple harmonic motions or complex harmonic motions. The latter, as we know, are nothing but combinations of sine waves according to the theorem of Fourier. However, as was stated in the introduction, long lasting vibrations (a basic requirement of true sine-wave motions and their analysis by Fourier series) are not the rule in the production of sound. More typically they are short lasting. Consider, for example, all plosive speech sounds. Even the voiced consonants and the vowels of running speech are not really "long lasting."

We have seen that a generator that has very little damping, a tuning fork, for example, will execute free vibrations for a long time after a stimulating force is withdrawn. It is evident, then, that short lasting sounds can be produced only by generators that have high damping. If one taps the diaphragm of a good quality loudspeaker, i.e., one that is well damped, one hears a short "plop." Although the output of a smaller speaker activated the same way sounds somewhat higher in pitch (such sounds are generally referred to as "clicks"), it is hard, and practically impossible, to assign real pitch values to such short lasting sounds, ordering them along a musical scale, for example. Their character is not that of a tone but rather of a short lasting *noise*.

Fourier Analysis. When forming the Fourier spectrum of such transient sounds, one will find a fundamental difference with respect to sine-wave events. Spectra of long lasting periodic events were said to consist of discrete lines, each line representing one sine-wave component. Spectra of short lasting events are *continuous*, consisting of frequency *bands* of varying widths. (Mathematically the two cases are also different from each other. With steady-state events, one forms a *Fourier series*, i.e., one considers one single period of an event that is understood never to change and to last infinitely long. With transients, one forms a *Fourier* integral, i.e., one considers the event as a whole.) The relation between time duration ($\Delta\tau$) and frequency band width (Δf) is given by the following equation:

$$\Delta\tau \times \Delta f \cong 1. \qquad (5)$$

In other words, the shorter the duration, the wider the band width, and vice versa. For a hypothetical transient of zero duration, the

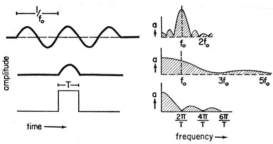

Figure 9. Time courses and associated spectra of some transient events. Top, Short section of a sine wave limited to three cycles; middle, a pulse representing half a cycle of the event shown on top; bottom, a square pulse of time duration (T). Note that all spectra are continuous, although they show nodes at multiples of the nominal frequency (f_0) or at multiples of the reciprocal time duration ($1/T$), respectively. (From Glorig, A. (ed.): Audiometry Principles and Practice. Baltimore, The Williams & Wilkins Co., 1965, Chapter II.)

band width would be unlimited. Figure 9 contains some examples of transients. It shows that a short section of a sine wave does not actually have a line spectrum. It has a composite band spectrum, and as its duration is increased the component around the nominal frequency, f_0 gains more and more prominence. A true line spectrum is not established until the duration becomes infinite. For this reason the point was made repeatedly in the foregoing that genuine sine-wave events are of very long (theoretically, infinite) duration. Actually the ear does not note any change in quality of a "tone" once it is held longer than for a few seconds, a fact justifying the use of the word "sinusoidal events."

It is noted that the two events—a pulse of zero duration, having an infinite band width, and an infinitely long sine wave, having a band width of zero cycles—are reciprocally related to each other, representing the two extremes of eq. (5). What is the waveform of one case, represents the spectrum of the other.

In extreme cases (examples 2 and 3 of Figure 9), transient signals may become *aperiodic*, that is, their waveform does not even show a single zero crossing, as shown in the middle tracings of Figure 9, for example. Such events are then known as *aperiodic*, since there is no periodic repetition.

When a sinusoidal event is suddenly started or ended or even when only the amplitude is stepped up or down from one level to another, one hears a click; that is to say, the sudden change involved produces a transient. Once more, the longer the transient, i.e., the more gradually one lets the change take place, the

narrower is the band width of the transient. It is this relationship that makes it possible to eliminate the click as an audible signal. Band width limitation usually takes place at the expense of the high frequency portion of the band, and it is in the higher frequencies (around 3000 Hz) that the human ear is most sensitive. Toward low frequencies its sensitivity falls off with about 12 dB/octave. Thus, increasing the duration of the transient by letting the signal grow (or decline) gradually will shift its acoustic energy into the low frequency region, making it essentially inaudible. For this reason, the ANSI standards for audiometers specify the duration of signal onset and decay (the signal envelope).

Acoustic transients produced during the onset or termination of tones have importance in another respect. They are characteristic of different musical instruments. Earlier, the quality of the tones produced was said to be different from instrument to instrument, and this quality was said to depend upon the number, relative amplitude, and distribution of higher harmonics. Actually it turns out that the initial (or terminal) transients are even more important criteria for telling one instrument apart from another when both of them are playing the same note.

Interestingly enough, when the initial transient was removed from the recording of notes played by various instruments and the mutilated recording presented to a panel of musical experts, they were unable to tell instruments apart, such as a cello and a trumpet which ordinarily (i.e., when their transients are present) are easily distinguished. Another way of demonstrating the importance of the initial transient is to listen to a tape recording of piano music while the tape is being rewound. Piano tones, being produced by a mallet hitting a string, have strong initial transients. When played backward, the tones cannot be recognized as those of a piano at all.

Noise. So far we have considered only single transients. The question is what type of sound will be produced when such transients are repeated. There are two possibilities: (1) The transients, e.g., pulses, are repeated in a periodic manner. In that case the spectrum is of the discrete line variety, having numerous harmonics. The repetition rate gives rise to the fundamental. The output of the human larynx producing a sustained sound in the voiced mode as was described earlier may serve as an example for this case. (2) The transients are repeated in a random manner, i.e., their repetition rate, their duration, and their amplitude are completely randomized. In that case, when there is no periodicity, the spectrum remains of the broad band type, and what one hears is a "whooshing," noiselike sound. The hissing of steam and, above all, the sound of jet engines are good examples. Because of their broad frequency content, the analogy to white light has suggested the term *white noise*, an expression that has found wide acceptance. Because of its ability to mask tones of any frequency, white noise is used in audiometry for masking purposes. Actually, since it is only a narrow band of frequencies around that of the test tone which is required for masking (the so-called critical band), more recently narrow bands of white noise are being employed. The total energy the patient is exposed to depends upon both amplitude and frequency band width. Thus, by limiting the band width the patient is exposed to less sound energy and has a lesser overall loudness sensation.

IMPEDANCE

We have learned that free vibrations (and also maintained vibrations) are associated with low damping and with narrow tuning, that is to say, devices such as tuning forks are capable of vibrating only within a narrow range around their natural frequency. Forced vibrations for which the frequency can be varied over a wider range (broad tuning), are associated with higher damping (usually less than critical).

When a tuning fork is driven at its natural frequency (maintained vibrations), a minimal effort is needed. In other words, the fork offers only a small "opposition" to such a driving signal. However, if one tries to drive the same fork at a frequency that is only moderately different from its natural one, the opposition to such an effort has risen very sharply. This opposition, which is thus shown to be frequency-dependent, is known as the *impedance (Z)* or, more specifically, the mechanical impedance *(Z_m)* in the case under consideration.

Mechanical Impedance. Resistance, in the sense just described, is only one component of the mechanical impedance. It is designated by the letter *R*, and it is a frequency-independent entity. The other frequency-dependent component is known as the *reactive* component and designated by the letter *X*. Like the natural frequency, it is determined by the elastic and inertial properties of the vibrating structure. The elastic force was said to be proportional to displacement, and inertial properties proportional to acceleration. Since these two factors are in phase opposition with respect to each other (Fig. 7), their resultant effect can be determined simply by forming their numerical difference. The total reactance is thus either mass dominated (by convention then considered positive) or stiffness dominated (then considered negative).

Once more, according to Figure 7, the phase relation between the two reactive factors (corresponding to displacement and acceleration, respectively) and the resistance (corresponding to velocity) is 90 degrees. Numerically such two components can be added by *vectorial summation*, which for this special case follows the well-known theorem of Pythagoras, i.e.,

$$Z = \sqrt{R^2 + X^2} \qquad (6)$$

In the case of a simple vibrating system (for example, a tuning fork, in which all masses, elastic components, and frictional factors may be conceptually lumped into one mass, etc., each) the impedance (Z_m) may be written in detail as follows:

$$Z_m = \sqrt{R^2 + \left(2\pi fM - \frac{E}{2\pi}\right)^2} \qquad (7)$$

(f = frequency; M = mass; E = elasticity; R = resistance). As was the case with the definition of the natural frequency [eq. (4)], it is seen that frequency is inversely related to mass and directly to the elastic property. We now solve eq. (7) for the case of the natural frequency by substituting eq. (4) into it and obtain

$$Z_m = \sqrt{R^2 + \left(M\sqrt{\frac{E}{M}} - E\sqrt{\frac{M}{E}}\right)^2}. \qquad (8)$$

The reactance part (X) of eq. (7), after appropriate simplification, can be rewritten as

$$X = \sqrt{EM} - \sqrt{EM} = 0. \qquad (9)$$

In other words, when the frequency is equal to the resonant frequency, the reactive component becomes zero, and the impedance is determined solely by the resistive component. This explains why tuning forks offer a minimal impedance when driven at their natural frequency, as was stated previously.

It also follows from eq. (7) that for all $f > f_o$ the impedance increases with the mass of the system as frequency goes higher, whereas for all $f<f_o$ it increases with the elasticity as frequency becomes lower. In other words, it is mass controlled above the natural frequency and stiffness controlled below that point. In either case it is always higher than that at the exact point of resonance.

Tuning forks were said to be narrowly tuned, and this was found to be associated with low damping. Inspection of equation (7) indicates that when the resistance R is small, the reactance X will become dominant, making the impedance Z_m strongly dependent upon frequency f.

The way one assesses such a situation quantitatively is to determine, frequency by frequency and for a constant input, the output of the system under consideration. The results are then plotted as amplitude *vs.* frequency. Figure 10 gives some examples of such *frequency response curves*, as they are called. In particular, Figure 10 shows that when damping is low the system is very narrowly tuned. As damping is increased, the tuning becomes broader and broader. (Thereby, the resonant point moves slightly to the left, as was mentioned previously.) When damping is critical, the curve does not display a resonant point anymore, sloping gradually as frequency goes higher. In the region of the former resonant point, it is already 6 dB down from its initial value. The flattest curve (which is obviously the most desirable from the standpoint of an optimal transducer) is reached when damping is somewhat less than critical, specifically at a logarithmic decrement of 3.14. Above the resonant point, all curves, regardless of damping,

slope down approximately with the square of frequency. This fact follows once more from eq. (7). When mass M becomes dominant, and elasticity E can be neglected, the impedance Z must vary with f^2, resistance R then being a constant for a given decrement. In order to have a good high frequency response, one has to push the resonant point of a system as high as possible, and this means low mass and relatively high stiffness.

The mechanical impedance may be defined as the complex ratio (complex because of the phase relationship between the resistive and reactive components) between the effective force acting upon a given area and the resulting linear velocity of displacement through that area. Its unit is the mechanical ohm (dyne $\times$ sec. $\times$ cm.$^{-1}$). (The term "effective" in this context is the same as the root-mean-square (RMS) value described previously.)

Acoustic Impedance. So far we have considered only the mechanical impedance which manifests itself when a system is driven mechanically in some form or another. The situation is slightly, but not principally, different when a system is considered that is driven acoustically or has an acoustic output. In both of the latter cases, one can determine the *acoustic impedance*, either "looking in" (system being driven) or "looking out" (system having an output). The unit is the acoustic ohm (dyne $\times$ sec. $\times$ cm.$^{-5}$). The exact definition is, "the complex ratio between the effective sound pressure averaged over the surface of the system to the effective volume velocity through it."

The reason one may be interested in the outgoing (looking out) impedance lies in the problem of *impedance matching* with the system the acoustic energy is being fed into (e.g., the surrounding air). The problem of impedance matching will be discussed later.

Characteristic Impedance. There is a third kind of impedance which is exhibited by large (theoretically unbounded) media, e.g., air or water. The mass of such large bodies is, at least theoretically, infinitely large. Consequently, according to eq. (4), their resonant frequency must approach zero Hz; that is to say, this type of impedance, which is known as the *characteristic impedance*, is frequency independent. The unit is the mechanical ohm/cm. (dyne $\times$ sec. $\times$ cm.$^{-3}$). It is more simply determined as the product of the sound velocity (c) within the particular medium (see later) and its density (ρ),

$$Z = c \cdot \rho \qquad (10)$$

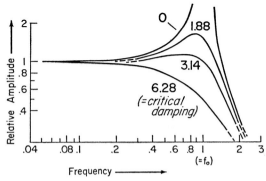

Figure 10. Frequency response curves of a system under various degrees of damping. Damping factors are as indicated. Note the slight shift of the resonance point to the left as damping is increased. When damping is critical (damping factor of 6.28) the response curve slopes off even before reaching the natural frequency f_o. (From Glorig, A. (ed.): Audiometry Principles and Practice. Baltimore, The Williams & Wilkins Co., 1965, Chapter II.)

The characteristic impedance of air is quite low. At 0° C. and at a barometric pressure of 760 mm. Hg it is 42.86 ohms/cm., varying slightly with atmospheric pressure and with temperature. At 20° C. it is approximately 41.5 ohms/cm. For water, the characteristic impedance is much higher. At 25° C. it is 149,000 ohms/cm. In sea water (salinity of 3.6 per cent), also at 25° C., it is 157,000 ohms/cm., the increase being due to the minerals in solutions. In solids it reaches its highest value. In steel, for example, it has a value of 4,570,000 ohms/cm. As its definition (ohms/cm.) implies, the total value of the characteristic impedance increases linearly, with the depth of penetration of the energy into a given medium.

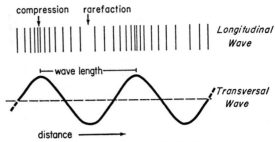

Figure 11. Waveforms of longitudinal waves and transversal waves, respectively. Both events have the same wavelength. (From Glorig, A. (ed.): Audiometry Principles and Practice. Baltimore, The Williams & Wilkins Co., 1965, Chapter II.)

SOUND TRANSMISSION

Before continuing our discussion on impedance and impedance matching, we must first describe how sound is being transmitted within a given medium, especially through air. Consider a loudspeaker diaphragm vibrating under the effect of an electrical signal applied to its voice coil. The speaker will radiate energy into the surrounding air. The underlying mechanism is as follows: As the speaker diaphragm moves out, it pushes the adjacent air particles forward, thus raising the air pressure very slightly above its static value, typically one atmosphere. As the diaphragm moves back again, and then beyond its resting position, it pulls the adjacent air particles with it, thus creating an equally slight decrease of the air pressure. In other words, alternating compressions and rarefactions of the surrounding air are being set up. These latter disturbances do not stay put within a continuous medium, but move away from their source. Let us for a moment consider the speaker as a point-shaped source radiating in all directions, a hypothetical case known as a "pulsating sphere." For such a case, the two-dimensional pattern created along the surface of a large pond into which a stone has been dropped provides a good illustration. Circular wave crests emerge from the site of excitation and, as they move outward away from the source, their diameters continually increase with time and distance. Each crest is followed by a trough and that, in turn, by another crest, and so forth, until eventually a whole system of concentric crests and troughs is established, continually moving away from the source.

The speed of propagation of such a disturbance, the velocity of sound in our case, is uniform and, as we have seen, a characteristic property of the medium in question. (Incidentally, this is not correct for surface waves on water; their speed of propagation increases with distance.)

There is another difference between sound waves in air and other types, and that concerns the *mode* of particle motion. We have seen that acoustic energy is propagated through air in the form of alternating compressions and rarefactions. As schematically shown in Figure 11 (top), these pressure changes take place in the same plane as that in which the waves are being propagated. Therefore, this mode is known as a *longitudinal* form of particle motion. A *transversal* mode (Fig. 11, bottom) is found in the propagation of light if one considers its wave property. (Polarization means to restrict the transversal motion to one particular plane.) Incidentally, surface waves on water move transversally and longitudinally at the same time, so-called *trochoidal* wave motion. That means a particle, as it is bobbing up and down, is simultaneously moving to and fro.

The parameters of Figure 11 are amplitude and distance, indicating that an event that is sinusoidal in time (Fig. 1) propagates also as a sinusoidal system of waves. The distance from crest to crest, or from any other points to its nearest equivalent, is called a *wavelength*. The information conveyed by Figure 11, top and bottom, is essentially the same, except for the difference in the mode of particle motion. For purposes of illustration, the transversal form (Fig. 11, bottom) is usually preferred both for temporal and spatial representation. It is easier drawn and recognized.

Sound Velocity. The propagation velocity of sound can be measured. In air it is relatively slow, varying somewhat with temperature. At 20° C. (68° F.), for example, it is 344 meters

(1120 ft.) per sec. Everyone has made the following observation: When watching a man from a distance who is cutting a tree, one *first* sees him swinging his ax and sometime *later* *hears* the impact. In water (fresh water of 30° C. [68° F.]), the velocity is higher (as was also the characteristic impedance), namely, 1493.2 m./sec. (4554.3 ft./sec.), that is, roughly four times the velocity in air. In steel it is about 16 times that in air, or four times that in water, namely, 5000 m./sec. (16,200 ft./sec.).

The following two statements are pertinent to the present problem: (1) When forced vibrations are being propagated, their frequency remains constant; and (2) within a given medium the wave propagation is independent of frequency. It follows from those two statements that in a given situation the wavelength (λ) must be in a reciprocal relation to the frequency (f) with respect to the propagation velocity (c):

$$c = f \times \lambda. \tag{11}$$

In air, then, wavelengths of sound waves between 100 Hz and 10,000 Hz vary from 3.44 m. (11.2 ft.) to 3.44 cm. (1.36 in.). Compared to the wavelength of visible light (4000 to 8000 Å.) the wavelength of sound waves is much larger, because of the difference in propagation velocity.

Inverse Square Law. The example of a stone being dropped into water may help to illustrate another point. We may say that each crest carries a certain amount of energy away from the source. Disregarding frictional losses for the time being, we see that this amount of energy is spread thinner and thinner as the circumference of the crest increases with distance from its source. It is recalled that intensity is a measure of "power density." Since the circumference of a circle varies as the square of the radius, it follows that the "*power density*" must vary as the square of the distance. This *square-of-the-distance law* is a good approximation of the attenuation of sound in a *free field* situation, i.e., when there are no obstacles in the way of a propagating sound wave. Even when the distribution is not strictly spherical, it still holds reasonably well.

Reflection of Sound, Diffraction, and Refraction. When the medium is not unbounded, as would be the case in all real situations, the energy cannot be propagated away from its source in an unlimited manner. (For the time being we are still disregarding frictional losses.) Sooner or later it will meet an obstacle—a wall, for example. In such a case some of the energy will be bounced off the obstacle, i.e., it will be reflected very much like a beam of light is reflected from a given surface under comparable circumstances. Reflections of sound produce echos. The same principles apply to acoustical as well as to optical reflections, i.e., the angle of reflection must be equal to the angle of incidence, etc. Moreover, it is the ratio of the magnitude of the surface roughnesses to the wavelength that determines whether the energy is reflected as a beam or is scattered (i.e., diffracted). To be optically flat, a surface must be planed and polished to a high degree of perfection. To be acoustically flat, tolerances can be less by many orders of magnitude. On the other hand, it is the ratio of the size of the obstacle to the wavelength that determines whether all energy is reflected or some of it is *refracted* around the obstacle.

For visible light, obstacles that cause refractions are very small; for example, dust particles suspended in the air. For sound, obstacles that are much larger still cause refraction. Moreover, the range of wavelengths of audible sound (3.4 cm. to 3.4 m. for a range of 100 to 10,000 Hz; see above) is several orders of magnitude larger than that of visible light (4000 to 8000 Å.), which represents only a range of a factor two. Consequently, for sound waves there must be a pronounced frequency-dependent effect with respect to diffraction and refraction. Low frequencies (long wavelengths) are more easily refracted, i.e., "heard around corners," than high frequencies. The latter are reflected in toto and, hence, prevented from going around corners. In general, it is the magnitude of the wavelengths of sound waves which causes refraction and diffraction to such a degree that it is virtually impossible to "beam" sound, except at very high frequencies.

Standing Waves. There is one special phenomenon we must mention. Whenever the path lengths between the walls of a room, into which sound is being fed, are an integral multiple of the wavelength, a sort of spatial resonance phenomenon is set up. The reflected sound returns in a direction opposite to that of the incident sound. At a hard reflecting surface, the sound pressure is maximal at the wall and changes phase abruptly by 180 degrees, so that the incident wave and the reflected one are in phase opposition. This does not lead to a cancellation of amplitude as in the time-domain situation of Figure 3, but to a *cancellation of wave travel*. The result is a system of so-called *standing waves.* (For the sake of illustration, they can be easily reproduced in a bathtub.) At some point along their pathway the sound pressure changes with time from maximal positive to maximal negative (this value being twice than that of the incident wave alone) in a sinusoidal fashion. The first such point is located directly at the wall. With distance from the wall, these points alternate with others at which the pressure is held constant at its resting value. The latter points are known as pressure *nodes* and the former as pressure *antinodes*. The particle velocity is shifted by 180 degrees with respect to the pressure. That is, antinodes of sound pressure correspond to nodes of velocity, and vice versa.

Standing waves are easily noticed in an enclosed room into which a high frequency sound is being transmitted, for example, the 9 kHz interference tone produced by two radio stations on adjacent frequency bands. On hearing such a tone one has only to move his head slightly ($\lambda = 3.8$ cm.; $1/2 \lambda = 1.9$ cm.) in order to go from an antinode where the tone sounds loud to a node where it may vanish altogether. Standing wave situations may also be used to tell whether a given microphone responds to sound pressure or to its velocity. Both types are being used. Such microphones will indicate in an opposite manner, either directly on the wall (where there is a velocity antinode) or at $1/2\lambda$ in front of it (where there is a pressure antinode).

Strange as it may sound, reflection (or formation of standing waves if conditions are right) takes place not only when the walls are hard (e.g., when aerial sound hits the water surface), but also when they are completely yielding (e.g., when sound propagating in water hits a water/air boundary). In the latter case there is a pressure node at the wall, i.e., a velocity antinode, the latter changing phase by 180 degrees on reflection.

In all other cases, when only some energy is being reflected and some is admitted into the second medium, *partial* standing waves will develop.

Impedance Matching. The condition for reflection is given whenever there is a large ratio between the impedances on both sides of the boundary, e.g., 41.5 ohms/cm. to 149,000 ohms/cm. for the case of an air-to-water boundary. The point must be made once more that it does not matter whether the energy goes from the medium of the lower impedance to that of the higher, or vice versa. A large impedance ratio, which is of course detrimental to the transmission of sound energy from one medium to another (or from one structure to another), is referred to as an *impedance mismatch.* One way of assessing the degree of impedance match or mismatch is to measure the ratio of the incident energy to the reflected energy and their relative phase angle. Especially when the impedance of one system is known, that of the other can be determined in this fashion. *Impedance bridges* that are built upon this principle have been in use for some time. One special, and quite promising, application is in the clinical assessment of the impedance of the tympanic membrane.

One might think of compensating for the loss at the boundary by delivering a large amount of energy to assure that a sufficient amount is transmitted into the second medium in spite of the high rate of rejection at the boundary. The example of the air/water boundary will serve to illustrate the futility of such an effort. In this particular case approximately 0.1 per cent of the incident energy is admitted into the second medium, while 99.9 per cent is being reflected. For small mismatches, say in the order 1:2 or 1:3, such strategy may be defensible, but with large mismatches it is simply too wasteful to be even considered.

There is a better way, one that does not waste energy, i.e., the use of an *impedance-matching transformer.* Electrical power transformers which serve exactly the same purpose in electrical or electronic circuits are well known illustrations of this method of transferring power in analogous situations. Mechanical and acoustical transformers are also used. The middle ear is a good example of a mechanical transformer. Its operating principles rely upon simple leverage systems.

Acoustic transformers are employed by musical instruments and also by loudspeakers. The horn of a trumpet is an impedance matching device from the mouthpiece (high impedance) to the surrounding air (low impedance). Here the matching is achieved by the gradually increasing inner diameter of the horn, which flares out in an exponential fashion, that is, an increasing wider volume of air is being driven as distance increases in the mouth of the horn. Megaphones, bullhorns, and horn-type loudspeakers apply the same principles. A man cupping his hands in front of his mouth improves the transmission of his voice in the same manner.

Acoustic Radiation Patterns. An acoustic horn may achieve an efficient power transfer from a loudspeaker into the surrounding air.

Yet most conventional loudspeakers create a "hole-in-the-wall" effect from which the sound appears to eminate. To make matters worse, speakers do not radiate all frequencies evenly in all directions. As long as the wavelength is large compared to the diameter of the speaker, the radiated pattern is evenly distributed as a result of the phenomenon of refraction (see earlier discussion). As this ratio becomes smaller with increasing frequency, the pattern becomes gradually pointed like a beam. In addition, side lobes begin to form so that a listener moving parallel to the speaker's axis goes repeatedly from maximum to minimum, back to a maximum, and so forth. For the same reason a complex tone will sound different from different listening angles. One way to overcome this deficiency is to mount smaller *high frequency tweeters* "co-axially" into the larger *woofer*. The woofer then produces a broad low frequency radiation and the tweeter (or tweeters) do the same for the high frequencies.

There is another point we must consider. Loudspeakers have definite low frequency limitations. With respect to the power radiated by them, we are concerned only with the *resistive* components of their impedances. (It is only in resistive elements that power is dissipated, i.e., in the form of heat.) When one starts out at a high frequency (although at one below the resonant point) and goes down in frequency, the resistive component of the output impedance of a given speaker is reasonably flat down to a point that is determined by the ratio of wavelength to the circumference of the speaker ($\lambda/2\pi R$). At this point it drops precipitously, i.e., with the square of inverse frequency (12 dB/oct).

The so-called *reciprocity theorem* of Helmholtz states that mechano-acoustic and other similar events, in which no power is permanently lost, i.e., dissipated, may also occur in a *reversed* manner. Loudspeakers can act as microphones, for example. From this viewpoint the consideration concerning loudspeakers has importance for the case of the tympanic membrane which receives acoustic power to transmit it to the inner ear. As with the power radiated off by loudspeakers, and essentially for the same reason, the power admitted by the tympanic membrane becomes less with inverse frequency below a cut-off frequency of approximately 2000 Hz, a phenomenon that accounts for the well-known low frequency attenuation of the threshold curve of hearing. This fact is not at all obvious when one neglects power considerations, i.e., when one

treats the ear as if it were simply a microphone that does not consume power. As was briefly mentioned in the introduction, microphones are analogous to voltmeters in electrical circuits. Neither of them must disturb the existing situation by drawing power. They measure sound pressure (microphone) or voltage (voltmeters), respectively. Sound pressures and voltages are analogous to each other.

Displacement Pattern of Vibrating Membranes. There is one additional point we must discuss with respect to vibrating membranes such as the tympanic membrane. For an example we shall consider the flat circular diaphragm of a magnetic earphone, the reason being that this is the only type of membrane which has been studied in sufficient detail both mathematically and experimentally. The membrane shall be assumed to be clamped around its edge. As long as $f \leq f_0$ the membrane will vibrate as a whole, bulging, of course, at its center.

Beyond their first resonant points, such systems usually display a number of additional resonant points. At the first additional one, the membrane ceases to vibrate as a whole, moving instead in opposite phases on its right and left as shown in Figure 12. The membrane is said to have changed its *mode* of vibrations, this particular one being the first *radial* mode. As further shown in Figure 12, there are a

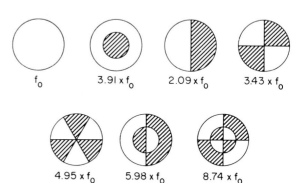

Figure 12. Displacement patterns of a circular membrane clamped around its edge. These different patterns occur at various multiples of the fundamental frequency. The white areas and the shaded ones move in phase opposition. At and below the first resonant point (f_0), the whole membrane vibrates in phase. Note that the multipliers determining the higher nodes are not exact integral multiples of f_0; therefore, the higher nodes do not occur precisely at higher harmonics of the fundamental frequency. The resultant patterns are either circular (for example, $3.9 \times f_0$), or radial (for example, $2.09 \times f_0$), or combinations of the two (for example, $5.98 \times f_0$). The patterns shown are only some examples of a much larger series. (From Glorig, A. (ed.): Audiometry Principles and Practice. Baltimore, The Williams & Wilkins Co., 1965, Chapter II.)

large number of higher modes, some radial, some circular, and some combinations of these two. (Figure 12 is by no means exhaustive in this respect.) It is evident, then, that when the membrane ceases to operate as a whole, its efficiency must drop. This is especially true for the radial modes. As a matter of fact, the resonance points for radial modes are typically very small, those of the first mode and of the second circular one being usually the highest. This is an additional reason for the fact that the efficiency of a membrane when acting as a radiator of a sound or as a receiver must drop beyond its first resonance point. Principally the same considerations will apply to the tympanic membrane.

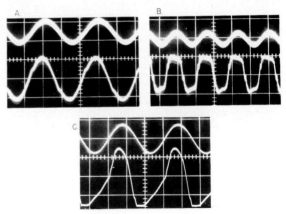

Figure 14. Examples of distorted waveforms. In each case an undistorted waveform is added for the sake of comparison. These waveforms were produced by deliberately overdriving an amplifier. (From Glorig, A. (ed.): Audiometry Principles and Practice. Baltimore, The Williams & Wilkins Co., 1965, Chapter II.)

DISTORTION—AMPLITUDE DISTORTION

It was mentioned in the section on generation of sound that the elastic restoring force is proportional to the displacement only as long as Hook's law applies, which means only as long as displacement amplitudes are relatively small. If such limits are exceeded (limits which will, of course, differ from system to system), the linear relation between the applied force and the resulting displacement will no longer be maintained. (This is equally true for unidirectional [dc] as well as alternating [ac] forces.) Figure 13 shows what is known as an *input/output function* of a typical case. Both axes are given in dB. It is seen that at higher driving amplitudes the output increases at a lesser rate

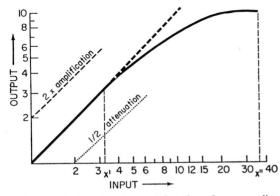

Figure 13. Input and output function of a system limited to an output of 10 arbitrary units. Note that both ordinates are given in a logarithmic manner. When the output is either amplified or attenuated, the curve is shifted to the left or to the right accordingly. At an input of $\times'$ the relationship ceases to be linear, and at $\times''$ the saturation value, 10 output units, is reached. (From Glorig, A. (ed.): Audiometry Principles and Practice. Baltimore, The Williams & Wilkins Co., 1965, Chapter II.)

than the input until it finally becomes independent of the input, i.e., it becomes flat. Thus, the function, which was originally linear, eventually becomes *nonlinear*. Since the result is a *distorted waveform* (as will be shown presently), the process is also known as distortion or, more exactly, *nonlinear distortion*. The particular kind described here is known as an *amplitude distortion* because of the dependence upon signal amplitude. Distortion in the *frequency* and *time* domains (i.e., frequency and phase distortion as well as "hangover" effects) will be discussed later.

Harmonic Distortion. Suppose the input has a simple sinusoidal waveform. After the limits of linearity are exceeded, the output waveform may become "distorted," as shown in the examples of Figure 14. While in Figure 14 *A* there are only two little wiggles opposite each other along either slope, in *B* the peaks on either side of the waveform are clipped off, so-called bilateral *peak clipping*. In *C* the peak clipping occurs only unilaterally in addition to further alterations of the waveform. Peak clipping means, of course, a definite limit of displacement amplitudes. In Figure 13 bilateral peak clipping would occur in the flat portion of the input/output function. Unilateral peak clipping is seen when the displacement is limited in one direction long before the other one becomes affected. In a badly designed loudspeaker, for example, the voice coil may hit the bottom of the slot it is moving in, but may still have leeway in the opposite direction.

We already know what a distorted waveform means. When it is analyzed according to the Fourier theorem, it will reveal the presence of *higher harmonics that were not part of the original signal.* For this reason, amplitude distortion is also known as *harmonic distortion.* For example, the two wiggles opposing each other in waveform *A* of Figure 14 indicate a relatively strong third harmonic. Needless to say, the situation becomes more complex as the driving amplitude gets higher.

Intermodulation Distortion. An additional form of distortion is observed in nonlinear systems. Ordinarily one can feed any two sinusoidal signals into a linear system, and the resultant will simply be a linear superposition of the two, i.e., the sum of the amplitudes of both systems at any instant of time, in the manner of Figures 3 and 4. An analysis will reveal nothing but the two original signals. By contrast, when fed into a nonlinear system the two signals will interact, that is, the lower signal will *modulate* the higher one in a similar way a program signal will modulate the carrier signal of an AM radio station. In this latter case, new frequencies are created, the so-called *combination tones:* The sums and differences between the primaries (first order combination tones), but also second order sums and differences. Let the primary frequencies be 300 and 1000 Hz. The first order sum and differences are $1000 \pm 300 = 1300$ Hz; and 700 Hz. Second order combinations are $1300 + 300 = 1600$ Hz; $700 - 300 = 400$ Hz; and so forth. There is no limit to such a process, although the relative magnitude of these distortion products decreases rapidly with rank order. This type of distortion, which has basically the same cause as harmonic distortion, is called *intermodulation distortion.*

It cannot be emphasized enough that any system will eventually show distortion after certain limits are exceeded. Commercial power amplifiers, for example, are rated in watts, that is, the amount of power they are capable of dissipating. It is customary to list the magnitude of distortion occurring at the level of maximal power rating. The result can be conveniently expressed as the percentage energy of the original signal that goes into the production of higher harmonics or, similarly, as per cent intermodulation distortion.

One can, of course, hear the results of either form of distortion. Most people when listening to running speech or music find any distortion exceeding 1 to 3 per cent very objectionable. The ear is quite sensitive in this respect, a fact that is somewhat strange since the ear has a low threshold of distortion of its own. Distortions in the frequency and time domains are a different matter.

FREQUENCY DISTORTION

Actually we have already touched upon frequency distortion without mentioning it by name. Whenever a receiving system has a usable frequency range (given by its frequency response curve as defined earlier) that is narrower than the range of signals it is supposed to transmit we call this *frequency distortion.* AM radio stations with their 9 KHZ band width "distort" music by cutting off its high frequency components. Hearing-aid earphones also have a limited frequency range. There are many more examples of this kind. An ideal system for good reproduction of sound should have at least a flat frequency response from 20 to 20,000 Hz. The significance of the high frequencies lies not so much in the reproduction of high frequency tones (there are no musical notes that reach that high, and hardly any important higher harmonics), but in the correct reproduction of fast transients which require wide frequency bands (see earlier discussion). It is for this reason that piano music is hard to reproduce in a really good manner in any but the best systems.

DISTORTIONS IN THE TIME DOMAIN

Phase Distortion. Phase distortion is actually a corollary of frequency distortion. By this is meant that a band width-limited system cannot reproduce complex signals with the same intercomponent phase relationship they originally had. Throughout the frequency range of such band-limited systems, phases change continually. (The reason for this will be discussed later in the section on filters.) Formerly the ear was thought to be insensitive to phase distortion. This erroneous conclusion was based upon a misinterpretation by other writers of one of Helmholtz' original experiments. A change in phase relationship between components of a complex signal affects the waveform (Fig. 5), and the ear is indeed sensitive to such changes, a fact that was well known to Helmholtz.

Hangover Effects. In systems that have insufficient damping, each signal is followed by some free vibrations, an effect which lends a "mushy" sound to reproduced speech. Since these hangover effects may interfere with subsequent signals, intelligibility must decrease. Most cheap systems suffer from this kind of distortion to varying degrees.

Noise Interference. There is no system in

which signals are transmitted that does not have *some noise,* either from internal or external sources, although the noise may be quite low with respect to the magnitude of the signal. Since there is interest only in the relative amount of noise, one defines the *signal to noise ratio.* (In fact, a branch of pyscophysics called *signal detection theory* considers the signal S/N ratio one of the most important determinants of the detection of auditory signals by listeners.) However, noise must not necessarily be equated with "distortion." It exists in linear systems as well, and then its effect is a mere *interference,* i.e., the noise is superpositioned upon the signal. Psycophysically the result is masking, which will not be discussed further in this chapter. If, on the other hand, the system acts nonlinearly, intermodulation distortion will occur, and the result may be very detrimental to the perception of the signal. Cheap tube-type radios with an audible 60 Hz power line hum often show intermodulation distortion between the hum and the signal, especially when the signal is weak and requires a large amount of amplification. In that case, of course, such a radio distorts.

FILTERING OF SOUND

A limitation of frequency band width can be introduced deliberately in a process that by analogy (sorting out of particles beyond a given size) is called *filtering.* There are *low pass* filters, *high pass* filters, *band pass* filters, and *band rejection* filters. Filters, depending upon their construction, attenuate frequencies outside their path band to varying degrees. Very simple filters may only attenuate 6 dB/oct, whereas very sharp filters attenuate 30 to 40 dB/oct. and more. Although with today's instrumentation it is easier to convert acoustic signals first into electrical ones and then use electric or electronic filters, mechano-acoustic filters are still in use.

Let us consider one common example of low-pass and high-pass filters and, finally, a variable filter, the upper respiratory tract.

Low Pass Filter. A car muffler is designed as a low pass filter. Since the ear is more sensitive to high frequencies (peak sensitivity around 3 KHZ) than to low ones, shifting the energy into the low frequency band must reduce the apparent loudness of the exhaust noise. Practically, this filter effect is achieved by having a large number of small, completely closed, side chambers along the main duct.

These side chambers act like springs, cushioning the sharp impact of the exhaust pulses, that is, limiting their high frequency content.

It may be added here that all transmission systems are essentially low pass filters. High frequency energy is lost as a result of absorption and scattering, and low frequency energy is transmitted farther.

High Pass Filter. Suppose one is listening via the telephone to somebody talking. As long as there is good contact between one's ear and the receiver, the voice quality is all right. However, if one moves the receiver only slightly away, thus breaking its seal with the ear, the speaker's voice becomes "tinny." It is lacking in low frequency components. One has produced a high pass filter effect. The explanation is as follows: At the leak the line is "loaded" with masses, i.e., the volumes of air which must be moved to and fro through such leaks as the pressure changes because the signal is passing along the line. Mass effects, as we recall, always affect the high frequencies. The cutoff point of such a high pass filter system is determined by the size of the holes. The resistance to sound varies with particle velocity. Thus, low frequencies are easier dissipated than high frequencies.

Filter Properties of the Upper Respiratory Tract. The steady-state output of the larynx was said to be either a noise (whispered voice) or a periodic pulse (normal voice). First of all, this generator can be switched on and off, and such switching can be accomplished in a sudden manner (vocal attack) or in a more gradual manner (breathy attack). Thus, the initial and terminal transients can be manipulated. But then the output of a human larynx does not sound very pleasant. It sounds rough, i.e., highly distorted, which is not surprising in view of its waveform. As a matter of fact, it does not sound like the voice of a human being at all. What determines the final sound quality is the action of the upper respiratory tract which, from the acoustic standpoint, may be considered a variable set of filters, mainly of the low pass and band pass types. The nasopharynx, for example (a side chamber) serves for low pass filtering. The mouth, being in essence a resonating cavity in series, represents a band pass filter. The cut-off frequencies of both of them can be varied over a fairly wide range simply by changing the enclosed air volume. In addition, changes in the widths of the passages, mainly the throat and the mouth, will affect the damping properties as a narrow channel increases the resistance to the passing air stream. This, in turn, affects the slopes of the filters.

The mouth especially, by virtue of the great mobility of the tongue and lips, can change its filter properties in a rapid manner and to an almost unlimited degree, allowing the generation of a great variety of speech sounds. This includes the production of transients as in plosive consonants.

The way the upper respiratory tract affects the laryngeal output is by favoring some frequency bands and attenuating others as a result of its filter properties at a given time. This is what makes the voice of a trained speaker or singer pleasant sounding. In this latter respect, the lower respiratory tract also has its effect. The upper and lower tracts and the larynx form what is known as a coupled system in which one part affects the performance of the others.

This brief account of voice production is by no means exhaustive and is given here only as an illustrative example.

Phase Effects of Filters. Filters do not affect only the frequency response, but shift the phase/frequency as well. It is for this reason that frequency distortion is invariably accompanied by phase distortion as was outlined previously.

In transmission lines, which in general act like low pass filters, the inherent phase distortion produces another effect. The transmission velocity decreases with frequency so that the high frequency components of a complex signal arrive at the terminal noticeably later than the low frequencies. Before it was learned how to compensate for this occurrence (simply by delaying the low frequencies proportionally), this phenomenon was the source of the so-called "birdies" heard in long distance telephone lines, that is, high frequency sounds that had become entirely separated from their original signals.

MAGNITUDE CONSIDERATIONS

In the discussion of the dB concept the reference levels for sound measurements, 10^{-10} watts/cm.^{2} or 0.0002 dynes/cm.^{2} were cited (1 dyne/cm.^{2} = 1 μbar; 1 μbar = 0.001 millibar, the unit in which barometric pressures is measured). The reader has perhaps wondered about their small magnitudes; 10^{-10}, after all, is 1/10 of 1/1,000,000,000! These values were originally chosen because they are reasonably close to sound intensity and pressure, respectively, at the hearing threshold of a human ear at 1000 Hz. (Actually, at the time the agreement was made, it was thought that they represented this threshold accurately.) The level of conversational voice in an enclosed room is approximately 60 dB SPL (sound pressure level); this is still only 10^{-4} watts/cm.^{2} or 0.2 dynes/cm.^{2} (0.2 mbar. is less than a barometer is capable of indicating). One hundred twenty decibels is a noise level that may already be considered as fairly high; but it is a mere 100 watts/cm.^{2} or 200 dynes/cm.^{2} These two examples may suffice to show that the power and pressures involved in acoustics are quite small when compared to those involved in other fields, such as electricity, mechanics (automotive power!), and others. By the same token, they indicate that the ear is an extremely sensitive detector of sound. The displacement amplitudes of structures in the ear, such as the tympanic membrane, the stapes, and the basilar membrane, are submicroscopic even at fairly high sound pressure levels.

REFERENCES

*1. Beraneck, L. L.: Acoustics. New York, McGraw-Hill Book Co., Inc., 1954.
2. Van Bergeijk, W. H., Pierce, J. E., and David, E. E., Jr.: Waves and the Ear. Garden City, N.Y., Science Study Series, Anchor Books, Doubleday & Co., Inc., 1960.
3. Davis, H., and Silverman, S. R.: Hearing and Deafness. New York, Holt, Rhinehart, and Winston, Inc., 1960, pp. 29–60.
4. Pierce, J. R., and David, E. E., Jr.: Man's World of Sound. New York, Doubleday & Co., Inc., 1959.
5. Olson, H. F.: Music, Physics, and Engineering. New York, Dover Publications, Inc., 1967.
*6. Stephens, R. W. B., and Bate, A. E.: Acoustics and Vibrational Physics. London, Edward Arnold, Ltd., 1966.
7. Stevens, S. S., and Davis, H.: Hearing. New York, John Wiley & Sons, Inc., 1938, pp 1–41.
8. Wever, E. G., and Lawrence, L.: Physiological Acoustics. Princeton, New Jersey, Princeton University Press, 1954, pp. 16–34.

*Contains a considerable amount of mathematics; should be reserved for advanced reader.

Chapter 8

PHYSIOLOGY OF THE EAR

PHYSIOLOGY OF THE MIDDLE EAR INCLUDING EUSTACHIAN TUBE

by

Ichiro Kirikae, M.D.

PHYSIOLOGY OF THE EUSTACHIAN TUBE

Three important muscles for the function of the eustachian tube are the tensor palatini, levator palatini and salpingopharyngeus muscles. The tensor palatini is innervated from the mandibular division of the trigeminal nerve and possibly from the glossopharyngeal nerve; the levator palatini, from the facial, vagus, and pharyngeal plexus. Though still unconfirmed, the motor innervation of the salpingopharyngeus is attributed to the pharyngeal plexus. The contraction of these muscles results in the opening movement of tubal lumen. The tensor palatini muscle plays the major role (Figs. 1 and 2).

Because of the elastic properties afforded by the cartilage and surrounding tissues, the cartilaginous portion of the tube is normally collapsed, its walls folded parallel with its long axis. Such actions as swallowing, yawning, sneezing, and shouting loudly will cause temporary opening of the closed pharyngeal orifice of the eustachian tube.

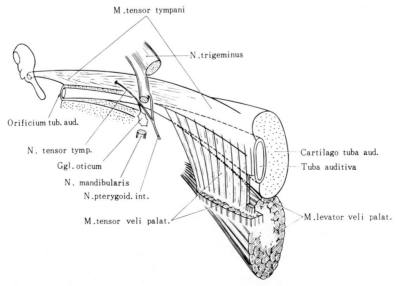

Figure 1. Relation between auditory tube and palatal muscles (right side).

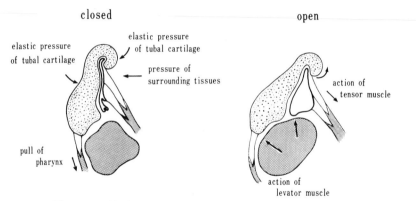

closed   open

Figure 2.   Closing and opening of the auditory tube (Zöllner).

Ventilatory Function of Middle Ear Cavity

The primary biological functions of the eustachian tube are to permit middle ear pressure to equalize with external air pressure and to protect the ear from large and rapid pressure changes. Such actions as swallowing and yawning result in (1) raising the pressure in the nasopharynx, and (2) temporary opening of the collapsed eustachian tube. When the air pressures inside and outside the tympanic cavity are different, they are equalized by the opening of the tube. When the pressure in the nasopharynx rose to 5 cm. water, the eustachian tube opened in 68 per cent of patients with normal ears.

Acoustic stimulus during tubal opening makes it possible to record transmission of the sound through the middle ear to the external canal. The resultant change in the envelope of the acoustic signal showed that the duration of the tubal opening varies at about a value of 0.3 sec. (Gyergyay, 1932). The shape of the sound envelope varies with the subject, and in the same subject from one swallow to the next, and depends on the materials to be swallowed.

Ingelstedt and Örtegren (1963 a and b) studied the relationship between the pressure changes in the nasopharynx and the tubal opening by Toynbee maneuvers or swallowing with the nose closed. The type and degree of middle ear ventilation is entirely dependent on the amount and the type of the pressure changes actually taking place in the nasopharynx during the tubal opening period. Figure 3 shows the recorded types of nasopharyngeal pressure complexes to the left and the resulting tubal air passages to the right. Because of biphasic movement of the palatine velum, the nasopharynx pressure complex is mostly biphasic (+2.5 to −7.5 mm. Hg). The commonest type

is number 4 followed by 5, both resulting in a final negative middle ear pressure.

The passage of the air from the tympanic cavity to the nasopharynx occurs with ease, but the passage in the opposite direction is difficult. This was proved by experiments done by Ingelstedt and Örtegren (1963 b). Raising or lowering the pressure with the "snorkel" chamber, they studied the ventilatory function of the tube during swallowing.

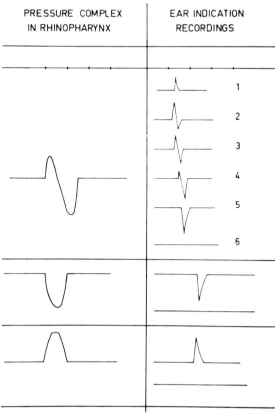

PRESSURE COMPLEX IN RHINOPHARYNX   EAR INDICATION RECORDINGS

1
2
3
4
5
6

Figure 3.   Various types of pressure change and air passage indication recordings obtained during Toynbee maneuvers (Ingelstedt and Örtegren).

TABLE 1.

	Air	Normal	Tubal Stenosis
O_2	20.9	14–17	9–15
CO_2	0.03	0	0
N_2	79.04	86–83	91–85

The values are in volume per cent. Air is the atmospheric air; normal is the air contained in the tympanic cavity of the normal subjects; and tubal stenosis, of the patients with tubal stenosis (Matsumura).

When the eustachian tube opens, it begins from the middle ear end and then proceeds to the nasopharyngeal orifice. The mucous film breaks toward the nasopharynx, and this might be the click that one hears in swallowing. Even in normal ears, when swallowing does not take place for a long period and the middle ear remains closed, the middle ear pressure becomes negative as a result of the resorption of oxygen into the capillaries of the mucous membrane. Table 1 by Matsumura (1955) shows the results of analysis of the composition of the air in normal subjects and in patients with tubal stenosis. The major resorbed component is oxygen, and the fall in the middle ear pressure parallels the decrease in per cent of oxygen.

When the negative pressure in the tympanic cavity increases and stays unchanged, hydrops ex vacuo is seen. Retraction of the tympanic membrane, edema of the mucosa of the tympanic cavity, and production of transudate compensate negative pressure and thus narrow the middle ear cavity. When negative pressure, resorption of oxygen, and hydrops ex vacuo are well balanced, negative pressure reaches a maximum of −30 mm. Hg.

Drainage Function

The mucous blanket of the eustachian tube is produced from the goblet cells and the mucous glands in the mucous membrane of the tube. The mucus is carried by ciliary movement directed toward the nasopharynx. In rabbits, the minute particles powdered into the 1.0 to 1.2 cm. long auditory tube take as long as six hours to reach the nasopharyngeal orifice. In the recovery period of otitis media, secretions are resorbed from the tympanic mucosa and, in part, excreted to the nasopharynx through the tube.

Tubal Patency

The cartilaginous portion of the eustachian tube is normally collapsed and its walls are folded. A slight increase in the nasopharyngeal pressure will pass the air from the nasopharynx to the tympanic cavity. This increase of pressure is called pressure for tubal patency. The normal value of this pressure is 20 to 30 mm. Hg by catheterization of the tube.

PHYSIOLOGY OF THE MIDDLE EAR

In vertebrates it has been shown that fish can hear or perceive vibration of surrounding water by means of the lateral line organ. Sensory hair cells soaked in sea water in the lateral line canal are stimulated directly by the movement of the surrounding water. Highly developed vertebrates which live temporarily or permanently on land have to hear air-conducted sound; consequently they must have developed receptors to profit by the vibration of air, because it is necessary that air vibrations be introduced from outside the body to the inner ear fluid. We call such receptors, which contribute to the matching of impedance between air and fluid, the middle ear.

Physiology of the Tympanic Membrane

Property of the Tympanic Membrane

The cross-sections of the tympanic membranes vary in shape according to classes of animals. In amphibians and reptiles the tympanic membrane is flat. In birds it is convex, whereas in mammals it is concave. The degree of the deflection is smaller in birds than in mammals, and the tympanic membrane in birds is almost flat. Let us take the diaphragm of a loudspeaker as an example. The tympanic membrane in amphibians, reptiles, and birds corresponds to a flat cone type of diaphragm. The cross-section of this type is a cone with a straight line (Fig. 4). The tympanic membrane in mammals, on the other hand, corresponds to a curved cone type whose cross-section is a cone with a curved line. As a diaphragm, a curved cone affords less distortion and broader frequency characteristics than a flat cone. This, in analogy, adds to the fact that the tympanic membrane in mammals is superior to those of other classes in its function.

Vibration of the Human Tympanic Membrane

Vibration Mode at Lower Frequencies. Many workers have studied the dynamics of

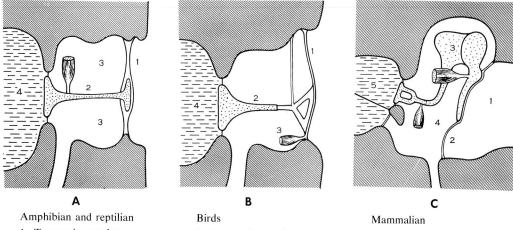

A

Amphibian and reptilian

1. Tympanic membrane
2. Columella
3. Tympanic cavity
4. Inner ear

B

Birds

1. Tympanic membrane
2. Columella
3. Tympanic cavity
4. Inner ear

C

Mammalian

1. External auditory canal
2. Tympanic membrane
3. Ossicles
4. Tympanic cavity
5. Inner ear

Figure 4. Schematic view of middle ear apparatus.

the tympanic membrane.* There are many methods for observing and measuring the movements of the membrane resulting from a change of pressure in the meatus. Classic experiments were done by optical methods using minute pieces of gold foil attached to the surface of the tympanic membrane (Mach and Kessel, 1874; and Wada, 1924). Stroboscopic or cinematographic observations have also been done (Kobrak, 1941, 1953; Perlman, 1945; and Kirikae, 1960). Others used the electronic condenser method which consists in evaluating the minute displacement of the tympanic membrane by capacitative probe (Wilska, 1935; Békésy, 1941).

The vibration mode of the human tympanic membrane differed at three zones; central, intermediate, and peripheral. The central or conic zone is situated around the umbo and is 1.2 to 1.5 mm. in radius. The peripheral zone is surrounded by the annulus tympanicus and is 2.0 to 3.0 mm. in width. The intermediate is the zone between the central and peripheral and is 0.7 to 2.0 mm. in width.

During vibration the central zone moves back and forth like a piston and its conic shape is retained. The peripheral zone makes a hinge-like movement, and the angular deflection takes place at its junction with the annulus

tympanicus. The intermediate zone moves in greater amplitude than the other two and its mode of vibration corresponds to that of the membrane with freely mobile boundaries. Figure 5 summarizes the results of various measurements of the human tympanic membrane; the membrane does not show a strictly concentric arrangement of zones, and the width of a zone differs in various tympanic portions.

The mode of vibration of the tympanic membrane should be analyzed not only by cross-sections (Figs. 5 and 6) but also by areal observations. Békésy (1941) used a very sensitive electrical probe to measure the linear displacement of the membrane. Figure 6 *B* shows the areas of equal excursion during acoustic stimulation by a tone of 2000 Hz. The largest excursion is seen along the line extended from the handle of malleus and is near the bottom. According to our observation, this portion corresponds to the intermediate zone. Figures 5 and 6 *B* and *C* show different ways of explaining the same situation, and the results are in accordance with each other.

There is a close relationship between the arrangements of fibers and the movement of the membrane. The fact that radial and circular fibers cross each other and that the membrane is thick around the umbo makes the membrane ready to vibrate as a stiff cone. During vibration the surface of the membrane rotates around the axis at the edge near the tympanic sulcus. The parabolic fibers which originate from the portion near the short process of the malleus are mainly suitable to strengthen the periphery of the membrane (Fig. 6 *A*).

Vibration Mode at Higher Frequencies. The

---

*Elasticity of human tympanic membrane is evaluated by two kinds of methods, namely, static and dynamic. Young's modulus, as determined by these methods, is 2.0 × 10⁸ dyne/sq. cm. (v. Békésy, 1960) in case of the former and 4.0 × 10⁸ dyne/sq. cm. (Kirikae, 1960) in case of the latter. The value of the latter was obtained by applying the vibrations within the audible range. These values are similar to those of rubber.

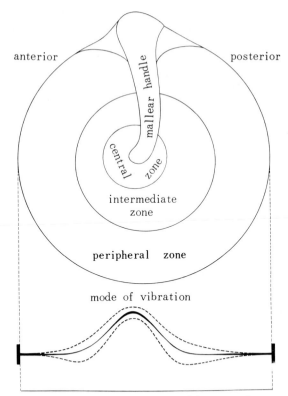

like a piston and this movement involves the whole area as long as the frequency of vibration is low or medium. Békésy (1941) observed by using his capacitative probe that above 2400 Hz the tympanic membrane starts to vibrate in segments and loses its stiffness.

Physiology of the Ossicular Chain

The function of the ossicles is to transmit the vibration of the tympanic membrane to the cochlea. If simple transmission alone were the function, all that would be needed would be a single intermediate structure between the membrane and the cochlea. This is true in the evolution of the hearing organ, and the ossicle up to the level of birds is, in fact, a single structure called columella which corresponds the stapes of mammals (Fig. 4). The three ossicles, the malleus, incus, and stapes, were first seen in mammals. The middle ear of the mammals reached the highest stage of development with increasing complexity in structure and function. Helmholtz in 1868 first studied in detail the function of the ossicles as a sound transmitter. Subsequent periods saw many important works in this field done by such notable persons as Dahmann (1930), Stuhlman (1943), and Fumagalli (1949).

Structure and Function of the Ossicles

The dynamic structure of the ossicles was learned from study of the thickness of the bony

Figure 5. Three sectional parts of the tympanic membrane and mode of vibration.

mode of membrane vibration, as proved in general physics, becomes segmental as the frequency becomes higher. This is true also in the tympanic membrane. Figures 5 and 6 *B* and *C* show that the membrane moves back and forth

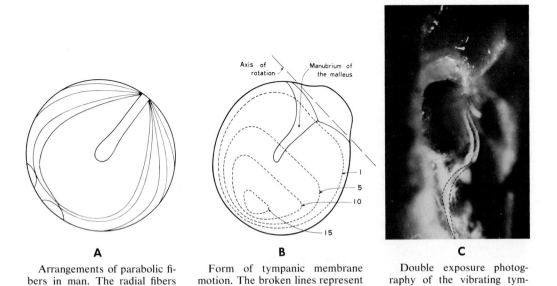

A	B	C
Arrangements of parabolic fibers in man. The radial fibers are not illustrated (Kirikae).	Form of tympanic membrane motion. The broken lines represent contours of equal amplitudes whose relative magnitudes are indicated by the numbers (Békésy).	Double exposure photography of the vibrating tympanic membrane (profile view) (Kirikae).

Figure 6. Relation between vibration and fiber arrangement of the tympanic membrane.

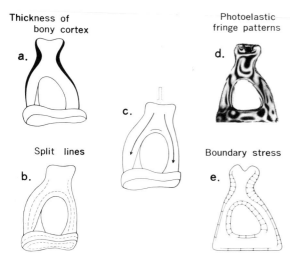

Figure 7.   Dynamic structure of the stapes.

cortex and the arrangement of the bony fibers or split lines. These studies explain to a certain degree the mode of the working forces. Another approach is a photoelastic experiment using three dimensional models of ossicles made from a plastic material called diallyl phthalate.

When force or pressure is applied, photoelastic fringe patterns are visualized. Let us take the stapes as an example. The cortex is thick at the head and at the lateral aspects of the neck. The bony fibers or split lines run from the neck, diverging into the two crura, down to the footplate. Photoelastic experiments showed that boundary stress is large where the cortex is thick. The structure of the stapes is in accordance with the dynamics of the force which is first applied to the head, passes the neck and, hence, is divided symmetrically into the two crura (Fig. 7). Similar experiments which were performed on the malleus and incus also show that the structure is in accordance with the dynamics of the force applied to the ossicles.

Mode of Vibration of the Ossicular Chain

This is best explained from the sphere of kinetics. The ossicular chain is taken as a mechanical transformer of sound energy. Let us take, as an example, the relationship between the center of gravity and the axis of rotation. If by the ossicular chain the center of gravity falls on the axis of rotation, the inertial moment of the system would be nought. As the principles of kinetics show, this system becomes a very effective transformer.

Center of Gravity and Axis of Rotation of the Ossicles.   The classic teaching has been that the axis of rotation of the ossicles matches the line drawn between the extremity of the long process of the malleus and the short process of the incus (Helmholtz, 1868; Dahmann, 1930; Bárány, 1938) (Fig. 8). It is ascertained that the axis of rotation of the ossicular chain coincides with the center of gravity of the whole sound conducting system. This mechanical system is very effective with the minimal inertial moment.

Incudomalleolar Articulation.   Helmholtz (1868) interpreted the joint as a kind of tooth-edged wheel or cog mechanism which makes an articulatory movement in only one direction. Bárány (1938) holds, on the other hand, that the joint does not make an articulatory movement. Recent studies are in favor of the latter view. The incudomaleolar joint is rigidly rocked under the intensity of ordinary sounds. Only when the intensity exceeds a certain level does the joint make an articulatory movement, the amplitude of vibration of the incus being held within a certain limit. This is interpreted as a protective mechanism for the inner ear.

Motion of the Stapes.   Vibratory motion of the stapes varies in two ways, according to the intensity of the sounds. Békésy (1936, 1939) showed that in sounds of moderate intensity the anterior end of the footplate oscillates with an amplitude greater than that of the posterior end (Fig. 9 *A*). In other words, a rocking motion occurs at the transverse axis near the posterior end.

According to our observation, the footplate also shows a pistonlike back and forth move-

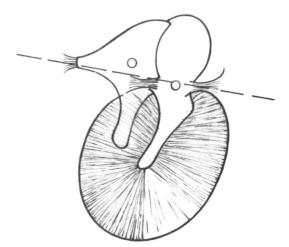

Figure 8.   The axis of rotation passes through the center of gravity of the ossicles (Dahmann, modified from Kostelijk). o = Centers of gravity of malleus and incus.

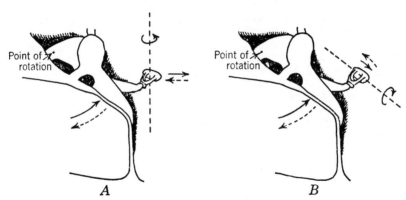

Figure 9. Mode of vibration of the stapes. For moderate sounds the stapes rotates about a vertical axis (*A*), for intense sounds it rotates about an anteroposterior axis (*B*). The point of rotation of the peripheral part of the ossicular system is shown (Békésy).

ment and, in this case, the rocking motion is accompanied by a pistonlike component (Fig. 10). The actual movement of the stapes is quite complex, as shown in Figure 10. This is because the annular ligament around the footplate is unequally distributed. The footplate is more rigidly fixed posteriorly than it is anteriorly, and the stapes rocks around the axis near the posterior edge.

With high sound levels the mode of action changes and a side-to-side rocking movement is seen around the axis running longitudinally through the length of the footplate (Fig. 9 *B*). As a result, the cochlear fluid flows only from one edge of the footplate to the other, with much less fluid displacement than when the

mode of vibration is through a vertical axis and the footplate is acting like a piston. This rotational shift of the axis is a protective mechanism for the inner ear.

Ossicular Chain as a Transformer

The outer end of the ossicular chain faces the air by the tympanic membrane and the inner end is connected to the inner ear by the oval window. The ossicular chain in the intermediate structure connects two different kinds of substances, namely, air and fluid. According to the well known principle in acoustics, sound waves traveling in a medium of some given

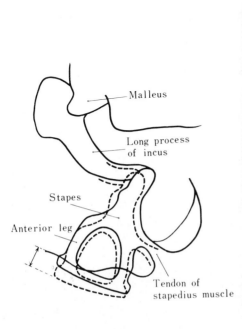

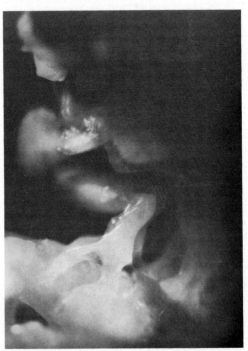

Figure 10. Vibration of the stapes seen from below (double exposure photography).

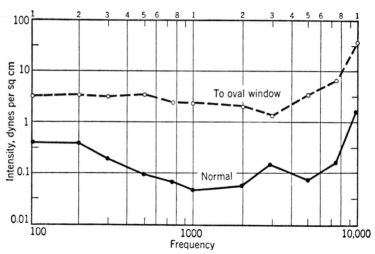

Figure 11. Sensitivity in the cat, expressed as the sound intensity required to produce a cochlear response of 10 microvolts. The solid line is for an ear with the middle ear intact, and the dashed line is for an ear with this structure removed and the sounds delivered directly to the oval window (Wever and Lawrence).

elasticity and density will not pass readily into a medium with a different elasticity and density but, rather, most of the sound will be reflected away. Thus, only one tenth of 1 per cent of the sound in the air will pass into water, while the remaining 99.9 per cent is reflected back. Figure 11 shows the results obtained from experiments on cats (Wever, Lawrence and Smith, 1948). The average transmission loss calculated from the graph is around 20 to 35 dB. In other words, the total mechanical advantage afforded by the middle ear is 20 to 35 dB. This value is comparable to the theoretical figure for the human ear, as calculated from the transformation ratio of 22:1. (The product of the areal and lever ratios will be discussed in the following sections.)

Ossicular Chain Lever. Helmholtz measured the amplitudes of displacement of the stapes and the manubrium of the malleus. He reported that the movement of the stapes is two thirds that of the manubrium and that their lever ratio is 1.5:1. He concluded that the force exerted upon the manubrium was increased by 1.5 and the amplitude reduced correspondingly. Dahmann's (1929) optical method revealed that the lever ratio as calculated from the length of the arms is 1.31:1. Stuhlman's (1943) model study showed the ratio to be 1.27:1. Wever's (1954) experiments on cats using cochlear microphonics showed that the lever ratio of the manubrium and the long process of the incus is 3:1 to 1:1. These comparable results show that the ossicular chain lever ratio is near 1 and its functional significance is not so great.

Areal Ratio of Tympanic Membrane and Oval Window. The difference in areas of the tympanic membrane and the stapes footplate results in a transformer action by hydraulic principle. Helmholtz (1868) measured the areas and he gave 64.3 sq. mm. for the tympanic membrane and 3.2 sq. mm. for the footplate. The areal ratio is 20:1. Subsequent studies of the ratio give slightly different values; 18.2:1, 19.1:1 (Wever et al., 1948), 21:1 (Fumagalli, 1949) and 26.6:1 (Békésy, 1951). The average of these five values is about 21:1 (Fig. 12). This is the anatomical ratio.

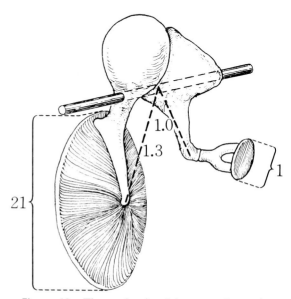

Figure 12. The areal ratio of the tympanic membrane and oval window, and the lever ratio of the ossicular chain.

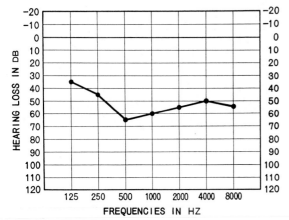

Figure 13. Hearing loss caused by disrupted ossicular chain (cat) (Wever and Lawrence).

As we have seen, the tympanic membrane does not vibrate as a whole because it is fixed all around the periphery. Wever and Lawrence (1954) deduce that the effective area for the tympanic membrane lies between 60 and 72 per cent of the anatomical area in the cat. Thus, the effective areal ratio will be 14:1. If we accept Dahmann's figure of 1.31 for the ossicular chain lever ratio, we obtain the overall ratio for the middle ear as the product, 14 × 1.31 = 18.3.

By means of the transformer action of the middle ear, the amplitude is greatly reduced at the oval window as compared with the amplitude at the tympanic membrane, and the force (pressure) at the oval window is increased in the same proportion, or 18.3 times.

Disturbance of the Ossicular Chain. When the ossicular chain is disrupted by causes such as head trauma and infection, a hearing loss of about 50 dB is seen even if the tympanic membrane is left intact. This hearing loss is caused by loss of the ossicular chain (28 dB) and by the existence of the tympanic membrane, which interferes with the sound conduction to

the inner ear (Fig. 13). On the other hand, even if the ossicular lever is lost by type III tympanoplasty, the hydraulic principle is restored because the head of the stapes is in contact with the tympanic membrane, as in the columella of birds. Loss of hearing in this case would be only 10 to 20 dB (Fig. 14).

Role of the Round Window

The area of the round window is 2 sq. mm. The window seals off the scala tympani and is situated at a right angle to the oval window. The round window is a relief opening to the labyrinth that permits the contained fluid to move under the influence of the stapes. As an entrance of sounds this is a very poor path and the sounds traveling by this route would be seriously attenuated because the tympanic membrane is in the way. The phase of sounds entering this window differs from that of the oval window because the two windows are not situated in the same plane.

This normal condition will change if the middle ear transformer is lost. The oval window is no more superior to the round window and the sound wave will strike the two windows simultaneously. The sound waves in the labyrinth, however, travel from both ends and will cancel each other. The loss of energy is about 12 dB and this is called the cancel effect (Fig. 15).

When we protect the round window with a small piece of wet cotton or tissue, the sound will not strike the window directly. This results in the improvement of hearing by 20 dB over low and middle frequencies. This is called the sound protection of the round window (Fig. 15). A similar effect is expected when we close the perforated membrane or make a small tympanum (curtain action of the tympanic membrane).

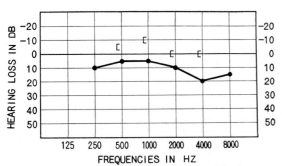

Figure 14. Audiogram of type III tympanoplasty by nature.

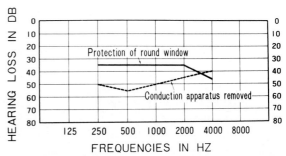

Figure 15. Protection effect of the round window upon cochlear microphonics in cat.

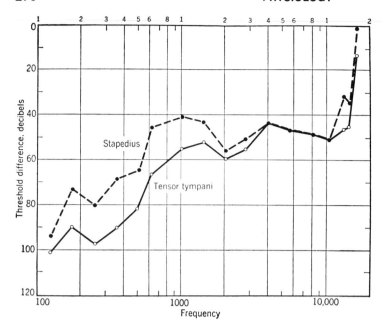

Figure 16. Reflex excitability of the tensor tympani and stapedius muscles in response to sounds. The ordinate values represent differences between reflex thresholds in the rabbit and tonal thresholds in man. For the low tones the stapedius reflex is more sensitive (Lorente de Nó and Harris).

Function of the Intrinsic Muscles of the Middle Ear

The middle ear structure includes two muscles, the tensor tympani and the stapedius, which are the smallest muscles in the body. The tensor tympani is the larger of the two.

Both are pennate muscles consisting of many short striated and nonstriated muscle fibers. They make involuntary contraction during acoustic stimulation. The reflex contraction starts first in the striated muscles, and the contraction is kept tense by nonstriated muscles.

Acoustic Reflex Contraction of the Intratympanic Muscles

This reflex contraction depends upon the frequency and intensity of stimulating sounds. Results obtained by experimenting with rabbits are shown in Figure 16. (Lorente de Nó, 1933). The threshold for the reflex contraction in a rabbit is about 40 to 100 dB. When the sounds are of frequencies less than 1500 Hz, the threshold of the stapedius reflex is lower than that of the tensor tympani muscle; at above the frequencies of 4000 Hz, similar thresholds are seen in both muscles.

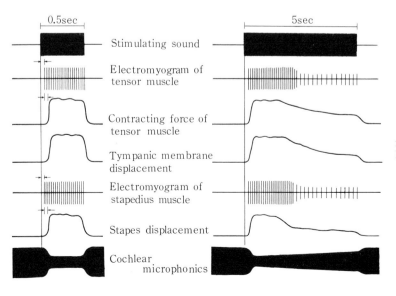

Figure 17. Tympanic muscle reflex contraction evoked by short and long sound stimulation.

Because of technical limitations, separate observation of thresholds for the two muscles is hardly possible in man. Two muscles are grouped together, and the threshold of this group in man is 70 to 90 dB above the thresholds of hearing in frequencies ranging from 250 to 4000 Hz.

Electromyographic study of cats showed that the latency time for the burst of action current of the muscle is 6 ~ 8 msec. in case of the tensor and always shorter in case of the stapedius. In addition, effective muscle contraction takes place after 2 to 3 msec., and maximal tension is obtained after a few more milliseconds (Kirikae, 1960) (Fig. 17).

The maximal tension of the tensor is 1.2 g. in case of a rabbit (Lorente de Nó, 1933), 3.5 g. in case of a cat (Wever et al., 1955), and about 50 g. in man. The constant tension as seen by electromyograms lasts for about 2 sec. after the sound stimuli and gradually decreases.

Effects of the Intratympanic Muscle Contraction

According to the experiments made on cats, the contraction of the tensor by sound stimuli produces inward displacement of the tympanic membrane accompanied by decrease in the amplitude of vibration (Fig. 17). Contraction of the stapedius exerts a force on the head of the stapes and draws it posteriorly. This displacement is not accompanied with a long process of the incus followed by a shift seen between the head of the stapes and the long process of the incus. Contraction of the stapedius alone does not cause any displacement of the tympanic membrane.

The effect of the reflex contraction upon the cochlear microphonics was studied in cats. A great decrease of amplitude was seen in the contraction of the stapedius and the tensor (Møller, 1964) (Fig. 18). According to a de-

tailed study made by Wever et al. (1955), the effect of the strong contraction of the tensor or the stapedius is a reduction in transmission. Being frequency selective in lower tones, this attenuation was only 5 to 10 dB.

To summarize, both muscles exert a force at right angles in the direction of ossicular movement and act as a damping mechanism which suppresses the degree of ossicular movement.

Tympanic Muscle Reflex in Man

Kawata (1958) measured the inward displacement of the manubrium mallei caused by reflex contraction of the muscles. Kobrak (1948) made direct measurement of the tilting of the footplate caused by reflex contraction of stapedius in a patient with a radical mastoid cavity. An experiment was done by Kobrak (1948) who made an optical perforation, i.e., the superior portion of the tympanic membrane was made transparent but not perforated. Maximal contraction was seen at maximal sensitivity of the human ear in frequencies ranging from 2500 to 3000 Hz. Møller (1962) observed in man the change in the acoustic impedance caused by tympanic muscle contraction. The change was measured in the external auditory canal. Figure 19 shows the results obtained from measurements of the impedance change of contralateral stimulation at various intensities. Sensitivity of muscle contraction is defined as the sound intensity required to give a certain percentage of maximal impedance change.

Attenuation of reflex contraction in man is said to be about 10 dB at low frequencies (Wever et al., 1954), or 5 to 10 dB (Békésy, 1951). Nakamura and Okamoto (1956) reported the value to be less than 5 dB in man, which coincided with the value of Metz' (1946) experiments on man, using the measurement of the impedance, which show that the reduction

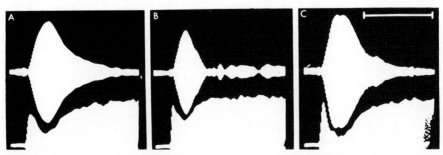

Figure 18. Upper curves: Change in acoustic impedance at 800 Hz recorded simultaneously with the cochlear microphonics (lower curves) in a cat. *A* represents contraction of the tensor tympani muscle; *B,* the stapedius muscle; and *C,* simultaneous contraction of both muscles. Time calibration: 100 msec. (Møller).

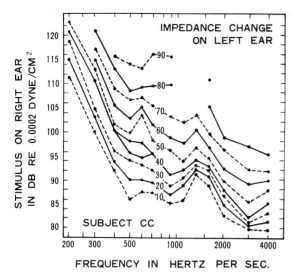

STIMULUS ON RIGHT EAR IN DB RE 0.0002 DYNE/CM²

IMPEDANCE CHANGE ON LEFT EAR

SUBJECT CC

FREQUENCY IN HERTZ PER SEC.

Figure 19. The sound intensity required for a constant degree of contralateral muscle contraction as a function of frequency. Percentage of maximal impedance change is indicated by numbers (Møller).

of sound absorption of 5 dB can be demonstrated at the maximal.

Physiological Role of the Tympanic Muscle Reflex

The stapedius and tensor tympani muscles exert force in directions opposite to each other (anatomical antagonists) but perpendicular to the primary rotational axis of the ossicular chain (functional synergists). Several functions have been attributed to the tympanic muscle reflex.

Protective Intensity Control Theory. The effect of the muscle reflex upon the performance of the ear, as stated previously, is reduction of transmission which is frequency selective in lower tones. This reflex mechanism serves to protect the cochlea from excessive stimulation caused by loud noises. In man, however, actual attenuation afforded by this mechanism is small, or its intensity control is not great.

Accommodation or Frequency Selection Theory. This is a theory which supposes that in certain frequencies muscle contraction selectively increases hearing sensitivity. But evidences, which actually show the degree of augmentation afforded by reflex contraction, are lacking.

Prevention of Aural Harmonics. Wiggers (1937) showed that the masking effect of low frequencies by muscle contraction and elimination of harmonics actually improves auditory acuity in higher tones.

Fixation Theory. The tympanic muscles have a simple and obvious function to provide stability of suspension for the ossicular chain. This is more than obvious when a surgeon divides the tendons of the tympanic muscles.

Acoustic Impedance of the Middle Ear

The main function of the middle ear is to facilitate the transmission of sound waves from air to the cochlear fluids. If sound waves act directly on the cochlear fluids, there will be a significant transmission loss of about 30dB. This is because the values of acoustic resistance (or impedance), which are determined by elasticity and density, are widely different between two media such as air and the inner ear fluid. In an example given previously, we speak of impedance mismatching, in which most of the sound energy is reflected. When the impedances are similar, or approximated by an intervening mechanical device, sound energy is transmitted effectively from one medium to the other, and this is called impedance matching. Thus, the middle ear acts as a transformer which "matches" the low impedance of air to the high impedance of the cochlear fluids.

The middle ear is a vibrating mechanical system whose acoustic impedance is determined by three factors: mass, stiffness (elasticity), and frictional resistance. We might draw our analogy from the principles of electronics which state that the flow in an electrical circuit is determined by three factors: resistance, inductance, and capacitance. The relation between the acoustic impedance (Za) and the mechanical impedance (Zm) is expressed by the following formula:

$$Za = Zm \, / \, A^2$$

in which A is the area of the piston.

If the acoustic system shown in Figure 20 is compared to the middle ear, the piston represents the tympanic membrane; M, the mass; S, the stiffness; and Rm, the friction of the middle ear mechanism. M represents the total weight

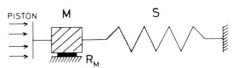

PISTON   M   S

Figure 20. An acoustic system consisting of mass (M), stiffness (S) and frictions (Rm) of the middle ear mechanism equipped with rigid piston (Møller).

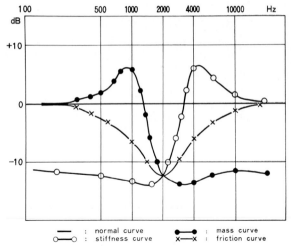

— : normal curve   ●—● : mass curve
○—○ : stiffness curve   ×—× : friction curve

Figure 21. A calculated curve demonstrating the frequency zones in which either the mass, the stiffness or the friction dominates and determines the auditory threshold (Johansen).

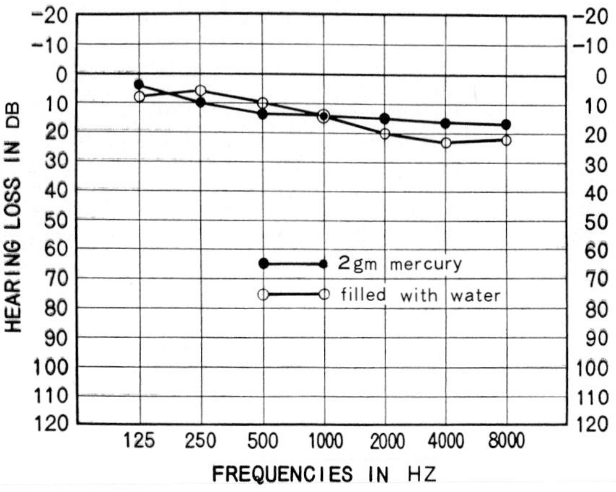

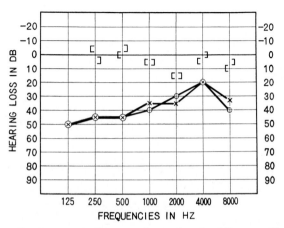

Figure 22. Loading of the tympanic membrane by pouring water or mercury into the external auditory meatus. (Lüscher).

of the tympanic membrane, the ossicular chain, and the inner ear fluids. The effective M would be less than the actual M since the center of gravity for the ossicular chain falls upon the axis of rotation. S consists of the ligaments of the middle ear, the incudostapedial joint, the tension of the tympanic membrane, the tension of the tympanic muscles, and the air in the tympanic cavity.

The concept of acoustic impedance will facilitate understanding of various kinds of hearing loss seen in the pathological middle ear.

Pathophysiology of the Middle Ear

According to Johansen (1948), the acoustic impedance of a vibrating system having mass, stiffness, and frictional resistance is calculated from the formula:

$$I = \sqrt{r^2 + (mf - s/f)^2}$$

where I is the impedance; r, the frictional resistance; m, the mass; s, the stiffness; and f, the frequency.

From the formula, calculated threshold value curves are obtained as shown in Figure 21. The natural resonance point of the middle ear is said at around 800 Hz although Békésy (1936) showed the value of 1000 Hz and Perlman (1947), 750 Hz. High values of f will exaggerate the effect of changes in mass.

When the mass is increased, the transmis-

sion of higher frequencies is impaired and the resonance point is shifted toward low tones. Low frequency values emphasize the effect of changes in stiffness. When the stiffness is increased, transmission of lower frequencies is impaired and the resonance point is shifted toward higher tones. These give rise to "mass curve" and "stiffness curve." When the mass is increased by loading the tympanic membrane with water and mercury, the thresholds for higher tones are elevated (Fig. 22). Similar audiograms will be seen by accumulation of fluids in ears with otitis media. The stiffness is increased by such causes as negative pressure in the tympanic cavity, eustachian tube stenosis, ossicular chain adhesion, and otosclerosis (Fig. 23).

Figure 23. Audiogram of otosclerosis (32 year old woman).

Acoustic Properties of the Air Spaces of the Middle Ear

The middle ear cavity consists of the tympanic cavity, tympanic antrum and mastoid cells, and the auditory tube. The tympanic cavity communicates with the tympanic antrum and mastoid cells by the tympanic aditus postero-superiorly, and with the auditory tube ante-roinferiorly.

These communicating air spaces are regarded as an entity in the sound conducting system. This closed air cavity has the physical effect of acting as a damping body. At low frequencies the air cavity of the middle ear affects vibration of the tympanic membrane, but at high frequencies only the tympanic cavity operates as an acoustic impedance. The larger the volume of the air space, the smaller the acoustic impedance or the less effect on the vibration of the tympanic membrane. The air spaces of tympanic antrum and mastoid cells add to the enlargement of the middle ear cavity, which corresponds to about 2 ml. of air in acoustic impedance. The middle ear cavity has resonance at 1800 Hz and antiresonance at 2600 Hz.

REFERENCES

Bárány, E.: A contribution to the physiology of bone conduction. Acta Otolaryng. Suppl. 26, 1938.

Békésy, G. v.: Zur Physik des Mittelohres und über das Hören bei fehlerhaftem Trommelfell. Akust. Ztschr. *1*:13, 1936.

Békésy, G. v.: Über die mechanisch akustischen Vorgänge beim Hören. Acta Otolaryng. *27*:281–296; 388–396, 1939.

Békésy, G. v.: Über die Messung der Schwingungsamplitude der Gehörknöchelchen mittels einer kapazitiven Sonde. Akust. Ztschr., *6*:1, 1941.

Békésy, G. v.: Experiments in Hearing. New York, Mc-Graw Hill Book Co., Inc., 1960.

Békésy, G. v., and Rosenblith, W. A.: The mechanical properties of the ear. *In* Stevens, S. S. (ed.): Handbook of Experimental Psychology. New York, John Wiley & Sons, Inc., 1951.

Dahmann, H.: Zur Physiologie des Hörens: experimentelle Untersuchungen über die Mechanik der Genörknöchelchenkette, sowie über deren Verhalten auf Ton und Luftdruck. Ztschr. f. Hals-, Nasen-, u. Ohrenheilk. *24*:462–497, 1929; *27*:329–368, 1930.

Dishoeck, H. A. E.: Theorie und Praxis des Pneumophons. Arch. Ohr. Nas. Kehlkopfheilk. *146*:5, 1939.

Dishoeck, H. A. E.: Tubal disorders and the pneumophone. Acta Otolaryng. *41*:196, 1952.

Feldman, A. S.: Acoustic impedance studies of the normal Ear. J. Speech Hear. Res. *10*:165, 1967.

Fumagalli, Z.: Ricerche morfologische sull apparats di transmissione del suone [Sound conducting apparatus: A study of morphology]. Arch. Ital. Otol. *60*: Suppl. 1, 1949.

Gyergyay, A.: Neue Wege zur Erkennung der Physiologie und Pathologie der Ohrtrompete. Mschr. Ohrenheilk. *66*:769, 1932.

Helmholtz, H. v.: Die Mechanik der Gehörknöchelchen und des Trommelfells. Arch. ges. Physiol. (Pflüger) *1*:1–60, 1868.

Ingelstedt, S., and Örtegren, U.: Qualitative testing of the eustachian tube function. Acta Otolaryng. Suppl. *182*:7–23, 1963a.

Ingelstedt, S., and Örtegren, U.: The ear snorkel–pressure chamber technique, Volumetric determination of tubal ventilation. Acta Otolaryng. Suppl. *182*:24–34, 1963b.

Johansen, H.: Relation of audiograms to the impedance formula. Acta Otolaryng. (Suppl.) *74*:65, 1948.

Kawata, S.: Judgment of recruitment by means of measuring the retraction grade of the tympanic membrane. Acta Otolaryng. *49*:517, 1958.

Kirikae, I.: Structure and Function of the Middle Ear. Tokyo, The University of Tokyo Press, 1960.

Klockhoff, I.: Middle ear muscle reflexes in man. Acta Otolaryng. Suppl. *164*, 1961.

Kobrak, H. G.: Zur Physiologie der Binnenmuskeln des Ohres. I. Untersuchungen zur Mechanik des Schalleitungskette. Passow-Schaeffer Beitäge. *28*:138, 1930; Ztschr. Hals. Heilk. *27*:386–402, 1930.

Kobrak, H. G.: Utilization of the tensor tympani muscle reflex in the analysis of the function of the middle and internal ear structures. Ann. Otol. *45*:830, 1936.

Kobrak, H. G.: Cinematographic study of the conduction of sound in the human ear. J. Acoust. Soc. Amer. *13*:179–181, 1941.

Kobrak, H. G.: Acoustic movements of the human sound conduction apparatus. Arch. Otolaryng. *36*:162, 1942.

Kobrak, H. G.: Direct observation of the acoustic oscillations of the human ear. J. Acoust. Soc. Amer. *15*:54, 1943.

Kobrak, H. G.: The present status of objective hearing tests. Ann. Otol. *57*:1018, 1948.

Kobrak, H. G.: Experimental observations on sound conduction in the middle and inner ear. Ann. Otol. *62*:748–756, 1953.

Kobrak, H. G.: The Middle Ear. Chicago, The University of Chicago Press, 1959.

Kostelijk, P. J.: Theories of Hearing. Universitaire pers Leiden, 1950.

Lawrence, M.: Recent investigation of sound conduction. Ann. Otol. *59*:1020–1061, 1950.

Lawrence, M.: Applied physiology of middle ear sound conduction. Arch. Otolaryng. *71*:132, 1959.

Lorente de Nó, R.: Experimental studies in hearing. Laryngoscope *43*:315, 1933.

Lüscher, E.: Untersuchungen über die Beeinflussung der Hörfähigkeit durch Trommelfellbelastung. Acta Otolaryng. *27*:250, 1939.

Mach, E., and Kessel, J.: Beiträge zur Topographie und Mechanik des Mittelohres. Sitzungsber. Akad. Wien. Math. Naturw. Klasse, Abt. III, *69*:221, 1874.

Matsumura, H.: Studies on the composition of air in the tympanic cavity. Arch. Otolaryng. *61*:220, 1955.

Metz, O.: The acoustic impedance measured on normal and pathological ears: Orientating studies on the applicability of impedance measurement in otological diagnosis. Acta Otolaryng. Suppl. *63*, 1946.

Møller, A. R.: Intra-aural muscle contraction in man, examined by measuring acoustic impedance of the ear. Laryngoscope *68*:48–62, 1958.

Møller, A. R.: The sensitivity of contraction of the tympanic muscles in man. Ann. Otol. *71*:86, 1962.

Møller, A. R.: Effect of tympanic muscle activity on movement of the eardrum, acoustic impedance and cochlear microphonics. Acta Otolaryng. *58*:525–534, 1964.

Møller, A. R.: The acoustic impedance in experimental studies on the middle ear. Int. Audiol. *3*(No. 2):1, 1964.

Møller, A. R.: An experimental study of the acoustic impedance of the middle ear and its transmission properties. Acta Otolaryng. *59*:1, 1965.

Nakamura, K., and Okamoto, M.: Study on sound transmission efficiencies of human ears with acoustic reflex contraction of middle ear muscles. Jap. J. Otol. (Tokyo) *59*:1933, 1956.

Onchi, Y.: Mechanism of the middle ear. J. Acoust. Soc. Amer. *33*:794, 1961.

Perlman, H. B.: The eustachian tube. Arch. Otolaryng. *30*:212, 1939.

Perlman, H. B.: Quantitative tubal function. Arch. Otolaryng. *38*:453, 1943.

Perlman, H. B.: Stroboscopic examination of the ear. Ann. Otol. *54*:483, 1945.

Perlman, H. B.: Physics of the conduction apparatus. Laryngoscope *55*:337, 1945.

Perlman, H. B.: Some physical properties of the conduction apparatus. Ann. Otol. *56*:334, 1947.

Perlman, H. B.: Normal tubal function. Arch. Otolaryng. *86*:632, 1967.

Schmitt, H.: Über die Bedeutung der Schalldrucktransformation und der Schallprotektion für die Hörschwelle. Acta Otolaryng. *49*:71, 1958.

Stuhlman, O.: An Introduction to Biophysics. New York, John Wiley & Sons, Inc., 1943.

Totsuka, G., Nakamura, K., and Kirikae, I.: Electromyographic studies of the acoustic-auricular reflex. Ann. Otol. *63*:935–945, 1954.

Toynbee, J.: On the muscles that open the eustachian tube. Proc. Roy. Soc. Med. *6*:286, 1853.

Wada, Y.: Beiträge zur vergleichende Physiologie des Gehörorganes. Arch. Ges. Physiol. (Pflüger) *202*:46, 1924.

Wever, E. G., and Lawrence, M.: The functions of the round window. Ann. Otol. *57*:579–589, 1948*b*.

Wever, E. G., and Lawrence, M.: The transmission properties of the middle ear. Ann. Otol. *59*:5–18, 1950.

Wever, E. G., and Lawrence, M.: Physiological Acoustics. Princeton, New Jersey, Princeton University Press, 1954.

Wever, E. G., Lawrence, M., and Smith, K. R.: The middle ear in sound conduction. Arch. Otolaryng. *48*:19–35, 1948*a*.

Wever, E. G., and Vernon, J. A.: The threshold sensitivity of the tympanic muscle reflexes. Arch. Otolaryng. *62*:204–213, 1955*a*.

Wever, E. G., and Vernon, J.A.: The effect of the tympanic muscles upon sound transmission. Acta Otolaryng. *45*:433–439, 1955*b*.

Wever, E. G., and Vernon, J. A.: The control of sound transmission by the middle ear muscles. Ann. Otol. *65*:5–14, 1956.

Wever, E. G., Vernon, J. A., and Lawrence, M.: The maximum strength of the tympanic muscles. Ann. Otol. *64*:383–391, 1955.

Wigand, M. E.: Steuerung, Reflexverhalten und funktionelle Bedeutung der Mittelohrmuskeln, Würzberg, Habil. Schrift, 1965.

Wiggers, H. C.: The functions of the intra-aural muscles. Amer. J. Physiol. *120*:771–780, 1937.

Wilska, A.: Eine Methode zur Bestimmung der Hörschwellenamplituden des Trommelfells bei verschiedenen Frequenzen. Skand. Arch. f. Physiol. *72*:161, 1935.

Wullstein, H.: Principles of tympanoplasty. Arch. Otolaryng. *71*:329, 1960.

Zöllner, F.: Anatomie, Physiologie, Pathologie und Klinik der Ohrtrompete. Berlin, Springer Verlag, 1942.

Zwislocki, J.: Acoustic measurement of middle ear function. Ann Otol. *70*:599, 1961.

Zwislocki, J.: An acoustic method for clinical examination of the ear. J. Speech Hear. Res. *6*:304, 1963.

INNER EAR PHYSIOLOGY

by

Merle Lawrence, Ph.D.

It is difficult to study the physiology of the inner ear because the tissues that make up the auditory labyrinthine system are suspended in fluid, and any attempt to enter the fluid system causes the different kinds of fluids to mingle, thus destroying the normal function. Fortunately some of the lower forms, especially the guinea pig, have a bony capsule for the inner ear which protrudes into the middle ear space. The bone of this capsule is thin and somewhat transparent, which has made this particular animal a favorite one for experimental work, and, although there are gross structural differences related to the nature of skull design, there is probably little species difference as far as the basic physiology is concerned. Many of the experiments upon which our present knowledge of inner ear physiology is based have been carried out on the lower forms but, for the most part, the results can safely be inferred as true for man.

A consideration of the physiological processes of the ear is essentially a consideration of the properties of the fluids that surround the various tissues, and there are at least four purposes that these fluids serve:

1. The fluids provide the nutrients to, and remove the catabolic products from, those cells whose only contact with the blood is through the surrounding fluids.

2. The fluids provide the proper chemical (ionic) environment for the energy transformation (vibration to nerve impulse) to take place.

3. The fluids are responsible for the relay of vibrations from the footplate of the stapes to the energy transforming elements.

4. The fluids control the pressure distribution within the system, if, indeed, there is any pressure.

A careful consideration of these purposes raises many questions of a more specific nature. What is known about the chemical constituents of the various fluids and what is the nature of exchange between blood and the fluids? What are the dynamic properties of these fluids? How do they circulate and does a hydrostatic pressure difference exist? In what way do these fluids contribute both to the mechanical properties of the inner ear and to the energy conversion process?

Actually, there are as yet no clear-cut answers to these questions, but progress is being made.

FLUID COMPONENTS AND THEIR SOURCE

Fluid Components

If there is any area concerning the physiology of the inner ear about which more facts are known it is probably that concerning the chemical composition of the fluids, despite the fact that the area occupied by these fluids is extremely small and methods of analysis without contamination are difficult. There are many reviews in which listings of the various components in endolymph and perilymph can be found. Two of the most recent are by Fernandez (1967) and Maggio (1966).

Electrolytes. The most numerous investigations are those determining the electrolytes of the fluids. The earliest work was carried out by Kaieda (1930), who pooled the fluids of freshly killed sharks and found sodium, potassium, and chloride to be about twice as concentrated in endolymph as in perilymph.

In 1954 microchemical methods specifically adapted for the purpose were employed by Smith, Lowry, and Wu in determining the electrolytes of the labyrinthine fluids as well as of serum and of cerebrospinal fluid in guinea pigs. Perilymph was withdrawn by piercing the round window with a Pyrex micropipette. Endolymph was taken from both the utriculus and cochlea. Samples of cerebrospinal fluid were taken from the fourth ventricle, and blood was removed from the heart for serum analysis. The results are shown in Table 1.

The remarkable thing about these findings is that endolymph with its relatively high potassium content resembles intracellular more than extracellular fluid. However, Rauch and Köstlin (1958) describe parotid gland secretions as also having a high potassium content.

Smith et al. were able to confirm their microchemical analyses by flame photometry in a few of the larger endolymph samples, although they state that the precision of measurements was less than with the chemical measures. These classic experiments were followed by others, and with some variation they have now been confirmed many times (Rauch and Köstlin, 1958; Rauch, 1963; Silverstein, 1966; Ulrich et al., 1966).

Rauch and Köstlin (1958) reported, for the first time, the concentration of electrolytes in the inner ear fluids of man. These do not differ in any great respect from the values given for the guinea pig. Rauch (1964) later reported these figures for living man in greater detail and added values for other electrolytes not previously determined. The histograms of Figure 24 summarize the results.

Proteins. In many different animals it has been shown that the protein content of perilymph is less than in blood serum and more than in endolymph and cerebrospinal fluid (Jensen and Vilstrup, 1954; Smith et al., 1954; Vilstrup and Jensen, 1954; Citron et al., 1956; Antonini et al., 1957; Miyake, 1960; Brosch, 1964). For man, Rauch and Köstlin (1958) reported total protein in mg. per 100 ml. as: serum, 7000; spinal fluid, 10 to 25; perilymph, 70 to 100; and endolymph, 20 to 30. As techniques were improved many analytic methods were applied to determine the specific proteins

TABLE 1. *Electrolytes in Fluids of Guinea Pig (mEq./L.)*

	PERILYMPH	ENDOLYMPH (UTRICULAR)	CSF	SERUM
Na	150.3	15.8	152	138.6
K	4.8	144.4	4.2	–
Cl	121.5	107.1	122.4	93.9

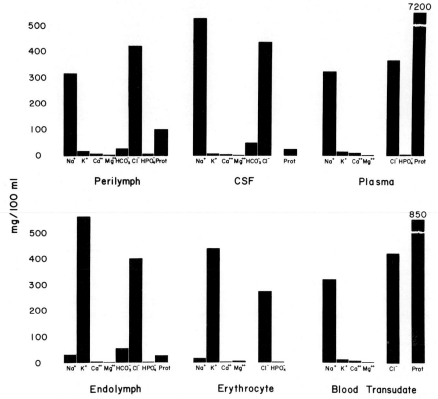

Figure 24. The distribution, in mg. per 100 ml., of electrolytes in labyrinthine and selected body fluids. Data for endolymph and perilymph were taken from Rauch (1964); the rest of the data were taken from Dittmer (1961) and converted where necessary.

present; Chevance et al. (1960) have summarized a series of their reports. Fritsch and Jolliff (1966), Palva and Raunio (1967 a and b), and Beck and Holz (1965) also reported on human perilymph and endolymph. Recently the techniques have been applied to man in diseased states (Silverstein and Schuknecht, 1966). The problem of contamination with erythrocytes and serum is a major one, and the results are not specific enough to give a concise list.

Other Characteristics

Some time before satisfactory methods were developed for analyzing the chemical constituents of the inner ear fluids some of the more readily determined characteristics were measured. Generally the interest was not based on curiosity concerning the measured physical attribute but on a desire to learn more about the metabolic processes occurring through the medium of the inner ear fluids, and to establish the characteristics by which these fluids differ. The major difficulty in working with the inner ear fluids is the paucity of material available. Maggio (1966) gives volume measures for cat,

dog, and man estimated by calculating the area of cochlear partitions in histological preparations. He reports for the cat that the volume of perilymph is 24.9 cu. mm. and the volume of endolymph is $2.91^{\pm} 0.1$ cu. mm. It is interesting to note, however, that by sampling all the perilymph and endolymph that could be extracted by means of the capillary action of glass tubing, the quantities were very much smaller. From the cat he was able to withdraw only 6.77 cu. mm. of perilymph and 1.46 cu. mm. of endolymph. From the dog he was able to withdraw considerably more: 17.8 cu. mm. of perilymph and 6.1 cu. mm. of endolymph.

The total calculated volume of perilymph in man is given as 78.3 cu. mm., with only 2.76 cu. mm. for endolymph (two specimens).

Despite the small volumes of fluid, such characteristics as osmotic pressure, refractive index, specific gravity, viscosity, pH, and certain electrical properties have been determined.

Osmotic Pressure. Aldred, Hallpike, and Ledoux (1940) determined the osmotic pressure of blood, cerebrospinal fluid, perilymph, and endolymph by using a thermoelectric method employing especially small thermocouple loops. The round window of the cat was exposed and a sample of perilymph collected by piercing the membrane with a micropipette maneuvered by a micromanipulator. The round window membrane was then removed and another micropipette inserted through the basilar membrane after cerebrospinal fluid flowing into the area through the cochlear aqueduct was sucked away and the basilar membrane left dry. The fluid then rising in the pipette was considered to be endolymph.

Cerebrospinal fluid was collected from the cisterna magna, and a sample of blood was collected from the carotid artery.

The total osmotic pressure recorded by this method was expressed in equivalent percentages of NaCl (gm. NaCl per 100 gm. H_2O), subject to error of ± 0.005 per cent. The figures obtained were: blood, 0.994; cerebrospinal fluid, 1.017; perilymph, 1.046; and endolymph, 1.058.

Ledoux (1941a) later used what was considered to be an improved thermoelectric method for very small samples with results somewhat less than above when expressed relative to the osmotic pressure of plasma.

Refractive Index. The first measures of the refractive index of the labyrinthine fluids were made by Szász (1923), who compared the refractive index of samples of cerebrospinal fluid obtained by cisternal puncture with that of perilymph samples obtained from inside the round window of dogs. The values he obtained were 1.335147 for labyrinthine fluid (perilymph) and 1.334270 for cerebrospinal fluid. From these results he considered perilymph and cerebrospinal fluid to be different, but there is sufficient overlap in the spread of readings from his 17 tests to indicate chance alone could account for the differences in the means.

Ledoux (1941b) also measured the refractive index in both dogs and cats, but his samples were too few and the overlap in readings too great to be of any significance.

Miyake (1953), in a study of the refractive index of cerebrospinal fluid in nerve-deaf patients, found it to be somewhat different from normal in all cases. The refractive index as determined by "Pulfrich's refractometer" was said to be 1.33409 in the normal individual. He also made determinations in healthy rabbits of the refractive index of labyrinthine fluid, presumably perilymph, but this is not stated. This value he gives as 1.33546, not much different from the earlier measures. On the basis of his results Miyake decided perilymph and cerebrospinal fluid are not the same.

Specific Gravity and Viscosity. So far these characteristics have been determined only for pigeons, and the results do not agree very well (Rossi, 1914; Money et al., 1966). The specific gravity and viscosity appear, within the limits of the experiments, to be greater for endolymph than for perilymph.

pH. Kaieda (1930) measured the pH of the inner ear fluids of the shark and obtained a value of 7.41 for perilymph, 7.23 for cerebrospinal fluid and 7.36 for endolymph.

Ledoux (1943) determined these values in the cat as: endolymph, 7.82; perilymph, 7.87; cerebrospinal fluid, 7.45; and plasma, 7.33.

Because the transfer of the minute volumes of fluid, as carried out by Ledoux, could lead to diffusion of carbon dioxide out of the fluid, resulting in slightly high pH determinations, Misrahy et al. (1958a) developed an electrochemical microelectrode technique to determine the pH of guinea pig endolymph and perilymph in situ. The active microelectrode was made by drawing soft glass capillary tubing to a tip of 10 to 12 μ and filling this with a specially prepared mixture of an antimony-Cerroseal alloy. The reference electrode was a glass micropipette with a 3 μ tip filled with a 0.9 per cent KCl solution into which a silver-silver chloride wire was placed. The pH of the perilymph exposed to the atmosphere was found to be 7.8 to 8.0 and that of the endolymph in situ 7.3 to 7.5. These values are lower and opposite to those found by Ledoux but are probably more reliable. Misrahy et al. found the pH to be very sensitive to changes in carbon dioxide tension, suggesting to them the possible presence in the endolymph of a bicarbonate buffer system.

Rauch and Köstlin (1958) give the pH in man as: perilymph, 7.2; endolymph, 7.5; serum, 7.35; spinal fluid, 7.35.

Blood-Endolymph Relationship

Until the chemical analyses of endolymph and perilymph were made it appeared entirely logical to assume that the stria vascularis is a special structure secreting endolymph. Corti, in 1851, made the statement, "One will be tempted to suppose a certain relationship between the vascular band [stria vascularis] in question and the secretion of endolymph." The supposition was further encouraged by the thought that one function of the fluids must be to separate the organ of Corti, sensitive to the slightest vibration or pulse, from its blood supply; and, consequently, the fluid must convey the necessary nutrients to the sensory cells. But when it was found that endolymph has a high potassium content it was suggested that perilymph would be a more suitable solution for surrounding the hair cells and unmyelinated fibers within the organ of Corti, and then it was suggested that this must be an entirely different fluid. Engström suggested the name "cortilymph" (1953, 1960).

Whatever the specific nature of these fluids may be, it is obvious that, somehow, a source of nutrients and oxygen must move from a blood supply through fluid to the sensory cells. Complicating the possibilities for metabolic exchange in the vicinity of the hair cells, however, is the fact that two of these vascular areas, the stria vascularis and spiral prominence, border the endolymph, while the third lies beneath the basilar membrane as an arcade of capillaries within the tympanic lamella. The artery to the cochlea arises from the basilar artery within the cranial posterior fossa. It is, therefore, as Anson et al. (1966) have noted, completely separate from the blood supply of the otic capsule.

The arterial supply and venous drainage have been described, along with a review of the early literature, by Smith (1951) and Scuderi and Del Bo (1952). Smith gives the description for the guinea pig ear. The cochlear artery (*a. cochleae propria*), along with the nerve fibers, enters the modiolus and gives off many branches as it spirals through the loose connective tissue between the nerve and bony wall to the apical turn. Relatively large primary branches give rise to coiled secondary branches that radiate either out over the scala vestibuli in the bone between two turns, or radiate toward the limbus and spiral osseous lamina as shown in Figure 25.

The arteriole passing out over the scala vestibuli does not divide into terminal branches until it enters the spiral ligament. Except for one or two branches from each arteriole that turn in a spiral direction, all others descend into the spiral ligament where they divide into four groups.

Group 1. Small branches given off from the arteriole as it enters the spiral ligament course in a spiral direction, usually above Reissner's membrane, and leave the area either by descending through the spiral ligament to the venules below or turn upward to join the collecting vein from the turn above.

Group 2. There is usually one of the branches from the arteriole that provides the capillary network of the stria vascularis. These capillaries follow a twisting course spirally between the epithelial cells with considerable interconnection and finally drain into a large ven-

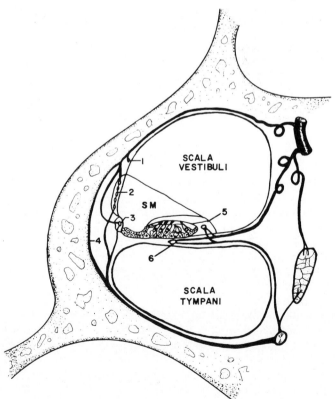

Figure 25. Blood supply to the membranes of the cochlea. SM = Scala media. See text for description of vessel groups.

ule that descends to the collecting venous system at the lower edge of the spiral ligament.

Group 3. A main branch descends behind the stria vascularis to enter the spiral prominence. It continues as a small vessel coursing in a spiral direction just beneath the epithelial cells. As it proceeds in this spiral course it is drained by many vessels that descend into the collecting venules.

Group 4. The rest of the terminal branches descend in the depths of the spiral ligament to the collecting venules, making some interconnections in the region below the attachment of the basilar membrane.

The secondary branches coiling toward the spiral osseous lamina usually divide into two groups: one going to the limbus (Group 5), and the other to the plexus below the basilar membrane (Group 6).

The vessels entering the limbus remain in the connective tissue base of the limbus. After a succession of loops they descend to the upper bony plate of the spiral lamina continuing toward the vein.

The vessels making up the plexus below the basilar membrane are extensions of vessels coursing outward either through the bone of the osseous lamina or directly on the surface of the nerve. After descending through the nerve they continue out below the fibers of the basilar membrane. Here they turn in a spiral direction, first, to form an interrupted group below the inner pillars. There are many radial connections that eventually either descend directly to the posterior spiral vein or join the limbus vessels. A second group of vessels extends out in a spiral path below the tunnel. In some animals, and in some turns, these "outer" spiral vessels may not be present (Smith, 1954). The two spiral groups may be connected by capillary bridges, but each has direct arterial and venous connections from the modiolus. Both groups of spiral vessels remain below the basilar membrane and are separated from the perilymphatic space by cells of the tympanic lamella and a thin layer of basilar membrane cells. Pericapillary spaces around these vessels have been described (Hawkins, 1968).

The various branches return to the modiolus after traversing either the bone or nerve channel and collect together in venules receiving branches from the spiral ganglion to end in the posterior spiral vein.

There are, then, three areas supplied with sufficient capillaries to provide nutrients and oxygen to the hair cells: the stria vascularis, the spiral prominence, and the basilar membrane vessels. A recent description of this vascular system in man has been presented in a monograph by Axelsson (1968).

Perlman and Kimura (1955) reviewed earlier work (Krejci and Bornschein, 1951a; Seymour and Tappin, 1951; Scuderi and Del Bo, 1952; Weille et al., 1954 a and b) involving histological and direct observation of the vessels of the spiral ligament and stria vascularis during stimulation of the cervical sympathetic ganglion, during direct application of adrenalin and noradrenalin, and following anaphylactic shock, all of which had varying results.

Their own technique for studying the vessels of the stria vascularis was an improvement over those of earlier workers. The bone over the spiral ligament of the fourth turn of the guinea pig was removed and the area was illuminated by an air-cooled 1000 watt light through a quartz rod. The animal's head was held rigidly and motion pictures were taken through a microscope with magnifications of from 90 to 165 times. Occasionally magnifications of 260 and 390 were used.

The blood flow appeared remarkably stable, and no spontaneous constriction or dilatation could be observed. Cutting the cervical trunk above the stellate ganglion or electrical stimulation of the stellate ganglion, cervical trunk, superior cervical ganglion, vertebral artery, basilar artery, and anterior inferior cerebellar artery did not produce visible changes in the observed strial vessels or in the rate of blood flow. Asphyxia and anaphylactic shock did produce changes.

Kimura and Perlman (1956, 1958) demonstrated, histologically, profound degeneration in the structures of the scala media following surgical obstruction of the inferior cochlear vein and the anterior inferior cerebellar artery. The hair cells were most vulnerable and, interestingly, the inner hair cells degenerated before the outer with arterial obstruction, whereas the outer hair cells showed disintegration before the inner hair cells following venous obstruction. Structures of the spiral ligament also degenerated. In a later experiment Perlman, Kimura, and Fernandez (1959) showed a decrease in the electrical response of the cochlea on temporary obstruction of the internal auditory artery.

Alford et al. (1965) showed that the injection of small plastic beads produced microscopic intravascular occlusion of the terminal branches of the arterial supply. These occasionally produced loss of hair cells in the presence of an apparently normal stria vascularis.

Although arterial and venous obstruction experiments have shown a direct relationship between blood flow to the structures of the spiral ligament and degeneration of the sensory epithelium, they do not show how the vascular areas are related to the fluids of the scala media.

Lawrence (1966) carried out an experiment, the results of which indicate the capillary area responsible for the fluid exchange necessary for the maintenance of the hair cells. With the aid of an operating microscope and using asceptic conditions, entrance high up in the scala vestibuli of a selected turn was made by a sterile hand-held drill honed to a triangular point of less than 100 μ. A small probe of approximately 25 μ at the tip was then inserted by hand through the opening and through the bony modiolar wall in those instances where interruption of blood supply to the vessels of the basilar membrane was desired. By back lighting the cochlea, the vessels descending into the spiral ligament were seen and avoided. In other animals these latter vessels alone were interrupted.

A period of recovery of from four to 16 weeks followed the above procedure, at which time the animals were killed and prepared for histological examination. It was found that occlusion of the vessels passing from the modiolus over the scala vestibuli to the stria vascularis resulted in its degeneration but had no effect upon the organ of Corti. Occlusion of only the modiolar vessels going to the capillary loops beneath the basilar membrane resulted in loss of hair cells in the presence of a histologically normal stria vascularis and spiral prominence, indicating these vessels as the source of nutrients for the organ of Corti. Cortilymph is most likely supplied by these vessels. The structures on the endolymphatic wall of the spiral ligament may maintain the ionic content of the endolymph essential to the energy transformation process.

Some supporting evidence for the importance of these spiral vessels in maintaining the organ of Corti is found in the examination of the cochleas of newborn Shaker-1 mice that are known to lose their auditory function in a few days after the third to fourth week following birth (Gruneberg et al., 1940). Kikuchi and Hilding (1967) noted in these mice that the spiral vessel beneath the tunnel of Corti undergoes involution and loses its lumen along with subsequent degeneration of hair cells and neural elements in the organ of Corti. At this stage, and until well into the second month after birth, the stria vascularis appears almost normal by electron microscopy.

It is also interesting to note that vasomotor innervation is supplied to the spiral vessels by unmyelinated fibers that accompany the myelinated cochlear fibers. These unmyelinated fibers descend to pierce the basilar membrane and terminate on the vessels (Hawkins, 1968). Somewhat similar observations have been made by Terayama, Holz, and Beck (1966).

Balogh and Koburg (1965) describe a special arrangement of cochlear blood supply in the *tractus arteriosus,* which spirals about the cochlear nerve in the modiolus. In this region the cochlear artery supplies a number of capillary twigs to a band of tissue containing epithelial cells resembling those of the choroid plexus. Because of this similarity they have called this region the *cochlear plexus* and have ascribed to it a secretory role in the formation of fluid of the perivascular spaces of the modiolus passing along the nerve fibers to the spiral ganglion and possibly reaching the interior of the organ of Corti. There are other papers concerning this cochlear plexus (Müsebeck, 1965 a and b).

Many attempts have been made to trace substances from the blood capillaries into the fluids of the inner ear in order to determine the possible pathway from blood to fluid. Yamamoto and Nakai (1964) have reviewed some of the earlier papers appearing in Japanese journals and refer to the assertion that neither the stria vascularis nor the spiral ligament constitutes a pathway for metabolites from blood vessels to the endolymphatic or perilymphatic spaces. They cite the experimental work of Nomura (1961), who observed the small vessels of the spiral ligament and stria vascularis after intracardial injection of 5 to 10 ml. of 1 per cent trypan blue solution and concluded that in the stria vascularis a barrier exists between it and blood.

Yamamoto and Nakai (1964) attempted to determine whether such a barrier exists. Iron dextran particles (100 Å.) were injected into the blood vessels and into the endolymphatic and perilymphatic spaces of guinea pigs. Following injection the animals were allowed to survive for various periods of time. They were then decapitated and the ears examined by electron microscopy.

The dextran iron particles injected into the blood vessels appeared in the stria vascularis and the spiral ligament in 10 minutes after injection and remained there for a subsequent 10 hours, but no particles were observed in the endolymph. Thus, there appears to be a barrier to the passage of these small particles even though, when used in the glomerular infiltration test, they easily enter glomerular cells through endothelial cells and the basement membrane.

These authors offer a nice discussion of related works, many of which are not referred to here, and conclude that this barrier probably exists for some specific substances but not for all substances. They bring out the observations made by others that the radioactive form of several elements has been observed to move into the fluid spaces from the blood (Hayashido, 1950; Ledoux, 1950; Rüedi, 1951; Portmann et al., 1960).

From the experimental results described so far, certain conclusions seem to have evolved. It would appear that the organ of Corti does have a blood supply, the arcade of spiral vessels beneath the tunnel and basilar membrane, and that this supply serves at least one function: providing for the exchange of metabolites within the sensory epithelium. The structures along the wall of the spiral ligament serve other purposes, the most likely of which, and the one for which there is the most evidence, being control of ions and perhaps other substances like water and other inorganic substances necessary for the energy transforming properties of the sensory epithelium.

Blood-Perilymph-Cerebrospinal Fluid Relationship

Interestingly many of the studies on blood-endolymph relationship employing the movement of radioactive ions indicated considerable difference between perilymph and cerebrospinal fluid in the accumulation of this material. Choo and Tabowitz (1964) noticed that 16 to 24 hours following intraperitoneal injection of radioactive sodium (^{22}Na), the rise of concentration in the perilymph was somewhat less than that in the cerebrospinal fluid, an observation that had also been made by Rüedi (1951). In another report (1965) they found, following intraperitoneal injection of radioactive potassium ^{42}K, that for up to 15 hours following the injection, the ^{42}K concentration was slightly higher in perilymph than in cerebrospinal fluid. During the period of 15 to 48 hours the perilymph concentration increased fivefold, whereas the cerebrospinal fluid concentration increased twofold.

Schreiner (1966), using radioactive substances, shows evidence that perilymph originates from the perilymphatic space itself. These observations introduce the possibility

that the blood-perilymph exchange is more predominant than the cerebrospinal fluid-perilymph exchange. Kley (1951) has emphasized this on the basis of his results from accumulation of fluorescein in perilymph after injection into the blood stream.

The many differences in chemical and physical characteristics between perilymph and cerebrospinal fluid are themselves sufficient evidence that these are not the same fluids, even though the cochlear aqueduct is a channel connecting cerebrospinal fluid to the perilymphatic space of the scala tympani in the region of the round window. Those investigators collecting samples of perilymph from behind the round window in the guinea pig and cat have always mentioned the necessity of taking a sample quickly before cerebrospinal fluid flowing through the cochlear aqueduct contaminated the area. And yet these samples showed the two fluids to be chemically different.

Studies of radioactive electrolyte concentration in the two fluids after injection into the blood or intraperitoneally have also shown a difference.

There seem to be, then, several possibilities for the source of perilymph: (1) It can be an ultrafiltrate of blood arising from some appropriate vascular area in the inner ear itself. (2) It can arise from endolymph, its chemical constituents being determined by the properties of the membranes separating the two fluids. (3) It can be a direct product of cerebrospinal fluid, perhaps acquiring a different chemical nature because the exchange between the two fluids is slow.

The commonly accepted view is that the aqueduct provides an open connection between the two fluids. This stems primarily from early anatomical studies, especially in the lower animals. in which there is no doubt about the patency of the duct. (For review see Grünberg, 1922; Karlefors, 1924; Gerlach, 1939.) However, this has been difficult to establish in primates in which the duct is long and narrow; in some places in the course of the duct, especially near its junction with the scala tympani, the membranous lining almost fills the entire space. Karlefors (1924) reported patients in whom hearing was present before death, but in whom subsequent histological examination of the temporal bone showed places where the lumen of the aqueduct was occluded. Uyama (1933) blocked the aqueduct in rabbits and, although he found a bulging of Reissner's membrane into the scala vestibuli, the organ of Corti was everywhere present and of good appearance. Although he concluded that the bulging of Reissner's membrane indicated that perilymph comes from cerebrospinal fluid and that the aqueduct was the pathway, one could reason that the bulging was produced by an overproduction of endolymph resulting from his method of occluding the duct.

The most frequently used method of investigating the communication of perilymph with cerebrospinal fluid is that of injecting into the perilymphatic space or the subarachnoid space identifiable material so that later histological examination would reveal the distribution of this foreign matter. The use of the method is over 100 years old, dating back to Schwalbe (1869), who used techniques similar to those employed today, although Cotugno reported in 1774 the patency of the bony canal which he demonstrated by forcing mercury through it. Subsequent investigations are reviewed by Lempert et al. (1952). The results of present-day experiments seem to depend on the species of animal used.

The experiments of Altmann and Waltner (1947) demonstrate this difference. They injected a mixture of iron ammonium citrate and potassium ferrocyanide solution into the cisterna magna of rabbits, cats, and monkeys. Immersing the tissues that had been removed from the killed animal for a period of time in hydrochloric acid produced a precipitation of particles of ferric ferrocyanide. In the rabbits and cats the particles were found in the scala tympani and often in the scala vestibuli, whereas in only one of nine monkeys was the precipitate found in the cochlea itself, although it was present in the cranial end of the cochlear aqueduct. Svane-Knudsen (1958) has recently carried out similar experiments on guinea pigs with results comparable to non-primates.

Schuknecht and Seifi (1963) injected avian erythrocytes into the subarachnoid space of the posterior fossa of cats. Subsequent histological examination of the temporal bones of these animals, which were allowed to live for progressive periods of time following injection, revealed many erythrocytes caught in large quantities in the connective tissue network of the cochlear aqueduct and, in many ears, in the perilymphatic spaces. From these results the investigators concluded that there is a flow of fluid from the subarachnoid space to the perilymph. It is to be noted, however, that when they blocked the aqueduct for periods up to 10 months no changes appeared in the cochlea, from which they conclude that the aqueduct is not necessary for maintenance of perilymph volume.

That there is some exchange between perilymph and cerebrospinal fluid, and that this exchange is in either one or both directions in animals lower than primates, is attested to by what has come to be known as the "Schreiner phenomenon" (1961). Schreiner found that after introducing radioactive phosphorus into the perilymph of one ear, the radioactivity of the perilymph of the opposite ear one hour later was considerably higher than that of either serum or cerebrospinal fluid obtained by suboccipital puncture. This phenomenon has been further investigated by Krochmalska et al. (1967).

Experiments with primates give different results, as Altmann and Waltner have shown. Lempert et al. [1952] injected an aqueous suspension of colloidal carbon into the cisterna magna of seven monkeys. These animals were sacrificed at various periods of time following injection and none was found to have carbon particles in the perilymph.

Ritter and Lawrence (1965) reported a study in humans. Eighteen patients, scheduled to undergo stapes surgery for deafness due to otosclerosis, had injected into their spinal fluid, at various time periods before surgery, indigo carmine dye or a radioactive protein (radioiodinated serum albumin). In none of these patients did the perilymph, at the time of surgery, show detectable coloring by the dye or any radioactivity. On the other hand, there are occasional reports of excessive amounts of cerebrospinal fluid escaping from the oval window when the stapes is removed during human stapes surgery.

It is glaringly evident that the patency of the cochlear aqueduct varies considerably among the species, within a species, and even at various stages of life in man (Lawrence, 1965a). During fetal life and in the newborn the aqueduct is wide open, whereas in adult man and the monkey the duct passes through a long bony channel. Considering these anatomical variations and the inconsistency of experimental evidence, it would seem most likely that the actual passage of fluid through this duct is not what gives perilymph its chemical and physical characteristics.

There is a vascular area associated with the perilymphatic spaces that has been suggested as a possible source of at least the special properties of perilymph. This area (Group 1 in Fig. 25) is to be found in the thin portion of the spiral ligament "above" the attachment of Reissner's membrane, in which the capillaries branching from the radial arterioles arching over the scala vestibuli run more or less longitudinally. Hawkins (1968) gives this serious consideration founded on his excellent microscopic studies. He describes these capillaries as being surrounded by well defined pericapillary spaces often interconnected by avascular channels, with the capillary pressure high enough to move fluid by filtration outward into the perilymph.

This is not a new idea. Just about every investigator who has compared perilymph with cerebrospinal fluid has come to this conclusion, and Mygind (1948) has been one of the earlier writers to insist that perilymph arises from the inner ear. The perilymph is presumably resorbed in the lower spiral ligament near the basilar membrane in the scala tympani (Svane-Knudsen, 1958; Kirikae et al., 1961).

Perilymph appears to be a unique fluid, acquiring its properties from the blood but connected with the cerebrospinal fluid through a duct which need not necessarily be patent in the sense of a direct fluid flow through it. Perhaps the connective tissue system is one for regulating pressures and controlling the slow circulation of the fluids, which brings up the consideration of the mechanical relationships of the fluids.

DYNAMIC PROPERTIES OF THE FLUIDS

There are tissues in the inner ear such as Reissner's membrane and cells of the organ of Corti that are immersed in fluids and could not survive if there were not replenishment of fluid contents and removal of waste. Also, study has shown the concentrations of various electrolytes and proteins to be very different on opposite sides of the separating membranes, so there must be movement of water or transport of ions to maintain the normal condition. The fluids, in a sense, must flow, but this need not necessarily be in the sense of a source, a conduit, and a sink. There may be constant exchange throughout the fluid system, but this must always be in delicate balance so that there is no build-up of pressure or failure in the circulation. There has been much speculation concerning pressure and circulatory relations in the fluids of the inner ear, and there has also been considerable contradictory evidence. Some patterns of significance are beginning to emerge, however.

Fluid Pressure

Except for those ducts that extend into the cranial cavity, and the round window membrane exposed to the middle ear, the entire fluid system of the inner ear is encased in bone. If the fluids were under any pressure other than that necessary to fill the inner ear, one might expect an excessive bulging of the round window membrane or perhaps a distention of the endolymphatic sac. Capillary pressures would have to be high to interact with fluid, or the capillaries would be taking in fluid. If relative pressure difference within the inner ear fluids is necessary, one might expect deviations from this normal situation to result in a change in function (hearing level).

Hansen (1968) took up the question of the relation between cerebrospinal fluid and hearing for pure tones. His material consisted of consecutively selected patients from the Department of Neurosurgery on whom, for a period of about three years, the pressure of the cerebrospinal fluid in the lateral ventricles of the hemispheres was measured in connection with intracranial ventriculography. Otological and audiometric examinations were carried out in the Department of Otolaryngology. The distribution of cerebrospinal fluid pressures ranged from the categories 0–200 to 1000–2000 mm. H_2O. In 108 patients no correlation between hearing and a raised intracranial pressure could be established.

Klockhoff et al. (1966) have reported changes in the acoustic impedance of the middle ear with what the investigators have described as increases in craniolabyrinthine pressure. This increase in intracranial pressure was produced by compressing the cervical veins by a pressure cuff around the neck of the subject. As the pressure in the cuff reached 30 mm. Hg the impedance shift reached a maximum and the subject usually reported an attenuation of the carrier tone (550 Hz), presumably indicating a diminished sound transmission. Further observations on this type of impedance change were made on cats and guinea pigs, and the authors felt that the effect was due to a direct transmission of intracranial pressure to the fluids of the inner ear. It is unfortunate that hearing tests were not carried out in these animals and that careful observations were not made of the blood vessels of the tympanic membrane and intratympanic muscles which might affect impedance.

Many investigators have demonstrated that intracranial pressure can be transmitted to the labyrinthine fluids in animals lower than the primate (Szasz, 1926; Meurman, 1929; Hughson, 1932; Kobrak et al., 1933, 1940; Ahlén, 1947; Filippi, 1950; Krejci and Bornschein, 1951b). Most of these have been experiments in which the changes in labyrinthine pressure were measured by a capillary manometer, by changes in the round window, or by similar observations.

Following the lead of Hughson (1932), Allen and various associates carried out a series of experiments in which the effects of cerebrospinal fluid pressure changes were determined by observing the changes in the magnitude of the cochlear potentials.

Allen and Habibi (1962) recorded, by means of a silver wire foil electrode on the edge of the round window, the electrical potentials arising from the cat's ear when it is stimulated by sound. Alterations in the cerebrospinal fluid pressure were produced by inserting a fine polyethylene tube into a small dural slit made through a lumbar laminectomy. They observed a quickly reversible reduction in the amplitude of the electrical response with increases of cerebrospinal fluid pressure. After prolonged pressure the electrical response sustained a small permanent loss. The reversible loss was attributed to an impairment in the sound transmission system, whereas the permanent loss, they thought, might be caused by changes in some metabolic factor such as anoxia resulting from compression of blood vessels.

On the other hand, Gulick et al. (1962) found the decrease in the electrical response of the cochlea to be very slight when up to 50 cu. mm. of perilymph was removed from the scala tympani. However, there was a slow progressive degeneration in the response if the perilymph was allowed to leak out continuously.

Later Kerth and Allen (1963) compared the perilymphatic fluid pressure changes with those made in the cerebrospinal fluid. They attempted to verify the observations of Kley (1951), who exposed the cochlear aqueduct in guinea pigs and observed the flow of fluid into the scala tympani. The flow, although very slow, still continued after plugging of the aqueduct. Kerth and Allen, however, observed no increase in perilymphatic pressure with increases in cerebrospinal fluid pressure after blockage of the aqueduct.

Feldman and Allen (1966) made a histological examination of the cochlear structures of seven cats which had been intravitally perfused while the cerebrospinal fluid pressure was elevated 11 cm. Hg above normal. There was no evidence of injury or alteration in any cochlear structure as a result of the pressure increase. Because of this they contend that the electrical changes seen in earlier experiments must have been the result of reversible mechanical alterations.

Following these observations Allen (1964) proposed a theory of pressure balance which seems quite reasonable (Lawrence, 1965). He suggests that the endolymphatic sac functions to transmit the increased intracranial pressure to the endolymph so as to equalize pressure increase to the perilymph through the cochlear aqueduct, thus preventing changes in position of Reissner's or the basilar membrane (Fig. 27). He points out that this kind of mechanism must be operating to account for the constancy of auditory function during changes in cerebrospinal fluid pressure accompanying the many shifts in bodily position during man's normal activities. However, as described later, other experiments in primates and in human temporal bones indicate that changes in perilymphatic pressure may not have a very profound effect.

In freshly removed human temporal bones Békésy (1960, p. 433) determined the effects of static pressure increase of the perilymph on the movement of the stapes. A needle was cemented into an opening made in the bony wall of a semicircular canal and the pressure of the perilymph was increased through a water-filled tube connected to the needle and to a syringe, the plunger of which was weighted and continuously rotated so as to produce a smooth pressure. He found that at a pressure of four to seven atmospheres the round window would break but that the stapes was not visually affected. After the preliminary measurements, the volume displacement of the round window for frequencies of 300 to 1000 Hz was measured. No changes were observed as the pressure was increased until damage occurred to the inner ear and bone, allowing fluid to escape.

The effect of increases in perilymphatic pressure has been determined in the monkey, with the electrical potentials of the ear serving as an indicator. Lempert et al. (1949) sealed a No. 25 hypodermic needle into an opening made in the external semicircular canal so that measured air pressure could be applied to the fluid. The electrical response of the ear was recorded from a platinum foil electrode in contact with the round window membrane. Increases of perilymphatic pressure up to 50 mm. of mercury had no effect on the magnitude of the cochlear potentials.

As pointed out before, there is quite a species difference in the size of the lumen of the cochlear acqueduct. Allen's measurements were made in the cat, and pressure increases went directly through the aqueduct to the scala tympani. In these instances increases in perilymphatic pressure had an effect on the electrical response of the ear. Perilymphatic pressure increases through the semicircular canals may be a different situation. Békésy's measurements may not have been sensitive enough, and the pressure may have been more evenly applied or more equally distributed in the Lempert experiments than in the Allen experiments. Any interference that might occur in inner ear function must come about through unequal pressure within the fluid systems of the inner ear, but it is unlikely that such a condition can occur naturally; Reissner's membrane is much too delicate to sustain much of a pressure gradient.

However, there are studies that have reported differences in static pressure between the endolymph and perilymph in normal ears. Weille et al. (1958, 1961) used a specially designed electromanometer, monitored the position of the tip by recording the DC potential within the scala media, and obtained measurements indicating that the pressure of perilymph in the living guinea pig is greater than pressure of the endolymph, but the results are much too variable to be quantified.

It is of interest that Henriksson et al. (1966 a and b), in a study of the effects of pressure variations on the frog labyrinth, noted that when the bony perilabyrinthine capsule was removed, the perilymphatic wall could be seen bulging somewhat outward, regaining its shape after having been slightly compressed by some instrument. When the membrane was penetrated and the perilymphatic fluid sucked away, the saccule seemed to lose its shape and become flatter, indicating a small or nonexistent pressure gradient between endolymph and perilymph.

Circulation

So far it has become evident that the fluids are engaged in a process vital to the function of the organ of Corti, that the fluid chemicals are in constant exchange with the tissues, and that they are in intimate relationship with the blood and cerebrospinal fluid. The number of articles reporting experiments and offering theories on the circulation of these fluids are much too numerous to report completely. About the best that can be done is to classify some of the more predominant ideas and cull from this what seems to be the trend of experimental evidence.

The earliest and simplest concepts of endo-lymph movement are probably those that we have classified as longitudinal flow theories (Lawrence et al., 1961a). Very little experimental work had been done on the circulation of endolymph until that of Guild (1927). Through a small pipette Guild injected a solution of potassium ferrocyanide and iron ammonium citrate into the scala media of several living guinea pigs. After the lapse of various time intervals the animals were sacrificed and preserved for histological examination. The acid in the fixation fluid precipitated Prussian blue granules in sites along the scala media. The temporal bones of these animals were then sectioned and mounted serially so that the location of the granules could be studied with the microscope. In 16 of 20 animals the blue granules were found in the walls of the endolymphatic sac. From this Guild concluded that the flow of endolymph was from the stria vascularis down the scala media through the ductus reuniens to the sacculus, ending finally in the endolymphatic sac after passing through the endolymphatic duct.

Some time later Anderson (1948) carried out an experiment in which he injected trypan blue intraperitoneally into a series of guinea pigs. This dye was later found in the endolymphatic sac but never in the endolymph, a condition which he explained as resulting from a concentration of stain too low to be observable. The dye is gradually absorbed in the sac, and this investigator felt the longitudinal flow of endolymph was indicated. It is possible, of course, that trypan blue did not show up in the endolymphatic fluids for other reasons.

Altmann and Waltner (1950), like Guild, injected iron salt solutions of various concentrations into the subarachnoid space of rabbits and monkeys. The iron salts were later found in the endolymph, in various areas of the scala media, and in the endolymphatic sac. The authors consequently favored a longitudinal flow.

Lundquist, Kimura, and Wersall (1964) injected a colloidal solution of 0.25 per cent silver into the basal turn of the cochlea of guinea pigs. These animals were killed 24 hours after the injection and the endolymphatic sac was prepared for electron microscopic examination. The silver granules were found in significant amounts only in the endolymphatic sac, where the cells of the epithelial wall appeared to have a considerable capacity to act as macrophages.

Ishii, Silverstein, and Balogh (1966) injected foreign protein (peroxidase) into the cochlear duct; after two days this material was found phagocytized in cells floating free in the endolymphatic sac but not in the lining cells or elsewhere in the membranous labyrinth. They made other observations with radioactive carbon-labeled foreign protein and felt all were in agreement with the concept that endolymph flows from the cochlear duct to the endolymphatic sac. Koburg, Haubrich, and Kernbach (1967), following similar experiments, came to the same conclusion.

These experiments, however, have not gone without their critics. Seymour (1954), in a lengthy report, said that his studies on the histology of the saccus endolymphaticus in human and animal specimens had convinced him that the function of the sac is to secrete endolymph.

Van Egmond and Brinkman (1956) injected guinea pigs subcutaneously with a 0.5 per cent trypan blue. This was later found in the endolymphatic sac. In two animals a small quantity of blue mucous fluid was found in the vicinity of Bast's utriculo-endolymphatic valve. They claimed that this filling of the ductus endolymphaticus was an indication that the flow of endolymph is in the direction of sac to sacculus—a longitudinal flow in the opposite direction from that of Guild.

Controversy of equal magnitude has concerned the other end of the system. Smith (1957) says that morphological evidence, including her electron microscopic observations, leaves little doubt that the stria vascularis and spiral prominence participate in the production of endolymph. Johnson and Spoendlin (1966) support this view, and they add that there may be several exchange mechanisms between endolymph and stria vascularis.

Chou and Rodgers (1962) determined by Cartesian diver respirometry the rate of oxygen consumption by tissues lining the membranous labyrinth and came to the conclusion that the stria vascularis, and the walls of the utriculus and sacculus, are all involved in the formation and maintenance of endolymph.

That the situation is not simply a secretion of endolymph within the scala media with a flow toward the endolymphatic sac was questioned by many investigators, and theories of more complicated flow patterns evolved. Borghesan (1957) has said that the stria vascularis cannot secrete endolymph because its histological structure is inadequate. However, he does infer that perhaps the stria secretes crystalloids while the spiral prominence secretes the plasma which, when these substances get together, make up endolymph. He proposes a

theory of circulation that falls in the category we have called radial flow theories (Lawrence et al., 1961). Borghesan believes that the endolymph, once formed as described, is absorbed by Hensen's cells, where it is transferred to the hair cells. This endolymph, containing catabolites, pours into the tunnel of Corti, flowing into the internal spiral sulcus where it is absorbed through the interdental furrows of the limbus. Borghesan has published many other papers supporting this idea with histological observations.

It is fairly safe to say that just about every separate structure found along the walls of the membranous labyrinth has been allotted by many different investigators the attribute of either secreting or absorbing endolymph. These are all listed in table form in Rauch (1964, pp. 287 and 292) and need not again be reviewed.

The problem of longitudinal flow was further complicated by the observation made by several investigators that blockage of the endolymphatic duct did not produce any evidence of accumulated endolymph in the scala media, nor did it it produce any other changes. Lindsay (1947) found no changes in the scala media of the monkey after obliteration of the endolymphatic sac and duct. Lindsay et al. (1952) and Schuknecht and Kimura (1953) found that cats suffered no histological or functional injury following loss of the endolymphatic duct and sac. Whereas these observations were rather disconcerting to those interested in determining the pattern of circulation of the endolymph, they did promote investigation into other possibilities. And then, recently, blocking the endolymphatic duct in the guinea pig has been found to produce a hydrops in the labyrinth (Kimura and Schuknecht, 1965), and combined theories have evolved.

Of all the radial flow theories, that of Naftalin and Harrison (1958) has been the most thorough in considering the necessity of accounting for the unique distribution of cations within the fluids. Their theory of fluid exchange is shown in Figure 26. These authors suggest that the fluid flow proceeds from perilymph through Reissner's membrane to endolymph, with the stria vascularis acting as a selective absorbing site. A function of Reissner's membrane is to prevent the flow of potassium from the scala media to the scala vestibuli. The stria vascularis, by an ion exchange system analogous to that of the renal tubular cell, extracts sodium and exchanges potassium for it. Potassium cannot pass Reissner's mem-

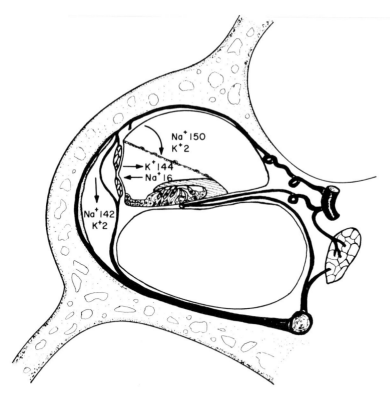

Figure 26. The theory of ion exchange proposed by Naftalin and Harrison (1958).

brane except by relatively slow equimolar exchange for sodium so that the amount of potassium builds up in the scala media until the required concentration is reached. The concentration of potassium in the endolymph is dependent upon the ratio of the volume of endolymph to the plasma flow through the stria vascularis per unit time, and equilibrium is determined by the structural characteristics of Reissner's membrane. Support for these speculations was later provided by Rauch and associates (1962, 1963) in experiments to be reported shortly.

These contrasting points of view, the longitudinal flow and the radial flow theories, typify the confusion regarding the circulation of inner ear fluids just 10 years ago. In 1961 Dobbing wrote a review on the blood-brain barrier in which he recommended that the use of foreign material for determining such things as the direction of cerebrospinal fluid flow be discarded. He arrived at this conclusion after a review of all the relevant experimental evidence which seems to show that such procedures do not give valid results. These substances, injected into the body tissues, are not normal solutions and the reaction of the tissues may be different from what it would be under normal conditions.

With this in mind Lawrence and co-workers attempted in a series of experiments to obtain some indication of direction and rate of endolymph flow without introducing any foreign matter. It was first necessary to determine whether the *pars superior* (semicircular canals and utriculus) and *pars inferior* (cochlea and sacculus) are capable of surviving alone; i.e., whether the flow of endolymph from both parts is toward the endolymphatic duct so that each system can exist without the other, and to determine to what extent restricted parts of the system are independent of others.

It had already been reported by Wever et al. (1956) that single semicircular canals in the monkey can be destroyed without the remainder of either the vestibular or cochlear portion degenerating. Kristensen (1960) reported the same results. Actually, such evidence dates back to 1842 when Flourens demonstrated that when separate parts of the vestibular labyrinth were destroyed the others remained functional.

In the Lawrence experiments (1961b) sensitivity to vibrations of the organ of Corti in cats and guinea pigs was determined by recording cochlear potentials before and after various time lapses following selective rupture of the membranous walls of the labyrinth. The animal's internal ears were then examined histologically. The experiments demonstrated that surgical injury to particular parts of the scala media did not result in complete deterioration of the organ of Corti either toward the apex or toward the base. In fact, the region of injury seems to remain confined to that particular spot unless damage is done to the bone of the walls of the cochlea or vestibule, in which case the entire area may fill with bone. There are also indications from earlier work (Lawrence and Yantis, 1957) that, in the case of injury to Reissner's membrane, it can repair itself, thus re-establishing the continuity of the scala media.

Because perilymph is toxic to the organ of Corti one might expect a general deterioration following a breakdown of Reissner's membrane. Davis et al. (1955) showed that injections of artificial perilymph into the scala media abolish, in the region of injection, the electrical response of the organ of Corti. And Békésy (1960) has indicated that, as he looked through Reissner's membrane into the organ of Corti, should perilymph flow through a break in Reissner's membrane thus contaminating the endolymph of the scala media, the hair cells, normally appearing as oil-like droplets, become opaque and the organ of Corti nonfunctional. On the basis of this evidence, and assuming a longitudinal flow of endolymph, one would expect that a tear in Reissner's membrane would allow the perilymph to flow toward the base within the scala media, destroying the organ of Corti from the region of the Reissner's membrane tear all the way basalward to the ductus reuniens.

There is very clear evidence that, should Reissner's membrane break, perilymph enters the scala media rather than endolymph flowing out into the scala vestibuli. By means of a special stain (Lawrence and Clapper, 1961), which stains endolymph darker than perilymph, Lawrence has shown (1960, 1964) that a rupture in Reissner's membrane allows perilymph to flow into the scala media, and that the area of fluid mingling remains confined to the region of the rupture which had been produced from within by excessive vibration of the cochlear partition.

Another set of experiments was performed (Lawrence, 1961a) to measure the flow of fluids by recording the cochlear potentials through time, by means of implanted electrodes, as a small surgical tear was produced in Reissner's membrane of the second turn of the guinea pig cochlea. No marked decrease in the electrical response to high frequencies, that have their locus of maximum activity in the basal turn, was observed in the basal turn over a period of four hours following rupture of Reissner's membrane in the second turn. This would indicate that perilymph, in toxic concentration, was not carried basalward over the organ of Corti by a longitudinal flow of endolymph.

This evidence suggests that the circulation of endolymph is local and radial and that any specific area of the organ of Corti is nutritionally independent of adjacent areas. Secretion and absorption of nutrient and waste material appears to take place continuously along the length of the scala media. Of interest is how specific this local circulation might be.

Small local surgical lesions were made in Reissner's membrane in a series of guinea pigs and the animals allowed to recover for from one to 10 weeks, at which time they were killed and their inner ears examined histologically (Lawrence, 1966a). All the animals showed very localized degeneration of the hair cells of the organ of Corti. The smaller the opening in Reissner's membrane the more restricted the extent of degeneration. These observations were confirmed and the degenerated areas studied by electron microscopy by Duvall (1967, 1968). It has also been shown that vital stains injected into the scala media through a small opening in Reissner's membrane remain localized (Duvall and Tonndorf, 1962; Tonndorf et al., 1962).

There was some question as to whether these exposures through the bone, to provide access to Reissner's membrane so it could be slit, might not have interferred with the blood supply crossing the bony bridge between turns to the stria vascularis of the operated turn. Further experiments (Lawrence, 1966b), however, demonstrated that it is actually the toxicity of perilymph that causes the hair cells to degenerate. These same experiments revealed the importance of the basilar membrane spiral vessels to the maintenance of the hair cells.

Since Kimura (1965, 1967) reported that he had successfully produced an overaccumulation of endolymph, a hydrops, in guinea pigs by blocking the endolymphatic duct, one must now interpret the normal flow of endolymph as being very slow toward the endolymphatic duct and sac. But there is constant chemical exchange between endolymph and the structures of the spiral ligament as well as with perilymph across Reissner's membrane. The organ of Corti has its own lymph provided by

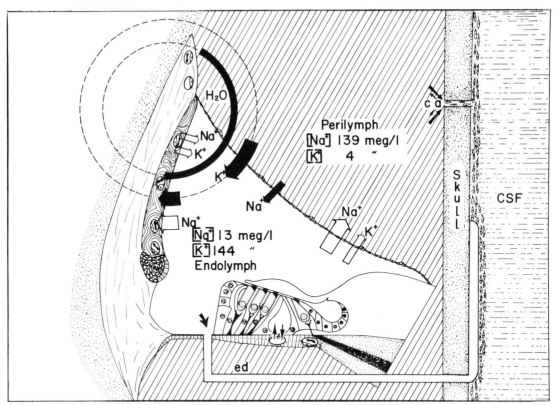

Figure 27. A schematic summary of the transfer of electrolytes and the flow of inner ear fluids. Filled arrows are based on experimental evidence; unfilled arrows represent speculative events. That part of the figure portraying ion transport has been adapted from Rauch (1964). ca= Cochlear aqueduct; ed= endolymphatic duct; CSF= cerebrospinal fluid.

the spiral vessels of the basilar membrane. This supplies the needed oxygen and nutrients to the structures between the tectorial membrane and the basilar membrane. These substances are supplied continuously over the length of the basilar membrane from base to apex, so the flow of cortilymph may be said to be localized in the manner of any fluid bathing a body tissue.

The function of endolymph is most likely that of providing the proper ionic content for the electrochemical functions of the organ of Corti. The exchange responsible for the balance of components within the endolymph also takes place throughout the scala media all along the surfaces of Reissner's membrane and the spiral ligament, with a slow drainage of this fluid toward the endolymphatic duct. So the flow is longitudinal, but the exchange or balance of chemicals is radial or continuous along the scala media. The flow of fluids is summarized schematically in Figure 27.

Specifically, the exchange between endolymph and stria vascularis and spiral prominence on the wall of the spiral ligament may be for the maintenance of the potassium and sodium content of the endolymph. Through a series of excellent studies Rauch and his associates (1962, 1963) have demonstrated the transport role of Reissner's membrane. When ^{42}K is injected into the scala vestibuli it rapidly appears in endolymph, exceeding the concentration of ^{42}K in the perilymph of the scala vestibuli in about two minutes. After injection of ^{42}KCl into the scala tympani, virtually no ^{42}K appears in the endolymph as long as the isotope does not diffuse into the scala vestibuli. After injection of ^{24}NaCl into the scala vestibuli there is a moderate increase of ^{24}Na in the endolymph, but this does not reach more than one third to one half the concentration in the perilymph of the scala vestibuli. The ^{42}K in exchange is four to five times more rapid. Reissner's membrane, therefore, is permeable to certain ions: potassium can enter endolymph from perilymph against the concentration gradient at a rate which is four to five times higher than that of sodium. A review of these results is shown in Figure 27.

After injection of ^{42}K into the endolymph it

not only appears in the endolymph but also in considerable quantity in the stria vascularis; apparently potassium is resorbed back through the stria vascularis (Rauch, 1963). This is in contrast to the interpretation of Johnson and Spoendlin (1966) as to the function of the stria vascularis. These investigators based their work on observations of Erulkar and Maren (1961), who showed that tissues of the cochlear partition possess a very high concentration of carbonic anhydrase. This chemical is best known for its activity in the kidney, where it accelerates the reversible reaction between carbon dioxide, water, and carbonic acid. Erulkar and Maren gave cats Diamox, which inhibits carbonic anhydrase and decreases the rate of the above reaction. The dosage was sufficient to cause great inhibition of cochlear carbonic anhydrase along with a marked decrease in potassium concentration in the endolymph.

Johnson and Spoendlin examined by electron microscope the cochleas of guinea pigs after Diamox administration. They found a decreased number of vacuoles in the stria vascularis and a decrease in potassium in the endolymph, which suggested that the stria vascularis serves to secrete potassium, with the observed vacuoles acting in some unknown fashion as carriers.

Studies of adenosine triphosphatase activity within the stria vascularis support the notion that this structure is important in endolymph metabolism and active in sodium and potassium transport (Nakai and Hilding, 1966; Iinuma, 1967). And Hilding (1965) has demonstrated what he has called "cochlear chromaffin" cells deep in the spiral ligament which he believes may influence the production of endolymph through control of the blood supply by release of adrenalin or no adrenalin.

The role of endolymph appears to be the control of ions in fluid "above" the tectorial membrane. These ions, and the associated resting potentials, are probably there to make possible the conversion of vibratory energy into a nerve impulse. In addition to this, the fluids must convey the vibrations to the right spot for this conversion to take place.

FLUID-DEPENDENT MECHANICAL PROPERTIES OF THE INNER EAR

Mechanical Response to Vibration

The conveyance of vibrations to the basilar membrane is obviously a property of the fluids.

The nature of interaction between the membrane and the fluids is complicated and has been the subject of debate for many years. In fact, this problem has been one of considerable importance because Helmholtz (1885), invoking Mueller's doctrine of specific energies of nerves (1838) to account for frequency analysis in the peripheral ear, set up the requirement that the fluids conduct the vibrations to the right spot or, as Helmholtz described it, that the right spot be activated by the vibrations in the fluids. An excellent review of the interplay between fluids and place of energy conversion can be found in E. G. Wever's book *Theory of Hearing* (1949) and in a later review of the traveling wave theories by Wever and Lawrence (1954).

Wever describes an early theory proposed by Lux, reported by Budde (1917), in which movements of the basilar membrane are supposed to be associated with double columns of fluid, one extending from the oval window to the vibrating segment and the other from this area to the round window. These bands are not supposed to exist as such, but the effective mass involved is presumed to be equivalent to such a band. Segments that are a greater distance from the footplate of the stapes have longer fluid columns, so the loading becomes greater. But, as Wever points out, this is like the "fabulous feat of lifting yourself by your own bootstraps." If there actually were separate fluid columns this view might be reasonable, but because the fluid is common to all parts of the basilar membrane any portion of it will be reinforced by sound through the fluid as well as any other portion of the basilar membrane. Fluid columns themselves cannot be responsible for frequency differentiation along the basilar membrane.

Wever prefers to consider fluid loading as a consequence of differential tuning of the basilar membrane rather than a cause of it. The effect is to influence the sensitivity of that particular segment of the basilar membrane that is put into vibration by virtue of its own characteristics. Thus, the mass of the fluid that moves along with the sensory structures contributes to the ease with which a particular segment can be put into vibration by a certain tone.

Békésy (1960, p. 443) classifies the theories that involve the fluids as a part of the vibrations along the basilar membrane into three classes. The first class, which he calls the "U-tube," is characterized by there being a distinct separation between the stiffness of the basilar membrane (he includes the structures between Reissner's membrane and the basilar membrane as the cochlear partition) and the mass of the vibrating fluid column.

In the second class, "the vibrating-plate type," the basilar membrane and its structures consist of a series of resonators and the mass of the fluid column serves to lower the resonant frequency of the responding element.

The third class, "the hydrodynamic type," takes into account the hydrodynamics of the fluid, with the cochlear partition having only the properties of volume elasticity.

Békésy performed a series of experiments to determine which of these types comes the closest to natural conditions. First, he removed all the fluid from a simplified model of the cochlea in which the helicotrema was blocked and introduced sound into this closed channel through an opening at one end. With no fluid the "basilar membrane" vibrated in phase over its entire length, but if a long drop of fluid were in contact with the membrane the vibratory pattern of this part became the same as when conditions were normal. Thus, the "U-type" of vibration cannot be very important because, in the middle frequency range, only the fluid in contact with the membrane influences its vibratory pattern. Further experimentation showed that of the three simplified classes of theories "the best approach is to conceive of the cochlear partition as a membrane with known volume elasticity and to take into consideration the hydrodynamic aspects of the vibrations near the place of maximum amplitude." Békésy's traveling wave is dependent upon the interplay of the hydrodynamic properties of the fluids and the forces of the vibrating cochlear partition.

There have been theories which have considered the fluid-filled cochlea as a tube with partially elastic walls. Ranke (1942) conceived of a wave of pressure traveling through the fluids and setting up a complex pattern of movement on the basilar membrane. This complicated wave is supposed to have characteristics that determine the location of the area that will be activated most vigorously by different tones.

Reboul (1938) also regarded the cochlea as an elastic-walled tube. The theory he proposed is a complicated one involving fluid mechanics in which the sound wave set up in the scala vestibuli moves through the flexible basilar membrane to the scala tympani. The frequency and velocity of wave propagation are important factors, the latter depending upon properties of the fluid, the diameter of the fluid-filled tube, and the thickness and elasticity of the basilar membrane.

The latest of these tube-resonance theories has been proposed by Naftalin (1967). He first constructed a very sensitive vibration-detecting probe using a Rochelle salt piezoelectric bimorph wrapped in layers of silicone rubber copying the structure of a pacinian corpuscle. By means of a small filter paper strip attached by a special arrangement to this structure he could determine the acoustic energy distribution in small cavities. He then constructed several models, each a modification of an earlier one, so as finally to imitate the essential characteristics of the internal geometry of the cochlea. For fluid he used tapwater. His experimental results showed that sounds of various frequencies were distributed along the "basilar gap." He found further that this differentiation with frequency became sharper when a thin wedge-shaped gel, in imitation of the tectorial membrane, was added to the model.

In these tube resonance theories it is the geometry of the fluid-filled tubes and the characteristics of the walls that determine the linear analysis of sound, whereas in Békésy's theory it is the hydrodynamic action of the fluids on the basilar membrane at the area of maximum vibration. In any case, there is one more act to follow: that of transforming this differentiated vibration into a stimulus for the dendrites of the complexly distributed cochlear nerve fibers. Békésy describes a shearing motion between the tectorial membrane and the hair cells acting upon the hairs, presumably to trigger an energy conversion process. There are many theories, but we do not yet know what this process may be, although it is becoming obvious that the electrical characteristics of the fluids play an important part.

Energy Conversion

Up through the time of Helmholtz it was thought that the nerve fibers were stimulated directly by the mechanical action of some element put into vibration by a sound wave. Although Helmholtz knew of Corti's description of the cellular elements on the basilar membrane, he attached no importance to the hair cells, probably because Corti, himself, thought they were attached to small rods and beat on the nerve endings like drumsticks on a drumhead. And Helmholtz described the hair cells as grouped "like a pad of soft cells on each side of Corti's arches" serving only as a "peculiar auxiliary apparatus."

In 1892 Gustav Retzius described the termination of the nerve fibers on the base of the hair cells and suggested that the fibers receive their stimulation from these cells, which are the final receptors of vibrations conveyed through the fluids. Then in 1930 Wever and Bray described the electrical AC potentials that arise from the cochlea when it is stimulated by sound, and subsequent experimentation has shown that this response is absent when the hair cells are not present. Although we do not yet know specifically what the stimulus to the nerve endings is, the evidence seems to point to this electrical AC output as part of the transduction process that most likely is related to the triggering action. Most of the theories that relate the fluids and the hair cells in the conversion process include the electrical AC potentials as the final concern.

Of great importance has been the discovery by Békésy (1960, pp. 647–654) of the DC resting potentials within the cochlear partition. He described the endolymph as normally resting at +50 mv. and the organ of Corti at −40 mv. with respect to the perilymph. These have subsequently been shown both to be at a value of near 80 mv. These resting potentials are essential to many theories but not to all.

Davis (1953) has proposed, as one possible model, that the DC voltages provide a current flow through hair cells of the organ of Corti and through the tissues outside the scala media. Bending of the hairs causes a change in the electrical resistance at the hair-bearing end of the hair cells, modulating the current flow to produce the recorded AC potentials.

Another type of theory, proposed by Dohlmann (1959) and based on his observation of mucopolysaccharides in the endolymph and tectorial membrane, suggests a release of potassium ions as the membrane is pushed up and down by the vibratory motion. Dohlmann objects quite strenuously to the notion that bending hairs, through shearing action, can produce an alternating electric current. He believes that the mucopolysaccharides with bound potassium ions are the most likely source of electric changes. Reviewing some of the work on electron microscopy, Dohlmann concludes that the hairs of the sensory cells protrude into fine canals in the substance of the tectorial membrane and that this meshwork is soaked through with a secretion containing sulfomucopolysaccharides and potassium. Upon movement of the membranes the positive potassium ions move in the direction of displacement. The hairs of the hair cells (which

Dohlmann calls antennae), surrounded by the large molecules and the freed ions, are exposed to the electrical charges so that movement toward the hairs increases the positive charge and movement away from the hairs increases the negative charge. Dohlmann further assumes that there is high concentration of potassium inside and outside the cell so that varying charges could not change the permeability of the cell membrane because this would overload the cell with potassium and kill it.

There are other theories of this nature (Lawrence, 1967b) but they do not involve the fluids to any great extent other than as a conveyor of the vibratory motion. Vinnikov and Titova (1964), for example, have proposed an elaborate cytochemical theory in which the energy transformation takes place by chemical activity within the hair cell.

One of the problems of great concern recently has been that of reconciling the conventional present-day view of traveling waves along the basilar membrane and shearing forces within the organ of Corti with the small amplitudes of vibration encountered at the threshold of hearing. Békésy combined the calculated amplitude of stapes vibration with figures from his experiments on the volume displacement of the round window to show that, at the threshold of hearing, the amplitude of movement of the basilar membrane is 10^{-11} cm. (0.001 Å.). Naftalin (1965a) points out that the thickness of the membrane of the hair process is 25 to 30 Å. for the outer layer. He continues:

"From X-ray diffraction studies the axis repeat unit of a protein backbone is of the order of 3.6 Å. The H atom has a radius of, on the average, 0.53 Å., but we are now in the realm of probabilities. The 'front' of a membrane, having as its outside layer a peptide or C-chain backbone, is a cloud of electron orbitals. If we draw this 'front' and give the outside C-chain a definite position we have a probability cloud extending outwards from any fixed part of the structure a distance of at least 0.5 Å., but to complicate matters this electron fog will be more or less extensive at any given point varying rapidly with time. This minimum fog depth of 0.5 Å. to the 'front' is *at least* 50 times greater than the specified, calculated, distance for the whole body movement of the ossicles acting as *mechanical levers* or of the movement of the basilar membrane to make the hair processes bend mechanically. . . . A whole body, even of microscopic size like a hair process, can never be said to have moved translationally through less than the average distance of the electron fog which constitutes its front." For this reason Naftalin has looked for a molecular process and has pinned his attention on the tectorial membrane.

From a careful analysis of the constituents of the tectorial membrane, Naftalin et al. (1964) conclude that this membrane does not simply lie in endolymph, bathed and permeated by the substances found in the endolymph, but is an independent medium with its own ionic composition. Compared with endolymph, the potassium content is low, but magnesium is high in the tectorial membrane. However, the ease with which magnesium can be washed out from fresh tectorial membrane suggests that the magnesium concentration gradient between endolymph and tectorial membrane may be maintained by metabolic activity in the scala media and, further, that this gradient allows for a mobility of distribution of electric charges. Furthermore, the tectorial membrane is sensitive to hydration changes, indicating that it is osmotically sensitive—a gel with a very high water content held in water structured form. The possibility is suggested that the acoustic-wave energy within the fluids produces a transient change in pressure within the tectorial membrane, causing oscillatory-osmotic pressure changes by "ion shuttling." The metastable state of the protein-metal complex in the tectorial membrane gel is probably maintained by the endolymphatic DC potential, and because this membrane is in direct contact with the hairs of the sensory cells, "the orientation of otherwise random molecular vibrations by the acoustic compression-relaxation wave provides the trigger for the transfer of the signal from the gel to the hair processes." Presumably the hair cells relay this to the nerve endings.

Naftalin has elaborated on this theory (1965b) and Lawrence (1965b) has searched for physiological evidence. It does not seem too improbable that the tectorial membrane may act as a polarized piezoelectric semiconductor to amplify the acoustic signal. Lawrence (1965b, 1967a, 1968) has reported a plateau of zero potential between the negative of the organ of Corti and the positive of the endolymph and has localized this to the tectorial membrane. The importance of the tectorial membrane as an acoustic amplifier such as described by Gibson (1965) is obvious in the face of the concern over the amount of energy available at auditory threshold levels. Davis (1957) has also discussed the necessity for such an amplifier.

The resting DC potential of the inner ear may not, then, just be a consequence of ion distribution but may be very important for the energy conversion process of the ear. The situation is unique in biological systems because endolymph has a high K^+ content much like intracellular fluid, yet it has a high positive potential quite unlike the interior of a cell. And it is not yet clear whether the negative potential found in the ogan of Corti is intracellular or interstitial or a combination of both. No doubt, the fluids play an important part in the maintenance and distribution of these potentials, but nothing very certain has yet been established.

There is, first of all, the question of whether the DC resting potentials are the same in all turns. Misrahy et al. (1958b) reported a DC potential near the round window as high as 120 mv. but near zero in the upper turns. Gisselsson (1960) and Suga et al. (1964) report that the endocochlear DC potentials are almost equal in all turns from base to apex.

Tasaki and Spyropoulos (1959) observed that the DC endolymphatic potential was of normal magnitude in waltzing guinea pigs which have no organ of Corti. They also drained the fluids from the ear and found a strong positive DC potential on the surface of the stria vascularis from which they conclude that the stria vascularis is the source of the positive DC potential and that is is maintained by some oxidative process. Davis et al. (1955) and Smith et al. (1958) arrived at the same conclusion.

On the other hand, Johnstone (1965), following a study of the effects of anoxia on the endolymphatic potential with subsequent microanalysis of the endolymph, concluded that the endolymphatic potential is a function of the differential K^+ gradient between scala media and plasma. However, earlier Johnstone et al. (1963), following an analysis of the fluids, had decided that the sodium concentration in the endolymph is low enough to allow the possibility that the positive endolymphatic potential is a Na^+ diffusion potential.

Actually the source and method of maintenance of the resting potentials are still a mystery. Wever (1966) has discussed the various viewpoints.

The possibility that the negative potential of the organ of Corti may be extracellular is suggested by Butler (1965), who was able to record negative potentials as high as −90 mv, with relatively large electrodes of 25 μ. This potential was also found to decrease linearly with the log K^+ in the scala tympani. Many studies have shown that a high K^+ in the scala tympani is detrimental to the negative potential, which implicates the basilar membrane in maintaining the potential. Microelectrode studies following perforation of the basilar membrane support this (Lawrence, 1967a). It has also been shown that the high K^+ of the endolymph is necessary for the generation of the AC potentials (Konishi and associates, 1966, 1968a and b).

Obviously there is still much that is unknown about the inner ear. Chemical microanalysis, techniques with microelectrodes, and electron microscopy are revealing more and more of the answers to problems presented here.

The author is greatly indebted to Miss Linda Lawrence for her persistence in obtaining and her meticulous checking of references.

This work was supported by grants NB-03410 and NB-05785 from the National Institute of Neurological Diseases and Blindness, United States Public Health Service.

REFERENCES

Ahlén, G.: On the connection between cerebrospinal and intralabyrinthine pressure and pressure variations in the inner ear. Acta. Otolaryng. 35:251–257, 1947.

Aldred, P., Hallpike, C. S., and Ledoux, A.: Observations on the osmotic pressure of the endolymph. J. Physiol. 98:446–453, 1940.

Alford, B. R., Shaver, E. F., Rosenberg, J. J., and Guilford, F. R.: Physiologic and histopathologic effects of microembolism of the internal auditory artery. Ann. Otol. 74:728–748, 1965.

Allen, G. W.: Endolymphatic sac and cochlear aqueduct. Arch. Otolaryng. 79:322–327, 1964.

Allen, G. W., and Habibi, M.: The effect of increasing the cerebrospinal fluid pressure upon the cochlear microphonics. Laryngoscope 72:423–434, 1962.

Altmann, F., and Waltner, J. G.: The circulation of the labyrinthine fluids. Ann. Otol. 56:684–708, 1947.

Altmann, F., and Waltner, J. G.: Further investigations on the physiology of the labyrinthine fluids. Ann. Otol. 59:657–686, 1950.

Andersen, H. C.: Passage of trypan blue into the endolymphatic system of the labyrinth. Acta Otolaryng. 36:273–283, 1948.

Anson, B. J., Winch, T. R., Warpeha, R. L., and Donaldson, J. A.: The blood supply of the otic capsule of the human ear (with special reference to that of the cochlea). Ann. Otol. 75:921–944, 1966.

Antonini, E., Casorati, V., and Crifó, S.: The proteins of the perilymph. Ann. Otol., 66:129–134, 1957.

Axelsson, A.: The vascular anatomy of the cochlea in the guinea pig and in man. Acta Otolaryng. Suppl. 243, 1968.

Balogh, K., and Koburg, E.: Der Plexus chochlearis. Arch. Ohr. Nas. Kehlkopfheilk. 185:638–645, 1965.

Beck, C., and Holz, E.: Versuche und kritische Betrachtungen zur immuno-elektrophoretischen Untersuchung der Innenohrflüssigkeiten. Arch. Ohr. Nas. Kehlkopfheilk. 184:411–418, 1965.

Békésy, G. V.: Experiments in Hearing. New York, McGraw-Hill Book Co. 1960.

Borghesan, E.: Modality of the cochlear humoral circulation. Laryngoscope 67:1266–1285, 1957.

Brosch, E.: Biochemische Festellung des Grundgesamteiweisses der Perilymphe und der zerebrospinalen Flüssigkeit im Tierexperiment bei Hunden. Deutsch. Gesundh. 19:2418–2420, 1964.

Budde, E.: Über die Resonanztheorie des Hörens. Phys. Zeits. 18:225–236; 249–260, 1917.

Butler, R. A.: Some experimental observations on the DC resting potentials in the guinea-pig cochlea. J. Acoust. Soc. Amer. 37:429–433, 1965.

Chevance, L. G., Galli, A., and Jeanmaire, J.: Immunoelectrophoretic study of the human perilymph. Acta Otolaryng. 52:41–46, 1960.

Choo, Y. B., and Tabowitz, D.: The formation and flow of the cochlear fluids. 1. Studies with radioactive sodium (Na^{22}) Ann. Otol. 73:92–100, 1964.

Choo, Y. B., and Tabowitz, D.: The formation and flow of the cochlear fluids. 2. Studies with radioactive potassium (K^{42}). Ann. Otol. 74:140–145, 1965.

Chou, J. T. Y., and Rodgers, K.: Respiration of tissues lining the mammalian membranous labyrinth. J. Laryng. 76:341–351, 1962.

Citron, L., Exley, D., and Hallpike, C. S.: Formation, circulation and chemical properties of the labyrinth fluids. Brit. Med. Bull. 12:101–104, 1956.

Corti, A.: Recherches sur l'organe de l'ouie des mammifères. Z. Wiss. Zool. 3:109–169, 1851.

Cotugno, D.: De aquaeductibus auris humanae internae. Vienna, 1774.

Davis, H.: Energy into nerve impulses: Hearing. Med. Bull. St. Louis University 5:43–48, 1953.

Davis, H.: Biophysics and physiology of the inner ear. Physiol. Rev. 37:1–49, 1957.

Davis, H., Tasaki, I., Smith, C. A., and Deatherage, B. H.: Cochlear potentials after intracochlear injections and anoxia. Fed. Proc. 14:35–36, 1955.

Dittmer, D. S. (ed.): Blood and Other Body Fluids. ASD Technical Report 61–199. Ohio, Wright-Patterson Air Force Base, June, 1961.

Dobbing, J.: The blood-brain barrier. Physiol. Rev. 41:130–188, 1961.

Dohlmann, G.: Modern concept of vestibular physiology. Laryngoscope 69:865–875, 1959.

Duvall, A. J., III: Ultrastructure of the lateral cochlear wall following intermixing of fluids. Ann. Otol. 77:317–331, 1968.

Duvall, A. J., III, and Rhodes, V. T.: Ultrastructure of the organ of Corti following intermixing of cochlear fluids. Ann. Otol. 76:688–708, 1967.

Duvall, A. J., III, and Tonndorf, J.: Vital staining of the cochlea in guinea pigs: A preliminary report. Laryngoscope 72:892–901, 1962.

Engström, H.: The cortilymph, the third lymph of the inner ear. Acta Morph. Neerl. Scand. 3:195–204, 1960.

Engström, H., and Wersäll, J.: Is there a special nutritive cellular system around the hair cells of the organ of Corti? Ann. Otol. 62:507–512, 1953.

Erulkar, S. D., and Maren, T. H.: Carbonic anhydrase and the inner ear. Nature (London) 189:459–460, 1961.

Feldman, R. M., and Allen, G. W.: Effects of cerebrospinal fluid pressure on the cat cochlea. Arch. Otolaryng. 84:422–425, 1966.

Fernandez, C.: Biochemistry of labyrinthine fluids (inorganic substances). Progress report. Arch. Otolaryng. 86:222–233, 1967.

Filippi, P.: Sui rapporti fra pressione del liquor e pressione endolabirintica nel Gatto. Soc. Ital. Biol. Sper. Boll. 26:661–663, 1950.

Flourens, J. P. M.: Recherches expérimentales sur les propriétés et les fonctions du système nerveux dans les animaux vertébrés. Paris, J. B. Baillière, 1842.

Fritsch, J. H., and Jolliff, C. R.: Protein components of human perilymph. 1. Preliminary study. Ann. Otol. 75:1070–1076, 1966.

Gerlach, H.: Über die Durchgängigkeit des Aquaeductus cochleae. Arch. Ohr. Nas. Kehlkopfheilk. 146:17–22, 1939.

Gibson, A. F.: A new method of amplifying sound. Discovery 26:34–38, 1965.

Gisselsson, L.: Die elektrischen Potentiale des Innenohres. Archiv. Ohr. Nas. Kehlkopfheilk. 177:45–56, 1960.

Grünberg, K.: Zur Frage der Existenz eines offenen Ductus perilymphaticus. Z. Hals.-Nasen.- Ohrenheilk. 2:146–151, 1922.

Grüneberg, H., Hallpike, C. S., and Ledoux, A.: Observations on the structure, development and electrical reactions of the internal ear of the Shaker-1 mouse (Mus musculus). Proc. Roy. Soc. (Series B) 129:154–173, 1940.

Guild, S. R.: The circulation of the endolymph. Amer. J. Anat. 39:57–81, 1927.

Gulick, W. L., Patterson, W. C., and Myers, D.: The effects of perilymph loss upon the electrical activity of the ear. Ann. Otol. 71:573–584, 1962.

Hansen, C. C.: Perceptive hearing loss and increased intracranial pressure. Arch. Otolaryng. 87:45–47, 1968.

Hawkins, J. E., Jr.: Vascular patterns of the membranous labyrinth. Third symposium on The Role of Vestibular Organs in the Exploration of Space, Pensacola, Florida, 1968.

Hayashido, H.: Studies on track autoradiography of the cochlea and auditory central pathway by using S^{35} and P^{32}. Oto-Rhino and Laryng. Clin. (Jibi-Inkoka Rinsho, Kyoto) 53:688, 1960.

Helmholtz, H. L. F.: On the Sensations of Tone. Second English edition, translated by A. J. Ellis, 1885.

Henriksson, N. G., and Gleisner, L.: Vestibular activity at experimental variation of labyrinthine pressure. Acta Otolaryng. 61:380–386, 1966a.

Henriksson, N. G., Gleisner, L., and Johansson, G.: Experimental pressure variations in the membranous labyrinth of the frog. Acta Otolaryng. 61:281–291, 1966b.

Hilding, D. A.: Cochlear chromaffin cells. Laryngoscope 75:1–15, 1965.

Hughson, W.: A note on the relationship of cerebrospinal and intralabyrinthine pressures. Amer. J. Physiol. 101:396–407, 1932.

Iinuma, T.: Evaluation of adenosine triphophatase activity in the stria vascularis and spiral ligament of normal guinea pigs. Laryngoscope 77:141–158, 1967.

Ishii, T., Silverstein, H., and Balogh, K., Jr.: Metabolic activities of the endolymphatic sac. (An enzyme histochemical and autoradiographic study.) Acta Otolaryng. 62:61–73, 1966.

Jensen, C. E., and Vilstrup, T.: Protein studies of endolymph and perilymph of the inner ear. Acta Chem. Scand. 8:399–401, 1954.

Johnson, R. L., and Spoendlin, H. H.: Structural evidence of secretion in the stria vascularis. Ann. Otol. 75:127–138, 1966.

Johnstone, B. M.: The relation between endolymph and the endocochlear potential during anoxia. Acta Otolaryng. 60:113–120, 1965.

Johnstone, C. G., Schmidt, R. S., and Johnstone B. M.: Sodium and potassium in vertebrate cochlear endolymph as determined by flame microspectrophotometry. Comp. Biochem. Physiol. 9:335–341, 1963.

Kaieda, J.: Biochemische Untersuchungen des Labyrinthwassers und der Cerebrospinalflüssigkeit der Haifische. Z. Physiol. Chem. 188:193–202, 1930.

Karlefors, J.: Die Hirnhautraume des Kleinhirns, die Verbindungen des 4. Ventrikels mit den Subarachnoidalräumen und der Aquaeductus cochleae bei Kindern und Erwachsenen. Acta Otolaryng. Suppl. 4, 1924.

Kerth, J. D., and Allen, G. W.: Comparison of the perilymphatic and cerebrospinal fluid pressures. Arch. Otolaryng. 77:581–585, 1963.

Kikuchi, K., and Hilding, D. A.: The spiral vessel and stria vascularis in Shaker-1 mice. Acta Otolaryng. 63:395–410, 1967.

Kimura, R. S.: Experimental blockage of the endolymphatic duct and sac and its effect on the inner ear of the guinea pig. Ann. Otol. 76:664–687, 1967.

Kimura, R., and Perlman, H. B.: Extensive venous obstruction of the labyrinth. A. Cochlear changes. Ann. Otol. 65:332–350, 1956.

Kimura, R., and Perlman, H. B.: Arterial obstruction of the labyrinth. Part 1. Cochlear changes. Ann. Otol. 67:5–24, 1958.

Kimura, R. S., and Schuknecht, H. F.: Membranous hydrops in the inner ear of the guinea pig after obliteration of the endolymphatic sac. Pract. Otorhinolaryng. (Basel) 27:343–354, 1965.

Kirikae, I., Nomura, Y., Nagakura, M., Matsuba, Y., and Sugiura, S.: A consideration on the circulation of the perilymph. Ann. Otol. 70:337–343, 1961.

Kley, E.: Zur Herkunft der Perilymphe. Z. Laryng. Rhinol. Otol. 30:486–502, 1951.

Klockhoff, I., Änggård, G., and Änggård, L.: Recording of cranio-labyrinthine pressure transmission in man by acoustic impedance method. Acta Otolaryng. 61:361–370, 1966.

Kobrak, M.: Untersuchungen über den Labyrinthdruck. Z. Hals.- Nasen.- Ohrenheilk. 34:456–463, 1933.

Kobrak, H. G., Lindsay, J. R., and Perlman, H. B.: The next step in auditory research. Arch. Otolaryng. 31:467–477, 1940.

Koburg, E., Haubrich, J., and Kernbach, B.: Autoradiographische untersuchungen zum Stoffwechsel des Ductus und Saccus endolymphaticus. Acta Otolaryng. 64:146–156, 1967.

Konishi, T., and Kelsey, E.: Effect of sodium deficiency on cochlear potentials. J. Acoust. Soc. Amer. 43:462–470, 1968a.

Konishi, T., and Kelsey, E.: Effect of tetrodotoxin and procaine on cochlear potentials. J. Acoust. Soc. Amer. 43:471–480, 1968b.

Konishi, T., Kelsey, E., and Singleton, G. T.: Effects of chemical alteration in the endolymph on the cochlear potentials. Acta Otolaryng. 62:393–404, 1966.

Krejci, F., and Bornschein, H.: Sul problema del meccanismo d'azione della simpaticectomia cervicale nelle affezioni dell' orecchio interno. Arch. Ital. Otol. 62:1–7, 1951a.

Krejci, F., and Bornschein, H.: Tierexperimentelle Untersuchungen über die Cochlearfunktion bei endokranieller Drucksteigerung. Pract. Otorhinolaryng. 13:146–166, 1951b.

Kristensen, H. K.: Acoustic-vestibular and histologic examinations in guinea pigs after interruption of membranous labyrinth in semicircular canals or cochlea. Acta Otolaryng. *51*:382–402, 1960.

Krochmalska, E., Mnich, Z., and Lupinski, T.: The Schreiner phenomenon in the light of new investigations. Acta Otolaryng. *64*:174–178, 1967.

Lawrence, M.: Some physiological factors in inner ear deafness. Ann. Otol. *69*:480–496, 1960.

Lawrence, M.: Endolymph-perilymph diffusion after barrier breakdown. Arch. Otolaryng. *79*:366–372, 1964.

Lawrence, M.: Fluid balance in the inner ear. Ann. Otol. *74*:486–499, 1965a.

Lawrence, M.: Dynamic range of the cochlear transducer. Cold Spring Harbor Symp. Quant. Biol. *30*:159–167, 1965b.

Lawrence, M.: Histological evidence for localized radial flow of endolymph. Arch. Otolaryng. *83*:406–412, 1966a.

Lawrence, M.: Effects of interference with terminal blood supply on organ of Corti. Laryngoscope *76*:1318–1337, 1966b.

Lawrence, M.: Electric polarization of the tectorial membrane. Ann. Otol. *76*:287–312, 1967a.

Lawrence, M.: Energy conversion in the peripheral ear. In Graham, A. B. (ed.): Sensorineural Hearing Processes and Disorders. Boston. Little, Brown and Co., 1967b.

Lawrence, M.: Electrophysiology of the organ of Corti. In Paparella, M. M. (ed.): Biochemical Mechanisms in Hearing and Deafness. Springfield, Ill., Charles C Thomas, 1968.

Lawrence, M., and Clapper, M.: Differential staining of inner ear fluids by Protargol. Stain Tech. *36*:305–308, 1961.

Lawrence, M., Wolsk, D., and Litton, W. B.: Circulation of the inner ear fluids. Ann. Otol. *70*:753–776, 1961a.

Lawrence, M., Wolsk, D., and McCabe, B. F.: Fluid barriers within the otic capsule. Trans. Amer. Acad. Ophthal. & Otolaryng. *65*:246–259, 1961b.

Lawrence, M., and Yantis, P. A.: Individual differences in functional recovery and structural repair following overstimulation of the guinea pig ear. Ann. Otol. *66*:595–621, 1957.

Ledoux, A.: Concentration moléculaire totale des liquides céphalo-rachidiennes et labyrinthiques du chat. Acta Biol. Belg. *1*:504–506, 1941a.

Ledoux, A.: Indice de réfraction des liquides céphalo-rachidiennes et labyrinthiques du chat. Acta Biol. Belg. *1*:506–508, 1941b.

Ledoux, A.: Le pH des liquides labyrinthinques (chat). Bull. Soc. Roy. Sci. Liege. *12*:254–256, 1943.

Ledoux, A.: Les liquides labyrinthiques. Acta Otorhinolaryng. Belg. *4*:216–223, 1950.

Lempert, J., Meltzer, P. E., Wever, E. G., Lawrence, M., and Rambo, J. H. T.: Structure and function of the cochlear aqueduct. Arch. Otolaryng. *55*:134–145, 1952.

Lempert, J., Wever, E. G., Lawrence, M., and Meltzer, P. E.: Perilymph: Its relation to the improvement of hearing which follows fenestration of the vestibular labyrinth in clinical otosclerosis. Arch. Otolaryng. *50*:377–387, 1949.

Lindsay, J. R.: Effect of obliteration of the endolymphatic sac and duct in the monkey. Arch. Otolaryng. *45*:1–13, 1947.

Lindsay, J. R., Schuknecht, H. F., Neff, W. D., and Kimura, R. S.: Obliteration of the endolymphatic sac and the cochlear aqueduct. Ann. Otol. *61*:697–716, 1952.

Lundquist, P-G., Kimura, R., and Wersäll, J.: Experiments in endolymph circulation. Acta Otolaryng. Suppl. *188*: 198–201, 1964.

Maggio, E.: The humoral system of the labyrinth. Acta Otolaryng. Suppl. *218*, 1966.

Meurman, Y.: Observations on some pressure phenomena accompanying artificial labyrinthine fistula. Acta Otolaryng. *13*:552–571, 1929.

Misrahy, G. A., Hildreth, K. M., Clark, L. C., and Shinabarger, E. W.: Measurement of the pH of the endolymph in the cochlea of guinea pigs. Amer. J. Physiol. *194*:393–395, 1958a.

Misrahy, G. A., Hildreth, K. M., Shinabarger, E. W., and Gannon, W. J.: Electrical properties of wall of endolymphatic space of the cochlea (guinea pig). Amer. J. Physiol. *194*:396–402, 1958b.

Miyake, H.: The refractive index of cerebrospinal and labyrinthine fluids in the nerve deafness. Nagoya J. Med. Sci. *16*:89–91, 1953.

Miyake, H.: Biochemical study of labyrinthine fluids. Jap. J. Otolog. *63*: (Suppl. 2) 1–4, 1960.

Money, K. E., Sokoloff, M., and Weaver, R. S.: Specific gravity and viscosity of endolymph and perilymph. Second symposium on The Role of the Vestibular Organs in Space Exploration (NASA SP-115), 91–98, 1966.

Mueller, J.: Handbuch der Physiologie des Menschen. II, Book 5, 1838.

Müsebeck, K.: Lichtmikroskopische Untersuchungen über den Plexus cochlearis. Arch. Ohr. Nas. Kehlkopfheilk. *184*:550–559, 1965a.

Müsebeck, K.: Die perivasculären Lymphspalten des Innenohres. Arch. Ohr. Nas. Kehlkopfheilk. *184*:560–570, 1965b.

Mygind, S. H.: Experimental histological studies on the labyrinth. Acta Otolaryng. *33*:86–116, 1945. Also, further labyrinthine studies. Acta Otolaryng. Suppl. *68*, 1948.

Naftalin, L.: The Transduction of Acoustic Energy in the Receptor Organ of the Cochlea. Paper Read at Cardiff Symposium, January 7–9, 1965a.

Naftalin, L.: Some new proposals regarding acoustic transmission and transduction. Cold Spring Harbor Symp. Quant. Biol. *30*:169–180, 1965b.

Naftalin, L.: The cochlear geometry as a frequency analyser. J. Laryng. *81*:619–631, 1967.

Naftalin, L., and Harrison, M. S.: Circulation of labyrinthine fluids. J. Laryng. *72*:118–136, 1958.

Naftalin, L., Harrison, M. S., and Stephens, A.: The character of the tectorial membrane. J. Laryng. *78*:1061–1078, 1964.

Nakai, Y., and Hilding, D. A.: Electron microscopic studies of adenosine triphosphatase activity in the stria vascularis and spiral ligament. Acta Otolaryng. *62*:411–428, 1966.

Nomura, Y.: Capillary permeability of the cochlea. Ann. Otol. *70*:81–101, 1961.

Palva, T., and Raunio, V.: Disc electrophoretic studies of human perilymph. Ann. Otol. *76*:23–36, 1967a.

Palva, T., and Raunio, V.: Disc electrophoretic studies of human perilymph and endolymph. Acta Otolaryng. *63*:128–137, 1967b.

Perlman, H. B., and Kimura, R. S.: Observations of the living blood vessels of the cochlea. Ann. Otol. *64*:1176–1192, 1955.

Perlman, H. B., Kimura, R., and Fernandez, C.: Experiments on temporary obstruction of the internal auditory artery. Laryngoscope *69*:591–613, 1959.

Portmann, G., Geraud, J., Morin, G., Kaneko, T., and Blanquet, P.: A propos de l'étude des liquides labyrinthiques par les substances radioactives. Acta Oto-laryng. *51*:373-381, 1960.

Ranke, O. F.: Das massenverhältnis zwischen Membran und Flüssigkeit im Innenohr. Akust. Zeits. 7:1-11, 1942.

Rauch, S.: Biochemische Studien zum Hörvorgang. Pract. Otorhinolaryng. 25:81-88, 1963.

Rauch, S. (ed.): Biochemie des Hörorgans. Stuttgart, Georg Thieme Verlag, 1964.

Rauch, S., and Köstlin, A.: Aspects chimiques de l'endo-lymphe et de la périlymphe. Pract. Otorhinolaryng. 20:287-291, 1958.

Rauch, S., and Köstlin, A.: Biochemische Studien zum Hörvorgang. Z. Laryng. Rhinol. Otol. *41*:56-69, 1962.

Rauch, S., Köstlin, A., Schnieder, E., and Schindler, K.: Arguments for the permeability of Reissner's mem-brane. Laryngoscope 73:135-147, 1963.

Reboul, J. A.: Théorie des phénomènes mécaniques se passant dan l'oreille interne. J. Physique Radium 9:185-194, 1938.

Retzius, G.: Die Endigungsweise des Gehörnerven. Biol. Unters *3*:29-36, 1892.

Ritter, F. N., and Lawrence, M.: A histological and ex-perimental study of cochlear aqueduct patency in the adult human. Laryngoscope 75:1224-1233, 1965.

Rossi, G.: Sulla viscosità della Endolinfa e della Perilinfa. Arch. Fisiol. *12*:415-428, 1914.

Rüedi, L.: Some animal experimental findings on the func-tions of the inner ear. Ann. Otol. 60:993-1018, 1951.

Schreiner, L.: Untersuchungen zum Stoffwechsel und Herkunft von Perilymphe. Arch. Ohr. Nas. Kehlkopf-heilk. *178*:140-145, 1961.

Schreiner, L.: Experimentelle Untersuchungen über die Bildungsstätten und den Stoffaustausch der Peri-lymphe. Acta Otolaryng. Suppl. *212*, 1966.

Schuknecht, H. F., and Kimura, R.: Functional and histo-logical findings after obliteration of the periotic duct and endolymphatic sac in sound conditioned cats. Lar-yngoscope 63:1170-1192, 1953.

Schuknecht, H. F., and Seifi, A. E.: Experimental obser-vations on the fluid physiology of the inner ear. Ann. Otol. 72:687-712, 1963.

Schwalbe, G.: Der Arachnoidalraum, ein Lymphraum und sein Zusammenhang mit dem Perichoroidalraum. Cen-tralbl. Med. Wiss. 7:465-467, 1869.

Scuderi, R., and Del Bo, M.: La vascolarizzazione del labirinto umano. Arch. Ital. Otolog. Suppl. *11*:1-90, 1952.

Seymour, J. C.: Observations on the circulation in the cochlea. J. Laryng. Otol. 68:689-711, 1954.

Seymour, J. C., and Tappin, J. W.: The effect of sympathet-ic stimulation upon the cochlear microphonic poten-tials. Acta Otolaryng. 42:167-174, 1952; Proc. Roy. Soc. Med. 44:755-759, 1951.

Silverstein, H.: Biochemical studies of the inner ear fluids in the cat. Ann. Otol. 75:48-63, 1966.

Silverstein, H., and Schuknecht, H. F.: Biochemical studies of inner ear fluid in man. Arch. Otolaryng. 84:395-402, 1966.

Smith, C. A.: Capillary Areas of the cochlea in the guinea pig. Laryngoscope 61:1073-1095, 1951.

Smith, C. A.: Capillary areas of the membranous laby-rinth. Ann. Otol. 63:435-447, 1954.

Smith, C. A.: Structure of the stria vascularis and the spiral prominence. Ann. Otol. 66:521-536, 1957.

Smith, C. A., Davis, H., Deatherage, B. H., and Gessert, C. F.: DC potentials of the membranous labyrinth. Amer. J. Physiol. 193:203-206, 1958.

Smith, C. A., Lowry, O. H., and Wu, M-L: The electro-lytes of the labyrinthine fluids. Laryngoscope 64:141-153, 1954.

Suga, F., Morimitsu, T., and Matsuo, K.: Endocochlear DC potential: How is it maintained along the cochlear turns? Ann. Otol. 73:924-933, 1964.

Svane-Knudsen, V.: Resorption of the cerebro-spinal fluid in guinea-pig. Acta Otolaryng. 49:240-251, 1958.

Szász, T.: Beitrage zur Labyrinthliquorfrage. Z. Hals.- Na-sen.- Ohrenheilk. 6:256-260, 1923.

Szász, T.: Experimentelle untersuchungen über den Innen-ohrdruck. Z. Hals.- Nasen.- Ohrenheilk. *14*:237-255, 1926.

Tasaki, I., and Spyropoulos, C. S.: Stria vascularis as source of endocochlear potential. J. Neurophysiol. 22:149-155, 1959.

Terayama, Y., Holz, E., and Beck, C.: Adrenergic inner-vation of the cochlea. Ann. Otol. 75:69-86, 1966.

Tonndorf, J., Duvall, A. J., III, and Reneau, J. P.: Per-meability of intracochlear membranes to various vital stains. Ann. Otol. 71:801-841, 1962.

Ulrich, M. T., Mundie, J. R., Jr., and Margen, S.: Biochemi-cal properties of inner ear fluids: methods of micro-chemistry and fluid withdrawal. AMRL-TR-65-177, 1966, pp. 1-23.

Uyama, Y.: Histopathologische Veränderungen im Innen-ohre, bedingt durch den experimentellen Verschluss des Aquaeductus Cochleae. Okayama-Igakkai-Zasshi. 45:1128-1150, 1933.

van Egmond, A. A. J., and Brinkman, W. F. B.: On the function of the saccus endolymphaticus. Acta Otolar-yng. 46:285-289, 1956.

Vilstrup, T., and Jensen, C. E.: Three reports on the chemical composition of fluids of the labyrinth. Ann. Otol. 63:151-163, 1954.

Vinnikov, Y. A., and Titova, L. K.: The organ of Corti; Its Histopathology and Histochemistry. New York, Consultants Bureau, 1964.

Weille, F. L., Gargano, S. R., Pfister, R., Martinez, D., and Irwin, J. W.: An experimental study of the circu-lation of the spiral ligament and stria vascularis of the living guinea pig. Trans. Amer. Acad. Ophthal. Otolaryng. 58:466-477, 1954a.

Weille, F. L., Martinez, D. E., Gargano, S. R., and Irwin, J. W.: An experimental study of the small blood ves-sels of the spiral ligament and stria vascularis of living guinea pigs during anaphylaxis. Laryngoscope 64:656-665, 1954b.

Weille, F. L., Irwin, J. W., Jako, G., Holschuh, L. L., Weille, A. S., Stanley, C. A., and Rappaport, M. B.: Pressures of the labyrinthine fluids. Ann. Otol. 67:858-868, 1958.

Weille, F. L., O'Brien, H. F., Clark, L., Rahn, P., Jako, G., Anderson, A., and Irwin, J. W.: Pressures of the labyrinthine fluids. Ann. Otol. 70:528-540, 1961.

Wever, E. G.: Theory of Hearing. New York, John Wiley & Sons, Inc., 1949.

Wever, E. G.: Electrical potentials of the cochlea. Physiol. Rev. 46:102-127, 1966.

Wever, E. G., and Bray, C. W.: Auditory nerve impulses. Science 71:215, 1930; also, Action currents in the auditory nerve in response to acoustical stimulation. Proc. Nat. Acad. Sci. (USA) 16:344-350, 1930.

Wever, E. G., and Lawrence, M.: Physiological Acoustics. Princeton, New Jersey, Princeton University Press, 1954.

Wever, E. G., Lempert, J., Meltzer, P. E., and Rambo, J. H. T.: The effects of injury to the lateral semicircular canal. Trans. Amer. Acad. Ophthal. Otolaryng. 60:718-725, 1956.

Yamamoto, K., and Nakai, Y.: Electronmicroscopic studies on the functions of the stria vascularis and the spiral ligament in the inner ear. Ann. Otol. 73:332-347, 1964.

NEUROPHYSIOLOGY OF THE CENTRAL AUDITORY SYSTEM

by

John F. Brugge, Ph.D.

Sound reaching the ear sets up a chain of mechanical and neural events which eventually result in volleys of nerve impulses in the auditory nerve. These volleys are relayed over afferent pathways to cell groups of the pons, midbrain, and thalamus and invade the cerebral cortex. Some impulses are transmitted to the cerebellum.

This chapter deals with ascending pathways linking the cochlea and auditory receiving areas of the cerebral cortex. It thus encompasses a major portion of the central auditory system now considered to be directly, though not exclusively, involved in processes of auditory perception. We first consider briefly some methods commonly used in studying the physiology of the auditory system and then move on to a description of ascending connections and topographic organization of major cell groups. Auditory areas of the cerebral cortex of animals and of man are described in some detail. Finally an account is given of functional properties of single auditory neurons. There are gaps in the discussion and some topics are given more weight than others. The reader may wish to refer to review articles that have appeared in recent years (Galambos, 1954; Ades, 1959; Hawkins, 1964; Katsuki, 1965; Schwartzkopff, 1967; Goldberg and Lavine, 1968; Grinnell, 1969; Eldredge and Miller, 1971).

ELECTROPHYSIOLOGICAL METHODS FOR STUDYING THE AUDITORY SYSTEM

An electrode placed in or on an appropriate region of the brain records electrical activity evoked by acoustic stimulation or by electrical stimulation of the auditory nerve or a small region on the auditory pathway. In such experiments one must take into account the anesthetic agent and the type of electrode used as well as the variables of the acoustic stimulus.

Barbiturates have been widely used for general anesthesia. Under these conditions synaptic transmission in auditory nuclei linking the cochlea with the cerebral cortex is in many respects resistant to the depressing effects these drugs have in many other areas of the brain. Thus, despite drawbacks in studying the physiology of the auditory system in anesthetized animals, this method has proved particularly useful for mapping the extent and pattern of the central representation of the cochlea. By contrast, the use of chloralose results in a highly excitable brain, and experiments under these conditions have revealed foci of auditory evoked potentials not seen under barbiturates. Some workers have avoided the use of anesthesia by immobilizing the animal with a neuromuscular blocking agent or by rendering the animal decerebrate by midcollicular transection of the brain stem. In recent years methods have become available for recording from awake animals with chronically implanted electrodes (Evarts, 1968a). Whereas these methods have been employed successfully in studies of single units in visual cortex of wake and sleeping cats (Evarts, 1963; Wurtz, 1969) and in the pyramidal tract of trained monkeys (Evarts, 1968b), few studies of the auditory system have been reported (Katsuki et al., 1959, 1960; Hubel et al., 1959; Miller et al., 1971).

Microelectrodes that are insulated except for a few microns at the tip record extracellularly action potentials of a single neuron or cluster of neurons (Fig. 28). Electrodes with considerably greater tip exposures are usually unable to record isolated action potentials but are particularly suited for recording the slow positive and negative potentials evoked by acoustic stimulation (Fig. 29). Despite the uncertainty attached to the interpretation of the evoked slow wave, this method has proved especially useful in mapping the auditory areas of the cerebral cortex. A drawback in the use of large electrodes lies in the uncertainty of the size and extent of the population of neural elements around the electrode tip which contribute to the slow wave potentials. This uncertainty is overcome, at least partially, when microelectrodes are employed for mapping purposes, since the criterion for an evoked response is the activation of single neurons which are not likely to be more than a few hundred microns from the electrode tip.

Microelectrodes have been employed in studies of single neurons in virtually all known major cell groups in the corticopetal pathway

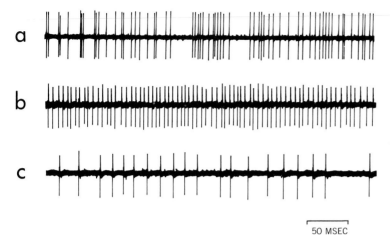

Figure 28. Action potentials recorded from three neurons in the superior olivary complex of the cat in response to acoustic stimulation. (From Goldberg, J. M., et al.: J. Neurophysiol. *27*:706, 1964. Courtesy of Charles C Thomas, publisher.)

of the auditory system. Metal electrodes etched to a fine tip and insulated with varnish or glass and micropipettes filled with indium and tipped with platinum and gold are commonly used. Because action potentials can be recorded with the electrode tip at some distance from the cell body, stable records can be obtained for several hours without damaging the neuron. Glass pipettes drawn to tip diameters of less than 1 μ and filled with an electrolyte have been employed for recording from inside a single auditory neuron (Nelson and Erulkar, 1963; Starr and Britt, 1970). The special techniques for the manufacture and use of microelectrodes have been described in some detail by Frank (1959), Nastuck (1964) and Lavallée et al. (1969).

A proper interpretation of electrophysiological data derived from studies of the central auditory system requires not only an understanding of the acoustic stimulus but also some comprehension of the way in which air-borne vibrations are transformed into mechanical motion by the action of middle and inner ear

structures. The mechanical events brought into play by sound vibrations have already been discussed in some detail, and the reader interested in the characteristics of the acoustic stimulus is directed to a discussion of the subject by Licklider (1951).

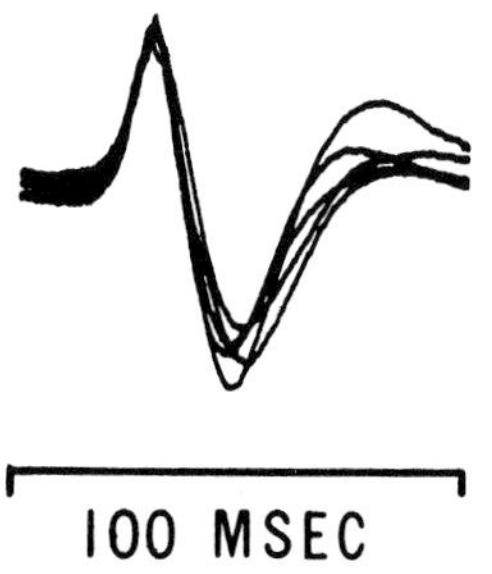

ANATOMY AND TOPOGRAPHY

Major auditory nuclei and ascending pathways connecting them are shown in Figure 30. Details of some of these connections are well known. For others the data indicate only that connections do exist. Pathways illustrated here are only those linking the cochlea with the cerebral cortex. There is anatomical and physiological evidence that parallel descending connections exist which may serve as feedbacks to successively lower auditory structures. Connections with some cranial and spinal motor nuclei no doubt exist also to subserve acoustic reflexes; these have been omitted.

Cochlear Nuclear Complex

Essentially all afferent fibers of the auditory nerve terminate in the cochlear nuclei, a complex of cell groups forming a brain stem protuberance lateral to the descending root of the trigeminal nerve and posterior and dorsal to the brachium pontis (Powell and Cowan, 1962; Osen, 1970). Neurons of the cochlear nuclei differ in their morphology, and the entire complex can be subdivided on the basis of the distribution of cell types. As many as 40 to 50 cell types have been identified in Golgi preparations (Lorente de Nó, 1933), whereas in sec-

100 MSEC

Figure 29. Evoked potentials recorded from auditory area I of the cerebral cortex of a cat under barbiturate anesthesia. Responses to five consecutive click stimuli are superimposed to show the regularity of the waveform.

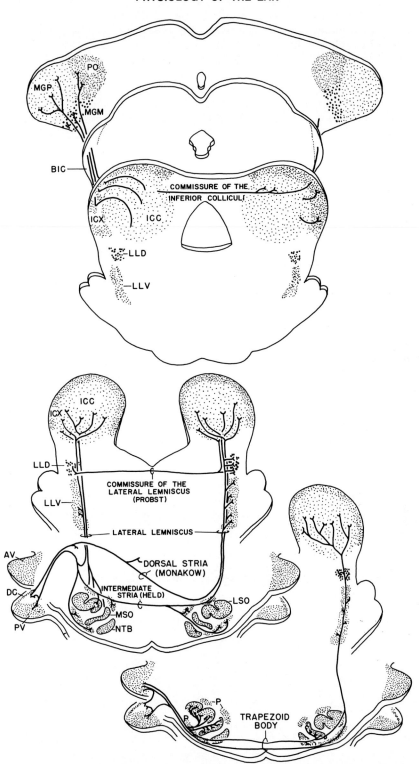

Figure 30. Ascending pathways of the central auditory system. P = periolivary cell groups; MSO = medial superior olivary nucleus; LSO = lateral superior olivary nucleus; NTB = nucleus of the trapezoid body; PV = posteroventral cochlear nucleus; AV = anteroventral cochlear nucleus; DC = dorsal cochlear nucleus; LLD = dorsal nucleus of the lateral lemniscus; LLV = ventral nucleus of the lateral lemniscus; ICC = central nucleus of the inferior colliculus; ICX = external nucleus of the inferior colliculus; BIC = brachium of the inferior colliculus; MGM = magnocellular division of the medial geniculate body; MGP = principal division of the medial geniculate body; PO = posterior nucleus of the thalamus.

tions stained for Nissl substance (Osen, 1969) and in protargol-stained material (Harrison and Irving, 1965, 1966) the number of categories is somewhat smaller. In addition to variants in cell morphology there exist great differences in the structure of the terminals of auditory nerve fibers. Of particular interest are the calycine endings (end bulbs of Held) that arise in the anteroventral nucleus from the ascending branch of the cochlear nerve. Assuming that nerve cells which differ in morphology also differ functionally, some very interesting questions arise as regards the way in which information transmitted along auditory nerve fibers is transformed at the first synapse. We will return to some of these questions in a later section.

In Nissl-stained preparations three major cell groups are seen: the dorsal nucleus (DC) and two subdivisions of the ventral ganglion, the anteroventral nucleus (AV) and the posteroventral nucleus (PV). Entering auditory nerve fibers divide in an orderly fashion, distributing branches to each of the three primary nuclei. Electrophysiological studies of single neurons have demonstrated a triple representation of the cochlear partition in the cochlear nuclear complex (Rose et at., 1959, 1960). Single neurons in the cochlear nuclei, and in all other cell groups of the auditory system, are excited by acoustic stimulation within a re-

stricted domain of frequency and intensity. The frequency which activates a neuron at the lowest sound intensity is called the "best" or "characteristic" frequency of the neuron, and this frequency can be considered the central representation of a restricted region of the cochlear partition. The results of an experiment in which the distribution of best frequencies was studied are illustrated in Figure 31. A microelectrode penetrating DC encounters neurons whose best frequencies make up an orderly high to low sequence. Similar sequences are apparent in PV and AV and, on the basis of a large number of similar experiments, it is clear that precise tonotopic arrangements exist and that in each of the three major subdivisions high frequencies are represented dorsally and low frequencies ventrally.

Axons of second order neurons in the cochlear nuclei, in addition to making connections with cells within the complex itself, form three main bundles; the stria of Monakow or dorsal acoustic stria, the stria of Held or intermediate stria, and the trapezoid body. The dorsal stria is essentially a crossed pathway by which cells in the dorsal nucleus project to the nuclei of the lateral lemniscus and inferior colliculus and possibly to cell groups of the superior olivary complex. The intermediate stria originates largely in PV and projects to periolivary nuclei of both sides, while the trapezoid body, arising

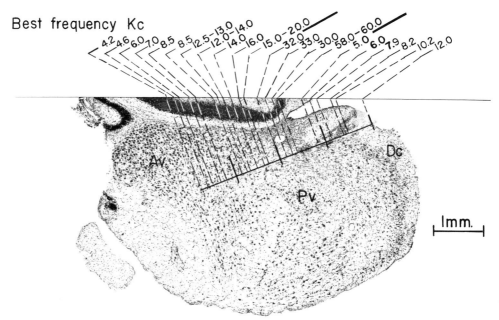

Figure 31. Sagittal section through the cochlear nuclear complex of the cat. Orderly sequences of best frequencies were encountered when a microelectrode penetrated the anteroventral nucleus (AV), the posteroventral nucleus (PV), and the dorsal cochlear nucleus (DC). Numbers refer to best frequencies of single neurons or clusters of neurons. Dashed lines indicate positions along the electrode path where the neurons were encountered. Heavy lines separate the sequences found in each division. (From Rose, J. E., et al.: Bull. Johns Hopkins Hosp. *104*:211, 1959.)

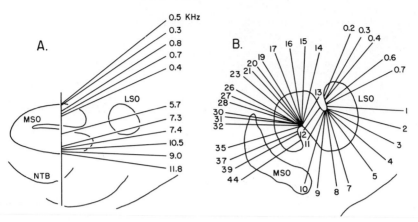

Figure 32. Distribution of best frequencies of single neurons in the superior olivary complex. *A,* Outline drawing of the medial nucleus in the dog showing the sequence of best frequencies obtained in one microelectrode penetration. MSO = medial superior olivary nucleus; LSO = lateral superior olivary nucleus; NTB = nucleus of the trapezoid body. (From Goldberg, J. M., and Brown, P. B.: J. Neurophysiol. *31*:639, 1968). *B,* Outline drawing of the lateral nucleus in the cat showing a map of best frequencies assembled from data of many experiments. (From Tsuchitani, C., and Boudreau, J. C.: J. Neurophysiol. *29*:684, 1966. Courtesy of Charles C Thomas, publisher.)

from cells in AV and PV, reaches major cell groups of the superior olivary complex. Some fibers from both striae terminate in or send collaterals to the nuclei of the lateral lemniscus. The remainder terminate in the central nucleus of the inferior colliculus (Barnes et al., 1943; Warr, 1966, 1969; Fernandez and Karapas, 1967).

Superior Olivary Complex

Anatomical studies of Goldberg and Brown (1968) and Warr (1966) suggest that projections to different cell groups of the superior olivary complex may be topographically organized. Electrophysiological experiments on two of the groups, the medial and lateral superior olivary nuclei, confirm the existence of separate tonotopic organizations (Goldberg and Brown, 1968; Tsuchitani and Boudreau, 1966). It might be pointed out here that whereas these two cell groups are both prominent in carnivores, in monkeys and humans the medial nucleus constitutes a major part of the complex and the lateral nucleus is relatively small.

In the dog the medial nucleus is folded into a U-shaped structure. Neurons with high best frequencies are located in the ventral limb, and those with low best frequencies are found in the dorsal limb (Fig. 32 *A*). Cells in this nucleus possess two primary dendrites. Ipsilateral afferent fibers terminate on one of these, contralateral afferents terminate on the other. The majority of these cells are sensitive to binaural

stimulation. Most of them receive convergent excitatory inputs from the two ears, whereas others are excited by stimulation of one ear and inhibited by stimulation of the other (Goldberg and Brown, 1968, 1969). The discharge characteristics of neurons affected by binaural stimulation are discussed in a later section.

The lateral superior olivary nucleus in the cat and dog forms a distinct S-shaped structure in the brain stem. Neurons are oriented with their long axes perpendicular to the S-shaped axis of the nucleus and receive a massive projection from the ipsilateral cochlear nucleus. A direct contralateral projection is small or nonexistent. In the cat, cells in the ventromedial limb are selectively responsive to high frequency tones, whereas those in the dorsolateral limb are most sensitive to low frequencies. Intermediate frequencies are represented in an orderly and progressive arrangement that follows the curvature of the nucleus (Fig. 32 *B*). The great majority of neurons in the lateral nucleus are excited by stimulation of the ipsilateral ear. Inhibition of the response by contralateral stimulation constitutes evidence for a projection, with a possible intermediate link, from the cochlear nuclei of the opposite side (Boudreau and Tsuchitani, 1968).

Nuclei of the Lateral Lemniscus

The lateral lemniscus is a complex pathway made up of axons arising from second and third order neurons of the cochlear nuclei and superior olivary complex and representing the

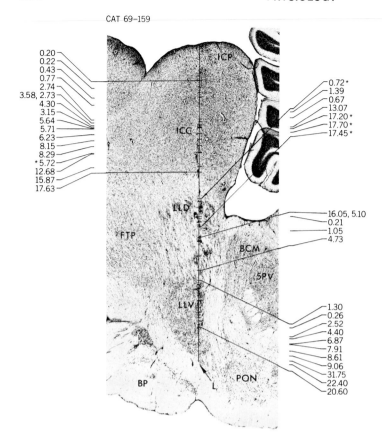

CAT 69–159

0.20	0.72*
0.22	1.39
0.43	0.67
0.77	13.07
2.74	17.20*
3.58, 2.73	17.70*
4.30	17.45*
3.15	
5.64	
5.71	
6.23	16.05, 5.10
8.15	0.21
8.29	1.05
*5.72	4.73
12.68	
15.87	1.30
17.63	0.26
	2.52
	4.40
	6.87
	7.91
	8.61
	9.06
	31.75
	22.40
	20.60

Figure 33. Sagittal section through the midbrain of a cat. Orderly sequences of best frequencies were recorded when a microelectrode penetrated the central nucleus of the inferior colliculus and the dorsal and ventral nuclei of the lateral lemniscus. Best frequencies of neurons encountered in the region between the dorsal and ventral nuclei did not make up an orderly sequence. ICP = pericentral nucleus of the inferior colliculus; ICC = central nucleus of the inferior colliculus; LLD = dorsal nucleus of lateral lemniscus; LLV = ventral nucleus of the lateral lemniscus; FTP = paralemniscal tegmental field; BCM = marginal nucleus of the brachium conjunctivum; 5PV = principal sensory trigeminal nucleus, ventral division; PON = preolivary nucleus; BP = brachium pontis; L = site of a small lesion marking the end of the electrode tract. (From Aitkin, L. M., et al.: J. Neurophysiol. *33*:421, 1970. Courtesy of Charles C Thomas, publisher.)

cochlea of the same and opposite side. Lying along the course of and intermingled with fibers of this pathway are two distinct cell groups, the dorsal and ventral nuclei of the lateral lemniscus. Aitkin et al. (1970) have shown that the great majority of neurons in the dorsal nucleus are affected by binaural stimulation, whereas most cells in the ventral nucleus are affected only by stimulation of the contralateral ear. Both the dorsal and ventral nuclei are organized tonotopically. Within each nucleus, cells with low best frequencies are located dorsally and those with high best frequencies, ventrally (Fig. 33).

Axons of neurons in the dorsal cochlear nucleus which cross the brain stem in the dorsal acoustic stria occupy a medial position in the lateral lemniscus. Some of these terminate on cells in the ventral nucleus, whereas others, on their way to the inferior colliculus, give off collaterals to cells in the dorsal nucleus. Both nuclei receive terminal fibers or collaterals from the intermediate stria and trapezoid body, whereas other components of the lateral lemniscus which apparently make afferent connections with lemniscal nuclei (and thus provide

an ipsilateral input) are of third order, arising from cells in the nuclei of the superior olivary complex. Along with axons of some cells in the dorsal nucleus, fibers of the lemniscus cross the midline in the commissure of Probst to end in the dorsal nucleus or inferior colliculus of the opposite side (Woollard and Harpman, 1940; Goldberg and Moore, 1967).

Inferior Colliculus

The majority of fibers in the lateral lemniscus terminate in the central nucleus of the inferior colliculus (Goldberg and Moore, 1967). The external nucleus may receive a few lemniscal fibers, but its major input stems from fiber tracts emerging from the central nucleus. Microelectrode studies of Rose et al. (1963) and Aitkin et al. (1970) have demonstrated an orderly tonotopic projection to the central nucleus (Fig. 33). A similar organization exists in the external nucleus (Rose et al., 1963).

Ascending projections of the inferior colliculus can be divided into two major components (Woollard and Harpman, 1940; Barnes et al.,

1943; Moore and Goldberg, 1963, 1966; Tarlov and Moore, 1966). The large ipsilateral component is the brachium of the inferior colliculus, which runs from the inferior colliculus to the medial geniculate body, giving off fibers that terminate in the external nucleus of the inferior colliculus, the parabrachial region of the lateral midbrain tegmentum, and the interstitial nucleus of the inferior colliculus. The principal division of the medial geniculate body receives a massive projection from the inferior colliculus by way of this pathway. The principal division is considered the main thalamic auditory nucleus; it degenerates severely following lesions restricted to the primary auditory area of the cerebral cortex (Rose and Woolsey, 1949, 1958; Neff et al., 1956; Diamond and Neff, 1957). The anatomical studies of Moore and Goldberg (1963, 1966) indicate that fibers of the inferior brachium distribute to cells in the principal division in an orderly fashion consistent with the electrophysiological findings which suggest an orderly tonotopic organization (Rose and Woolsey, 1958; Aitkin and Webster, 1971). The magnocellular division of the medial geniculate body also receives a projection from the inferior colliculus, and in the cat some brachium fibers terminate in the lateral part of the posterior thalamic group. Although Rose and Galambos (1952) failed to record click-evoked potentials outside of the principal division, Poggio and Mountcastle (1960) were able to isolate single neurons in the magnocellular division and posterior thalamus responsive to acoustic stimulation.

A second component of the ascending projection of the inferior colliculus is the intercollicular commissure. Fibers arise mainly from the dorsal part of the central nucleus of the inferior colliculus and many terminate in the dorsal part of the central nucleus of the opposite side, whereas others enter the contralateral inferior brachium.

Auditory Areas of the Cerebral Cortex

Auditory areas of the cerebral cortex have been mapped by the evoked potential method in a large number of animals. However, much of our knowledge of cortical organization has come from more detailed electrophysiological, behavioral, and anatomical studies conducted for the most part on cats. Some of the major contributions to the present knowledge of the cortical auditory system have been reviewed by Woolsey (1960, 1961, 1971).

The central auditory region of the cat can be parcelled into at least four areas and each, on the basis of evoked potential mapping experiments, has been shown to have complete representation of the cochlea (Fig. 34 *A*). These areas correlate to some degree with the four principal cytoarchitectural divisions described by Rose (1949). Auditory area I (AI) lies just ventral to the suprasylvian sulcus on the lateral aspect of the hemisphere. It is the only cortical auditory area known to receive essential projections from the principal division of the medial geniculate body (Rose and Woolsey, 1949, 1958; Diamond and Neff, 1957). High frequencies (B) are represented rostrally in the field, whereas the low frequencies (A) are rep-

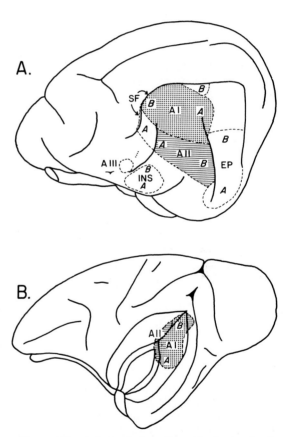

Figure 34. *A,* Lateral view of a cat brain showing the extent and organization of auditory areas of the cerebral cortex. AI = auditory area I: AII = auditory area II; AIII = auditory area III; SF = suprasylvian fringe area; EP = auditory area of the posterior ectosylvian gyrus; INS = insular area; *A* = representation of the cochlear apex (low frequencies), *B* = representation of the cochlear base (high frequencies). (From Woolsey, C. N. *In* Rasmussen, G. L. and Windle, W.: Neural Mechanisms of the Auditory and Vestibular Systems. Springfield, Ill., Charles C Thomas, 1960.) *B,* Lateral view of the monkey brain with the sylvian fissure spread to expose auditory areas I and II. (From Walzl, E. M.: Laryngoscope *57:*778, 1947.)

resented caudally. Auditory area II (AII) lies between the ectosylvian sulci just ventral to AI. Here low frequencies are found represented rostrally and high frequencies caudally. The lower two thirds of the posterior ectosylvian gyrus is occupied by area EP. In this region the cochlear apex is represented low in the field and the base is represented above. Areas AII and EP receive sustaining (collateral) projections from the principal division of the medial geniculate body. The suprasylvian fringe area (SF) begins on the anterior ectosylvian gyrus where low frequencies are represented, disappears in the depth of the suprasylvian sulcus, and emerges again above the posterior ectosylvian sulcus where representation of the high frequencies is found. The insular area (Ins) is located outside of this central region; in it there is some suggestion of tonotopic organization. The third auditory area (AIII), described by Tunturi (1945) in the dog, overlaps the head division of the second somatic area. This area apparently receives connections from the posterior thalamic group of the dorsal thalamus.

The primary auditory receiving area in Old World monkeys, apes and man is located on the superior temporal plane of the superior temporal gyrus (Fig. 34*B*). Low frequencies are represented rostrolaterally in this area; high frequencies are represented caudomedially (Walzl, 1947; Kennedy, 1955; Brugge and Merzenich, 1971; Woolsey, 1971). This area is confined to the region of koniocortex which was shown by Walker (1938) to receive its afferent input from the principal division of the medial geniculate body. Surrounding AI is a belt of auditory cortex that extends onto the upper bank of the sylvian fissure (AII) and laterally onto the surface of the superior temporal gyrus.

Despite a large body of electrophysiological and anatomical evidence for a highly ordered auditory cortex, studies of isolated single neurons have raised questions regarding the extent to which the organization of this region can be viewed simply as a two-dimensional representation of the cochlear partition. The cerebral cortex is a complex structure made up of nerve fibers and a variety of cell types disposed in six fairly definite layers. Axons reaching sensory areas of the cortical mantle from the thalamus form a dense terminal plexus, chiefly in layer four that makes synaptic contact with cells located in this and other laminae. Within the cerebral cortex, cells with short axons relay impulses vertically to cells in different laminae and provide horizontal con-

nections with other cortical areas. Lorente de Nó (1949), from his studies of synaptic connections in the cerebral cortex, suggested that a vertically linked group of cells is the elementary unit of cortical function. Mountcastle (1957), studying discharge characteristics of cells in somatosensory cortex, and Hubel and Wiesel (1962) in their studies of single neurons in the visual cortex have provided electrophysiological evidence supporting this view. Hind et al. (1960) and Goldstein et al. (1970) studied the discharge properties of single cortical neurons in unanesthetized and barbiturate-anesthetized cats and found that

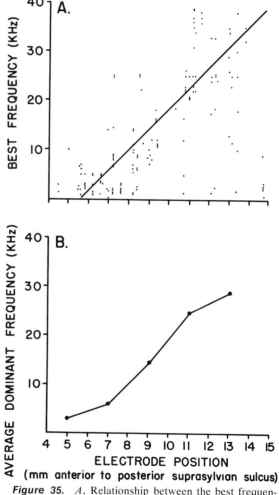

Figure 35. *A*, Relationship between the best frequencies of 131 single neurons in cortical area A1 and the position of the electrode penetration measured from the suprasylvian sulcus. Points in the lower right-hand corner of the graph may have been located outside of A1. Data were fitted best by a straight line. *B*, Best frequencies in graph A were averaged and plotted against electrode position. (From Hind et al., *In* Rasmussen, G. L., and Windle, W. F. (eds.): NEURAL MECHANISMS OF THE AUDITORY AND VESTIBULAR SYSTEMS. 1960. Courtesy of Charles C Thomas, publisher, Springfield, Illinois.)

neurons with low best frequencies were, for the most part, located caudally in AI, whereas high best frequencies were more likely to be found in the rostral portions of the field (Fig. 35). However, in any small sector of the first auditory field it is possible to record from neurons with very different best frequencies and with very different discharge characteristics. Likewise, neurons occupying the same vertical column may have the same or very similar best frequencies (Fig. 36) even though they may have very different functional properties (Hind et al., 1960; Abeles and Goldstein, 1970).

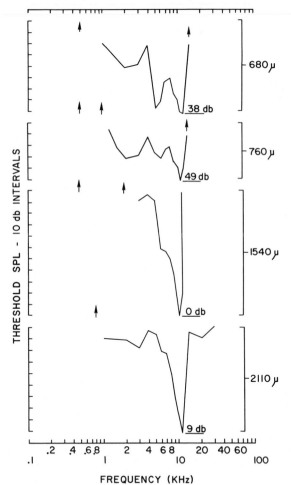

Figure 36. Tuning curves obtained for four neurons encountered in a single penetration of AI in the cat. Curves obtained by plotting the lowest sound pressure level required to evoke a discharge against the frequency of the tone. Threshold sound pressure level given for the best frequency tone. Numbers to the right of each curve indicate the depth in microns from the surface of the brain where the neuron was encountered. (From Hind, J. E., et al., *In* Rasmussen, G. L., and Windle, W. F. (eds.): NEURAL MECHANISMS OF THE AUDITORY AND VESTIBULAR SYSTEMS. 1960. Courtesy of Charles C Thomas, Springfield, Illinois.)

Auditory Areas in the Cerebral Cortex of Man

It has been known for a long time that auditory hallucinations sometimes accompany seizures resulting from lesions of the temporal lobe. The patient will describe them as resembling the ringing of bells, the escape of steam, the blowing of a whistle, or the rumbling of a train. They may be elaborate and extensive, including the sight and sound and the accompanying emotion of a period of time, and the patient usually recognizes them spontaneously as coming from his past. Penfield and Perot (1963) speak of these latter hallucinations as "experiential hallucinations," and many of them have been reproduced by electrically stimulating small regions of the temporal lobes of humans undergoing neurosurgical operations under local anesthesia. Penfield and Perot have summarized data from a large number of patients studied in this way and have found evoked auditory experiential responses limited to the lateral and superior surfaces of the first temporal convolution (Fig. 37). In the right hemisphere the responses extended more posteriorly along the lateral aspect of the gyrus than in the left, and none were found within the most anterior of the transverse temporal gyri (Heschl's gyrus), a region believed to be the primary auditory area in man. The most frequent types of experiential responses were a voice, voices, music, or a meaningful sound. Furthermore, the responses tended to occur more often with stimulation of the nondominant temporal lobe than with the dominant one.

It is generally believed that the auditory area in man occupies Heschl's gyrus since this region is known to receive fibers from the medial geniculate body (Walker, 1938). Celesia and Puletti (1969), using computer averaging techniques, recorded evoked responses from this region in patients under local or light general anesthesia (Fig. 38). Waveforms recorded from Heschl's gyrus have two major peaks: the first peak has an amplitude of 3 to 30 microvolts and latency of 12 to 22 msec.; the second is larger, 30 to 75 microvolts, and has a latency of 23 to 55 msec. The early components show little change in waveform during wakefulness, sleep, and light general anesthesia. Evoked responses from points on the lateral surface of the temporal lobe have relatively long latencies (20 to 45 msec.) and small amplitudes and are variable in waveform.

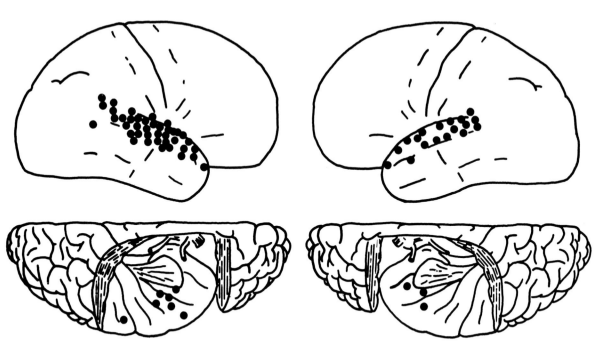

Figure 37. Lateral and dorsal views of the right and left hemispheres of the human brain showing the regions where electrical stimulation evokes auditory hallucinations. The dorsal view shows the upper bank of the first temporal convolution exposed. (From Penfield, W., and Perot, P.: Brain *86*:595, 1963.)

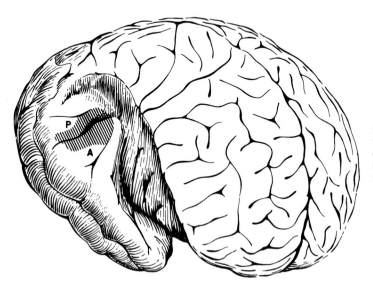

Figure 38. View of the upper bank of the first temporal convolution in the human temporal lobe showing auditory area I as defined by the evoked potential method. (From Celesia, G. G., and Puletti, F.: Neurology *19*:211, 1969.)

Scalp-evoked Auditory Responses in Man

Auditory evoked potentials, presumably of neural origin, can be recorded from electrodes placed on the scalp, particularly at the vertex. Often these potentials are so small that they are obscured by normal background activity of the EEG, especially when an auditory stimulus is presented at low intensity levels. In recent years computers have been used to extract the small evoked responses from the background activity through the process of signal averaging and have provided the audiologist with a potentially powerful tool for assessing the hearing of children who are too young to respond to conventional audiometric tests, or of individuals who are unable or unwilling to cooperate, such as the mentally retarded, the emotionally disturbed, and those with nonorganic hearing involvement (Price and Goldstein, 1966; Barnet and Lodge, 1967; McCandless, 1967; McCandless and Lentz, 1968; Rapin and Bergman, 1969; Rapin et al., 1969).

The average electroencephalic response (AER) is usually recorded with one electrode at the vertex and the other on the pinna, mastoid or nose. It is a complex waveform that can be divided, somewhat arbitrarily, into three time periods that contain, respectively, the early components, late components and contingent negative variation (CNV). Little clinical use has been made of the early components, those waves occurring within about 40 msec. after the onset of the stimulus. These potentials are smaller than the later ones but have properties (e.g., long-term stability, resistance to habituation, persistence during sleep) that may in the future prove useful in clinical electroencephalic audiometry (Goldstein, 1972). Most descriptions of the late components focus upon peaks or troughs occurring around 100, 180 and 300 msec. after the onset of the stimulus (Davis, 1968). Both early and late components grow in amplitude to a maximum, and the latencies of major peaks decrease with increased stimulus magnitude. Both are evoked by visual and somatic stimulation as well as by sound. In contrast to the relatively stable configuration of the early components, the late components habituate to repetitive stimulation and are greatly affected by drugs, sleep, and the attentiveness of the listener. In some subjects this may limit the certainty with which responses can be identified for threshold audiometry. The contingent negative variation is essentially a dc change that trails off after the late components. A conditioning stimulus is required to develop the CNV. The amplitude of the CNV seems unrelated to either stimulus modality or magnitude but is usually larger when a voluntary response to the stimulus is required. These properties, along with the fact that it is not clearly seen in children under five years of age, limit its use in clinical audiometry.

The AER is not a unitary response but rather the electrical sign of events occurring in different areas of the brain at different times in response to the stimulus. At present one can only speculate on the origin and functional significance of each of the components. When these become known the audiologist will be able to develop a powerful tool for evaluating peripheral and central auditory disorders.

RESPONSE PROPERTIES OF SINGLE NEURONS

Timing of Peripheral Afferent Volleys

Everything we perceive in our auditory environment is derived from the temporal and intensive cues of the sound coded in all-or-none action potentials in a population of auditory nerve fibers. As we have already seen, the vibration pattern set up on the cochlear partition is a function of the frequency components transmitted to the inner ear and their relative amplitudes. At low frequencies at least, the timing of single auditory nerve discharges is, in turn, governed by the unidirectional motion of the cochlear partition (Brugge et al., 1969a). When a single tone of low frequency (below about 5000 Hz) is employed, the discharges are locked to a particular portion of the sine wave stimulus and occur at time intervals that correspond to integral multiples of the period of the stimulating sinusoid (Rose et al., 1967, 1968; Hind et al., 1967). When complex stimuli are presented, the action potentials occur at times corresponding to the relative times of occurrence of the peaks of the complex waveform (Brugge et al., 1969a; Rose et al., 1969). Thus, information regarding low frequency sounds may be transmitted to the brain in a time code. This view of the way low frequency information is transmitted is not new. Wever (1949), on the basis of evidence available to him at that time, put forward in his volley theory the idea that low frequency information is coded by the periodicity of nerve impulses generated in a population of auditory nerve fibers. Viewed in this way the data of Rose and his colleagues were able to account for cochlear mechanisms involved in auditory masking and in the generation of certain combination tones.

It is of interest to consider what these results may imply for the interpretation of hearing loss that accompanies auditory nerve damage. Dandy (1934) sectioned the eighth nerve in man to relieve symptoms of Meniere's disease and noted that when a portion of the cochlear division of the nerve remained intact, the result was often a high frequency hearing loss. In no case was there selective hearing loss for low frequencies. Neff (1947) later found that lesions involving approximately one half or more of the auditory nerve of the cat produced hearing losses for frequencies of 1000 Hz and above and stated that it does not appear possible to produce marked hearing loss at frequencies below 1000 Hz without destroying almost the entire cochlear nerve. Johnson and House (1964) and Johnson (1968) have reviewed case histories of over 200 patients operated on for acoustic neuromas of various sizes and have found that the majority of patients suffered postoperatively from a high tone loss that sloped from low to high frequencies, with a loss of at least 25 db through the speech frequencies, or a total loss of hearing beyond 3000 Hz, or both. Recall that as the frequency of a tone is lowered, a greater extent of the cochlear partition is set in motion and, thus, a greater proportion of auditory nerve fibers is activated to discharge volleys of action potentials phase locked to the cycles of the stimulating sinusoid. Although damage to a sizeable proportion of auditory nerve fibers would reduce the number of afferents reaching the brain, it is likely that many of those remaining would still be activated by low frequencies and the timing of the discharges, and thus the ability of those fibers to transmit low frequency information would be unaffected by the lesion.

Discharge Characteristics of Central Auditory Neurons

A central auditory neuron receives inputs from many cells located in lower, and perhaps higher, auditory stations and probably from neighboring cells within the same cell group. These afferents may be excitatory or inhibitory, and the response of a neuron to converging volleys of impulses will be determined by the temporal and spacial interactions of these inputs. The fact that both inhibitory and excitatory pathways are activated by acoustic stimulation has been recognized in studies of single neurons at all levels of the auditory system in animals under barbiturate anesthesia.

Auditory neurons in the brain stem commonly discharge spikes throughout the duration of the tonal stimulus. For some cells, however, the spike train is interrupted by a brief pause, and for others the response is no more than a single spike or short burst of spikes at the onset of the stimulus (Greenwood and Maruyama, 1965; Pfeiffer, 1966; Goldberg and Greenwood, 1966; Goldberg and Brown, 1968; Aitkin et al., 1970). At the level of the midbrain a variety of firing patterns are seen. The usual response to a brief tonal stimulus is an onset burst of spikes followed by a period of relative quiesence, after which the neuron resumes firing (Rose et al., 1963; Geisler et al., 1969). The response of neurons in the thalamus and cerebral cortex is often no more than a single onset spike or short burst of spikes regardless of the tone duration (Erulkar et al., 1956; Adrian et al., 1966; Goldstein et al., 1968; Dunlop et al., 1969; Brugge et al., 1969b). For any given cell at all levels these patterns may change with changes in frequency and intensity of the tone.

Responses from cortical neurons similar to those seen under barbiturate anesthesia have been obtained in unanesthetized preparations (Katsuki et al., 1959, 1960; Goldstein et al., 1968; Miller et al., 1971). The question of the effects of anesthesia on the response of single auditory neurons is still not settled, however, and the extent to which the balance between excitation and inhibition is altered by changes in the conscious state of the animal will not be entirely known until more extensive studies of single neurons are performed on awake animals.

Responses to Changes in Intensity

A question of interest to auditory physiologists is how intensity is coded in the discharges of all-or-none action potentials in a population of neurons. The answer to the question is incomplete, but it is likely to involve the rates at which cells discharge and the temporal ordering of the discharges, as well as the absolute number of neural elements activated by the stimulus.

Characteristically, the number of spikes evoked during a given period of time is an increasing monotonic function of sound intensity over a range of about 20 to 40 db. The function may become sigmoid in shape, reaching a plateau and remaining there at higher intensities, or the number of spikes may actually fall significantly as sound intensity is raised (Fig. 39). This nonmonotonic behavior,

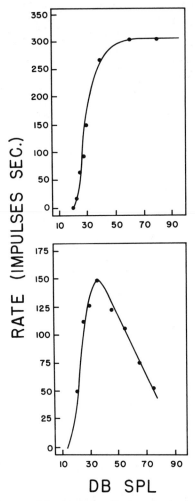

Figure 39. Monotonic and nonmonotonic spike-count functions obtained from two neurons in the cochlear nuclear complex of the cat. (From Goldberg, J. M., and Greenwood, D. D.: J. Neurophysiol. *29*:72, 1966. Courtesy of Charles C Thomas, publisher.)

which has been seen in all central auditory nuclei so far studied but not in auditory nerve fibers, has been attributed to a central inhibitory effect that begins to dominate the response at higher intensities. The terms monotonic and nonmonotonic are conveniently used to describe the general shapes of the curves relating spike counts to intensity. The functions may vary from one cell to the next and also may vary for any given neuron, depending upon the frequency of the tone.

Great differences exist among neurons in any auditory region and between cells from one region to the next with regard to the temporal distribution of spikes in a discharge train and the changes in this distribution that occur when intensity is varied (Rose et al., 1963;

Greenwood and Maruyama, 1965; Pfeiffer, 1966; Goldstein et al., 1968; Aitkin et al., 1970). Figure 40 illustrates the effect of raising stimulus intensity on the firing patterns for two neurons in the dorsal nucleus of the lateral lemniscus.

Even though the discharge pattern and the spike-count function may vary considerably, the latent period to the first spike, as a rule, decreases in a nonlinear monotonic fashion as intensity is raised (Erulkar et al., 1956; Hind et al., 1963; Brugge et al., 1969b; Aitkin et al., 1970). Hind et al. (1963) have suggested that these changes in latency of the first discharge may provide information for coding sound intensity.

Responses to Changes in Frequency

The sensitivity of a single auditory neuron to frequencies within a restricted range has been discussed briefly already. When the threshold response of a neuron is plotted as a function of stimulus frequency and intensity, the resultant curve encloses the "response area" of the cell; the frequency to which the neuron is most sensitive is called its "best" or "characteristic" frequency (Fig. 36). Katsuki (1961) has called attention to the variety of shapes these functions can take, and the data of Greenwood and Maruyama (1965) suggest that inhibitory areas, located on either side of the excitatory region of the frequency spectrum, may in some neurons give shape to the response area. Response areas can be quite narrow or they may span several octaves, and it does not appear likely that this response characteristic alone can account for the capacity of a listener to make fine frequency discrimination.

It is now well known that within the response area of some neurons the discharge patterns change when the frequency of the tone is varied (Rose et al., 1963; Greenwood and Maruyama, 1965; Goldstein et al., 1968; Aitkin et al., 1970). The effect of varying frequency at a constant sound pressure level on discharge patterns is shown in Figure 41.

In order to determine the transformations that take place within any synaptic station along a sensory pathway it is essential that both the input and the output of the individual neurons be well known. Nowhere in the auditory system is there a more favorable place to study these transformations than the cochlear nuclear complex, and several recent studies have begun to shed light on the functional implications of a few of the anatomical arrangements that are

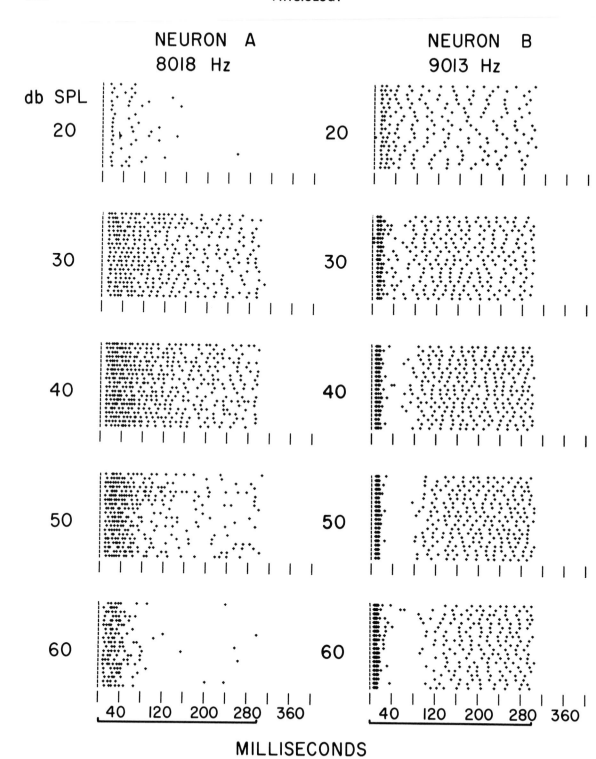

Figure 40. Temporal discharge patterns recorded from two neurons in the dorsal nucleus of the lateral lemniscus of the cat. Data taken at the best frequency of the neuron. Sound pressure level was varied and is shown to the left of each pattern. The column of short vertical dashes to the left of each pattern indicates the time the tone was turned on. Each pattern is made up of 20 consecutive stimuli. Stimulus duration was 300 msec. and is shown by the horizontal bars below each column of dot patterns. Each dot indicates the occurrence of an action potential. (From Aitkin, L. M., et al., 1970, unpublished figure.)

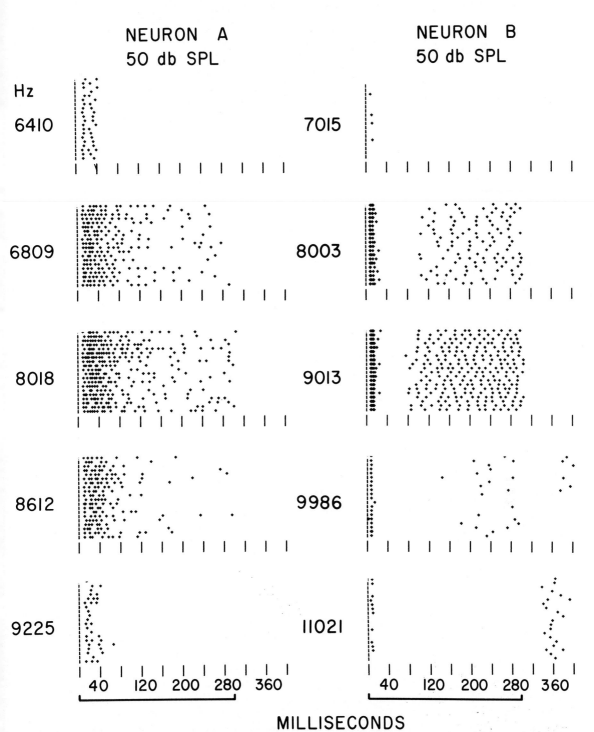

Figure 41. Temporal discharge patterns recorded from two neurons in the dorsal nucleus of the lateral lemniscus of the cat. Data were obtained from same neurons as shown in Figure 40. Sound pressure level was held constant and frequency was varied. See legend of Figure 40 for explanation of dot patterns. (From Aitkin, L. M., et al., 1970, unpublished figure.)

known to exist in this region (Lavine, 1971; Goldberg et al., 1971).

The dorsal cochlear nucleus contains a rich variety of cell types and has a complex synaptic organization reflecting direct innervation from the cochlea, indirect inputs from interneurons, and projections from higher centers. Accordingly, the discharge characteristics of these cells are complicated. Receptive fields may include prominent inhibitory sidebands, and contralateral ear stimulation produces inhibition of spontaneous discharges and of the response to ipsilateral stimulation. The response to tone bursts shows a complex interplay of converging inhibitory and excitatory inputs. By contrast the oral pole of the anteroventral nucleus consists almost exclusively of spherical shaped cells upon which five to eight auditory nerve fibers terminate as end bulbs of Held. There may be additional inputs from higher centers and from other parts of the cochlear complex, but the discharge patterns of these cells are very similar to those of first-order fibers, at least at low frequencies. The discharges may be phase-locked for tonal frequencies exceeding 3 kHz. Thus, these cells behave as simple relays to transmit to the superior olivary complex, and perhaps other cell groups, the precise timing information from each ear that is employed in localizing the source of a sound in space. In the superior olivary complex, as well as in the dorsal nucleus of the lateral lemniscus and inferior colliculus, discharges in response to frequencies below 1000 Hz are locked to the cycles of stimulating sinusoid, indicating rather secure synaptic transmission of time information to levels at least as high as the midbrain. To what extent phase-locking is maintained at all frequencies for which it is routinely obtained in auditory nerve fibers and whether it can be seen at levels of the auditory system higher than the midbrain is presently unknown.

Responses to Binaural Stimulation

Both temporal and intensive cues are utilized to localize the source of a sound in space. Psychophysical observations indicate that at low frequencies (below about 1000 Hz) the time of arrival (phase difference) of sounds at the two ears is an important cue, whereas at higher frequencies it is the difference in sound intensity at the two ears created by the acoustic shadow of the head and pinna which is most useful in localizing a sound. A number of workers have shown that discharges of neurons in the superior olivary complex, the dorsal nucleus of the lateral lemniscus, the inferior colliculus, and the auditory cortex are very sensitive to variations in interaural intensity and, when low frequency tones are employed, to differences in the time of arrival of the stimulus at the two ears.

One of the first sites in the auditory system where the inputs from both ears converge is the medial nucleus of the superior olivary complex. Goldberg and Brown (1969) have shown that at low frequencies the discharge rate of some cells in this region and in adjacent nuclei of the complex is a periodic function of the interaural phase relations between the stimuli delivered to the two ears; the period of the function is equal to the period of the stimulating sinusoids. Thus, a change in the time of arrival of the tone at one ear with respect to the other by as little as 200 μsec. can result in a change in cell discharge from essentially no spikes to maximal firing. Similar observations have been made in the dorsal nucleus of the lateral lemniscus (Brugge et al., 1970), inferior colliculus (Rose et al., 1966; Geisler et al., 1969), and auditory cortex (Hirsch, 1968; Brugge et al., 1969b). Figure 42 shows the effect on spike count of varying the interaural time delay at several frequencies. There exists for some cells a particular interaural delay time, a "characteristic delay," at which the relative discharge rate is the same regardless of the frequency to which the neuron is sensitive (Rose et al., 1966; Geisler et al., 1969; Brugge et al., 1969b, 1970). Thus, some neurons are capable of detecting an absolute time difference between sounds arriving at the ears.

When pure tones are employed the average discharge rate of cells receiving convergent input from the two ears is a function of the relative times of arrival of periodic sequences of excitatory and inhibitory events that are phase locked to the stimulating sinusoids (Goldberg and Brown, 1969; Brugge et al., 1970). When the excitatory inputs from the two ears arrive at a cell at the same time, the discharge rate is maximal. The rate falls to a minimum when these afferent volleys arrive at the site of convergence 180 degrees out of phase. Geisler et al. (1969) obtained similar periodic rate functions when band-pass noise was employed and noted that the functions could be approximated by cross-correlating two linearly filtered sinusoids of the same frequency.

A listener reports that a sound moves away from the median plane when a signal to one ear is reduced in intensity. Neurons at several lev-

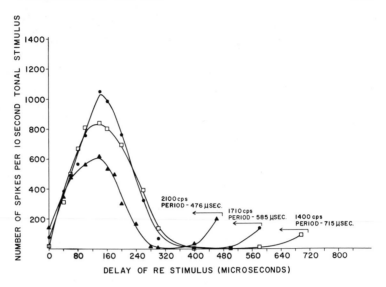

Figure 42. Response of a single neuron in the central nucleus of the inferior colliculus to low frequency binaural stimulation. Curves show the effect on spike count of delaying the arrival time of the tone to the right ear. Three frequencies were studied, and in each case the maximal number of spikes was obtained at a delay of about 140 μsec. (From Rose, J. E., et al.: J. Neurophysiol. 29:288, 1966. Courtesy of Charles C Thomas, publisher.)

els of the auditory system which receive a predominant excitatory input from one ear and inhibitory input from the other are very sensitive to changes in interaural intensity difference, and raising or lowering the intensity at one ear by only a few db can have a dramatic effect on the discharge rate, as is illustrated in Figure 43 (Rose et al., 1966; Goldberg and Brown, 1969; Brugge et al., 1969b, 1970). These cells are affected over a range of some 20 to 30 db and have been implicated as playing a role in detecting intensity cues created by the acoustic shadow of the head and pinna.

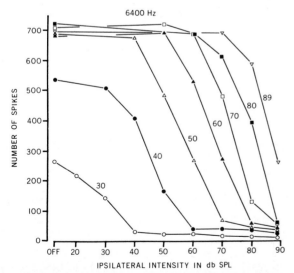

Figure 43. Response of a single neuron in the dorsal nucleus of the lateral lemniscus to binaural stimulation. Each curve shows the effect of raising the sound pressure level at the ipsilateral ear when the level at the contralateral ear is held constant. Number beside each curve indicates the constant sound pressure level at the contralateral ear. (From Brugge, J. F., et al.: J. Neurophysiol. 33:441, 1970. Courtesy of Charles C Thomas, publisher.)

REFERENCES

Abeles, M., and Goldstein, M. H.: Functional architecture in cat primary auditory cortex: Columnar organization and organization according to depth. J. Neurophysiol. 33:172, 1970.

Ades, H. W.: Central auditory mechanisms. In Magoun, H. W. (ed.): Handbook of Physiology. Vol. 1. Baltimore, Md., The Williams & Wilkins Co., 1959.

Adrian, H. O., Lifschitz, W. M.; Tavitas, R. J., and Galli, F. P.: Activity of neural units in medial geniculate body of cat and rabbit. J. Neurophysiol. 29:1046, 1966.

Aitkin, L. M., Anderson, D. J., and Brugge, J. F.: Tonotopic organization and discharge characteristics of single neurons in nuclei of the lateral lemniscus of the cat. J. Neurophysiol. 33:421, 1970.

Aitkin, L. M., and Webster, W. R.: Tonotopic organization in the medial geniculate body of the cat. Brain Res. 26:402, 1971.

Barnes, W. T., Magoun, H. W., and Ranson, S. W.: The ascending auditory pathway in the brain stem of the monkey. J. Comp. Neurol. 79:129, 1943.

Barnet, A. B., and Lodge, A.: Diagnosis of hearing loss in infancy by means of electroencephalographic audiometry. Clin. Proc. Child. Hosp. 23:1, 1967.

Boudreau, J. C., and Tsuchitani, C.: Binaural interaction in the cat superior olive S segment. J. Neurophysiol. 31:442, 1968.

Brugge, J. F., and Merzenich, M. M.: Representation of frequency in auditory cortex in the macaque monkey. In Sachs, M. (ed): The Physiology of the Auditory System. Proceedings of a workshop sponsored by the Information Center for Hearing, Speech and Disorders of Human Communication, Baltimore, Md., June 26–27, 1971. Baltimore, National Educational Consultants, 1971.

Brugge, J. F., Anderson, D. J., and Aitkin, L. M.: Responses of neurons in the dorsal nucleus of the lateral lemniscus of cat to binaural tonal stimulation. J. Neurophysiol. 33:441, 1970.

Brugge, J. F., Anderson, D. J., Hind, J. E., and Rose, J. E.: Time structure of discharges in single auditory nerve fibers of the squirrel monkey in response to complex periodic sounds. J. Neurophysiol. 32:386, 1969a.

Brugge, J. F., Dubrovsky, N. A., Aitkin, L. M., and Anderson, D. J.: Sensitivity of single neurons in auditory cortex of cat to binaural tonal stimulation; effects of varying interaural time and intensity. J. Neurophysiol. 32:1005, 1969b.

Celesia, G. G., and Puletti, F.: Auditory cortical areas of man. Neurology 19:211, 1969.

Dandy, W. E.: Effects on hearing after subtotal section of the cochlear branch of the auditory nerve. Bull. Johns Hopkins Hosp. 55:240, 1934.

Davis, H.: Auditory responses evoked in the human cortex. In DeReuck, A. V. S., and Knight, J. (eds.): Hearing Mechanisms in Vertebrates. London, J. & A. Churchill, Ltd., 1968.

Diamond, I. T., and Neff, W. D.: Ablation of temporal cortex and discrimination of auditory patterns. J. Neurophysiol. 20:300, 1957.

Dunlop, C. W., Itzkowic, D. J., and Aitkin, L. M.: Toneburst response patterns of single units in the cat medial geniculate body. Brain Res. 16:149, 1969.

Eldredge, D. H., and Miller, J. D.: Physiology of hearing. Ann. Rev. Physiol. 33:281, 1971.

Erulkar, S. D., Rose, J. E., and Davies, P. W.: Single unit activity in the auditory cortex of the cat. Bull. Johns Hopkins Hosp. 99:55, 1956.

Evarts, E. V.: Photically evoked responses in visual cortex units during sleep and walking. J. Neurophysiol. 26:229, 1963.

Evarts, E. V.: A technique for recording activity of subcortical neurons in moving animals. J. Electroenceph. Clin. Neurophysiol. 24:83, 1968a.

Evarts, E. V.. Relation of pyramidal tract activity to force exerted during voluntary movement. J. Neurophysiol. 31:14, 1968b.

Fernandez, C., and Karapas, F.: The course and termination of the striae of Monakow and Held in the cat. J. Comp. Neurol. 131:371, 1967.

Frank, K.: Identification and analysis of single unit activity in the central nervous sytem. In Magoun, H. W. (ed.): Handbook of Neurophysiology. Vol. 1. Baltimore, Md., The Williams & Wilkins Co., 1959.

Galambos, R.: Neural mechanisms of audition. Physiol. Rev. 34:497, 1954.

Geisler, C. D., Rhode, W. S., and Hazelton, D. W.: Responses of inferior colliculus neurons in the cat to binaural acoustic stimuli having wide-band spectra. J. Neurophysiol. 32:960, 1969.

Goldberg, J. M., Adrian, H. O., and Smith, F. D.: Response of neurons of the superior olivary complex of the cat to acoustic stimuli of long duration. J. Neurophysiol. 27:706, 1964.

Goldberg, J. M., and Brown, P. B.: Functional organization of the dog superior olivary complex: An anatomical and electrophysiological study. J. Neurophysiol. 31:639, 1968.

Goldberg, J. M., and Brown, P. B.: Response of binaural neurons of dog superior olivary complex to dichotic tonal stimuli: Some physiological mechanisms of sound localization. J. Neurophysiol. 32:613, 1969.

Goldberg, J. M., and Greenwood, D. D.: Response of neurons of the dorsal and posteroventral cochlear nuclei of the cat to acoustic stimuli of long duration. J. Neurophysiol. 29:72, 1966.

Goldberg, J. M., and Lavine, R. A.: Nervous system: Afferent mechanisms. Ann. Rev. Physiol. 30:319, 1968.

Goldberg, J. M., and Moore, R. Y.: Ascending projections of the lateral lemniscus in the cat and monkey. J. Comp. Neurol. 129:143, 1967.

Goldberg, J. M., Brownell, W. E., and Lavine, R. A.: Discharge characteristics of single units of the anteroventral and dorsal cochlear nuclei. In Sachs, M. (ed.): The Physiology of the Auditory System. Proceedings

of a workshop sponsored by the Information Center for Hearing, Speech and Disorders of Human Communication, Baltimore, Md., June 26–27, 1971. Baltimore, National Educational Consultants, 1971.

Goldstein, M. H., Abeles, M., Daly, R. L., and McIntosh, J.: Functional architecture in cat primary auditory cortex: Tonotopic organization. J. Neurophysiol. 33:188, 1970.

Goldstein, M. H., Hall, J. L., and Butterfield, B. O.: Single-unit activity in the primary auditory cortex of unanesthetized cats. J. Acoust. Soc. Amer. 43:444, 1968.

Goldstein, R.: Electroencephalic audiometry. In Jerger, J. (ed): Modern Developments in Audiology. New York, Academic Press, 1972.

Greenwood, D. D., and Maruyama, N.: Excitatory and inhibitory response areas of auditory neurons in the cochlear nucleus. J. Neurophysiol. 28:863, 1965.

Grinnell, A. D.: Comparative physiology of hearing. Ann. Rev. Physiol. 31:545, 1969.

Harrison, J. M., and Irving, R.: The anterior ventral cochlear nucleus. J. Comp. Neurol. 124:15, 1965.

Harrison, J. M., and Irving, R.: The organization of the posterior ventral cochlear nucleus in the rat. J. Comp. Neurol. 126:391, 1966.

Hawkins, J. E.: Hearing. Ann. Rev. Physiol. 26:453, 1964.

Hind, J. E., Anderson, D. J., Brugge, J. F., and Rose, J. E.: Coding of information pertaining to paired low-frequency tones in single auditory nerve fibers of the squirrel monkey. J. Neurophysiol. 30:794, 1967.

Hind, J. E., Goldberg, J. M., Greenwood, D. D., and Rose, J. E.: Some discharge characteristics of single neurons in the inferior colliculus of the cat. II. Timing of the discharges and observations on binaural stimulation. J. Neurophysiol. 26:321, 1963.

Hind, J. E., Rose, J. E., Davies, P. W., Woolsey, C. N., Benjamin, R. M., Welker, W. I., and Thompson, R. F.: Unit activity in the auditory cortex. In Rasmussen, G. L., and Windle, W. F. (eds.): Neural Mechanisms of the Auditory and Vestibular Systems. Springfield, Ill., Charles C Thomas, 1960.

Hirsch, J. E.: Effect of interaural time delay on amplitude of cortical responses evoked by tones. J. Neurophysiol. 31:916, 1968.

Hubel, D. H., Henson, C. O., Rupert, A., and Galambos, R.: "Attention" units in the auditory cortex. Science 129:1279, 1959.

Hubel, D. H., and Wiesel, T. N.: Receptive fields, binocular interaction and functional architecture in the cat's visual cortex. J. Physiol. 160:106, 1962.

Johnson, E. W.: Auditory findings in 200 cases of acoustic neuromas. Arch. Otolaryng. 88:598, 1968.

Johnson, E. W., and House, W. F.: Auditory findings in 53 cases of acoustic neuromas. Arch. Otolaryng. 80:667, 1964.

Katsuki, Y.: Neural mechanism of auditory sensation in cats. In Rosenblith, W. A. (ed.): Sensory Communication. New York, John Wiley & Sons, 1961.

Katsuki, Y.: Comparative neurophysiology of hearing. Physiol. Rev. 45:380, 1965.

Katsuki, Y., Murata, K., Suga, N., and Takenaka, T.: Electrical activity of cortical auditory neurons of unanesthetized and unrestrained cat. Proc. Jap. Acad. 35:571, 1959.

Katsuki, Y., Murata, K., Suga, N., and Takenaka, T.: Single unit activity in the auditory cortex of an unanesthetized monkey. Proc. Jap. Acad. 36:435, 1960.

Kennedy, T. T. K.: An electrophysiological study of the auditory projection areas of the cortex in monkey (Macaca mulatta). Doctoral dissertation, University of Chicago, 1955. Reported by Neff, W. D.: Neural mechanisms of auditory discrimination. In Rosenblith, W.

A. (ed.): Sensory Communication. New York, John Wiley & Sons, 1961.

Lavallée, M., Schanne, O. F., and Hébert, N. C.: Glass microelectrodes. New York, John Wiley & Sons, 1969.

Lavine, R. A.: Phase-locking in response of single neurons in cochlear nuclear complex of the cat to low-frequency tonal stimuli. J. Neurophysiol. 34:467, 1971.

Licklider, J. C. R.: Basic correlates of the auditory stimulus. In Stevens, S. S. (ed.): Handbook of Experimental Psychology. New York, John Wiley & Sons, 1951.

Lorente de No, R.: Anatomy of the eighth nerve. III. General plan of structure of the primary cochlear nuclei. Laryngoscope 43:327, 1933.

Lorente de No, R.: Cerebral cortex: Architecture, intracortical connections, motor projections. In Fulton, J. F. (ed.): Physiology of the Nervous System. New York, Oxford University Press, 1949, Chapter 15.

McCandless, G. A.: Clinical application of evoked response audiometry. J. Speech Hear. Res. 10:468, 1967.

McCandless, G. A., and Lentz, W. E.: Evoked response (EEG) audiometry in nonorganic hearing loss. Arch. Otolaryng. 87:123, 1968.

Miller, J. M., Kimm, J., Clopton, B., and Fetz, E.: Sensory neurophysiology and reaction time performance in nonhuman primates. In Stebbins, W. C. (ed): Animal Psychophysics: The Design and Conduct of Sensory Experiments. New York, Appleton-Century-Crofts, Inc., 1971.

Moore, R. Y., and Goldberg, J. M.: Ascending projections of the inferior colliculus in the cat. J. Comp. Neurol. 121:109, 1963.

Moore, R. Y., and Goldberg, J. M.: Projections of the inferior colliculus in the monkey. Exp. Neurol. 14:429, 1966.

Mountcastle, V. B.: Modality and topographic properties of single neurons of cat's somatic sensory cortex. J. Neurophysiol. 20:408, 1957.

Nastuk, W. L.: Physical Techniques in Biological Research. Vol. 5. New York, Academic Press, 1964.

Neff, W. D.: The effects of partial section of the auditory nerve. J. Comp. Physiol. Psychol. 40:203, 1947.

Neff, W. D., Fisher, J. E., Diamond, I. T., and Yela, M.: Role of auditory cortex in discrimination requiring localization of sound in space. J. Neurophysiol. 19:500, 1956.

Nelson, P. G., and Erulkar, S. D.: Synaptic mechanisms of excitation and inhibition in the central auditory pathway. J. Neurophysiol. 26:908, 1963.

Osen, K. K.: Cytoarchitecture of the cochlear nuclei in the cat. J. Comp. Neurol. 136:453, 1969.

Osen, K. K.: Course and termination of the primary afferents in the cochlear nuclei of the cat. An experimental anatomical study. Arch. Ital. Biol. 108:21, 1970.

Penfield, W., and Perot, P.: The brain's record of auditory and visual experience—A final summary and discussion. Brain 86:595, 1963.

Pfeiffer, R. R.: Classification of response patterns of spike discharges for units in the cochlear nucleus: Toneburst stimulation. Exp. Brain Res., 1:220, 1966.

Poggio, G. F., and Mountcastle, V. B.: A study of the functional contributions of the lemniscal and spinothalamic systems to somatic sensibility. Bull. Johns Hopkins Hosp. 106:266, 1960.

Powell, T. P. S., and Cowan, W. M.: An experimental study of the projection of the cochlea. J. Anat. (Lond.) 96:269, 1962.

Price, L. L., and Goldstein, R.: Averaged evoked responses for measuring auditory sensitivity in children. J. Speech Hear. Dis. 31:248, 1966.

Rapin, I., and Bergman, M.: Auditory evoked responses in uncertain diagnosis. Arch. Otolaryng. 90:307, 1969.

Rapin, I., Graziani, L., and Lyttle, M.: Summated auditory evoked responses for audiometry. Experience in 51 children with congenital rubella. Intern. Audiol. 8:371, 1969.

Rose, J. E.: The cellular structure of the auditory region of the cat. J. Comp. Neurol. 91:409, 1949.

Rose, J. E., Brugge, J. F., Anderson, D. J., and Hind, J. E.: Phase-locked response to low-frequency tones in single auditory nerve fibers of the squirrel monkey. J. Neurophysiol. 30:769, 1967.

Rose, J. E., Brugge, J. F., Anderson, D. J., and Hind, J. E.: Patterns of activity in single auditory nerve fibers of the squirrel monkey. In DeReuck, A. V. S., and Knight, J. (eds.): Hearing Mechanisms in Vertebrates. London, J. & A. Churchill, Ltd., 1968.

Rose, J. E., Brugge, J. F., Anderson, D. J., and Hind, J. E.: Some possible neural correlates of combination tones. J. Neurophysiol. 32:402, 1969.

Rose, J. E., and Galambos, R.: Microelectrode studies on medial geniculate body of cat. I. Thalamic region activated by click stimuli. J. Neurophysiol. 15:343, 1952.

Rose, J. E., Galambos, R., and Hughes, J. R.: Microelectrode studies of the cochlear nuclei of the cat. Bull. Johns Hopkins Hosp. 104:211, 1959.

Rose, J. E., Galambos, R., and Hughes, J. R.: Organization of frequency sensitive neurons in the cochlear nuclear complex of the cat. In Rasmussen, G. L., and Windle, W. F. (eds.): Neural Mechanisms of the Auditory and Vestibular Systems. Springfield, Ill., Charles C Thomas, 1960.

Rose, J. E., Greenwood, D. D., Goldberg, J. M., and Hind, J. E.: Some discharge characteristics of single neurons in the inferior colliculus of the cat I. Tonotopical organization, relation of spike-counts to tone intensity and firing patterns of single elements. J. Neurophysiol. 26:294, 1963.

Rose, J. E., Gross, N. B., Geisler, C. D., and Hind, J. E.: Some neural mechanisms in the inferior colliculus of the cat which may be relevant to localization of a sound source. J. Neurophysiol. 29:288, 1966.

Rose, J. E., and Woolsey, C. N.: The relations of thalamic connections, cellular structure and evocable electrical activity in the auditory region of the cat. J. Comp. Neurol. 91:441, 1949.

Rose, J. E., and Woolsey, C. N.: Cortical connections and functional organization of the thalamic auditory system of the cat. In Harlow, H. F., and Woolsey, C. N. (eds.): Biological and Biochemical Bases of Behavior. Madison, University of Wisconsin Press, 1958.

Schwartzkopff, J.: Hearing. Ann. Rev. Physiol. 29:485, 1967.

Starr, A., and Britt, R.: Intracellular recordings from cat cochlear nucleus during tone stimulation. J. Neurophysiol. 33:137, 1970.

Tarlov, C. E., and Moore, R. Y.: The tecto-thalamic connections in the brain of the rabbit. J. Comp. Neurol. 126:403, 1966.

Tsuchitani, C., and Boudreau, J. C.: Single unit analysis of cat superior olive S segment with tonal stimuli. J. Neurophysiol. 29:684, 1966.

Tunturi, A. R.: Further afferent connections to the acoustic cortex of the dog. Amer. J. Physiol. 144:389, 1945.

Walker, A. E.: The Primate Thalamus. Chicago, Ill., University of Chicago Press, 1938.

Walzl, E. M.: Representation of the cochlea in the cerebral cortex. Laryngoscope 57:778, 1947.

Warr, W. B.: Fiber degeneration following lesions in the anterior ventral cochlear nucleus of the cat. Exp. Neurol. 14:453, 1966.

Warr, W. B.: Fiber degeneration following lesions in the posteroventral cochlear nucleus of the cat. Exp. Neurol. *23*:140, 1969.

Wever, E. G.: Theory of Hearing. New York, John Wiley & Sons, 1949.

Woollard, H. H., and Harpman, J. A.: The connexions of the inferior colliculus and of the dorsal nucleus of the lateral lemniscus. J. Anat. *74*:441, 1940.

Woolsey, C. N.: Organization of cortical auditory system: A review and synthesis. *In* Rasmussen, G. L., and Windle, W. F. (eds.): Neural Mechanisms of the Auditory and Vestibular Systems. Springfield, Ill., Charles C Thomas, 1960.

Woolsey, C. N.: Organization of cortical auditory system. *In* Rosenblith, W. A. (ed.): Sensory Communication. New York, John Wiley & Sons, 1961.

Woolsey, C. N.: Tonotopic organization of the auditory cortex. *In* Sachs, M. (ed): The Physiology of the Auditory System. Proceedings of a workshop by the Information Center for Hearing, Speech and Disorders of Human Communication, Baltimore, Md., June 26–27, 1971. Baltimore, National Educational Consultants, 1971.

Wurtz, R. H.: Visual receptive fields of striate cortex neurons in awake monkeys. J. Neurophysiol. *32*:727, 1969.

VESTIBULAR PHYSIOLOGY: ITS CLINICAL APPLICATION IN UNDERSTANDING THE DIZZY PATIENT

by

Brian F. McCabe, M.D.

This chapter is designed and written for the clinical practitioner who is at times bewildered by the dizzy patient and the multitude of causes that his problem might represent. It does not purport to inform the reader in depth concerning what is known of vestibular neurophysiology today, but it hopes to give him a qualitative conceptualization of vestibular mechanisms in health and disease and, to the degree it does so, make the patient with such a problem an interesting challenge. The dizzy patient may be a perplexing diagnostic problem because he presents himself very often for treatment without any objective sign or test result of diagnostic value. Even audiometric data may be absent or nonrevealing. A thorough and practical knowledge of how the vestibular system works as it relates to the symptom of vertigo may be then the physician's best diagnostic tool.

Some initial points need to be made for this particular appreciation of vestibular function in understanding the dizzy patient.

The first is that all that is dizzy is not vestibular. Many body systems can produce dizziness—the cardiovascular system, the extravestibular tracts, the cardiopulmonary system, the metabolic system, the oculomotor system, the hormonal system, etc. Herein lies the first big fork in the flowsheet to diagnosis—the distinction between nonvestibular dizziness (an altered sensation of awareness of environment or self) and vestibular dizziness (vertigo or a specific alteration of orientation which involves motion of either the subject or his environment).

The second point is that a knowledge of the minute structure of the end-organ is not clinically essential. It can be simplified in a conceptual manner for the purpose of understanding the dizzy patient. The endolymphatic system consists of the coiling cochlear duct at one end, the three semicircular ducts on the other, and three specializations of this continuous tube in between—the utricle, the saccule and the endolymphatic duct and sac. Any movement of the head in which there is some angular acceleration causes a piling up of endolymph on one side of the cupulae of two or more of the six semicircular canals (they are orthogonally paired structures), and the brain is signaled. The density of the cupula and endolymph is probably the same, since their refractive indices are the same. Hence, gravity cannot affect the cupulae. The utricle and the saccule contain flat sensory areas, the maculae, overlain by a gelatinous coat studded with calcified bodies, the otoliths. These organs seem best equipped to sense linear acceleration, of which gravity is one variety.

The third important point is that the vestibular end-organs are dynamic structures. They are dynamic in three ways:

(1) They respond to linear and radial accelerations.

(2) They are not silent until stimulated, but

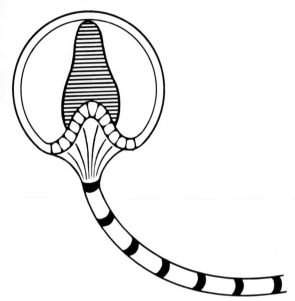

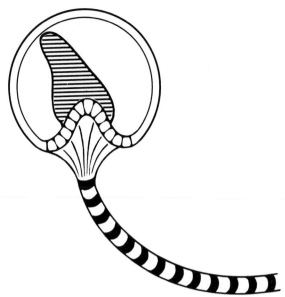

Figure 44. Diagrammatic representation of the ampullated end of one semicircular canal, showing the crista capped by its cupula and the vestibular nerve branch supplying it. The black bars represent impulse bursts along the nerve. Each end-organ has a resting discharge so that it is not silent at rest but has an "open line" to the central nervous system.

Figure 45. The crista is a frequency modulator of the resting discharge of its vestibular nerve. Here the cupula is deviated left, and the resting frequency is modulated upward to the *exact degree* of the deviation. When the cupula is deviated right in this canal, the resting frequency will be modulated downward, always proportionate to the degree of deviation.

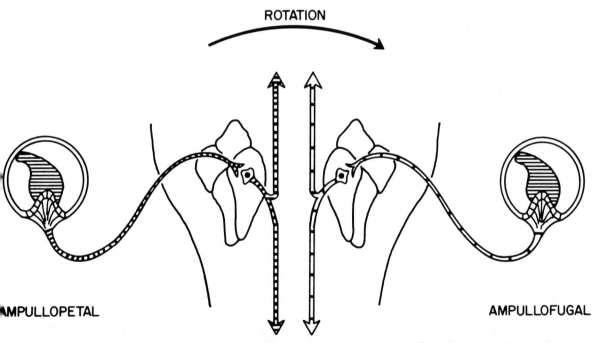

Figure 46. It is important to conceive of the vestibular system as being two-sided, constantly discharging a proportionately equal and opposite message to the central nervous system. The modulation of the discharge above resting level on the left is of a specific quantity; its paired canal on the other side experiences an opposite endolymph flow of the same magnitude, resulting in a modulation of discharge below resting level. This equal-and-opposite pattern is distributed to the brain and interpreted.

constantly discharge a resting pattern of signals to the brain (Fig. 44). Acceleration or a change in acceleration deviates the cupula and produces a change in this pattern of signals (Fig. 45), and it is this change that is distributed to the brain and interpreted.

(3) There are two sets of vestibular systems, each constantly signaling. A difference in the signal pattern between right and left is produced by an acceleration, and it is this difference that is the relevant quantity to the brain (Fig. 46).

THE BALANCE THEORY

The vestibular system, being a very old system phylogenetically, has diffuse connections with the central nervous system (Fig. 47). Some of the important areas upon which the vestibular system discharges are illustrated here (Fig. 48), but the illustration is on a conceptual rather than on an anatomic basis. On normal stimulation there is brought about a change in impulse patterns of a precise and specific nature on the two sides. On one side the resting potential is modulated downward, and on the other side the resting discharge is modulated upward. As far as we know, the difference between the downward modulation on one side and the upward modulation on the other side is precisely the same. Thus the two sides of the brain are informed in an equal but opposite manner. This polarity is important in understanding the system; the equality is even more important. The numerous areas to which the vestibular system discharges respond in recognition. The cerebral cortex interprets the change as a movement of specific direction and speed. The eye muscle nuclei move the eyes compensatorily to retain the field of last gaze, opposite to the motion of the head, as a protective mechanism in retaining orientation to environment. The anterior horn cells in the spinal cord adjust trunk and limb muscles, and the cerebellum adjusts muscle tonus to meet the new situation. These processes are probably partly instinctual and partly learned. The cortex, for example, likely underwent a prolonged period of training while the organism was learning to stand and walk. It learned to match a certain degree of cupula displacement in response to sudden head motion to a specific degree of alteration of the surrounding environment by matching a number of modalities against it, e.g., the eyes informed the brain that the body had moved so far, the proprioceptors informed the brain that

the body had moved so far, and tactile modalities informed the brain when the organism had hit the floor. Over the years, then, the brain had learned exactly what to expect from its vestibular end-organs in combination with other modalities. Being a superb computer, by childhood the brain has integrated these sensations to a high degree.

Again it is important to conceive of the vestibular apparatus as two systems, right and left, in constant dynamic balance, one checking against the other, working as a team to inform the organism of movements and head positions, and adjusting the body to meet these new conditions.

Last, it is important to conceive of each vestibular system, right and left, as a complete system from end-organ to cortex, and not as an isolated end-organ on one side.

DISEASE STRIKES

When there occurs a sudden pathologic diminution of function of one vestibular system (and vestibular crises are usually of the diminution or destructive variety rather than the irritative variety), as by, for example, a Meniere's spell of one end-organ, there exists a major imbalance (Fig. 49). The involved side is no longer able to deliver its equal and opposite fund of information to the brain. The two systems are discharging at rest at an unequal intensity, and unequal intensity of discharges has a specific meaning to the brain. The sequelae of this imbalance are manifestations of a relative hyperfunction of the intact side; thus, uncontrolled and prolonged vestibular reflexes result.

The disparate message arrives at the cerebral cortex, and the cortex interprets this unbalanced information from two sides in the only way it can: in the light of past experience. The cortex interprets it as a condition of constant motion—and this is our definition of vertigo. This misinterpretation of the actual state of affairs is a rotary sensation when the whole end-organ is involved because the six semicircular canals predominate in their overall effects over misinformation from the four otolith organs alone, simply by the law of mass action. Thus the sensation is of a rotary nature. It may be of a pitching, yawing or rolling character, but always of a rotational nature because of this predominance of innervation.

The same massive imbalance in discharges arrives at the eye muscle nuclei and the reticu-

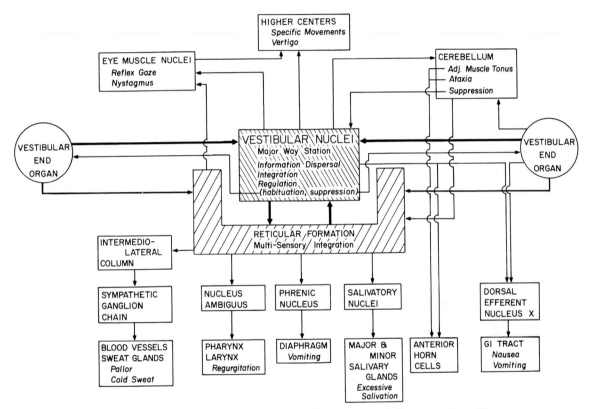

Figure 47. Schematic representation of some of the more important vestibular connections. The arrows represent known tracts. This indicates the high degree to which the vestibular system is integrated into the neuraxis. Under normal circumstances the vestibular system is principally a proprioceptive one (upper half of schema), but under abnormal circumstances it initiates considerable motor activity (lower half of schema).

lar formation. The imbalance, interpreted as before in the light of past information and training, directs the eye muscle nuclei to deviate the eyes in the direction of last gaze to retain orientation; the slow component of nystagmus is born. The eyes, however, cannot continue to track indefinitely in any single direction because of their anatomic limitations, so after a deviation specific to the number of motoneurons has transpired, inhibitor neurons in the reticular formation cut off the incoming flow from the vestibular nuclei and, at the same time, reticular activating neurons direct the ocular muscle nuclei to return the eyeballs to the point of gaze at which the slow component began the deviation (across the midline). This second phase of eye deviation is a much faster one because it is a compensatory or recovery phase. The quick component of nystagmus is

thus generated. The reticular activating neuron, having fired, enters into its refractory period, and the end-organ inflow from the vestibular nuclei resumes its effect upon the eye muscle tracts—the eyeballs are directed again to retain the field of last gaze. This repetitive attempt to retain last field of gaze by a conjugate movement of the eyes and a rapid reflex return of the eyeballs across the midline in compensation is our definition of vestibular nystagmus.

The same imbalance of information is transmitted from the vestibular nuclei down the spinal cord to anterior horn cells, instructing the postural and locomotor muscles to meet a new situation that never comes; staggering and ataxia result.

The imbalance in impulses also plays upon the dorsal efferent nucleus of X. At first this

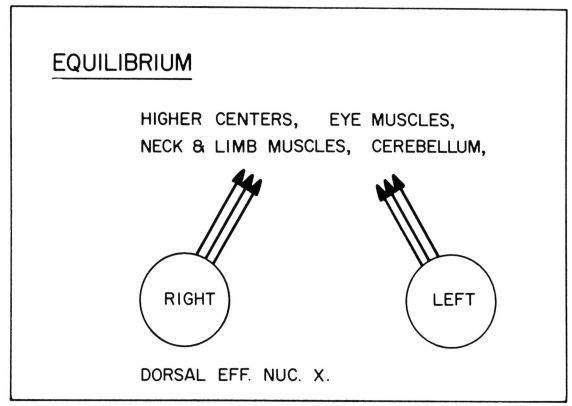

EQUILIBRIUM

HIGHER CENTERS,   EYE MUSCLES,
NECK & LIMB MUSCLES, CEREBELLUM,

RIGHT   LEFT

DORSAL EFF. NUC. X.

Figure 48. The Balance Theory of vestibular function. There are two end-organs, constantly discharging at a steady state when at rest. On their actuation the brain receives impulses from both sides simultaneously, weighs one against the other, interprets the equal and opposite difference in discharge strength in the light of past experience, and transmits this information. Each effector organ responds to its particular ability (an awareness of motion, deviation of the eyes to retain the field of last gaze, and so forth).

nucleus effects only a cessation of peristalsis. Gut activity is not needed in an emergent situation. If the imbalance is massive and continuous, however, this nucleus is heavily stimulated, and reverse peristalsis occurs with resultant nausea and vomiting.

The effects mediated by the cerebellum in response to a massive imbalance on the two sides is only beginning to be understood. In a matter of minutes the cerebellum imposes a virtual shutdown of electrical activity of the vestibular nuclei (at least the medial nucleus, the major way station for incoming canal impulses) by virtue of its profound inhibitory influence on vestibular activity (Fig. 50). The cerebellum does not eliminate the great imbalance by this shutdown because not all information from the end-organs distributes to the brain through these nuclei—some fibers from the end-organ distribute straight to numerous other parts of the brain stem and cerebellum (Fig. 47) without vestibular nuclear synapse. The nuclear shutdown does not then eliminate the problem, but does serve to render the imbalance at a lower level of magnitude so that the full effects of the imbalance do not distribute through all available vestibular pathways.

THE PHYSIOLOGY OF REPAIR AND COMPENSATION

The organism then sets about trying to restore the situation. It cannot long endure it; the organism will eventually die through dehydration and fluid and electrolyte imbalance. Restoration of equilibrium between the two centers brings about resolution of the uncon-

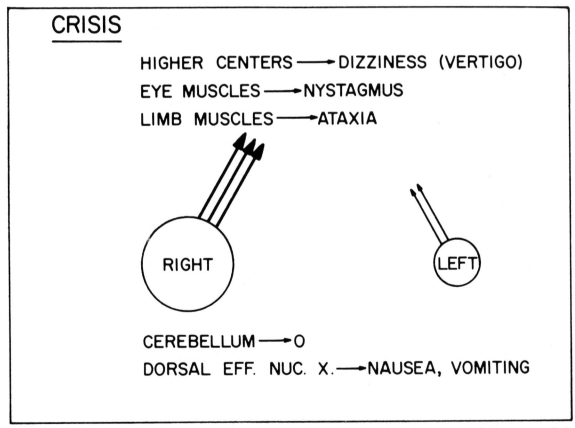

Figure 49. When disease strikes one labyrinth (here the left), resulting in sudden diminution of discharge strength, it is unable to match the normal side in providing its equal and opposite discharge flow. The brain, still able to interpret only in the light of past learned responses, distributes a false stream of impulses to its effector organs. Thus the cortex is informed the organism is in a constant state of motion (vertigo), the eyes seek repetitively to retain the field of last gaze (nystagmus), limb muscles prepare to meet a situation that never comes (ataxia), and the gut is stopped and reverse peristalsis begins (nausea and vomiting).

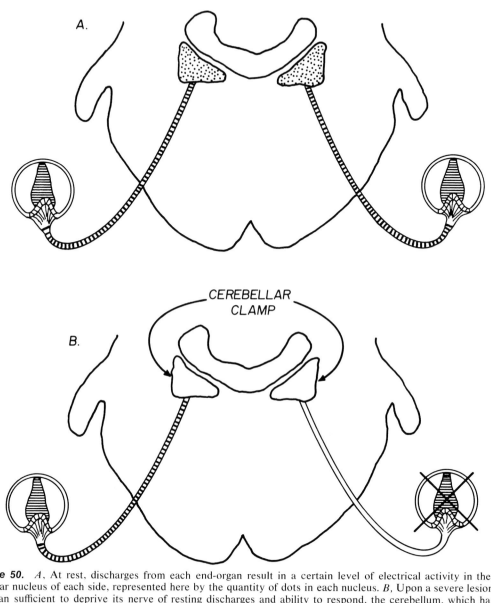

Figure 50. *A*, At rest, discharges from each end-organ result in a certain level of electrical activity in the medial vestibular nucleus of each side, represented here by the quantity of dots in each nucleus. *B*, Upon a severe lesion of one end-organ sufficient to deprive its nerve of resting discharges and ability to respond, the cerebellum, which has direct connections not only with the nuclei but with each end-organ, applies a clamp that during the critical period of recovery or compensation renders *each* nucleus electrically silent. This does not eliminate symptoms (vestibular interconnections are too widespread for that) but does serve to somewhat redress the situation by rebalancing part of the vestibular system on a lower level of activity. This lessens the impact of a massive imbalance on the rest of the neuraxis. The clamp will be slowly released as a new resting activity is generated in the deprived nucleus.

trolled reflexes. This can be done in three ways, 1) restoration to health of the diseased system, which may take hours to days, 2) central suppression of the intact side by invocation of inhibitory tracts in the central nervous system, and 3) generation of a new electrical activity in the underdischarging system to balance the normal but now relatively hyperactive side. These include probably all theoretical mechanisms involved. In practice it is very likely that all three mechanisms go on at once in varying degrees. For example, in the crisis of Meniere's disease the end-organ heals itself in a few hours, and a normal or near normal discharge pattern from the end-organ resumes. The cerebellar "clamp" is not needed, or at least only temporarily. Reflexes then revert to normal as equal and opposite reactions are signaled from the two end-organs. Another example would be acute suppurative labyrinthitis. In this disease the end-organ is destroyed and, since it cannot rebuild itself, restoration must be a central process. Very quickly the cerebellum imposes vestibular and nuclear shutdown, and this provides a barely tolerable situation for the organism as long as there is no or at least minimal stimulation of the opposite end-organ to accentuate the great imbalance. For this reason patients in vestibular crisis remain perfectly still with as little head motion as possible. Motion of the head results in accentuation of the imbalance, with waves of vertigo and vegetative symptoms. Then, over a matter of days and possibly weeks a new resting electrical activity is generated in the denervated vestibular nuclei. As this new activity builds, symptoms begin to abate and the cerebellar shutdown is slowly released. When the activity is full and matches the other side, symptoms disappear except for varying degrees of motion intolerance. Motion interpretation involves integration, and this must gradually be built up following regeneration of resting activity in the nuclei.

We do not know what stimulates the generation of the new resting activity in the denervated nuclei, but we know of certain essentials for it. Certainly there must be a chronic vestibular input imbalance or, more simply, a vacuum stimulating its need. The speed at which it is brought about is dependent upon the severity of the imbalance stimulating it, and the ability of the central nervous system (CNS) to respond. This ability is a function of the vigor of the whole organism—age of the patient, availability of neuron arcs, efficiency of the central nervous system vascular supply, and so forth.

CLINICAL APPLICATIONS OF THE BALANCE THEORY

From such a consideration of the balance theory of vestibular function, we arrive at two axioms:
  (1) In vestibular crises of any severity, there will always be labyrinthine nystagmus.
  (2) If the symptoms last continuously for more than two or three weeks, the cause is not vestibular.

These axioms can be applied clinically. The first can be helpful if the patient, while dizzy can be observed by the physician or, indeed, any instructed person. *If the patient in a significant spell does not have spontaneous labyrinthine nystagmus, the disease is not vestibular.* The physician may not often have opportunity to observe a spell because the patient presents usually between spells. However, the patient's spouse can oftentimes be a surprisingly good observer once instructed. The physician can instruct the spouse in the office at the initial visit by pointing out carefully the features of the nystagmus produced by the simple caloric test he performs in the course of his workup. The author has come across some people who have become surprisingly astute observers after little instruction. This may seem at first self-evident, but it is an important starting point because it may clearly establish the disease as vestibular or extravestibular early in the diagnostic workup. If the otolaryngologist is able to establish its nature as nonvestibular, this alone is helpful to the referring physician. If he can establish the disease as vestibular, he can proceed to the next important fork in the flowsheet, that of central or peripheral causation.

The second axiom is also helpful in this regard. If on close questioning the patient states that his dizziness has been nonepisodic and continuous for, say, two or three months, then his disease cannot be vestibular. As we have previously pointed out, the vestibular system does not work in this way. There are virtually no clinical exceptions to this axiom.

VESTIBULAR FUNCTION TESTS—WHAT WE CAN LEARN FROM THEM

The goal of vestibular function tests in the present state of the art should be primarily to distinguish a vestibular disease as either end-organ or central. If this can be determined with satisfaction, this alone will be a laudable achievement. It is frequently an immense relief to a patient to be told that his disease is end-organ and that, whatever follows in the way of symptomatology, his condition will not shorten his life by one day. Even if his disease is not directly treatable, he can at least be assured of eventual relief. If, on the other hand, the disease can be recognized as central, the patient can be put in the hands of the proper specialist until it is diagnosed or time and the emergence of new symptoms make it diagnosable.

Rotation Tests

Rotation tests are the oldest of vestibular tests and have advantages and disadvantages. The major advantage is that cupula deviation can be produced to a precise degree, but this takes sophisticated and expensive equipment. The major disadvantage is that it stimulates both ears at once and gives no laterality information. It should not be considered purely a research test, however, because some clear and useful information can at times be adduced. If for example a gross difference (more than 30 per cent) in nystagmus duration is produced by equal spins in the two directions, there either *is* or *has been* a significant vestibular incident. This is not specific, but it helps one along the flowsheet to diagnosis. This rotation test can be done rather simply by putting the patient in any chair that will rotate, turning the patient up by hand ten turns in ten seconds, and then stopping him suddenly. After a few minutes, the turns can be repeated in the opposite direction.

Another example of the utility of this test is in the very young child brought in by his parents because of apparent severe deafness. Very young children require special audiometric equipment and skills for hearing quantification, such as EEG audiometry, available for the most part only in large medical centers. The child can be positioned on the lap of a parent, who holds the head of the child under his own chin so that the heads are on nearly the same axis. The rotation test is done, and if the child's nystagmus is grossly less than the parent's, particularly if there is little or no nystagmus, it can be accepted that there is a severe derangement of the inner ears; immediate and extensive referral is warranted. Although there may seem little urgency, experts in education of the deaf are placing hearing aids on children at an increasingly early age.

Electrical Tests

In this category we have only the faradic and galvanic variety, with the electrode placed over the mastoid cortex. This produces a depolarization of the vestibular nerve and precipitates gross movement of the body. The electrical charge necessary to penetrate the skin and temporal bone to the nerve is so large that it is a painful and, thus, impractical test. Some form of electrical stimulus will be the test of the future, however, for it is precisely quantifiable in terms of strength. Some future investigator will give us an electrical stimulus which can be driven without significant pain, much like square wave testing of the facial nerve.

Postural Tests

Postural tests are performed for the detection of positional nystagmus. They can be performed with and without visual fixation. With visual fixation the patient fixes his eyes at a point in each test position with the eyes in cardinal position of gaze. Testing without visual fixation is done with Frenzel glasses, or preferably by electronystagmography. The usual test positions are: (1) upright with head erect, (2) recumbent with left ear down, (3) recumbent with right ear down, and (4) head hanging, with vertex pointed at the floor. Whether the head is moved with the body or the head moved on the body with neck torsion is not important unless one is seeking to distinguish between gravity actuated nystagmus and nystagmus produced by vascular embarrassment or from torsion of neck vessels.

The important features of the provoked nystagmus to note are latency, fatiguability, direction changing or direction fixed, and perversion. No latency, or a very short one, is indicative of a central lesion; a long latency is indicative of a peripheral lesion. In the latter case, the latency may be as long as 15 or 20 seconds; hence, the position must be held for that period in search of nystagmus. A nonfatiguable nystagmus (that lasting as long as the position is held) is indicative of a central lesion, fatiguable nystagmus is indicative of a peripheral lesion.

Direction-changing nystagmus is nystagmus which changes in direction from one head position to another, or one examination to another (Aschan Type II). Direction-fixed nystagmus is in the same direction regardless of position or time (Aschan Type I). Direction-fixed positional nystagmus is virtually always end-organ in origin. The majority of patients with direction-changing nystagmus will also have their lesion in the end-organ, but a significantly high percentage will be central in origin. For that reason, a direction-changing positional nystagmus should be a red flag of warning.

Perverted nystagmus is defined as that which is unexpected in terms of the stimulus. For example, a rotatory nystagmus upon stimulation of the horizontal semicircular canal would be a perverted one. Positional nystagmus of the end-organ variety produces a horizontal-rotatory nystagmus and, less often, a pure rotatory or pure horizontal nystagmus. Thus, a vertical nystagmus on positional testing would be a perverted one. Perverted nystagmus almost always means a central lesion.

Postural vertigo is a disease characterized by positional nystagmus. Repeated examinations may be necessary to elicit the nystagmus, but they are essential to a definitive diagnosis. There is a specific and relatively common form of this disorder termed "benign paroxysmal postural vertigo" (Aschan Type III). With the involved ear undermost, after a definite latent period there appears a rapid labyrinthine nystagmus of brief duration (fatiguable) accompanied by intense vertigo. It is direction fixed. It is thought to be of peripheral origin, but this is not known with certainty. Physiologically it appears to be an otolithic defect, with consequent loss of otolith organ governing or modulating influence over the semicircular canals. It is a self-limited disease.

Caloric Testing

There are a great variety of caloric tests used clinically; they vary essentially only in volume and temperature of water used. The important features of caloric testing of the labyrinth are twofold, a) enough stimulus should be provided to compare the two sides, and b) enough stimulus should be provided to evoke all the sequelae of cupula deflection. Unless these are done, much valuable information may be missed. Threshold tests are of limited value as they provide only part of the picture. A suitable screening caloric examination is the injection of 5 ml. of ice water over a 5 sec. period directed at the posterosuperior quadrant of the tympanic membrane under direct vision. If this does not drive each labyrinth to the desired degree as indicated previously, 10 ml. of ice water may be used or, if this is not adequate, 20 ml. of ice water. If this does not

produce nystagmus or vertigo, that vestibular apparatus is said to be inactive.

The important initial questions to be answered by the caloric test are: (1) does the labyrinth work or not, and (2) does the caloric qualitatively (not quantitatively) reproduce the patient's spell?

At a minimum the above information should be provided by the caloric test. By following these principles the discriminating observer can, at times, adduce significant information that may pinpoint the lesion. If enough stimulation is given to evoke all the sequelae of cupula deflection routinely, a missing component may be highly significant. For example, if there is nystagmus and vertigo but no nausea upon adequate stimulation, this may be indicative of a low pontine or medullary lesion with a cutoff of impulses to the dorsal efferent nucleus of X. If there is nystagmus and nausea but no vertigo, this may indicate a midbrain lesion with a cutoff of impulses to higher centers where vertigo is interpreted. If there is vertigo and nausea but no nystagmus, this may indicate a median brain stem lesion with cutoff of impulses to eye muscle nuclei such as in syringobulbia or multiple sclerosis.

ELECTRONYSTAGMOGRAPHY

The technique of electronystagmography (ENG) and interpretation of electronystagmograms is not within the purview of this chapter, but some comments must be made upon this relatively new study for the sake of completeness. (See Chapter 39.)

There is no question that ENG has moved out of the research laboratory and is now properly a clinical neuro-otologic test. It allows us to determine the intensity of vestibular response (eyeball speed in the slow component), to detect latent nystagmus (that present with the eyes closed, or the eyes open in the dark), and to detect the gaze nystagmus characteristic of some central lesions and late peripheral lesions. It allows us to perform positional tests with a higher degree of yield since optic fixation can be eliminated, and it provides us with a permanent record for analysis and comparison. Finally, it allows us to observe some of the provoked features of nystagmus, such as secondary phase nystagmus (or provocation nystagmus), which might otherwise be missed.

ENG, by providing us with the precise intensity of the nystagmic response, also gives

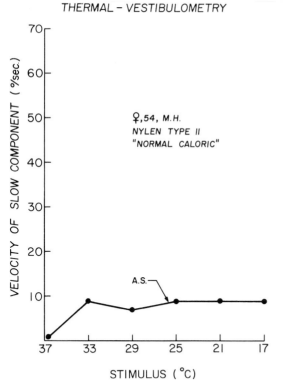

Figure 51. An adaptation curve, seen with end-organ lesions. The system is unable to respond incrementally to an increasing stimulus beyond a certain level.

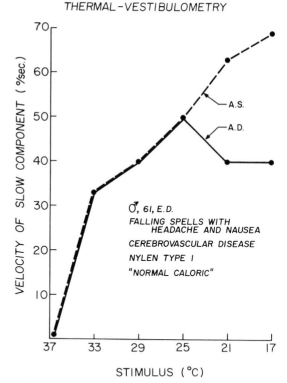

Figure 52. A fatigue curve, seen with central lesions. Not only is the system unable to respond incrementally to an increasing stimulus, but at high stimulus levels a falling response occurs, presumably as a result of an accumulation of chemical mediator in a depleted and overloaded neuron system.

opportunity to add another dimension to nystagmus analysis. By comparing the intensities of response (slow component speed) to varying stimulus intensities of an incremental nature, we are able to construct an intensity-function curve of vestibular response for that system. The intensity of response should be incremental to each succeeding rise in stimulus, such that the graphic representation would be a straight line, as long as all stimuli are within physiologic limits. This is neurophysiologically true in all sensory systems. And, indeed, normal individuals do respond in a linear fashion, with serial intensities varying by three degrees each from body temperature. In pilot studies peripheral lesions tend to show an increasing response to incremental stimuli up to a limit and then to level off, so that no further increase in stimulus strength provides any further increase in response. This has been termed an "adaptation curve" (Fig. 51). Central lesions, on the other hand, tend to show a normal buildup of response to incremental in-

creases in stimulus strength to a certain level, then an actual diminution in intensity response to high levels of stimulation strength. This has been termed a "fatigue curve" (Fig. 52).

The interpretation of an "adaptation curve" is that of an end-organ lesion and a hair cell depopulation. The increasing stimulus gets all hair cells working and, when they are finally doing so, no additional neurons can be recruited to fire into the central nervous system, so that the response stays at that level regardless of the stimulus strength. In the case of the "fatigue" curve, an adequate hair cell population drives a depleted neuron population adequately at low stimulus strength, but at high stimulus levels the overdriving of available neurons causes buildup of chemical mediator, cutting out many of the neurons available so that final response levels fall below early maximum response levels. This test is tedious and difficult to perform but has some promise of pointing the way to a test which is a discriminator of the site of the lesion.

Chapter 9

NASAL PHYSIOLOGY

by Henry L. Williams, M.D., M.S.

The nasal pyramid, as was pointed out by Schaeffer (1920), is a uniquely human attribute, not being possessed by any other primate. Being large and centrally placed, it is an individual's chief characterizing facial feature and, according to Groner (1963), is of basic importance in the formation and preservation of the body image.

For these reasons questions as to why there is a nose, what does it do, and how does it do it. were among the earliest physiologic interests of the physician.

In the beginning, like all physiology, the physiology of the nose was based on intuition. It was eventually realized that intuition is not enough. There must be rigorous scientific validation if the factual is to be separated from the merely fanciful. The rhinologist became the first respiratory physiologist. We should not be astonished that Rohrer, who was, according to Mead, the father of respiratory mechanics, was the son of a distinguished rhinologist.

Early primacy was, however, a misfortune to rhinology. The fact that air, below Mach 1, behaves like an incompressible fluid of low viscosity was lost on the rhinologic research that preceded explanation of the flow of fluid through round pipes, to say nothing of flow through twisting conduits of irregular circumference and varying section. The experiments of the rhinologist were inconclusive and frustrating.

Mathematics and physics are basic for study of driving pressure, resistance, conductance, and flow rate, as Reynolds (1883) demonstrated in deriving the criterion of whether turbulent flow can be sustained by fluid flowing through a round pipe. The mathematics of hydrodynamics, however, proved to be difficult for the rhinologist.

The doctrine developed that intuitive hypothesis, particularly the concept of final purpose, is scientifically inadmissable. This, it was said, is "teleology" or armchair science. This dogma conceals the fact that the roots of nasal physiology, as of any science, lie in intuitive reality. Disregard for application and intuition, as Courant and John (1965) point out, leads to an introverted science, isolation, atrophy of the imagination, and a smug purism.

Rhinologic physiology was undone by the rush of enthusiastic hope for a "scientific" practice of medicine because it did not have the steadying and saving grace of a foundation in the basics. The rhinologist was also deprived of a normal impulse toward justification by a profound feeling of guilt, for indeed he had much in his past to regret. Therefore, since the rhinologist could not furnish valid laboratory research support for his claims, physiology and basic science in general began to ignore them and him. Much mention of the nose or of its possible respiratory activity was cleverly avoided in the formative undergraduate medical years. This resulted in an attrition of respect for rhinology as a discipline which has extended to otorhinolaryngology as a whole. This bland disregard has even, at times, persuaded the rhinologist himself that such nasal function as is generally conceded is of such minor importance as to scarcely warrant consideration.

With the present trend toward early integration of the laboratory and the clinic in the teaching of medicine this bodes ill for selection of otolaryngology as one of the junior or senior "pathways" by medical students of the future.

Without a properly developed nasal physiology there can be no advances in rhinology. It is high time that the limitation of nasal function

329

to the surface epithelium and ciliary streaming is corrected by realization that the present attitude of many otorhinolaryngologists must be abandoned for a thoroughgoing involvement of otolaryngology in basic rhinologic research.

THE NASAL CYCLE

The upper respiratory tract is a twisting, curving, closed conduit of varying section and irregular circumference stretching from the nares to the glottis. Its nasal portion is divided from nares to choanae by a wall termed the nasal septum.

The teleologic explanation for this division is that one nasal chamber may rest while the other carries on the functions of the nose. Although it is a well supported observation that in a normal nose one nasal airway opens up with secretion of serous and mucous glands while the opposite airway closes down with almost complete cessation of such activity and that passage of respiratory air is carried on in nearly its entirety through the open nasal chamber, no convincing explanation as to why such alternation of resting and functioning states of the nasal airway should be necessary for the well-being of the organism has been presented.

The normal presence of a cycle of congestion and decongestion of the cavernous tissues of the nasal conchae was observed by Kayser and termed the nasal cycle in 1895. He suggested that there is a continual shifting in autonomic balance between the two body halves which, in turn, causes a continually changing blood balance in the erectile tissues of the turbinate and septum.

The emptying of the turbinal and septal swell bodies by the continuously present recoil of the elastic fibers surrounding these structures was described by Wright (1910), while the mechanism of the filling of these structures was described by Burnham (1941).

Lillie (1923) related the complaint of alternating nasal obstruction of some patients to the nasal cycle. He was the first to associate the shrinking of the mucosa of one nasal chamber with the throwing off of its serous and mucus secretions while the mucosa of the opposite nasal chamber shows an increasing congestion approaching complete nasal respiratory obstruction with repression of secretions. Lillie's findings were confirmed by Heetderks (1927). The latter reported that there was a characteristic individual cycle of reaction in about 80 per cent of his test subjects. He found, in gener-

al, that the nasal cycle is most active during adolescence and youth and gradually decreases in activity with aging. He also found that damp cold atmosphere brought about the most marked mucosal congestion, warm dry air a somewhat less marked reaction, while optimum conditions in the ambient atmosphere (humidity 50 to 60 per cent and temperature 15 to 18° C.) caused cycles of the least degree. Although the same nose might respond somewhat differently at different times under apparently the same conditions, the cycles, including both filling and emptying on the same side, occurred characteristically for a given nose over periods of from 30 minutes to four hours. Heetderks suggested that activity of the nasal cycle might be related to the activity of secretion of the sex hormones. He believed this view is supported by the appearance of the so-called honeymoon coryza of marked edema, swelling, and increased serous secretion under the stress of unusual or excessive sexual activity.

Heetderks also examined the effect of sleeping posture on filling of the erectile tissue "swell bodies." He found that the turbinates in the dependent nasal chamber reached a maximum size in from 15 to 20 minutes. By turning the test subject to the opposite side, the superior side of the nose became open and the inferior congested in from 10 to 15 minutes. He concluded that changes in turbinate congestion as influenced by position must be produced by the effect of gravity.

Stoksted et al. (1953) also found the nasal cycle present in about 80 per cent of individuals tested. Guillerm et al. (1967) studied the nasal cycle by rhinometry and demonstrated that the total nasal resistance (using the formula $\frac{1}{R} = \frac{1}{R_1} + \frac{1}{R_2}$ in which R is the combined resistance of both nasal airways, R_1 the resistance to passage of air through one airway and R_2 the resistance to passage through the other) remains essentially constant in spite of continual cross-sectional changes caused by the congesting and decongesting of the turbinal and septal erectile tissues in the separate nasal airways. He stressed the functional importance of steadily maintained total resistance, despite the nasal cycle, in noses in which, owing either to trauma or developmental aberration, there is great inequality in the effective section of the two sides. This was further emphasized by Spoor's (1963, 1967) finding that the total conductance of the nasal airways tended to remain the same no matter what changes in conductance are found when each nasal airway is measured separately.

Ogura and Stoksted (1958) found that when one nasal cavity is anatomically wide and the other narrow, the respiration through the wide side runs parallel with and is about equal to the total nasal respiration. Owing to this, the cyclical changes on the wide side are not compensated for by reciprocal changes on the other. During the congested phase on the wide side they found that obstruction of the upper airway might produce hypoventilation. When very marked septal deflection was present they found regular and normal cyclic fluctuations on the wide side, but on the narrow side cyclic changes were irregular and appeared to be influenced by premature contact of turbinate with septum during the congested phase. When "vasomotor rhinitis" was present they found that both nasal cavities react synchronously to external irritants to an exaggerated degree, with interruption or disturbance of the normal nasal cycle and decrease of total nasal conductance. In the normal nose they found that bilateral synchronous turbinal reaction to external irritants took place to a limited degree and required but a short time for adaptation so that cyclical rhythm is not disturbed.

Keuning (1968) made cycle determinations on 17 males in their 20's who were found to have rhinoscopically normal noses and who gave no history suggesting hypersensitivity or recurring sinusitis. He found regular cycles in seven subjects which were individually characteristic and ranged from 2 to 7 hours; there were no patency reversals in six of the group and irregular cycles were found in four. The amplitudes of the curves were remarkably constant in a given individual, whether they had rhythmic cyclical congestion and decongestion, irregular cycles, or no reversals of patency. The total nasal conductance remained essentially constant whether regular or irregular cycles or no reversals were present.

In 19 children between four and ten years of age cyclic activity while sitting was investigated by use of Zwardemaakers nasal mirror. From his observations Keuning concluded, as had Kayser, (1895), that the nasal cycle appears to be initiated by a physiologic mechanism in which a sympathetic (adrenergic) predominance exists on one body half while a parasynthetic (cholinergic) predominance exists on the other, the predominances alternating from one side to the other. It is influenced neither by anesthetizing the nose or the larynx or by breathing through the mouth, but the cycle is absent after laryngectomy. These, he believes, are arguments against the cycle's originating in the nose, and yet a direct influence from the larynx seems improbable, as does a reflex from the bronchi.

From the fact that the cycle continues after anesthetization of the nasal as well as the laryngeal mucous membranes and during temporary prevention of nose breathing, it was Keuning's opinion that the initiating mechanism of the nasal cycle has not been identified. He believed, however, that the "receptor" structures in the nasal mucosa described by Temesrakasi (1959), Terracol (1958), Majer (1968), and Jabonero (1953), which are not affected by topical anesthesia, may be the structures responsible, since some balancing mechanism producing the nasal cycle must exist. From experiments on unilateral adrenergically or cholinergically denervated nasal cavities it appeared that while a nasal cycle may be present in the parasympathetically denervated side, one is not present on the sympathetically denervated side. This seemed to him to imply that an intact sympathetic supply is essential for the maintenance of the nasal cycle. He offers the "more or less teleological conclusion" that the nose maintains a constant respiratory resistance.

When sympathetic or parasympathetic denervation has been done unilaterally the patient may continue nasal breathing because respiratory resistance remains the same. If the situation is altered artificially, the nose adapts itself so as to again offer the same respiratory resistance. The assumption may be made that the nasal cycle is maintained through the peripheral vegetative centers, sphenopalatine, and stellate ganglia, with interconnections through which an increase of tonus in one set will result in a decrease of tonus in the others. The two peripheral centers must be regulated by a central autonomic "center," possibly located in the hypothalmus. By increasing or decreasing the tonus this center can produce increased or decreased nasal conductance in keeping with the requirements of the organism for intake of oxygen or discharge of carbon dioxide.

The conclusion and suggestions of Keuning seem to receive support from recent observations of Connell (1968).

INFERIOR AND MIDDLE NASAL CONCHAE (TURBINATED BONES)

In relation to the nasal cycle the vascularization of the nasal turbinates is of interest. Burnham (1935, 1941) found the arterial supply to the inferior and middle turbinates to be from the sphenopalatine artery and its branches, which run in the periosteal layer of the mucoperiosteum. The arterial supply divides into: (1) superficial, supplying the surface epithelium and the tissue immediately subjacent; and (2) deep, which enters canals in the bony skeleton of the turbinates which are lined with periosteum. The periosteum of these bony canals contains venous plexuses carrying blood away from the deep (true) layer of erectile tissue. Dilatation of the canalicular aterial vessel will, therefore, tend to produce distention of the erectile tissue.

Certain blocks of cavernous tissue react as units physiologically. The cavernous tissue of the inferior turbinate is divided into three functional areas; the first comprises the anterior two fifths of the turbinate; the second is comprised by the middle one fifth; and the third, the posterior two fifths. It was found that these areas of cavernous tissue do not contract systematically in an anteroposterior direction. Ephedrine applied to the posterior area caused shrinkage of the anterior but had very little effect on the middle area. Application of ephedrine to the middle area produced comparatively little effect on the anterior and posterior areas but exerted a powerful constricting effect on the plexus of vessels on the medial antral wall. It was suggested that the reaction is a vasomotor one acting through the vessels in the bony canals. Under normal circumstances reactions in the two anterior segments are carried on without any appreciable influence on the posterior. The influence of the area of the posterior tip on the anterior tip is called into play only when the first area is subjected to excessive stress. Removal of the anterior tip of the inferior turbinate produces much subsequent discomfort to the patient, the most annoying symptom being watering of the homolateral nose. Removal of a mulbery posterior tip of the inferior turbinate has not been found to produce symptoms.

The arterial supply (from the inferior turbinal) to the maxillary sinus gains entrance through the ostium and the bone immediately surrounding it. The veins accompany the arteries. On reaching the interior of the sinus the vessels form a collarlike plexus about the ostium a few millimeters in width and then radiate out in straight lines from the plexus "like the setting sun." Negus (1958) found that the arrangement of the vascular supply to the turbinal tissues and the nasal mucosa generally allowed four possible modes of reaction of the nasal mucosa and swell bodies: (1) Hyperemia of surface vessels with filling of erectile tissues. This is associated with an increase in mucosal temperature. This picture may be produced by exposure to cold dry air. (2) Ischemia of superficial vessels, shrinkage of cavernous tissues and decrease in mucosal temperature. This picture may be produced by exposure to warm moist air. (3) Ischemia and constriction of superficial vessels but congestion of cavernous tissues. This picture may be produced by breathing warm air of average relative humidity. (4) Superficial arterial dilation with increased mucosal surface temperature but without congestion of cavernous tissues. This picture may be produced by superficial irritation.

NERVOUS SUPPLY TO THE NOSE

Common sensation, according to Slome (1966), is carried from skin, mucosa, and subcutaneous and submucosal tissues by the fifth cranial nerve. The motor supply to the nasal respiratory muscles is through the seventh cranial nerve; integration of their contraction with the respiratory rhythm is carried to the seventh nerve through the vagus.

The physiologically important control of the circulation to the nasal airways is mediated by the autonomic system. The adrenergic nonmedulated postganglionic fibers pass through the sphenopalatine ganglion, without synapsing, to the serous and mucous glands of the respiratory epithelium. One preganglionic adrenergic fiber synapses in the outlying superior and middle cervical ganglia (the stellate ganglion) with about 30 postganglionic fibers. Sympathetic (adrenergic) action is, therefore, diffuse. The neuro-effector substance of the postganglionic adrenergic fiber is noradrenaline, or at least an adrenergic substance.

The cell bodies of the cholinergic or parasympathetic supply to the head and neck region lie in the brain stem. From the superior salivary nucleus cholinergic fibers form the nervus intermedius and join the facial nerve, passing to the middle meningeal artery by way of the greater superficial petrosal nerve. Through the nerve of the pterygoid canal parasympathetic fibers pass to the sphenopalatine ganglion. After synapsing they are distributed to the nasal structures.

In general, the effects of the sympathetic and parasympathetic nervous systems are antagonistic. On the other hand, in some areas both systems cause the same general effect but of a different quality. For example, parasympathetic stimulation causes an abundant, watery, salivalike flow, whereas sympathetic stimulation causes a mucinous, "enzymatic" secretion in the nose. The nonmedulated adrenergic fibers end in relation to the arterioles and do not supply metarterioles or capillaries. Following cervical sympathetic block (producing parasympathetic overaction) there is nasal hypersecretion, hyperemia, swelling, and obstruction. Following section of the greater superficial petrosal nerve, according to Gardner et al. (1947), the nasal mucosa becomes pale, dry, and shrunken from the effect of unapposed adrenergic activity.

Adrenergic Blockade

Disorders of nasal function associated with so-called autonomic imbalance can be explained by the hypothesis of Szentivanyi (1968) that block of the action of catecholamines on the effector substance, adenyl cyclase, is responsible for symptoms listed as being on the basis of allergic hypersensitivity.

LYMPHATICS OF THE NASAL CHAMBERS

Rouviere (1938) stated that the lymphatics of the maxillary sinus anastomose with one another and converge beneath the mucosa toward the sinal ostium. They pass through it and arrive at the middle meatus where they unite with the lymphatics of that region. The lymphatic trunks of the middle meatus join the lymphatic plexus lying above the pharyngeal orifice of the eustachian tube, which is also joined by the "paratubal lymphatics." From the plexus the lymphatics of the middle meatus drain to the lateral retropharyngeal nodes.

The lymphatics of the inferior meatus do not communicate freely with those of the middle meatus, nor at all with the lymphatic plexus above the torus, but drain to the deep cervical internal jugular nodes. This somewhat unexpected distribution of the lymph vessels has a definite influence on the production of serous otitis media in conjunction with chronic infection of the homolateral maxillary sinus. The products of inflammation block the lateral retropharyngeal nodes which also drain the lymph plexus above the torus into which the paratubal lymphatic trunks from the membranocartilaginous portion of the eustachian tube also drain. The resulting tubal lymphedema causes the serous otitis media.

The blood and lymph capillaries of the nasal mucosa lie in the superficial stroma; the larger blood and lymph vessels, in the deep. The mucous membrane as a whole rests on a periosteum of variable thickness. The fact that all the blood and lymph channels entering or leaving a sinus go through or close to the sinal ostium is of considerable clinical importance. In inflammation, with swelling of the mucosa in the region of the ostium, this arrangement leads to early edema and congestion of the sinal lining. This relationship also contraindicates instrumentation through the ostium because of the possibility of interfering with lymphatic and venous return flow from the sinus.

PARANASAL AIR SINUSES

The maxillary sinus, according to Schaefer (1932), is usually the largest and is always the most precocious of the paranasal sinuses. Both the maxillary antrum and some portion of the ethmoid labyrinth are usually present at birth. The ethmoid cells, from their beginning in the fetus, are divided into two primary groups by the attached border and lamina of the middle nasal (ethmoidal) concha. In Caucasians the expansion of the maxillary sinus into the alveolar process of the maxilla is often carried to an extreme degree, the roots of the molars and premolars all mounding into the antral floor.

From infancy to adult life the frontal sinuses vary greatly in size and shape, not only in different individuals but also in the same individual, and supernumerary frontal sinuses are common.

The anterior ethmoid cells also empty into the infundibulum, which is usually described as being continuous with the nasofrontal duct. Weille (1946) stated, however, that the classically described nasofrontal duct is frequently not found at operation, the frontal sinus presenting a simple round opening into the anterior aspect of the superior meatus.

The sphenoid sinus develops after birth. In the adult the sphenoid sinuses are usually asymmetrical and their walls are often very irregular and may be indented by the hypophysis, the pons, the optic nerve, the carotid artery, or any or all of them.

MAXILLARY OSTIUM

The maxillary sinus is described as communicating with the middle meatus by an opening of oval shape, and being from 1 to 2 mm. in size; accessory ostia are often present.

Ballenger (1925) and Myerson (1932) found that in life the maxillary ostium is sometimes supplemented by a tubular formation of the sinal mucosa having valvelike activity. This observation was confirmed by Drettner (1965), who found that such a structure is capable of maintaining peak expiratory pressures for considerable periods of time; as a rule, there is a lag between changes in intranasal and intraantral pressures. Although Drettner did not find correlations between the presence of obstructed sinal ostia and sinal infection, or even with subjective symptoms, it has been inferred from similar findings that subjective symptoms varying from vague discomfort to aching pain have been produced by blockage of the sinal ostial valve. Drettner (1965) found that partial or complete block of the sinal ostium is usually present in either acute or chronic disease, but he expressed no opinion as to whether such block is causative or resultant.

FUNCTION OF THE SINUSES

The "reason" for the existence of the paranasal air sinuses has never been satisfactorily explained. After an extensive review of the literature and experiments made on models, Mink (1915) concluded that there is no convincing evidence to suggest that the paranasal sinuses serve any purpose whatsoever. This was also the opinion of Negus (1958). Possibly the most interesting hypothesis as to sinal function is that of Semenov (1950). He suggested that since the paranasal air sinuses seem to bear a similar physical relationship to the nasal airway as the "surge tanks" do to the hydraulic braking system of an automobile, they also may serve to dampen the surge of pressure caused, in the instance of the nose, by bringing the air stream to a sudden stop twice during each respiratory cycle.

In sudden deceleration of flow, according to Streeter (1958), a sudden surge of pressure occurs known as "water hammer." With a surge tank, although surge will occur, the development of a high pressure intensity along the conduit is prevented. In an orifice tank (such as a paranasal sinus) the opening or orifice between tank and conduit is restricted and, hence, allows more rapid pressure changes in the conduit than would be allowed by an unrestricted orifice. The more rapid pressure change causes a more rapid adjustment of flow through the conduit, and dissipation of excess energy resulting from sudden stoppage of flow. Abruptly stopping and reversing the flow of

respiratory air might well be a sufficient stimulus for the development of the paranasal air sinuses.

OLFACTION

In discussing the primary function of the nose Negus (1958) stated that the observer has become confused as to what it is because of the secondary functions added to that for which the nose was originally designed.

In fish the olfactory organ has no other uses except for those of finding and recognizing food and for procreation. Various stages in olfactory elaboration can be observed in amphibia and reptiles and in various mammals, there being a multiplication of specialized turbinal bodies with great complexity in macrosmatic carnivores in whom there is extension of olfactory turbinals into frontal and sphenoidal sinuses. In the arboreal apes and in man reliance is placed on sight rather than on smell, and a regression of the olfactory area is observed.

Mucosal Division. In conformity with the path of the main air stream through the nasal chambers and the histological differences in the nasal mucous membranes, Negus stated that the nasal fossae are considered to have olfactory and respiratory portions. He called attention to the fact that in a nasal fossa the mucous membrane is unequally divided into two types of mucous membranes, the olfactory and the respiratory, in conformity with its multiple functions.

In the noses of mammals he found a correspondence between the olfactory and the respiratory areas. Both areas were small in species with feeble powers of scent and extensive in keen-scented animals. The primate microsmatic nose shows a regression from the nose of furred macrosmatic vertebrates. This has had important influence on some of the functions which will be considered under Nasal Respiratory Functions.

Hypotheses. Although it was stated earlier that olfaction is the most primitive of the special senses and at one time was considered the most important nasal function, Wenzel and Sieck in their review (1966) state: "Systematic research in olfaction continues to be hampered both by lack of an accepted working hypothesis for the basic receptive mechanism and by the lack of standardized equipment for the control of stimulus intensity. Consequently even basic research tends to be ahypothetical."

Anosmia as Compensible Disability. Interest

of the rhinologist in olfaction has been stimulated recently by the fact that in some states anosmia has become a compensible disability under workman's compensation laws. Therefore, most clinicians are more interested in tests that will demonstrate the presence or absence of osmation than in research as to its physiologic mechanism.

To be smelled, a substance must not only be volatile, but must also be soluble in water and lipids. It seems probable that the need for enough moisture to preserve the lipoliquid film over the surface of the olfactory epithelium was a factor in the development of the multiple purpose mammalian nose.

Embryology. The organ of smell, according to Morrison, is one of the first of the special sense organs to develop. The olfactory placodes are apparent as early as the fourth week of embryonic development. The bipolar olfactory cells send axons to the primitive brain as early as the fifth week, and this area later elongates to form the olfactory bulb and tract. A small region of the nasal mucous membrane over the upper part of the superior concha and the corresponding portion of the nasal septum is characterized by a yellow-brown color tone; it is somewhat thicker than the surrounding respiratory epithelium and contains the terminations of the nervi olfactorii in a specially constructed epithelium which constitutes the olfactory organ. This epithelium is made up of three types of cells and Bowmans glands, which supply the lipoliquid solution which covers the surface of the olfactory organ.

Anatomy. The three types of cells of the olfactory epithelium are the olfactory cells, the sustentacular cells, and the basal cells. The bipolar olfactory cells have a peripheral process extending toward the epithelial surface as the olfactory rod. This ends in a vesicle protruding about 2 μ above the surface of the surrounding cells. From this vesicle a number of cilia protrude and form a network above the epithelium with cilia from other cells. The function of cilia in osmation is not well understood. The central end of the olfactory cell tapers to a process of about 1 μ in diameter that penetrates the basement membrane as an unmyelinated axon. After leaving the olfactory cell the axon is sheathed by central projections, both from a sustentacular cell and from a basal cell. Many axons are then gathered into a bundle which is sheathed by a Schwann cell. These fascicles are assembled into small nerve bundles called filia olfactoria which pass through the cribriform plate of the ethmoid bone

to the olfactory bulb. There are no synaptic connections between the single axon of each receptor cell and any other cell until it reaches the bulb, and none between the receptor cells in the olfactory mucosa. It has been suggested, however, that the tight packing together of the unmyelinated axons in the olfactory fascicle may result in synchronization of discharge in the olfactory nerve. The afferent connections from the olfactory bulb appear to be extremely varied and complex and indicate integration of olfaction with a great many other sensory stimuli which reach higher centers, particularly the vegetative centers in the hypothalmus and brain stem.

The olfactory glands (Bowman's) secrete a lipolipid material that is spread evenly over the surface of the olfactory epithelium. This material is dissimilar to the secretion of other glands of the respiratory epithelium. It gives no reaction for mucin nor is it typically serous. Lipase and esterase are found in Bowman's glands. The ducts but not the acini are positive for alkaline glycerophosphatase. These same enzyme systems are found in the taste buds. This emphasizes the similarity and the association of these two systems of special sensation.

Olfactory Perception. Wenzel and Sieck (1966) pointed out that a precision olfactometer does not in itself guarantee the obtaining of valid and reliable threshold measurements. The results of comparison tests showed that threshold values are greatly affected by the method of stimulus presentation, and that care should be taken both in designing procedures for obtaining thesholds and in valuation of threshold results reported by others. They suggest that a concept of "the threshold" is untenable and that a range would be a more appropriate statement of sensitivity.

These remarks are more applicable to laboratory research in olfactometry and of less importance in clinical evaluation, in which the problem of the presence or absence of perceptual anosmia is usually the major concern.

Anosmia. Uncomplicated perceptual anosmia is rare. Congenital anosmia is very unusual and appears to be the result of agenesis of the olfactory bulb. Van Dishoeck classified anosmia as "conductive" when anatomical obstruction keeps inspired air from reaching the olfactory membrane and "perceptive" if there is dysfunction of the olfactory receptive or transmittive apparatus. He found that "conductive" anosmia is relative and, in reality, is nearly always hyposmia, since odor-bearing air usually reaches the olfactory mucosa to some degree. It has been found that, probably from their close relationship, taste and smell are readily confused by some patients. Using the stereochemical classification of odors of Amoore (1962), which will be considered later, van Dishoeck determined that some patients may be anosmic to certain primary odors but perceive others normally. He classified this as partial perceptive anosmia. The commonest cause of temporary obstructive anosmia is the common cold. A more persistant "conductive" anosmia may be produced by marked bilateral nasal polyposis. This is usually, but not always, relieved by medical or surgical elimination of the polyps.

Long-continuing or permanent anosmia may follow viral invasion of the olfactory epithelium or possibly result from the effects of viral or bacterial "toxins" by direct contact with the olfactory cells or through the circulation. Such loss may return rather quickly after the infection subsides, may persist for months or years (return of smell after five and one half years was reported by Morrison), or may be permanent.

Neurotoxic effects. Neurotoxic effects of some air-borne agents may also produce long-continued to permanent primary anosmia. Thus, anosmia may become a medicolegal problem. Control of odor and potentially damaging fumes is important in industries, particularly in regard to air conditioning and ventilation and also in the perfume industry. This latter industry illustrates the many subtle ways in which odor, by appeal to one of our most primitive senses, may affect our lives without our awareness.

Trauma. Severe trauma to the skull with fracture of the cribriform plate of the ethmoid and interruption of the olfactory fibers is becoming the commonest cause of perceptive anosmia. In trauma anosmia may be unilateral or bilateral but is nearly always complete and permanent.

Disability rating. The J.A.M.A. Guide to Evaluation of Permanent Impairment recommends a 3 per cent disability rating for permanent bilateral anosmia. Man is a microsmatic animal, a group which includes the primates and the whalebone whales. Except for the toothed whales, which are anosmic, all other mammals are macrosmatic, and in them the sense of smell has survival value. Microsmatic man, however, can exist comfortably without the sense of smell even though anosmia will interfere with the enjoyment of food and some social relationships. It has been found on test-

ing thresholds of "domiciled male veterans" from 49 to over 70 years of age that they showed an increase in absolute thresholds for odor until about the age of 60 years after which there appeared to be a constancy in thresholds. It was also found that some senile individuals have normal olfactory function.

Receptive Process. Wenzel and Sieck (1966) stated, "There is at present no adequate description of the transducing mechanism for either the quality or the intensity of olfactory sensations; nor, even worse, is there an understanding of what constitutes the critical feature of the olfactory stimulus."

The most popular current hypothesis is that of Amoore (1962), which has the heuristic value of being able to predict, "rather precisely," the odors of newly synthesized compounds. He categorized a large number of odorous compounds according to the type of odor generally ascribed to them, and then reduced the apparent multiplicity to seven distinct types. From an analysis of the structural configuration of the various molecules represented in this catalog he suggests that all the members of one class can be described by a single general outline form. By postulating seven different sites on the receptor cells that are appropriately shaped for reception of the seven different molecular configurations, the process of qualitative differences in olfactory sensations can be explained. Amoore's hypothesis has received support from a number of other investigators.

Receptors and central pathways. Most of the functions of cortical and subcortical and olfactory centers are beyond the scope of this chapter. Those interested are referred to the review of Wenzel and Sieck (1966).

Interconnections of Olfaction with Other Functions. The extensive interconnections between the primary olfactory centers and many other portions of the brain suggest that the sense of smell may influence several aspects of biological function.

The role of olfaction in the reproductive process has been emphasized in observations ranging from the ability of many insects to locate mates by means of odor to the psychic importance of odors in influencing the emotional life of the human being. Kloeck (1961) found the smell of some steroid sex hormones and their metabolites to have profound effects on the mutual relations of the sexes in man. The incorporation of musk as a base in the more expensive perfumes may be pointed out as a practical application of such observations. The effect of odors on appetite and, thus, on eating and drinking has been mentioned previously. The observations that have been made on the alterations of water metabolism caused by lesions of the olfactory bulb in rats and also their arousal by low dosage roentgen rays directed at the same area are interesting, but not understood as yet.

Bazarov, during experiments on human subjects in whom the vestibular mechanism was stimulated, found that vestibular and visceral reactions are increased by some odors but inhibited by others. The excitation of visceral reactions by certain odors is an everyday experience, but an inhibiting effect has not been previously recognized; the mechanism of neither reaction has been satisfactorily explained.

Clinical Testing of Human Olfaction. Morrison has devised a clinical olfactometer somewhat similar to the diffusion olfactometer used by Zwaardemaker. Both observers point out that there is marked deviation in the olfactory end point in normal individuals from minute to minute and from day to day. Morrison suggests that this difference may depend on many factors but mentioned especially the nasal cycle. Owing to this variability, Morrison concludes that the usefulness of olfactometry in a clinical situation is almost confined to testing for the presence or absence of anosmia, particularly when a medicolegal question is involved.

He found it impractical to make quantitative tests for olfaction for all the odors as classified by either Zwaardemaker or Amoore. He observed that few of his patients could identify by name any of the familiar odors such as cinnamon, vanilla, coffee or castor oil even though they perceived the odor of the test substance. His findings did not agree with those of van Dishoeck on "partial anosmia," mentioned previously. He found that if a patient could not smell one of the test odors he could not smell any of them, and if he could smell one odor he could smell them all. It, therefore, seemed reasonable to him to reduce the test substance to a single odor; after extensive testing he selected either oil of clove or oil of orange as the odorous substance to be used. Morrison stated: "The procedure is designed to test olfaction at the threshold of minimum perceptible odor. The test is dependent on the cooperation of the patient just as visual testing and audiometric testing are dependent upon patient responses. A single drop of an oily extract of an odorous substance (either oil of clove or oil of orange) is dropped into an ordinary 10 cc. syringe barrel. The plunger is inserted and twisted about so as to get an even distribution of the oil over the inside of the barrel and the surfaces of the plunger. Any excess oil is expelled from the tip of the syringe and the outside is carefully cleaned with alcohol or ether. After storage of the syringe with the plunger in place at $0°$ C. no odor can be detected about it. The instrument is now capable of delivering a measured amount of odorized air at a reasonably constant concentration. To use the instrument the plunger is slowly withdrawn to the number of cc. of odorized air it is desired to deliver. The nozzle of the syringe is then placed under the nostril to be tested, pointing it away from the other nostril to avoid minor bilateral cross stimulation. The patient is instructed to inhale and as he does so the dose of odorized air is delivered by pushing in the plunger at a constant rate. The patient indicates whether or not he has smelled an odor and identifies it if he can. Responses are recorded as positive or negative: a positive answer is regarded as the slightest acknowledgment that olfaction has taken place. Questionable responses are repeated until a definite answer is obtained."

The normal minimum identifiable odor was determined by delivering a smaller and smaller volume of odorized air until the patient's response became negative. It was determined that a patient should normally detect a dose of 0.1 cc. of odorized air (oil of clove). This is utilized as the standard normal. A dose of 10 cc. or larger which is not smelled is considered to place the patient in the classification of anosmic.

This appears to be a simple and reasonably accurate clinical method of testing for anosmia. More sophisticated tests of osmation await development.

NASAL CHAMBERS

The respiratory epithelium, in general, is a ciliated stratified or pseudostratified columnar type. The tunica propria is formed of fibroelastic tissues and contains mucus-secreting, purely serous, and "mixed" glands. Their secretions combine to form the moist mucous covering or "mucus blanket." Negus (1956, 1957) believed that the need of a covering of moisture over the nasal mucosa is the legacy of a pelagic origin. He found the epithelium generally known as respiratory to be of two types: one thick and ciliated, the other thin and permeable. The epithelium over the maxillary turbinal is only two cells in thickness, with freedom of passage for moisture; it responds to adrenaline, histamine, and sympathetic control in an active manner. This is in contrast to the reactivity of the remainder of the respiratory mucosa in which fluid transfer suffers at the expense of formation of the mucus blanket. As the result of his researchers, Negus stated that many of the ideas in regard to nasal function require readjustment.

Mucus Blanket

The mucus blanket is a product of goblet cells and serous and mucous glands. Unusual properties are ascribed to the mucus blanket. In association with ciliary streaming it is said to form a protective barrier over the underlying mucosa of the nose and paranasal sinuses. Lysozyme, an enzyme that disrupts some bacteria, was described by Fleming (1921–1922) as being present in the mucus blanket. It is now the consensus, according to Tomasi et al. (1965), that lysozyme is probably identical with immune globulin A (IgA) with an additional factor (immunological piece) added by the secreting cells, as at all body orifices. Some individuals, according to Smith et al. (1968) and Bellanti (1968), may inherit or develop a deficiency in IgA or a defect in the mechanism by which the immunologic piece is added. It is the addition of the "piece" that activates the immunizing power of this globulin. Either of these deficiencies may make an individual more susceptible to invasion of the upper respiratory tract by potentially pathogenic microorganisms.

Proetz (1953) estimated the secretion of mucus and serous fluid from the nasal epithelium to be about one liter in 24 hours. According to Lucas and Douglas (1934), there tends to be a viscosity gradient from the surface of the mucus blanket in contact with respiratory air and that in contact with the epithelium. Thus, the upper layer is highly viscous, elastic, and tenacious and normally forms a continuous, tough, and movable protective film. The lower layer is of lower viscosity and forms the medium for the recovery stroke of the cilium.

Speed of Mucus Flow. Hilding (1967) found that the speed of flow of the mucus blanket is not the same in all parts of the nose. The line between ciliated and nonciliated epithelium is not a definite boundary and differs between individuals and between the nasal chambers of the same individual. In the sinuses the direction of flow is spiral, centering at the natural ostium. If the continuity of cilia through a natu-

ral ostium is interfered with by scar formation, natural drainage of the sinus through the ostium may be very poor.

Hilding estimated that the mucus blanket in the nose is renewed every 10 to 20 minutes and in the sinuses every 10 to 15 minutes.

According to Proetz (1956), dryness is the natural enemy of a cilium; at 70 per cent relative humidity of inspired air (body temperature) there is no discernible effect on ciliary activity, but at 50 per cent relative humidity ciliary action stops after 8 to 10 minutes; at 30 per cent relative humidity, in from 3 to 5 minutes. The optimum temperature of the cilium itself for activity is between 18 and 37° C; between 7 and 12° C. ciliary action ceases.

NASAL RESPIRATORY FUNCTIONS

For both clarity and convenience, although there is considerable overlap, the respiratory functions of the nose have been considered to be: (1) the action of the nose as a mechanical, negative feedback control device to match the supply of air to the need for alveolar ventilation; (2) tempering of the inspired air and a role in the control of body temperature; (3) humidification of the inspired air; (4) cleaning of the inspired air of dust and microorganisms; and (5) as a practical consequence of the latter, the resistance of the nose and paranasal sinuses to invasion by pathogenic microorganisms.

Cleaning Inspired Air. An important function of the mucus blanket, according to Hilding (1967), is that of cleansing the inspired air. Foreign particles carried in the air sheets, which may be no more than a millimeter in thickness, while passing by the middle meatus adhere to the sticky mucus surface and are carried along to the pharynx and swallowed.

Waterproofing. Negus (1957, 1964 a and b) believes that the most important function of the mucus blanket is often ignored. From the evidence of comparative biology he concluded that mucus has a waterproofing function, both on the surface of animals such as earthworms, slugs, and eels, and on mucosal surfaces. Its presence prevents excessive passage of water inward by osmosis and outward by transudation by virtue of its very long molecules of mucopolysaccharide (hyaluronic acid) which form a meshwork and act like a sponge in restricting the escape or absorption of water. This makes it necessary to re-examine the relation of mucus to ciliary streaming in the air passages. Instead of mucus being present for the benefit of cilia, and for the protection of the underlying mucosa from invading bacteria, the cilia are present primarily for the removal of excess mucus and transudate. Comparative anatomy and histology demonstrate that, as seen in the nose and paranasal sinuses, cilia are present only in those body cavities open to the ambient atmosphere and incapable of closure by muscular contraction (peristalsis) (Adams, 1964; Negus, 1964b). The "protective effect" of the mucociliary mechanism is thus seen to be certainly fortuitous and probably of minor importance.

Nose as Respiratory Control Mechanism. Goodale (1896) concluded after his study of respiration that, inasmuch as the manner of breathing of each individual is dependent upon a natural or acquired habit peculiar to the person in question, absolute figures of nasal pressure indicating that the respiratory function of the nose under consideration is normal or abnormal are out of the question even under wholly physiologic conditions. "Experiments instituted, therefore, for the purpose of comparing abnormal with normal pressure changes, must inevitably include considerable error, owing to the fallacy involved in attempting to obtain absolute results from relative and variable factors." This statement was true in 1898 and it remains true today. No progress was made toward the assessment of the hypothesis of nasal respiratory control function until Ogura and Stoksted (1958), realized that, to have any meaning, measurements of nasal pressure, flow, and conductance must be correlated in some manner with respiratory function as a whole.

Although for more than 100 years the rhinologist has based many of his therapeutic guidelines on the hypothesis that the valvular structures of the nose, pharynx, and glottis composed, in a "fail safe" series, an inlet valve for a central effector mechanism, he has been frustrated in getting "scientific proof" of this idea because of his inadequate understanding of fundamental physical facts. As a result, he has quailed before the icy statement of an occasional academician: "I am aware of no data that support the theory that the nasal chambers can have a significant influence on alveolar ventilation and on oxygenation of the cells of the body."

Nasal respiratory physiology has also suffered from an overeagerness on the part of some rhinologists to devise a "scientific" method of measuring isolated nasal function that not only would support the hypothesis of the nose as a control mechanism for respiration but that also would tell them what sort of a surgical manipulation should be done and upon what part of the nasal chamber it should be practiced.

Cybernetics. In discussing the cybernetics of respiration Defares (1966) compared its effector organization to a negative feedback mechanical control mechanism for maintaining a "steady-state" level of water in a tank, with inflow and outflow pipes permitting variations. The control mechanism adjusted the width of the inlet valve in relation to increased outlet flow to produce a new steady state level. He stated that from physiological experimentation it is apparent that, primarily, the control system involved in respiration operates like a system designed to keep alveolar (and thus arterial) carbon dioxide tension within narrow limits under varying conditions. Ultimately, of course, it is not the alveolar gas tension that is important but the resulting concentration in the tissues.

Rhinomanometry. Without hydrodynamics the rhinologist cannot subject his hypothesis of a relationship between nasal conductance and cellular metabolism to rigorous scientific tests for support or invalidation by rhinomanometry. Without such testing there can be no valid nasal respiratory physiology. Without valid understanding of nasal respiratory function it is extremely difficult, if not impossible, to soundly base either a medical or surgical therapeutic attack on those nasal diseases or disorders which seem to be associated with problems of air flow.

It is possible that lack of interest in understanding the physics of nasal respiration may have been a major factor in the decline of the relative position of rhinology in the former "triumvirate" of otology, rhinology, and otolaryngology? Can patient care be inadequate because of this information gap? Yet, at present, rhinomanometry is an investigative not a clinical tool (Wenzel and Sieck, 1966).

Inefficiency of Mouth Breathing. The cliché that mouth breathing compensates for all dysfunction caused by nasal airway obstructions seems to be a hardy but misleading half truth. Although mouth breathing is effective as an emergency measure to compensate for an extraordinary demand over a short period, for normal respiration over a long period mouth breathing is inefficient and leads to an increased expenditure of energy for a given alveolar ventilation. Hellman (1927) stated that the physiologic superiority of nose over mouth breathing lies in the slower deeper respiration that he found associated with the former. He suggested that inadequate mixing and mass transfer of inspiratory gas might interfere with maximum diffusion of O_2 in the pulmonary alveoli and that the slower deeper respiration associated with nasal breathing gives more and needed time for this process. This opinion has received support recently from Arnott, Cumming and Horsfield (1968). It has also been suggested by Pattle (1963) and by Williams, Tierney and Parker (1966) that deeper breathing dilates the more peripheral alveoli better and allows distribution of surfactant in them, both processes tending to prevent the development of micro-atelectasis.

Haldane, Meakins and Priestly (1919) found that shallow breathing causes anoxemia and that anoxemia causes shallow breathing, the body being in a vicious cycle which, if not broken, must inevitably cause death.

Manchioli (1942) found that more severe fatigue and exhaustion appeared more rapidly in laborers with relative inspiratory obstruction. Yasa (1939) found in tests on healthy boys before and after artificial occlusion of the nasal air passages that mouth breathing tends to produce dyspnea and early exhaustion on exertion.

Lüscher (1930) found a decrease in the alkali reserve of the blood from respiratory acidosis following occlusion of the nasal airway both by hypertrophied tonsils and in artificial occlusion of the nasal airways.

Noonan (1965) reported the presence of reversible cor pulmonale in patients in whom the nasopharyngeal airway was obstructed by the superiorly mounding upper roles of hypertrophied tonsils and by hypertrophied adenoids. This finding soon received confirmation from Luke and her associates (1966) and other pediatric groups.

The evidence seems adequate to support the statement that mouth breathing is unphysiologic under ordinary circumstances and can be considered normal only under conditions of emergency ventilatory demand.

Alar Collapse. Although it has been said that the cartilaginous skeleton of the lobule prevents the drawing in of the nasal wings except under "extreme conditions," this suggests both inadequate anatomical knowledge and lack of clinical observation.

The effect of the nasal respiratory muscles in maintaining nasal section was demonstrated by van Dishoeck. He called attention to the collapse of the homolateral ala on inspiration in Bell's palsy, in which the effect of absence of normal tonus in the nasal respiratory muscles may be plainly seen.

Bilateral alar collapse has been seen as a genetic trait in certain families. In son, father, and grandfather, although the crura of both lower lateral (lobular) cartilages appeared to be present on both sides, the alae nasi were equally drawn in on inspiration even in quiet respiration, producing subjective nasal obstruction and forcing mouth breathing. This type of maldevelopment may be more frequent than has been reported since the cause of difficulty has so frequently been unrecognized.

Resistance of the Nasal Airways to Invasion by Pathogenic Microorganisms. In considering the resistance of the airways to invasions by pathogenic microorganisms, is the abstraction "rhinosinusitis" a term which validly includes the nasal airways with the paranasal sinuses as a unit in this function or may some confusion be produced by ignoring differences and favoring similarities for increased taxonomic simplicity?

There seems to be some evidence that the latter may be the case.

Acute rhinosinusitis. As Negus (1958) pointed out, many bacteria which strike the mucus blanket become caught in its viscous surface and are transported to the pharynx and swallowed. Hilding (1967) assumes that most of them are destroyed in the stomach and intestines. Davison (1944, 1963, 1967) has found that deficiency in immune globulin (IgG) may favor recurring acute infection. Recurring infection is also found in the lethal granulomatous disease of children recently described by Smith and his associates (1968), in which there is a defect in the immunologic mechanism of the bursal-derived polymorphonuclear leukocyte. Recently this disorder has been described in the adult. These serious developmental deficiencies may also be associated with chronic disease in the airway.

Virologists point out, as Green (1968) stated, that a viral disease is a disease of cellular necrosis. Necrotic cells form excellent culture media for bacteria. Viruses also appear to stimulate the virulence of dormant or commensal bacteria that may be present. Therefore, in a viral rhinosinusitis, a bacterial factor is usually evident in from 24 to 48 hours. Even so, acute coryzas, generally conceded to be viral in origin, in most instances run an acute course and rarely result in chronic disease, either in the nasal chambers, the paranasal air sinuses, or elsewhere in the respiratory tract. In those patients in whom they become subacute, the use of antibiotics should be considered.

Chronic rhinosinusitis. After a series of experiments on dogs supplemented by observations on chronic disease of the paranasal sinuses in the human, Wilson (1915) stated that there are three elementary facts in regard to chronic bacterial inflammation of a sinus that should be so generally accepted that they become axiomatic: (1) no chronic bacterial inflammation can occur in a sinus unless its physiologic defense mechanisms are disturbed or destroyed; (2) it is not the physical presence of bacteria in the sinal lumen or even in its lymph or blood vascular system that induces chronic infection, but it is the functional condition of the tissue on which the bacteria are implanted that influences the future course of disease; and (3) the mucous membranes of the nasal chambers and sinuses are associated in their reaction to stress by a common mechanism, the nervous control of which is through the sphenopalatine ganglion.

Air Conditioning or the Effect of Passage Through the Nasal Airways of the Respired Air with Regard to Heat and Moisture

From the standpoint of physics the alveolar membrane may be considered a water film for the diffusion of the respiratory gases. The preservation of this water film is necessary for respiration and for life. Therefore, the air that reaches the alveolus must be saturated with water vapor. This need, as was mentioned previously, is evidence of our marine origin and from a teleologic viewpoint can be considered a major factor in the development of the human nose. As was also said before, the primate nose appears to have regressed to a point at which it cannot supply sufficient water for saturation of the inspired air even under average conditions.

Goodale (1896) pointed out, however, that many estimations of the humidifying power of the nose were made without regard to the conditions of temperature and humidity of the ambient air, "although it will readily be seen that the consideration of these two factors is important." He found, in general, that while the nose nearly saturates the inspiratory stream that passes through it, owing to the fact of intranasal temperature being cooler than body temperature, it contributes only about two thirds of the water necessary to maintain the alveolar water film intact.

On computing the energy expended by the nose he found that about 11.05 gm./cal. were used during each respiratory cycle in raising the temperature of inspired air from 1 to 27° C. He also drew attention to the antipyretic effect of breathing cold dry air, stating that there is not only a continuous abstraction of heat without disturbance of the patient but also one of primary affection of a portion of the body which it is particularly desirable to cool in febrile conditions. He believed that the relation of pathological conditions within the nose to changes in heat and moisture of the respiratory current were of importance in those affections in which the nose performs *less* than its customary share of work. Atrophy of luminal mucosa from disease or surgical manipulation and nasal disorders that produced mouth breathing are unfortunate in setting "the normal functions of the nose in abeyance."

The findings of Goodale have been repeatedly confirmed, although there has been some disagreement as to the relative importance of the nose in supplying moisture to the inspired air. Cramer (1957) stated that his experiments indicated that under ordinary conditions of relative humidity in ambient air a laryngectomized patient can humidify inspired air as efficiently as a person breathing through a normal nose. This was not true, however, when central heating which had not been corrected had created an atmosphere detrimental to the respiratory tract.

Effect of Dry Ambient Air

Because of the obvious inability of these structures to cope with the added stress of dry air, Cramer proffered the generalization that the nasal mucosa functions chiefly as a regulator of body heat, humidification being a local factor of minor importance to the airway as a whole. Scott (1954) suggested that the regression of the primate nose mentioned by Negus might be explained by the substitution of the sweat glands and subepithelial capillaries of the primate skin for the nasal structures in temperature control.

Ballenger (1925) observed that the nose reacts to the environmental insult of dry air by decrease of conductance because of bilateral engorgement of the turbinal erectile tissues. This may result in mouth breathing. Then the increased demand on the tissues of the mouth, pharynx, larynx, and trachea will produce chronic irritation and inflammation.

Holmes (1914) stated that when for any reason the middle turbinate and lower wall of the ethmoid are sacrificed "there results a deformity which practically produces all the ill effects of mouth breathing. The inspired air is not sufficiently warmed or moistened and there almost always follows a chronic dry pharyngitis and a chronic laryngitis." Koch and his associates (1958) stated that most pulmonary complications following tracheostomy appear during the postoperative period and are favored by the insufficient humidification of the inspired air produced by exclusion of the nasal airway. This results in impaired ciliary activity, increased viscosity of secretion, and decreased resistance to bacterial invasion.

Brown (1951) advocated that a relative humidity of 35 to 45 per cent be maintained in the homes of asthmatic children. He mentioned that the state of our health is a very subtle evaluation, and we are usually not aware of not being in full health unless a derangement or alteration occurs which is of considerable magnitude or degree. Also, that we tend to forget or ignore the differences in the adaptive capacities of different individuals or different groups of people whose bodies cannot take the punishment of a hostile, arid environment. Some must leave a frigid, sere environment, control it adequately, or suffer from disease and shortened lives.

It seems evident, therefore, that even if the nose is not wholly competent to saturate the inspired air at body temperature, its role is still an important one. It should not, however, be asked to perform beyond its capabilities. Humidification of dry, centrally heated air should not only aid the recovery of those with infections of the respiratory tract but should be considered a prophylactic health measure.

RELATION OF INFECTION IN THE PARANASAL SINUSES TO THE INFECTIVE BRONCHITIC TYPE OF CHRONIC OBSTRUCTIVE PULMONARY DISEASE

The typical attitude of the rhinologist in the past toward the relationship of infections in the paranasal sinuses to those in the lung was expressed by Schenck (1941) in a paper on the etiology of bronchiectasis. He stated that the concept that sinus infection is primary and bronchial infection is secondary is supported by experimental evidence which shows that infectious material is readily carried from the upper to the lower respiratory tract. He concluded that treatment of chronic suppurative disease of the lower respiratory tract is doomed to failure if it does not include thorough treatment of sinus infection. However, he added that cure of the diseased sinuses will not always be followed by the arrest of the pulmonary lesions, and once the bronchial disease is well established, eradication of the sinusitis will not arrest the disease.

There were many other similar and equally ambiguous statements made which seemed to promise amazingly good results from sinal surgery, when chronic sinusitis and chronic bronchitis are associated, on the one hand, while warning that too much therapeutic effect on the pulmonary disease should not be expected from sinal surgery, on the other. This dichotomy in the opinions expressed resulted from the incomplete understanding of the rhinologist as to both the chronic "hyperplastic" type of sinusitis usually present and the semantics of pulmonary disease.

The latter fault usually resulted in the opinion that bronchiectasis and chronic bronchitis are in no respect synonymous and that bronchiectasis is a localized and never diffuse condition. Neither of these ideas appears to be consistent with the present thinking of most of those specializing in the diseases of the chest.

The matter was brought to a head when Dixon and Hoerr (1944 a and b) performed a series of experiments which they said demonstrated the invalidity of the experiments of Mullin (1919, 1926) and of Fenton and Larsell (1937), which Schenck had mentioned in support of his opinions. When this was added to the fact that in many patients with "bronchiectasis" chronic suppuration in the paranasal sinuses was apparently not present, grave doubts as to any relationship whatever was raised.

It was Davison's (1944) opinion that when bronchiectasis and chronic sinusitis coexist, the sinusitis and the bronchiectasis both started at the time of the initial combined upper and lower respiratory tract infection in infancy or childhood. In 45 patients with "bronchiectasis" he studied, Davison made a diagnosis of chronic sinusitis in 23. In 20 patients with extensive sinusitis of dental origin of from one to ten years' duration, none had any bronchopulmonary symptoms despite the fact that they had purulent discharge in the nasopharynx both by day and by night. It seemed apparent to him that some mechanism other than the mere presence of bacteria is required to produce bronchiectasis, and he thought this factor might well be mucosal edema on the basis of allergic hypersensitivity with obstruction of bronchi by gummy exudate from hyperplasia and hypersecretion of the mucus-secreting glands. Clerf (1934) noted that while sinal infection was infrequent in the cases of unilateral bronchiectasis he studied, 82 per cent of his patients with bilateral bronchiectasis also had chronic sinusitis.

It would seem that more progress might be made in considering the relationship of sinal disease to bronchopulmonary disease if the term and concept of bronchiectasis were excluded since it seems to mislead by obscuring the point at issue by distracting debate as to the definition, anatomical background, and pathology of this disorder. If we substitute chronic suppurative bronchopulmonary disease, the focus becomes clearer and resolution more definite. Feingold (1959) pointed out the role of infection in bronchial allergic disease in children. Diamond and Van Loon (1942) found chronic sinal disease in 64 per cent of children with bronchiectasis and 61 per cent of children with chronic trachobronchitis. Horesh believed that he had established a cause and effect relationship between "allergy" and infection in childhood. Voorhorst (1962) believed that chronic bronchopulmonary infection developed on the basis of lowered resistance produced by perennial atopies to house dust, mold spores, and human dander. The "allergic" edema so disturbed the resistance mechanism that it allowed the establishment of *Haemophilus influenzae* as the "resident flora" in an attenuated or commensal form. Van Dishoeck confirmed the relationship of allergic hypersensitivity with infection in sinuses in which, eventually, the "hyperplastic" sinusitis of Uffenorde was established.

The upper and lower respiratory tracts are a continuum, and debate as to which is first in showing evidence of the combination of chronic infection and hypersensitivity is as unrewarding as debate about the priority of chicken or egg. There can be little doubt that infection in one influences infection in the other. Of equal certainty is that both "hyperplastic" sinusitis and chronic suppurative bronchitis, in most instances, constitute a so-called spectrum disorder or disease sui generis termed "bronchosinusitis infection" by Wasson (1929), in which the final picture is made up of both hypersensitivity and infection, and probably endocrine factors also, which are present to different degrees in different patients.

Sasaki and Kirschner (1967) recently repeated the experiments of Mullin (1926) of Fenton and Larsell (1937), and of Dixon and Hoerr (1944). They supported the conclusions of Mullin and of Larsell and Fenton and added an additional pathway of infection from sinuses to lung. They concluded that the probable routes of infection involved in the sinobronchial syndrome are: (1) tracheal aspiration; (2) the lymphatic-hematogenous route of Mullin; and (3) a purely lymphatic pathway.

Recently Cowan (1968) stated: "Symptomatic relief of a patient with both paranasal sinus pathology and associated bronchopulmonary change can become almost complete with detailed, diligent and strict allergic management alone. However, this symptomatic relief is *not* attended by a reversal of chronic mucous membrane disease of the sinuses. Exacerbations recur and the persistent, latent, paranasal sinus pathology can and does continue to produce antigenic stimulation and the ultimate return of some relatively major broncho-sinusitis problems, whether it be some type of chronic bronchitis, broncho-spastic disease, obstructive emphysema or frank bronchiectasis."

From the available evidence an interrelation between hyperplastic sinusitis and chronic bronchopulmonary infections seems not only reasonable but obvious. Dissatisfaction has been the result of overenthusiasm for some single therapeutic approach, such as the idea that surgery alone can accomplish the impossible task of "curing" both the infection and the allergy. Dogged insistence that medical treatment alone will restore full health has also caused unnecessary invalidism. The facts seem to be that in some instances medical treatment will attain an essential cure. Too often, however, a dormant infection is present which will be repeatedly lighted up. A hypersensitivity, probably to breakdown products of the bacterial wall, will be set up which will gradually replace the initial perennial atopies. Surgical intervention may then be needed. Surgery, however, is not curative in itself. It merely affords an improved opportunity for a success from a combined specific and nonspecific treatment for both the hypersensitivity and the infection.

CONCLUSIONS

Our knowledge of the physiology of the nose and the upper respiratory tract as a whole is slowly approaching a closer approximation to reality, but there are still wide areas of challenge to rhinologic research. Progress was hobbled for a time by fashionable adoption of the doctrinaire position that clinical observation and experience is an unacceptable basis for laboratory research and that intuitive appreciation must of necessity be incorrect. The changing attitude of science, in general, toward this position is permeating research in rhinology, so that a healthier, less restrictive outlook has developed.

The doctrine which so gladdens the indolent sceptic, that only the proponent of an idea needs to find support for it while an antagonist need only present a smug nonacceptance, is becoming suspect as a mere intellectual stratagem. It is now incumbent on an opponent to produce nullifying data if he is to justify active opposition as something more than a "ploy" or fixation of thought in a well worn rut.

From the data now available, however, a number of reasonable assumptions and justified conclusions seem possible.

First: Because of its position at the entrance to the airway system and because of its valvular structure, the hypothesis that the human nose plays an important role in the control of respiration seems not without merit. Although some supporting data are at hand, more rigorous experimental validation is needed. Measurements of driving pressure, resistance, flow, and conductance, to have significance, must be correlated with alveolar ventilation and respiration of the entire organism. Second: It has been shown that the most important factor in resistance to nasal air flow is turbulence. Therefore, increased resistance to nasal air flow depends much more on interference with the stream lines in the nasal lumina than on the nasal cross-section. Testing the airway conductance before and after the use of nasal vasoconstrictors adds surprisingly little to the ability of a rhinologist to relieve a patient's nasal complaints. Third: the facts of resistance and conductance in the nasal airways have not received proper consideration in planning surgical and semisurgical procedures designed to improve the passage of air through the nasal chambers. Fourth: Undue emphasis has been placed on the air conditioning function of the nasal chambers and on the activity of the cilia. Although these functions are important, they are probably secondary. Fifth: It is important for the well-being of the specialty of otology-rhinology-laryngology that nasal physiology be recognized and developed. With new curricula in the medical schools the relationship of the specialty to the basic subject of respiration must be emphasized if the undergraduate medical student is to become aware that there is a "pathway" such as ours.

REFERENCES

Adams, F. H.: Functional development of the fetal lung. J. Pediat. 68:794–801, 1966.

Amoore, J. E.: Identification of the seven primary odors. Proc. Scient. Soc. Toilet Goods Association (Supplement) 37:1–12, 1962.

Arnott, W. M., Cumming, G., and Horsfield, K.: Alveolar ventilation. Ann. Intern. Med. 69:1–12, 1968.

Ballenger, W. L.: Diseases of the Nose, Throat and Ear. 5th ed. New York, Lea and Febiger, 1925.

Bazarov, V. G.: Quoted by Wenzel and Sieck.

Bellanti, J. A.: Role of loca gamma-A-immunoglobulins in immunity. Amer. J. Dis. Child. 115:239–246, 1968.

Brown, E. A.: Nasal function and nasal neurosis. Ann. Allerg. 9:563–567, 1951.

Burnham, H.: An anatomical investigation of blood vessels of the lateral nasal wall. J. Laryng. 50:569–595, 1935.

Burnham, H.: Clinical study of inferior turbinate cavernous tissue; its divisions and their significance. Canada Med. Ass. J. 44:477–481, 1941.

Clerf, L. H.: The interrelationship of sinus disease and bronchiectasis with special reference to prognosis. Laryngoscope 44:568–571, 1934.

Connell, J. T.: Reciprocal nasal congestion–decongestion reflex. Trans. Amer. Acad. Ophthal. Otolaryng. 72:18–25, 1968.

Courant, R., and John, F.: Introduction to Calculus and Analysis. Vol. I. New York, Interscience Publishers, 1965.

Cowen, D. E.: The relationship of allergic and infectious chest conditions to the upper respiratory tract. Trans. Amer. Acad. Ophthal. Otolaryng. 72:943–958, 1968.

Craig, A. B., Jr., Dvorak, M., and McIreath, F. J.: Resistance to airflow through the nose. Ann. Otol. 74:589–603, 1965.

Cramer, J. J.: Heat and moisture exchange of respiratory mucous membrane. Ann. Otol. 66:327–343, 1957.

Davison, F. W.: Does chronic sinusitis cause bronchiectasis? Ann. Otol. 53:849–854, 1944.

Davison, F. W.: Hyperplastic sinusitis—a five year study. Trans. Amer. Laryng. Ass. 84:75–90, 1963.

Davison, F. W.: Chronic sinus and bronchopulmonary disease: The relationship. Minnesota Med. 50:855–858, 1967.

Defares, J. G.: Principles of feedback control and their application to the respiratory control system. Chapter 26, pp. 649–680 in Hdbk Physiol. Section 3, Respiration Vol. II. Section editors, W. O. Fenn and H. Rahn. Washington, D.C., American Physiology Society, 1966.

Diamond, S., and Van Loon, E. S.: Bronchiectasis in childhood. J.A.M.A. 118:771–778, 1942.

Dishoeck, H.A.E., van: Modern olfactometry. Personal communication.

Dixon, F. W., and Hoerr, N. B.: The lymphatics of the nose and paranasal sinuses. Laryngoscope 54:165–175, 1944a.

Dixon, F. W., and Hoerr, N. B.: The lymphatic drainage of the paranasal sinuses. Trans. Amer. Laryng. Rhinol., Otol. Soc. 49:200–212, 1944b.

Drettner, B.: Pressure recordings in the maxillary sinus. Rhinol. Internat. 3:13–18, 1965.

Farrior, J. B.: Moderator, symposium on management of atelectatic middle ear. Arch. Otolaryng. 89:199–200, 1969.

Feingold, B.: Infection in bronchial allergic disease. Pediat. Clin. N. Amer. 6:709–718, 1959.

Fenton, R. A., and Larsell, O.: Defense mechanisms of the upper respiratory tract. Ann. Otol. 46:303–312, 1937.

Fleming, A.: On a remarkable bacteriolytic element found in the tissues and secretions. Proc. Roy. Soc. (Ser. B.) 93:306–317, 1921–1922.

Gardner, W. J., Stowell, A., and Duttinger, R.: Resection

of the greater petrosal nerve in the treatment of unilateral headache. Neurosurgery *4*:105–114, 1947.

Goodale, J. L.: An experimental study of the respiratory function of the nose. Boston Med. Surg. J. *135*:457, 487, 1896.

Goodale, R. L.: Management of sinusitis in cases of bronchiectasis. Arch. Otolaryng. *34*:792–796, 1941.

Green, R. N.: The role of viral infection in the etiology and pathogenesis of chronic bronchitis and emphysema with consideration of a naturally occurring animal model. Yale J. Biol. Med. *40*:461–476, 1968.

Groner, R.: The nose, relais of encounter and self image. Rhinol. Internat. *1*:58–64, (July), 1963.

Guillerm, R., Badre, R., Riv. R., Le Den, R., and Fallot, P.: La rhinorheographie. Rev. Laryng. (Bordeaux) *3* (Suppl.) 45–60, 1967.

Haldane, J. S., Meakins, J. C., and Priestly, J. G.: The response of anoxaemia. J. Physiol. *52*:433–453, 1919.

Hellman, K.: Untersuchungen zur normalen und pathologieschen Physiologie der Nase. Z. Laryng. *15*:1–25, 1927. Also, Investigation of the functions of the nose. J. Laryngol. Otol. *42*:413–422, 1927.

Heetderks, D. L.: Observations on the reactions of normal nasal mucous membrane. Amer. J. Med. Sci. *174*:231, 1927.

Hilding, A. C.: Experimental surgery of nose and sinuses. The effects of operative windows on normal sinuses. Ann. Otol. *50*:379–392, 1941.

Hilding, A. C.: The role of the respiratory mucosa in health and disease. Minnesota Med. *50*:915–919, 1967.

Holmes, E. M.: Clinical classification of ethmoiditis. J.A.M.A. *63*:2097–2100, 1914.

Jabonero, V.: Der anatomische Aufbau des peripheren vegetativen Systems. Vienna, Springer, 1953.

Kayser, R. L.: Über den Weg der Atmungluft durch die Nase. Arch. Laryngol. *3*:101–118, 1895.

Keuning, J.: On the nasal cycle. Rhinol. Internat. *6*:99–136, 1968.

Kloek, J.: The smell of some steroid sex hormones and their metabolites. Reflections and experiments concerning the significance of smell for the mutual relation of the sexes. Psychiat. Neurol. Neurochir. *64*:309–344, 1961.

Koch, H., Claes, A., Inglestedt, S., and Toremalm, N.Y.: A method for humidifying inspired air in post-tracheotomy care. Ann. Otol. *67*:991–1004, 1958.

Lillie, H. I.: Some practical considerations of the physiology of the upper respiratory tract. J. Iowa Med. Soc. *13*:403–408, 1923.

Lucas, A. M., and Douglas, L. C.: Principles underlying ciliary activity in the respiratory tract. II. A comparison of nasal clearance in man, monkey and other mammals. Arch. Otolaryng. *20*:518–541, 1934.

Luke, M. J., Mehrizi, A., Folger, G. M., and Rowe, R. O.: Chronic nasopharyngeal obstruction causing cor pulmonale. Pediatrics *37*:762–768, 1966.

Lüscher, E.: Die Alkalireserve des Blutes bei behinderter Nasenatmung und bei Tonsillen hyperplasie. Acta Otolaryng. *14*:90–101, 1930.

Majer, E. H.: Possible vascular regulating mechanisms in the mucous membrane of the upper respiratory tract. Acta Otolaryng. *65*:59–62, 1968.

Manchioli, G.: Importanza della respirazione nasale nei lavoratori. Rass. Med. Industry *13*:36–45, 1942.

Mink, P. J.: Das Speil der Nasenflügel. Arch. Ges. Physiol. *120*:210–218, 1907.

Mink, P. J.: Über die Funktion der Nebenhohlen der Nase. Arch. Laryng. Rhinol. *29*:453–461, 1915.

Mink, P. J.: Die Role des kavernosen Gewebes in der Nase. Arch. Laryngol. Rhinol. *30*:47–58, 1916.

Mink, P. J.: Physiologie der obern Luftwege. Leipzig, F. C. W. Vogel, 1920.

Morrison, L. E.: A Simple Accurate Method of Office Olfactometry. Unpublished data.

Mullin, W. V.: The lymph drainage of the accessory nasal sinuses. Trans. 25th Ann. Meet. Amer. Laryng. Rhinol. Otol. Soc. *73*:103, 1919.

Mullin, W. V.: Relationship of paranasal sinus infection to diseases of the lower respiratory tract. J.A.M.A. *87*:739–743, 1926.

Myerson, M. C.: The natural orifice of the maxillary sinus. Arch. Otolaryng. *15*:680–761, 1932.

Negus, V.: The airconditioning mechanism of the nose. Brit. Med. J. *4963*:367–371, 1956.

Negus, V.: Observations on the exchange of fluid in the nose and respiratory tract. Ann. Otol. *66*:344–363, 1957.

Negus, V.: The Comparative Anatomy and Physiology of the Nose and Paranasal Sinuses. London, E. & S. Livingstone, Ltd., 1958.

Negus, V.: The action of bronchial muscles. Acta Otolaryng. *57*:404–409, 1964.

Negus, V. E.: The function of mucus. Ann. Roy. Coll. Surg. *34*:400–403, 1964b.

Noonan, J. A.: Reversible cor pulmonale due to hypertrophied tonsils and adenoids: Studies in two cases. Trans. Amer. Pediat. Soc. (Abstract). *48*, 1965.

Ogura, J. H., and Stoksted, Paul: Rhinomanometry in some rhinologic diseases. Laryngoscope *68*:2001–2014, 1958.

Ogura, J. H., Unno, T., and Nelson, J. R.: Baseline values in pulmonary mechanics for physiologic surgery of the nose. Preliminary report. Ann. Otol. *77*:367–397, 1968.

Pattle, R. E.: The lining layer of the lung aveoli. Brit. Med. Bull. *19*:41–44, 1963.

Proetz, A. W.: Applied Physiology of the Nose. St. Louis, Annals Publishing Co., 1953.

Proetz, A. W.: Humidity: A problem in air conditioning. Ann. Otol. *65*:376–384, 1956.

Reynolds, O.: An experimental investigation of the circumstances which determine whether a motion of water shall be direct or sinuous and of the law of resistance in parallel channels. Philosophical Transactions, London. *174*:935–982, 1883.

Rouviere, H. (American translation by Mathias): Anatomy of the Human Lymphatic System. Ann Arbor, Edwards Bros., Inc., 1938.

Sasaki, C. T., and Kirchner, J. A.: A lymphatic pathway from the sinuses to the mediastinum. Arch. Otolaryng. *85*:432–444, 1967.

Schaeffer, J. P.: The Nose and Paranasal Sinuses. Philadelphia, Blakeston, Inc., 1920.

Schaeffer, J. P.: The anatomy of the paranasal sinuses in children. Arch. Otolaryng. *15*:657–659, 1932.

Schenck, Harry: Etiology of bronchiectasis. Arch. Otolaryng. *34*:958–968, 1941.

Scott, J. H.: Heat regulating function of the nasal mucous membrane. J. Laryng. *68*:308–312, 1954.

Semenov, H.: Personal communication.

Slome, D.: Physiology of nasal circulation. *In* Scott Brown, D. G. (ed.): Physiology of the Nose and Paranasal Sinuses in Diseases of the Ear, Nose and Throat. 2nd ed. London, Butterworth, Ltd., 1966.

South, M. A., Cooper, M. D., Wolheim, F. A., Hong, R., and Good, R. A.: IgA System. II. Clinical significance of IgA deficiency. Studies in patients with agammaglobulinemia and ataxia telangiectasia. Am. J. Med. *44*:168–178 (Feb.), 1968.

Spoor, A.: Aerodynamics. Rhinol. Internat. *1*:19–22, 1963.

Spoor, A.: Nasal conductivity. Proc. Otorhinolaryng. *29*:315, 1967.

Stoksted, P.: The physiologic cycle of the nose under normal and pathological conditions. Acta Otolaryng. *42*:175–179, 1952.

Stoksted, P.: Etude rhinometrique du cycle nasal. Acta Otolaryng. (Suppl.) *109*:143–181, 1953.

Stoksted, P.: Obstructions in the nose and their influence on pulmonary functions. Acta Otolaryngol. (Suppl.) *158*:110–132, 1960.

Stoksted, P., and Nielson, J. Z.: Rhinomanometric measurements of the nasal passage. Ann. Otol. *66*:187–197, 1957.

Stoksted, P., and Thomsen, K. A.: Changes in the nasal cycle under stellate ganglion block. Acta Otolaryng. (Suppl.) *109*:176–181, 1953.

Streeter, V. L.: Fluid Mechanics. 2nd ed. New York, McGraw-Hill Book Co., Inc., 1958.

Szentivanyi, A.: The beta adrenergic theory of the atopic abnormality in broncheal asthma. J. Allerg. *42*:203–232, 1968.

Temesrakasi, D. von: Neurohistologische Angaben zur Function der unteren Nasenmuschel des Menschen. Pract. Otorhinolaryng. *21*:254-263, 1959.

Terracol, J.: Les vaisseaux glomerulaires de la cloison nasale. Rév. Laryng. *79*:902, 1958.

Tomasi, T. B., Tan, E. M., Soloman, A., and Pendergast, R. A.: Characteristics of immune system common to certain external secretions. J. Exp. Med. *121*:101-124, 1965.

Voorhorst, R.: Basic Facts of Allergy. Leiden, Stenfert-Kroese, 1962.

Wasson, W. W.: Incipiency of disease. Radiology *13*:29-35, 1929.

Weille, F. L.: The problem of secondary frontal sinus surgery. Ann. Otol. *55*:372-397, 1946.

Wenzel, B. M., and Sieck, M. H.: Olfaction. Ann. Rec. Physiol. *28*:381-434, 1966.

Williams, H. L.: The nose as form and function. Ann. Otol. *78*:725-741, 1969.

Williams, J. A., Tierney, D. F., and Parker, H. R.: Surface forces in the lung, atelectasis and transpulmonary pressure. J. App. Physiol. *21*:819-827, 1966.

Wilson, J. G.: The etiology of pansinusitis. Laryngoscope *25*:823-831, 1915.

Wright, G.: The contractile elements in the connective tissue in the elastic fibers in the nasal mucosa in health and disease. J. Med. N.Y. *19*:729-735, 1910.

Yasa, K.: Atemphysiologische Untersuchungen über die. Störung der Nasenatmung III. Mitt. J. Orient. Med. *30*:122-131, 1939.

Chapter 10

PHYSIOLOGY OF THE THROAT

PHYSIOLOGY OF THE SALIVARY GLANDS

by
George A. Gates, M.D.

The primary function of the salivary glands is to generate an adequate volume of saliva, which serves to maintain oral and dental hygiene; to prepare food for mastication, taste sensation, and deglutition; and to initiate the preliminary phase of carbohydrate digestion. By their indirect influence upon thirst sensation, the salivary glands participate to a limited extent in fluid balance by regulating water intake. Although the appearance of certain substances in saliva (e.g., toxic chemicals, viruses) may occasionally be of clinical significance, excretion of metabolites into saliva occurs to a limited extent and is not a significant factor in the maintenance of body homeostasis. Absence of salivary gland function creates a serious oral disability without systemic effects.

Saliva is a nonhomogenous fluid whose volume and composition differ from gland to gland and even from the same gland, depending on the nature of the stimulus, the rate of salivary flow, the method of collection, and the prestimulus condition of the gland. Production of saliva is a complex process involving the secretion and resorption of water and electrolytes, as well as the synthesis and excretion of a variety of organic compounds. Although much is known about the physiology of the salivary glands, many basic questions about the production of saliva and the regulation of secretion remain unanswered.

PRODUCTION OF SALIVA

Secretory Structure. The functional salivary unit consists of an acinus, a secretory tubule, and a collecting duct. The structural relationships and secretory capabilities of these units within each salivary gland differ widely among the several salivary glands. The major salivary glands, which are located at some distance from the oral cavity, exhibit a specialized and branched ductal system. By contrast, the minor salivary glands have a short rudimentary ductal system. Both the parotid and submandibular glands have a single, elongated, large-caliber collecting duct with but a few major branches, the interlobular ducts. These are connected to many intralobular ducts, each of which transport saliva from several acini through the small intercalated ducts. The intralobular and proximal interlobular ducts are designated as the secretory tubules in this chapter in order to emphasize their important role in salt and water transport. The sublingual gland secretions are discharged through 10 to 12 separate collecting ducts. The parotid acini are composed solely of serous cells, the sublingual acini are predominantly mucous, and the submandibular acini contain both cell types. Myoepithelial cells surround the acini and proximal ducts and, like the contractile mammary myoepithelial cells, serve to

347

expel preformed secretions (Shear, 1966). The minor salivary glands are small groups of secreting units distributed throughout the submucosa of the oral cavity. Their acinar cells are serous, mucous, or both, and their collecting ducts are short and convoluted. Little is known about the secretory capabilities of the minor salivary gland ductal system.

Acinar cell ultrastructure exhibits cytoplasmic organelles common to secretory cells: a ribosomal-coated endoplasmic reticulum, Golgi bodies, and secretory vesicles. The secretory vesicles are intracellular containers of the protein which is manufactured by the ribosomes, transported apically by the endoplasmic reticulum, and packaged by the Golgi bodies. Ductal cells contain prominent basal striations formed by infoldings of the plasma membrane which enclose columns of mitochondria. The basal infoldings increase the absorptive surface of the plasma membrane across which active transport of electrolytes is effected by the ATP-enzyme system contained in the mitochondria (Tandler, 1963).

Secretory Processes. The earliest theories of saliva formation held that saliva was an acinar ultrafiltrate of plasma, a basically passive process. Present-day concepts recognize that saliva is formed by cellular synthesis and active transport, the energy for which is provided by oxidative reduction of monosaccharides, principally glucose. The pyruvic acid so formed enters the citrate cycle where it is aerobically converted to carbon dioxide, water, and energy by the cytochrome system. At low flow rates aerobic metabolism predominates, but at high flow rates anaerobic conversion of pyruvate to lactate occurs, resulting in an increase in the lactic acid and a decrease in the glucose content of saliva (Chauncey and Shannon, 1965).

Saliva formation proceeds at two distinct levels: the proximal or acinar level, and the distal or tubular level. Proximally a primary secretion is formed whose osmolality and major electrolyte composition are similar to plasma. In the tubule, hypertonic resorption of electrolytes secondarily modifies the primary secretion and a hypotonic fluid results. The common conception that the acinar cells are the principal source of salivary secretion is no longer tenable in view of considerable evidence that the events occurring in the tubule largely determine the final composition of saliva. In fact, salivation can occur in the absence of acinar cells; before acini develop in the newborn puppy and rat, ductal secretion alone produces as abundant a saliva as in the mature animal (Schneyer and Schneyer, 1961). The human salivary glands, like those of many species, elaborate a secretion which differs significantly from plasma in osmolality and electrolyte composition. In general, it is hypo-osmolar, low in sodium and chloride, and rich in potassium, iodide, bicarbonate, and phosphates.

Primary secretion. It is generally assumed that most of the organic components of saliva are secreted by the acinar cells, whose histologic characteristics resemble those of other protein-secreting cells. The products of the secretory cells have been identified by direct means in a few instances. The secretory granules of the parotid gland are rich in amylase and DNA-ase. (Schramm and Danon, 1961). Glynn and Holborow (1959) studied the distribution of blood group-specific substances in human salivary tissue by Coombs fluorescent antibody technique and demonstrated strong staining in the submandibular mucous acini and an absence of staining in serous acini or in duct cells. Glycoprotein molecules have been identified by electron microscopy in the submandibular acini of several species (Gallagher et al., 1969).

Autonomic stimulation results in the extrusion of the secretory granules into the acinar lumen, and for distal transport to occur the acini must also secrete a sufficient volume of fluid. This fluid, which is known as the primary secretion, is plasmalike in composition and is probably formed by the acini and the intercalated duct (Young et al., 1967). Theories regarding the formation of the primary fluid include pinocytosis (Lewis, 1931) and active ionic transport. Pinocytosis describes the process whereby interstitial fluid imbibed by basal pseudopods is transported through the cell in vesicle form, absorbing potassium and organic solutes along the way, and is expelled apically into the acinar lumen and intracellular spaces (Yoshimura, 1967). On the other hand, the electrical properties of the acinar cell indicate that active ion transport is involved in the secretory process. Unlike nerve or muscle cells which depolarize upon stimulation, salivary acinar cells respond to autonomic stimulation by hyperpolarization of the basal membrane (Lundberg, 1955). Lundberg explained this secretory potential by postulating the existence of a chloride pump which actively transports chloride ions into the cell, thereby increasing intracellular electronegativity (Lundberg, 1957). Sodium and water passively follow the electrochemical gradient and increase the intracellular hydrostatic pressure sufficiently to force the outward discharge of fluid at the apical end. More recent work, however, indicates that the secretory potential results from outward diffusion of potassium secondary to a stimulation-induced increase in cell membrane permeability (Yoshimura, 1967). This correlates with the observations of Burgen (1956a) concerning the marked depletion of intracellular potassium during stimulation and the hypertonic potassium concentration in primary saliva of certain glands.

The intracellular sodium and potassium concentration gradients of nearly all cells are maintained by an active cation transport system located in the cell membrane known as the sodium-potassium pump. The presence in parotid tissue of adenosine triphosphatase (ATPase), which is identified with this system (Filsell and Jarrett, 1965), supports the contention that active cation transport does occur in the salivary glands. Its role in the secretory process is indicated by the finding that saliva extruded from the stimulated gland pretreated with ouabain contains more potassium and less sodium than control glands (Schneyer and Schneyer, 1965). Ouabain, a cardiac glycoside, specifically inhibits active cation transport.

Although the mechanisms involved in acinar secretion are not fully delineated, it would appear that active transport of cations and anions, as well as stimulation-induced changes in cell membrane potassium permeability, are important determinants of salivary secretion. The dualistic effect of secretory stimuli upon the volume and solute concentration of saliva is mediated by the physiological differences in acinar and tubular secretion; net fluid transfer into the saliva probably occurs only into the primary secretion, which remains isotonic even at different flow rates (Young et al., 1967), whereas in the ductal system the principal effect is upon tonicity, which varies significantly with the flow rate.

Ductal secretion. The functional capabilities of the secretory tubule cells of the proximal ductal system are complex, varied, and only partially understood. Secretion of electrolytes, water, and organic solutes as well as resorption of electrolytes and water have been demonstrated by both direct and indirect means. The relationships between secretion and resorption, which presumably proceed simultaneously at varying rates in different levels of the ductal system, are not well defined and, in general, only the net effect on saliva has been measured. The net change in electrolyte concentration at the tubular level is closely related to the rate at which the precursor fluid flows past the luminal face of the striated cell. At low flow rates there is a relatively long time period in which ion transfer across the

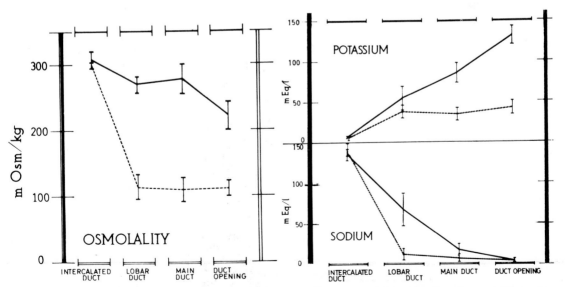

Figure 1. The salivary values of osmolality (left) and for potassium (upper right) and sodium (lower right) are shown at various levels in the ductal system of the rat's submandibular gland. Solid line = resting saliva; dashed line = pilocarpine stimulated saliva. (Young, et al.: Micropuncture and Perfusion Studies of Fluid and Electrolyte Transport in the Rat Submaxillary Glands. New York, Academic Press, 1967.)

tubular cell can alter the luminal fluid. At higher flow rates the contact time is shortened, thereby diminishing the effect of tubular cell secretion and resorption upon solute concentration. Whether the rate of ion transfer is constant or varies with the stimulus intensity can only be conjectured about at the present time.

Young et al. (1967) analyzed ductal fluid at several levels in the rat submandibular gland under resting and pilocarpine-stimulated conditions. Comparing the primary secretion to end saliva, they demonstrated that sodium concentration fell from 150 mEq./L. to 5 mEq/L., potassium rose from 10 mEq./L. to 40 mEq./L., and the total osmolality declined from 300 mOsm./μg. to 100 mOsm./μg. (Fig. 1). Hypertonic resorption of sodium occurred primarily in the intralobular duct and continued, at a lesser rate, in the main duct. Secretion of potassium into the intercalated duct fluid increased markedly following stimulation and continued in the larger ducts as well. The rise in sodium concentration at higher flow rates reflects the decreased contact time in the resorptive segments. The rise in potassium from 6 mEq./L. in the intercalated duct to 31 mEq./L. in the final saliva suggests that considerable ductal secretion of potassium occurs. At very low flow rates, steady state potassium concentration levels as high as 130 mEq./L. were seen; but at higher flow rates, the concentration decreased.

The secretory ability of the ductal epithelium was demonstrated by Burgen et al. (1960), who studied the salivary outflow patterns following the intra-arterial injection of radioactive isotopes. Minute quantities of labeled water (T_2O), chloride, bromide, iodide, sulfate, bicarbonate, sodium, potassium, urea, and four amino acids (valine, methionine, isoleucine, and tyrosine) were injected into the arterial supply of the dog parotid while the gland was secreting at a steady rate, and the times at which they appeared in the saliva were measured. Since the blood flow in the periductal capillaries, for the most part, runs countercurrent to the direction of saliva flow, the isotope reaches the distal ductal segments before the proximal ducts and acini. As the saliva column moves toward the exterior, it must displace outward the secretion already more distal to it. Therefore, isotopes which are extracted from the blood at the most distal sites appear earliest in the collected saliva. The appearance times and outflow patterns of water, sodium, potassium, chloride, iodide, and urea are shown in Figure 2. Neither sulfate nor

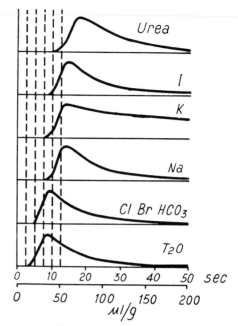

Figure 2. The concentration curves of labeled T_2O, Cl, Br, HCO_3, Na, K, I and urea in the dog parotid saliva following close intra-arterial injection are shown in relationship to the time of injection (0). (Burgen, A. S. V., and Emmelin, N.: Physiology of the Salivary Glands. London, Edward Arnold, Ltd., 1961.)

the amino acids entered the saliva in significant amounts.

It is apparent that water enters the saliva most distally, followed by the anions (chloride, bromide, bicarbonate), the cations (sodium and potassium), then iodide and, finally, urea. These data suggest that a considerable functional specialization of the intralobular ducts exists in spite of their uniform appearance in the light microscope. It should be stressed that although the outflow experiments demonstrate sites of ion transfer, they do not necessarily indicate that bulk ion transport occurs at these same sites in the intact animal. As chloride and bicarbonate concentrations vary inversely under the influence of the arterial pH, it is likely that the chloride-bicarbonate exchange occurs primarily in the distal duct segments where cation entry does not take place. Since anions can enter saliva at this point they must be also able to leave because, in the absence of cation entry, anion movement can occur only by anion exchange.

While the leading edge of the outflow curve indicates the most distal sites of ion entry, the slope of the trailing edge of the curve may indicate a more proximal process. The long duration of the potassium curve suggests that acinar secretion is also involved. A similar pattern could be expected for water, which is known to be excreted proximally. The radioactivity in the water outflow declines rapidly, however, because of rapid dilution or exchange of the labeled water in the proximal saliva by nonradioactive water from the blood stream. This would indicate that the ducts are freely permeable to water. Water resorption does occur in the distal ducts only during low rates of flow (Burgen, 1956b). Although the net effect of water secretion versus resorption in the ductal system remains unknown, it is likely that net water transfer into saliva occurs in the primary secretion and that a considerable portion of this volume is replaced by water accompanying ionic movements in the ductal system.

REGULATION OF SECRETION

General Aspects. Unlike the other glands whose secretions enter the digestive tract, the salivary glands do not depend upon specific hormonal stimuli to initiate or regulate their secretory processes. Under physiological conditions salivation results from an outflow of impulses along the secretomotor nerves. In the absence of stimuli, as during sleep, secretion from the parotid gland ceases entirely and submandibular-sublingual secretion approaches zero (and would probably stop altogether except for the mechanical stimulation from the bulky intra-oral collecting device) (Schneyer et al., 1956). This is in contrast to the minor salivary glands of the palate which, like the bovine and sheep parotid and cat sublingual glands, exhibit spontaneous secretion (Ostlund, 1953). Secretion from these glands is not affected by atropine or denervation and continues even after excision, if the glands are placed in a nutrient medium. The measured rate of salivation from subjects in the awake basal state varies from 0.33 ml./min. (Becks and Wainwright, 1943) to 0.65 ml./min. (Schneyer and Levin, 1955). Parotid resting secretion is approximately half that of the submandibular gland, but with vigorous stimulation the parotid flow is considerably greater (Enfors, 1962). Whole saliva flow rates of 8.13 ml./min. obtained by intra-oral chemical stimuli represent the upper limit of human salivary responses (Kerr, 1961). The daily saliva volume of normal humans is from 1000 to 1500 ml., which corresponds to an average

flow rate of 1 ml./min. Measurements of saliva volume and flow rate for clinical diagnosis have proved generally unsatisfactory because of the technical problems involved and because of the significant variance of these parameters in normal subjects. The values of stimulated flow rates are meaningful only to the extent that the stimuli can be quantitated.

Excitation of human salivary responses normally occurs through unconditioned reflexes initiated principally by gustatory and olfactory stimuli and, to a lesser extent, by chewing and by intra-oral tactile stimuli. The common experience that one's mouth waters at the sight or thought of food is not substantiated by the experimental observations of Kerr (1961) and Enfors (1962); rather, the sensation is one of awareness of saliva already present in the mouth. Salivation induced by olfactory stimuli also contributes. The studies of Pavlov (1928), who conditioned dogs to salivate in response to auditory and visual stimuli, are well known. Cortical impulses can modify the chemically stimulated rate of secretion through suggestion and hypnosis (Winer et al., 1965).

Even as the rate of secretion is influenced by the nature and intensity of the stimulus, so, too, is the composition of the secretion. Adaptation of the salivary response to the stimulus appears to be physiologically useful; e.g., meat placed in the mouth evokes a viscous mucin-rich secretion which facilitates deglutition, whereas inedible material such as sand results in a thin, water secretion which helps to irrigate the oral cavity. In general, foodstuffs elicit a protein-rich secretion while the response to nonfoods is a protein-poor fluid. The stimulus intensity of foods is proportional to their gustatory characteristics. The mechanisms that control this adaptability in composition remain an enigma. While changes in composition in whole saliva, which is a mixture of the products of many glands, or in the composition of submandibular saliva, which is a mixed gland, can be understood as a differential output from the individual units, the variation in parotid saliva is more difficult to understand because the parotid gland is histologically uniform in appearance.

Autonomic Innervation. The salivary glands contain both parasympathetic and sympathetic nerve fibers. The latter arise in the superior cervical ganglion and enter the gland with its arterial supply. The former arise in the salivary nuclei of the brain stem and enter the gland in sensory nerves—the auriculotemporal nerve to the parotid, the chorda tympani-lingual nerve to the submandibular and sublingual. (See the chapter, Embryology and Anatomy of the Salivary Glands.) The parasympathetic fibers are postganglionic from the otic ganglion, the sublingual fibers are postganglionic from the submandibular ganglion, but the submandibular fibers are preganglionic and synapse in ganglion cells within the hilum of the gland (Langley's ganglion). Garrett (1967) described the distribution of nerve fibers in the human parotid and submandibular glands, using cholinesterase and catecholamine stains. Cholinergic and adrenergic fibers of both the parotid and submandibular glands are distributed in a similar fashion about the acini, intercalated ducts, and striated ducts, with cholinergic fibers being more numerous. The collecting ducts are sparsely innervated; the myoepithelial cells are liberally innervated. Neuroeffector synapses or specialized nerve ends are not present; rather, bare axons frequently lie in close proximity to the secretory cells. He assumes that the neurohumoral transmitter is produced by these axons, many of which contain mitochondria and vesicles, and reaches the cells by diffusion.

It is well known that the salivary glands of many species liberate acetylcholine following parasympathetic stimulation and that true cholinesterase is present. The finding that intracellular electrical changes following acetylcholine administration and parasympathetic stimulation are identical (Lundberg, 1958) is further support that acetylcholine is the cholinergic chemical mediator. The sympathetic nerves are presumed to be adrenergic because both adrenaline and noradrenaline are released from the cat submandibular gland following sympathetic stimulation (Oborin, 1954). In man, stimulation of the chorda tympani nerve results in a lively secretion from the submandibular gland (Diamant et al., 1959); stimulation of the cervical sympathetics (Folkow and Laage-Hellman, 1961) and adrenaline administration (Emmelin and Stromblad, 1954) elicit secretion from the submandibular gland but not from the parotid. Both adrenaline and noradrenaline elicit as rapid a flow from the cat submandibular gland as does sympathetic stimulation, but adrenaline is more potent than noradrenaline (Emmelin, 1955). Amine oxidase activity is very high in human salivary glands (Stromblad, 1959).

In most species both parasympathetic and sympathetic stimuli result in saliva flow; the former is generally copious and watery and persists as long as the stimulus is applied, while sympathetic saliva is scant, rich in organic and nonorganic solutes, and ceases entirely with prolonged stimulation. It has been generally assumed that under physiological conditions true secretion results only from parasympathetic activity and that sympathetic stimuli expel preformed saliva by inducing myoepithelial cell contraction. It is clear, however, that the individual secretory cell responds to both parasympathetic and sympathetic stimuli and that the response differs in each case. Electrical responses from a single cell occur with either parasympathetic or sympathetic stimulation, although the responses to each differ in magnitude, latency, and duration (Lundberg, 1955). In the salivary glands parasympathetic and sympathetic stimuli are not antagonistic as they are in most other areas; the stimuli are complementary and, in some cases, synergistic. With the gland secreting at a steady rate from parasympathetic stimulation, simultaneous stimulation of the sympathetics changes the composition but does not increase the flow rate, and after a short period the flow rate actually decreases because of vasoconstriction (Emmelin, 1955). The response to sympathetic stimulation is increased, however, by previous excitation of the parasympathetic fibers, i.e., and augmented secretion (Langley, 1889). The supersensitivity of the gland cells to both adrenaline and acetylcholine that follows the removal of either the chorda tympani or the superior cervical ganglion is further evidence of the dual innervation (Emmelin and Muren, 1951). Although it is tempting to speculate that the dual innervation is responsible for the adaptability of the salivary reflex to various oral stimuli, Burgen and Emmelin (1961) point out that adaptation still occurs following section of the sympathetic fibers.

Antagonistic effects of autonomic stimulation are exerted upon the vascular bed of the gland, however, with the sympathetic causing vasoconstriction and the parasympathetic, vasodilatation. The vascular effect is such an integral part of the action of autonomic impulses upon the salivary glands that, under physiological conditions, it becomes difficult to distinguish between the purely vascular and the purely secretory components. Parasympathetic vasodilatation occurs even when secretion is blocked by atropine and results from stimulation of atropine-resistant dilator fibers (Schachter, 1967) rather than from the liberation of kinin-releasing enzymes as was previously postulated (Hilton and Lewis, 1956). Under special conditions—i.e., administration of physostigmine or large doses of acetylcholine—chorda stimulation results in vasoconstriction (Graham and Stavarky, 1953). Sympathetic vasoconstriction results from a direct effect upon the vessels and is followed by vasodilation after prolonged stimulation as a result of release of vasodilating enzymes from the secretory cell. Sympathetic after-dilatation may also result from beta-adrenergic stimulation as it is abolished by propanolol administration (Schachter, 1967). It is likely that the "dry mouth" associated with anxiety or fear states is secondary to vasoconstriction from increased sympathetic discharge.

Autonomic Denervation. Although reflex salivation ceases after section of the secretomotor nerves, secretion may still be observed. Mention has previously been made of the phenomenon of spontaneous secretion which is unaffected by denervation. Two other types of secretion, denervation secretion and paralytic secretion, occur only after secretomotor nerve interruption. Denervation secretion follows postganglionic section of the parasympathetics and, to a lesser extent, the sympathetics. This lasts only two days and is the result of leakage of transmitter substance from the degenerating nerve ends (Emmelin, 1967). Paralytic secretion occurs after either preganglionic or postganglionic denervation or following prolonged administration of blocking drugs such as atropine (pharmacologic denervation) and is the result of changes that occur in the nerve or the cell that render it more sensitive to circulating transmitter substances or their chemical analogues. Maximum supersensitivity develops at about three weeks (Cannon's law of denervation) and persists for years or until regeneration occurs (Emmelin, 1967). Section of either the sympathetic or parasympathetics causes the gland to become supersensitive to both epinephrine and acetylcholine. Under usual conditions paralytic secretion occurs only when the circulating level of catecholamines is increased; it disappears in the laboratory animal following adrenalectomy and is therefore closely related to the phenomenon of paradoxical pupillary dilation. Parasympathetic denervation usually results in partial atrophy of the gland, whereas the gland weight does not change after sympathetic denervation or after pharmacologic denervation (Stromblad, 1956). Atrophy is more pronounced following hypophysectomy or adrenalectomy (Kahlson and Renvall, 1956).

PHARMACOLOGY OF SECRETION

The salivary glands are sensitive to a variety of chemical agents which stimulate or inhibit the salivary reflex by their actions at the peripheral, ganglionic, or central levels. Stimulation of salivation results from agents that affect the sensory receptors, that act centrally, that mimic the pharmacological action of the autonomic neural mediators, or that prolong the action of these mediators. Inhibition results from certain central nervous system depressant drugs, peripheral autonomic blocking agents, or ganglionic blocking compounds.

Peripheral Agents. Chemical agents that irritate taste or pain receptors can initiate reflex secretion. Six per cent citric acid sprayed into the mouth is an effective salivary stimulant (Enfors, 1962). Inhalation anesthetics, like ether, chloroform, and cyclopropane, stimulate salivation by irritating the oral mucosa. Hypersalivation is a prominent feature of mercury poisoning; the mercury is excreted into the saliva in high levels and causes a chemical stomatitis. Topical anesthetization of the sensory receptors prevents reflex stimulation of salivation.

CNS Agents. Central stimulants, such as picrotoxin, induce salivation as a part of their generalized effect. Hypersalivation occurs in the nausea syndrome and may be induced by drugs that stimulate the chemoreceptor emetic trigger zone, such as apomorphine, morphine, cardiac glycosides, and Veratrum alkaloids (Goodman and Gilman, 1965a). General anesthetics and barbiturates depress salivation. Antiemetic drugs, such as the antihistamines and the phenothiazine compounds, reduce the hypersalivation component of the nausea syndrome by depressing the chemoreceptor zone.

Autonomic Agents. The maximum pharmacological stimulation of saliva occurs with those drugs which possess the muscarinic properties of acetylcholine, such as pilocarpine and methacholine. These drugs stimulate the secretory cell directly. The nicotinic properties of acetylcholine can induce salivation by ganglionic stimulation, but with the large doses required, muscarinic effects predominate. Adrenergic drugs induce salivation when administered intraductally, intra-arterially, or in large intravenous dosages, but are less effective than parasympathomimetic drugs. In clinical practice many of the sympathomimetic drugs used for nasal decongestion also slightly decrease salivation. Autonomic agents are seldom used in practice to induce salivation because of the widespread and often unpleasant side effects from stimulation of other receptor sites. Salivation occurs following anticholinesterases which prolong the action of endogenously generated acetylcholine, but this effect is not prominent. More important is the marked susceptibility of the salivary reflex to autonomic blocking agents acting at the cellular or at the ganglionic level. Atropine, which competes with acetylcholine for cell receptor sites, is widely used as an antisialogogue, although scopolamine and methscopolamine are more effective (Domino and Corssen, 1967). Ganglionic blocking agents used to control hypertension also depress salivation. Mood-elevating drugs such as the dibenzazepine derivatives, imipramine (Tofranil) and amitryptyline (Elavil), and, to a lesser extent, many of the monoamine oxidase inhibitors exert an atropinelike side effect on the salivary glands (Goodman and Gilman, 1965b), which occasionally precludes their usage because of a secondary stomatitis.

FUNCTIONS OF SALIVA

The various roles of saliva and its components in maintaining the health of the individual have been mentioned previously in this chapter and in the chapter, Biochemistry of the Salivary Glands and Saliva, but may be summarized here.

Digestive Functions. Saliva facilitates the passage of food into and through the oral cavity by its moistening and lubricating actions. Soluble food substances dissolved by saliva are able to act chemically upon the taste receptors. Subsequent taste stimuli can be detected because the flow of saliva from the minor salivary glands of the tongue continually irrigates the taste buds. Prolonged gustatory stimulation results from those substances like iodides and saccharine which are secreted into the saliva. Fortunately the salivary concentrations of glucose and sodium are normally below taste thresholds. Carbohydrate digestion is initiated by salivary amylase and continues for some time in the inner parts of the gastric bolus until inhibited by gastric acidity.

Protective Functions. Saliva cleans the oral cavity by dilution and irrigation of retained foodstuffs, epithelial debris, and bacteria. Similarly, hot foods are cooled and chemical agents are neutralized or buffered. Lysozyme and other salivary components inhibit bacterial growth in vitro but their in vivo efficacy is inhibited by salivary mucins. Prior to vomiting, hypersalivation occurs and acts to protect the oral cavity from gastric acidity.

Anticariogenic Functions. Rapid destruction of teeth usually accompanies xerostomia, but the cariogenic nature of the diet is of greater significance than the presence or absence of saliva; extensive caries develop in desalivated animals fed a sucrose diet, whereas caries are infrequent with carbohydrate-free diets (Klapper and Volker, 1953 a and b). Caries susceptibility decreases with posteruptive duration, and saliva is believed to be essential in the development of tooth maturation and caries resistance (Fanning et al., 1954). Incorporation of salivary inorganic ions such as calcium, fluoride, and phosphates by immature teeth contributes to the maturation of and subsequent decreased acid solubility of enamel (Leung, 1965). Incipient or early dental caries become filled with saliva-derived accumulations which tend to prevent further enamel dissolution. Whether these accumulations actually remineralize the defect or act as an occlusive plaque is debated, but that a reparative process occurs is well recognized. Attempts to correlate the concentration of inorganic compounds and enzyme substances in saliva with caries susceptibility and caries resistance have generally been inconclusive.

Thirst Regulation. With loss of body fluids by hemorrhage, evaporation, sweating, or from the lungs, gastrointestinal tract, urinary system, or from decreased water intake, the salivary glands—like other tissues—become dehydrated, and salivary flow becomes diminished or absent. Dryness of the mouth follows and leads to the sensation of thirst and the desire to replace fluid losses by ingestion of water.

Excretory Function. Many substances appear in saliva following ingestion: mercury, lead, sulfur, iodides, morphine, and many antibiotics. Salivary glucose may be elevated in severe diabetes, and urea in uremic patients. The viruses of rabies and poliomyelitis appear in the saliva and may be transmitted by this route. Salivary excretion of metabolites is not essential for maintenance of homeostasis. The deposit of lead in the gingiva and the stomatitis of mercury poisoning are manifestations of salivary secretion of these compounds.

Endocrine Function. An extensive literature exists describing the hormone, parotin, which is apparently elaborated by the parotid glands and which affects protein, carbohydrate, and calcium metabolism. The existence of salivary hormones or deficiencies following the removal of salivary glands has not been generally recognized.

REFERENCES

Becks, H., and Wainwright, W. W.: Human saliva; rate of flow of resting saliva of healthy individuals. J. Dent. Res. 22:391–396, 1943.

Burgen, A. S. V.: The secretion of potassium in saliva. J. Physiol. 132:20–39, 1956a.

Burgen, A. S. V.: The secretion of non-electrolytes in the parotid saliva. J. Cell Comp. Physiol. 48:113–138, 1956b.

Burgen, A. S. V., and Emmelin, N. G.: Physiology of the Salivary Glands. London, Edward Arnold, Ltd., 1961.

Chauncey, H. H., and Shannon, I. L.: Glandular mechanisms regulating the electrolyte composition of human parotid saliva. Ann. N.Y. Acad. Sci. 131:830–838, 1965.

Diamant, H., Enfors, B., and Hohmstedt, B.: Salivary secretion in man elicited by means of stimulation of the chorda tympani. Acta Physiol. Scand. 45:293–299, 1959.

Domino, E. F., and Corssen, G.: Central and peripheral effects of muscarinic cholinergic blocking agents in man. Anesthesiology 28:568–574, 1967.

Emmelin, N.: Innervation of the submaxillary gland cells in cats. Acta Physiol. Scand. 34:11–21, 1955.

Emmelin, N.: Secretion from denervated salivary glands. In Schneyer, L. H., and Schneyer, C. A.: Secretory Mechanisms of Salivary Glands. New York, Academic Press, 1967, pp. 127–140.

Emmelin, N., and Muren, A.: Sensitization of the submaxillary gland to chemical stimuli. Acta Physiol. Scand. 24:103–127, 1951.

Emmelin, N., and Stromblad, R.: A method of stimulating and inhibiting salivary secretion in man. Acta Physiol. Scand. 31:(suppl. 114):12–13, 1954.

Enfors, B.: The parotid and submandibular secretion in man. Acta Otolaryng. Suppl. 172:1–67, 1962.

Fanning, R. J., Shaw, J. H., and Sognnaes, R. F.: Salivary contribution to enamel maturation and caries resistance. J. Amer. Dent. A. 49:668–671, 1954.

Filsell, O. H., and Jarrett, I. G.: Adenosine-triphosphatase activity and nicotinamide nucleotide coenzymes in the parotid gland of the young lamb and adult sheep. Biochem. J. 97:479–484, 1965.

Folkow, B., and Laage-Hellman, J. E.: Quoted in Burgen, A. S. V., and Emmelin, N. G.: Physiology of the Salivary Glands. London, Edward Arnold, Ltd., 1961, p. 61.

Gallagher, J. T., Marsden, J. C., and Robards, A. W.: Electron microscopic investigations of submaxillary salivary gland glycoproteins. Arch. Oral Biol. 14:731–734, 1969.

Garrett, J. R.: The innervation of normal human submandibular and parotid salivary glands. Arch. Oral Biol. 12:1417–1436, 1967.

Glynn, L. E., and Holborow, E. J.: Distribution of blood-group substances in human tissues. Brit. Med. Bull. 15:150–153, 1959.

Goodman, L. S., and Gilman, A.: The Pharmacologic Basis of Therapeutics. 3rd ed. New York, The Macmillan Company, 1965, pp. 169a and 201b.

Graham, A. R., and Stavraky, G. W.: Reversal of the effects of chorda tympani stimulation, and of acetylcholine and adrenaline, as seen in the submaxillary

salivary gland of the cat. Rev. Canad. Biol. 11:446–470, 1953.

Hightower, N.: Salivary secretion. In Best, C. H., and Taylor, N. B.: Physiological Basis of Medical Practice. 8th ed. Baltimore, The Williams & Wilkins Company, 1966, pp. 1061–1080.

Hilton, S. M., and Lewis, G. P.: The relationship between glandular activity, bradykinin formation, and functional vasodilatation in the submandibular salivary gland. J. Physiol. 134:471–483, 1956.

Kahlson, G., and Renvall, S.: Atrophy of the salivary gland following adrenalectomy or hypophysectomy and the effect of DOCA in cats. Acta Physiol. Scand. 37:150–158, 1956.

Kerr, A.: The Physiological Regulation of Salivary Secretion in Man. New York, Pergamon Press, 1961.

Klapper, C. E., and Volker, J. F.: Influence of impaired salivary function on dental caries in Syrian hamster. J. Dent. Res. 32:219–223, 1953a.

Klapper, C. E., and Volker, J. F.: Effect of partial impairment of salivary gland function on dental caries in Syrian hamster. J. Dent. Res. 32:227–231, 1953b.

Langley, J. N.: On the physiology of salivary secretion. V. The effect of stimulating the cerebral sympathetic nerves upon the amount of saliva obtained by stimulating the sympathetic nerve. J. Physiol. 10:291–328, 1889.

Leung, S. W.: Saliva in relation to caries. Ann. N. Y. Acad. Sci. 131:795–801, 1965.

Lewis, W. H.: Pinocytosis. Johns Hopkins Hosp. Bull. 49:17–26, 1931.

Lundberg, A.: The electrophysiology of the submaxillary gland of the cat. Acta Physiol. Scand. 35:1–25, 1955.

Lundberg, A.: The mechanism of establishment of secretory potentials in sublingual gland cells. Acta Physiol. Scand. 40:35–58, 1957.

Lundberg, A.: Electrophysiology of salivary glands. Physiol. Rev. 38:21–40, 1958.

Oborin, P. E.: A Study on the Role of the Sympathomimetic Vasomotor Innervation of the Cat's Submaxillary Gland. M. Sc. Thesis, McGill University, Montreal, 1954.

Ostlund, S.: Palatine glands and mucin. Odont. T. 62:1–128, 1953.

Pavlov, I.: Conditioned Reflexes; An Investigation of the Physiological Activity of the Cerebral Cortex. London, Oxford University Press, 1928.

Schachter, M.: Control of blood flow. In Schneyer, L. H., and Schneyer, C. A.: Secretory Mechanisms of Salivary Glands. New York, Academic Press, 1967, pp. 209–217.

Schneyer, C. A., and Schneyer, L. H.: Secretion by salivary glands deficient in acini. Amer. J. Physiol. 201:939–942, 1961.

Schneyer, L. H., and Levin, L. K.: Rate of secretion by individual salivary gland pairs of man under conditions of reduced exogenous stimulation. J. Appl. Physiol. 7:508–512, 1955.

Schneyer, L. H., Pigman, W., Hanahan, L., and Gilmore, R. W.: Rate of flow of human parotid, sublingual, and submaxillary secretions during sleep. J. Dent. Res. 35:109–114, 1956.

Schneyer, L. H., and Schneyer, C. A.: Salivary secretion in the rat after ouabain. Amer. J. Physiol. 209:111–118, 1965.

Schramm, M., and Danon, D.: The mechanism of enzyme secretion by the cell. I. Storage of amylase in the zymogen granules of the rat-parotid gland. Biochem. Biophys. Acta 50:102–112, 1961.

Shear, M.: The structure and function of myoepithelial

cells in salivary glands. Arch. Oral Biol. *11*:769–780, 1966.

Stromblad, B. C.: Supersensitivity and amine oxidase activity in denervated salivary glands. Acta Physiol. Scand. *36*:137–153, 1956.

Stromblad, B. C.: Observations on amine oxidase in human salivary glands. J. Physiol. *147*:639–643, 1959.

Tandler, B.: Ultrastructure of the human submaxillary gland. II. Base of the striated duct cells. J. Ultrastruct. Res. *9*:65–75, 1963.

Winer, R. A., Chauncey, M. H., and Barber, T. X.: The influence of verbal or symbolic stimuli on salivary gland secretion. Ann. N. Y. Acad. Sci. *131*:874–883, 1965.

Yoshimura, H.: Secretory mechanism of saliva and nervous control of its ionic composition. *In* Schneyer, L. H., and Schneyer, C. A.: Secretory Mechanisms of Salivary Glands. New York, Academic Press, 1967.

Young, J. A., Fromter, E., Schogel, E., and Hamann, K. F.: Micropuncture and perfusion studies of fluid and electrolyte transport in the rat submaxillary gland. *In* Schneyer, L. H., and Schneyer, C. A.: Secretory Mechanisms of Salivary Glands. New York, Academic Press, 1967, pp. 11–31.

PHYSIOLOGY OF THE MOUTH, PHARYNX AND ESOPHAGUS

by

James F. Bosma, M.D.

The mouth, pharynx, nose, and larynx constitute the principal portal of the organism to his environment. These portal elements have a variety of functions which separately utilize their peripheral sensations and which employ their muscular and skeletal effectors in different coordination patterns, most of which are concerned with displacement of nutrient or of air from or into the environment. The portal area functions of feeding and of respiration are separately represented in the central nervous system, and each evolves separately in postnatal human maturation. Each of these functions is separately impaired, or achieves compensation by separate mechanisms, in the clinical circumstances of abnormalities of form, of peripheral motor mechanisms, of primary sensory inputs, or of the central representation of these functions in bulbar and in suprabulbar areas.

Pharynx

Within this portal area, the pharynx is central in anatomy and in functions. The constrictor musculature in its dorsal and lateral walls is in lamellar pattern, resembling the arrangement of the smooth muscle in the esophagus and gut. But in its ventral wall, where in embryologic development the foregut intersects with the stomodeum and the branchial arches, are the specialized structures of the soft palate, tongue, and larynx. During human postnatal development, the pharynx elongates and enlarges; and the soft palate, tongue, and larynx undergo changes in position and dimension. In a remarkable demonstration of integration in development, the upper pharynx enlarges as the soft palate acquires mobility within it (Fig. 3).

The pharynx performs in either of two major motor patterns. Pharyngeal swallow is a distinctive peristalsislike closure involving the constrictors and the more complexly arranged musculature in the ventral wall of the pharynx (Fig. 4). It is thus demarcated from the motor coordination in the alternative pattern of coincident function in agonist-antagonist synergies, comparable to those found generally in the branchial and segmental musculature. The pharyngeal actions in tidal respiration, in the respiratory adaptations of cough and cry, and in stabilizations of spatial position about the pharyngeal airway are in the pattern of agonist-antagonist coordinations. The pharynx continues in a central role during the postnatal development of other performances, including the speech adapations of respiration and the development of cervical posture.

Esophagus

The esophagus is more simple in its embryological formation, structure, and innervation. It is linked with the pharynx in its functions. In addition to nutrient swallow, the gut is inflated by air swallowing, a process initiated in the first postnatal minutes (Frimann-Dahl et al.,

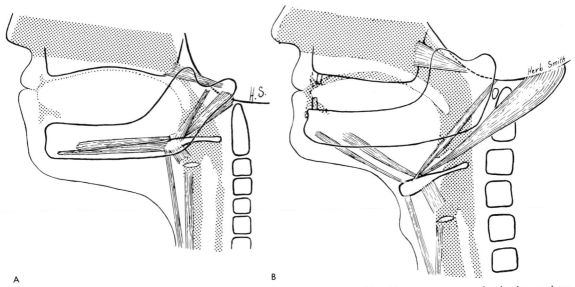

Figure 3. Schema of spatial orientation of mouth and pharynx and of hyoid suspensory muscles in the newborn infant (*A*) and in the adult (*B*).

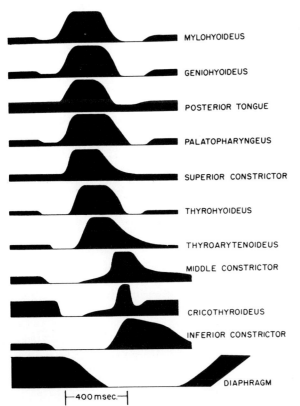

MYLOHYOIDEUS

GENIOHYOIDEUS

POSTERIOR TONGUE

PALATOPHARYNGEUS

SUPERIOR CONSTRICTOR

THYROHYOIDEUS

THYROARYTENOIDEUS

MIDDLE CONSTRICTOR

CRICOTHYROIDEUS

INFERIOR CONSTRICTOR

DIAPHRAGM

|—400 msec.—|

Figure 4. Schematic summary of electromyographic activity in deglutition for unanesthetized dog medulla. The activity is visually summated, and the height of line for each muscle indicates intensity of action observed, ranging from complete silence to maximum occurring in deglutition. In certain muscles, firing more intense than here represented was observed in other synergies. Action of diaphragm is that seen in eupnea. Contours of rise and fall of activity are not considered accurate. See text.

1954). The esophagus is also employed as a reservoir of air for esophageal speech. In this accessory speech maneuver, the esophageal air is expressed by thoracic expiration across one or more constrictions in the pharyngoesophageal segment to effect phonation.

Mouth

The anatomical arrangement of the infant mouth is that of a piston within a cylinder — the sucking mouth of the mammalian young. The superior portion of the cylinder is the concave hard palate. The lateral and ventral walls are mobile, the branchial musculature moving the mandible and hyoid. The tongue is suspended within this arrangement, from the mandible and from the hyoid and styloid cartilages. Its converging extrinsic and intrinsic musculature interweaves in all three anatomical planes and inserts upon a connective tissue lattice and median septum. Its muscular mass, stabilized by its connective tissue skeleton, is the piston of the sucking pump.

With the elongation of the facial skeleton in human postnatal development, the oral chamber enlarges, and the extrinsic tongue muscle origins descend along with the facial skeleton (Fig. 3). An open oral cavity results. Coincident with this anatomical development, the tongue elongates and acquires a variety of discrete lever and probe functions within the expanding oral space.

The mucosal surfaces of the mouth are a

distinctively rich and varied sensory receptor system. The histological variety of receptors has been reviewed by Seto (1963) and by Grossman and Hattis (1967). The oral mucosal sensory inputs constitute a major guiding mechanism of oral motor function, supplementing the proprioceptive inputs from oral musculature, skeleton, and teeth. In the tongue these sensory inputs are intimately related to the motions which affect their experience for, in the absence of an enclosing fascial layer, elements of the skeletal musculature extend into the lamina propria of the complexly papillated mucosa on its upper surface.

In the human infant the mouth is principally concerned with suckle feeding and the associated reflexes of approximating and orienting to the nipple and enclosing it. There is also generalized approximation of tongue and palate which supplements the stable approximation of the soft palate to the pharyngeal part of the tongue and the epiglottis, so that tidal respiration is normally via nasal portal. In infant cry these appositions are given up, as the mouth is widely opened at lips, jaw, and tongue.

Compared with the pharynx, the mouth is represented more extensively in the developing brain. Paralleling the postnatal anatomical development of the mouth and pharynx are central neurological changes related to each of the separate portal area functions. Therefore, in clinical studies of infants and children impaired by peripheral anomaly and/or by neurologic disease, we simultaneously evaluate oral and pharyngeal form and their several separate functions.

FEEDING

Deglutition

The swallow is the most elementary component of feeding.* It is also the earliest function of the pharynx, occurring at the twelfth week of fetal age (Hooker, 1952, 1954). In experimental preparations, swallow is elicitable by stimulation of either the superior laryngeal or the glossopharyngeal nerves (Doty and Bosma, 1956; Doty, 1968). In the adult human it may be elicited by touching upon the faucial pillars or adjacent areas of the soft pal-

---

*The history of investigations of swallow and current information about its neural organization and peripheral actions have been reviewed by Bosma (1957), Ingelfinger (1958), and Doty (1968).

ate, pharynx wall, and tongue (Pommerenke, 1928). It may be evoked voluntarily, but material appropriate to bolus formation is also necessary, for voluntary "dry swallows" cannot be accomplished in succession in the adult (Doty, 1968) or in the sucking infant (Peiper, 1963, p. 444).

As demonstrated by electromyography in cat, dog, or monkey, the swallow is a distinctive action with a set pattern of sequential participation of the upper, middle, and inferior constrictor (Fig. 4). The more complexly arranged musculature in the ventral wall of the pharynx is drawn into this synergy with activity in the adjacent parts of the constrictor (Doty and Bosma, 1956). There is little temporal coordination of firing of motor units in adjacent muscles. When once initiated, the reflexly elicited swallow coordination is unmodified by associated sensory phenomena. This activity is temporally surrounded by a zone of inhibition, demarcating it from preceding or succeeding respiratory actions of the pharynx (Fig. 4). Swallow is not only alternative to respiration, but is also "dominant" over respiration in the hierarchical arrangement of pharyngeal functions in the brain stem, so that the swallow action displaces respiration (Doty and Bosma, 1956). By successive sectioning of the brain stem of the cat, Doty et al. (1967) have located a discrete "swallowing center" in the medullary reticular formation 1.5 mm. from the midline and 1 to 3 mm. dorsal to the inferior olive.

The mechanisms of opening of the pharyngoesophageal (p-e) segment during swallow, and of its stable closure at other times, are uncertain. The varied observations and interpretations of those mechanisms are reviewed by Doty (1968). Stable closure of the p-e segment is facilitated by local anatomical adaptations of contour and structure, including a venous plexus in the human (Fyke and Code, 1955), a funnel-shaped mucosal fold in the cat (Bosma, 1956), or mucous glands in other carnivora, (Doty, 1968). The principal effectors of this closure must be the inferior pharyngeal constrictor and the musculature which positions the cricoid cartilage, upon which the inferior constrictor inserts. The closure is maintained in a variety of circumstances, probably in response to local elicitations. A considerable range of maintained pressure is described, depending upon the manner of testing, whether by air from within the pharynx, by liquid within the esophagus, by penetrating catheter or pressure transducer, or by resistance to a mass in traction through it. A continuing electrical

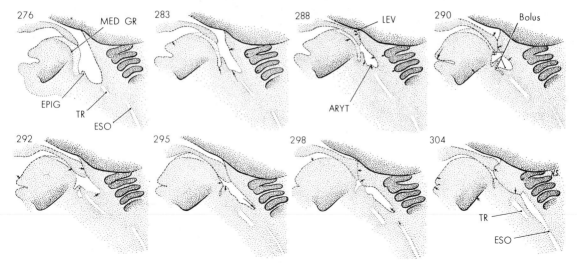

Figure 5. Motions of swallow of bolus accumulated generally in pharynx.

In frame 276 the pharynx is in inspiration contour. In frames 283 and 288 the palate is drawn dorsally and into contour, indicating levator traction. The pharynx wall is drawn ventrally at the level of palate body in frames 283, 288, 290 and 292 to accomplish an extensive apposition with the palate.

The dorsal portion of tongue moves dorsally and cephalically to general apposition with the soft palate and adjacent hard palate.

The lower portion of pharynx, hyoid and larynx are drawn progressively cephalad. In final elevation and constriction action, frames 295, 298 and 304, the bolus is expressed from mesopharynx and hypopharynx and larynx vestibule, into the esophagus. The larynx and cervical portion of trachea are moved ventrally and cephalically. The pharyngo-esophageal segment is opened between frames 292 and 295.

activity has not been demonstrated in the cricopharyngeus muscle (Doty, 1968).

With swallow, the p-e segment opens ahead of the descending bolus. Coordinated with this is a cephalad and ventrad movement of the hyoid and larynx. In clinical evaluation of swallow, the bolus may be stopped at the p-e segment if elevation of the larynx is prevented by the examiner's finger holding in the notch between hyoid and larynx. In the normal subject the larynx suspensory musculature is capable of elevating the larynx from between the holding fingers. But in subjects having weakness of the suspensory musculature, the p-e segment may fail to open in this circumstance. Similarly, if marginally adequate suspensory muscles are placed in mechanical disadvantage by partial extension at head and neck, the swallow bolus may be stopped at the p-e segment (Bosma, 1953).

The pharyngeal swallow actions of the newborn human and the route of the bolus are shown in Figure 5. Prior to onset of swallow, a liquid bolus is enclosed by the tongue in a primary bolus accumulation area near the junction of hard and soft palate. The bolus continues in contact with the soft palate as it is conveyed to the pharynx by the tongue at onset of swallow. During the infant's swallow, the dorsal pharyngeal wall is drawn ventrad, so that the route of the bolus is relatively ventral within the general pharyngeal area.

This convergence of the constrictor walls, tongue, and palate upon the penetrating liquid bolus in human infant swallow occurs despite variations in gross anatomy or in particular motor components of the action. For example, in a series of three infants having varied patterns of cleft of the soft palate, three patterns of compensatory motions of these components were observed, differing in displacements of the contrictor wall and/or of the tongue (Bosma, 1965c). Other patterns of compensatory or alternative motions have been found in infants having neurological impairment of the pharynx. Adequate swallow may be achieved by exceptionally greater motions of the constrictor walls or of the tongue without the usual motions of constriction and cephalad shortening of the pharynx. Adequate opening of the pharyngoesophageal segment may occur with little displacement of the hyoid and larynx: essentially the infant equivalent of the "pint-swallow" described in the mature human (see later).

Favorable experience with therapy of infant dysphagia has increased attention upon its diagnosis and its pathological mechanisms. By means of cineradiography in transverse projection it is possible to distinguish between three familiar mechanisms of dysphagia: penetration of bolus through the larynx during swallow, penetration through the palatopharyngeal isthmus, and incomplete emptying of the pharynx during swallow. Aspiration follows either the second or third mechanisms. Cineradiography in transverse projection with the infant tilted in head down position may demonstrate reflux of bolus into the pharynx from the esophagus and stomach. This is an important separate mecha-

nism of feeding-related respiratory disability; the infant may be more at risk from milk that it has successfully swallowed than from milk in process of swallow. Identification of mechanisms of pharyngeal dysphagia and of the compensatory mechanisms which the infant may employ is essential for design of appropriate therapy (Logan and Bosma, 1967). Feeding gastrostomy, with or without semirecumbent (chalasia) positioning, is employed with increas-

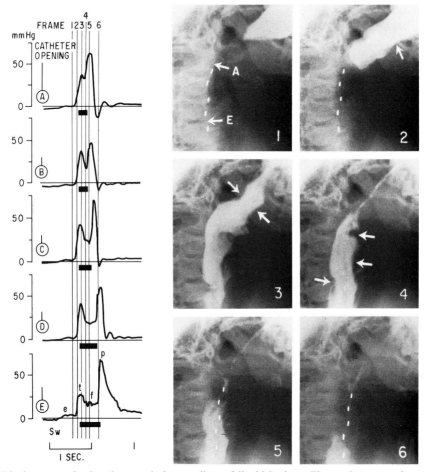

Figure 6. Displacements in the pharynx during swallow of liquid barium. Five catheter openings 1 cm. apart are marked by opaque clips (A-E). Pressures from each catheter opening are reproduced on the left. The moment of each selected cine frame (1 to 6) is indicated by a vertical line transversing the pressure tracings. Sw indicates the approximate time of onset of the swallow. Bar below tracings indicates the period of time during which barium is present at the level of the indicated catheter opening. The subject is prone and turned to permit a lateral projection of the neck.

Frame 1 shows barium beginning to pass through the fauces. The tongue moves backward between frames 1 and 2. Frame 2 shows continued filling of the oropharynx as the tongue (arrow) moves back. In frame 3 the bolus has left the mouth, and the uppermost peristaltic wave (between arrows) begins to empty the proximal pharynx. Frame 4 shows emptying almost to the level of the turned-down elevated epiglottis (upper right arrow). The onset of the peristaltic wave is being recorded at A. In this frame, the postcricoid impression (right lower arrow) and the posterior cricopharyngeal lip (left arrow) are well seen. Frame 5 shows complete emptying at A and B after the onset of the p wave. Emptying at C and D promptly follows. In frame 6 the stripping peristaltic wave is closing over opening E. Air returned to the oropharynx shortly after this frame at the end of the terminal negative wave in A, B, and C. The duration of barium filling and of flow increases from above downward as indicated by the progressive increase in the length of the black bars below each of the pressure curves.

(Figures 4 to 7 are used by permission of Cohen, B. R., and Wolf, B. S.: American Physiol. Soc. Handb. of Physiol. 6:1821, 1968.)

ing frequency. If the mechanisms of pharyngeal airway maintenance and of laryngeal valving are adequate, tracheostoma may usually be avoided.

In the mature swallow of children and adults, the displacements are in a different pattern, in accord with postnatal changes in the spatial arrangement of the pharynx. The displacement of the dorsal constrictor is less than in the infant swallow, and the displacements of the tongue and soft palate and the general motions of shortening of the pharynx are relatively greater. As a result, the path of the bolus is relatively dorsal within the general pharyngeal area. These patterns are well illustrated in the correlated cineradiographic and intraluminal pressure recordings of Cohen and Wolf (1968) (Fig. 6).

Particular patterns of convergence of pharynx walls about the descending bolus, and the associated shortening of the pharynx, vary among normal individuals, including variations with habitus. These differences have been noted by Rix (1946) and by Tulley (1953). Variations of compensation are found in pharyngeal anomaly, in postnatal excision of palate and/or tongue, and in neurological impairment. The most common compensation is an exceptional ventrad displacement of the constrictor wall about the penetrating bolus (Bosma and Brodie, 1968 a and b). Again, in the adult, the pharyngoesophageal segment can be opened without the usual elevation of the hyoid and larynx in relation to vertebrae or facial skeleton. This has been designated as "pint-swallow," from the ability of some normal persons to decant a large volume of liquid into the esophagus without separate or successive swallowing efforts.

Deglutition and the Esophagus. The esophagus is anatomically and physiologically simpler than the pharynx. Its musculature, like that of the intestine, is arranged as an inner circular and an outer longitudinal layer. The upper 2 to 6 cm. is striated in continuity with the constrictors (Arey and Tremaine, 1933). The upper end of the esophagus is held in position by its continuity with the pharynx, and its only specific skeletal-type support is a median band extending from its outer layer to the fascia on the dorsal aspect of the cricoid cartilages. Its lower end is positioned by its penetration through the diaphragm. The position and contour of the length of the esophagus are otherwise determined by its contents and by adjacent structures. With filling, the esophagus remains tubular (Cohen and Wolf, 1968). During

tidal respiration, the p-e segment is stably closed. The esophagogastric junction is closed less constantly at the penetration of the diaphragm, so that small amounts of air or fluid gastric content may reflux this junction during respiration. The cervical portion of the esophagus commonly contains a small amount of air, so that the closed portion of the p-e segment is outlined by pharyngeal air superiorly and esophageal air inferiorly.

The primary peristaltic wave is initiated as the bolus enters the esophagus, in continuity with pharyngeal swallow. A single swallow bolus is delivered into the esophagus and carried through in a continuous passage. Its penetration through the esophagogastric segment is by the same sequence of initial opening followed by constriction. A following "stripping" wave of peristaltic constriction normally empties the esophagus.

The esophagus of the human actively propels food and air only caudally. During emesis, it is a passive tract through which gastric contents may be expressed (Stevens and Sellers, 1960). This differs from the rumination of cud-chewing animals, in which the esophagus and pharynx actively propel the cud upward in the esophagus and pharynx into the mouth (Stevens and Sellers, 1960). Analogously the human belch is without activation of the esophagus (McNally et al., 1964). The eructation of the ruminant is effected by a rapid antiperistaltic wave in the esophagus (Stevens and Sellers, 1960).

Suckle Feeding*. Sucking is the definitive phenomenon of mammalian infant feeding. The full-term human infant demonstrates a composite feeding performance, including approximation to the nipple and its enclosure. The sucking action is distinctive in pattern. The tongue, lower lip, and skeletal elements of mandible and hyoid move in concert, approximating the palate and the firm upper lip of the infant. This motor complex of tongue, lower lip, mandible, and hyoid moves in an elliptical pistonlike action, initially ventrad-caudad and then dorsal-cephalad. The diphasic suckle cycle is repeated rhythmically and in consistent temporal relation to swallow and to respiration (Peiper, 1963). The detailed motion pattern and the strength of the suckle action, its rhythmicity (Kron, 1970) and its pattern of linkage with swallow and respiration (Peiper,

(Text continued on page 365)

*The reader is referred to Peiper, (1963, pp. 404–416) for a comprehensive review of rooting and other feeding–associated responses.

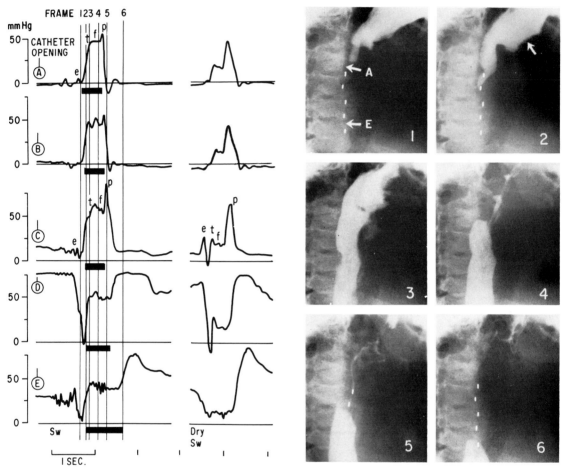

Figure 7. Displacements in the lower pharynx and pharyngo-esophageal segment during swallow. Maximum resting pressure is recorded from D; lesser elevations of resting pressure at C and E; and atmospheric pressure at A and B. Elevation and the e wave occur before frame 1. The onset of relaxation (tracings D and E) also occurs prior to frame 1. Backward movement of the tongue (arrow in frame 2 points to the root of the tongue) begins between frames 1 and 2 with the onset of the t wave. Frame 3 shows a prominent posterior cricopharyngeal tip indenting the barium column during continuous barium flow. Frames 4, 5 and 6 show sequential emptying coincident with the onset of the P wave (A to E). The catheter assembly and the posterior lip descend during emptying. The posterior lip is located immediately above the flattened tail of the barium column in frame 6, i.e., at the level of the D opening. The maximum height of the pressure curve in tracing D is probably underestimated owing to limitations of the measuring system.

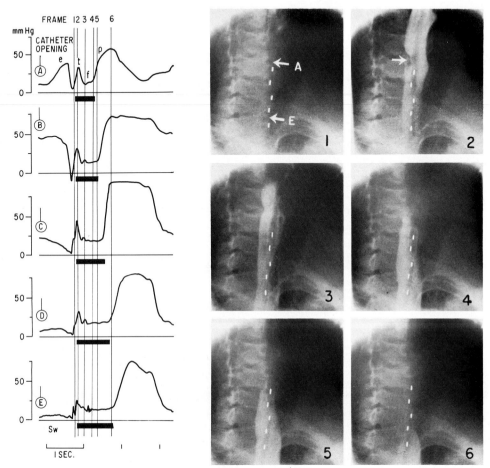

Figure 8. Simultaneous cinemanometric study of pharyngo-esophageal segment and cervical esophagus. Catheter A is in the hypopharynx; B at the level of the cricopharynx; C and D, in the cervical esophagus; and E, at the cervicothoracic esophageal junction. The hyoid bone and catheter assembly rise during inscription of the e wave prior to frame 1. Relaxation at B, C and D is completed before frame 1. This frame shows maximum elevation of the hyoid and of the catheters at the end of the e wave. Barium fills the pharynx and cervical esophagus between frames 1 and 2 during inscription of the t wave. The posterior lip (arrow) is located at the C4–5 vertebral interspace during barium flow. Frame 3 shows stripping of the oropharynx while flow continues distally. In frame 4 stripping extends down to the level of the posterior lip, which has now descended a distance equal to half the vertebral body. Further descent occurs during sequential stripping of the cervical esophagus evident in frames 5 and 6. The region of the lip, therefore, ends up in the region between the C5 and C6 vertebral bodies adjacent to opening B. Note the relatively longer barium flow period in the cervical esophagus and that pressures throughout the entire region are approximately equal during the flow plateau period (f).

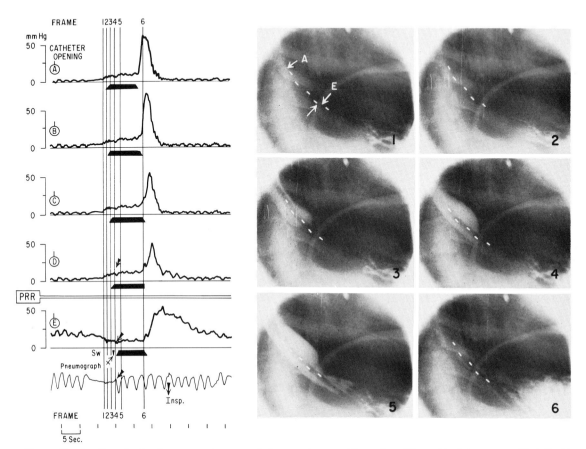

Figure 9. Swallow in the lower esophagus and the esophagogastric region. The subject is prone with left side elevated. Respiration is recorded in the lowermost (pneumograph) tracing in which inspiration is indicated by a downward displacement of the curve. Resting end-expiratory pressures at A, B, C and D are atmospheric. Resting pressure at E is elevated above fundic pressure by about 10 mm. Hg. Respiration is suspended with barium in the mouth and during the pharyngeal phase of swallowing. Relaxation at E begins prior to frame 1, well before the arrival of any barium. Pressure increases ("first positive wave") shortly before frame 2 to flow pressure level at the catheter openings above the PRR. Barium appears in the distal esophagus after frame 2. Pressure below the PRR begins to diminish immediately before frame 1. Flow through the hiatus begins between frames 3 and 4 (+ in tracing E) but is interrupted by an inspiration (arrows in D, E and pneumograph tracings). Free flow through the hiatus and filling of the submerged segment occurs immediately after frame 4 and continues until the esophagus is stripped (frame 6). The junction between the phrenic ampulla and submerged segment, evident in frame 5 between D and E, corresponds to the site of the PRR demonstrated before the swallow.

1963) are characteristic of the individual infant.

That the infant suckle is fully represented in the medulla and midbrain is indicated by the observation that fully competent suckle is accomplished in anomalous infants having little significant organized neural structure above the midbrain (Catel and Krauspe, 1930; Kron, 1970). Hooker (1952, 1954) observed sucking movements in fetuses in the twenty-fourth week of fetal age. Basch (1894) located a sucking center in the medulla adjacent to the trigeminal nuclei.

Mastication

The apparatus and the motions of the mature patterns of biting, chewing, and bolus preparation of particulate food differ from those in infant suckle feeding. The mouth changes as a motor effector in postnatal maturation, with the acquisition of an oral cavity which is not entirely filled by the tongue, of a cupped glenoid fossa which aids in stabilizing the temporomandibular joint, and of teeth. The erupted teeth are a significant new sensory resource, pertinent to the mature functions of mastication. The most significant developmental change, however, is in the central representations of the mouth, by which it acquires its qualitative differences of function and its capacity for voluntary sensory motor functions. Its actions become varied and extensively adaptive to the physical character of the nutrients which it encounters.

The mature human patterns of biting and chewing develop in sequence. Bite is achieved at approximately seven months; at first it is a random or exploratory maneuver. Chewing is achieved at approximately 10 to 12 months. Development of these functions is in variable relation to the eruption of the incisor and molar teeth. Biting and chewing, voluntarily initiated and directed, proceed as a complex sensory-guided system with agonist-antagonist reciprocities comparable to those encountered in limbs. Its afferent resource is the proprioception from jaw muscles and the exteroception of oral mucosal surface sensors. Each of these is projected in pattern in the trigeminal nuclei (Cooper et al., 1953; Jerge, 1963). The integration of bulbar nuclei and thalamus and cerebrum has been well reviewed by Anderson (1968) and by Kawamura (1970).

The motions of mastication have been elegantly defined by the use of cinephotography with indicator bars protruding from the jaws (Anderson, 1968), cineradiography of the mandible and tongue (Kydd, 1958) and of the temporomandibular joint, strain gauge recordings, and electromyography. Chewing consists of individually characteristic small forward, backward and/or lateral rhythmic motions. The masticatory stroke is composed of an isotonic phase, followed by an isometric phase when the teeth make contact (Anderson, 1968). Definition of these phases varies with the consistency of food. Strength of the closing stroke varies over a wide range, to more than 200 pounds per square inch (p.s.i.) (Anderson, 1968). During all these movements the tongue and cheek muscles play an essential role in keeping the food between the masticatory surfaces. The sensory guidance and central regulation of these motions is precise, so that the large physical forces converged upon the teeth do not fracture them, and the adjacent soft tissues of tongue and cheeks are not damaged. Swallow associated with mature feeding is initiated voluntarily.

Relation of Feeding and Respiration

In the experimental model in which pharyngeal swallow is elicited by stimulation of the superior laryngeal nerve and is observed by electromyography, the swallow coordination is alternative to respiratory participation of the pharynx. Swallow is generally separated from respiration by a zone of inhibition. (See Figure 4.) This alternative utilization of the pharynx is essential in those species in which the pharynx is the common pathway for both feeding and respiration.

Nevertheless, these two coordinations also interact. In the experimental preparation, swallow is followed by a quick breath, a "schluck-atmung." In the suckle feeding composite of normal infants, as described by Peiper (1963), the associated respiration follows the swallow component (Halverson, 1944), and Pieper has found respiration paced with sucking in established feeding at a ratio of 1:1 or 1:2; sometimes respiration continued in its periodicity after suckle ceased. The temporal arrangement of the feeding elements of suck, swallow, and respiration is individually characteristic and recurs in established suckle feeding throughout infancy. Irregularities in this temporal patterning are a useful clue to immaturity or of acquired impairment of central neurological regulation of feeding and respiration.

Cervical auscultation is a useful method of observation of these associated actions. Swallows are acoustically characteristic and readily recognized (Bosma et al., 1965b). It is thus possible to evaluate the temporal arrangement of this composite of performances, clinically noting variability of the pattern during established feeding. It is also possible to recognize inadequate emptying of the pharynx by swallow, by the criterion of bubbling sounds of the next respiration through fluid.

Poliomyelitis patients with paralytic disability of the thoracic musculature may replace inspiration with a glossopharyngeal pumping action, consisting of pharyngeal expansion and cephalocaudal compression. This has been designated "frog breathing" because of its similarity to the lung-filling mechanism of the frog, which lacks a diaphragm. An analogous pharyngeal pumping of air into the lung was observed radiographically during natal transition (Bosma et al., 1960). This accessory mechanism of respiration is recognized as an emergency resource. Peiper (1963) comments, "Swallowing respiration is the last safeguard before death due to respiratory arrest."

Similar actions of the pharynx are employed in air-filling of the esophagus to produce esophageal speech (Weinberg and Bosma, 1970).

RESPIRATION

The pharynx and the intrinsic parts of the larynx, which are also derived from the foregut, perform as an upper respiratory chamber, distinguished from the lower, thoracic chamber. In it are the principal exteroceptive resources of respiration. And in it, also, the adaptive respiratory action of cough and infantile cry are defined. Comparison with lower order vertebrates affords perspective of this arrangement. In fish, the pharynx and the adjacent areas of the gill system are the only respiratory chamber. In the amphibia, the lungs are inflated by glossopharyngeal pumping.

Studies in experimental preparations demonstrate functionally separable systems of reflexes elicitable from the upper and from the lower pharynx which are accessory to the primary control of tidal respiration. Sniffing is elicitable by tactile stimulation of the upper pharynx or of the nose (Takagi et al., 1966a). Respiration may be accelerated by tactile stimulation of the palatopharyngeal mucosa. Forced expirations, on occasion accompanied by glottal occlusion or even the total action of coughing, result from tactile, chemical, or pressural stimulations of the lower pharynx or the

larynx (Lumsden, 1923; Takagi et al., 1966b). Sensations from pharyngeal surfaces probably modulate each respiration.

Upper Respiratory Mechanisms in the Infant. The contour of the infant pharynx is shown in Figure 3A; the epiglottis approximates the uvula and soft palate. The contours of the ventral wall of the pharynx (the "dorsal profile of the face") reflect the spatial relation of tongue, hyoid, and mandible to each other, to the basicranium and to the facial skeleton. As a part of their role of maintaining the pharyngeal airway, the tongue, hyoid, and larynx are held stably in this relative position. During dyspneic inspirations accompanying crying, the pharynx enlarges in both vertical and transverse diameters and, reciprocally, it contracts with expiration (Bosma et al., 1965a).

Upper Respiratory Mechanisms in the Mature Human. In the adult the pharynx is elongated and differentially enlarged in its upper portion (Fig. 3B). Though the tongue and hyoid and larynx are spatially farther from the supporting muscular origins of the basicranium and mandible, they are more stable as a reflection of the general maturation of cervical posture. The constrictor walls of the pharynx are also more stable. Essentially the only visible respiratory motion is in the vocal cord abduction and adduction with tidal inspiration and expiration, respectively.

Maintenance of Position

The Pharynx. The positional functions of the pharynx are closely linked with respiration. Muscular actions maintain the pharynx as a conduit in the respiratory tract between its skeletal enclosure at the nose and at the larynx and trachea. The anteroposterior diameters at mesopharynx are increased with extension at head and neck, but are not decreased in normal subjects by flexion at head and neck, because the tongue and hyoid are simultaneously moved ventrad in relation to the descending and dorsally displaced mandible and facial skeleton. Passive displacement of the tongue dorsalward with the examining finger inside of mouth, or of hyoid and larynx dorsalward by the finger upon the skin of the neck, elicits a response of ventrad displacement of the tongue and hyoid in the normal infant.

This ability to maintain the pharyngeal airway is present in viable premature infants, and the mandible, hyoid, and larynx are normally well stabilized in position at term birth. Infants with the Robin's syndrome (1923) have, in addition to a degree of hypoplasia and/or cleft of the palate, a characteristic impairment of this pharyngeal positioning function, evidence by pharyngeal respiratory obstruction with retrusion of the mandible and ptosis of the tongue (Takagi et al., 1966b).

This stabilization of the pharyngeal airway is the earliest positional or postural function of the developing human. It is the essential prologue of posture of head at neck, and of the sequential cephalocaudal development of upright posture in the vertebral stem. With postnatal elongation of the cervical vertebra and the facial skeleton, the pharynx elongates and enlarges and the contours of structures in the ventral wall of the pharynx are changed, particularly with the separation of the epiglottis and the soft palate by the tongue. (See Figure 3.) The phenomena of pharyngeal airway maintenance continue throughout this development, though after infancy the nasal portal is no longer "obligate." If the pharyngeal contour of an infant is distorted by a mass, such as a retropharyngeal abscess, the infant assumes a characteristic compensatory posture of extension at head and neck, thus ventrally displacing the structures of the ventral pharyngeal wall. If the suspensory musculature of the tongue, hyoid, and larynx are impaired, as in amyotrophic lateral sclerosis, the subject assumes the "swan neck" compensatory posture, with extension at head and neck and with the head displaced ventrally in relation to the upright trunk (Bosma and Brodie, 1969b).

Mouth. The young infant's mouth is closed, and the tongue is in general apposition to the hard palate as well as the soft palate, with the possible exception of a small space adjacent to the anterior palatine foramen. In early childhood, with the eruption of teeth and descent of the mandible, the mouth enlarges about the tongue. With descent of the hyoid, the tongue is withdrawn from its previous generalized apposition to the maxilla to produce the "open masticatory space."

SENSORY FUNCTIONS

In recent years there has been increasing study and appreciation of the role of the mouth and pharynx in man's communication with his environment. Sensations from the oral and pharyngeal surfaces, along with proprioception from muscles, joints, and teeth, elicit and modulate and guide the actions of feeding, respiration, and position maintenance. In addition, stimuli applied to the surface of larynx and adjacent pharynx may contribute to the complex neural mechanisms of bronchomotor and systemic arterial blood pressure control (Nadel and Widdicombe, 1962b). The effects are analogous to those of stimulation of the carotid sinus, which are also sensorily mediated by the glossopharyngeal nerve (Nadel and Widdicombe, 1962a).

Our subjective awareness of the *pharynx* is exceptional, as in the circumstance of pain associated with pharyngeal inflammation. Touch localization is crude. But Shelton and associates (1970 a and b) have demonstrated that, with attention and training, palate elevation could become an intentional performance, with local awareness.

Our subjective awareness is principally of the highly discriminate, conscious perceptions of *oral* touch and of taste. The mouth is in active motor participation in these receptive and perceptive processes. Sensations occasion relevant local motions. In the case of sensations with awareness, these motions of seeking and manipulating the stimulus are also voluntary.

The infant's mouth is engaged in the immediate regulation of the motions of feeding and position. Later in development his oral experiences are communicated to his thalamus and cerebral cortex, and integrated with his voluntary oral actions. These on-going, sensory-cued performances of the infant and young child are essential to the subsequent neurological development of function in the oral area. Humphrey (1970) describes continuing functions as the "matrix" upon which further developmental encephalization depends, and upon which it is built.

Touch functions of the mouth far exceed those of the skin in sensitivity and in discrimination. The distribution and degree of these discriminations were initially described by Sherrington (1910), who noted definition of two-point touch of 1 mm. on tongue tip and of 2 mm. on lower lip close to midline. These findings have been confirmed recently by Ringel (1970) and by Henkin (1967). But the sensory capacities of the mouth are more meaningfully described by criteria of sensory-guided oral motor functions. Tongue following of touch cues has been used in clinical evaluation of sensorimotor oral functions of infants and children. More recently tests of oral skills in recognition of shapes have been developed. A plastic "stereognosis form" held on a string or short handle is palpated by the tongue and lips and thus compared with forms seen, or palpated in hands, or recently palpated in mouth

(McDonald and Aungst 1967; Arndt et al., 1970; Weinberg, 1970; Ringel et al., 1970). Procedures of motions of tongue, lips, and jaw in this task of form recognition vary among subjects. But the achievement is basically the result of central integration of information from multiple spatial sites, by which dimension and contour are subjectively derived. This function of form recognition in the mouth is a late acquisition in neurological development, maturing rapidly in years 5 to 8 (Arndt et al., 1970). During these years, and subsequently, it affords an additional criterion of oral neurological function, reflecting neural afferent channels and central integrations of oral function.

The surface sensory function of *taste* is also an elegant, highly differentiated afferent specialization. This is principally an oral sensation, though Von Skramlich (1926) has demonstrated taste discriminations in the pharynx of cooperative subjects. In the newborn, taste buds are found on the epiglottis and elsewhere in the pharyngeal mucosa. These are not found in the adult pharynx; the schedule of their disappearance is not known. Peiper (1963, pp. 44–49) reviews extensive evaluations of taste in the young infant, noting both attracting and adversive responses. There is evidence of regression of taste sensitivity during postnatal development.

The detection and recognition of taste may be evaluated with high accuracy by well standardized testing routines in cooperative subjects (Henkin, 1970a). The local site of taste includes not only the taste buds, but also the oral mucosa more generally (Robbins, 1970). The taste modalities of salt and sweet are better discriminated on the tongue, and bitter and sour on the palate (Henkin and Christiansen, 1967). The heterogeneous multiple-factor taste capacities such as that of detection of phenylthiocarbamate (PTC) vary in genetic pattern (Chung et al., 1965). The acuity of taste varies with the time of day. Taste acuity also varies pathologically with endocrine abnormalities, becoming more acute than normal in hypocorticoadrenalism and less acute than normal in hypercorticoadrenalism (Henkin, 1970a), in hypogonadism (Henkin, 1967) and pseudohypoparathyroidism (Henkin, 1968). Taste sensitivity is reduced during active rickets (Lichtenstein, 1894), apparently on the basis of abnormalities of central neurological mechanisms (Czerny, 1921). Taste sensitivity is markedly diminished in familial dysautonomia (Henkin, 1967, 1970b) in association with absence of taste buds on the tongue (Smith et

al., 1965); taste and other sensory modalities are briefly achieved in these persons following the administration of methylcholine (Henkin, 1970b).

The role and contribution of the "special" sensation of taste is uncertain. It facilitates feeding by stimulation of secretion of saliva (Krasnogovski, 1931; Kapur, 1970); it defends against some noxious ingesta; and it contributes to the aura of satisfaction. Taste may be generally similar to oral touch in its capacity to elicit responsive motion at the bulbar level of integration, as well as eliciting voluntary exploratory motions in the familiar conscious tasting experience. It would thus differ from the touch sensory guidance of feeding and respiratory and positional functions only in the parameter of central representation in consciousness.

PHONATION

Infant Cry. The infant cry is essentially the phonatory correlates of the dyspnea and struggle of the young infant's generalized distress response (Bosma et al., 1965a). Like other infant portal area functions, it is repetitive in stereotypic pattern characteristic of the individual infant. Its respiratory pattern is that of dyspnea with exaggerated inspirations, partially by nasal portal, and exaggerated expirations with phonated glottal constriction, constriction of the pharynx in both longitudinal and transverse diameters, and constriction with or without closure at the palatopharyngeal isthmus. The mouth is open at the lips, jaw, and tongue, in a remarkable contrast with the usual apposition of the tongue with the hard and soft palate.

Speech. Speech differs qualitatively from infant cry in each of the parameters of performance which are achieved in postnatal human development. In the normal subject it is monitored not from direct exteroception but, in more sophisticated fashion, from the special sense of hearing. It is more complexly related to both current and past experience. It is complex in its volition and in its motor composition, in which it uses items chosen from a wide variety of separately established enunication patterns. Like cry it also utilizes the portal area generally, and also involves the whole of the respiration synergy. And, again like cry, mature speech articulation in the mouth can proceed without local area mucosal sensory support; the elimination of local surface sensation by anesthesia (Ringel and Steer, 1963) or by prosthetic covering does not notably impair speech articulation. In this latter respect speech is reciprocal to the neurologically mature organism's voluntary exploration of oral environment by surface sensations such as touch or taste.

REFERENCES

Anderson, D. J.: Mastication. Amer. Physiol. Soc. Handb. of Physiol. 4:1811, 1968.

Arey, L. B., and Tremaine, M. J.: The muscle content of the lower oesophagus of man. Anat. Rec. 56:315, 1933.

Arndt, W. B., Elbert, M., and Shelton, R. L.: Standardization of a test or oral stereognosis. In Bosma, J. F. (ed.): Second Symposium on Oral Sensation and Perception. Springfield, Ill., Charles C Thomas, 1970.

Basch, K.: Jb. Kinderhk. 38:68 (1894) in Peiper, p. 403.

Bosma, J. F.: Studies of disability of the pharynx resultant from poliomyelitis. Ann. Otol. 62:529, 1953.

Bosma, J. F.: Comparative myology of the pharynx of cat, dog and monkey, with interpretation of the mechanism of swallowing. Ann. Otol. 65:981, 1956.

Bosma, J. F.: Deglutition. Pharyngeal stage. Physiol. Rev. 37:275, 1957.

Bosma, J. F.: Human infant oral function. In Symposium on Oral Sensation and Perception. Springfield, Ill., Charles C Thomas, 1967.

Bosma, J. F.: Evaluation of oral function of the orthodontic patient. Amer. J. Orthod. 55:578, 1969.

Bosma, J. F.: Comment. In Second Symposium on Oral Sensation and Perception. Springfield, Ill., Charles C Thomas, 1970.

Bosma, J. F., and Brodie, D. R.: Cineradiographic demonstration of pharyngeal area myotonia in myotonic dystrophy patients. Radiology 92:104, 1969a.

Bosma, J. F., and Brodie, D. R.: Disabilities of the pharynx in amyotrophic lateral sclerosis as demonstrated by cineradiography. Radiology 92:97, 1969b.

Bosma, J. F., and Lind, J.: Roentgenologic observations of motions of the upper airway associated with the establishment of respiration in newborn infant. Acta Paediat. Scand. (Suppl.) 123:18, 1960.

Bosma, J. F., Truby, H. M., and Lind, J.: Cry motions of the newborn infant. Acta Paediat. Scand. (Suppl.) 163:61, 1965a.

Bosma, J. F., Truby, H. M., and Lind, J.: Studies of neonatal transition: Correlated cineradiographic and visual acoustic observations. Acta Paediat. Scand. (Suppl.) 163:95, 1965b.

Bosma, J. F., Truby, H. M., and Lind, J.: Distortions of upper respiratory and swallow motions in infants having anomalies of the upper pharynx. Acta Paediat. Scand. (Suppl.) 163:111, 1965c.

Catel, W., and Krauspe, C. A. Jb. Kinderhk, 129:1, 1930.

Chung, C. S., Witkop, C. J., Wolf, R. O., and Brown, K. S.: Dental caries in relation to PTC taste sensitivity, secretor status and salivary thiocyanate level. Arch. Oral Biol. 10:645, 1965.

Code, C. F., and Schlegel, J. F.: Motor action of the esophagus. Amer. Physiol. Soc. Handb. of Physiol. 6:1821, 1968.

Cohen, B. R., and Wolf, B. S.: Cineradiographic and intraluminal pressure correlations in the pharynx and esophagus. Amer. Physiol. Soc. Handb. of Physiol. 4:1841, 1968.

Cooper, S., Daniel, P. M., and Whitteridge, D.: Nerve

impulses in the brainstem of the goat. Short latency responses obtained by stretching the extrinsic eye muscles and the jaw muscles. J. Physiol. (London) 120:471, 1953.

Czerny, A.: Rachitis. In Handbuch von Kraus-Brugsch, Berlin and Vienna, 1921.

Dail, C. W., Affeldt, J. E., and Collier, C. R.: Clinical aspects of glossopharyngeal breathing. J.A.M.A. 158:445, 1955.

Doty, R. W.: Neural organization of deglutition. Amer. Physiol. Soc. Handb. of Physiol. 4:1861, 1968.

Doty, R. W., and Bosma, J. F.: An electromyographic analysis of reflex deglutition. J. Neurophysiol. 19:44, 1956.

Doty, R. W., Richmond, W. H., and Storey, A. T.: Effect of medullary lesions on coordination of deglutition. Exper. Neurol. 17:91, 1967.

Frimann-Dahl, J., Lind, J., and Wegelius, C.: Roentgen investigations of the neonatal gaseous content of the intestinal tract. Acta Radiol. 41:256, 1954.

Fyke, F. E., and Code, C. F.: Resting and deglutition pressure in the pharyngoesophageal region. Gastroenterology 29:24, 1955.

Grossman, R. C., and Hattis, B. F.: Oral mucosal sensory innervation and sensory experience. In Symposium on Oral Sensation and Perception. Springfield, Ill., Charles C Thomas, 1967.

Gryboski, J. D.: The swallowing mechanism of the neonate 1. Esophageal and gastric motility, Pediatrics 35:445, 1966.

Halverson, H. M.: Mechanisms of early infant feeding. J. Genet. Psychol. 64:185, 1944.

Henkin, R. I.: Sensory mechanisms in familial dysautonomia. In Symposium on Oral Sensation and Perception. Springfield, Ill., Charles C Thomas, 1967.

Henkin, R. I.: Neuro-endocrine control of sensation and perception. In Second Symposium on Oral Sensation and Perception. Springfield, Ill., Charles C Thomas, 1970a.

Henkin, R. I.: The role of unmyelinated nerve fibers in the taste process. In Second Symposium on Oral Sensation and Perception. Springfield, Ill., Charles C Thomas, 1970b.

Henkin, R. I.: Abnormalities of taste and olfaction in patients with chromatin negative gonadal dysgenesis. J. Clin. Endocrin. 27:1436, 1967.

Henkin, R. I.: Abnormalities of olfaction and tastes of sour and bitter in pseudohypoparathyroidism. J. Clin. Endocrin. 28:624, 1968.

Henkin, R. I., and Banks, V.: Tactile perception on the tongue, palate and the hand of normal man. In Symposium on Oral Sensation and Perception. Springfield, Ill., Charles C Thomas, p. 182, 1967.

Henkin, R. I., and Christiansen, R. L.: Taste localization on the tongue, palate, and pharynx of normal man. J. Appl. Physiol. 22:316, 1967.

Hooker, D.: The prenatal origin of behavior. Porter Lectures Ser. University of Kansas Press 18:143, 1952.

Hooker, D.: Early human fetal behavior, with a preliminary note on double simultaneous fetal stimulation. Assoc. Res. Nerv. Ment. Dis. 33:98, 1954.

Humphrey, T.: The development of mouth opening and related reflexes involving the oral area of human fetuses. Alabama J. Med. Sci. 5:126, 1968.

Humphrey, T.: Reflex activity in the oral and facial area of the human fetus. In Second Symposium on Oral Sensation and Perception. Springfield, Ill., Charles C Thomas, 1970.

Ingelfinger, F. J.: Esophageal motility. Physiol. Rev. 38:533, 1958.

Jerge, C. R.: Organization and function of the trigeminal mesencephalic nucleus. J. Neurophysiol. 26:379, 1963.

Kapur, K. K.: A study of food textural discrimination in persons with natural and artificial dentitions. *In* Second Symposium on Oral Sensation and Perception. Springfield, Ill., Charles C Thomas, 1970.

Kawamura, Y.: A role of oral afferents for mandibular and lingual movements. *In* Second Symposium on Oral Sensation and Perception. Springfield, Ill., Charles C Thomas, 1970.

Krasnogorski, N.: Erg. inn. Med. 39: 613, 1931.

Kron, R. E.: Studies of sucking behavior in the human newborn: The predictive value of measures of earliest oral behavior. *In* Second Symposium on Oral Sensation and Perception. Springfield, Ill., Charles C Thomas, 1970.

Kydd, W. L.: Rapid serial roentgenographic cephalometry for observing mandibular movements. J. Prosthet. Dent. 8:880, 1958.

Lichtenstein, A.: Jb. Kinderhk. 37: 76, 1894.

Logan, W. J., and Bosma, J. F.: Oral and pharyngeal dysphagia in infancy. Pediat. Clin. N. Amer. 14:47, 1967.

Lumsden, T.: Observations on the respiratory centres. J. Physiol. (London) 57:353, 1923.

McDonald, E. T., and Aungst, L. F.: Studies in oral sensorimotor function. *In* Symposium on Oral Sensation and Perception. Springfield, Ill., Charles C Thomas, 1967, p. 202.

McNally, E. F., Kelly, J. E., Jr., and Ingelfinger, F. J.: Mechanism of belching: Effects of gastric distention with air. Gastroenterology 46:254, 1964.

Moyers, R. E.: Temporomandibular muscle contraction patterns in angle class 2, division 1 malocclusions; an electromyographic analysis. Amer. J. Orthodont. 35:837, 1949.

Nadel, J. A., and Widdicombe, J. G.: Reflex effects of upper airway irritation on total lung resistance and blood pressure. J. Appl. Physiol. 17:6, 1962a.

Nadel, J. A., and Widdicombe, J. G.: Effect of change in blood gas tensions and carotid sinus pressure on tracheal volume and total lung resistance to airflow. J. Physiol. (London) 163:13, 1962b.

Peiper, A.: Cerebral function in infancy and childhood. New York, Consultants Bureau, 1963.

Pommerenke, W. T.: A study of the sensory areas eliciting the swallowing reflex. Amer. J. Physiol. 84:36, 1928.

Ringel, R. I.: Oral region two-point discrimination in normal and myopathic subjects. *In* Second Symposium on Oral Sensation and Perception. Springfield, Ill., Charles C Thomas, 1970.

Ringel, R. L., Burk, K. W., and Scott, C. M.: Tactile perception: Form discrimination in the mouth. Brit. J. Dis. Comm. 3:150, 1968.

Ringel, R. L., Burk, K. W., and Scott, C. M.: Tactile perception: Form discrimination in the mouth. *In* Second Symposium on Oral Sensation and Perception. Springfield, Ill., Charles C Thomas, 1970b.

Ringel, R. L., and Steer, M. D.: Some effects of tactile and auditory alterations on speech output. J. Speech & Hear. Res. 6:369, 1963.

Rix, R. E.: Deglution and the teeth. Dental Res. 66:103, 1946.

Robbins, N.: Are taste-bud nerve endings the site of gustatory transduction? *In* Second Symposium on Oral Sensation and Perception. Springfield, Ill., Charles C Thomas, 1970.

Robin, P.: La Glossoptose: Son diagnostic: ses conséquences, son traitement. J. Méd Paris. 43:235, 1923.

Seto, H.: Studies on the Sensory Innervation. 2nd ed. Springfield, Ill., Charles C Thomas, 1963.

Shelton, R. L., Harris, K. S., Sholes, G. N., and Dooley, P. M.: Study of non-speech voluntary palate movements by scaling and electromyographic techniques. *In* Second Symposium on Oral Sensation and Perception. Springfield, Ill., Charles C Thomas, 1970a.

Shelton, R. L., Knox, A. W., Elbert, M., and Johnson, T. S.: Palate awareness of non-speech voluntary palate movement. *In* Second Symposium on Oral Sensation and Perception. Springfield, Ill., Charles C Thomas, 1970b.

Sherrington, C. S.: Note on certain reflex action connected with the mouth. Brit. Dent. J. 31:785, 1910.

Smith, A., Farbman, A., and Dancis, J.: Absence of taste bud papillae in familial dysautonomia. Science 147:1040, 1965.

Stevens, C. E., and Sellers, A. F.: Pressure events in bovine esophagus and reticulorumen associated with eructation, degultition and regurgitation. Amer. J. Physiol. 199:598, 1960.

Takagi, Y., Irwin, J. V., and Bosma, J. F.: Effect of electrical stimulation of the pharyngeal wall on respiratory action. J. Appl. Physiol. 21:2, 1966a.

Takagi, Y., McCalla, J. L., and Bosma, J. F.: Prone feeding of infants with the Pierre Robin syndrome. Cleft Palate 3:232, 1966b.

Tulley, W. J.: Methods of recording patterns of behavior of the oro-facial muscles using electromyography. Dent. Rec. 73:741, 1953.

Weinberg, B.: A comparative study of visual, manual, and oral form identification in speech impaired and normal speaking children. *In* Second Symposium on Oral Sensation and Perception. Springfield, Ill., Charles C Thomas, 1970.

Weinberg, B., and Bosma, J. F.: Similarities between glossopharyngeal breathing and injection methods of air intake for esophageal speech. J. Speech Hear. Dis., 1970.

Von Skramlich, E.: Handbuch der niederen Sinne. Leipzig, G. Thieme, 1926.

PHYSIOLOGY OF THE LARYNX

by

John A. Kirchner, M.D.

The primary function of the larynx is to act as a sphincter which prevents the entrance of anything but air into the lung. Comparative anatomical studies indicate that this is as true of the highly refined larynx of man as it is of the primitive larynx of the lung-fish. Even in man phonation remains a secondary, although highly refined, function of the larynx.

COMPARATIVE ANATOMY AND PHYSIOLOGY

The most primitive larynx is found in the lung-fish (Dipnoea), a species inhabiting rivers which periodically become dry. As a protection for the lungs against the entrance of water, a simple circular group of muscle fibers constitutes a sphincteric band at the upper end of the trachea. When the sphincter is closed, the lower respiratory tract is isolated from the upper, so that ingested water cannot invade the lungs (Negus, 1949).

In this primitive larynx, consisting only of constricting fibers, dilation is brought about merely by relaxation of the muscle. In higher forms of lung-fish a separate group of dilator fibers appears, passing laterally from each side of the sphincter muscle (Lemere, 1934). These are eventually represented in man as the posterior cricoarytenoid muscle.

The sphincteric closure of the larynx ultimately came to serve other functions besides protection in higher animals. In man, for example, phonation, cough, and straining are functions of the sphincteric mechanism. Certain respiratory and circulatory effects are also related.

In macrosmatic species olfaction is a further function of the larynx. Some herbivorous animals, for example, defend themselves partly by their ability to sniff the air for the presence of enemies while grazing. In the deer the free edge of the epiglottis lies on the nasopharyngeal surface of the soft palate, so that a continuous isolated passage for air exists through the nose to the lungs. As the deer breathes, food is swallowed along the lateral food channels formed by the epiglottis and aryepiglottic folds medially and by the soft palate above (Negus, 1937). Man's analogue, the pyriform sinuses, do not provide much protection to the larynx. Further, the descent of the human larynx from a position higher up under the base of the skull where it is found in lower animals and in the human fetus, represents a regression in the efficiency of the human larynx as an olfactory, respiratory, and protective organ.

On the other hand, the low position of the human larynx results in a capacious pharynx, with an epiglottis free of contact with the soft palate, so that sounds can be emitted by both mouth and nose. The human larynx is not specialized for any one function, as we find in the apes (valvular action), the deer (olfaction), or the horse (respiration), but it is an extremely versatile and efficient organ.

Anatomy of the Intrinsic Laryngeal Muscles

The intrinsic laryngeal muscles comprise two groups, the adductors and abductors of the vocal cords. The adductors include: (1) the lateral cricoarytenoid muscle, which turns the vocal process inward; (2) the internal and external thyroarytenoid muscles, which form the bulk of the vocal cord and which serve as internal tensors of the cord; (3) the interarytenoid muscle, which extends between the two arytenoids and which pulls the arytenoids together, closing the posterior glottic chink (Fig. 10).

The abductor is a single muscle on each side, the posterior cricoarytenoid. By pulling dorsally on the muscular process of the arytenoid, it rotates the vocal process outward and abducts the vocal cord.

The internal portion of the thyroarytenoid muscle, known also as the vocalis, modifies the margins of the glottis by virtue of the innumerable attachments of its small fibers to one another and to the conus elasticus. It appears well suited to provide gradations of internal tension in very small steps and within single parts of the vocal folds (Zenker, 1964). These functions of fine, internal, isometric, vocal cord tension supplement the relatively crude isotonic tension provided by the externally located cricothyroid muscle (Luchsinger and Arnold, 1965).

Disturbances of innervation will be discussed

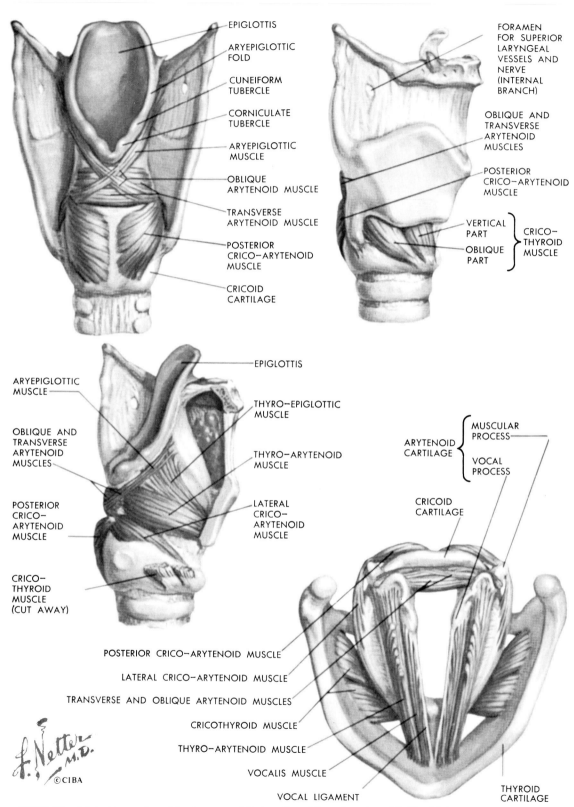

EPIGLOTTIS

ARYEPIGLOTTIC
FOLD

CUNEIFORM
TUBERCLE

CORNICULATE
TUBERCLE

ARYEPIGLOTTIC
MUSCLE

OBLIQUE
ARYTENOID MUSCLE

TRANSVERSE
ARYTENOID MUSCLE

POSTERIOR
CRICO–ARYTENOID
MUSCLE

CRICOID
CARTILAGE

FORAMEN
FOR SUPERIOR
LARYNGEAL
VESSELS AND
NERVE
(INTERNAL
BRANCH)

OBLIQUE AND
TRANSVERSE
ARYTENOID
MUSCLES

POSTERIOR
CRICO–ARYTENOID
MUSCLE

VERTICAL
PART

OBLIQUE
PART

CRICO–
THYROID
MUSCLE

ARYEPIGLOTTIC
MUSCLE

OBLIQUE AND
TRANSVERSE
ARYTENOID
MUSCLES

POSTERIOR
CRICO–
ARYTENOID
MUSCLE

CRICO–
THYROID
MUSCLE
(CUT AWAY)

EPIGLOTTIS

THYRO–EPIGLOTTIC
MUSCLE

THYRO–ARYTENOID
MUSCLE

LATERAL
CRICO–
ARYTENOID
MUSCLE

MUSCULAR
PROCESS

VOCAL
PROCESS

ARYTENOID
CARTILAGE

CRICOID
CARTILAGE

POSTERIOR CRICO–ARYTENOID MUSCLE

LATERAL CRICO–ARYTENOID MUSCLE

TRANSVERSE AND OBLIQUE ARYTENOID MUSCLES

CRICOTHYROID MUSCLE

THYRO–ARYTENOID MUSCLE

VOCALIS MUSCLE

VOCAL LIGAMENT

THYROID
CARTILAGE

Figure 10. Intrinsic muscles of the larynx and their action. (From Saunders, W. H.: Clinical Symposia, 1964. Ciba Pharmaceutical Company.)

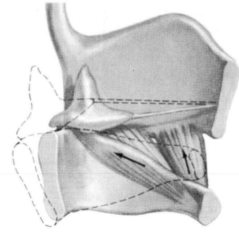

ACTION OF
CRICOTHYROID
MUSCLE

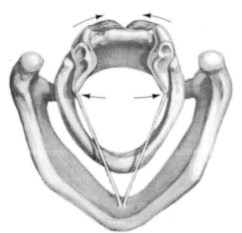

ACTION OF POSTERIOR CRICO–ARYTENOID MUSCLES

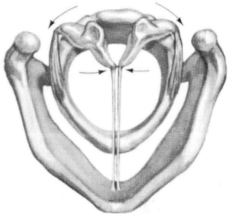

ACTION OF LATERAL CRICO–ARYTENOID MUSCLES

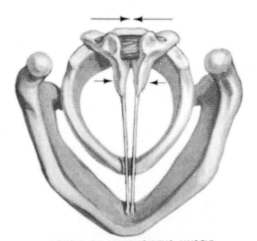

ACTION OF ARYTENOIDEUS MUSCLE

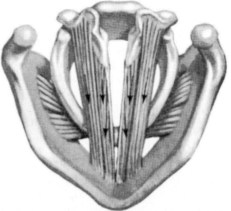

ACTION OF VOCALIS AND THYRO–ARYTENOID MUSCLES

Figure 10.   *Continued.*

under the section on paralysis. However, the observer should be cautioned about interpreting movements of the vocal cord after complete section of the recurrent laryngeal nerve of the same side. Such movements may be the result of the adducting and stretching action of the intact cricothyroid muscle; the action of the bilaterally innervated interarytenoid muscle; the passive motion elicited by the passage of air, especially on inspiration; the descent of the trachea on inspiration (Fink et al., 1956); or the action of the extrinsic laryngeal muscles (Sonninen, 1956).

Innervation of the Larynx

Recurrent Laryngeal Nerve. Each inferior or recurrent laryngeal nerve supplies motor innervation to all the intrinsic laryngeal muscles of the same side, and to the interarytenoid muscle of both sides. In addition, it carries sensory fibers from the infraglottic mucosa and the trachea (Sampson and Eyzaguirre, 1964; Suzuki and Kirchner, 1969). Another group of extravagal afferent fibers traveling in the recurrent laryngeal nerve trunk originates in the cardiopulmonary structures (v.i.), reaching the central nervous system by way of the ramus communicans, which joins the superior laryngeal nerve and which is present in most human subjects (Andrew, 1954; Suzuki and Kirchner, 1967; Bowden and Scheuer, 1961).

In the human recurrent laryngeal nerve there is no separation outside the larynx of nerve trunks into those supplying adductor and those supplying abductor muscles. A partial injury to the cervical portion of the recurrent laryngeal nerve trunk, for this reason, cannot selectively injure nerves destined for the abductor or the adductor muscles (Sunderland and Swaney, 1952).

Electrical stimulation of the recurrent laryngeal nerve of the dog produces abduction of the vocal cord at stimulus frequencies below 30 per second. If the stimulus is delivered faster than 30 per second, the vocal cord gradually moves to an adducted position, the degree of adduction depending on the frequency of stimulation. At 80 stimuli per second the cord is markedly adducted. This phenomenon is not related to intensity of stimulation (i.e., voltage), but to frequency. It demonstrates that tension of the posterior cricoarytenoid muscle becomes maximum at around 30 cycles per second, whereas higher frequencies are needed to produce maximum tension in the adductors (Nakamura, 1964).

Superior Laryngeal Nerve. The superior laryngeal nerve divides extralaryngeally into an internal and an external division. The inner branch is purely afferent, supplying sensation to those portions of the larynx above the glottis. The external branch is the motor nerve to the cricothyroid muscle, the extrinsic vocal cord tensor. The external branch also supplies sensation to the mucous membrane lining the infraglottic larynx at the level of the cricothyroid membrane (Andrew and Oliver, 1951; Lemere, 1932). In addition, it carries afferent impulses arising in mechanoreceptors in the fibrous capsule of the cricothyroid joint (Suzuki and Kirchner, 1968).

Action of the Larynx During Swallowing

The usual mechanisms which protect the laryngeal inlet during swallowing include: (1) reflex inhibition of respiration; (2) closure of the glottic sphincter; (3) elevation and anterior displacement of the larynx, bringing its inlet under the protection of the base of the tongue; and (4) clearing of ingested material from the pharynx before inspiration is resumed.

In man, unlike the deer, respiration ceases during deglutition. This is a reflex act resulting from stimuli arising in the pharynx as food enters, the stimuli being conducted centralward through the ninth and tenth cranial nerves. The reflex is involuntary, occurs in decerebrate animals, and is triggered by the receptor end organs which exist in great abundance in the mucous membrane of the pharynx and larynx (Ranson, 1921; Pressman and Kelemen, 1955; Doty and Bosma, 1956; Yamashita and Urabe, 1960). The most densely innervated regions of the laryngeal mucosa are those on the laryngeal aspect of the epiglottis, in the aryepiglottic folds, the ventricular bands, and the interarytenoid area (Koizumi, 1953; König and von Leden, 1961; van Michel, 1963).

Closure of the glottic sphincter is a reflex act, initiated by stimuli carried centrally in the internal branch of the superior laryngeal nerve. Electrical stimulation of the central cut end of the superior laryngeal nerve produces swallowing movements, closure of the glottic sphincter, and inhibition of respiration (Aldays, 1936; Murtaugh, 1945; Ogura and Lam, 1953; Doty and Bosma, 1956). Closure begins by approximation of the true vocal cords. Next, the false cords close against one another and against the base of the epiglottis. The posterior commissure is sealed off by an inward rotation and approximation of the arytenoid cartilages. When the false cords have been brought into by apposition, a squeezing effect results, occurring according to Pressman and Keleman (1955), as a result of intrinsic muscular activity within the mass of the false cords themselves. Passive forces may also contribute to the sphincteric closure of the supraglottic structures. Elevation of the larynx and increased intrapharyngeal pressure during swallowing, by compressing the pre-epiglottic body between the thyroid cartilage and hyoid bone, pushes the base of the epiglottis posteriorly against the elevated ventricular bands and helps to complete closure of the laryngeal inlet (Fink, 1956). The forward pull of the thyroepiglottic ligament may also help to approximate the vocal folds (Josephson, 1927).

In any event, the normal sphincteric action produces an uninterrupted tissue surface at the laryngeal inlet. If this barrier is rendered incomplete by loss of a part, as by malignant or other destructive disease, by surgical removal of a portion, or by paralysis which prevents close approximation of the surfaces, the sphincter becomes incompetent and aspiration may occur.

Individual variations in the anatomy of the larynx may explain why some individuals compensate better than others for loss of portions of the laryngeal sphincter mechanism. For example, removal of one vocal cord and arytenoid cartilage for glottic cancer usually results in no disability of deglutition. An occasional individual, however, continues to aspirate a part of the liquids he ingests, particularly when large mouthfuls are taken. This may be the result of several defects which occur in varying degrees as a result of surgical changes in the laryngeal anatomy. In the Som-type hemilaryngectomy, for example, in addition to removal of the arytenoid cartilage, the aryepiglottic fold is carefully thinned out so as to allow it to be brought down as a lining for the larynx over the area of resection. This maneuver produces two changes in the laryngeal anatomy which may cause aspiration. First, the cartilages of Wrisberg are removed in the thinning process so that their normal function of helping to fill the posterior gap is lost (Negus, 1937). Second, the downward mobilization of the mucous membrane remaining after removal of the arytenoid cartilage results in a flattening out of the pyriform sinus, since much of its medial wall has been brought into the laryngeal inlet. In this event, the sinus no longer lies below the level of the glottis but above it, particularly in

an individual whose pyriform sinus was relatively shallow to start with. Ingested fluids may thus be directed straight toward the glottis.

After supraglottic laryngectomy the base of the tongue affords the chief protection to the laryngeal inlet during swallowing. After removal of the epiglottis and both false cords, the true cords take over the entire function of the laryngeal sphincter mechanism. The cords must meet tightly in the midline and the posterior commissure must be closed by the arytenoids or, if their resection is required, by a suitable substitute.

The absence of the epiglottis produces only a minimal disability in these cases. Since the valleculae no longer exist after epiglottectomy, small residues of liquid after deglutition remain on the superior surface of the true cords. When the cords separate at the end of the swallow, the residual fluid must be cleared by a cough before inspiration is resumed or it will drop into the trachea. It is largely for this reason that normal pulmonary function is important in rehabilitating deglutition in patients subjected to supraglottic laryngectomy.

Anatomical structures which can be resected without destroying the laryngeal protective mechanism include the epiglottis, both aryepiglottic folds, the false cords, the pre-epiglottic space and the upper third of the thyroid cartilage (Staple and Ogura, 1966; Conley and Seaman, 1963). Loss of these structures still allows operation of the "squirt mechanism" produced by pressure of the tongue against the soft palate and faucial arches. If, on the other hand, the base of the tongue is resected so as to prevent contact with the soft palate, residual fluid can remain in the posterior part of the mouth and pharynx after swallowing and can flood the laryngeal inlet with the next inspiration (Shedd et al., 1960, 1961; Kirchner, 1967).

Similar flooding of the larynx and trachea may result from paralysis of the pharynx for several reasons. First, in the absence of a normal stripping wave by the constrictor muscles, liquids may accumulate in the atonic pyriform sinus until they spill over the laryngeal inlet. Second, the lesion high in the vagus or in the medulla which causes the paralysis also causes a paralysis of the vocal cord in the intermediate position. The open glottis thus allows intrusion by fluids and saliva.

Paralysis of the cervical portion of the recurrent laryngeal nerve usually produces no aspiration, partly because the true cord lies immobile in the paramedian position where the opposite cord can meet it. Paralysis of the recurrent laryngeal nerve in the thorax with cancer of the esophagus or lung may result in a nearly intermediate position of the cord with an incompetent glottis. In such a case the voice is weak and breathy and, more important, ingested liquids may pass into the trachea.

Action of the Larynx During Respiration

The glottis opens a fraction of a second before air is drawn in by descent of the diaphragm (Green and Neil, 1955). This opening is brought about by contraction of the posterior cricoarytenoid muscles. The recurrent nerve supply to this muscle provides a rhythmic burst of motor activity which begins just before that in the phrenic nerve (Bianconi and Raschi, 1964). It is driven by the respiratory center and, like the activity in the phrenic nerve, is accentuated by hypercapnia and ventilatory obstruction and is depressed by increases in arterial oxygenation and by hyperventilation. These rhythmic inspiratory bursts in the recurrent laryngeal nerve persist after respiratory movements have been arrested by succinylcholine paralysis (Suzuki and Kirchner, 1969). They persist after tracheostomy, indicating that the mechanism does not depend on stimulation of laryngeal receptors by passing air (Nakamura et al., 1958).

As a result of variations in the size of the glottic aperture during respiration, the larynx may be an important contributor to adjustments in the intrinsic airway resistance during respiration. Abduction of the vocal cords produces glottic dilation and reduction of resistance during inspiration. Adduction with constriction of the glottis produces increased expiratory pressures which may assist air mixing within the lungs (Otis et al., 1956). Rattenborg (1961) concluded from his studies that adjustments in the glottic aperture compensate for changes in total airway resistance arising in the nose and bronchi.

O'Neil (1959), in this regard, reported a lowered maximum breathing capacity and an impaired intrapulmonary mixing in laryngectomized subjects.

Cardiovascular Reflexes from the Larynx

Arrythmia, bradycardia and, occasionally, cardiac arrest may result from stimulating the larynx, particularly in infants, a fact well known to the bronchoscopist. The mechanism appears to be related to stimulation of nerve fibers which arise in aortic baroreceptors and, in some individuals, travel to the central nervous system by way of the recurrent laryngeal nerve, ramus communicans, and superior laryngeal nerve (Andrew, 1954). These nerve fibers, when stimulated within the larynx, slow the heart rate. They pass through the larynx in the deep tissues near the thyroid ala and, thus, are not influenced by topical anesthetics. They are most effectively stimulated when the larynx is dilated, as with a bronchoscope or a tight endotracheal tube. The reflex cardiac effects can be controlled by atropine (Suzuki and Kirchner, 1967) and are enhanced by morphine (Reid and Brace, 1940).

Burstein et al. (1950) reported electrocardiographic disturbances in 68 per cent of patients anesthetized with the common agents. With intravenous procaine, the incidence fell to 24 per cent. Factors which enhanced these disturbances include light anesthesia, prolonged laryngoscopy, repeated attempts at intubation, respiratory obstruction, or tracheal irritation. Hypoxia and hypercapnea are also thought to contribute to reflex cardiac disturbances (Converse et al., 1952; Denson and Joseph, 1954). These disturbances during intubation are generally transient and are unaccompanied by decreased cardiac output as reflected by the blood pressure.

PHONATION

Sound production originates in the larynx as a fundamental tone which is then modified by various resonating chambers above and below the larynx. The sound is ultimately converted into speech by actions of the pharynx, tongue, palate, lips, and related structures. The fundamental frequency of a tone is produced by vibrations of the vocal folds against one another as a result of the passage of an air stream from below. The vibrations are passive, for they occur in the paralyzed larynx (Froeschels, 1957; von Leden et al., 1960) or in the larynx of a cadaver upon application of a subglottic air stream (Müller, 1837). Similarly, they can be abruptly terminated by diverting the subglottic air stream through a tracheostomy cannula (Dunker and Schlosshauer, 1957).

This interpretation of vocal cord vibration is known as the myoelastic-aerodynamic theory, as contrasted with the "neurochronaxic" theory of Husson which enjoyed acceptance in some quarters for a time after it was proposed in 1950. Husson's theory explained vocal cord vibrations by rhythmic impulses in the recurrent laryngeal nerves corresponding, beat by beat, with the frequency of the sound produced (Husson, 1950). The theory is no longer accepted, having been shown to lack either physiological (Weiss, 1959) or acoustical merit (van den Berg, 1958).

Our understanding of vocal cord movement during phonation is derived from the high speed motion picture film made by the Bell Telephone laboratories in 1940. This classic film of vocal cord movements was made at 4000 frames per second and has been analyzed by many observers (Farnsworth, 1940). Other methods of observing vocal cord movements during phonation include frontal tomography (Hollien and Curtis, 1960; Fink and Kirchner, 1958) and electronic stroboscopy (Smith, 1954).

During phonation the vocal cord is adducted to near the midline by the cricothyroid muscle, which serves as a crude isotonic tensor of the cord. Finer isometric adjustments are then made by the thyroarytenoid muscle. Medial movement of the cord into contact with its fellow is brought about by three forces: (1) tension in the cord, as just described; (2) decrease in subglottic air pressure with each vibratory opening of the glottis; and (3) the sucking-in effect of the escaping air (Bernoulli effect) (van den Berg, 1958; Smith 1954). The result of this rapidly repeating cycle of opening and closing at the glottis is the release of small puffs from the subglottic air column which form sound waves.

During ordinary phonation the anterior two thirds of the vocal cords form the vibrating portion, the vocal processes of the arytenoids being held firmly in apposition (Pressman, 1942; Sonninen, 1954). Fink analyzed the Bell Telephone film and concluded that the axis of vibration of human vocal folds is not in the midline but is paramedian and appears bowed and elliptical. One possible advantage of a paramedian axis might be a minimum velocity at the time of impact, thereby lessening the risk of trauma (Fink, 1962).

If the glottis is observed in the frontal plane, it will be seen that the area of vocal cord surface in contact with its partner varies according to pitch. At low pitches the cross-sectional area of the vocal folds is large. As pitch is raised, the folds become thinner (Hollien and Curtis, 1960).

At low pitches, opening of the glottis begins from the inferior surface of contact, the opening proceeding upward between the two surfaces of the vocal folds. The lower portion is also the first to close. In other words, there is a phase difference in the motion between different vertical portions of the vocal folds. Smith compared the mechanism of vocal cord vibration to the passage of an air bubble between two soft, elastic pillows (Smith, 1954).

PITCH

The frequency of vocal cord vibrations depends upon: (1) the effective mass of the vibrating part of the vocal fold, and (2) the effective tension in the vibrating part of the vocal fold. Other related forces include (1) damping of the vocal folds, (2) subglottic pressure, and the (3) glottic area, which in turn influences resistance and which determines the value of the Bernoulli effect (van den Berg, 1958).

With rising vocal pitch the vocal cord is lengthened by the action of the cricothyroid muscle (Pressman, 1942; Sonninen, 1954). Although this would tend to lower the pitch, its effect is counteracted by contraction of the thyroarytenoid muscle, which thins the vocal cord and increases its inner tension (Fink, 1962). Because of its large number of extraordinarily thin, short fibers which can pull in various directions, the thyroarytenoid muscle appears to be well designed to produce a wide range of tension in many small steps (Zenker, 1964).

The extrinsic laryngeal muscles may lengthen or shorten the vocal cords in certain head positions by changing the relation of the thyroid to the cricoid cartilage. Sonninen cites four observers who reported lowering of the voice and loss in range along with failure of the glottis to close completely at high tone ranges after section of various extrinsic laryngeal muscles at thyroidectomy. He also reported an experiment performed during an operation under local anesthesia in which the patient sang a sustained note. In this experiment stimulation of the sternothyroid muscle lowered the note by a half tone when the neck was extended. When the head was held in the same plane as the body there was no change in pitch (Sonninen, 1954; Faaborg-Anderson and Sonninen, 1960).

PROPRIOCEPTION IN THE LARYNX

A challenging problem to students of laryngeal physiology is the source of control over the intrinsic laryngeal muscles during singing and speaking. Is the necessary degree of coordination between the central nervous system, the respiratory muscles, the extralaryngeal, pharyngeal, and oral musculature and the intrinsic muscles of the larynx monitored entirely by the auditory apparatus? The flat, unmodulated voice of the completely deaf person attests to the importance of hearing in regulating vocal performance (Proctor, 1968). On the other hand, the ability of a trained singer to produce a precise pitch at the moment the sound is emitted indicates that there exists in the laryngeal structures a monitoring receptor system which signals position, movement, and tension in the vocal cords and related structures and is therefore independent of any additional adjusting influence signaled by the hearing mechanism after the sound is emitted. Furthermore, the performance of a singer can be impaired by the application of a local anesthetic to the pharynx and larynx (Proctor, 1965).

The case for a feedback system of control originating within the larynx is supported by:

(1) The presence of receptor end organs in the laryngeal mucosa (Koizumi, 1953; König and von Leden, 1961; van Michel, 1963), muscles (Rossi and Cortesina, 1965; Lucas Keene, 1961; Rudolph, 1961), perichondrum (Jankovskaya, 1959; Gracheva, 1963), and joint capsules (Andrew, 1950; Kirchner and Wyke, 1964). (2) The recording of afferent nerve discharges in the superior and the recurrent laryngeal nerves in response to excitation of receptors by stimuli which occur during phonation. These include touch, vibration, pressure, passage of air across mucosal surfaces, changes in the length of the vocal cords, and stretching of the fibrous capsules of the cricothyroid joint (Sampson and Eyzaguirre, 1964; Suzuki and Kirchner, 1967, 1968; Martensson, 1964; Kirchner and Suzuki, 1965). (3) The demonstration that appropriate mechanical stimulation of these receptors gives rise to reflexly coordinated changes in the tone of the intrinsic laryngeal muscles (Kirchner and Wyke, 1965; Abo El-Enene and Wyke, 1966).

In summary, the "mechanism of the larynx" continues to challenge the ingenuity of the investigator today as surely as it did at the time of Negus' original and monumental contribution to the subject 40 years ago (Negus, 1929).

REFERENCES

Abo El-Enene, M. A., and Wyke, B. D.: Myotatic reflex systems in the intrinsic muscles of the larynx. Proc. Anat. Soc. *100*:926, 1966.

Aldaya, F.: Le controle réflexe de la réspiration par la sensibilité du larynx. Compt. Rend. Soc. Biol. (Paris) *123*:1001, 1936.

Andrew, B. L.: Proprioceptors at the joint of the epiglottis. J. Physiol. *111*:18, 1950.

Andrew, B. L., and Oliver, J.: The epiglottal taste buds of the rat. J. Physiol. *114*:48, 1951.

Andrew, B. L.: A laryngeal pathway for aortic baroreceptor impulses. J. Physiol. *125*:352, 1954.

Bianconi, R., and Raschi, F.: Respiratory control of motoneurones of the recurrent laryngeal nerve and hypocapnic apnoea. Arch. Ital. Biol. *102*:56, 1964.

Bowden, R. E. M., and Scheuer, J. L.: Comparative studies of the nerve supply of the larynx in eutherian mammals. Proc. Zool. Soc. (London) *136*(part 3):325, 1961.

Burstein, C. L., Woloshin, G., and Newmann, W.: Electrocardiographic studies during endotracheal intubation. II Effects during general anesthesia and intravenous procaine. Anesthesiology *11*:299, 1950.

Conley, J., and Seaman, W.: Function in the crippled laryngopharynx. Ann. Otol. *72*:441, 1963.

Converse, J. G., Landmesser, C. M., and Harmel, M. H.: Electrocardiographic changes during extubation. Anesthesiology *13*:163, 1952.

Denson, J. S., and Joseph, S. I.: Cardiac rhythm and endotracheal intubation—A clarification. Anesthesiology *15*:650, 1954.

Doty, R. W., and Bosma, J. F.: An electromyographic analysis of reflex deglutition. J. Neurophysiol. *19*:44, 1956.

Dunker, E., and Schlosshauer, B.: Hochfrequenzkinematographische untersuchungen des verhaltens der Stimmlippen bei unterbrechung der Anblaseluft. Arch. Ohr. - Nas. - Kehlk. - Heilk. *171*:225, 1957.

Faaborg-Andersen, K., and Sonninen, A.: The function of the extrinsic laryngeal muscles at different pitch. Acta Otolaryng. (Stockh.) *51*:89, 1960.

Farnsworth, D. W.: High speed motion pictures of human vocal cords. Bell Lab. Rec. *18*:203, 1940.

Fink, B. R.: The mechanism of closure of the human larynx. Amer. Acad. Ophthal. *60*:117, 1956.

Fink, B. R.: Tensor mechanism of the vocal folds. Ann. Otol. *71*:591, 1962.

Fink, B. R., Basek, M., and Epanchin, V.: The mechanism of opening of the human larynx. Laryngoscope *66*:410, 1956.

Fink, B. R., and Kirschner, F.: Observations on the acoustical and mechanical properties of the vocal folds. Folia Phoniat. *11*:167, 1958.

Froeschels, E.: The question of the origin of the vibrations of the vocal cords. A clinical contribution. Arch. Otolaryng. *66*:512, 1957.

Gracheva, M. S.: Sensory innervation of locomotor apparatus of the larynx. Fed. Proc. *22*:1120, 1963.

Green, J. H., and Neil, E.: The respiratory function of the laryngeal muscles. J. Physiol. *129*:134, 1955.

Hollien, H., and Curtis, J.: A laminographic study of vocal pitch. J. Speech Hear. Res. *3*:157, 1960.

Husson, R.: Étude des phénomènes physiologigues et acoustiques fondamentaux de la voix chantée. Thesis. Paris, June, 1950.

Jankovskaya, N. F.: Receptive innervation of the perichondrium of the laryngeal cartilages. Arkh. Anat. *37*(8):71, 1959.

Josephson, E. M.: The physiology of the "false" vocal cords and the anatomy of the thyro-arytenoid muscle and of the thyro-epiglottic ligament. Arch. Otolaryngol. *6*:139, 1927.

Kirchner, J. A.: Pharyngeal and esophageal dysfunction. Minnesota Med. *50*:921, 1967.

Kirchner, J. A., and Suzuki, M.: Laryngeal reflexes and voice production. Ann. N. Y. Acad. Sci. *155*(Art. 1):98, 1968.

Kirchner, J. A., and Wyke, B.: Innervation of laryngeal joints and laryngeal reflexes. Nature *201*(No. 4918):506, 1964.

Kirchner, J. A., and Wyke, B. D.: Articular reflex mechanisms in the larynx. Ann. Otol. *74*:479, 1965.

Koizumi, H.: On sensory innervation of larynx in dog. Tohoku J. Exp. Med. *58*:199, 1953.

König, W. F., and von Leden, H.: The peripheral nervous system of the human larynx: I. The mucous membrane. Arch. Otolaryng. *73*:1, 1961.

Lemere, F.: Innervation of the larynx. Amer. J. Anat. *51*:417, 1932.

Lemere, F.: Innervation of the larynx. IV. An analysis of Semon's law. Ann. Otol. *43*:525, 1934.

Lucas Keene, M. F.: Muscle spindles in the human laryngeal muscles. J. Anat. *95*:25, 1961.

Luchsinger, R., and Arnold, G. E.: Voice — Speech — Language. Belmont, Calif., Wadsworth Publishing Co., 1965.

Martensson, A.: Proprioceptive impulse patterns during contraction of intrinsic laryngeal muscles. Acta Physiol. Scand. *62*:176, 1964.

Müller, J.: Handbuch der Physiologie des Mensehen für Vorlesungen. 3rd ed. Coblenz, J. Hölscher, 1837.

Murtagh, J. A.: The respiratory function of the larynx. 1. Some observations on laryngeal innervation. Ann. Otol. *54*:307, 1945.

Nakamura, F., Uyeda, Y., and Sonoda Y.: Electromyographic study on respiratory movements of the intrinsic laryngeal muscles. Laryngoscope *68*:109, 1958.

Nakamura, F.: Movement of the larynx induced by electrical stimulation of the laryngeal nerves. *In* Brewer, D. W.: Research Potentials in Voice Physiology, 129. N.Y. State University Press, 1964.

Negus, V. E.: The Mechanism of the Larynx. London, William Heinemann, Ltd., 1929.

Negus, V. E.: The evidence of comparative anatomy on the structure of the human larynx. Proc. Roy. Soc. Med. *30*:1394, 1937.

Negus, V. E.: The Comparative Anatomy and Physiology of the Larynx. London, William Heinemann, Ltd., 1949.

Ogura, J. H., and Lam, R. L.: Anatomical and physiological correlations on stimulating the human superior laryngeal nerve. Laryngoscope *63*:947, 1953.

O'Neil, J. J.: The role of the vocal cords in human respiration. Laryngoscope *69*:1494, 1959.

Otis, A. B., et al.: Mechanical factors in the distribution of pulmonary ventilation. J. Appl. Physiol. *8*:429, 1956.

Pressman, J. J.: Physiology of the vocal cords in phonation and respiration. Arch. Otolaryngol. *35*:355, 1942.

Pressman, J. J., and Kelemen, G.: Physiology of the larynx. Physiol. Rev. *35*:506, 1955.

Proctor, D. F.: The physiologic basis of voice training. Ann. N.Y. Acad. Sci. *155*(Art. 1):208, 1968.

Proctor, D. F.: Personal communication, 1965.

Ranson, S. W.: Afferent paths for visceral reflexes. Physiol. Rev. *1*:477, 1921.

Rattenborg, C.: Laryngeal regulation of respiration. Acta Anaesth. Scand. *5*:129, 1961.

Reid, L. C., and Brace, D. E.: Irritation of respiratory tract and its reflex effect upon the heart. Surg. Gynec. Obstet. *70*:157, 1940.

Rossi, G., and Cortesina, G.: Morphological study of the laryngeal muscles in man. Acta Otolaryng. *59*:575, 1965.

Rudolph, G.: Spiral nerve-endings (proprioceptors) in the human vocal muscle. Nature (London) *190*:726, 1961.

Sampson, S., and Eyzaguirre, C.: Some functional characteristics of mechanoreceptors in the larynx of the cat. J. Neurophysiol. *27*:464, 1964.

Shedd, D. P., Scatliff, J. H., Chase, R. A., and Kirchner, J. A.: Observations on the function of the faucial isthmus in deglutition. J. Surg. Res. *1*:291, 1961.

Shedd, D. P., Scatliff, J. H., and Kirchner, J. A.: A cineradiographic study of postresectional alterations in oropharyngeal physiology. Surg. Gynec. Obstet. *110*:69, 1960.

Smith, S.: Remarks on the physiology of the vibrations of the vocal cords. Folia Phoniat. 6:166, 1954.

Sonninen, A.: Is the length of the vocal cords the same at all different levels of singing? Acta Otolaryng. (Suppl.)*118*:219, 1954.

Sonninen, A.: The role of the external laryngeal muscles in length-adjustment of the vocal cords in singing. Acta Otolaryng. (Suppl.):130, 1956.

Staple, T. W., and Ogura, J. H.: Cineradiography of the swallowing mechanism following supraglottic subtotal laryngectomy. Radiology *87*:226, 1966.

Sunderland, S., and Swaney, W. E.: The intraneural topography of the recurrent laryngeal nerve in man. Anat. Rec. *114*:411, 1952.

Suzuki, M., and Kirchner, J. A.: Laryngeal reflex pathways related to rate and rhythm of the heart. Ann. Otol. *76*:774, 1967.

Suzuki, M., and Kirchner, J. A.: Afferent nerve fibers in the external branch of the superior laryngeal nerve in the cat. Ann. Otol. *77*:1059, 1968.

Suzuki, M., and Kirchner, J. A.: Sensory fibers in the recurrent laryngeal nerve. Ann. Otol. *78*:21, 1969.

Suzuki, M., and Kirchner, J. A.: The posterior cricoarytenoid as an inspiratory muscle. Ann. Otol., 1969.

van den Berg, J.: Myoelastic-aerodynamic theory of voice production. J. Speech Hear. Res. *1*:227, 1958.

von Leden, H., Moore, P., and Timcke, R.: Laryngeal vibrations: Measurements of the glottic wave. Part III. The pathologic larynx. A.M.A. Archiv. Otolaryng. *71*:16, 1960.

Van Michel, C.: Considerations morphologiques sur les appareils sensoriels de la muqueuse vocale humaine. Acta Anat. *52*:188, 1963.

Weiss, D.: Discussion of the neurochronatic theory (Husson). Arch. Otolaryngol. *70*:607, 1959.

Yamashita, T., and Urabe, K.: Glottisschlussreflex und M. cricoarytenoideus posterior. Arch. Ohr. Nas. Kehlkopfheilk. *177*:39, 1960.

Zenker, W.: Vocal muscle fibres and their motor end-plates. *In* Brewer, D. W.: Research Potentials in Voice Physiology, 7. New York State University Press, 1964.

PHYSIOLOGY OF THE RESPIRATORY TRACT

by

Richard Witt, M.D.

The basic functions of the lung are to supply the blood with oxygen and to remove from it the waste products, carbon dioxide and water. The lung also helps to maintain acid-base equilibrium and acts as a filter to remove endogenous or foreign particles from the blood that passes through its capillary bed.

In order to provide these basic physiologic functions, the normal alveolar-capillary membrane of the lung is dependent upon many other activities of a physiologic nature. These dependencies include an adequately performing heart to pump blood through the lung, a properly flowing blood stream with adequate amounts of functioning hemoglobin, and a balanced distribution of blood flow and alveolar ventilation. Sufficient ventilation of the lung requires innervated muscles of respiration plus a suitably elastic pleura and lung parenchyma as well as a tracheobronchial tree which conducts air with a minimum of air flow resistance. Finally, a cleaned, warmed, and humidified volume of fresh air must be delivered into the tracheobronchial tree and, thence, the alveoli.

In order to accomplish these ends certain physiologic mechanisms have been supplied to the human body. Impairment of or interference with these physiologic functions will result in abnormalities which may be of only minimal annoyance to the patient or which may be of such magnitude as to cause his death.

PHYSIOLOGY OF THE UPPER RESPIRATORY TRACT AS IT PERTAINS TO RESPIRATION

The hairs found at the anterior nares serve as filters to remove larger foreign particles from the inhaled air. In addition, the air is baffled by the nasal turbinates, the pharyngeal wall, the tonsils, the adenoids and, in the case of mouth breathers, by the tongue, teeth, and oral mucosa. Larger size particles of foreign material in the inhaled air are effectively deposited on these mucous membranes (Proctor, 1964). The estimate is that virtually all particles over 40 μ in size are thus removed from the inhaled air.

The large surface of mucosa covering the nasal turbinates aided by the additional mucosa of the mouth and pharynx also serves to warm and humidify the inhaled air (Proctor, 1964). This air must be warmed to body temperature and must be 100 per cent humidified at that temperature. This means that if the air inhaled were absolutely dry, the body would have to supply over 40 mg. of water per liter of inhaled air or approximately 2½ L. of water in a 24 hour period. When a tracheostomy is required, the inhaled air bypasses the upper respiratory tract and must therefore be artificially warmed and humidified before being inspired. If care is not taken to do this the tracheobronchial tree will have to perform the function. If the latter occurs, the mucosa becomes dried and secretions become thickened. Crusts and bronchial plugs may develop. This is especially likely if the patient requires supplementary oxygen, which is delivered to the tracheal stoma as a desiccated gas.

Cold air has been known to cause bronchospasm (Comroe, 1965), which may well be significant to patients with chronic obstructive lung diseases such as chronic bronchial asthma, chronic bronchitis, and emphysema. In some parts of this country physicians are recommending that their patients wear a face mask during extremely cold periods in order to warm the inhaled air. It seems logical that humidified air being inhaled via a tracheostomy should therefore be warmed to body temperature before being allowed to enter the tracheobronchial tree.

A number of reflexes encountered in the upper respiratory tract are of extreme importance in protecting the lower respiratory tract from the aspiration of foreign material. The most obvious of these is the cough reflex, which occurs normally whenever the mucosa of the pharynx or the larynx is stimulated. The properly performed cough is dependent upon an intact functioning larynx. A very inefficient cough is produced by the patient whose larynx has been bypassed by a tracheostomy. The cough reflex also becomes greatly impaired by diseases of the neuromuscular system such as strokes, myasthenia gravis, muscular dystrophy, and infections of the central nervous system like poliomyelitis and the Guillain-Barré syndrome. Sedation and drug overdose are frequent causes of depressed reflexes. The swallowing and gag reflexes are also of importance in protecting the airway. A patient who is unable to swallow properly may well aspirate his own secretions, food particles, or emesis.

It is thus obvious that whenever the patient requires a tracheostomy, certain functions must be supplied for him. The air must be warmed to body temperature and humidified 100 per cent. The secretions must be removed from the trachea and bronchi, and care must be taken that secretions and gastric contents are not aspirated.

PHYSIOLOGY OF THE TRACHEA AND BRONCHI

The trachea and major bronchi are very similar in structure. They are rounded tubes whose inner surface is lined by tall, ciliated, columnar epithelial cells. Interspersed are goblet cells which are secreting mucus. Under the basement membrane are submucosal mucus-secreting glands. The trachea is supported by a crescent-shaped cartilaginous ring. Its posterior surface is membranous. The bronchi have a circular cartilaginous structure which is interrupted, forming a semirigid protective ring. There is, in addition, a "geodesic network" of smooth muscle which surrounds the trachea and the major bronchi (Miller, 1950). The vagus nerve supplies sensory endings to the mucosa of the bronchi. However, the lung is relatively insensitive beyond the first portion of the subsegmental bronchi.

During respiration the trachea and bronchi have a definite motion. They become greater in diameter and length during inspiration and shorter and narrower during expiration. This can be nicely seen by viewing cinebronchograms (Witt and Wiot, 1965). During a cough the bronchi become rather rapidly shorter and narrower in their circular form and the trachea becomes a slit-like crescent or c-shaped tube. This is brought about by the posterior membranous portion of the trachea invaginating into the cartilaginous c ring. This pronounced narrowing of the lumen of the tracheobronchial tree during the forced expulsion of air brings about a marked increase in the air flow velocity and allows the escaping gas to clean the

mucosa with a greater degree of efficiency (Comroe, 1965).

The cilia found lining the lumen of the trachea and bronchi beat rhythmically at a regular rate, 160 to 1500 times per minute. Their beat is such that they can waft the mucus coat with any embedded foreign material toward the larynx at a speed of approximately 16 mm. per minute (Proctor, 1964; Comroe, 1965). Such sweeping action is extremely important in keeping the tracheobronchial tree free of smaller particulate matter which may be inhaled. A great proportion of particles between 8 and 20 μ in size are caught in the bronchi and removed by the ciliary action. It should be noted that certain situations are harmful to this ciliary action. Hypoxia has been shown to slow or to stop the motion and, surprisingly enough, hyperoxia will do the same (Laurenzi et al., 1968). Cigarette smoking has also been shown to result in a cessation of action of the cilia (Ballenger, 1960).

Certain disease states affect the motion of the bronchi. Bronchial asthma is associated with a spasm of the smooth muscles of the bronchial musculature as a result of the allergic antigen-antibody reaction, producing a markedly narrowed airway. The bronchi of the emphysema patient are atrophic and, hence, flabby and tend to collapse quite easily (Wright, 1960; Petty et al., 1965). This is particularly so during forced expiration, at which time the intrathoracic pressure is sufficient to collapse the bronchi and cause obstruction to air flow. In chronic bronchitis the bronchi also have a tendency to collapse during expiration (Petty et al., 1965; Filley, 1967). In addition, the hypertrophied mucus glands further obstruct the air flow by impinging on the bronchial lumen (DeHaller and Reid, 1965; Mitchell et al., 1966; Reid, 1960, 1967).

MECHANICS OF BREATHING

In order to move air in and out of the lungs, two forms of resistance must be overcome; these are elasticity and friction.

In considering elasticity, the lung per se and the chest wall must both be included. The elastic tendency of the lung may be likened to a rubber band. When the lung tissue is stretched it tends to recoil toward a collapsed or emptied position. The chest cage, on the other hand tends, to act like a spring that is partially compressed. It tends to seek the expanded position of maximum inspiration. These opposite trends of elasticity may be fully realized if the chest x-ray of a patient who has a pneumothorax is studied. Here can be visualized the collapsed lung and the chest cage which is expanded toward the inspiratory position. If the work of breathing is related to the elasticity, it becomes apparent that the work on inspiration is done by expanding the lung, whereas the work during expiration is done to compress the rib cage. Furthermore, the larger the volume per breath the greater the work against elasticity.

Friction is encountered in two forms, tissue resistance and air flow resistance (Otis et al., 1950; Fenn, 1951). So-called tissue resistance is encountered in the friction of ribs moving in their joints, the diaphragm peeling off the chest wall and compressing abdominal viscera during inspiration, and the pulling apart of alveolar and respiratory bronchial walls as air enters previously nonused spaces. Some include here the various stages of mechanical advantage during contraction of muscles and moving of ribs and diaphragm.

Air flow resistance is encountered in two forms, laminar and turbulent air flow (Comroe et al., 1962). Laminar air flow is normally found in the trachea and larger bronchi. Such resistance is related to the viscosity of the gas. Turbulence occurs with high speed air flow and particularly around the bends such as the bifurcation of bronchi and segmental bronchi. This frictional resistance is related to the density of the gas. Both forms of frictional resistance are increased with increase in the rate of respiration. It should be noted that if one alters the radius of an airway, the work of breathing will vary inversely with the fourth power of the radius of that airway; thus, if one diminishes the radius of the airway to one half its previous size, it will now take 16 times the pressure to push the same amount of gas through the airway in the same period of time (Comroe, 1965).

If the work of breathing is plotted against the frequency of respirations, keeping the minute ventilation constant at 6 L., and if the work done against friction and elasticity are separated, a graph similar to Figure 11 is produced. If the patient breathes one breath of 6 L. in one minute, the work is maximum against elasticity and minimum against friction. Keeping the minute volume constant at 6 L. per minute and increasing the rate of breathing, the work per breath against elasticity diminishes while the work against friction increases. When the total work per breath is plotted, it

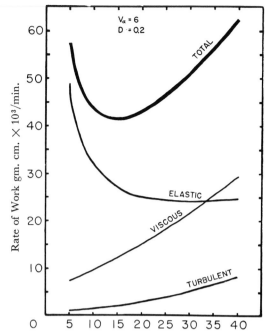

Figure 11. Relationship of elastic and frictional (viscous and turbulent) fractions of the total work of breathing at a rate of 6 L. per minute using different frequencies. Values calculated according to a modification of equation 5. (After Otis, A. B., Fenn, W. O., and Rahn, H.: J. Appl. Physiol. 2:592, 1950.

becomes obvious that while breathing 6 L. per minute the optimum rate of respiration is approximately 12 breaths per minute. This optimum value will shift to the right or left, depending on whether the disease increases work done against friction or elasticity (Fenn, 1951).

The compliance of the lung and chest wall, an expression of the elasticity, can be calculated in the laboratory. The determination is done by measuring the changes in intraesophageal pressure while simultaneously recording changes in pulmonary volume. By the method of Mead and Whittenberger (1953) the mean compliance is 0.22 liters per centimeter of water pressure change.

Air flow resistance may be measured by utilizing a total body plethysmograph. As done by the method of DuBois et al. (1956), the normal mean airway resistance is equal to 1.5 cm. of water per liter per second of air flow.

In order to evaluate the mechanics of breathing of an individual patient, certain pulmonary function studies may be done in the laboratory. The forced vital capacity is the maximum amount of air that can be exhaled from the lung after a maximum inspiration. This forced vital capacity will vary with the age, height and sex of the individual being tested (Kory et al., 1961; Baldwin et al., 1948). This measurement is useful in following the progress of an individual patient such as one in heart failure or one who has had a failure of his respiratory muscles such as in Guillain-Barré syndrome or poliomyelitis. It does not, however, give a very dynamic picture of the patient per se.

The forced expiratory volumes (FEV) in one, two, and three seconds are measurements expressed as a percentage of the forced vital capacity (FVC) which can be exhaled in the first second, the first two seconds, or the first three seconds of the effort. Normally the FEV_1 will be 75 to 80 per cent of the total FVC, while the FEV_2 will equal 85 to 90 per cent of the FVC; the FEV_3 will equal 95 to 100 per cent of the FVC. This determination was originally called the timed vital capacity by Gaensler (1951); many variations of such a study have been devised over the years. This particular determination is a much more dynamic study and gives the physician a closer evaluation of whether the air volume of the forced vital capacity is really available to the patient to use. A patient with a small forced vital capacity with 100 per cent available for use is much less likely to become dyspneic than a patient who has a very large forced vital capacity but only 30 or 40 per cent of it available to him.

The maximum voluntary ventilation (MVV) is defined as the maximum amount of air that a patient can voluntarily move in and out of his lungs per minute. This study is performed by having a patient breath as hard and as fast as he can under a coercsive cheer-leading effort by the technician. He breathes for 12 to 15 seconds, and the measured amount of air which moves in and out of the lungs is multiplied by four or five in order to obtain the minute value. The performance of this test will vary with age, sex, and body surface area (Kory et al., 1961; Baldwin et al., 1948). This evaluation adds the aspect of stamina to the FEV_1 and thus becomes much more valuable in the evaluation of a patient's ventilatory ability. It is especially valuable for preoperative evaluation of the patient (Woodruff et al., 1953).

It is particularly difficult to relate the subjective symptom of dyspnea to any pulmonary function study. However, Warring (1945) devised a dyspnea index which is the ratio of the required minute ventilation to the maximum voluntary ventilation. When this ratio exceeds 30 per cent the patient will usually be dyspneic. When it reaches 40 per cent the patient is usually quite uncomfortable. A dyspnea index of 50 per cent or higher indicates a person who is usually markedly and symptomatically impaired.

There are three major patterns of ventilation abnormalities; these are restrictive, obstructive, and neuromuscular.

The restrictive-type ventilation defect has a pattern which consists of a reduced FVC and relatively normal FEV and MVV performances. Many diseases and conditions will result in this type of ventilation abnormality. They include (1) conditions which occupy space in the thorax, such as a pleural effusion or a pneumothorax; (2) disease processes which replace normally functioning lung tissue (e.g., diffuse interstitial fibrosis, lobar pneumonia, and a large tumor mass; (3) the extensive operative removal of lung tissue as in a lobectomy or pneumonectomy, and (4) any situation which pushes the diaphragm up and immobilizes it, such as a multiple pregnancy at term or a massive tense ascites.

Obstructive-type ventilation defects are typified by the production of studies of the patient which consist of a normal or lowered FVC and very diminished FEV and MVV values. This type of ventilatory abnormality is the result of diseases which in some way narrow the airway or obstruct the flow of air from the lungs. Examples of conditions in which an obstruction to air flow is encountered are (1) laryngeal narrowing (e.g., edema or neoplasm); (2) tracheal obstruction by an endotracheal tumor or stricture or by compression from without as occurs often with aneurysm of the aorta; (3) bronchial narrowing as it occurs during the muscle spasm, mucosal edema, and mucus secretion of bronchial asthma (Comroe, 1965); and (4) bronchial obstruction when its lumen is impinged upon by hypertrophied mucous glands and their secretions in chronic bronchitis and by collapse of the walls of the bronchi during expiration in patients with chronic bronchitis and emphysema (Mitchell et al., 1966; Petty et al., 1966; Filley, 1967).

The ventilation abnormality of the neuromuscular type consists of a virtually normal FVC and FEV_1. Patients with neuromuscular insufficiency are not able to carry out the sustained effort necessary for performance of the MVV. Therefore, the MVV values are usually quite low. This pattern is most commonly seen in patients who have been bedridden with a chronic debilitating illness. However, patients with specific neuromusculature diseases such as muscular dystrophy, multiple sclerosis, and myasthenia gravis will very often display this particular pattern in their function tests.

ALVEOLAR PHYSIOLOGIC FUNCTION

The inner surface of the alveolus is made up of alveolar cells of two types: Type I cells are thin alveolar lining cells; Type II cells are more spheroidal and granular. They apparently secrete a surface actant material which coats the inside of the alveolus. The cells rest upon a basement membrane which is often in direct apposition to the basement membrane of the alveolar capillary.

The material which lines the alveoli is composed of phospholipids, neutral lipids, polysaccharides, mucopolysaccharides, and protein. Together they make up the surfactant system of the lung. The resulting surface action provides for increased surface tension during expansion and decreased surface tension during contraction of the alveolus.

During inspiration the surfactant material acts to further the complete expansion of lung by increasing in degree of surface tension with inflation (Scarpelli, 1968). A minimum pressure is needed to initiate inflation of the degassed lung. This minimum pressure is dependent on the surface tension and the radius of the terminal airway. Once underway, inflation of the alveolus increases the surface tension in the alveolus. The pressure required for enlarging the volume is a function of the La Place relationship for a sphere.

$$P = 2\ \gamma/r \qquad \begin{aligned} &P = \text{internal pressure} \\ &\gamma = \text{surface tension} \\ &r = \text{radius} \end{aligned}$$

Thus, the increasing surface tension plus the natural elasticity of the alveolus requires an increased pressure to continue the lung inflation. In addition, the smaller airways and their alveoli are progressively recruited by the increased pressure being applied.

The noted variability in surface tension brought about by the surfactant system provides for a stability of the lung during expiration. Such stability occurs because, as the alveolus becomes smaller, the surface tension becomes progressively less and, according to the La Place relationship ($P = 2\ \gamma/r$), when the surface tension is very low the internal pressure is minimal. Thus, the natural tendency for the smaller elastic alveoli to empty into the

larger ones is counteracted and the collapse of small alveoli is prevented.

The surfactant system of the lung may be altered by many abnormal or disease states. Among these are ischemia, hypoxia, hyperoxia, hypercarbia, pulmonary edema, inhalation of cigarette smoke and air pollutants, and the aspiration of hydrocarbons and surfactants (Scarpelli, 1968).

Inhaled gases enter the alveoli during inspiration and leave during expiration. At least a portion of the gas motion occurs by diffusion of the various gases within the air space itself. In this regard oxygen diffuses in a mixture of gases much better than carbon dioxide. Thus, if one introduces a high concentration of oxygen at the larynx, a goodly amount of the oxygen will diffuse through the gas all the way to the alveolus even though no respiratory motions are encountered. Carbon dioxide, on the other hand, does not diffuse in gas nearly so well as oxygen. If alveolar ventilation is not accomplished, the carbon dioxide tension in the alveolus, and hence in the capillary blood, will rise to high levels. Gases in the alveolus and in the capillary blood diffuse across the alveolar capillary membrane passively according to the pressure difference, the flow being from the area of high pressure to an area of low pressure; thus, oxygen diffuses from the alveolus into the capillary blood, and carbon dioxide diffuses from the blood into the alveolar space. Carbon dioxide is some 25 times more diffusable in water than is oxygen; hence, carbon dioxide diffuses through the capillary lining cell and the alveolar lining cell much more readily than does oxygen.

This difference has led to the description of an alveolar-capillary block syndrome in which a clinical state of respiratory alkalosis with a low partial pressure of carbon dioxide (PCO_2) in the blood coexists with low partial pressure of oxygen (PO_2). Such a state is said to exist when an alteration in the alveolar-capillary membrane occurs that will block the oxygen transfer but does not block the more readily diffusable carbon dioxide which is reduced by alveolar hyperventilation. This theory is being challenged by investigators who feel that there is really no situation that exists in which a functioning alveolar-capillary membrane is altered enough to really block the transfer of oxygen.

There is normally a balance that exists between the ventilation of the alveoli with air and the perfusion of the alveoli with blood. This occurs in a ratio of 4 L. of alveolar ventilation to 5 L. of blood flow in the normal resting lung. However, normally there are areas of a certain degree of imbalance, so that the apical portions of the lung in the upright position will receive smaller amounts of blood flow and ventilation than the basal portions of the lung. The ratio of ventilation to blood flow in the apex is such that the blood is relatively hyperoxic when it leaves the alveolus. The larger total amount of ventilation and perfusion occurs in the lower portions of the lung fields. The ratio, however, allows for slightly less oxygenation per unit of blood in this portion of the lung. The peripheral arterial blood gas levels are the result of the mixture of pulmonary venous blood from all parts of the lung (West, 1962).

One of the more common physiologic abnormalities that occurs is a condition which will produce a ventilation-perfusion imbalance. Many different diseases involving the pulmonary parenchyma will result in a ventilation-perfusion imbalance. Examples include chronic obstructive pulmonary diseases such as emphysema, chronic bronchitis, and prolonged severe asthma; diffuse lung diseases including sarcoidosis, pulmonary fibrosis, interstitial pneumonias, pneumonoconiosis and pulmonary edema; and areas of atelectasis including tiny widespread areas of micro-atelectasis. When such an imbalance occurs there will be areas of the lung which are overventilated and underperfused and other areas which are underventilated and overperfused. Such an imbalance will always result in at least a slight degree of hypoxia; large areas of ventilation-perfusion imbalance will result in more severe degrees of hypoxia. This hypoxia cannot be corrected by the overventilation of small areas of the lung breathing room air. This is because of the peculiar nature of the hemoglobin dissociation curve for oxygen.

The effect of ventilation-perfusion imbalance on the blood level of carbon dioxide, however, is considerably more varied. If the ventilation-perfusion imbalance is severe, there will most likely be retention of carbon dioxide. However, it must be pointed out that the hemoglobin dissociation curve for carbon dioxide in the physiologic range is virtually a straight line (Fig. 12). Therefore, a small area of lung being normally perfused and overventilated can account for a rather marked loss of carbon dioxide from the blood of that area. When this particular bit of blood is mixed with the blood returning from other areas which are underventilated, the mixture may well balance to produce a normal amount of CO_2 in the blood

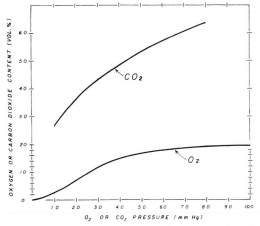

Figure 12. O_2 and CO_2 dissociation curves plotted on the same scale to illustrate the important point that the O_2 curve has a very steep and a very flat portion and the CO_2 curve does not. Therefore, hyperventilation breathing air cannot raise the PO_2 or the O_2 saturation beyond a certain point. However, the PCO_2 can decrease to a very low level as a result of the hyperventilation. (From Comroe, J. H., Jr.: Physiology of Respiration. Chicago, Year Book Medical Publishers, 1965.)

or an even lower than normal amount. A ventilation-perfusion imbalance then, while most often associated with hypoxia, may also be associated with either an elevated PCO_2 (respiratory acidosis), normal PCO_2 or, on occasion, a lowered PCO_2 (respiratory alkalosis).

There are several methods available for evaluating the alveolar function. The determination of the amount of lung volume, hence alveolar volume, is relatively easily done by the helium dilution method as described by Meneely and Kaltreider (1949). The diffusing capacity of the lung is also rather easily determined in the laboratory during either the single breath diffusing capacity test for carbon monoxide as described by Ogilvie et al (1957) or by doing a steady-state diffusing capacity test according to the method of Filley et al. (1954). For practical purposes, however, the simplest and most reliable clinical evaluation of the moment is derived from an analysis of the arterial blood gas contents. Arterial puncture is safely and easily performed (Petty et al., 1966). This can be done either on the radial, brachial, or femoral artery; in adults no complications have been reported to date. A sample of arterial blood obtained anaerobically in a heparinized syringe can be analyzed quickly and inexpensively for pH, PO_2, PCO_2, and oxygen saturation. This can be done either by using the method devised by Siggaard-Anderson (1965) on the Astrup-type equipment or by utilizing

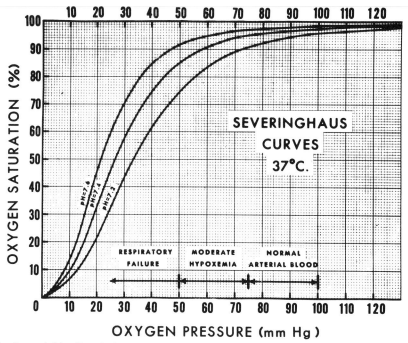

Figure 13. Oxyhemoglobin dissociation curves, based on the data of Severinghaus (1966). The range of arterial oxygen pressure values encountered in respiratory failure is indicated. (From Filley, G. F.: Pulmonary Insufficiency and Respiratory Failure. Philadelphia, Lea & Febiger, 1967.)

the Clark and Severinghaus (1960) electrodes and the Instrumentation Laboratories type equipment. These determinations take only moments and can be repeated frequently during the day or night to evaluate the status of a patient who is having a respiratory problem.

Figure 13 illustrates the hemoglobin dissociation curve for oxygen and carbon dioxide according to Severinghaus. It should be noted that the dissociation curve for oxygen is a sigmoid-shaped curve; the lower ranges of PO_2 and O_2 saturation on the straight line ascending portion of the curve are probably better determined using an oximeter and determining the O_2 saturation, as this portion of the curve occurs with a minimum of pressure change. However, on the top flat portion of the curve where the saturation changes very little but the partial pressure of the oxygen is widely variable, a direct PO_2 type determination is probably much more informative and reliable. For extremely accurate oxygen content determination, the method of Peters and Van Slyke should be used (Peters and Van Slyke, 1932).

Breathing air at sea level, a patient should have a partial pressure of oxygen in his arterial blood in the range of 80 to 110 mm. Hg. If the PO_2 falls below 75 mm. Hg the patient is hypoxic and in a state of respiratory failure; a

PO_2 below 50 mm. Hg is indicative of severe respiratory failure. Reference to the hemoglobin dissociation curve shows that when the hemoglobin is normal and the pH is 7.4, blood under a PO_2 of 50 mm. Hg will be 85 per cent saturated with oxygen. Most clinicians cannot detect cyanosis until the O_2 saturation of the blood is below 80 per cent. Therefore, a patient can be in severe hypoxia and respiratory failure and still appear pink to the clinician. One must have a high index of suspicion and analyze arterial blood gas whenever there is a possibility that the patient is in a state of respiratory failure.

The normal partial pressure for carbon dioxide in the arterial blood should not exceed 45 mm. Hg. When the PCO_2 is 50 mm. Hg or higher, this also is considered respiratory failure. If the PCO_2 exceeds 80 mm. Hg, this represents severe respiratory failure. It is not unusual to find the patient with a PCO_2 of 80 mm. Hg or more in a lethargic state. Coma may occur if the PCO_2 rises rapidly or to a level of 100 or more, particularly if the pH is below 7.25 and the patient is also hypoxic (Sieker and Hickam, 1956; Refsum, 1963). The clinician must have a high index of suspicion for CO_2 retention because the patient may exhibit no signs or symptoms of elevated PCO_2

until the level has reached near lethal proportions. The patient who is a candidate for respiratory failure should have periodic determinations of his arterial blood PCO_2, PO_2, and O_2 saturation as well as pH. Management may then be based on these findings.

CONTROL OF RESPIRATION*

There is no one respiratory center in the brain. There are a number of areas in the medulla and pons which correlate incoming stimuli and generate efferent integrated and correlated nervous responses of simple or complex type. Such are necessary to effectively alter the respiratory action of the organism in an appropriate manner.

A pneumotaxic center has been identified in the upper pons. This center is related to rhythmic respiration, apparently by the action of inhibiting inspiration and stimulating expiration.

An apneustic center located in the lower pons appears to be the center of the vagal inflation reflex, although the vagal efferents have not been traced to it. If the pneumotaxic center and the vagi are ablated, respiration will cease in the inspiratory position (apneusis).

In the lower medulla the medullary center receives impulses from the higher respiratory centers. Stimuli also come from the hypothalamus, cortex, and reticular-activating system. Efferent impulses from this center stimulate a coordinated pattern of alternating inspiration and expiration.

The medulla also has two chemoreceptor areas on the lateral aspect of its upper portion. These are hydrogen ion receptors. At one time these receptors were thought to respond to increases in the PCO_2. Now it is considered more likely that the stimulus is an increment in the hydrogen ion concentration in the spinal fluid which is brought about by the elevation of the arterial PCO_2. Carbon dioxide then diffuses quite easily into the cerebral spinal fluid to form carbonic acid. The latter dissociates and raises the hydrogen ion concentration. This increased concentration of hydrogen ion goes unbuffered because the cerebral spinal fluid has no hemoglobin and is low in protein; also, the meninges are relatively impermeable to bicarbonate, which can only slowly enter the cerebral spinal fluid. Impulses from these

central chemoreceptors are transmitted to the medullary center for coordination with other stimuli and subsequent action.

Other chemoreceptors are found in the aortic and carotid bodies. These chemoreceptors also react to the stimulus of increased hydrogen ion concentration to reflexly cause an increase in the rate and volume of respiration. They also respond to large increments of arterial PCO_2.

The aortic and carotid body chemoreceptors are also sensitive to a lack of oxygen. This sensitivity is considerably less than that to hydrogen ion concentration or PCO_2. The amount of oxygen in the inspired air must drop to the 8 to 10 per cent level before stimulation to respiration is noted in normal man. Further decrease causes a large increase in ventilation. The actual stimulus to these chemoreceptors is more likely a decreased oxygen supply rather than a simple drop in arterial PO_2. This is seen to be true during a time of diminished or absent blood flow to the receptors.

Other reflexes enter more or less into the control of respiration in man. These include the Hering-Breuer reflexes which are mediated via the vagus nerve. One stimulus is the stretch of the lung tissue which occurs during inflation. The action is to inhibit further inspiration. Another stimulus is deflation of the lung, which stimulates inspiration.

The paradoxical reflex of Head described in rabbits is of interest. According to Comroe, Head cooled the vagi to 0° C. and noted that inflation of the lung did not inhibit inspiration. Further, as the nerves were being warmed, inflation of the lungs produced a paradoxical further inspiration rather than the usual inhibition of inspiration. Such a reflex if present in man could be of value in the newborn and in opening up atelectatic areas in the adult.

A number of other reflexes exert their control over respirations in animals and perhaps in man. The stretch reflex of skeletal muscle is familiar to everyone. In this reflex a muscle is stretched, for example, by tapping the tendon, and the skeletal muscle contracts reflexly. The same or a very similar reflex occurs in the muscles of respiration wherein stretching brings about contraction. This reflex may well have to do with interpreting stimuli from the respiratory center into the necessary rate and depth of respiration. It may also be responsible for the adaptation of response in the situation in which there is obstruction to air flow.

Reflexes arising in the carotid sinus and aortic arch influence respiration in addition to

---

*For a more complete description and more detailed references the reader should consult Comroe (1965), from which this topic was abstracted.

their effect on the cardiovascular system. An elevation of blood pressure inhibits the respiratory centers. A fall in blood pressure stimulates an increase in ventilation. This response may also serve the cardiovascular needs by lowering the mean intrathoracic pressure and helping to increase venous return to the heart. The improved ventilation would also tend to improve oxygenation and removal of carbon dioxide.

Certain chemoreflexes arising in the thorax of animals are of great theoretical importance to man. Following the intravenous injection of certain chemicals or the inhalation of irritant gases, a triad of bradycardia, hypotension, and apnea has been observed in animals. Such chemoreflexes may be of importance in man in regard to the ill effects, similar to the triad, which have been known to occur during the rapid intravenous injection of medication, during anesthesia or the inhalation of irritant fumes, at the time of pulmonary embolism, and as a result of thoracic surgery procedures about the hilum of the lung.

Reflexes arising in somatic and visceral tissue may increase the rate and depth of breathing. These reflexes may be originated by stimulation of pain, temperature, or mechanoreceptors. Well known examples include the hyperventilation which accompanies the application of cold water to the skin and the response of the apneic infant to spanking, cold water, or even stretching of the anal sphincter.

Finally, there is the variation of the influence of sensory stimuli which is dependent upon the state of wakefulness. Wakefulness is a powerful stimulus to respiration and may well override other types of stimuli. During sleep certain reflexes are depressed; for example, ventilation is diminished and the PCO_2 rises without its usual effect on respiration. Other stimuli, however, are unaffected (Comroe, 1965).

REFERENCES

Baldwin, E. deF., Cournand, A., Richards, D. W., Jr.: Pulmonary insufficiency I: Physiological classifications, clinical methods of analysis, standard values in normal subjects. Medicine 27:243, 1948.

Ballenger, J. J.: Cigarette smoke and respiratory cilia. New Eng. J. Med. 263:832, 1960.

Comroe, J. H., Jr.: Physiology of Respiration. Chicago, Year Book Medical Publishers, Inc., 1965.

Comroe, J. H., Jr., Forster, R. E., II, DuBois, A. B., Briscoe, W. A., and Carlsen, E.: The Lung: Clinical Physiology and Pulmonary Function Tests. 2nd ed. Chicago, Year Book Medical Publishers, Inc., 1962.

DeHaller, R., and Reid, L.: Adult chronic bronchitis—Morphology, histochemistry and vascularization of the bronchial mucous glands. Med. Thorac. 22:549, 1965.

DuBois, A. B., Botelho, S. Y., and Comroe, J. H., Jr.: A new method for measuring airway resistance in man using a body plethysmograph: Values in normal subjects and in patients with respiratory disease. J. Clin. Invest. 35:327, 1956.

Fenn, W. O.: Mechanics of respiration. Amer. J. Med. 10:77, 1951.

Filley, G. F.: Pulmonary insufficiency and generalized obstruction of the airways. In Pulmonary Insufficiency and Respiratory Failure. Philadelphia, Lea & Febiger, 1967, Chap. 2.

Filley, G. F., MacIntosh, D. J., and Wright, G. W.: Carbon monoxide uptake and pulmonary diffusing capacity in normal subjects at rest and during exercise. J. Clin. Invest. 33:530, 1954.

Gaensler, E. A.: Analysis of the ventilatory defect by timed vital capacity measurements. Amer. Rev. Tuberc. 64:256, 1951.

Kory, R. C., Callahan, R., Boren, H. G., and Syner, J. C.: Clinical spirometry in normal men. Amer. J. Med. 30:243, 1961.

Laurenzi, G. A., Yin, S., and Guarneri, J. J.: The adverse effect of oxygen on tracheal mucus flow. New Eng. J. Med. 279:333, 1968.

Mead, J., and Whittenberger, J. L.: Physical properties of human lungs measured during spontaneous respiration. J. Appl. Physiol. 5:779, 1953.

Meneely, G. R., and Kaltreider, N. L.: Volume of lung determined by helium dilution: Description of method and comparison with other procedures. J. Clin. Invest. 28:129, 1949.

Miller, W. S.: The Lung. 2nd ed. Springfield, Ill. Charles C Thomas, 1950.

Mitchell, R. S., Ryan, S. F., Petty, T. L., and Filley, G. F.: The significance of morphologic chronic hyperplastic bronchitis. Amer. Rev. Resp. Dis. 93:720, 1966.

Ogilvie, C. M., Forster, R. E., Blakemore, W. S., and Morton, J. W.: A standardized breath holding technique for the clinical measurement of diffusing capacity of the lung for carbon monoxide. J Clin. Invest. 36:1, 1957.

Otis, A. B., Fenn, W. O., and Rahn, H.: Mechanics of breathing in man. J. Appl. Physiol. 2:592, 1950.

Peters, J. P., and Van Slyke, D. D.: Quantitative Clinical Chemistry, Volume II (Methods). Baltimore, The Williams & Wilkins Co., 1932. (Reprinted 1956.)

Petty, T. L., Bigelow, B., and Levine, B. F.: The simplicity and safety of arterial puncture. J.A.M.A. 195:693, 1966.

Petty, T. L., Mercort, R., Ryan, S., Vincent, T., Filley, G. F., and Mitchell, R. S.: The functional and bronchographic evaluation of postmortem human lungs. Amer. Rev. Resp. Dis. 92:450, 1965.

Proctor, D. F.: Physiology of the Upper airway. Handbook of Physiology Section 3, Respiration, Volume I, Chapter 8. Editors, W. O. Fenn and H. Rahn. American Physiological Society, Washington, D.C. 1964.

Refsum, H. E.: Relationship between state of consciousness and arterial hypoxemia and hypercapnea in patients with respiratory insufficiency, breathing air. Clin. Sci. 25:361, 1963.

Reid, L.: Measurement of the bronchial mucous gland layer: A diagnostic yardstick in chronic bronchitis. Thorax 15:132, 1960.

Reid, L.: The Pathology of Emphysema. Chicago, Year Book Medical Publishers, Inc., 1967.

Scarpelli, E M.: The Surfactant System of the Lung. Philadelphia, Lea & Febiger, 1968.

Severinghaus, J. W.: Respiratory system: Methods of gas analysis. *In* Glasser, O. (ed.) Medical Physics. Vol. 3, pp. 550, 559. Chicago, Year Book Publishers, Inc., 1960.

Sieker, H. O., and Hickam, J. B.: Carbon dioxide intoxication: The clinical syndrome, its etiology and management with particular reference to the use of mechanical respirators. Medicine *35*:389, 1956.

Siggaard-Anderson, O.: The Acid-Base Status of the Blood. Baltimore, The Williams & Wilkins Company, 1965.

Warring, F. C., Jr.: Ventilatory function. Experiences with a simple procedure for its evaluation in patients with pulmonary tuberculosis. Amer. Rev. Tuberc. *51*:432, 1945.

West, J.: Regional differences in gas exchange in the lung of erect man. J. Appl. Physiol. *17*:893, 1962.

Witt, R. L., and Wiot, J. F.: Cinebronchography. *In* Tice-Harvey Practice of Medicine, Volume II. Hagerstown, Maryland, W. F. Prior Company, Inc., 1965.

Woodruff, W., Merchel, C. G., and Wright, G. W.: Decisions in thoracic surgery as influenced by the knowledge of pulmonary physiology. J. Thorac. Surg. *26*:156, 1953.

Wright, R. R.: Bronchial atrophy and collapse in chronic obstructive pulmonary emphysema. Amer. J. Path. *37*:63, 1960.

Section Three

BIOCHEMISTRY

Chapter 11

BASIC PRINCIPLES OF CELLULAR METABOLISM

by James F. Koerner, Ph.D.

DEFINITIONS AND BASIC ASSUMPTIONS

The word "metabolism" refers to the chemical reactions that occur in living organisms. It is now a fundamental assumption of biochemists that these reactions conform to the same laws of chemistry and physics that also govern the reactions of nonliving matter. This assumption has far-reaching consequences. One consequence is that matter is conserved in living things. Every carbon, nitrogen, or any other atom that enters an organism can, at all times, be accounted for in one compound or another within the organism until it is finally released to the environment. Living things must balance their chemical equations. Another consequence is that energy is conserved and the laws of thermodynamics are applicable. Converting simple precursors to complicated proteins, polysaccharides, lipids, and other constituents inevitably requires energy, and this energy must come from somewhere. Along with anabolic (synthetic) energy-requiring reactions, organisms must carry out catabolic (degradative) energy-yielding reactions that provide the necessary energy. In addition, catabolism must furnish the energy expended by the organism as mechanical work and also the heat energy and entropy that inevitably must be expended during the operation of essentially irreversible processes. This energy ultimately comes from the sun. Photosynthetic plants are capable of utilizing solar energy to perform anabolic reactions, and it is the resulting plant-produced organic compounds that are, directly

or indirectly, the source of energy for animals. These organic compounds are also the precursors or "building blocks" for all the protein, nucleic acids, polysaccharides, lipids, and other constituents synthesized by the animal.

DISTINGUISHING FEATURES OF METABOLIZING ORGANISMS

It seems impossible to devise an adequate definition that unequivocally differentiates between all forms of life and all natural or contrived nonliving chemical and mechanical systems. However, living things do possess certain distinguishing features which, when considered together, display a pattern that is found nowhere else. It seems reasonable to believe that this is true because life originated only once, or perhaps a limited number of times by similar events, and then developed through an unbroken chain of evolution and diversification that must establish a kinship between all individual organisms, living or dead, and all species, extant or extinct.

Some of the distinguishing features pertaining to the metabolism of all organisms will now be reviewed.

Enzyme Catalysis

One distinguishing feature of living organisms is that almost all their metabolic reactions are catalyzed by enzymes. The constituents of living things are quite stable under physiological conditions, that is, in dilute

393

aqueous salt solutions, at pH near neutrality and a range of temperatures whose absolute extremes for a few organisms are near the freezing point or somewhat below the boiling point of water. In fact, stability under these conditions was probably a prerequisite for selection as a component of living matter, and compounds of biological origin with half-lives as short as a few hours under these conditions in the absence of enzymes are definitely exceptional. All enzymes are proteins (Dickerson and Geis, 1969). Each kind of enzyme has a definite molecular structure with a unique amino acid sequence and a unique three-dimensional conformation of the peptide chain. Each kind of enzyme molecule possesses the necessary specific structure to interact with and catalyze a reaction of a specific compound or group of related compounds. During enzyme catalysis, the reactants (substrates) interact with specific functional groups of the enzyme molecule (the active site). This binding brings the reactants into precise juxtaposition and also alters the chemical reactivity of their functional groups in such a way that a specific reaction takes place that otherwise would occur only rarely under physiological conditions. The products of the reaction are released from the active site; the free enzyme molecules then have the same structure they had before the reaction, and they can participate in the conversion of additional molecules of the substrate. Each enzyme shows a remarkable specificity not only for the kind of reaction which it will catalyze but also for the structure and stereochemistry of nonreacting portions of the substrate molecules. This specificity is not necessarily absolute; closely related analogues to the natural substrate sometimes can be found that participate in the enzymatic reaction. However, such analogues often are not present in the living system in which the enzyme operates; the combination of highly specific enzymes and a limited number of natural substrates together make metabolism in vivo remarkably free from wasteful and purposeless side-reactions.

Coupled Reactions

A feature of living systems that baffled biologists for decades is how these systems derive the energy necessary to conduct their intricate biosynthetic and physiological feats. Before it was established that total energy is indeed conserved in living things, this problem provided a fruitful area for invoking the intervention of speculative "vital forces." Later it made possible the proliferation of elegant hypothetical mechanisms for energy transfer. The distinctive manner in which this is now known to take place is by pairs of chemical reactions that share a common intermediate, that is, coupled reactions. In order to participate efficiently in energy transfer, the common intermediate must possess certain properties, and during evolution a limited number of substances were selected for this role. These include the high-energy phosphate compounds, typified by ATP* (Lipmann, 1941). It happens that the free energy for hydrolysis of either of the two phosphate anhydride linkages in ATP, one yielding ADP and P_i, the other AMP and PP_i, is much greater than the free energy change involved in formation of many biologically important phosphate ester linkages and other linkages. If an anabolic reaction such as the formation of glucose-6-phosphate from glucose, occurs by a reaction involving hydrolysis of ATP, such as the reaction catalyzed by the enzyme hexokinase,

glucose + ATP → glucose-6-phosphate + ADP,

the equilibrium constant of this reaction will be strongly favorable to synthesis of glucose-6-phosphate. Now if this reaction is coupled with a reaction of a catabolic process that derives sufficient energy from breakdown of some compound to produce ATP with favorable equilibrium, the catabolic process will effectively "drive" the formation of glucose-6-phosphate through participation of the common intermediate, ATP. Examples of systems which produce ATP in mammals include the familiar glycolytic pathway and the mitochondrial electron transport system. In the latter system, reduced coenzymes such as NADH and $FADH_2$, formed during catabolism of acetyl CoA by the citric acid cycle or during catabolism of fatty acids by the fatty acid degradative cycle, are reoxidized, and the energy for this is utilized for formation of ATP. The hydrolysis of this ATP, in turn, "drives" a large number

---

*The abbreviations used are those accepted by the Journal of Biological Chemistry and include: ATP, ADP, AMP, adenosine tri-, di-, and monophosphate; GTP, guanosine triphosphate; UTP, uridine triphosphate; CDP, cytidine diphosphate; P_i, PP_i, inorganic orthophosphate and pyrophosphate; NAD, NADH, nicotinamide adenine dinucleotide and its reduced form; NADP, NADPH, nicotinamide adenine dinucleotide phosphate and its reduced form; CoA, coenzyme A; DNA, deoxyribonucleic acid; RNA, ribonucleic acid.

of metabolic processes, including polysaccharide synthesis, muscle contraction, and nucleic acid and protein synthesis.

Although ATP occupies a key role in the economy of the cell, it is not the unique intermediary between anabolism and catabolism. In some cases other high energy phosphate compounds (e.g., GTP or phosphoenolpyruvate), nucleotide-sugars (e.g., UDP-glucose), coenzyme A derivatives (e.g., palmityl CoA) or nucleotide-lipids (e.g., CDP-choline) are used. In other cases reduced coenzymes (e.g., NADPH) are directly involved instead of being used for ATP synthesis as mentioned previously. In all cases the basic principle is the same: the intermediate is synthesized by thermodynamically favorable catabolic reactions; it is degraded to provide energy for an anabolic process.

In reality all so-called anabolic processes run "down-hill." A process like the abundant, spontaneous biosynthesis of lactose, for example, was formerly observed with awe because the equilibrium for the reaction is, as shown, strongly in favor of hydrolysis:

$$glucose + galactose \rightleftharpoons lactose + H_2O.$$

However, the actual biochemical process is now known to be:

$$glucose + UDP\text{-}galactose \rightarrow lactose + UDP.$$

This reaction occurs with a free energy change favoring lactose synthesis. The high energy intermediate necessary for this process, UDP-galactose, was synthesized by reactions involving the catabolism of ATP; the ATP, in turn, was derived from a catabolic process.

The Genetic Code

A feature of living things that has long been recognized to be unique is the system for their not-quite-perfect self-duplication: the genetic system. Achieving a general description of the chemical basis for this system has recently revolutionized biological knowledge, and, in fact, all human thought in a manner analogous to the revolution wrought near the beginning of this century by the physicists' theories of relativity and quantum mechanics. At the center of the system for heredity is the molecule on which is imprinted the genetic code, DNA (Watson, 1965). The position of every amino acid residue in every peptide chain of every protein of an organism is encoded in its molecules of DNA. The sequence of purine and pyrimidine bases of three adjacent nucleotides of a DNA chain provides the code for each amino acid residue. The entire code sequence is arranged in a linear fashion on the DNA chain, with the triplet code "words" arranged in the same sequence as the sequence of amino acids of the protein. At the end of the code for one peptide chain, a terminating codon is present in the DNA molecule; then the code for another peptide chain starts.

The DNA molecule is constructed of two nucleotide chains rigidly bound together in a helical structure. One chain is complementary to the other in that an adenine base on one chain is always opposite to a thymine on the other, and a guanine on one to a cytosine on the other. During multiplication of the cell the DNA is replicated by a process which involves unwinding of the complementary chains and simultaneous synthesis of two daughter chains, each complementary to its parental chain (Kornberg, 1962). During protein synthesis the nucleotide code sequence of one of the DNA chains is specifically *transcribed* to a newly synthesized molecule of messenger RNA. The messenger RNA code is *translated* into the correct amino acid sequence during protein synthesis by a biochemical system in which the participants include ribosomes, enzymes and their cofactors, amino acids, high energy phosphate compounds, and a number of different kinds of transfer RNA, each kind capable of "recognizing" the messenger RNA code for one amino acid (Watson, 1965). All the components of the nonspecific "factories" for replication, transcription, and translation must be allocated to the daughter cells from the parent so that the DNA code passed on can be interpreted. Given this, the cell can multiply all its protein components, including those of the genetic apparatus itself, and these proteins, in turn, are responsible for synthesis and integration of all other metabolic and structural features of the cell.

Metabolic Controls

Another feature common to all living systems is the group of mechanisms by which metabolism is controlled. The rate of flow of metabolites through each individual enzyme pathway must always be in adjustment to provide the proper balance of materials for the momentary requirements of the organism.

Either overproduction or underproduction of intermediates is pathological or fatal. The demand of the system for a certain metabolite may fluctuate rapidly with changing physiological circumstances, and the systems must accomodate these changes. Rapid advances in understanding control systems in living things have been made only in the past 10 to 15 years. A detailed description of the control mechanisms of mammalian metabolism is not yet available. However, several distinctive mechanisms of control are now known and these probably all play a role in mammalian metabolism.

One such control mechanism operates on the system for synthesis of enzyme protein under the direction of the genetic code. The DNA code of an organism embodies the complete recipe for the amino acid sequence of every protein that the organism can ever make. However, by the two related mechanisms of induction and repression (Jacob and Monod, 1961), this code is read selectively. Certain specific proteins, called repressor proteins, have sites included in their structure for binding to specific regions, the operator genes, in the DNA molecule. Each of the many different kinds of repressors can attach only to its own specific operator gene.

The affinity of a given repressor protein for its operator gene is modified by the presence or absence of certain specific metabolites. In some cases the molecule of a metabolite, when present in excess, binds to the repressor protein, and the structure of the repressor-metabolite complex is altered so that the protein portion does not readily attach to its operator gene. In this case the operator gene is free to initiate expression of a specific part of the genetic message, and certain enzyme proteins are synthesized. This is called *enzyme induction*. Enzyme induction may occur when an excess of some potential nutrient, for example, lactose, triggers the synthesis of enzymes for its utilization, like β-galactosidase. In other cases the molecules of metabolite, when present in excess, bind to the repressor protein, and the structure of the repressor-metabolite complex is altered so the protein more readily attaches to its operator gene than when the metabolite is absent. In this instance the operator gene is blocked and cannot initiate expression of the portion of the genetic message which it controls. This is called *enzyme repression*. Enzyme repression may occur when an end product of metabolism, for instance, an amino acid, accumulates to a level greater than

needed. At that time the production of enzymes for its synthesis may be repressed.

In microorganisms, in which this system is now best understood, growth and multiplication of the cells soon effectively dilute the biosynthetic enzymes that are still present. In nongrowing tissues, such as those found in mammals, the mechanism for removing unneeded enzymes is less clearly understood. In these organisms there may be a system for the destruction, at a controlled rate, of the enzyme proteins and a system of induction and repression for control of their formation (Schimke et al., 1963).

Another system for metabolic control is by *allosteric effectors* (Monod et al., 1963). This mechanism operates by regulating the activity of the enzyme protein that is present rather than governing the synthesis of protein. Certain key enzymes in metabolism possess *allosteric sites* in addition to their catalytically *active site*. The allosteric sites selectively bind certain metabolites, termed allosteric effectors, when these metabolites attain sufficient intracellular concentration. The three-dimensional structure of the entire enzyme molecule is reversibly altered by attachment or removal of these metabolites from the allosteric sites, and these structural changes alter the capability of the active site to catalyze the enzymatic reaction. Allosteric effectors may either be positive (i.e., stimulatory) or negative (i.e., inhibitory) effectors to the enzyme reaction. In many cases the key enzyme involved in this process catalyzes the first reaction of a unique metabolic pathway, and one of end products of the pathway serves as an allosteric effector. Then, when the end product attains an excess concentration, it effectively inhibits production of its starting material and, thus indirectly, of all its intermediates.

Another mechanism for metabolic control is by *enzyme conversion*. Enzyme molecules subject to such control possess specific chemical moieties that can be modified by specific enzyme reactions; that is, enzymes modify these enzymes. At least two systems for conversion are present, one to convert the enzyme to its active form, the other to convert it to its inactive form. A notable feature of these systems is that they are sensitive to the presence of hormones and may provide an explanation at a molecular level of the action of hormones on metabolic processess. The system for enzyme conversion that has been studied best involves enzymes for glycogen synthesis and degradation (Larner, 1966).

EXPERIMENTAL APPROACHES TO STUDY OF METABOLISM

Physiology

A number of different experimental approaches have been fruitful in elucidating metabolism. One general type of methodology may be termed the physiological approach. This is characterized by the experimental philosophy of dealing with an intact animal or an isolated organ, homogenate, or other metabolizing system as a "black box." This approach involves supplying various well defined nutrients and perhaps subjecting the system to the action of various drugs. temperature changes, or other controlled inputs and then measuring various outputs either during the experiment or post mortem. From this information an attempt is made to deduce what is taking place inside the "black box." Some of the earliest meaningful physiological experiments involved feeding large amounts of a specific nutrient or feeding a material with distinctive chemical properties and isolating the products of metabolism. An early triumph was the work of Knoop who, in 1904, used this approach to deduce that fatty acids are degraded into two-carbon fragments. More recently, techniques using isotopic tracers and the entire modern armamentarium of procedures for tissue culture, cell disruption and fractionation, quantitative separation and analysis of a host of biologically important compounds, and antimetabolites and drugs with high specific action against a single enzyme or enzyme system has given the physiological approach great power.

Enzymology

Another approach to metabolism is by the technique of enzymology. The enzymes are isolated and separated and the specificity of each individual enzyme is studied in vitro. From this, the nature of the metabolic pathway in which these enzymes participate in vivo is deduced. It is because of certain favorable characteristic features of living systems that this approach has proved to be uniquely powerful. One is the unique and sometimes almost singular specificity of each of the biological catalysts. Another is that, although the cell is subdivided into a number of separate regions or compartments, these compartments seem to be relatively few in number. Therefore, much of the routing of metabolites through specific pathways is the result of the specificity of the enzymes; and the carefully prepared cell-free homogenate, especially one derived from a specific subcellular fraction, seems in many respects to duplicate the events occurring within the living cell.

Much experience has indicated that physiological experiments alone are usually ill-suited to the task of elucidating an unknown metabolic pathway. The alternative possible explanations that are consistent with the experimental data are too numerous, and the correct pathway has rarely been included among the list of postulated ones because of the remarkable and still largely unpredictable types of reactions catalyzed by enzymes. On the other hand, the techniques of enzymology, although capable of clarifying the reactions that do take place, cannot often give good insight into the importance of these reactions under specific physiological conditions. However, physiological studies, when applied to systems with known enzymology, often can do this, and a judicious use of well designed physiological experiments, performed on systems with known enzymology, seems to be one of the most promising approaches to learning what is actually going on inside a living cell.

Biochemical Genetics

A third approach to the study of metabolism is with the techniques of biochemical genetics. Ever since Beadle and Tatum, in 1941, demonstrated that specific mutants of the mold *Neurospora crassa* lacked the ability to catalyze specific enzymatic reactions, this approach has been refined and its use has been broadened (Beadle, 1946). Today such studies are often made on bacterial systems because of the ease with which the one significant mutant can be selected from the millions of normal individuals. Surprisingly, human mutants have played an increasingly prominent role in elucidating both the nature of baffling pathological conditions and normal human metabolism. This is because a human mutant of a specific kind, although rare, often displays a syndrome of grave concern to his physician and, because of the excellent communication that has developed between specialists, this patient eventually is frequently evaluated by the person most qualified to study his particular condition. It has always been important to select a favorable organism for enzymatic or physiological study. Today the best choice is often not some exotic species but a carefully selected mutant of practical importance or of a species commonly used for basic research.

METABOLIC PATHWAYS OF MAMMALS

The experimental knowledge of metabolism that has been obtained can be conveniently summarized in the form of metabolic maps. It is not the purpose of this chapter to present any of these in detail; they can be seen in any modern biochemistry textbook. Only the interrelationships of some major pathways in mammals will be pointed out. These are diagrammed in Figure 1.

Glycolysis is a central pathway of carbohydrate catabolism. The net effect of this pathway is to convert hexose phosphates to pyruvate aerobically or to lactate anaerobically. This process is practically irreversible, and it is coupled to the synthesis of ATP. In addition, certain intermediates of glycolysis serve as the starting materials for important processes, including amino acid and lipid synthesis.

Another pathway for catabolism of hexoses is the hexose monophosphate shunt. Enzymes for both glycolysis and the shunt are present in the cytoplasm of many kinds of cells. In addition to providing intermediates such as the ribose-5-phosphate needed for nucleic acid synthesis, a major role for the shunt is the production of NADPH. This compound acts as the reducing agent for a wide variety of important anabolic reactions and thus rivals ATP as a source of energy for anabolism.

The pyruvate produced by catabolism of hexoses may be oxidized to acetyl CoA, a compound with important roles for both carbohydrate and lipid metabolism. One important fate of the two-carbon acetyl group of acetyl CoA is its oxidation to carbon dioxide by the mitochondrial enzymes of the citric acid cycle. The reduced coenzymes produced by the stepwise oxidation of acetyl CoA are reoxidized by the mitochondrial electron transport system. The terminal step of this chain of oxidation-reduction reactions is the reduction of molecular oxygen to water. A major role for oxygen in mammals and other aerobic organisms is in the

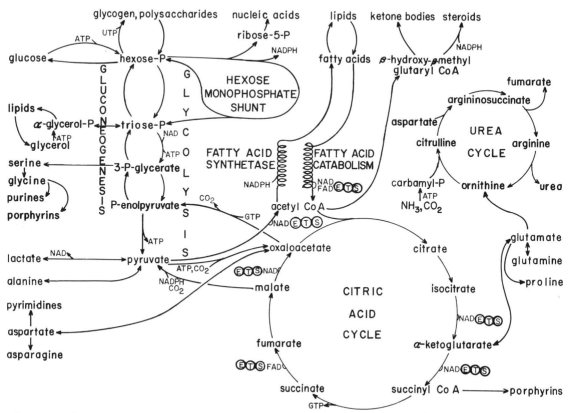

Figure 1. Central pathways of mammalian metabolism. In this diagram only a limited number of key intermediates are shown. Some mitochondrial processes that are thought to be major sources of reduced coenzymes for operation of the electron transport system for synthesis of ATP are designated ETS.

operation of this system. Coupled to the electron transport system is the apparatus for oxidative phosphorylation, a biochemical process for which the mechanism remains to be elucidated. The system for oxidative phosphorylation utilizes the free energy changes which accompany the oxidation-reduction reactions of the electron transport system for synthesizing ATP from ADP plus inorganic phosphate. The oxidation of acetyl CoA is thus a primary source of ATP in mammals.

A major source of acetyl CoA, in addition to carbohydrate metabolism, is fatty acid catabolism. The stepwise process of fatty acid degradation occurs in the mitochondria, and the reduced coenzymes formed by this oxidation are reoxidized by the electron transport system. Thus, both carbohydrates and fatty acids can furnish energy for ATP synthesis by oxidative phosphorylation.

A third source of acetyl CoA is from catabolism of the ketogenic amino acids.

There are three major fates of acetyl CoA besides its oxidation by the citric acid cycle. These are for biosynthesis of fatty acids, ketone bodies, and steroids. Certain metabolic disturbances, including diabetes and starvation, result in an excessive rate of production of acetyl CoA in comparison to its rate of utilization. In these circumstances, ketone body synthesis by the liver, which ordinarily is an important but not major source of energy for extrahepatic tissues, is greatly augmented and the condition of ketosis occurs.

Fatty acid synthesis and steroid synthesis are examples of anabolic processes that require NADPH, whereas polysaccharide synthesis, nucleic acid synthesis and protein synthesis are examples of processes that require ATP. It seems reasonable to suppose that the supply of NADPH and ATP in the cell may be adjusted by control of the relative rates of flow of carbohydrates through glycolysis and the hexose monophosphate shunt (Landau et al., 1965).

Although the same two compounds that are the key starting material and product for anabolism may also have the reverse roles for catabolism, nevertheless the reactions linking these compounds may have no enzymes or intermediates that are common to the two pathways. Such is the case for the metabolism of saturated fatty acids. The process for degradation of fatty acids to acetyl CoA by a mitochondrial enzyme system involves CoA intermediates and is coupled to the electron transport system. On the other hand, the process

for synthesis of fatty acids from acetyl CoA by a cytoplasmic system utilizes acyl carrier protein intermediates and requires NADPH. A similar situation is seen for the metabolism of polysaccharides. In this case the biosynthetic pathways involve high-energy phosphate reactions utilizing nucleotide-sugar intermediates while the degradative pathways involve hydrolytic or phosphorolytic reactions. The processes of glycolysis and gluconeogenesis are not completely distinct but proceed through some reactions common to both pathways and some that are different. In general, for those steps of glycolysis that are practically irreversible, an alternative gluconeogenic reaction is available. This is known to be true for three steps. One is the glycolytic conversion of phosphoenolpyruvate to pyruvate. This irreversible step is circumvented during gluconeogenesis by conversion of pyruvate to oxaloacetate which, in turn, is converted to phosphoenolpyruvate. Both these reactions utilize high energy phosphate compounds and have favorable equilibria for gluconeogenesis. Similarly, the hexokinase and phosphofructokinase reactions of glycolysis are not used for gluconeogenesis. Instead, thermodynamically favorable hydrolytic reaction catalyzed by glucose-6-phosphatase and fructose-1,6-diphosphatase are used to produce glucose and fructose-6-phosphate, respectively. It is evident that these reactions are of critical importance for establishing the rate and direction of carbohydrate metabolism. It is therefore not surprising that the enzymes involved are controlled by mechanisms that serve to adjust the flow of metabolites through glycolysis and gluconeogenesis in response to the momentary requirements of the cell (Scrutton and Utter, 1968).

Closely related to the pathways of carbohydrate metabolism are those for synthesis of amino acids. Of the 11 amino acids that are not required in the diet for adequate human nutrition (nonessential amino acids), the origin of the carbon skeletons of nine are shown in Figure 1. The other two, cysteine and tyrosine, are derived from dietary methionine and phenylalanine, respectively.

Catabolic pathways are also needed to dispose of excess dietary amino acids, both essential and nonessential. The catabolism of some nonessential amino acids is by reversal of the reaction used for anabolism. Special degradative pathways are provided for some nonessential amino acids and all essential amino acids. These are discussed in biochemistry textbooks. The bulk of the excess amino acid nitrogen that is released by catabolism is converted to urea by the urea cycle and eliminated in the urine. Once the nitrogen has been removed from an amino acid, the carbon skeleton remaining undergoes catabolism. An appreciable fraction of the energy of humans is derived from dietary amino acids. The carbon skeletons of many amino acids, the glycogenic amino acids, can also undergo gluconeogenesis because they are converted to intermediates of the glycolytic pathway or of the citric acid cycle.

CONCLUSION

The status of biochemistry at the beginning of this decade is that of a mature science with a large body of factual knowledge. This knowledge is securely based on the laws of chemistry and physics and it also has proved to be effective in explaining a great variety of biological phenomena. However, it is still of limited value as a predictive tool for deciding what events will occur if a certain physiological stress is imposed on an organism. It is also of limited value for devising rational therapeutic procedures for most pathological conditions. Although there are still some blank areas on the metabolic maps, it appears that the greatest limitations of this science now are in understanding the control mechanisms that regulate the various enzymatic pathways. Hopefully, greater knowledge in these areas will convert biochemistry from a descriptive to a predictive science, and this, in turn, may lead to rational therapy for many common disorders.

REFERENCES

Beadle, G. W.: Genes and the chemistry of the organism. Amer. Sci. *34*:31, 1946.

Dickerson, R. E., and Geis, I.: The Structure and Action of Proteins. New York, Harper & Row, 1969.

Jacob, F., and Monod, J.: On the regulation of gene activity. Cold Spring Harbor Symp. Quant. Biol. *26*:193, 1961.

Kornberg, A.: Enzymatic Synthesis of DNA. New York, John Wiley & Sons, Inc., 1962.

Landau, B. R., Katz, J., Bartsch, G. E., White, L. W., and Williams, H. R.: Hormonal regulation of glucose metabolism in adipose tissue *in vitro*. Ann. N. Y. Acad. Sci. *131*:43, 1965.

Larner, J.: Hormonal and nonhormonal control of glycogen metabolism. Trans. N.Y. Acad. Sci. *29* (2):192, 1966.

Lipmann, F.: Metabolic generation and utilization of phosphate bond energy. Advances Enzym. *1*:99, 1941.

Monod, J., Changeux, J. P., and Jacob, F.: Allosteric proteins and cellular control systems. J. Molec. Biol. *6*:306, 1963.

Schimke, R. T., Brown, M. B., and Smallman, E. T.: Turnover of rat liver arginase. Ann. N. Y. Acad. Sci. *102*:587, 1963.

Scrutton, M. C., and Utter, M. F.: The regulation of glycolysis and gluconeogenesis in animal tissues. Ann. Rev. Biochem. *37*:249, 1968.

Watson, J. D.: Molecular Biology of the Gene. New York, W. A. Benjamin, 1965.

Chapter 12

BIOCHEMISTRY OF THE SALIVARY GLANDS AND SALIVA

by George A. Gates, M.D.

The production of saliva and its role in the oral phase of digestion have been the subject of extensive study since the 19th century when such great physiologists as Mueller, Baylis, Bernard, Pavlov, Ludwig, and Heidenhain made their historic contributions to the knowledge of cellular biology based on their investigations of the salivary glands. Although considerable knowledge about the composition of saliva has accrued from the works of subsequent investigators, much remains to be known about the mechanisms of saliva production. Elucidation of these mechanisms is made difficult because of the nonhomogenous nature of saliva and because of the differences in cellular composition of the several salivary glands. Furthermore, the composition of saliva varies not only from gland to gland but from the same gland, depending upon the nature of the stimulus, the flow rate, and the methods of collection and chemical analysis.

Saliva is formed in the paired parotid, submandibular, and sublingual glands, and in the minor salivary glands scattered throughout the oral cavity. Secretion of saliva results from tactile, mechanical, and gustatory stimulation of intraoral reflexes and from olfactory stimuli from direct stimulation of the parasympathetic and sympathetic secretomotor nerves. Direct chemical stimulation of the gland and the postganglionic neurons may be obtained with adrenergic and cholinergic drugs. Resting saliva refers to the flow of saliva in the absence of specific stimulation. Whole or mixed saliva refers to secretions obtained by expectoration. Saliva from the individual glands is collected by direct cannulation of the ducts or by various appliances positioned over the ductal orifice, such as the Carlsen-Crittenden cup or the Pickerill segregator. Saliva collected by cannulation or intra-oral devices cannot be considered resting saliva because of the inherent mechanical stimulation produced by the insertion and presence of the collecting device.

The 24 hour volume of human mixed saliva is 1000 to 1500 cc. The solid components of saliva consist of the electrolytes normally found in extracellular fluid and a variety of organic materials, some of which are unique to saliva. The organic constituents of saliva are formed principally by acinar epithelium. The active transport of water and electrolytes into the saliva occurs mainly through the cells of the intralobular ducts.

INORGANIC CONSTITUENTS

Osmolarity

Human saliva is slightly hypotonic compared to plasma. The osmolarity of human parotid saliva increases with the rate of salivary flow (Kostlin and Rauch, 1957). Loss of body water results in an increase in salivary osmolarity; overhydration, in a decrease. The mechanisms that maintain this osmotic gradient are not known. Specific gravity of whole saliva varies from 1.002 to 1.012.

pH – Bicarbonate

Intraductal saliva is slightly acid and rapidly becomes alkaline upon entering the oral cavity where the dissolved CO_2 leaves solution. Schmidt-Nielsen (1946) found that the pH of resting parotid saliva averages 5.81 (range, 5.45 to 6.06) and that of the submandibular saliva averages 6.59 (range, 6.02 to 7.14). Stimulation increases the pH 1 to 2 units. Bicarbonate is the principal buffer in saliva and is derived both from plasma and from glandular metabolism (Weschler 1959). The pCO_2 of saliva varies directly with the arterial pCO_2, although it is some 20 to 30 per cent higher and is independent of secretion rate (Sand, 1949). Parotid and submandibular bicarbonate concentrations exceed that of serum, except at very low flow rates; and as the flow rate increases, parotid bicarbonate stabilizes at about 60 mEq./L. (Thaysen et al., 1954). Sublingual saliva in man and other species contains little bicarbonate. Fluctuations of arterial pCO_2 alter salivary pH to only a limited extent because bicarbonate and CO_2 concentrations change proportionately. Studies of the effect of a carbonic anhydrase inhibitor (Diamox) upon the salivary pH and bicarbonate are contradictory, showing either no effect in parotid saliva (Chauncey et al., 1958) or a reduction in bicarbonate, sodium, buffer content, and flow rate of mixed saliva (Niedermeier et al., 1955). Carbonic anhydrase activity is greater in submandibular than in parotid saliva and increases as the flow rate approaches 0.8 ml./min., after which no further increase is noted (Szabo et al., 1966).

Sodium

The concentration of sodium in human saliva, as in all species which produce a hypotonic saliva, is less than the serum sodium. It varies from 5 mEq./L. at low rates of flow to 100 mEq./L. at maximum rates. Sodium concentrations in unstimulated or resting saliva are fairly constant, however. In normal children, resting saliva contains 2 to 15 mEq./L. of sodium as opposed to children with mucoviscidosis, in whom values of 20–45 mEq./L. are seen (Prader and Gautier, 1955). In isotonic saliva, such as is produced by the rat parotid gland, sodium is the predominant cation and is present at concentrations of 140–160 mEq./L. (Schneyer and Schneyer, 1959). Salivary sodium levels are depressed by the administration of ACTH (Grad, 1952) and to a lesser degree by desoxycorticosterone (White et al., 1955). The diminished sodium concentration and flow rates noted in the stimulated saliva of hypertensive patients may be due to an aldosterone effect (Wotman et al., 1967).

Potassium

Whole saliva, as well as saliva from each of the major salivary glands, contains potassium in concentrations of 1.5 to 4.0 times that of serum (Kostlin and Rauch, 1957). The relationship of potassium concentration to salivary flow is U shaped, being elevated at both high and low rates (Burgen, 1956). Salivary potassium is elevated in hyperkalemic states by ACTH (Grad, 1952) and by adrenocortical hormones (White et al., 1955). Sympathetic stimulation produces saliva richer in potassium than does parasympathetic stimulation. The mean salivary Na/K ratio in stimulated mixed saliva is 1.47 (range, 0.6 to 3.4) and is less than 0.25 in patients with primary or secondary aldosteronism (Lauler et al., 1962). The extreme dependency of salivary electrolyte concentration upon flow rates must be considered in interpreting the results of such tests.

Chlorides

Salivary chloride concentration is less than that of serum, ranging from 5–70 mEq./L., and shows a linear relationship to the flow rate. Sublingual saliva contains more chloride than does parotid or submandibular saliva. Salivary chloride concentration is independent of serum levels and shows a moderate decrease along with sodium levels following the administration of adrenocorticoids (White et al., 1955). Bicarbonate and chloride concentrations in saliva vary inversely in response to changes in arterial pCO_2 (Burgen and Emmelin, 1961c).

Phosphates

Like potassium, phosphate concentration in saliva is hypertonic at all flow rates and increases with the flow rate (Shannon and Prigmore, 1960 b). Phosphates are important buffers of acid metabolites in saliva, and along with bicarbonate, sodium, potassium, and chloride constitute the main electrolytes found in saliva. The total phosphate of saliva is usually about twice that of plasma; approximately 80 per cent is present in organic form (Chauncey and Weiss, 1958).

Iodide

Unlike most other inorganic components of saliva, iodide is hypertonic to plasma by a factor of from 10 to 40 (Schiff et al., 1947). The ability to concentrate iodide varies among different species and is highest in man. Iodoproteins are found in dog parotid saliva but not in the human. Iodide concentration is virtually independent of flow rate and varies with the plasma levels. Salivary secretion of iodide is not affected by thyroxin or TSH (Brown-Grant, 1961), but is depressed by the administration of thiocyanate, perchlorate, and nitrate, presumably by competitive inhibition at a common transfer site. The intralobular ductal cells appear to be the principal site of iodide transfer and concentration (McGee et al., 1967). The metallic taste following administration of iodide compounds is due to the excretion of iodide into the saliva. Xerostomia following the administration of therapeutic doses of ^{131}I is a not uncommon clinical observation. Technetium-99m pertechnetate, which is used for salivary gland scanning, is presumed to be concentrated by the salivary ductal epithelium in the same manner as iodide (Gates and Work, 1967).

Other Electrolytes

Bromine, calcium, fluoride, magnesium, lithium and other ions are detectable in saliva. Their concentrations tend to vary with the salivary flow rate and are, in general, increased by sympathetic stimulation.

ORGANIC CONSTITUENTS

Salivary Proteins

Much remains to be known about the complex structure and function of salivary proteins, although the use of modern methods of analysis such as electrophoresis, ultracentrifugation, and immunochemical techniques has added considerable knowledge. Proteins are the largest group of salivary organic compounds and they impart to the saliva its physical characteristics. For example, the viscous nature of submandibular, sublingual, and palatine saliva results from the abundance of mucoproteins in these secretions. The internal molecular configuration of the protein molecule influences its viscosity. Proteins having a coiled lattice structure like hyaluronic acid trap large amounts of solute within the coils and readily form mucin clots, whereas those proteins with long polypeptide chains do not. Total protein output is dependent upon the flow rate; with prolonged stimulation the protein concentration falls exponentially with duration and reaches a steady state at which a balance between synthesis and secretion is presumed to exist (Burgen and Emmelin, 1961). The total protein output of stimulated saliva rises with time and is a direct function of cellular stimulation rather than volume output; at maximal rates of flow, an increase in the stimulation rate applied to the dog parotid gland raises the output and concentration of protein without any further increase in saliva flow (Burgen et al., 1956). Protein content is higher following sympathetic than parasympathetic stimulation and, in addition, differs in physical and chemical properties. Whether these differences are the result of changes in the proportions of proteins or in their composition is not clear. Total protein content of human parotid saliva averages 200 mg. per 100 ml. (depending on the analytical procedure used), of which amylase constitutes 30 per cent; serum proteins, 20 per cent; glycoproteins, 35 per cent; and lysozyme, 10 per cent; whereas human submandibular saliva total protein content is about 100 mg. per 100 ml. (Mandel and Ellison, 1965).

Amylase

The major electrophoretic peak in parotid saliva is amylase which, like pancreatic amylase, is an alpha-1,4-glucan 4-glucanohydrolase which splits the alpha-1,4-glucosidic bonds of starch in a random fashion to produce maltose and a variety of dextrins. Amylase is the major protein fraction of parotid saliva and its concentration is independent of flow rates (Ferguson et al., 1958). Amylase is also present in submandibular saliva. It is a carbohydrate-free protein with an optimum pH of 6.9 (Muus, 1954) and requires chloride ions for full enzymatic activity. Salivary amylase can be readily crystallized by successive acetone and ammonium sulfate precipitation. Electrophoresis of crystaline salivary amylase shows from four to eight bands of amylolytic activity which represent isoenzymes of amylase (Lamberts et al., 1967; Muus and Usenchak, 1964; Wolf and Taylor, 1967). The number of salivary isoamylases is probably under genetic control. The sensitivity of the separation and the staining techniques and the method of pretreatment of saliva also influence the number of bands detected (Wolf and Taylor, 1967). Using gel filtration fractionation (Sephadex G-100), Wilding (1963) found that serum, saliva, and pancreatic juice amylases have a molecular weight of about 45,000. The nonidentity of pancreatic and salivary amylase was demonstrated by Norby (1964), who found that pancreatic amylase is a single rapidly moving band compared to the several heavier bands of salivary amylase. Most of the electrophoretic studies of amylase depend upon the decolorization of a starch-iodine paste for identification of amylolotic activity. These amyloclastic staining methods are not specific for amylase because hemoglobin, protein, dilution, and heating effects can influence the decolorization reaction. Inasmuch as the principal action of amylase upon starch is the liberation of maltose, quantitative measurement of liberated maltose (saccharogenic method) is a more specific method of measuring amylase activity. With this technique normal serum amylase has been demonstrated to be electrophoretically identical to liver amylase and distinguishable from both salivary and pancreatic amylase (Joseph et al., 1966). Serum amylase may be transiently elevated in patients with mumps, parotid trauma, salivary ductal obstruction, and suppurative infection of the parotid gland.

The importance of salivary amylase to carbohydrate breakdown has been debated. The rapid transit time of ingested food through the mouth and the inactivation of amylase activity by low pH suggests that salivary degradation of starch can occur to only a limited extent. The absence of carbohydrate nutritional problems in patients without saliva suggests that sufficient pancreatic amylase is available for this purpose. Digestion of starch by salivary amylase does continue in the stomach up to several hours after ingestion, however, because the inner layers of the gastric bolus remain alkaline. Under these circumstances conversion of starch to maltose in the stomach may be 75 per cent complete. (Bergheim, 1926). The commonly observed hypertrophy of the salivary glands of patients with excessive carbohydrate intake (starch eaters) indicates that salivary amylase does play an active role in starch digestion.

Other Enzymes

The other enzymes present in saliva have not been so extensively studied as has amylase. Their origins and metabolic importance are incompletely understood. The presence (Hightower, 1966) and absence (Fenton and Cowgill, 1956) of maltose in saliva have been reported. Acid phosphatase, esterases, cholinesterase, lipase, and beta-glucuronidase have been detected in isolated parotid saliva and, in addition, alkaline phosphatase, beta-d-glactosidase and hyaluronidase are present in whole saliva. Many of these enzymes appear to originate from oral bacteria as well as from glandular secretion or synthesis (Chauncey et al., 1954). Parotid and submandibular saliva contains an enzyme, kallikrein, which produces a fall in blood pressure after intravenous injections (Werle, 1955). The hypotensive effect of kallikrein appears to result from its action upon a plasma protein with the release of the vasodilator polypeptide, bradykinin.

Blood coagulation factor activity comparable to that of antihemophiliac globulin (VII), Christmas factor IX, and platelet factor has been identified in whole human saliva (Nour-Eldrin and Wilkinson, 1957). Saliva may be substituted for platelets in the thrombin generation test but not in the thromboplastin generation test.

Lysozymes are a group of substances found in saliva, tears, serum, nasal mucus, egg white, and certain plant materials which have the ability to hydralize bacteria of the genera Bacillus, Micrococcus, Staphylococcus, Streptococcus, Proteus, and Brucella (Burgen and Emmelin, 1961a). The enzyme is present in human parotid and submandibular saliva but is difficult to measure quantitatively because of chemical interactions with other salivary constituents. Electrophoretic separation of lysozyme is possible because it behaves as a cation at the usual pH employed (Kinersley and Hogberg, 1955). The clinical importance of antibacterial properties of salivary lysozyme is not clear.

Mucoproteins

. The chemical identification of salivary mucoproteins is made difficult because of the anomalous precipitation reactions of the carbohydrate fractions when separation is attempted. Many studies of salivary mucoproteins have been based on incomplete and impure mucoprotein fractions and have led to conflicting results. Ultracentrifugation, gel filtration, dialysis, and electrophoresis are more reliable methods of separation of the protein fractions. Many substances separated by these techniques still remain unclassified as to structure and function, however. Although the total submandibular protein is lower than that of the parotid, it is more complex, exhibiting up to 20 bands on acrylamide gel electrophoresis; and, in addition, the submandibular proteins are anionic rather than cationic and contain a different spectrum of carbohydrates (Mandel and Ellison, 1965). The largest electrophoretic band is a low mobility neutral glycoprotein (Kostlin and Rauch, 1957).

Salivary mucoproteins may be classified as (1) fucomucins, which are composed of equal parts of fucose, glucosamine, and galactose; and (2) sialomucins, which are probably composed entirely of sialic acid N-acetylglucosamine. The third general class of mucoproteins, mucoitin sulfuric acid, appears to be absent from saliva.

The blood group-specific substances found in submandibular saliva are typical fucomucins in their chemical composition (Morgan and Watkins, 1959). The amount of blood group substances in saliva is small, in the order of 10-20 mg./L. These substances are present in the submandibular saliva from all individuals tested and may be A, B, or O, unless the red cells have the Le[a] antigen, in which case the saliva contains Le[a] substance rather than the other antigens. Fluorescent antibody studies reveal heavy staining in the mucous acinar cells of the submandibular gland and an absence of staining in the parotid gland (Glynn and Holborow, 1959). It would appear that secretion blood group substances in man occur only in the mucous acini of the submandibular gland.

Sialic acid is present in many of the glyco- and mucoproteins of nasal, trachobronchial, intestinal, and gastric mucus as well as in submandibular saliva (Gottschalk, 1960). It appears to be an aldol condensate of N-acetyl-D-glucosamine and pyruvate and is designated, in its unsubstituted form, as neuraminic acid (R1=R2=H). It is the major component of the high mobility submandibular acid mucoprotein fraction and appears to be the active substance in mucin which inhibits the ability of certain viruses to agglutinate red blood cells. These viruses, such as the influenza virus, produce a enzyme, neuraminidase, which hydrolyzes the glucosidic linkage of terminal neuraminyl groups in cell membranes. The sialic acid in mucin inhibits the enzyme by competing with the cellular neuraminyl groups for the virus neuraminidase. This enzyme is also found in submandibular-sublingual saliva, but not in parotid saliva (Pertlish and Glickman, 1966a). The sialic acid produced by salivary neuraminidase is rapidly destroyed by oral bacteria. Desquamated cells of the oral cavity and oral bacteria also appear to produce neuraminidase (Pertlish and Glickman, 1966b).

Immunoglobulins and Serum Proteins

Saliva contains many proteins that are found in serum, of which some are transudates and others are synthesized in the salivary gland. In addition, certain proteins in saliva are not found in serum and appear to be synthesized locally. Immunoelectrophoresis of the culture fluid produced by human parotid and submandibular tissue slices incubated with ^{14}C-labeled amino acids (L-isoleucine and L-lysine) and mixed with specific antisera showed local synthesis of an alpha-1-globulin, a beta- 1-globulin, IgG, IgM and IgA (Hurlimann and Zuber, 1968a). Albumin, transferrin, and hepatoglobulin, on the other hand, did not appear on the tissue culture medium, indicating the lack of synthesis of these proteins by the salivary tissue. Furthermore, the IgA so produced was immunologically distinct from serum IgA, but the salivary IgM and IgG were immunologically identical to their serum counterparts. By substituting rabbit antisaliva antisera, other proteins were identified: large amounts of lactoferrin were produced by both parotid and submandibular tissue; six proteins specific to saliva were synthesized by the submandibular gland (amylase and five other nonclassified electrophoretic components), and three proteins specific to saliva were synthesized by the parotid gland (amylase and two nonclassified components) (Hurlimann and Zuber, 1968b). An acid-resistant glycoprotein with a molecular weight of that of gastroferrin is present in whole saliva and presumably accounts for its iron binding capacity (Reilly et al., 1968). Being acid resistant, this glycoprotein presumably contributes to the iron binding capacity of gastric juice as well.

Amino Acids

Many free amino acids have been identified in human saliva, but their concentrations are, in general, only 10 to 20 per cent of the plasma levels. Most of the alpha amino acids are derived from plasma amino acids, although three gamma amino acids (gamma amino glutamate, taurine, and o-phosphoethanolamine) appear to be synthesized locally. Dreyfus et al., (1968) measured the concentration values of 20 amino acids in whole saliva and found delta-amino valeric acid (DAVA), glycine, proline, and taurine were present in greatest amount. The concentration of proline and DAVA increases markedly upon standing, presumably as a result of bacterial action. The concentration of salivary amino acids increases proportionately with increases in the free plasma amino acids (Rose and Kerr, 1958).

Urea

At average secretion rates the urea concentration in whole saliva is 20 mg. per 100 ml., being higher in parotid than in submandibular fluid, and it varies directly with the serum concentration and is inversely proportional to the flow rate (Shannon and Prigmore, 1960a). About one third of the urea enters through the acini and the remainder by ductal secretion (Burgen and Seeman, 1958). Salivary urea levels have been used to monitor blood levels in hemodialysis patients (Forland et al., 1964).

Glucose

Glucose and other reducing sugars are normally absent from human saliva when the Somogyi technique is used. Salivary glucose levels are very low in diabetes; the salivary threshold for glucose appears to be at a blood sugar of 300 mg. per 100 ml. (Hebb and Stavraky, 1936). Using ultramicro techniques, Campbell (1965) found glucose levels in unstimulated whole saliva of nondiabetic patients to vary from 0.24 to 0.33 mg. per 100 ml. and in diabetic patients, from 0.44 to 6.33 mg.

SUMMARY

Saliva is a complex fluid consisting of water and varying amounts of electrolytes and organic compounds. The concentration of these constituents varies with the nature and intensity of the stimulus; but, in general, salivary osmolarity and sodium, chloride, glucose, and protein concentrations are less than in plasma, while salivary potassium, bicarbonate, urea, and iodide levels are higher. Although many metabolic disorders are revealed in the saliva, the use of salivary biochemical analysis has not been widely adopted because of technical difficulties in standardizing the rate of secretion. The value of salivary biochemistry in the diagnosis of salivary gland disorders remains largely unexplored.

REFERENCES

Bergheim, O.: Intestinal chemistry, III. Salivary digestion in the human stomach and intestines. Arch. Intern. Med. 37:110–117, 1926.

Brown-Grant, K.: Extrathyroidal iodide concentrating mechanisms. Physiol. Rev. 41:189–213, 1961.

Burgen, A. S. V.: The secretion of potassium in saliva. J. Physiol. 132:20–39, 1956.

Burgen, A. S. V., and Emmelin, N. G.: Physiology of the Salivary Glands. London, Edward Arnold, Ltd., 1961, a–p. 179; b–p. 182; c–p. 219.

Burgen, A. S. V., and Seeman, P.: The role of the salivary duct system in the formation of saliva. Canad. J. Biochem. Physiol. 36:119–143, 1958.

Burgen, A. S. V., Weiss, P., and Seeman, P.: The dynamics of protein secretion in the formation of saliva. Canad. J. Biochem. Physiol. 36:119–143, 1956.

Campbell, M. J.: Glucose in the saliva of the non-diabetic and the diabetic patient. Arch. Oral Biol. 10:197–205, 1965.

Chauncey, H. H., Lionetti, F., Winer, R. A., and Lisanti, V. F.: Enzymes of human saliva; The determination, distribution and origin of whole saliva enzymes. J. Dent. Res. 33:321–334, 1954.

Chauncey, H. H., and Weiss, P. A.: Composition of human saliva; parotid gland secretion: Flow rate, pH and inorganic composition after oral administration of a carbonic anhydrase inhibitor. Arch. Int. Pharmacodyn. 113:377–383, 1958.

Cohen, B., Logothetopoulos, J. H., and Myant, N. B.: Autoradiographic localization of I-131 in the salivary glands of the hamster. Nature (Lond.) 176:1268–1269, 1955.

Dreyfus, P. M., Levy, H. L., and Efron, M. L.: Concerning amino acids in human saliva. Experientia 24:447–448, 1968.

Fenton, R. F., and Cowgill, G. R.: Salivary glands. In Fulton, J. R.: Textbook of Physiology. 17th ed. Philadelphia, W. B. Saunders Company, 1956, pp. 987.

Ferguson, M. H., Krahn, K. P., and Hildes, J. A.: Parotid secretion of protein in man. Canad. J. Biochem. 36:1001–1008, 1958.

Forland, M., Shannon, I. L., and Katz, F. H.: Parotid-fluid urea nitrogen for the monitoring of hemodialysis. New Eng. J. Med. 271:37–38, 1964.

Gates, G. A., and Work, W. P.: Radioisotope scanning of the salivary glands. A preliminary report. Laryngoscope 77:861–875, 1967.

Glynn, L. E., and Holborow, E. J.: Distribution of blood-group substances in human tissues. Brit. Med. Bull. 15:150–153, 1959.

Gottschalk, A.: The Chemistry and Biology of Sialic Acids and Related Substances. London, Cambridge University Press, 1960.

Grad, B.: The influence of ACTH on the sodium and potassium concentration of human mixed saliva. J. Clin. Endocr. 12:708–718, 1952.

Hebb, C. O., and Stavraky, G. W.: The presence of glucose in the salivary secretion after the administration of adrenalin. Quart. J. Exp. Physiol. *26*:141–153, Oct., 1936.

Hightower, N. W., Jr.: Salivary secretion. *In* Best, C. H., and Taylor, M. D.: The Physiological Basis of Medical Practice. Baltimore, The Williams & Wilkins Company, 1966.

Hurlimann, J., and Zuber, C.: In vitro protein synthesis by human salivary glands I: Synthesis of salivary IgA and serum proteins. Immunology *14*:809–817, 1968a.

Hurlimann, J., and Zuber, C.: In vitro protein synthesis by human salivary glands II: Synthesis of proteins specific to saliva and other excretions. Immunology *14*:819–824, 1968b.

Joseph, R. R., Olivero, E., and Ressler, N.: Electrophoretic study of human isoamylases. Gastroenterology *51*:377–382, 1966.

Kinersly, T., and Hogberg, O.: An antibacterial effect of saliva demonstrated with use of paper electrophoresis. Yale J. Biol. Med. *28*:145–147, 1955.

Kerby, G. P., and Taylor, S. M.: Salivary kallikrein levels in normal and rheumatoid individuals. J. Lab. Clin. Med. *71*:704–708, 1968.

Koslin, A., and Rauch, S.: Zur Chemie des ruhespeichels einzelner Speicheldrusen. Helv. Med. Acta *24*:600–621, 1957.

Lamberts, B. L., and Meyer, S. J.: Amylolytic fractions of salivary secretion. *In* Schneyer, L. H., and Schneyer, C. A.: Secretory Mechanisms of Salivary Glands. New York, Academic Press, Inc., 1967, pp.313–324.

Lauler, D. P., Hickler, R. B., and Thorn, G. W.: The salivary sodium-potassium ratio. New Eng. J. Med. *267*:1136–1137, 1962.

Mandel, I. D., and Ellison, S. A.: Organic components of human parotid and submaxillary saliva. Ann. N.Y. Acad. Sci. *131*:802–811, 1965.

McGee, J. O., Mason, D. K., and Duguid, W. P.: The site of iodide concentration in hamster salivary glands as demonstrated by autoradiography. Arch. Oral Biol. *12*:1189–1194, 1967.

Morgan, W. T., and Watkins, W. M.: Some aspects of the biochemistry of the human blood-group substances. Brit. Med. Bull. *15*:109–113, 1959.

Muus, J.: The amino acid composition of human salivary amylase. J. Amer. Chem. Soc. *76*:5163–5165, 1954.

Muus, J., and Vnenchak, J. M.: Isozymes of salivary amylase. Nature (Lond.) *204*:283–285, 1964.

Niedermeier, W., Stone, R. E., Dreizen, S., and Spies, T. D.: The effect of 2-acetylamino-1, 3, 4 thiadiazole-5-sulfonamide (Diamox) on sodium, postassium, bicarbonate and buffer content of saliva. Proc. Soc. Exp. Biol. Med. *88*:273–295, 1955.

Norby, S.: Electrophoretic non-identity of human salivary and pancreatic amylases. Exp. Cell. Res. *36*:663–666, 1964.

Nour-Eldin, F., and Wilkinson, J. F.: The blood clotting factors in human saliva. J. Physiol. *136*:324–332, 1957.

Perlitsh, M. J., and Glickman, I.: Salivary neuraminidase I: The presence of neuraminidase in human saliva. J. Periodont. *37*:368–373, 1966a.

Perlitsh, M. J., and Glickman, I.: Salivary neuraminidase II: Its source in whole human saliva. J. Dent. Res. *45*:1239, 1966b.

Prader, D., and Gautier, E.: Die Na-und-K-Konzentration im gemischten Speichel. Helv. Paediat. Acta *10*:56–62, 1955.

Reilly, P. L., Davis, P. S., and Deller, D. J.: Iron binding properties of saliva. Nature (Lond.) *217*:68, 1968.

Rose, G. A., and Kerr, A. C.: The amino acids and phosphoethanolamine in salivary gland secretions of normal men and of patients with abnormal calcium, phosphorus and amino acid metabolism. Quart. J. Exp. Physiol. *43*:160–168, 1958.

Sand, H. F.: The Carbonic Acid Content of Saliva and Its Role in the Formation of Dental Calculus. Thesis, University of Oslo, 1949.

Schiff, L., Stevens, C. D., Molle, W. E., Steinberg, H., Kumpe, C. W., and Stewart, P.: Gastric and salivary excretion of radioiodine in man. J. Nat. Cancer Inst. *7*:349–354, 1947.

Schmidt-Nielsen, B.: Micro-determination of pH in saliva. Acta Physiol. Scand. *11*:97–103, 1946.

Schneyer, C. A., and Schneyer, L. H.: Electrolyte levels of rat salivary secretions. Proc. Soc. Exp. Biol. Med. *101*:568–569, 1959.

Shannon, I. L., and Prigmore, J. R.: Parotid gland flow rate and parotid fluid urea concentration. Oral Surg. *13*:1013–1018, 1960a.

Shannon, I. L., and Prigmore, J. R.: Parotid flow rate. Its relationship to pH and chemical composition. Oral Surg. *13*:1488–1500, 1960b.

Szabo, I., Mason, D. K., and Harden, R. M.: Carbonic anhydrase activity in saliva in man. Quart. J. Exp. Physiol. *51*:202–206, 1966.

Thaysen, J. H., Thorn, N. A., and Schwartz, I. L.: Excretion of sodium, potassium, chloride and carbon dioxide in human parotid saliva. Amer. J. Physiol. *178*:155–159, 1954.

Werle, E.: The Chemistry and Pharmacology of Kallikrein and Kallidin in Polypeptids Which Stimulate Smooth Muscle. Edinburgh, E. & S. Livingstone, Ltd., 1955.

Weschsler, A.: The Secretion of Bicarbonate in Saliva. Thesis, McGill University, Montreal, 1959.

White, A. G., Entmacher, P. S., Rubin, G., and Leiter, L.: Physiological and pharmacological regulations of human salivary electrolyte concentrations. J. Clin. Invest. *34*:246–255, 1955.

Wilding, P.: Use of gel filtration in the study of human amylase. Clin. Chem. Acta *8*:918–924, 1963.

Wolf, R. O., and Taylor, L. L.: Isoamylases of human parotid saliva. Nature (Lond.) *213*:1128–1129, 1967.

Wotman, S., Mandel, I. D., and Thompson, R. H., Jr.: Salivary electrolytes and salt taste thresholds in hypertension. J. Chronic Dis. *20*:833–840, 1967.

Section Four

MICROBIOLOGY

Chapter 13

BACTERIOLOGY: BASIC AND APPLIED TO OTORHINOLARYNGOLOGY

by K. Gerhard Brand, M.D.

It is not the intention in this chapter to provide comprehensive coverage of the field of bacteriology. Instead, those aspects have been selected which appear relevant to problems of the otorhinolaryngological practice. It is assumed that the reader is reasonably acquainted with the fundamental facts, concepts, and methods of bacteriology. For gathering supplementary information a number of excellent textbooks are availabe, e.g., Burrows' *Textbook of Microbiology* (Saunders, 1968), Davis et al., *Microbiology* (Hoeber, 1967), and others.

BACTERIAL STRUCTURES AND FUNCTIONS

Capsule. Many bacteria carry a capsule as an outermost structure, and this is usually composed of polysaccharides or, in some instances, of polypeptides. The ability to form a capsule is a genotypic property which may be lost by mutation. However, the environment often has a determining influence on whether the capsule is produced.

The capsule serves as a means of protection against a variety of adverse conditions. In the body most notably it inhibits or prevents phagocytosis; hence, the presence of the capsule is often associated with the pathogenic properties of the bacterium.

Cell Wall. The cell wall is a firm, rigid structure which provides and preserves the shape of a bacterial cell. In gram-positive bacteria the major chemical component is a peptidoglycan (a polymer of amino sugars and peptides). Also, mucopolysaccharides and a polymer of phosphate compounds (teichoic acid) are found. In gram-negative bacteria teichoic acid is missing. The outer layer of the gram-negative cell wall is composed of lipopolysaccharides and lipoproteins; the inner surface consists of the same muco-complex as that present in gram-positive bacteria. Cocci and rod-shaped bacteria possess a thick, rigid cell wall, whereas in spirochetes the wall is thin and flexible.

Bacteria may lose their cell walls under experimental as well as natural conditions and remain viable in this state. A bacterium devoid of a cell wall is called a protoplast. Protoplasts can be produced experimentally by treatment with lysozyme. This enzyme weakens the cell wall of gram-negative bacteria and dissolves that of gram-positives by cleaving the muco-peptide complex. Protoplasts take on spherical shape, being held together only by the cytoplasmic membrane. They can be maintained in this form when suspended in hypertonic solutions such as 10 to 20 per cent sucrose, which is equivalent to the osmotic strength of the cytoplasm.

Antibiotics that block cell wall synthesis such as penicillin, as well as antibodies and a variety of adverse environmental factors, may lead to "natural" formation of protoplasts. These are also called "L-forms." Since traces of cell wall material remain on the surface of L-forms, a distinction from true protoplasts which are void of any cell wall material is made by defining them as "spheroplasts." All cellular functions proceed normally. The cell is even able to divide and can resume cell wall synthesis. In this case it reverts back to the original bacterial form. In one genus of bacteria, the mycoplasmas, absence of a cell wall is a fixed genetic property.

Cytoplasmic Membrane. The cytoplasmic membrane is involved in the active transport mechanism of the bacterial cell. It also is the site of enzyme systems such as the cytochromes and serves a function similar to mitochondria in mammalian cells. Membrane invaginations into the cytoplasm enlarge the active surface. These specific areas with condensed invaginations and concentrated enzyme activity are called mesosomes, which also seem to play a role in chromosome separation. Numerous submicroscopic particles, the ribosomes, are found in connection with membrane invaginations throughout the cytoplasm. They are involved in protein synthesis, as will be discussed later in more detail.

Cytoplasm. The cytoplasm in its basic composition is not much different from other living cells. Structures such as mitochondria or chloroplasts, however, do not exist in bacterial cells. Various types of storage granules may be present and are often characteristic for certain genera or species; for instance, the metachromatic granules in corynebacteria.

The Genetic Apparatus. Bacteria belong to the category of procaryotic cells. This means they possess neither a mitotic apparatus nor a nuclear membrane. The entire genetic information of a bacterial cell is inscribed in a single circular ring chromosome. Usually several such identical chromosomes are present in one bacterial cell. The sites (nuclear regions) where these chromosomes are located can be demonstrated by DNA-specific stains such as the Feulgen reaction. The replication of the chromosome is semiconservative. The strands of the DNA-helix separate and each one acts as template for a duplicate complementary strand. In this way two new chromosomes are formed which are identical with the original. Attachment of the double chromosome to a mesosome, which seems to be a prerequisite for their separation, occurs prior to cell division.

The function of bacterial chromosomes is in no way different from that of chromosomes in mammalian cells. The DNA serves as template for single-stranded messenger RNA (mRNA) with a nucleotide sequence complementary to one of the DNA strands. Another class of RNA molecules, soluble or transfer

RNA (sRNA or tRNA), is present in the cytoplasm and upon enzymatic activation binds with specific amino acids. Ribosomes, mRNA, and the tRNA-amino acid complexes join, whereby the latter line up corresponding to the nucleotide sequence in the messenger RNA molecule. According to this sequence, which actually represents the code of information as it was inscribed into the mRNA by chromosomal DNA, the amino acids are hooked together to form specific polypeptide chains. Hence, it is ultimately the structural gene in the chromosome which determines the structure of the product. Next to structural genes, the chromosome carries operator genes which turn the structural genes on. Their activity is controlled by a third class of genes, the regulator genes, which direct production of a repressor substance to block the operator gene. Occasionally mutations occur which make the operator genes unable to bind repressor substance, or which affect regulator genes so that they are no longer able to mediate production of repressor substance. In either situation the operator genes are continuously turned on or, as it is called, "derepressed."

Bacterial as well as animal or plant cells may contain autonomous cytoplasmic DNA in the form of plasmids or episomes besides chromosomal DNA. Plasmid-DNA, for instance, seems to carry the genetic information which renders staphylococci resistant to penicillin. The term "episome" is used if autonomous cytoplasmic DNA alternates between a free cytoplasmic state and a state of attachment to the chromosome.

Endospores. Spores are produced by the aerobic genus Bacillus and the anaerobic genus Clostridium. Only one spore can be produced by one individual bacterial cell. Genus and species differences exist according to size, shape, and location of the spore within the cell. Sporulation usually occurs when the environment is depleted of certain nutritional components. Germination of spores is seen as soon as conditions again favor growth of the vegetative bacterial cell. These processes are not yet fully understood. Obviously the spore preserves the complete genetic information content of the bacterium. Characteristic for the spore is its extreme state of dehydration, which is presumably maintained by a high concentration of calcium dipicolinate. However, the spore does not appear to be metabolically inert since enzyme functions have been demonstrated, at least at a low level.

Thanks to the high degree of dehydration,

spores are highly resistant to desiccation and heat, especially dry heat. The ability to form spores is obviously a great ecological advantage.

Flagella. Flagella are found in motile bacteria, apparently associated with locomotion, although the mechanism of their function is unclear. The number and arrangement of flagella aid in the classification of bacteria.

BACTERIAL GROWTH

Growth Arrangements. Bacteria show characteristic growth arrangements which reflect different manners of cell division. If cells divide in irregular planes with subsequent adherence of cells, the result is a cluster typical for staphylococci. Cell division in parallel planes with sister cells adhering to each other occurs in streptococci and streptobacteria. If cell adherence persists for only one or two generations, short chains or diplococci will be seen. Some bacteria divide at an angle of 90 degrees and subsequently adhere to each other, forming flat quadruplets (tetragena) or cubical bundles (sarcina). In corynebacteria sister cells turn around the point of division by 180 degrees, leading to a parallel "palisade" arrangement.

Such characteristic patterns are observed only in nonmotile bacteria. If motile, they move actively away from each other after cell division.

Growth Requirements The biochemical requirements for growth are very similar to those of animal or plant cells. Oxidizable substrates are necessary as hydrogen donors and sources of energy. Hydrogen acceptors are required as the terminal phase of energy yielding oxidation-reduction reactions. Molecular oxygen serves this purpose in aerobic bacteria; inorganic or organic compounds are utilized by anaerobic bacteria, which for various reasons cannot exist in the presence of oxygen.

Carbon, nitrogen, and minerals are required for biosynthesis of organic substances. If a bacterium needs a certain organic compound for its growth, but is unable to synthesize this compound, it must be provided as a "growth factor." Characteristic differences exist between genera or species with regard to the requirement of growth factors.

Bacteria also have specific demands as to the range of pH, temperature, and gas composition, particularly regarding the ratio of oxygen to carbon dioxide.

Differences exist between bacteria in their ability to carry out specific metabolic or catabolic reactions, e.g., the breakdown of certain carbohydrates or bacterial genera and species is largely based on such reactions.

Growth Curve. After seeding of bacteria into a growth medium it takes some time (*lag phase*) for the microbes to adapt themselves to the new environment. Enzymes and metabolites are formed and accumulated as they are needed for cell division. Individual bacterial cells may swell before they divide. This might result in a slight increase of turbidity of fluid growth medium without actual increase in cell number.

Then the bacteria enter into the *exponential* or *log phase*. During this time the growth rate is constant and the cell number doubles per unit of time. There are great differences among bacteria regarding the length of the generation time, which might range from a few minutes to several days. It is obvious that fast-growing microbes reach gigantic population sizes numbering billions and trillions within less than a day. This has to be remembered when considering the likelihood of mutations occurring in bacterial populations, e.g., in the development of drug resistance.

Eventually the rate of replication levels off and leads into the *stationary phase*. Nutrients are exhausted, and toxic metabolic products begin to accumulate. The rate of cell multiplication is low and approximately equals the rate of cell death. Finally, the number of bacteria dying exceeds the number of those dividing. This *death phase* is characterized by gradual diminution of viable cells. Rarely, however, will the culture become entirely sterile. A few viable cells may persist for months or even years, either in a state of complete dormancy or with intermittent division cycles utilizing organic substrates released from disintegrating cells as nutrients.

Familiarity with the specific features of a bacterial growth curve is important for understanding the kinetics of sterilization and disinfection procedures as well as chemotherapy.

ANTIBACTERIAL AGENTS

This discussion relates to antibacterial agents suitable for topical use as well as those for internal administration. Many topical chemotherapeutic substances such as alcohol, dyes, heavy metals, and so forth, act on bacteria as disinfectants do, mostly by directly destroying somatic matter, particularly proteins. A number of antibiotics are also applicable in this way, specifically those which are not suitable for internal use or require great caution because of systemic toxicity. Among these are the antibiotics tyrocidin and gramicidin, nystatin, amphotericin B, bacitracin, neomycin, and polymyxin B.

Chemotherapeutic Drugs: Mode of Action. The effect of sulfonamides is based on competitive antagonism with an essential metabolite, para-aminobenzoic acid (PABA). This metabolite is needed for synthesis of folic acid, which serves as a coenzyme in bacterial cells. Sulfonamides are structurally quite similar to, and can therefore take the place of, PABA, a substitution which places a roadblock in the pathway of folic acid synthesis. Animal cells are unable to synthesize folic acid and have to rely on exogenous sources; therefore, animal cells are not affected by sulfonamides. Certain bacteria are also unable to synthesize folic acid and require this substance as a vitamin; hence, these bacteria are naturally sulfonamide-resistant. The action of this drug is reversible. It can be overcome by increasing the supply of PABA. Obviously, the effect of sulfonamides is bacteriostatic, not bactericidal.

A number of antibiotics act on bacteria by blocking cell wall synthesis. These include penicillin, which acts on gram-positive bacteria, and cephalosporin, which acts on both gram-positive and gram-negative bacteria. Bacitracin, vancomycin, novobiocin, cycloserine and others also affect cell wall synthesis, at least in part. These antibiotics are bactericidal because if no cell walls are synthesized the usual fate of a bacterium is osmotic rupture. Naturally these antibiotics can act only on dividing cells, i.e., at the time when new cell walls have to be synthesized in sister cells.

A number of antibiotics have been shown to interfere with the selective permeability of the cytoplasmic membrane. Among these drugs are polymyxin, which affects mainly bacteria, and polyene, an antifungal drug, as well as streptomycin.

Two widely used classes of antibiotics inhibit protein synthesis. Chloramphenicol, erythromycin, and the tetracyclines interfere with the amino acid assembly on the ribosomes, although in different ways; streptomycin and neomycin cause misreading of the messenger RNA code at the ribosomal level.

Other antibiotics inhibit nucleic acid synthesis. Actinomycin binds to DNA and in this way blocks formation of messenger RNA.

Bacterial Death. Chemotherapy aims for destruction of the bacterial population. Bactericidal drugs have an immediate killing effect on bacteria. Under bacteriostatic treatment, bacterial cells undergo a slow process of aging and eventually die because they are prevented from entering into a new generation cycle. While aging, the bacteria may lose some of their virulence factors and can then be eliminated actively by the body's defense mechanisms.

The criteria for death of a bacterium are uncertain unless the cell appears visibly degraded. In testing for viability the judgment of whether a bacterium is "dead" depends in great measure on the method employed and on a variety of biological factors. In practice, bacterial "death" is meaningful only at the population level, e.g., in chemotherapy or in the evaluation of sterilization or disinfection procedures, chemotherapeutic drugs, killed bacterial vaccines, and the like. In order to determine death of a bacterial population by means of laboratory examination, relatively small test samples must be used for practical reasons. This presents a statistical problem and additional factors of uncertainty. The death process of a bacterial population proceeds at an exponential rate; the point of zero viability is reached mathematically only after an infinite time period. Therefore, one has to measure death of a bacterial population in terms of probability, the calculation of which is based on extrapolation from actual measurements as obtained on small samples. However, the slope observed in the range of the actual measurements does not necessarily continue as a straight line through the range of extrapolation because the number of survivors may be larger than expected statistically. The state and fate of individual bacterial cells become increasingly important as the extrapolation approaches zero. Penicillin, for instance, kills only dividing bacteria. A few cells that happen not to divide during the time of drug exposure would survive. Such cells are called "persistors" and may explain many instances in which chemotherapy fails.

Mechanisms of Drug Resistance. Various mechanisms have been described which operate in bacteria, permitting them to escape the action of chemotherapeutic agents. Sulfonamide resistance is acquired by increasing production of para-aminobenzoic acid, which lessens the capacity of the drug to compete as a substitute. Microbes resistant to penicillin frequently achieve this by producing penicillinase. Also, the permeability of the cytoplasmic membrane for chemotherapeutic drugs may decrease so that lesser amounts are permitted to enter the cell. Increased synthesis or chemical alteration of a drug-inhibited enzyme may offset the capacity of the drug quantitatively or qualitatively. Some bacteria are able to circumvent the metabolic pathway blocked by the chemotherapeutic drug altogether by developing an alternate metabolic pathway. In streptomycin-resistant bacteria the structure or functioning of ribosomes may change so that messenger RNA is no longer misread. On the whole there seems to be no chemotherapeutic mode of action for which bacteria could not develop an escape mechanism.

DEVELOPMENT OF DRUG RESISTANCE

Development of drug resistance is a result of mutations. For this genetic event to occur, presence of the drug is not required. However, presence of the drug quickly leads to selection of the resistant mutants and elimination of the sensitive nonmutant population. On the other hand, the property of drug resistance may spread from mutants to nonmutants. This phenomenon is based on transfer of DNA from one cell to another by various mechanisms. It has been demonstrated to occur within bacterial species and even among different bacterial genera, provided a certain degree of relationship exists. This phenomenon has become increasingly important. Since pathogenic as well as saprophytic bacteria readily spread from person to person, especially in hospital environments, specific drug resistance patterns may be transmitted along with them.

Mutation and Selection. Mutation takes place in DNA often as the consequence of an error during DNA replication. Presumably a tautomeric shift of electrons makes nucleotides change from the keto to the enol form. This leads to wrong base pairing, "point mutation," and may happen spontaneously. The mutation rate (the probability that a cell will mutate) can be increased experimentally by the use of mutagens. Some of these agents have been shown to increase the incidence of tautomerization or they cause chemical alteration of bases. Also, deletions or additions of single nucleotides may occur so that the frame of triplet reading shifts by one notch.

Mutations take place in chromosomal as well as extrachromosomal (cytoplasmic) DNA. For instance, the production of penicillinase in penicillin-resistant staphylococci seems to be based on a mutation of plasmid-DNA.

TRANSFER OF DRUG RESISTANCE

The transfer of DNA (either of chromosomal, episomal, or plasmid origin) from one bacterial cell to another is a relatively frequent occurrence. Most recipient cells destroy the foreign DNA, but in a few (less than 1 per cent) the donor DNA becomes an integral part of the recipient DNA. If this happens the properties inscribed in the transferred DNA segments (e.g., resistance to chemotherapeutic drugs) are acquired by the recipient. Three mechanisms have been discovered by which DNA is transferred: transformation, conjugation, and transduction.

Transformation. Transformation is, for the most part, an experimental system but also seems to occur spontaneously under natural conditions. Experimentally DNA is extracted from one bacterial population and directly added to the culture medium of a recipient cell population. The cells may take up small segments of donor DNA and incorporate one strand of the double helix into their own DNA, whereas the other strand is usually degraded. A prerequisite for successful transformation is a state of "competence" on the part of the recipient cell and a close relationship (homology) in base sequence between donor and recipient DNA.

Conjugation. Conjugation occurs normally between related bacteria such as the enterobacteriaceae which comprise the genera: Escherichia, Salmonella, Shigella, and others. In this process two cells make direct physical contact and a piece of DNA is transferred from one to the other.

The usual kind of DNA transferred in this way is cytoplasmic in nature and fits the definition of an episome. It has been described as "fertility factor" (F-factor). Cells which contain the F-factor are called F^+ cells or male cells. These cells transfer their F-factor at high frequency to cells that lack the F-factor (F^- cells) but become F^+ cells after conjugation. The F-factor itself carries the gene that determines the structural surface property of a male cell to engage in conjugation.

The F-factor DNA tends to undergo a specific mutation at a rate of approximately 10^{-4}. This mutation causes the F-factor to attach to the "nuclear" chromosome of the bacterial cell. (Hence, the F-factor is defined as an episome.) At the site where the F-factor has attached itself, the bacterial ring chromosome breaks open. One end of the broken chromosome holds onto the F-factor. The other end starts replicating while the cell is in conjugation. One newly formed sister chromosome moves over into the conjugated cell, whereas the other sister chromosome stays back in the male cell. Normally the conjugation process is mechanically interrupted before the entire chromosome with the trailing F-factor has moved over. This would take roughly two hours. Therefore, the recipient cells usually remain F^-. The frequency at which chromosomal DNA is transferred by way of conjugation is no higher than the frequency with which the cytoplasmic F-factor acquires by mutation the property of chromosomal attachment, namely 10^{-4} or less. (It is experimentally possible to grow clonal bacterial populations consisting entirely of cells with the F-factor in the state of chromosomal attachment. Such strains are designated "H fr," indicating that chromosome transfer to F^- cells occurs with high frequency.)

F-factor mutants can back-mutate so that they detach themselves from the chromosome. Occasionally the detachment is not "clean," and a piece of chromosomal DNA may stick to the F-factor when it returns to the cytoplasmic state. Both the F-factor DNA and the contaminating chromosomal DNA-segment replicate simultaneously. Whenever the cytoplasmic F-factor is transferred to a female cell, and this occurs with high frequency, it is accompanied by the contaminating chromosomal DNA-piece. Accordingly, the genetic information inscribed in the chromosomal DNA-segment is conveyed to the receptor cell.

Resistance Transfer Factor. The resistance transfer factor is probably also an episome, although it is usually found in the cytoplasmic state like a plasmid. This particular DNA entity determines resistance to a wide range of antibiotics and is able to transfer a complete pattern of resistance against multiple drugs to previously drug-sensitive recipient cells. The exact mechanism of this phenomenon is still largely obscure. However, its practical importance is obvious, although it has so far been observed only in enterobacteriaceae.

Transduction. Viruses of bacteria (bacteriophages) can be demonstrated in two states. When in their lytic or virulent phase, infection of a bacterial cell results in prompt phage propagation and cell destruction. Temperate bacteriophages, on the other hand, do not reach complete maturation in a large percentage of host cells but persist as "prophages" with a relatively low rate of spontaneous lytic activation. In this state of "lysogeny" phage DNA is demonstrable in the bacterial host cell. It may happen that segments of bacterial DNA adhere to phage DNA. When such a prophage is activated spontaneously or upon stimulation with chemical, physical, and even medicinal agents, phage progeny together with adhering bacterial DNA is released to infect new host cells as temperate phages. The specific genetic information inscribed in the bacterial DNA segment is transmitted as well. It appears that antibiotic resistance patterns of staphylococci which are determined by plasmid DNA are transferred in this way.

MEASURES TO PREVENT DEVELOPMENT OF DRUG RESISTANCE

Chemotherapy is often a race against the statistical chance of a mutation which could increase resistance of the etiological agent against the drug in use. Therefore, therapy aims for elimination of the bacterial population from the body as quickly and as completely as possible in cooperation with the body's own defense mechanisms. This may be achieved by (1) reaching and maintaining sufficiently high drug levels; (2) drug administration for a sufficient length of time to prevent recovery of survivors and to catch persistors; and (3) combined drug therapy. The rationale for the latter recommendations is based on the following: If the frequency of resistant mutants to either one of two drugs is expected to be 10^{-6}, the likelihood that a mutant will arise that is resistant to both drugs simultaneously would be 10^{-12}. However, in practice this simple statistical calculation turns out to be somewhat overoptimistic, because the possibility of transfer of drug resistance as discussed in the previous section is not taken into account. There is ample evidence that two mutants, one resistant against drug A, the other resistant against drug B, may recombine by way of DNA transfer, breeding a line that is resistant against both drugs.

In general, chemotherapeutic drugs used in combination should be synergistic. However, certain drugs are known to cancel each other out. For instance, bacteriostatic sulfonamides prevent multiplication; nondividing cells, however, would not be affected by penicillin. Yet incompatible drugs such as sulfonamides and penicillin may be useful in combination under special circumstances, since they reach their peak concentrations in different parts of the body. Sulfonamides, for instance, reach high levels in spinal fluid, in contrast to penicillin which accumulates in blood and vascularized tissues.

Drugs which are chemically related should not be combined because mutants often exhibit cross-resistance.

A more general yet probably the most important way to prevent appearance of drug-resistant mutant strains is, of course, avoidance of indiscriminate use of chemotherapeutic drugs.

CONSIDERATION OF HOST FACTORS IN CHEMOTHERAPY

Influence of Host Factors on Drug Efficiency. One of the main problems in chemotherapy is to reach effective drug levels at the site where drug action is needed. Distribution and concentration of drugs in tissues and body fluids varies considerably under normal conditions and may be entirely unpredictable in pathological situations. Dosage and route of drug administration are not without influence and must be carefully considered, but host-related factors such as degree of vascularization or natural anatomical barriers also play an important role. Fibrinous or connective tissue encapsulation of inflammatory processes can make it difficult or impossible for a drug to reach the etiological agent. Pus and necrotic tissue have a strong absorptive effect on a number of drugs, so that their therapeutic power may be severely impaired. Bacteria that tend to grow intracellularly are protected against certain drugs such as streptomycin, whereas other antibiotics such as oxytetracycline have less difficulty in penetrating effectively into tissue cells.

Considerations along these lines are particularly important when results of antibiotic sensitivity tests are used as a basis for a therapeutic regimen. The growth conditions as well as the metabolic state of the bacterial population are far more constant and uniform in laboratory tests than in pathological *in vivo* situations. The growth curve of a bacterial population in an infected host will rarely show the even logarithmic shape of that seen in an 18-hour laboratory culture. Many important clinical factors can hardly be simulated *in vitro*. For example, the temperature is kept at 37° C in in vitro tests, not taking into account that the patient might run a high fever. Furthermore, antibiotic-induced L-forms may find compatible osmotic conditions in diseased tissue, whereas they would rupture osmotically in a laboratory medium. Therefore, discrepancies between in vitro and in vivo effectiveness of drugs must always be anticipated.

Adverse Drug Effects on the Host. There is practically not a single chemotherapeutic drug without a certain degree of toxicity for specific organ systems; also, any drug may cause allergization.

Another serious adverse effect is that on the normal bacterial flora, particularly in the respiratory, intestinal, and genital tracts. Antibiotic attack on normal organisms of the body can lead to disease by itself, especially if drug-resistant pathogens or opportunists such as staphylococci, Proteus, coliform bacteria, or fungi fill the vacancies left by the extermination of parts of the normal flora.

If the causative agent of an infection develops drug resistance, the disease may become chronic. On the other hand, it is possible that after elimination of a sensitive pathogen (e.g., streptococci in otitis), it is replaced by a different but drug-resistant organism (e.g., pseudomonas). In this situation the etiological agent changes while the disease persists.

THE NORMAL BACTERIAL FLORA OF THE UPPER RESPIRATORY TRACT

Numerous microbial species reside in the respiratory tract of man under normal conditions. Some are regularly demonstrable as major permanent constituents, including alphahemolytic *Streptococcus viridans* and unclassified anaerobic streptococci, several aerobic and anaerobic species of corynebacteria ("diphtheroids"), a variety of neisseria species (*N. catarrhalis*, *N. pharyngis*) and the morphologically similar but anaerobic Veillonella group. Frequently also present, although in lower percentage, are staphylococci (*Staphylococcus albus*, *Sarcina lutea*, *Gaffkya tetragena*, as well as the potentially pathogenic *Staphylococcus aureus*). Furthermore, we find vibrios, spirochetes, and symbiotic anaerobic fusobacteria, the genus bacterioides (small anaerobic gram-negative rods), and leptothrix. Other microbes are present only occasionally as transient visitors; for instance, potentially pathogenic beta-hemolytic streptococci, pneumococci, and hemophilus organisms, also coliform bacteria, Proteus, Pseudomonas, and others which are known as predominant constituents of the normal intestinal flora. Even obligate pathogens may exist within the normal flora of persons who have recovered from infection and have established, mainly by means of immune mechanisms, an equilibrium with the organism. Such persons are, of course, a possible source of infection for the nonimmune population.

Thorough knowledge and understanding with regard to the normal bacterial flora appears to be important for many reasons. For instance, in the evaluation of laboratory reports concerning bacteriological examination of clinical specimens the physician is often faced with the necessity of judging whether the isolated organisms can be disregarded as saprophytes, or whether they may be of etiological significance in an individual patient. Marked differences may be observed among normal persons regarding the composition of their normal microbial flora. This depends on numerous factors. Various degrees of compatibility are known to exist among groups of bacteria, based on differences in metabolic activities and growth requirements. On the other hand, host factors are even more important in creating a specific ecological composition and equilibrium of the bacterial flora. Living habits, food preferences, hormonal or metabolic peculiarities, and other factors exert specific influences.

The existence of an ecological balance makes it plausible that the normal flora serves as a strong natural barrier against invading pathogens. In many instances the invader encounters an environment which does not permit a foothold within the biosystem of the existing flora. Any disturbance of the normal flora, however, can create conditions which could give invading pathogens a chance to establish themselves. Even an imbalance among the regular members of the normal flora can lead per se to a pathological situation, since some of them are typical opportunistic pathogens.

Disturbances of the normal flora occur from many causes, local as well as general. Chemical or physical irritation, allergic inflammation, anatomical or physiological changes, such as mucosal atrophies or functional defects, may have a direct local effect on the bacterial flora. Causative factors of systemic nature include nutritional deficiencies, avitaminosis, unbalanced metabolic disorders (for instance, diabetes), and other similar pathological situations.

However, the most noteworthy and also the most dangerous cause is chemotherapy, especially the application of antibiotics. For whatever reason and in whatever form antibiotics are administered to a patient, they necessarily exert an effect on the normal bacterial flora because any drug-susceptible microbe will be attacked. Very often no overt consequence is noted, and upon termination of therapy the flora shifts back to its previous composition and equilibrium. Yet the danger of a disease complication resulting from a breakdown of the normal bacterial flora must not be underestimated. This peril demands no less vigilance than possible development of drug resistance.

DISEASE-PRODUCING PROPERTIES OF BACTERIA

Some organisms, especially fungi, cause disease more or less simply by their presence in the tissue, which may respond with foreign body reactions and formation of granulomas. As the microbes multiply and consume nutrients, inadequate nourishment of the tissue may lead to reversible damage or even necrosis.

Many gram-negative bacteria possess endotoxins. These are complex molecules consisting of a protein portion and lipopolysaccharide which carries the toxicity. The endotoxin molecules are closely associated with the bacterial cell wall. They are released only upon death and disintegration of the bacterial cells. Free endotoxin causes local edema, hemorrhage and, possibly, necrosis; general symptoms include fever, diarrhea, and shock in various degrees dependent on the amount of endotoxin liberated into the circulation.

Other bacteria excrete actively into their environment metabolic products with toxic properties (exotoxins) or enzymes which aid in the invasiveness of the organisms. Most exotoxin producers are gram-positive, including *Corynebacterium diphtheriae* and the clostridia of tetanus and botulism. Minute amounts of exotoxin are sufficient to cause severe damage to specific organ or cell systems often distant from the focus of infection. Some exotoxins can be converted by treatment with formaldehyde to toxoids which have lost toxicity but not their specific antigenicity. Immunization with toxoids elicits humoral antibodies which specifically bind to and neutralize the exotoxin in case of infection.

PATHOGENIC BACTERIA ENCOUNTERED IN OTORHINOLARYNGOLOGICAL INFECTIONS

A great variety of pathogenetically important bacterial enzymes have been described in organisms ranging from streptococci to the etiological agents of gas gangrene. These include hyaluronidase, proteinases, fibrinolysin, collagenase, and numerous others, most of which facilitate spread of infection in the tissue (Fig. 1).

Streptococci

Streptococci are found in man and animals alike. They are grouped on the basis of antigenic properties, and these groups possess a certain degree of host specificity. Group A streptococci cause 90 per cent of streptococcal infections in man. The natural reservoir of these human pathogenic streptococci is the respiratory tract of persons who have developed an immunologic equilibrium with the organisms. Other groups of streptococci are found normally under similar conditions in various animal species. Certain groups of streptococci are saprophytes and members of the normal human bacterial flora, among them the ungroupable *Streptococcus viridans* in the mouth and pharynx, group D-streptococci (enterococci) in the intestinal tract, and ungroupable anaerobic streptococci in the respiratory tract and in the vagina. Any of these strains can occasionally become pathogenic; for instance, when the equilibrium of the normal flora is upset or when the organisms are displaced into other areas of the body. Typical examples are enterococcal cystitis, puerperal sepsis from anaerobic streptococci, endocarditis caused by *Streptococcus viridans*. Other streptococcal groups are normally present in the human environment, e.g., *Streptococcus lactis* (group L) in milk.

About half the human population develops a delayed type of hypersensitivity against strep-

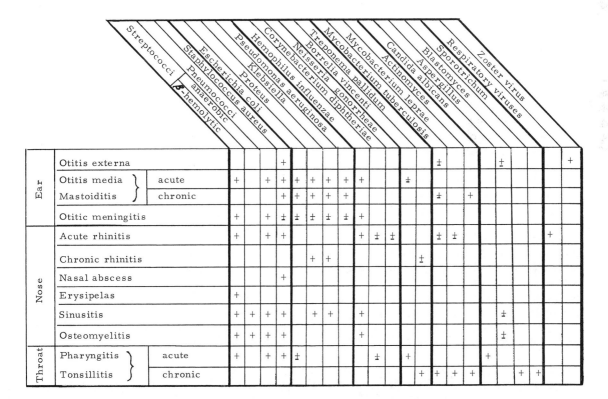

			Streptococci β-hemolytic	Pneumococci	anaerobic	Staphylococcus aureus	Escherichia coli	Proteus	Klebsiella	Pseudomonas aeruginosa	Hemophilus influenzae	Corynebacterium diphtheriae	Neisseria gonorrheae	Borrelia vincenti	Treponema pallidum	Mycobacterium tuberculosis	Mycobacterium leprae	Actinomyces	Candida albicans	Aspergillus	Blastomyces	Sporotrichum	Respiratory viruses	Zoster virus
Ear	Otitis externa					+													±			±		+
Ear	Otitis media	acute	+			+	+	+	+	+	+	+						±						
Ear	Mastoiditis	chronic				+	+	+	+	+								±		+				
Ear	Otitic meningitis		+			+	±	±	±	±	±	+												
Nose	Acute rhinitis		+			+	+				+	±	±						±	±			+	
Nose	Chronic rhinitis										+	+						±						
Nose	Nasal abscess					+																		
Nose	Erysipelas		+																					
Nose	Sinusitis		+	+	+	+			+	+		+										±		
Nose	Osteomyelitis		+	+	+	+				+												±		
Throat	Pharyngitis	acute	+			+	+	±				+		±		+						+		
Throat	Tonsillitis	chronic																+	+	+	+		+	+

+ = frequent

± = less frequent

blank = not reported or rare

Figure 1. Pathogenic microbes in otorhinolaryngological infections.

tococcal substances, as can be demonstrated by skin testing with streptococcal extract.

Bacteriological Characterization. Streptococci are gram-positive cocci in chains. No spores and no flagella are formed. Virulent strains are invariably encapsulated. The capsule consists of hyaluronic acid and proteins. Presence of the capsule makes streptococci grow in more opulent, sometimes confluent, mucoid colonies.

Streptococci, in general, have high nutritional requirements for cultivation. Blood or serum has to be added to the medium to promote growth. On blood agar most streptococci produce hemolysis. Beta-hemolytic streptococci digest the stroma of red blood cells as well as the hemoglobin, so that ·complete clearing of the medium ensues. Alpha-hemolytic strains digest only erythrocyte stroma, not the hemoglobin which is oxidized and creates a greenish discoloration around the colonies. Some streptococci do not hemolyze at all and are called gamma-hemolytic.

Antigens of streptococci have been extensively studied and are useful for diagnostic and epidemiological purposes. The cell wall contains the group-specific carbohydrate antigens which permit differentiation of about a dozen groups. The human pathogenic group A, which is comprised of beta-hemolytic strains, can be broken down further into some 40 to 50 types on the basis of proteinaceous antigens, specifically the M protein which is located throughout the surface layers of the organism. (Only in heavily encapsulated strains might the M protein be hidden under the cover of hyaluronic acid.)

Virulence Factors. A basic prerequisite for pathogenicity is the presence of the capsule. Streptococci without the capsule are readily phagocytized by polymorphonuclear leukocytes and destroyed. The pathogenic streptococci produce a great number of exotoxic enzymes in varied amounts and combinations which largely determine the clinical course of a streptococcal infection. The most important exotoxins are the following: several proteinases; fibrinolytic streptokinase which converts plasminogen to plasmin; hyaluronidase, one of the most powerful spreading factors which destroys intercellular ground substance; erythrogenic toxin causing skin rash in scarlet fever; and DPNase (diphosphopyridine nucleotidase) which interferes with intracellular respiration. This latter enzyme is toxic for polymorphonuclear leukocytes and may be lethal because of its effect on the heart muscle cells.

Two enzymes, streptolysin S and O, are responsible for the hemolytic property of the organism. Streptolysin O is used for demonstrating streptococcal antibodies (antistreptolysin O reaction).

Pathogenesis. The kind of extracellular enzymes found in group A beta-hemolytic streptococci explains the tendency of streptococcal infections to spread rapidly. However, strains of streptococci differ with regard to types and amounts of toxins actually produced. Therefore, considerable variability in the degree of virulence is generally observed.

Probably some form of presensitization of the host is required for some of the virulence factors to become fully effective. This is indicated by the observation that very young children up to the age of about three years are usually not so severely sick from streptococcal infections as older children.

The organisms are transmitted by air-borne droplets from carriers or directly in food, e.g., milk. The infection may spread rapidly, causing carbuncles, cellulitis, and phlegmons. Streptococcal tonsillitis or pharyngitis often involves the sinuses, the middle ears, the mastoids, and the meninges.

Erysipelas is a special form of streptococcal infection and pathogenetically not fully understood. The microbes are found packed in lymph spaces some 2 to 3 cm. ahead of the demarcation of the infected area. Erysipelas tends to reoccur at the same site.

Endocarditis can be caused by various bacteria, among them *Streptococcus viridans* and enterococci. Prerequisites for the development of this disease are (1) an endocardial defect, and (2) bacteremia. Invasion of the blood stream by bacteria may occur through lesions in the mouth or in the pharynx as a consequence of surgery or tooth extraction, and even through minute punctures of the mucosa from brushing the teeth too forcefully.

Systemic sequelae of streptococcal infections are rheumatic fever and glomerulonephritis. The pathogenic development of these complications is still a matter of controversy. Two mechanisms are being discussed: (1) some form of hypersensitivity reaction; (2) antigenic cross-relationship between streptococcal antigens and tissue antigens so that streptococcal antibodies would cross-react with components of the body's own tissue.

Immunity. Antistreptococcal immunity is based on two mechanisms: First, on the presence of opsonic antibodies which are directed against capsular antigens, especially against the M protein. With antibodies bound to their capsules, the organisms can readily be phagocytized by polymorphonuclear leukocytes. Since there are numerous types of group A streptococci with as many different M protein antigens, type-specific opsonic immunity has only a limited effect on the general susceptibility of a person to streptococcal infections. However, with progressing age an increasing number of types will have been encountered and, accordingly, opsonic immunity will gain in protectiveness.

More important in streptococcal immunity are antibodies that neutralize the various streptococcal enzymes and toxins. They do not prevent infection as such but break the invasive power of the microbes. In this way they render streptococcal diseases less severe and less dangerous, irrespective of the type of the causative organism.

Laboratory Diagnosis. Usually no technical difficulties are to be expected in obtaining specimens and sending them to the laboratory. If swabs are taken they should be inserted in transport tubes containing a few drops of bacteriological medium to keep the material moist. The part of the applicator that was touched with the fingers should be broken off while inserting the swab into the tube in order to prevent contamination of the specimen. Blood samples for blood culture should be sent in special tubes prefilled with an anticoagulant and special medium.

Streptococci can be cultured easily on blood agar plates. If the physician suspects anaerobic streptococci as the etiological agent, e.g., in cases of sinusitis, he should specifically request anaerobic cultivation. Tentative identification of group A beta-hemolytic streptococci is possible by means of bacitracin discs which inhibit growth of group A beta-hemolytic streptococci directly on the culture plate. More precise group or type diagnosis involves the extraction of antigens and a precipitation reaction with specific reference sera. These methods are employed mainly in epidemiological investigations.

Antistreptococcal antibodies in patients' sera can be identified by means of the antistreptolysin O reaction. In this test the antibodies inhibit the lysis of red blood cells by streptolysin O. Inhibition by normal sera may be noted in dilutions of up to 1:200. Higher titers have diagnostic significance, e.g., in cases of rheumatic fever. Other more complicated serological tests are also available and are based on the ability of antibodies to inactivate the various enzymes listed previously, specifically hyaluronidase and streptokinase.

Antibiotic sensitivity tests are usually not necessary because penicillin is the drug of choice in treating infections caused by group A beta-hemolytic streptococci. Susceptibility to penicillin appears to be a stable property. *Streptococcus viridans* and enterococci are less susceptible to penicillin than group A streptococci and need higher doses. All streptococci may develop resistance to other antibiotics.

Pneumococci

Pneumococci are closely related to streptococci. Natural infections are observed in man, guinea pigs, rats, and monkeys. These microbes are part of the normal bacterial flora of man, especially in the respiratory tract, from where they may ascend into the eustachian tubes and the lacrimal ducts.

Bacteriological Characterization. Pneumococci are gram-positive cocci in pairs or short chains with the distal ends slightly pointed. As in streptococci, no spores or flagella are formed. Virulent pneumococci carry a capsule and grow as smooth colonies on solid medium in contrast to the rough colonies of nonencapsulated strains. Slight alpha hemolysis is produced on blood agar. The organisms are delicate and tend to autolyze. While a colony grows and expands peripherally, the microbes in the center part of the colony die and disintegrate. As a result, such colonies appear crater-shaped. Growth is favored by low redox potential. Pneumococci obtain their energy from anaerobic glycolysis with an accumulation of lactic acid, which is a growth-limiting factor. Some virulent pneumococcal strains are obligate anaerobes.

All pneumococci possess an antigenetically identical carbohydrate in their cell wall. Some 80 pneumococcal types are distinguished on the basis of a capsular carbohydrate antigen, the so-called specific soluble substance (SSS). Type-specific reference sera give precipitation reactions with extracts of homologous SSS. If such sera are applied to whole encapsulated organisms, a microscopic "Quellung" reaction is obtained: specific binding of antibody to the capsule changes light diffraction so that the capsule appears to swell.

Virulence Factors. The capsule prevents phagocytosis in nonimmune patients who lack type-specific antibodies; otherwise, no toxins or extracellualr enzymes of proved importance have been demonstrated in amounts large enough to explain the virulence of pneumococci. Since the organisms are usually found in abundant numbers in infected tissues, damage might be inflicted by competition for essential nutrients or metabolites.

Pathogenesis. Genotypic constitution is believed to explain the predisposition of certain patients for repeated pneumococcal infections, especially pneumonia. Conditioning factors, however, seem to be more important, e.g., irritation of the respiratory organs by chemical dust or gases, functional or circulatory impairment of the lung, aspiration, heart failure, viral precursor infection, and others.

Immunity. Immunity is entirely based on anticapsular opsonic antibodies. If present in the body, they bind to the capsules of invading pneumococci and make them phagocytizable for polymorphonuclear leukocytes. The appearance of such type-specific antibodies in the course of pneumococcal infections is the basis of spontaneous termination of the disease. Since there are some 80 different types of pneumococci, this mechanism of immunity has little effect on the general susceptibility to pneumococcal infections.

Laboratory Diagnosis. The organisms are very delicate and fragile; therefore, quick transport of clinical specimens to the laboratory is essential. Cultivation of pneumococci also presents some technical problems and is not always successful. Differentiation from alphahemolytic streptococci may become necessary and requires special tests. Pneumococci are virulent for mice; they are dissolved in solutions of bile, deoxycholate, or certain detergents; and their growth on solid medium is inhibited by Optochin discs.

Antibiotic sensitivity tests are not necessary. If pneumococci are incriminated as etiological agents of an infectious process, the drug of choice is penicillin. It must be kept in mind, however, that the heavily encapsulated pneumococcus type 3 ("pneumococcus mucosus") presents great therapeutic difficulties, even in respect to treatment with antibiotics.

Staphylococci

A number of saprophytic micrococcaceae, e.g., *Staphylococcus albus, Gaffkya tetragena, Sarcina lutea* and others, are part of the permanent or transient normal flora of the body. They rarely play a role as causative agents of infections. When isolated from clinical specimens, they most likely represent contaminants. The important pathogenic member in this group of organisms is *Staph. aureus,* which causes purulent infections in animals and man alike. It is ubiquitously present on the skin, in the nose, in the gastrointestinal tract, and in other parts of the body. Most persons (at least 65 per cent of the population) have developed delayed hypersensitivity against staphylococcal substances, as can be demonstrated by skin tests with staphylococcal extracts. Usually a well-balanced equilibrium exists between host and microbe. The microbe is held in check by means of various host factors, e.g., the pH of continuous keratinization and shedding of superficial cell layers, as well as specific immunity. This equilibrium may be disturbed in numerous possible ways: mechanical or allergic irritation of the skin, traumatic lesions, nutritional or hormonal imbalance such as diabetes, and so forth. If the resident strain of *Staph. aureus* is antibiotic-resistant, any application of this antibiotic would give the organism a growth advantage. Especially in hospital environments, patients may pick up antibiotic-resistant staphylococci and incorporate them into their normal bacterial flora.

Bacteriological Characterization. The grampositive nonmotile staphylococci grow in grapelike clusters and do not form spores or capsules. Their metabolic requirements are modest so that growth proceeds aerobically or anaerobically under a wide range of conditions with a minimal nutritional supply and even in high salt concentrations. *Staphylococcus aureus* produces a golden yellow pigment, a lipochrome, particularly in the presence of oxygen and at room temperature. The pigment does not diffuse out into the medium; therefore, only the colonies appear yellow. In contrast, the pigment is soluble in tissue fluid or exudate, so that staphylococcal pus can be recognized because of its yellow tint.

On blood agar medium, red blood cells and hemoglobin are completely digested. This results in complete clearing of the agar.

Virulence Factors. *Staphylococcus aureus* produces a number of toxins. The so-called lethal toxin causes shock; the dermonecrotic toxin is responsible for tissue necrosis; leukocidin destroys polymorphonuclear leukocytes; heat-stable enterotoxin accumulates in contaminated foodstuffs and causes food poisoning. In addition, numerous extracellular enzymes may be produced by *Staph. aureus,* including hyaluronidase, proteinases, fibrinolysin, coagulase, and many others. Demonstration of coagulase is used in the diagnostic laboratory as the most regular criterion of staphylococcal pathogenicity.

Pathogenesis. Staphylococcal disease often begins with invasion of skin follicles, wound-infection, or ascending expansion into areas which are normally free of bacteria, e.g., the eustachian tubes. The purulent character of staphylococcal inflammation is the result of attraction of polymorphonuclear leukocytes and their destruction by leukocidin. The tendency to form abscesses can be explained at least partly by the action of the enzyme coagulase. By gelling the inflammatory exudate the organism seems to protect itself against antibacterial components in serum and tissue fluid. The host supports this process with firbroblastic proliferation around the focus of inflammation. However, if the infection is not stopped at this stage spontaneously or by therapy, the organisms will eventually break through the abscess wall with the help of their enzymes: hyaluronidase, proteinase, and fibrinolysin. In this way, abscesses enlarge in repeated steps until internal or external fistulas provide drainage. Erosion of blood vessels, particularly in areas of strong vascularization (e.g., in the nasal area), may lead to hematogenic dissemination, toxemia, or septicemia with metastatic abscesses.

Chronic staphylococcosis is often seen in conjunction with a pronounced state of allergy against staphylococcal substances.

Immunity. Most persons build up a certain degree of immunity during early life based on antitoxic antibodies against the various virulence factors. However, opsonic antibodies seem to play a minor role. Therefore, man has no sufficient means to protect himself against invasion of his body by *Staph. aureus*, but he is capable of fighting its establishment, its toxic manifestations, and the spread of infection.

Laboratory Diagnosis. *Staphylococcus aureus* is quite resistant against adverse environmental conditions; therefore, no special precautions are required for sending specimens (swabs, purulent discharge, necrotic tissue, etc.) to the laboratory. The organism can easily be cultured and identified. Demonstration of coagulase activity indicates virulence. Saprophytic coagulase-negative cocci are often isolated from clinical specimens as contaminants from skin, mouth, or nose. Before attributing any etiological significance to such findings it is recommended that the bacteriological examination be repeated. Special care should be taken to avoid contamination from the normal resident flora, and the site for taking the specimen should be carefully selected.

Antibiotic sensitivity testing is most important in *Staph. aureus* infections. The resistance pattern is unpredictable and may change rapidly. The physician has to watch for clinical indications of increasing antibiotic resistance. Repeated cultivation of the agent and antibiotic-sensitivity testing are advisable, especially in chronic or slowly responding cases.

Neisseria

Several species of Neisseria are part of the normal flora in the respiratory tract such as *N. catarrhalis* and *N. pharyngis*. Only occasionally must they be incriminated as etiological agents of infection. *Neisseria pharyngis* is known to cause occasional problems in tracheostomies by forming crusts.

The pathogenic members of this genus, *N. meningitidis* and *N. gonorrhoeae*, cause disease exclusively in man. *Neisseria gonorrhoeae* is found in otorhinolaryngological diseases only under unusual circumstances, e.g., gonorrheal rhinitis of the newborn, in contrast to *N. meningitidis*, the meningococcus. This organism inhabits the pharynx of about 5 per cent of normal persons but shows little tendency to spread to noncarriers. Restricted outbreaks of meningococcal meningitis occur in special epidemiological situations, usually among people who live in crowded conditions and under physical stress, such as armed service recruits or inhabitants of camps for displaced persons or refugees.

The species of meningitidis can be subdivided into three serological types: Type B is presently encountered most often in epidemics, whereas one or two decades ago type A was more prominent. Type C is occasionally found in sporadic infections.

Bacteriological Characterization. Neisseriae are gram-negative diplococci with their adjoining sides slightly flattened. They neither possess flagella nor form spores. With the exception of *N. meningitidis* types A and C, these organisms are not encapsulated.

Saprophytic neisseriae grow readily on ordinary media, even on plain nutrient agar, and at room temperature. Colonies are of firm consistency, so that emulsification for staining is accomplished with difficulty. Pathogenic neisseriae need enriched media, high humidity, increased CO_2 tensions and a strict incubation temperature of 37° C. for cultivation. Even then the colonies remain small and tend to autolyze.

Neisserial species can be biochemically distinguished on the basis of differential breakdown of sugars. All neisseriae produce oxidase, which causes a color reaction with tetramethylparaphenylenediamine. However, oxidase is also found in other bacteria, so that a negative oxidase reaction excludes neisseriae, whereas a positive reaction requires additional confirmation.

The only antigens of diagnostic importance are those associated with capsules of *N. meningitidis* types A and C.

Virulence Factors and Pathogenesis. Pathogenic neisseriae excrete neither exotoxins nor toxic enzymes. Their virulence is probably caused by endotoxins.

The primary site of infection is usually the nasopharynx. From there the organisms reach the blood stream through the lymph channels. Target organs are the meninges and other parts of the body, specifically the skin, which responds with a characteristic hemorrhagic rash, and the adrenal cortex, a condition which leads to the Waterhouse-Friderichsen syndrome.

Immunity. The body has little if any capacity to build up immunity against meningococci, and actually no protection is acquired to subsequent infections. If untreated and not fatal, a meningococcal infection may become chronic.

Laboratory Diagnosis. It is often possible to demonstrate *N. meningitidis* directly microscopically in clinical specimens, e.g., in spinal fluid sediment. Negative gram staining, typical morphology, and frequently intracellular location of organisms in polymorphonuclear leukocytes permit rapid etiological diagnosis. For successful cultivation the clinical specimen should reach the laboratory as quickly as possible and be kept warm in transport.

Corynebacteria

Saprophytic corynebacteria (diphtheroids) are found ubiquitously and constitute a large portion of the normal flora of skin and mucous membranes. The medical importance of the pathogenic species, *Corynebacterium diphtheriae*, has been drastically reduced, first, by the introduction of antiserum treatment, and even more so later by active immunization with diphtheria toxoid. However, there are still several hundred cases per year in the United States with a fatality rate of 20 to 25 per cent.

Corynebacterium diphtheriae is one of the best studied pathogenic microbes. Its ability to produce toxin is connected with the presence of a lysogenic bacteriophage. The phage nucleic acid is actually integrated into the bacterial nucleic acid and replicates with it. This state is associated with the "abnormal" property of the bacterium to synthesize and excrete diphtheria toxin (lysogenic conversion). Activation of phage nucleic acid occurs at any time in a few of these infected organisms (10^{-4} to 10^{-5}), followed by phage maturation, lysis of the bacterial cells, and release of phage progeny. In this manner the bacterial population is continuously reinfected.

Bacteriological Characterization. Corynebacteria are club-shaped, gram-positive rods with agglomeration of polyphosphoric acid at the poles. This material stains selectively (metachromatic granules) and is characteristic for this group of bacteria. Spores are not produced; flagella or capsules are not present.

The organisms are microscopically arranged, either parallel to each other (palisades) or completely irregular. Some correlation between pathogenicity and morphologic features exists but cannot be relied upon. Pathogenic corynebacteria usually show irregular arrangements and a larger number of metachromatic granules. Colonial and metabolic differentiation is possible between saprophytic and pathogenic corynebacteria. Moreover, three types of *C. diphtheriae* have been distinguished, namely, gravis, mitis, and intermedius. A correlation between type, toxicity, and severity of illness was suggested but is no longer considered meaningful with regard to prophylaxis, prognosis, or therapy.

The medium of choice for cultivation of corynebacteria is blood-tellurite-agar, which inhibits most other bacterial genera. It has the additional advantage that corynebacteria are able to reduce tellurite to tellurium so that the colonies are conspicuously blackened.

Virulence Factors and Pathogenesis. There is only one virulence factor in *C. diphtheriae*: the toxin. It affects the tissue locally, particularly the mucous membranes, leading to inflammation, cell death, necrosis, and formation of pseudomembranes. In addition, the toxin has an affinity for various other organs such as the heart, nerves, and adrenals.

Convalescents may carry and spread *C. diphtheriae* for a long time after recovery. But the bacterial strain may gradually lose its toxicity and, hence, its pathogenicity. This can probably be attributed to the appearance in the host of antibodies against the bacteriophage. Any free bacteriophages will be neutralized by the antibodies, so that reinfection of the bacterial population is prevented.

Immunity. Immunity is based entirely on toxin-neutralizing antibodies (antitoxin). The immune status of individual persons can be determined by means of the Schick test which, therefore, has some epidemiological importance. The test is performed by intradermal injection of a small amount of active toxin. In the absence of antibody a local toxic reaction is observed, with its peak between the third and seventh day. Hypersensitivity reactions to somatic substances of corynebacteria must be excluded in a control test with heat-inactivated toxin. The peak of hypersensitivity reactions is reached within two days and fades quickly.

Laboratory Diagnosis. The organisms are quite resistant, and no special precautions are necessary for transporting material to the laboratory. Swabs must not be taken after application of local disinfectants.

Direct microscopic examination is of little diagnostic value. Cultivation of the organism and demonstration of toxin production by immunodiffusion or in laboratory animals such as the guinea pig is needed to affirm the diagnosis of diphtheria.

Haemophilus Influenzae

Haemophilus influenzae is frequently found in the respiratory organs of normal persons. However, in this situation the organism is usually avirulent and lacks a capsule.

Primary infections are seen, especially in children. In cases of meningitis *H. influenzae* is almost as frequently isolated as pneumococci or meningococci. It also causes otitis media in 25 per cent of affected children under three years of age. Other primary infections include sinusitis, laryngotracheitis, and pneumonia.

Haemophilus influenzae, similar to streptococci, pneumococci, or staphylococci, may play a role in secondary bacterial infections of viral diseases such as influenza-pneumonia. In fact, it was considered by its discoverer to be the etiological agent of influenza.

Bacteriological Characterization. *Haemophilus influenzae* is a small pleomorphic gram-negative rod. In its virulent form it carries a capsule. Spores are not produced and flagella are not present. In culture the organism is extremely fastidious and needs various growth factors. These can be provided with heated blood (chocolate agar) or by growing them as satellite colonies in a mixture with "nursing" bacteria such as staphylococci, from which the growth factors diffuse out into the medium. The so-called X-factor was identified as hemin, the V-factor as diphosphopyridine nucleotide. These are needed for biosynthesis of cytochromes, co-enzymes, and certain other enzymes such as catalase. Six serological types of *H. influenzae* can be distinguished. Type B is most frequently involved in hemophilus infections of children.

Laboratory Diagnosis. The microscopic finding of gram-negative pleomorphic bacteria can be of some significance with regard to choice of therapeutic drug: *H. influenzae* is penicillin resistant and so are most other gram-negative rods. Further bacteriological identification and typing of the organism is possible microscopically by capsular quellung reaction or by immunofluorescence with type-specific reference sera. When attempts are made to cultivate the organism, its requirements for growth factors must be taken into account.

Opportunistic Gram-negative Bacteria (Enterobacteriaceae and Others)

This general group of organisms includes a large variety of ubiquitous microbes, some of which regularly inhabit the human body, particularly the intestine but also the skin and the pharynx. As opportunistic pathogens they play an important role in every medical specialty, including otorhinolaryngology. *Escherichia coli* (the predominant member of the intestinal flora), Proteus, Klebsiella, Aerobacter, *Pseudomonas aeruginosa*, and others may be encountered in otitis, sinusitis, pneumonia, and meningitis. Klebsiella species are thought to cause, or at least to participate regularly in, conditions such as ozena and rhinoscleroma. Since these organisms are resistant to penicillin and many other antibiotics, they are often seen in hospital infections and in disorders which require prolonged antibiotic therapy. Genetic resistance transfer is common among these bacteria and involves also obligate pathogens (Salmonella, Shigella, and others).

Bacteriological Characterization. These gram-negative rods do not produce spores, but most of them possess flagella (except Klebsiella, and a few species or variants of other genera). Capsules are found regularly only in Klebsiella, Aerobacter, and some types of *Escherichia coli*. Identification is based partly on a variety of biochemical properties, e.g., degradation of sugars with development of gas and/or acidity. A characteristic blue-green pigment is produced and liberated into the medium by *Pseudomonas aeruginosa*. A serological breakdown of types within the genus Escherichia has been worked out similar to the procedure for the differentiation of Salmonella species.

Virulence Factors. If the organisms reach areas of the body which are normally free of bacteria, this usually results in highly purulent and stubborn inflammations. Local and systemic effects are caused by endotoxin, whereas exotoxins, as a rule, are not produced by these organisms.

Laboratory Diagnosis. Direct microscopic examination is of no value. However, cultivation is easy on routine media and selective indicator plates which are commonly used for examining fecal specimens. Growth may be so abundant that in cases of mixed infections with more fastidious bacteria the latter are rapidly outgrown and go undetected, although they might have been predominant in the original specimen. Even such organisms as staphylococci may lose ground beyond detection if overgrown by a swarming Proteus. Therefore, whenever isolation of these organisms is reported to the physician he has to evaluate such findings critically with the above viewpoints in mind.

Mycobacteria

Main diseases caused by mycobacteria are tuberculosis and leprosy. Both are encountered in otolaryngology. However, these manifestations are usually part of a systemic infection. Therefore, this group of organisms will be discussed here only briefly; the reader is referred to the appropriate literature.

Bacteriological Characterization. The organisms of this group are slender acid-fast rods. (Dyes penetrate only slowly, or when heated, through the cell wall and bind to the cytoplasmic membrane. Once the dye has been taken up it is retained despite washing in acid alcohol. Almost all other genera of bacteria are non-acid-fast.) *Mycobacterium tuberculosis* can be cultivated in special solid or fluid media. However, it usually takes several weeks before growth becomes visible. A very sensitive laboratory animal for diagnostic infection with *M. tuberculosis* is the guinea pig.

The demonstration of acid-fast organisms in clinical specimens of suspected tuberculosis permits only a presumptive diagnosis. Saprophytic mycobacteria must be excluded on the basis of cultural characteristics. However, certain saprophytic mycobacteria have been shown with increasing frequency to cause infections similar to tuberculosis.

Spirochetes

We distinguish three genera of human pathogenic spirochetes: Borrelia, Treponema, and Leptospira. Only the first two are of special interest to the otolaryngologist. In both genera we find saprophytic and pathogenic species. Saprophytic spirochetes live in natural waters. and also in the oral cavities of man and animals. Here they can become opportunistic pathogens like *B. vincenti* which causes Vincent's angina, stomatitis gangrenosa, and gangrenous processes in other parts of the respiratory tract. *Treponema pallidum*, the causative agent of syphilis, must be of interest to the otolaryngologist insofar as respiratory organs may be involved in any stage of syphilis.

Bacteriological Characterization. Treponema and Borrelia are distinguished mainly on morphological grounds, particularly when observed alive under the darkfield microscope. Their basic form is a three-dimensional coil wound around an axial filament. Treponema has eight to twenty-four rigid permanent coils and moves by bending and rotating back and forth. Borrelia is thicker and has four to eight coils which change position and size.

Pathogenic borreliae and treponemata cannot be cultivated on artificial media.

Borrelia vincenti, the opportunistic pathogen in the human oral cavity, lives in close symbiosis with so-called fusobacteria. These are slightly bent rods, pointed at the ends, that stain with varying intensity so that they appear striped transversely.

Virulence Factors. The basis of spirochetal virulence is not fully understood. Treponemata seem to possess endotoxins and to evoke strong hypersensitivity, which appears to be one of the decisive factors in the pathogenesis of syphilis. *Borrelia vincenti* is able to produce proteolytic enzymes which are supposedly responsible for gangrenous tissue necroses.

Laboratory Diagnosis. Laboratory diagnosis of Vincent's angina and other manifestations of infections with Borrelia and fusobacteria are limited to microscopic demonstration of the organisms involved. Since they are normally present in the oral cavity, the diagnosis of Vincent's angina hinges on the relative number of organisms seen in microscopic preparations.

Laboratory diagnosis of syphilis is twofold. Direct demonstration in the darkfield microscope of the living organism can be performed on exudate or tissue fluid of lesions during the primary or secondary stages. If the specimen is taken from the oral region, morphological distinction of *T. pallidum* from Borrelia can be crucial in avoiding misdiagnosis of Vincent's angina.

Serological diagnosis of syphilis is based on antibodies of various specificities. One type of antibody is directed against nonspecific lipid antigens (cardiolipin) and determined by complement fixation or flocculation reactions (e.g., VDRL). These tests are easily executed and inexpensive. The strength of the reaction (the antibody titer) closely parallels the course of the disease in that it drops in correlation to the effect of treatment and rises again preceding an imminent relapse. This prognostic advantage is somewhat offset by the fact that false positive reactions have been recorded in many nonsyphilitic diseases.

Other serological methods make use of specific treponemal antigens. These tests (treponemal immobilization, agglutination, immunofluorescence) are more expensive, since for antigen preparation the organism must be propagated by elaborate procedures, e.g., in rabbit testes. Results obtained with these tests are highly specific. However, once an antibody titer has developed, it will remain at a constant height for the rest of the patient's life.

Mycoplasma and Bacterial L-forms

Absence of a cell wall is characteristic for these organisms. Many bacteria may develop into L-forms under adverse conditions such as exposure to osmotic imbalance, humoral antibodies, or chemotherapeutic drugs. L-forms can revert back to their original bacterial form when normal environmental conditions have been restored. This phenomenon may explain the tendency of certain infectious diseases to relapse or to become chronic. L-forms of penicillin-susceptible bacteria are, in the absence of cell walls, no longer affected by this drug since penicillin inhibits cell wall synthesis. It is also important to realize that bacteriological examinations of clinical specimens may yield negative results if the causative organism is camouflaged as a temporary L-form.

Mycoplasma organisms are structurally very similar to L-forms. However, their origin from known bacterial forms is unlikely. No mycoplasma has ever been demonstrated to revert back to a complete bacterial form. Also, there are no antigenic relationships between mycoplasma and known bacteria in contrast to L-forms. Furthermore, the cytoplasmic membrane of mycoplasma is somewhat stronger against osmotic pressure than that of L-forms. This makes mycoplasma fitter for survival as a free living microbe despite the permanent absence of a cell wall.

Mycoplasma species are commonly found as saprophytes in all kinds of habitats, including the respiratory tract of man and animals. Several species have been confirmed as pathogens, among them *Mycoplasma pneumoniae*, which causes the Eaton type of atypical pneumonia in man.

Chapter 14

VIRAL DISEASE IN OTOLARYNGOLOGY

by Gilbert Schiff, M.D.

The number of otolaryngeal diseases for which viruses are responsible is indeed great. Mere consideration of the incidence of the common cold provides proof for the statement. Consider further the incidence of overall upper and lower respiratory diseases, and the role of viruses in this specialty becomes even more appreciated. Yet relatively little has been said about viral etiology in textbooks on otolaryngology in the past. The reasons for this state of affairs are probably the regard of virology more as a basic science, the reluctance of the physician to obtain a laboratory diagnosis, and the lack of specific treatments for viral disease.

Clinical virology has developed rapidly during the past decade. This has been accompanied by concomitant development of laboratory diagnostic facilities and antiviral drugs. Interest in learning the viral etiology of diseases in all specialties has been and will become intensified. Because of this, a chapter on viral disease in otolaryngology has been included in this textbook. The purpose of the chapter is to familiarize the student and the practitioner with virological principles and the various viruses or viral groups that cause the diseases they will study and treat. The initial portion of the chapter deals with background information on general virological considerations, including viral diagnosis and viral therapy. The remaining portion of the chapter discusses otolaryngeal viral diseases from the viewpoint of individual viruses or viral groups or clinical entities.

GENERAL CONSIDERATIONS

What Is a Virus?

Viruses are microorganisms consisting of genetic material (nucleic acids) surrounded by a protective protein or lipoprotein coat. They require living cells for successful self-replication. To accomplish this, viruses have achieved a parasitic status in relation to the living cells. The virus commandeers the reproductive apparatus of the living cell to produce the various parts of the virus and to assemble these parts into a mature virus. Viral replication can occur without obvious detrimental effects to the host cell; can increase host cell rate of reproduction as the virus itself reproduces; can transform host cells; or can divert the genetic reproductive pathways of the host cells so that quality host cell reproduction ceases, with ultimate cell death, while viral multiplication occurs. In addition, a lysogenous state can be created between virus and host cell in which host cells reproduce while the virus remains latent in the cell and in cell progeny.

There are animal, plant, and bacterial viruses. Every virus contains either RNA or DNA nucleic acids; never both. Viruses have been seen by electron microscopy and vary in size and shape. Viruses range in size from 15 to several hundred millimicrons in diameter. There are a number of systems for classifying viruses that are based on their physical, chemical, and biologic characteristics.

Viral Diagnosis

The diagnosis of viral disease requires laboratory assistance, except for a few diseases such as varicella, mumps, measles, and herpes zoster in which dependence on clinical diagnosis is reliable. A good general rule is that most human viruses are capable of producing a variety of clinical syndromes; and most viral-associated clinical syndromes can be caused by a multiplicity of viruses. Thus, coxsackie B viruses have been linked etiologically to aseptic meningitis, upper respiratory illness, lower respiratory illness, gastrointestinal illness, myocarditis, pericarditis, central nervous system disease, and subclinical infections; upper respiratory viral syndromes can be caused by enteroviruses (echoviruses, coxsackie A and B viruses, polioviruses), adenoviruses, rhinoviruses and myxoviruses.

The laboratory diagnosis of viral infection is made by detection of the virus or demonstration of a significant change in serum antibody titer to a particular virus. Viral detection is accomplished by use of tissue culture systems, embryonated eggs, or laboratory animals. In the sensitive tissue culture cell, egg, or animal the virus multiplies to a level at which host cell alteration occurs. In the tissue culture cell this is usually the production of a cytopathic effect (CPE) in the cell, which can be observed under the light microscope. Some viruses cause red blood cells to adhere to cells infected by the virus. This is called hemadsorption. In the egg the viral effects are localized growth in membranes, embryo death, or production of hemagglutinins in various fluids. Viral effects in animals are varied. These may be muscle paralysis, central nervous system (CNS) lesions, pancreatitis, hepatitis (as caused by coxsackie viruses); death (caused by many viruses); or keratitis (as caused by herpes simplex). Once a viral effect is detected, the offending agent is identified by "neutralization" of the effect with known type-specific antisera. Cell sensitivity to different viruses varies, so that the diagnostic laboratory must have available multiple "detection" systems to achieve a wide spectrum of viral diagnostic capability. Viruses can be isolated from many types of specimens collected from the patient: nasopharyngeal swabs or washes, aspirates of lesions (such as herpetic sores, chickenpox), conjunctival and keratitic scrapings, middle ear aspirates, blood, spinal fluid, stool, urine, tissue biopsies, and postmortem materials. Specimens should be collected as early as possible in the course of the infection. Collecting media and containers must be sterile and should be stored at −20 to −70° C (with some exceptions) until tested. The reader is referred to the numerous textbooks which detail the various aspects of specimen collection and viral detection.

Serological diagnosis is accomplished by the documentation of a significant (four-fold or greater) rise in the antibody titers between acute (collected early in the illness) and convalescent (two to three weeks later) serum specimens. The antibody levels are measured by neutralization, hemadsorption inhibition, hemagglutination inhibition, complement fixation, or immunofluorescent antibody techniques.

It can be appreciated that definitive laboratory diagnosis of viral infection involves a relatively complex and expensive operation. For these reasons, availability of viral diagnostic services are scarce, or so inefficient that test results are reported long (if at all) after submission of specimens, so that practical assistance to the physician becomes negligible. At most, the physician has become accustomed to making a diagnosis of "viral disease," depending on certain laboratory events such as leukopenia, or absence of leukocytosis, and a negative bacterial culture report. Exact diagnosis of viral etiology is regarded as an academic exercise or, at best, of "public health" importance. However, two facts should be emphasized: practical ("helpful") viral diagnosis can be accomplished; and exact viral diagnosis will become a necessity within the next several years as antiviral chemotherapy becomes a reality.

Therapy of Viral Infections

Current treatment of viral infections primarily involves active and passive immunoprophylaxis. Table 1 lists the current status of vaccines developed for the prophylactic treatment of viral infections associated with otolaryngeal disease.

Live, attenuated adenovirus vaccines have been developed utilizing selected strains which cause morbidity in military recruits and result in subsequent economic loss. The vaccines appear to be effective, but it has been shown that suppression of certain strains of endemic adenoviral infection among military populations is accompanied by increased incidence of other adenoviral strain infections which apparently fill the ecological void created by mass vaccination. In addition, the proved oncogenic association of certain adenovirus strains has been a detriment to the development of a polyvalent adenovirus vaccine for general use.

TABLE 1

VACCINE	TYPE	REMARKS
Adenovirus	Live, attenuated	Used by military only; contains a limited number of strains
Influenza	Killed, egg-grown	Effective if vaccine contains contemporary or prevalent strains of influenza viruses
Mumps	Live, attenuated	Duration of immunity unknown
Rubeola	Live, attenuated	"Further" attenuated vaccines superior
Rubella	Live, attenuated	Duration of immunity unknown
Para-influenza	Killed or live, attenuated	Experimental status
Respiratory-syncytial	Killed or live, attenuated	Experimental status

Influenza Vaccines. Influenza vaccines are in general use. Although the overall effectiveness of the vaccines is controversial, there are certain factors which correlate directly with their effectiveness. The influenza virus types (A and B) have a tendency to periodically change their antigenic configuration, so that essentially new viruses evolve. This evolution results in a generally unprotected population, as immunity developed from previous experience with influenzal infection or vaccination becomes ineffective against the newer antigenic strains. Therefore, to be effective, influenza vaccine preparations must contain the prevalent, or contemporary, strains of influenza virus. Type A influenza viruses undergo major antigenic shifts approximately every ten years, i.e., 1947, 1957, and 1968. Another factor is the amount of antigenic mass contained in a vaccine. Antibody response and, hence, protection varies directly with the amount of antigenic mass of a particular strain of vaccine. Since total antigenic mass is also directly proportional to degree of reactions to or side effects of influenza vaccination, a limit to the antigenic mass has been placed on vaccine preparations. If an influenza vaccine contains more than one strain of influenza virus (bivalent, polyvalent) the antigenic mass for the individual strains is reduced.

Reactions to influenza vaccines are relatively frequent and, in themsevles, result in considerable morbidity. Reactions include discomfort at the site of vaccination as well as constitutional signs and symptoms (fever, myalgia, malaise). Reactions are usually due to the impurities in the vaccine preparations. Newer methods for production of influenza vaccines have partially solved this problem.

Initial vaccination with a particular strain of influenza virus should include two inoculations one month apart to achieve adequate levels of circulating antibody. Frequent (annual) booster shots are required to maintain the desirable levels of circulating antibody.

Recently the intranasal administration of influenza vaccination has been advocated by some investigators. They rationalize that this procedure results in a greater production of "local" or respiratory tract antibody (secretory IgA immunoglobulin). The local antibody is more effective in preventing influenza, which is primarily a respiratory tract infection.

Mumps Vaccine. Mumps vaccine is a live, attenuated vaccine produced in embryonated chick tissue culture. Significant levels of serum antibody develop in over 95 per cent of mumps-susceptible children and adults who receive a single 0.5 ml. subcutaneous dose of vaccine. Very few side effects or untoward reactions to the vaccine have been reported. Because the duration of vaccine-induced immunity to mumps has not been determined, it is felt by some that mumps vaccination should be reserved for only those children approaching puberty who have no clinical and/or laboratory evidence of prior mumps infection. In this way, natural lifelong immunity acquired during childhood will not be altered by artificially-induced immunity which might disappear post puberty. Others feel that avoidance of mumps infection and its complications during childhood justifies vaccination. Determination of the duration and effectiveness of mumps vaccination lies in the future.

Rubeola Vaccine. Rubeola (measles) vaccination has benefited from a decade or so of experience. Initial confusion about immunizing schedules has disappeared. The early recommendations for multiple inactivated vaccines, or inactivated vaccine followed by live, attenuated vaccine, or live vaccine with simultaneous administration of gamma globulin have given way to advocacy of a single inoculation with "further" attenuated rubeola vaccine strains. Morbidity associated with rubeola vaccination has also decreased. Communitywide inoculation programs accompanied by routine rubeola inoculation in well-baby care clinics and private physicians' offices have resulted in dramatic reduction in the incidence of rubeola.

Rubella Vaccines. Rubella vaccines have recently been developed. The rubella vaccines are live, attenuated preparations which are highly effective stimulations of serum antibody when administered in a single subcutaneous 0.5 ml. dose. Vaccination is accompanied by little illness and few side effects in children, although care should be exerted if known allergies to vaccine-containing materials are known (eggs, dog dander, rabbit fur, neomycin). Determination of the duration of vaccine-induced immunity awaits the future, although preliminary studies indicate that it will be long lasting.

Because of potential teratogenicity of the vaccines themselves, the vaccines should not be given to a pregnant female. A nonpregnant woman who needs the vaccine should delay any comtemplated pregnancy until at least eight weeks after vaccination. Careful vaccination of postpubertal women who have been shown to lack rubella immunity, and are on an effective contraception program, is possible. However, temporary arthralgia or arthritis occurs in a significant percentage.

Para-influenza and Respiratory-syncytial Vaccines. Experimental vaccines, both inactivated and live, have been developed for the para-influenza and respiratory-syncytial viruses. In general, these vaccines have been disappointing in that they are either poor antigens or are associated with serious hypersensitivity phenomena.

Immunoprophylaxis. Passive immunoprophylaxis has limited application in the prevention of the viral infections and complications seen by the otolaryngologist. Use of immune globulin in association with rubeola infection has been mostly supplanted by effective rubeola vaccination. Even in children exposed to rubeola, vaccine can be effective. However, in the case of the chronically ill individual, or perhaps the pregnant woman, postexposure administration of immune globulin preparations can ameliorate or completely prevent the infection, depending on the promptness and the size of dose. Use of hyperimmune globulin in the adult exposed to mumps is effective in reducing some of the complications (orchitis, oophoritis).

More controversial is the role of immune globulin in the pregnant woman exposed to rubella. Several factors are undoubtedly responsible for the conflicting reports on immune globulin effectiveness against rubella. These factors include immune status of the woman, dosage of immunoglobulin used, time of administration of the immune globulin in relation to time of viral exposure, and correct diagnosis of rubella. Immune globulin can convert clinical rubella to subclinical rubella. Such a situation is not sufficient to avoid congenital rubella. It is felt by some that large doses (20 ml.) of a high-titered immunoglobulin preparation given within six days of exposure to rubella virus is effective in preventing subsequent rubella viremia.

There are some types of viral infections in which prevention of infection by immunoprophylaxis is impractical. Hence, an effective "common cold" virus vaccine would have to include over a hundred strains of virus. In addition, some viral infections occur in the presence of circulating antibody, i.e., recurrent herpes, cytomegalic inclusion disease virus. Stimulation of antibody production or administration of gamma globulin to prevent these infections would appear worthless. The need for chemotherapeutic agents for some viral infections is obvious.

Chemotherapy. Viral chemoprophylaxis and chemotherapy are in the embryonic stage of development. Although there are many compounds shown to be effective in vitro or in animals, there is a paucity of compounds approved for human use or in the human evaluation stage. Methasone has been shown to be effective against smallpox and vaccine reactions. Antimetabolites such as 5-idoxuridine (5-IDU, Stoxil) and cytosine arabinoside have been shown to be effective against herpes keratitis, and are questionably effective against herpes encephalitis. Amantadine hydrochloride (Symmetrel) is effective prophylactically against several strains of influenza A-2. Despite the limited experience with antiviral drugs, several things have become evident. The compounds have disappointingly narrow antiviral spectra, viral resistance will become a problem, and the drugs are relatively toxic.

A promising approach to effective antiviral treatment involves the role of interferon and interferonlike substances. Interferon is a protein with antiviral activity which is liberated or synthesized by cells following multiple types of cell injury, including viral infection. The antiviral activity is relatively nonspecific and covers a wide spectrum. Attempts to develop practical methods to supply exogenous or induce endogenous interferon to the site of viral infection have encountered numerous problems, primarily toxicity. However, many feel that interferon will prove to be the panacea of viral infection.

THE VIRUSES AND CLINICAL ENTITIES

This portion of the chapter has been divided into consideration of viral diseases of the oral cavity, ear, and respiratory system. It must be kept in mind that there is much overlapping and that the division is quite arbitrary.

Viruses Causing Disease of the Oral Cavity and Oropharynx

Viruses mentioned in this category include the coxsackie A, herpes, infectious mononucleosis, and mumps viruses. Additional viruses which primarily cause acute pharyngitis are discussed under the respiratory virus section.

Coxsackie A Virus

Several strains of coxsackie A viruses have been associated with lesions of the oral cavity and oropharynx. The coxsackie A viruses are members of the picornavirus family; hence, they are small and contain an RNA nucleic acid. They have a striking pathogenicity for newborn mice and hamsters, which is used to distinguish them from coxsackie B viruses. There are at least 23 immunologically distinct coxsackie A types. The coxsackie A viruses have been shown to cause aseptic meningitis, paralysis, exanthems, hepatitis, and respiratory disease.

Nine strains of coxsackie A viruses have been implicated as the etiological agents for herpangina; the strains are types 1, 2, 3, 4, 5, 6, 8, 10, and 22. Herpangina is a clinical syndrome which occurs in the summer season and mainly affects children. The illness is featured by an acute onset of fever, sore throat, and dysphagia, sometimes accompanied by abdominal pain, myalgia, headache, and vomiting. The characteristic feature of the syndrome is the presence of small scattered vesicles in the oropharynx, each surrounded by an erythematous zone. They are commonly located on the anterior pillars of the fauces, but can also occur on the palate, uvula, tonsils, and tongue. They do not occur on the gingival or buccal mucosa. The individual lesion appears first as a grayish white papule or vesicle about 1 to 2 mm. in diameter and surrounded by a red areola. Within several days the areola becomes more intensely red and the vesicles enlarge and become shallow grayish ulcers. Both vesicles and ulcers may be present at the same time. Usually there are four to five lesions, but as many as 14 have been seen. The course of the illness is usually benign. There have been reports of parotitis complicating herpangina.

Coxsackie A-10 has been associated with an epidemic of acute lymphonodular pharyngitis in children. The patients had fever, headache, and sore throat from four to 14 days. The distinct lesions were discrete whitish or yellowish nodular papules on the uvula, anterior pillars, and posterior pharynx which did not vesicate. Histological examination of the nodules revealed the papules to be formed of tightly packed lymphocytes.

Coxsackie A-16 virus has been associated with hand-foot-and-mouth disease. The illness runs a febrile course, with oral blisters and a maculopapular rash of the hands and feet which progresses to vesicles.

The laboratory diagnosis of coxsackie A virus disease involves the inoculation of suckling mice, which subsequently suffer paralysis. Mice are also utilized for neutralization tests for antibody. There is no specific treatment for coxsackie A disease.

Herpesvirus Infections (Herpes Simplex)

Herpesvirus infections are very common and widely disseminated. The herpes simplex virus is a DNA-containing virus of 100 to 200 $m\mu$ in size. Cells infected by the herpes virus contain intranuclear, eosinophilic inclusion bodies and assume a multinucleated, giant-cell appearance. The cytoplasm of infected cells becomes edematous and produces a ballooning degeneration. Intercellular edema occurs among adjacent infected cells, with fluid accumulation and development of a vesicle. Lesions occurring on mucous membranes usually present as shallow ulcers. The superficial epithelium collapses and sloughs.

An unusual "life cycle" of human infection

by herpes simplex virus exists. Infection is presumably spread by intimate contact. A susceptible host, without antibodies, reacts by developing a primary infection, which 99 per cent of the time is inapparent. When the primary infection takes an overt form, several types of clinical syndromes may result. These syndromes include acute herpetic gingivostomatitis, acute herpetic oculovaginitis, eczema herpeticum (Kaposi's varicelliform eruption), traumatic herpes infections, acute herpetic keratoconjunctivitis, and acute herpetic infection. Primary infection usually occurs in infants and preschoolers, although it can occur later in life. Following primary infection, antibodies develop which persist for life. The virus apparently persists in a latent stage. A number of excitants, such as fever, ultraviolet irradiation, trauma, other infections, menstruation, and psychic or psychological upsets may subsequently provoke a recurrent infection which is characterized by an overt lesion and a boost in antibody level, followed by a return to the latent stage.

The commonest primary infection is acute herpetic gingivostomatitis. The onset is abrupt, with high fever, irritability, anorexia, and lesions of the oropharynx. The gums become swollen, reddened and friable and bleed easily. White plaques or shallow ulcers 2 to 3 mm. in diameter, surrounded by red areolae, appear on the buccal mucosa, tongue, palate, and fauces, usually in that order. A regional, tender anterior cervical lymphadenopathy occurs. The disease may be mild or very severe. Severe cases can be accompanied by dehydration and electrolyte imbalance caused by the child's reluctance to eat or drink. The duration of the illness varies from five to 14 days. In herpetic vulvovaginitis, the lesions appear in the genital area.

Primary infection may take the form of eczema herpeticum or Kaposi's varicelliform eruption. Eczema herpeticum is characterized by the abrupt onset of high fever, irritability, and restlessness, followed by the appearance of vesicular or crusting eruptions superimposed on the site of atopic eczema or chronic dermatitis. The lesions may appear over the course of a week. Soon after they appear, the lesions rupture and become crusted. After the crusts fall off, the eczematous skin remains. The duration of the constitutional symptoms may be up to two weeks. The disease varies in severity, at times assuming a rapidly fatal course. Frequently superinfection with bacteria occurs in the area of the oozing and crusted

skin. Traumatic herpetic infections of the skin are similar to eczema herpeticum, except that the lesions are restricted to the area of previous burn, abrasion, and laceration.

Rarely the primary herpes infection occurs as an acute herpetic keratoconjunctivitis or as an acute meningoencephalitis. In the former there are fever and constitutional symptoms accompanied by a unilateral keratoconjunctivitis and preauricular adenopathy. The cornea assumes a hazy appearance, with formation of typical dendritic ulcers. Deeper involvement of the cornea and iris may follow, with residual sight impairment. The conjunctiva becomes reddened and edematous, with a purulent exudate. The eyelid becomes swollen shut. The surrounding skin may be the site of discrete vesicles. Acute herpetic meningoencephalitis may produce a relatively mild aseptic meningitis or a rapidly fatal encephalitis. The patient develops fever, headache, lethargy, and convulsions. The spinal fluid shows a pleocytosis with a predominance of lymphocytes.

Disseminated visceral herpetic infection occurs in premature or newborn infants. During the first week of life the infants develop fever or hypothermia, progressive icterus, hepatosplenomegaly, vomiting, lethargy, respiratory distress, cyanosis, and shock. Death invariably results. Disseminated visceral herpetic infection has also been seen with increasing frequency in adult patients on immunosuppressive medications.

Recurrent herpetic infections are very common. The most common lesion is the well known fever blister or herpes labialis, although the recurrent lesions may appear elsewhere on the skin or mucous membranes. Recurrent herpes lesions are usually not accompanied by any constitutional symptoms or signs.

The diagnosis of herpes simplex infection can be confirmed in the laboratory by isolation of the virus from a primary or recurrent lesion and by detection of a rise in serum antibody level. Herpesvirus isolation is achieved by the inoculation of infected material into the scarified cornea of a rabbit, into the chorioallantoic membrane of the chick embryo, or into a variety of primary or continuous tissue culture cell lines. The cornea of the rabbit will become the site of a keratoconjunctivitis; in embryonated eggs the chorioallantoic membrane will become the site of small oval plaques; in tissue culture a cytopathic effect occurs rapidly in which the cells become multinucleated giant cells containing intranuclear, eosinophilic inclusion bodies. Serological diagnosis is accomplished by use of paired samples of acute and convalescent sera tested for a change in neutralizing or complement-fixing antibodies.

The treatment of herpetic infections is primarily supportive. Appropriate antibiotic therapy for secondarily infected lesions is used. Topical 5-iodo-2-deoxyuridine (5-IDU) is effective in the treatment of herpes keratitis. Use of systemic 5-IDU in cases of herpes encephalitis has reportedly been effective.

Infectious Mononucleosis

Infectious mononucleosis (IM) is an acute infectious disease of presumed viral etiology which occurs predominantly in children and young adults. The search for the viral etiology of IM had been one of disappointment and frustration. It now appears that IM is closely associated with the Epstein-Barr (EB) virus. The EB virus is a member of the herpes group and was first detected in cultures of Burkitt's lymphoma cells. The association of the virus with IM is based on a serological relationship. Individuals with IM develop antibody to EB virus in their serum.

The incubation period for IM has been estimated to range from several days to two weeks. The disease varies in severity and duration, being generally mild in children and more severe and protracted in adults. The disease is characterized by fever, exudative or membranous pharyngitis, generalized lymphadenopathy, splenomegaly, a peripheral blood picture with an increase in atypical lymphocytes, and the development of a high titer of heterophil antibody in the serum. The disease may begin abruptly or insidiously, with headache, fever chills, anorexia, and malaise followed by lymphadenopathy and severe sore throat. The fever rises to 103 to 105° F. and gradually falls by lysis over a period of a week or more. The lymph nodes enlarge rapidly to a variable size, are tender, tense, discrete, and firm to the touch. Any chain of lymph nodes may become involved, although the cervical groups are usually included. The adenopathy remains for weeks. In approximately 50 per cent of the patients there is a detectable splenomegaly. Occasionally the splenic enlargement may be followed by spontaneous rupture resulting in hemorrhage, shock, and death if not promptly recognized. A cardinal symptom of the disease is the sore throat. The tonsils become enlarged and reddened, with or without exudate. Thick, white membranous tonsillitis occurs commonly. The membrane gradually peels off after a week or so. Petechiae are often seen on the palate.

Other clinical manifestations which might occur include hepatitis, an erythematous maculopapular eruption, pneumonitis similar to atypical pneumonia, and central nervous system involvement. In the latter, the neurologic findings may present as an aseptic meningitis, encephalitis, or infectious polyneuritis.

The diagnosis of IM is made on the basis of the clinical factors, a typical peripheral blood picture, the development of a positive heterophil agglutination titer, or a rise in EB virus antibody. The peripheral blood picture characteristically contains an absolute increase in the number of atypical lymphocytes during some stages of the disease. The white blood count is variable. A leukopenia may occur during the first week of the disease, but most commonly there is a leukocytosis with a predominance of lymphocytes. Frequently the diagnosis is confused with leukemia. Anemia is rare, and occasionally a thrombocytopenia may complicate the illness.

During the course of IM, patients develop positive heterophil antibodies in the serum. The heterophil usually becomes positive by the end of the first week of the disease, peaks within three weeks, and falls off at variable rates. Occasionally there is a delay of two weeks in the development of a positive heterophil antibody test. Newer slide agglutination test kits have simplified the test for IM serology.

Treatment for infectious mononucleosis is chiefly supportive. Steroids have been used in severe cases with beneficial effects. The most serious complication is rupture of the spleen; this requires immediate surgery.

Mumps Virus

The mumps virus is the commonest cause of viral infection of the salivary glands. Although it usually affects the parotids, the other salivary glands may be involved with mumps virus infection. The mumps virus is a myxovirus containing a nuclear protein core of RNA surrounded by a lipoprotein envelope with numerous spikelike projections, is 90 to 135 mμ in size, has only one serotype, and has an antigenic relationship to other members of the myxovirus family, including Newcastle disease virus and para-influenza viruses. Infection with the mumps virus is followed by formation of complement-fixing antibodies and a delayed hypersensitivity state in the skin of humans. The former is the basis for a serological diagnostic test; the latter, for a skin test to measure immunity for mumps infection. Mumps is an endemic disease in most urban populations, occurring most commonly in the five- to ten-year age group. There is a higher incidence of mumps during the winter and spring, but cases occur on a year-round basis. The source of infection is the saliva or other secretions of an infected person spread by direct contact or by droplet.

Mumps infection is acquired via the oropharynx, with subsequent proliferation of the virus in the parotid gland and/or the respiratory epithelium. This followed by a viremia and localization of virus in the glandular or nervous tissue.

The incubation period is 16 to 18 days. In approximately 30 to 49 per cent of the patients the infection is subclinical. In the majority of the remaining 60 to 70 per cent of patients clinical mumps is characterized only by a uni- or bilateral, painful parotitis. Classically, fever, headache, anorexia, malaise, and "earache" precede the enlargement of the parotids by 24 hours. The parotids enlarge over a period of three days to maximum size and then gradually decrease over a period of seven days. Usually one parotid enlarges a few days earlier than the second. Unilateral parotitis occurs in approximately 25 per cent of the patients. The skin over the enlarged glands is tense, and frequently the orifice to Stensen's duct is inflamed. Submaxillary and sublingual swellings may also occur with or without parotid enlargement. With extensive salivary gland enlargement, presternal edema develops as a result of obstructed lymphatics.

The mumps virus may cause orchitis, meningoencephalitis, or pancreatitis with or without salivary gland involvement. Unilateral orchitis occurs in 20 to 30 per cent of postpubertal males who develop mumps infection. Bilateral orchitis occurs in 2 per cent of postpubertal males. The orchitis usually develops during the first week of infection. It rarely is the cause of sexual impotence or sterility. Mumps meningoencephalitis occurs in about 10 per cent of all patients. It usually follows the parotitis by three to ten days, although it may precede or occur in the absence of the parotitis. There are typical signs and symptoms along with pleocytosis and elevated proteins in the spinal fluid. The course is usually benign, with no sequelae. Pancreatitis is uncommon but is severe when it occurs. Oophoritis, thyroiditis, and mastitis occur but are quite rare. There has been some association between mumps during pregnancy and fetal abnormalities; there is strong evidence that endocardial fibroelastosis may be so induced.

A serious but rare complication of mumps is deafness. There is usually a sudden onset of vertigo, tinnitus, ataxia, and vomiting followed by permanent deafness. The cause is probably auditory nerve neuritis. Other complications are postinfectious encephalitis, facial neuritis, trigeminal neuritis, arthritis, hepatitis, and myocarditis.

The diagnosis of mumps can usually be made on clinical grounds. Occasionally laboratory confirmation is required, especially in adults. Mumps virus can be recovered from mouth washings, saliva, and urine for a period ranging from several days before onset of symptoms to two weeks after onset. The greatest incidence of viral recovery occurs in specimens collected within the first five days of illness. The specimens are inoculated into HeLa cells or rhesus monkey kidney cells and observed for cytopathic effect or positive hemadsorption effect, respectively. More practical than viral isolation is serologic diagnosis. The test of choice is the complement-fixing antibody test. As with most serologic tests, a definite diagnosis can be made only when a significant rise in antibody titer is demonstrated by the examination of paired specimens of serum taken at appropriate intervals (two weeks or more apart) following the onset of disease.

Elevated serum amylases have been found in most cases of mumps in which parotitis occurs, in addition to cases of mumps pancreatitis. Serum amylase determination is a worthwhile ancillary diagnostic test.

Contrary to common belief, recurrent mumps infection is uncommon, estimated to be 4 per cent. Inapparent infection and unilateral parotid infection provide as solid immunity as bilateral parotid infection. Confusion over reinfection probably reflects missed diagnosis of parotitis. Immunity can be determined by testing for the presence of complement-fixing antibody or by positive skin test. It becomes desirable to determine immune status of adults (usually after exposure to their infected children) because of the possible occurrence of orchitis. Reliance on past history is unreliable because of the frequency of inapparent infection. Of the two tests for immunity, the assay for complement-fixing antibody is the most reliable.

The treatment for active mumps infection is usually entirely supportive. In cases of mumps orchitis, surgical intervention is sometimes required to relieve pressure. Use of hyperimmune gamma globulin has been effective in reducing the incidence of orchitis but not in prevention of mumps infection. Inactivated mumps vaccines proved to be poor antigens and have been discarded. There is now available an effective live, attenuated mumps vaccine. There has been some reluctance to use the live vaccine routinely until more information on duration of immunity is obtained. The vaccine should be used in children about to enter puberty who have not had mumps and in susceptible adults.

Coxsackie B viruses have been associated with salivary gland disease. They are discussed under the section on respiratory viruses.

Viral Infections of the Ear

Acute middle ear disease caused by viruses is most often an extension of inflammation from the nasopharynx. Therefore, the viruses implicated are those which cause respiratory tract disease (see section on viral respiratory diseases). In addition, otitis media is frequently encountered during measles and mumps. Two viruses are discussed in detail in this section: herpes zoster and rubella.

Herpes Zoster Virus

Herpes zoster virus is the cause of herpetic or vesicular eruption in the external auditory canal and on the auricle. This is called Ramsay Hunt's disease and involves viral infection of the geniculate ganglion of the facial nerve with paralysis. The virus which causes herpes zoster also causes chickenpox, or varicella, and is referred to as the V-Z virus. It is a member of the herpesvirus family, a DNA-containing virus 200 mμ in size, and causes a typical cytopathology in human fibroblastic tissue culture cells. In herpes zoster infections there is an eruption, usually to one or more dermatomes, corresponding to involved dorsal root or extramedullary cranial nerve ganglia. The eruption consists initially of erythematous maculopapules, which develop into vesicles. The vesicles become pustular and crust; ulcers may form. The lesions are painful and pruritic. Regional lymphadenopathy occurs. There may be some constitutional symptoms. The lesions remain from one to several weeks. The most commonly involved of the cranial nerves is the trigeminal, especially its ophthalmic division. Lesions appear on the upper third of the head unilaterally, with a keratoconjunctivitis. With cranial nerve involvement there is frequently paralysis.

Laboratory diagnosis of herpes zoster infection is accomplished by isolation of the virus from fresh vesicles. The specimens are inoculated into human fibroblastic tissue cultures with subsequent development of foci of cytopathology of the cells. Serologic diagnosis is accomplished by testing paired serum specimens for a rise in complement-fixing antibody titer.

There is no specific treatment for herpes zoster infection.

Hearing loss can result from viral-caused otitis media or from central nervous system lesions which occur during the course of viral encephalitis. Hearing loss is frequently associated with mumps and measles, and is also a complication of respiratory tract viral illness caused by any of numerous viruses.

Congenital Rubella

Rubella virus has tentatively been assigned to the myxovirus group of viruses, primarily because of its electron microscopic appearance. Rubella virus is medium in size, contains RNA nucleic acid, and causes hemagglutination of various fowl species red blood cells.

Acquired or noncongenital rubella is a childhood disease highlighted by a three-day maculopapular rash, cervical (usually pre- or postauricular) lymphadenopathy and low-grade fever. There is frequently a slightly injected pharynx and a fleeting enanthem consisting of Forschheimer spots on the palate. Rubella occurs 50 per cent of the time without the rash, and the combination of pharyngitis and prominent lymphadenopathy due to rubella is frequently presented to the otolaryngologist.

The most frequent involvement of the otolaryngologist with rubella is because of hearing deficiencies caused by congenital or intrauterine rubella infection. The existence of congenital rubella was first pointed out by Gregg in 1941. There have been many investigations into this problem in an effort to determine its scope, to define the teratogenic mechanisms, and to devise methods of prevention. The development of laboratory methods for rubella in 1962 and the occurrence of a widespread epidemic of rubella in 1964-1965 provided much new information about congenital rubella. The risk to a woman of giving birth to an infant with significant defects varies with the time in the gestational period when infection occurs: first month's gestation, 50 per cent; second month's gestation, 20 per cent; and third month's gestation, 4 per cent. Overall risk for the first trimester is about 18 per cent. There has been some evidence for the association of congenital birth lesions with maternal rubella which occurred past the first trimester.

The pathogenic mechanisms have not been fully elucidated. Rubella virus has been shown to invade the fetus and to be widely disseminated in the fetal tissues. Invasion, dissemination, and effect in the fetus appear to depend on the time in gestation of viral infection. Chronic infection follows viral invasion of the fetus, so that effects are not restricted to the exact time of the teratogenic insult. Fetal damage may reflect direct cellular damage by the virus, hypersensitivity effect, or compromised blood supply caused by viral invasion of endothelial vascular tissue. The presence of the virus in fetal tissue has been shown to exert an inhibition or multiplication of certain human cells.

Intrauterine rubella infection may result in a wide spectrum of clinical manifestations. Spontaneous abortion, stillbirth, live birth with single or multiple anomalies, or subclinical infection may result from rubella in utero. Rubella viruses have been recovered from virtually every organ.

The hearing loss resulting from congenital rubella infection may be severe or mild, unilateral or bilateral, but it is permanent. Inflammatory changes in the vascular stria and degenerative changes in the cochlear duct and organ of Corti are probably the commonest causes of deafness. Defects in the middle ear have also been reported. Central nervous system lesions may also play a role in hearing loss. At times deafness may be the only manifestation of congenital rubella, especially if maternal infection occurs after the first eight weeks of pregnancy. Vestibular dysfunction frequently occurs, as determined by water caloric testing.

Other congenital rubella affections include neonatal disorders, which are more or less self-limited, and permanent anomalies. The former include thrombocytopenic purpura, hemolytic anemia, bone lesions, hepatosplenomegaly, hepatitis, pneumonitis, myocarditis, and meningoencephalitis; the latter include cardiovascular anomalies, eye defects, neurological defects, and mental retardation.

The diagnosis of acquired and congenital rubella may be made in the laboratory by isolation of the virus and serological tests. Isolation of the virus can be accomplished by tissue culture systems using monkey kidney or rabbit kidney cells. The patient with acquired rubella sheds the virus in the nasopharynx for a period of three weeks, bracketing the time of overt symptoms. Serological diagnosis is best done by the hemagglutination-inhibition antibody test, documenting a rise in antibody titer in acute and convalescent serum specimens.

The recent development of several live, attenuated rubella vaccines has provided an optimistic forecast toward the eventual eradication of rubella.

Viral Respiratory Diseases

Although exact data are difficult to obtain, it is generally agreed by most authorities that acute respiratory disease is the greatest cause of morbidity in the United States. Surveys conducted by the National Health Survey in the United States and England indicate that citizens experienced three to six acute respiratory infections annually, which result in three and a half days of restricted activity per illness per person. Economically, acute viral respiratory illnesses account for millions of dollars for medications and in wasted work days.

Viral respiratory illnesses are caused by several groups of viruses. The viruses produce a variety of clinical syndromes; any individual virus group is capable of causing a multiplicity of syndromes, and a particular syndrome can be caused by various groups of viruses.

There appears to be a difference in the morbidity caused by some of these viruses between children and adults; children are apt to develop more severe disease than adults. This phenomenon is probably the result of acquired immunity, which is present by adulthood.

The diagnosis of viral etiology of the respiratory disease most often is wholly dependent on the laboratory.

In this section several viruses or viral groups are discussed separately. But once again the reader is reminded to consider the great degree of overlap which exists.

Adenoviruses

The adenoviruses were first isolated by Rowe and co-workers in 1953 by culturing adenoid tissue from children undergoing adenoidectomy. There are now 31 immunologically distinct adenoviruses of human origin, nine of which have been associated with respiratory infections. Synonyms are adenoid degeneration (AD) agents, acute respiratory disease (ARD) viruses, and adenoidal-pharyngeal-conjunctival (APC) viruses. The adenoviruses are DNA viruses, 70-90 mμ in diameter, which grow in a variety of tissue culture cell lines. For the isolation of the virus, primary human embryonic kidney cells are preferred. The cytopathogenic effect produced in tissue culture cells by adenoviruses is typical and consists of marked rounding and clumping of cells. Serological diagnosis of adenoviral infection is performed by use of the complement fixation and hemagglutination-inhibition antibody assays.

The clinical syndromes associated with adenovirus infections include undifferentiated acute respiratory disease, pharyngoconjunctival fever pharyngitis, and pneumonia. In undifferentiated acute respiratory disease clinical signs include sore throat, pharyngitis, cervical lymphadenopathy, cough, chills, malaise, and headache. Coryza and fever may be present. In pharyngoconjunctival fever pharyngitis, fever, conjunctivitis and, frequently, gastrointestinal pain occur. In pharyngitis there is febrile pharyngitis. Pneumonia or severe lower respiratory tract involvement occasionally occurs.

There are several interesting features associated with adenoviral infections. Some types (types 4 and 7) are almost solely restricted to military groups, differing from the types responsible for civilian population disease. Children under four years of age tend to have more severe illnesses. Seasonal variation occurs. Pharyngoconjunctival fever occurs during the summer and is associated with irritation to the conjunctiva by swimming. However, the highest incidence of overall adenovirus infection occurs during the winter and spring. It is generally thought that adenoviruses account for 2 to 6 per cent of all respiratory viral disease.

Adenoviruses are of particular concern to the military as an economic and logistic problem in recruit populations. This has prompted the development of vaccines against the types prevalent in the military populations. The vaccines have shown some effectiveness but, because of the oncogenic properties of some adenovirus types, general use has not received widespread support.

Influenza Viruses

Influenza viruses have had a profound effect on mankind. Pandemics of influenza have taken severe tolls in morbidity and mortality throughout history. The severest pandemic occurred in 1918-1919 and is thought to have been responsible for over 20,000,000 deaths. Alteration in the antigenic makeup of influenza viruses has resulted in pandemics approximately every 10 years for the last 30 years.

The influenza viruses are members of the myxovirus family. The viruses have a nucleoprotein core surrounded by a lipoprotein envelope and numerous spikelike projections. The inner core contains RNA as the nucleic acid. The viruses are medium size (100 to 150 mμ), are ether sensitive, and will agglutinate erythrocytes from several species.

The influenza viruses are divided into three types, A, B, and C, on the basis of the presence of a common soluble antigen associated with the inner core. Each type is further divided into subtypes, which are assigned numbers. Hence, there are subtypes A^0, A^1, A^2, B^0, B^1, B^2, etc. The subtypes differ from each other by the antigenic makeup of their lipoprotein envelope. It is the seemingly continuous shifting in the antigenic configuration of the viruses that creates "new" viruses to which the population has no antibody or immunity, resulting in new pandemics of influenza.

Influenza viruses can cause a wide spectrum of respiratory tract disease, ranging from subclinical infection to fulminating pneumonia. Influenza viruses have caused diseases featuring predominantly croup, bronchitis, or bronchiolitis in children and adults. However, the typical case of influenza, which is familiar to all physicians, is characterized by respiratory tract involvement accompanied by systemic symptoms. After a short incubation period of one to three days, coryza, cough, sore throat, headache, fever, malaise, anorexia, and frequently nausea and vomiting occur, accompanied by an apathetic appearance. Abnormal physical findings and laboratory studies are usually rare. The illness persists for a week to ten days and is usually followed by a prolonged period of convalescence in which the patient is somewhat lethargic or "not up to par." Pneumonia, either purely viral or caused by a secondary bacterial invader, or of mixed viral and bacterial etiology, is the commonest complication but in itself occurs less than 10 per cent of the time. Other complications are meningoencephalitis and myocarditis, but both are quite rare.

There appears to be no difference between the clinical syndromes caused by types A and B, but there is considerable variation in the severity of "virulence" of the influenza virus strains. Type C disease is relatively uncommon.

There are definitely high-risk groups in which influenza complications are likely to develop. These high-risk groups include individuals with known cardiovascular or chronic pulmonary disease, young infants, individuals on immunosuppressive drugs, and diabetics. In certain influenza epidemics, increased morbidity and mortality have occurred among pregnant women. Efforts should be exerted to provide protection to the high-risk groups during outbreaks or impending outbreaks of influenza.

Immunity of varying degree follows active influenza infection or vaccination. Immunity is greatest against the influenza viruses which caused the illness or were included in the vaccine given. There also results some immunity to closely related influenza viral strains. However, the immunity is relatively short-lived and requires boosting re-exposure to the influenza virus by vaccination or natural exposure.

Influenza virus infection is primarily an infection of the respiratory tract epithelium, with the systemic symptoms caused by liberation of toxic products from injured cells. For this reason, immunity is closely related to the presence of secretory immunoglobulin, IgA, at the site of infection, the respiratory tract.

The diagnosis of influenza depends on the recovery of the virus from nasopharyngeal specimens and/or the demonstration of a rise in antibody levels in acute and convalescent paired serum specimens. Influenza virus can be detected by the inoculation of nasopharyngeal washings into embryonated eggs. Presence of virus is determined by death of the embryo, foci of infection on the chorioallantoic membranes, or the production of hemagglutinins in the chorioallantoic fluids. An alternative method is by the hemadsorption method using monkey kidney or human embryonic kidney tissue culture cells and guinea pig or human O-type erythrocytes. Growth in eggs and tissue culture varies from strain to strain of influenza viruses, and a prudent laboratory will use both the embryonated egg and hemadsorption techniques to isolate the virus. A more rapid technique to detect influenza viruses is to flood a smear of nasal epithelial scrapings with fluorescent-labeled specific antisera and to search for fluorescence under a fluorescent microscope. Serological diagnosis is accomplished by using the complement fixation, hemagglutination-inhibition, or hemadsorption-inhibition antibody techniques. Paired serum specimens collected at the time of symptoms and at least two weeks later are required for the diagnosis.

Once a laboratory diagnosis of influenza has been established in a community undergoing an influenza epidemic, reliance on clinical findings for diagnosis of additional cases is justified. However, it should be kept in mind that other respiratory viruses can flourish in the presence of an influenza epidemic.

There is no specific treatment for influenza. Active infection is treated by supportive measures and the appropriate antibiotic if secondary bacterial infection occurs. Prophylaxis is available through vaccines. To be effective, the vaccine should contain the influenza viral strains which are currently prevalent. Protection does not occur until at least ten days after administration of the vaccine. Primary vaccination with new influenza strains requires two inoculations, one month apart. Booster inoculations are needed to maintain effective protection. There is a reluctance to obtain routine annual influenza vaccination because of uncomfortable reactions frequently associated with the vaccines and a lack of understanding of their need. Because of this reluctance and the periodic antigenic shift in the influenza viruses themselves, influenza vaccination programs have been only 65 per cent effective in civilian populations.

Amantadine hydrochloride (Symmetrel) is an anti-influenzal drug shown to be an effective prophylactic agent for several strains of influenza type A viruses. However, the drug must be taken daily to maintain an effective body level. If used during an epidemic of influenza, this might mean six to eight weeks of daily medication. Central nervous system side effects to the drug have been described. The drug has value during an influenza epidemic for use in persons at high risk who have not been properly vaccinated.

Para-influenza Viruses

The para-influenza viruses were first isolated during the 1950's. There are four distinct serologic types which have been recovered from humans. The viruses are members of the myxovirus family, have an inner nucleoprotein core surrounded by lipoprotein spikes, contain RNA, are ether sensitive, and are of medium-size (150 to 250 mμ). They have common antigens which they do not share with influenza viruses but do share with other members of the myxovirus family (measles, distemper, respiratory-syncytial viruses). Hence, there are frequently cross-serological reactions among them and with other myxoviruses following active infection.

The para-influenza viruses are usually detected by means of the hemadsorption technique, using primary monkey kidney tissue culture cells and guinea pig erythrocytes. Serological diagnosis is accomplished by hemagglutination-inhibition or hemadsorption-inhibition tests.

The para-influenza viruses are capable of causing a wide spectrum of diseases which range from subclinical infection to pneumonia. Their greatest importance in human disease is that they are most commonly responsible for viral infectious laryngotracheitis, or croup, in young children. Type 3 has frequently been associated with lower respiratory infection. Antibody surveys have indicated that initial experience with the para-influenza viruses occurs early in life. Reinfection with an individual type of para-influenza virus is common and usually results in a milder illness than the original infection and a serum antibody booster effect. Immunity to para-influenza viruses is dependent on the presence of local respiratory tract antibody, or secretory IgA immunoglobulin rather than circulating IgG antibody. In adults para-influenza virus infection usually results in mild upper respiratory disease. The mild nature of the disease is probably a reflection of existing partial immunity created by earlier experience with the viruses during childhood.

Para-influenza types 1, 2, and 3 have a worldwide distribution and exist endemically in certain communities. Type 4 has been found only in the United States. Infection with type 4 sometime during life appears to be common, as determined by antibody surveys, but the exact role that type 4 plays in human disease remains to be elucidated. There appears to be some cross-protection from mumps virus, which might serve as a limiting factor to human infection by the type 4 virus.

The fact that para-influenza types 1, 2, and 3 account for relatively serious disease in young children makes preventive measures for these viruses desirable. Inactivated and live, attenuated, experimental vaccines have been developed, but early evaluations have failed to show the vaccines to be effective. However, additional vaccine development is underway using temperature-sensitive mutant strains of para-influenza viruses.

Respiratory Syncytial (RS) Virus

The RS virus was first isolated in 1956 from chimpanzees with coryza. A synonym for RS virus is "chimpanzee coryza agent." There now appear to be more than one antigenic type of RS virus, although all strains are closely related. The RS virus has been classified as a myxovirus, has RNA as its nucleic acid type, is medium size, and is sensitive to ether. Unlike some other myxoviruses, the RS virus will not grow in embryonated eggs, will not hemagglutinate erythrocytes, and will not hemadsorb chicken, guinea pig, or human type O erythrocytes in tissue culture.

The laboratory isolation of RS virus is made by inoculation of nasopharyngeal or sputum specimens into heteroploid continuous tissue culture cell lines such as HeLa, KB, or Hep-II cells, with subsequent production of prominent syncytial cells. The RS virus is relatively unstable, so that direct inoculation of specimens into tissue culture is recommended, avoiding storage at even −60° C temperature. Serological diagnosis utilizes complement fixation or neutralization antibody tests.

In adults and children RS infection is usually associated with mild upper respiratory symptoms that are indistinguishable from those caused by many other respiratory viruses. However, RS virus infection is most important for its ability to cause the severe lower respiratory diseases bronchiolitis and bronchopneumonia in infants. RS has also been associated with croup in children.

The RS virus is found in the upper respiratory tract shortly after onset of symptoms and remains for several days. In infants with bronchiolitis, isolation of the virus is possible for as long as ten days.

Active infection has been shown to be possible in the presence of serum neutralization antibodies. This might account for the relatively mild disease caused by RS virus in adults.

Much work has been devoted to the development of vaccines, both live and inactivated, against RS virus because of the lower respiratory illness caused by the virus in infants. However, experimental vaccines have not only been ineffective but in some instances have appeared to set the stage for severe hypersensitivity reactions when vaccinees were exposed to the natural virus. Further vaccine development has involved work with temperature-sensitive mutants of the RS virus.

Rhinoviruses

The rhinoviruses are the most recent viruses to be referred to as the "common cold virus." The initial rhinovirus isolates were made in 1954 from afebrile individuals with coryza, sore throat, and cough. There are probably over 100 distinct serological strains of rhinoviruses. Currently some 60 specific serological types have been classified.

Synonyms for the rhinoviruses include coryzaviruses, muriviruses, ERC viruses, and unclassified common cold viruses.

The rhinoviruses are characteristic of the picornavirus group to which polio, coxsackie and echo viruses belong. The rhinoviruses have RNA-type nucleic acid, are small, and are ether resistant. They are distinguished from other picornaviruses by their acid lability.

The laboratory diagnosis of rhinoviruses depends on viral isolation and assay for serum neutralization antibody. Viral isolation is best conducted in human diploid tissue culture cells in which a characteristic cytopathogenic effect occurs. Neutralization antibody tests are conducted in the same tissue culture system.

The rhinoviruses are clearly established as a cause of acute coryza (the common cold) in man. This is especially true in adults. The incubation period is one to three days. The most frequent symptoms are coryza, sore throat, cough, and malaise. Fever is usually absent, but if present is low grade and of short duration. No pharyngeal exudates are present, although at times cervical adenopathy may occur. The symptoms usually disappear within one week. In children rhinoviruses sometimes cause more severe respiratory disease such as croup, bronchitis, or bronchopneumonia. It has not been possible to distinguish between illnesses caused by the individual serological types of rhinoviruses on clinical grounds.

The rhinoviruses probably account for only 15 per cent of mild upper respiratory illnesses in man. Rhinovirus-associated illnesses have their peak in autumn, occur less frequently in the midwinter, and increase in prevalence in the spring.

Treatment for rhinovirus infections is entirely symptomatic. Some effort has been devoted to vaccine development, but the multiplicity of strains makes immunoprophylaxis impractical.

"Coronaviruses"

The "coronaviruses" are a relatively new group of viruses which have been associated with the common cold. "Coronavirus" is still placed in quotes because the term has not officially been assigned by the nomenclature committees. The term is derived from the fact that the electron micrograph of the human "coronavirus" resembles a crown.

"Coronavirus" resulted from the application by English workers of organ culture techniques as a means of detecting viruses. These workers were intrigued by the fact that some 70 per cent of the typical common colds studied by orthodox techniques failed to reveal rhinoviruses or other known respiratory viruses. By explanting sections of human respiratory epithelium, a system was devised to detect the presence of viruses from some of these rhinovirus-negative specimens. The end point in the system is the cessation of the beating of cilia and destruction of the ciliated respiratory epithelial cells. Apparently a whole group of viruses will emerge from use of this detection system.

The "coronaviruses" have a three to four day incubation period and cause acute rhinitis characterized by a copious rhinorrhea of relatively short duration. At the end of a few days there is less catarrh, nasal secretion, and cough than seen with rhinoviruses. The patients are usually afebrile.

Enteroviruses

The enteroviruses are members of the picornavirus family and are ordinarily thought of as etiological agents for gastrointestinal upsets, aseptic meningitis, and pericarditis. However, several enteroviruses have been associated with acute respiratory disease. Undoubtedly other members besides those mentioned here can cause respiratory illness.

The coxsackie B viruses, of which there are six serotypes, have been associated with colds (rhinorrhea and cough), pharyngitis, and tonsillitis. The pharyngitis-tonsillitis were frequently associated with other signs and symptoms such as exudate, cervical adenitis, otitis media, rhinorrhea, cough, and exanthem. Patients were usually febrile. The associated signs and symptoms were more likely to occur in children. When exudative pharyngitis-tonsillitis occurred it was clinically confused with streptococcal disease. Coxsackie B viruses have also caused croup and pneumonia in younger children.

Coxsackie A-21 virus, or Coe virus, has been associated with febrile pharyngitis, febrile or afebrile common colds, influenzalike syndromes, and atypical pneumonia. The signs and symptoms are sore throat, coryza, cervical adenitis, hoarseness, mild conjunctivitis, headache, and muscle pain. The coxsackie A viruses are further described in the oral cavity and oropharyngeal section of this chapter.

Echo-II virus has been associated with acute rhinitis, pharyngitis, and croup. Fever was variable. The virus has been isolated from both throat and rectal swabs taken from patients with echo-11 respiratory disease.

These enteroviruses are usually most prevalent during the summer months. However, infection can occur any month of the year.

The coxsackie B's, coxsackie A-21, and echo-11 are easily detected in tissue culture, and this might account for their being most prominently associated with illnesses. Coxsackie B's and Echo-11 are best cultured in primary monkey kidney or primary human cell lines, whereas coxsackie A-21 grows best in continuous heteroploid cell lines (HeLa, KB, Hep-II) or primary human embryonic kidney cells. Serological tests are best done by neutralization techniques in tissue culture, although coxsackie A-21 antibody can be tested by a hemagglutinin-inhibition test.

REFERENCES

Conference on Newer Respiratory Disease Viruses, Loosli, C. G. (ed.). Amer. Rev. Resp. Dis., Oct. 1962.

Cooper, L. Z., and Krugman, S.: The Rubella Problem. Disease-a-Month, Year Book Medical Publishers, Inc., Chicago, Feb. 1969.

Goodheart, C. R.: An Introduction to Virology. Philadelphia, W. B. Saunders Company, 1969.

Hable, K., O'Connell, E. J., and Herrmann, E. C., Jr.: Group B coxsackie viruses as respiratory viruses. Mayo Clin. Proc. 45: 170–176, 1970.

Henle, G., and Henle, W.: Observations on childhood infections with the Epstein-Barr virus. J. Infect Dis. 121: 303–310, 1970.

Horsfall, F. L., Jr. and Tamm, I.: Viral and Ricksettsial Infections of Man. Philadelphia, J. B. Lippincott Co., 4th ed. 1965.

Jackson, G. G., and Muldoon, R. L.: A Manual of Newer Viruses and Nonbacterial Agents Causing Respiratory Illness in Man. 2nd ed. Sponsored by Commission on Acute Respiratory Diseases of the Armed Forces Epidemiological Board, 1969.

Kibrick, S.: Current status of coxsackie and ECHO viruses in human disease. Progr. Med. Virol. 6: 27–70.

Krugman, S., and Ward, R.: Infectious Diseases of Children. 3rd ed. St. Louis, The C. V. Mosby Co., 1964.

Lennette, E. H., and Schmidt, N. J.: Diagnostic Procedures for Viral and Rickettsial Diseases. 3rd ed. New York, American Publishers Health Association, 1964.

Chapter 15

MYCOSES

by Jan Schwarz, M.D.

Mycoses play an increasingly important role in otolaryngology for several reasons: (1) there is greater awareness of their presence; (2) better diagnostic facilities are available; (3) the incidence is increased because of therapeutic interference (antibiotics, immunosuppressive drugs, radiation); and (4) there is increased longevity in such diseases as lymphomas, other neoplasms, and hematologic disorders.

Conditions favorable to the development of mycoses prevail in the upper respiratory tract and cranial sinuses, where a moist, warm environment and such crevices as tonsillar crypts and periodontal spaces encourage growth. Such conditions as obstructive lesions, deviated nasal septa, blocked eustachian tubes, and abscesses around teeth favor the development of fungi and related organisms. Mycoses are caused by fungi; however, Actinomyces and Nocardia, now universally accepted as bacteria, are traditionally discussed with fungi because of the close resemblance between the symptomatology and course of the diseases they cause.

The diagnosis of mycosis rests on a low threshold of suspicion by the physician, a (mentally) well equipped laboratory, and the use of modern immunologic and staining procedures. Contrary to widespread belief, the biopsy and not culture is the most rapid and commonly successful diagnostic tool. However, biopsy material should be divided into two specimens, one for cultural studies and one for staining. The selection of proper media by the laboratory can be greatly aided by positive suggestions from the clinician, since, for instance, *Actinomyces israelii* requires strictly anaerobic conditions, whereas certain fungi have specific temperature or other requirements.

The tissue section should be studied with the help of fungus stains; the present method of choice is the methenamine-silver method of Grocott, which brings out even isolated and small organisms in excellent contrast and which is strikingly photogenic. The method of Gridley scores second, the widely used PAS procedure a poor third. Gram stains may be helpful in the diagnosis of actinomycosis, and acid-fast stains for the demonstration of nocardias. If animal inoculation is needed—for instance, from contaminated material (ulcers, sputum)—the white mouse and the hamster (*Cricetus auratus*) are the preferred species. After four weeks the animal will have suppressed contaminating fungi, leaving in its tissues just the pathogen, which can then be recovered by culture, smear, or tissue sections from the animal organs. Fluorescent antibody stains, when available and applicable, can give rapid and accurate information, but frequently fail to react in fixed material (tissue sections).

HISTOPLASMOSIS

Histoplasmosis will produce ulcerations about and in the oral cavity. Laryngeal, tracheobronchial, and esophageal lesions, perforation of the nasal septum, and involvement of tonsils and neck nodes are among the conditions caused by *Histoplasma capsulatum*, especially in endemic areas. In large areas of Indiana, Illinois, Missouri, Kansas, Ohio, Kentucky, and Tennessee 80 to 90 per cent of the population will show a positive skin test with

443

histoplasmin, indicating past or present infection. In recent years the organism has reportedly been found increasingly in the soil of other areas.

Histoplasma capsulatum is a biphasic organism, appearing in tissues as a small yeast (2 to 5 μ) and in culture at room temperature as a whitish mold. The culture mount from the latter is characterized by the development of tuberculate spores about two weeks after the growth first becomes apparent. The disease is acquired by inhalation of spore-containing dust, a primary complex regularly being formed in the lungs. Most primary infections are subclinical, and the only sign of past infection may be calcified lesions in the lung parenchyma and in the draining lymph nodes. If the skin test with histoplasmin is applied, it will be positive and remain so forever in most individuals; the use of the skin test should be judicial, since adequate conclusions will become available only in a given set of circumstances. Recent infection will be demonstrable by skin test alone if a previously (known) negative reaction turns positive. In any other constellation a positive skin test will signal only past or present infection, without revealing whether the infection is recent and active or burned out and quiescent. It is also well to consider that a positive skin test in a fair number of patients will elevate the complement fixation titer, depriving us of a most important diagnostic tool; complement fixation is available through most State Health Departments or in a few selected laboratories, particularly in the endemic areas. This test should be performed with antigens derived from the mycelial and yeast phase of the organism; in acute disease the titer of the yeast phase is generally elevated, whereas in chronic, particularly cavitary, pulmonary diseases the mycelial phase (histoplasmin) is elevated.

Commercially available latex particles, sensitized with histoplasmin, may give an answer, but not necessarily the right one—at least in comparison with results obtained with complement fixation. Agar gel diffusion tests are valuable in the hands of some investigators.

The primary infection almost always produces a self-limited, benign, hematogenous dissemination, which even after years is demonstrable in the form of granulomas (generally calcified) in the spleen and, to a lesser degree, in the liver. However, other organs are also occasionally involved. Ulcers about the lips, tongue, or oral mucosa can be found in the course of the disease, ranging from completely nonspecific, shallow, and superficial "aphthous" lesions to deep crateriform ulcers at the base or on the borders of the tongue or tonsils. Often syphilis is suspected (a suspicion that is quite far-fetched in view of the infrequent occurrence of gummas in our time and location, as compared with the incidence of histoplasmosis). Differentiation can be made rapidly by culture of a portion of the biopsy material, particularly when histiocytic proliferation is found, often with innumerable intracellular organisms. On hematoxylin and eosin slides the organism appears as a small dot surrounded by a halo, which has been shown, on electron microscopy, to represent an artifact of fixation. The cells, especially if few in number, are more easily picked up with the Grocott silver stain. If deep ulcers are present in the tongue and larynx, and deeper in the passages, granulation tissue with true epithelioid cell tubercles and caseation may be found.

In some instances leishmaniasis has been mistaken for histoplasmosis in biopsies (Zinneman et al., 1961).

An important cause of spastic cough and

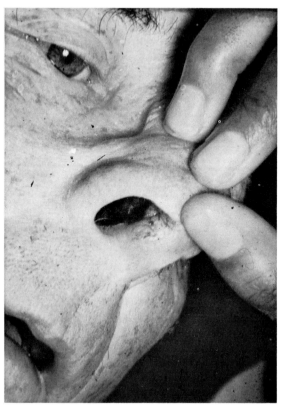

Figure 1. Apparently minor, slightly elevated lesion in nasal septum in case of chronic, widely disseminated histoplasmosis.

hemoptysis is perforation of calcified lymph nodes into the trachea or bronchial tree (Baum et al., 1958; Weed and Anderson, 1960). The mechanism is well explained by adhesion formation between the acutely inflamed lymph node and the wall of the airway. When the lymphadenitis subsides, the lymph node becomes firmly attached to the trachea or bronchus and, after calcification, each respiratory movement grinds away minute tissue particles until an ulcer is formed, the base of which forms calcific particles. The irritation of the mucosa produces the cough, the ulceration, the hemorrhage. Multiple fragments of the calcified lymph node may fall into the bronchial tree and cause great discomfort until expelled by the patient. Such perforation may cause bleeding which results in anything from blood-flecked sputum to hemoptysis. The larynx may show nonspecific infiltrates and superficial or deep ulcers in almost any location, and papillomatous lesions may produce actual obstruction of the airway (Bennett, 1967). Extension from the larynx into the mucosa of the pyriform sinuses is on record (Hulse, 1951). Downward extension involving the trachea or even main bronchi has been described (Sones et al., 1951; King and Cline, 1958).

The concept of the primary pulmonary origin of histoplasmosis establishes that involvement of oral, laryngeal, pharyngeal, and similar sites is secondary to the pulmonary lesions and does not represent the portal of entry. Proper management of the patient depends on an understanding of this concept; since the lesions are only manifestations of a generalized disease, therapy must be directed toward arrest of the pulmonary lesion and of its dissemination, as well as palliation of the otolaryngologic lesions.

The only available therapy at present is the antifungal antibiotic, amphotericin B. This drug is quite effective in most cases, but is hard to administer, harder to tolerate, and severely toxic to many patients. These facts call for the most circumspect diagnostic workup, as the drug should be given only if the diagnosis is firmly established, preferably by cultural as well as microscopic proof or by demonstration of the organisms in tissues, and only if there seems good clinical evidence of progressive disease or metastasis.

Like most granulomatous diseases, histoplasmosis may follow an unpredictable course, with temporary or permanent arrest or with relapses and sudden acute episodes. Cooperation with an experienced chest physician is well advised in treating such patients. Broncholiths will obviously require attempts at removal through bronchoscopy, and obstructive lesions in the larynx may require emergency procedures; outside of this, surgical intervention is of little avail. Excision of even circumscribed tumorlike lip or tongue lesions will rarely be curative, since these represent merely systemic localizations. Steroid therapy and broad-spectrum antibiotics are not indicated; the former because it may precipitate dissemination, the latter because it is ineffective.

NORTH AMERICAN BLASTOMYCOSIS

North American blastomycosis is caused by the dimorphic organism *Blastomyces dermatitidis*. It occurs mainly in North America; although its exact incidence outside North America is not known, rare cases have been reported from Africa and Latin America. The organism has been isolated from soil (Denton et al., 1961) and enters the lungs with dust. The pulmonary origin of the lesions is well established. Laryngitis, from superficial to ulcerative, with hoarseness and occasionally with space-consuming papillomatous proliferation, is a frequent complication of the chronic pulmonary form of the disease. Extension into the trachea and bronchi can become quite prominent in the clinical picture (cough!) and may determine the spread and outcome of the condition.

Lesions on the lips and around the nose are seen commonly in this disorder, and ulcerative and verrucous appearance of the lesions is quite characteristic (de Palma et al., 1958). Sometimes the borders of the ulcers are indurated and elevated and may contain tiny abscesses, which are most important for diagnosis; aspiration of even one drop from such abscesses reveals thousands of round yeast cells 8 to 24 μ in size, characterized by thick walls and single buds. Culture of this material at room temperature grows a whitish mold, with rather uncharacteristic microscopic findings consisting of septate hyphae with microconidia varying in size from 2 to 8 μ but without any specific spore forms that facilitate the recognition of the species. When grown on blood or cottonseed agar at 37° C., a waxy yeastlike colony develops, consisting of the same round budding yeast cells observed in tissues. The disease can easily be induced in experimental animals and is quite frequently found spontaneously in dogs.

In a fair number of patients solitary skin lesions are found which give the false impression that this represents a primary cutaneous disease. This misconception has been dispelled (Schwarz and Baum, 1951), and the presence of the solitary skin lesion must be explained by isolated metastases from a lung lesion which has become arrested or, at least, inactive.

Clinically it may not be easy to demonstrate in each instance the presence of pulmonary lesions, but thorough radiological and cultural search will generally reveal their presence. Even so, occasionally surgical removal of isolated lesions about the ala nasi, the lip or periorbital areas may shorten the hospital stay. If for several months patients do not develop mucocutaneous lesions, one can assume that the pulmonary source of the metastases has dried up, and it may be easier on the patient to submit to excisional therapy than to take the toxic amphotericin, which requires prolonged infusions and, frequently, hospitalization of several weeks or months. Excision, if decided upon, must be performed with wide borders, avoiding scrupulously inoculation of Blastomyces into the excisional wound.

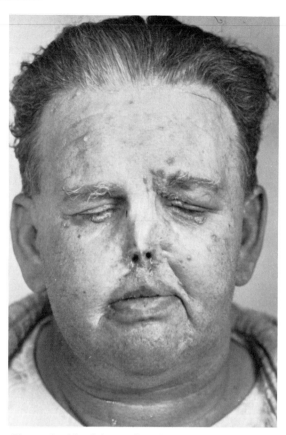

Figure 3. Nasal destruction after facial blastomycosis.

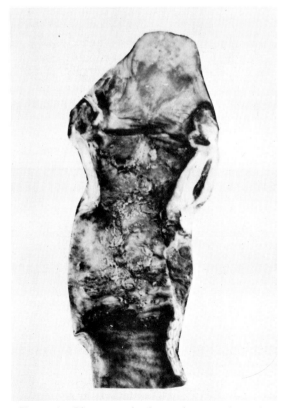

Figure 2. Blastomycotic destructive, pseudomembranous and ulcerative laryngotracheitis. (Courtesy Dr. E. Chick.)

Untreated lesions can lead to considerable mutilation of the face, and recurrences in damaged tissue around the mouth or nose have frequently been seen in our patients. Involvement of the oral mucosa is not common in North American blastomycosis but can be most treacherous, occurring first as superifical aphthous lesions, to extend subsequently in diameter and depth; mere removal of diseased tissue is not necessarily curative. Here, as in histoplasmosis, we are dealing with a disorder originating in the lung, with sometimes protracted and sometime acute pneumonitis. Cavitary pulmonary lesions are on record but are not common. Metastasis from the pulmonary lesions to skin and mucosae may easily be mistaken for squamous cell carcinoma, especially when seen around the facial orifices.

Microscopically the mucocutaneous lesions of blastomycosis produce a pseudoepitheliomatous hyperplasia, which can be quite extensive and confusing to the point that it, too, is misread as squamous cell carcinoma. The presence of microabscesses in the epithelium (often with organisms in the exudate) aids recognition of the true nature of the disorder. Furthermore, the maturation of the proliferating squamous epithelium is such that it precludes interpretation as malignant neoplasm.

All mucocutaneous lesions must be carefully evaluated in reference to the activity of the pulmonary lesions and their own aggressiveness. Frequently solitary lesions are self-limited and seem to improve in spite of, rather than because of, therapy. Little wonder that "cures" have been reported with a series of procedures that would not be expected to be effective. Indirect methods (serology, skin tests) are of little, if any, help in the diagnosis of blastomycosis. In addition to amphotericin B, 2-hydroxy-stilbamidine has been found effective in the management of blastomycosis. Iodine—an old standby—has no place in rational therapy.

CRYPTOCOCCOSIS

Cryptococcosis (torulosis, European blastomycosis) is caused by *Cryptococcus neoformans*, a yeastlike organism commonly surrounded by a polysaccharide capsule. The capsule can easily be demonstrated on India-ink mounts, showing the yeast cell surrounded by a clear halo on a black background. The organism has been isolated from pigeon nests and dried pigeon droppings, and there is good evidence to assume that, like most of the deep fungi, it enters the human body by way of the respiratory tract.

Cryptococcosis neoformans is definitely neurotropic, and many clinical cases present with central nervous disease—meningitis or meningoencephalitis. However, localizations of interest to the otolaryngologist have been observed in the paranasal sinus (Kohlmeier, 1955), in the nasopharynx (Jones), and as membranous inflammation (Norris and Armstrong, 1954). Lesions on the face affecting the skin and mucocutaneous borders of nose and ear occur as parts of disseminated infection.

Widely disseminated cryptococcosis is seen as a terminal complication of lymphomatous disorders and should be sought especially in Hodgkin's disease when sudden febrile illness or meningitis develops. Steroid therapy, cytotoxic drugs, and therapeutic irradiation are common predisposing factors for the development of cryptococcosis.

In short, this disease seldom affects man as a primary infection. It develops in individuals with defective globulin mechanisms and can considerably accelerate a lethal outcome of other disorders; diagnosis is, therefore, mandatory, since therapy with amphotericin B is effective and, unless the underlying disease is irreparable, can be curative.

Diagnosis is best established by morphological and cultural demonstration of the organisms (which often grow within 1 or 2 days), or by serologic means; a latex particle test demonstrating the antigen in spinal fluid or serum of the patient is probably the most reliable. Direct meningeal involvement from intranasal experimental infection has been demonstrated in hamsters (Herrold, 1965). About 10 per cent of patients with cryptococcosis show cutaneous involvement, about 3 per cent mucosal lesions (Karcher, 1963). Lesions on or close to nose, ear, or mouth sometimes result from minor injuries or, as in a patient of Symmers (1953), from a scratch by the patient's fingernail. In addition to ulcers, pimples, papules, and hemorrhagic lesions are on record.

As the cutaneous ulcers may have all the characteristics of basal cell cancer (rodent ulcer), needless surgery or radiotherapy can be prevented by smear, biopsy, or culture. Microscopically the tissue response can vary from no response to true granuloma formation, with epithelioid cell nodules and multinucleated giant cells. The mucocutaneous surfaces may, rarely, show pseudoepitheliomatous reaction. The demonstration of *C. neoformans* in tissues can be made easier with mucicarmine, which almost specifically stains the organism pink to red, whereas other yeast cells remain unstained.

CANDIDIASIS

Disease caused by the yeastlike organism *Candida albicans* covers a wide gamut. Candidiasis is most often found about the oropharynx. The small yeast (2 to 5 μ) is ovoid, appears intensely blue with the Gram stain, and can be demonstrated with any of the numerous stains for fungi. Broad hyphae can be seen in association with the yeast cells. Often it is quite obvious that the hyphae are just elongated yeast cells when budding takes place at the point of constriction. *Candida albicans* grows easily on all standard culture media used for bacteriologic isolation (blood agar, heart brain infusion, and so forth) and on Sabouraud's glucose agar overnight. A few cells from the culture introduced into sterile serum produce germ tubes within 1 to 3 hours, and for all practical purposes this clinches the diagnosis of *C. albicans*. The incidence of *C. albicans* in the oral cavity varies from country to country (in Cincinnati in adults about 30 per cent [Baum, 1960]) and depends on age, hygiene, diabetes, broad-spectrum antibiotic therapy, and so forth (Bartels, 1937; Burnett and Scherp, 1968).

A mild form of candidiasis is thrush, a white to grayish membranous formation over tonsils or adjacent mucosae, which either occurs in discrete or confluent specks and which can often be removed with a swab, with or without provoking bleeding. Smears of such membranes are most revealing and rule out differential diseases like diphtheria, the ulceration of mononucleosis, or acute leukemia. Thrush is seen most often at both extremes of life, in the (often premature) newborn who acquire the disease in the maternal birth canal, and in the geriatric patient, dying of old age or from tumors. Thrush, therefore, is often a warning signal of some profound abnormality existing in the body and does not itself require energetic therapeutic measures.

The only rational therapy is with topical nystatin, obtainable as an oral suspension or for incorporation into a gelatin base for sustained release. Crystal or gentian violet is popular but certainly not specific, messy, destructive to pillows and bedding, and, in any case, of questionable benefit to the patient. It has been our experience that nystatin eliminates thrush within a few days. (When it is given for at least a week, the number of failures and recurrences decreases markedly.) Obviously other supportive measures (oral hygiene, interruption of broad-spectrum antibiotic therapy) may be necessary to prevent recurrence. Since nystatin is practically unabsorbable, toxicity is no problem; 100,000 units can be given several times in suspension, even to newborns. Enteric-coated tablets of nystatin are useless for the topical therapy of oropharyngeal lesions, since they dissolve in the duodenum and may lower the intestinal candida count; however, since nystatin is not absorbed, they do nothing to better the oral lesions.

Oral candidiasis, if unattended, can spread to the gums and buccal mucosa and may extend, particularly in the elderly, to one or both angles of the mouth (perlèche). Spread to the larynx (sometimes with hyperkeratosis) (Tedeschi and Cheren, 1968), trachea, and esophagus can be seen in marantic patients. Oral candidiasis in the infant can be associated with candida diaper rash.

In addition to the maternal birth canal, thrush in the newborn has two other main sources: nipples of mother or bottles; skin of mother and nurses (Winner and Hurley, 1964). In the neonate the presence of *C. albicans* on oral smear is almost regularly followed by clinical thrush (66 times in 67 patients) (Taschdjian and Kozinn, 1957), and prophylactic use of nystatin may be considered in such setting.

Another much more severe but fortunately rare form of pediatric candidiasis is the granulomatous and destructive mucocutaneous form. Such children (mostly female) often have a background of hypothyroidism or hypoparathyroidism; candidiasis can lead to severe ulcerative involvement of the nasopharynx, with complete destruction of facial tissue unless specific treatment and proper care are given early in the disease (Goldman and Schwarz, 1962). Diabetics also have a predisposition to candidiasis, particularly on intertriginous areas of the skin, from which it can be transmitted upon the hands to form buccal lesions.

Candidiasis of the middle ear in a premature infant after considerable antibiotic and steroid therapy has been described by McLellan et al. (1965).

Candida endocarditis is fortunately a rare complication but does occur after prolonged intravenous infusions, particularly with plastic materials; it has been seen after open-heart surgery and in drug addicts, but occasionally seems to find its way to the endocardium from superficial lesions of skin or mucosae. Prompt diagnosis, elimination of candida-infested indwelling catheters, and intense intravenous amphotericin B therapy are essential; even so, the prognosis of candida sepsis with or without endocardial localization is poor (Utz et al., 1961).

Hairy tongue, a harmless hypertrophy of filiform papillae, of unknown etiology, is often associated with positive cultures of Candida species; there is no evidence pointing toward a casual relationship.

In addition to *C. albicans*, other Candida species may also be isolated from oropharyngeal lesions. Differentiation between the species is, however, a task requiring a high degree of expertise.

COCCIDIOIDOMYCOSIS

The organism *Coccidioides immitis* appears in tissues, exudates, and body fluids as a rounded large structure called a spherule. By cleavage of the cytoplasm, endospores are formed which, when few in number, are large and decrease in size with numerical duplication. The spherule is generally between 20 and 200 μ in size, while the endospores can be up to 40 μ in size. On culture media a comparatively fast-growing mold develops, often with a "bald" center surrounded by a grayish cottony growth. A culture mount from such colonies reveals septate hyphae which break into smaller structures (arthrospores). These are easily air-borne and are responsible not only for natural infection, but also for laboratory accidents. Accidental infection is most common with this fungus, and extraordinary precautions should be taken to avoid such a problem. We autoclave the cultures before they are examined on culture mounts, since the morphology does not change and diagnosis can be established in the context of the clinical picture, the gross and microscopic appearance of the colony, geographic history, and serologic reactions. The disease is common in the southwest section of the United States and with lesser frequency in Mexico, Argentina (where it was discovered), and other Latin American countries. In the endemic areas the disease is widespread, up to 90 per cent of the population reacting positively to the skin test with coccidioidin. Numerous clinical cases are described in a great variety of development and degree of gravity. The overwhelming majority of cases are either subclinical or very minor in symptomatology, but *C. immitis* as an agent of meningitis in Caucasian man and of widespread dissemination, especially in pigmented races, should be considered seriously in any differential diagnosis in an endemic area (Fiese, 1958).

Facial lesions with ulcerative destruction or papillomatous granulomas about the oronasal orifices are common and should be considered in any native of or visitor to the endemic area. Long intervals between primary infection and development of granulomatous forms, while unusual, do occur and make the recognition of the disease even more complex. Biopsy, preferably with special stains, affords the fastest and most conclusive confirmation. Such lesions may also affect the pinna and the external ear canal. Lesions of the oropharyngeal mucosae and of the larynx (Mumma, 1953) are seen as part of progressive pulmonary coccidioidomycosis and should not be mistaken for primary localizations of the disease. Laryngeal destruction can be considerable but is amenable to treatment with amphotericin B

(Lyons, 1966). Perforation of lymph nodes into the bronchus is an unusual complication (Forbus and Bestebreurtje, 1946). Here again management and prognosis must be geared to the pulmonary lesion, representing almost without exception the primary site and the source of dissemination. The disease—even advanced cases—responds as a rule to amphotericin B therapy; empirically a rising titer in the complement fixation test (CFT) suggests progressive disease, whereas a falling titer is generally of good prognostic significance.

PARACOCCIDIOIDOMYCOSIS

Perioral and, in general, periorificial localization of several deep mycoses is quite common and most frequently seen in paracoccidioidomycosis. Generally seen in Latin America, occasional cases occur also in North America (Furtado et al., 1954; Fountain and Sutliff, 1969). The lesions may be tumorlike, with areas of breakdown and ulceration, or may surround the lips as an oozing ulcerated rim. Both the cutaneous and mucosal areas of the lips may also be involved.

The tongue and oral mucosa in general often show superficial hemorrhagic lesions or deep ulcers. Gingival lesions and periodontal granulomas are quite common in this disease and may lead to extensive ulceration of the gingiva, often with periodontal involvement leading to loosening of teeth (Fonseca, 1957).

All evidence points to the lungs as the site of primary infection (as will be repetitiously mentioned in most other deep mycoses). The organisms *Paracoccidioides (Blastomyces) brasiliensis* presents, in tissues, a large yeast, often with multiple buds surrounding the mother cell, measuring from 10 to 60 μ in diameter. In culture at room temperature a mold of creamy color develops slowly; the diagnosis can be reliably established by transfer of the mold into the tissue phase by growth at 37° C. on blood agar or Kurung's egg medium until the dimorphic character of the organism is demonstrated.

The disease responds to sulfa therapy and also to amphotericin B treatment. Local measures may become necessary for cosmetic reasons or because of mechanical obstruction, but the underlying pulmonary disease should never be neglected. Without arrest of the pulmonary lesion, all other measures become of little avail. Superficial, ulcerative, and granulomatous laryngitis may occur, and the vocal cords are sometimes destroyed beyond repair.

No indirect methods are available for the diagnosis (serology or skin tests). This disorder has not been reported in lower animals.

PHYCOMYCOSIS

(Mucormycosis — Zygomycosis)

The class Phycomycetes is characterized by coenocytic (nonseptate) hyphae and includes the genera Mucor, Rhizopus, Absidia, and others which attack diabetic patients particularly, especially those in diabetic acidosis. A favorite localization is the nose and paranasal sinuses. Extension of the infection to the brain has been observed repeatedly and seems to take place directly through the cribriform plate or through the ethmoid sinus. Cellulitis is found in the course of the disease in the retro-orbital tissue; clinically the "orbital apex cuff" syndrome, with total internal and external ophthalmoplegia, is observed. The exudate is foul smelling, of greenish dark color, and abundant (McBride et al., 1960; Berk et al., 1961; Bank, 1962; Straatsma et al., 1962; LaTouche et al., 1963; Prockop and Silva-Hutner, 1967; Abramson, 1967; Battock, 1968).

In addition to acidotic diabetics, patients on immunosuppressive therapy or after extensive antibiotic therapy have also been known to acquire the disease. In the years 1943 to 1967 about 160 cases of phycomycosis were reported, with 45 patients having cephalic involvement. Bank et al. (1962) report the use of skin test and CFT for diagnosis, but no large series of patients has been screened by immunologic methods.

Therapy consists in correction of the acidosis and surgical debridement, which should be as thorough as possible, and extensive use of amphotericin B, either daily or on alternate days. The use of iodine is probably not rational.

Lately — particularly in tropical countries — nose and paranasal sinuses have been found infected by fungi of the order Entomophthorales, with spectacular tumefactions arising in these sites (Williams et al.).

MYCOSES ABOUT THE NOSE

Several other fungi can be found producing damage to the skin or mucosa of the nose. The common periorificial involvement by *P. brasiliensis* has been mentioned; *B. dermatitidis* also may infect the ala nasi and destroy considerable parts of the nose. Rarely *Sporotrichum*

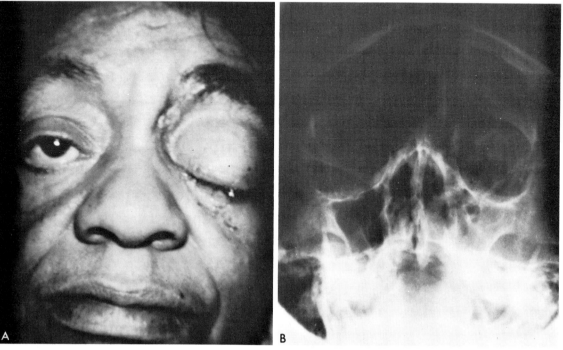

Figure 4. *A*, Severe swelling of left half of face (phycomycosis). *B*, Maxillary sinusitis (same case). (Battock, D.J.: Ann. Intern. Med. *68*:122, 1968.)

schenckii invades the skin of the nose when patients are scratched or otherwise injured by spore-containing thorns or sharp leaves.

Sporotrichum schenckii is a dimorphic organism, found especially on barberry bushes, roses, and a sphagnum moss; by traumatic inoculation it produces a chancre at the portal of entrance with regularly developing lymphangitis; in the lymphangitic streaks are found nodules that do not represent lymph nodes but rather inflammatory infiltrates.

The lymphangitis leading to preauricular lymph nodes creates a typical picture and should be kept in mind for differential diagnosis. In the older literature, descriptions are found of extension of sporotrichosis to mucosae of mouth, pharynx, and nose from cutaneous facial involvement (Hodara, 1923). Claims of "primary" pharyngitis, presumably caused by grains, and of involvement of the palate and nose (Philipp, 1921) have been made. Ulceration of the larynx involving the epiglottis and vocal cords was interpreted as a complication of pharyngitis in the case of one authority.

The organism grows easily within three to four days at room temperature, first as a waxy, creamy colony which, with age, becomes dark brown or black. Mounts reveal thin, segmented hyphae with conidiophores with terminal, mostly pyriform conidia giving the appearance of daisies. The yeast—seldom demonstrable in tissues—is about 5 μ in greatest diameter and quite elusive to routine hematoxylin and eosin stains; even in the best hands and with adequate staining, the microscopic demonstration of *S. schenckii* in tissues is capricious. This is the rare instance when culture is an absolute necessity and superior to simple microscopic methods.

Histoplasmosis can produce perforation of the nasal septum. The finding of such a defect in our environment should always lead to attempts at culture, complement fixation, and adequate tissue biopsy. In the endemic area, perforation of the septum is more likely to be of histoplasmic than of luetic origin. Cryptococcosis occasionally involves the skin and mucosa of the nose or lips; the diagnosis rests entirely on demonstration of the organism in the lesion. As a rule, this is simple in view of the broad capsule of the organism and because *C. neoformans* selectively stains with mucicarmine. In all these instances—except in sporotrichosis resulting from traumatic local inoculation—the fact must be recalled that the primary lesion is pulmonary and that the mucocu-

taneous lesions are metastatic. The importance is self-evident for the management of the patient and highlights the futility of topical measures if not combined with systemic therapy.

Rhinosporidiosis

Another rare disorder to be mentioned, even if there is no absolute proof that we are dealing with a fungal organism, is rhinosporidiosis. This disease is common in India and Ceylon, less frequent in Africa, rare in America, exceptional in Europe; it produces granulomatous papillary lesions about the nose, unilateral or bilateral, sometimes reaching obstructive proportions. The commonest sites of origin are the mucosae of the septum, inferior turbinate, and nasal floor. Less common localizations are the middle turbinate, middle meatus, and the nasal roof, followed by involvements, including lacrimal duct and sac. Rare sites are the hard palate, inner end of the eustachian tube, tonsils, epiglottis, outer ear, and oropharynx. Combinations also occur.

The polypous lesions vary in color from pink to strawberry red. The growth is friable and vascular and bleeds readily on touch. Exceptional and apparently unrelated association with squamous cell carcinoma has been observed. Infectious associations on record include leprosy, leishmaniasis, and molluscum contagiosum. Epistaxis is the commonest clinical symptom, all the way to life-threatening hemorrhage, and obstructive lesions may cause breathing difficulty.

In the tissues the organism *Rhinosporidium seeberi* produces large saclike structures filled with endospores that are released through a porus in the sac. No culture has ever been obtained from clinical material, but the biopsy is quite characteristic and specific. No treatment except debridement seems effective (Karunaratne, 1964).

EXTERNAL OTITIS

The importance of fungi in the etiology of external otitis is hard to assess. On the one hand, a great variety of fungi can be recovered from normal-looking outer ears, so that the recovery of similar species from an inflamed external canal may pose a problem of interpretation, open to guess rather than to evidence.

Aspergillus species are frequently found in the ear canal and are especially troublesome after fenestration and mastoid operations (Smyth, 1961). The same author found increased numbers of fungi after topical applications of broad-spectrum antibiotics. A meaningful decision will be possible if biopsy demonstrates tissue invasion. Moisture and high temperature seem to contribute to the proliferation of fungi in the outer canal (Sharp et al., 1946), as illustrated by the increase in frequency of external otitis from 2 per cent in winter to 11 per cent in summer.

Underlying eczematous conditions are accepted as contributory causes in fungal otitis, as is poor hygiene with accumulation of debris. Topical application of antiseptic and antibiotic solutions may be necessary, but none can be considered as specific therapy unless the suspected fungus fulfills the mentioned criteria. When *C. albicans* is isolated, it will react promptly and unmistakably to nystatin. Should dermatophytes be isolated from the skin of the outer ear, griseofulvin (oral) is the treatment of choice.

ASPERGILLOSIS

Aspergillus species are often found in the external auditive canal, but this finding is not synonymous with etiologic diagnosis. Meningitis has been reported after aspergillosis of the cranial sinuses (Saversky and Waltner, 1961), or supposedly originating from the orbit or the region of the pharynx (Watjen, 1928; Finegold et al., 1959).

The genus Aspergillus comprises a large array of species, the differentiation of which may require considerable skill and time. As a rule, the organisms can be described as fast growing, generally with development of abundant pigment which is formed in practically all shades of the rainbow. The colonies are generally cottony, with a dry, powdery surface resulting from the abundant development of spores, often in long chains. The spores are formed on the tip of sterigmata which, in turn, are crowded together on the heads of the fungus.

Aspergilli are the commonest cause of death in birds in captivity; hence, bird fanciers are especially likely to develop aspergillosis.

This fungus is so widespread in nature that there is no dearth of source material. We have occasionally seen casts obstructing the trachea or some of the larger bronchi, mostly or entirely composed of mycelia of aspergilli. The invasion of pre-existing pulmonary cavities

(bronchiectatic, histoplasmic, tuberculous) by Aspergillus is well known, producing a classic x-ray picture and resulting in the formation of the so-called intracavitary fungus ball (Schwarz et al., 1961). Pseudomembranous tracheitis and bronchitis with coagulation necrosis of the underlying tissue occurs in association with aspergillus infection (Okudaira and Schwarz, 1962).

Invasion of bronchiectatic structures by Aspergillus is not uncommon. Isolated reports indicate that nebulization of nystatin is useful (Vedder and Schorr, 1969).

ACTINOMYCOSIS

Actinomycosis occurs most commonly about the mandible and is caused by Actinomyces species lodging in tonsils, tooth pockets, and other oropharyngeal areas. Tooth extraction, tonsillectomy, or comparable surgical trauma can precipitate introduction of the organism into soft tissue, with inflammatory response of the host. Numerous species of Actinomyces have been described, but *Actinomyces israelii* and *bovis* are the best studied and universally accepted species (Howell et al., 1962).

In tissues the sulfur granule is formed, a structure of 1 to 2 mm. in size, composed of interlacing hyphae arranged with club-shaped radial projections in the periphery of the granule, which is often kidney shaped. The granule, visible to the naked eye, can be found in the exudate draining through sinuses to the skin covering the mandible. If the drainage is scant, a few layers of gauze applied for a few hours over the fistula will trap the escaping granules.

A simple microscopic preparation stained with methylene blue or by the Gram procedure reveals the nature of the organism. More sophisticated and specific is staining with fluorescent antibody. Culture of the organism is difficult for several reasons: (1) the organism is anaerobic; and, (2) the organism is exquisitely sensitive to most antibiotics, which precludes addition of antibiotics to the media, leading in turn to overgrowth of Actinomyces by associated bacteria. Biopsy is the fastest and frequently most reliable and most rewarding method of obtaining a diagnosis. Purists claim (rightly) that granules are not sufficient proof for the diagnosis of actinomycosis, particularly for establishing the species. But for all practical purposes, the finding of a granule surrounded by lipid-laden white cells is acceptable (albeit not strictly scientific) proof of actinomycosis. Sometimes numerous sections are necessary before a granule can be found.

To start with the abortive forms, abscesses in the cervicofacial region (sometimes as low as the thyroid and sometimes as high as the region of the upper jaw) that heal after simple incision or after breaking through the skin may be shown to contain species of Actinomyces, generally associated with *Staph. aureus*. How many such lesions heal without medical interference is anybody's guess.

Similar abscesses may, however, continue draining either after incision or after spontaneous fistulization. It must be stressed that any fistula about the jaw should immediatley be suspected to be actinomycosis until proved otherwise. From these simple draining sinuses the next step leads to grave osteomyelitis of the jaw, with or without sequestration of bone or swelling of bone and surrounding soft tissue. Such cases are rarely seen except in neglected patients or in underdeveloped countries. The infiltrate is remarkably firm; diffuse cellulitis may persist for an indefinite period. Osteomyelitis, even in the age of antibiotics, may require surgical cleansing of the cavity, particularly in the presence of a sequestrum.

The therapy of choice is penicillin, but most other antibiotics have their supporters. In view of the proteolytic activity of the organisms, unexpected subcutaneous tunnels may lead far away from the point of origin; fistulization is the most outstanding and constant feature of actinomycosis.

NOCARDIASIS

Nocardiasis in the United States is caused most frequently by *Nocardia asteroides* and south of the border by *N. brasiliensis*. It is not commonly found about the upper respiratory tract, but subcutaneous infiltrates and fistulas frequently found on the chest and back sometimes extend into the neck region. Both organisms are acid fast and hard to differentiate from Mycobacteria.

Nocardia asteroides is found with some frequency in sputa; both nocardiae grow aerobically more easily than their close cousin, *A. israelii*. *Nocardia brasiliensis* frequently creates multiple and recurrent subcutaneous lesions, particularly on the trunk and extremities; the localization on the lower limbs is known as mycetoma pedis.

Few laboratories are able to establish speciation of Nocardias, and consultation with a reference laboratory is generally necessary. Nocardia species and the closely related Streptomyces are common laboratory contaminants; this creates an additional problem, since even a positive culture of these organisms does not necessarily confirm their pathogenetic importance.

Sulfadiazine has been reported as curative (Hildick-Smith et al., 1964), but personal experience with this drug has been somewhat less than impressive.

REFERENCES

Abramson, E., Wilson, D., and Arky, R. C.: Rhinocerebral phycomycosis in association with diabetic ketoacidosis; report of two cases and review of clinical and experimental experience with amphotericin B therapy. Ann. Intern. Med. 66:735, 1967.

Bank, H., Shibolet, S., Gilat, T., Altmann, G., and Heller, H.: Mucormycosis of head and neck structures. Brit. Med. J. 1:766, 1962.

Bartels, H. A.: Significance of yeastlike organisms in denture sore mouth. Amer. J. Orthodont. 23:90, 1937.

Battock, D. J., Grausz, H., Bobrowsky, M., and Littman, M. L.: Alternate-day amphotericin B therapy in the treatment of rhinocerebral phycomycosis (mucormycosis). Ann. Intern. Med. 68:122, 1968.

Baum, G. L.: The significance of Candida albicans in human sputum. New Eng. J. Med. 263:70, 1960.

Baum, G. L., Bernstein, I. L., and Schwarz, J.: Broncholithiasis produced by histoplasmosis. Amer. Rev. Tuberc. 77:162, 1958.

Bennett, D. E.: Histoplasmosis of the oral cavity and larynx. Arch. Intern. Med. 120:417, 1967.

Berk, M., Fink, G. I., and Uyeda, C. T.: Rhinomucormycosis. J.A.M.A. 177:121, 1961.

Burnett, G. W., and Scherp, H. W.: Oral Microbiology and Infectious Disease. Baltimore, The William & Wilkins Company, 1968.

Denton, J. F., McDonough, E. S., Ajello, L., and Auscherman, R. J.: Isolation of Blastomyces dermatidis from soil. Science 133:1126, 1961.

DePalma, A. T., Hardy, S. B., and Erickson, E. E.: Blastomycotic ulcer of the lower lip. Amer. Surg. 24:919, 1958.

Fiese, M. J.: Coccidioidomycosis. Springfield, Ill., Charles C Thomas, 1958.

Finegold, S. M., Will, D., and Murray, J. F.: Aspergillosis; a review and report of 12 cases. Amer. J. Med. 27:463, 1959.

Fonseca, J. B.: Blastomicose sul-americana. Estudo das lesoes dentarias e paradentarias sob o ponto de vista clinico e histopatologico. Tesis, São Paulo, 1957.

Forbus, W., and Bestebreurtje, A. M.: Coccidioidomycosis. A study of 95 cases of the disseminated type, with special reference to the pathogenesis of the disease. Milit. Surg. 99:653, 1946.

Fountain, F. F., and Sutliff, W. D.: Paracoccidioidomycosis in the United States. Amer. Rev. Resp. Dis. 99:89, 1969.

Furtado, T. A., Wilson, J. W., and Plunkett, O. A.: S.A.

blastomycosis or paracoccidioidomycosis. Arch. Derm. & Syphil. *70*:166, 1954.

Goldman, L., and Schwarz, J.: Chronic muco-cutaneous candidiasis in children. Acta Dermatovener. *42*:314, 1962.

Gridley, M. F.: A stain for fungus in tissue sections. Amer. J. Clin. Path. *23*:303, 1953.

Grocott, R. G.: A stain for fungi in tissue sections and smears. Amer. J. Clin. Path. *25*:975, 1955.

Herrold, K. McD.: Cryptococcus neoformans: Pathogenesis of the disease in Syrian hamsters. Fed. Proc. *24*:492, 1965.

Hildick-Smith, G., Blank, H., and Sarkany, I.: Fungus Diseases and Their Treatment. Boston, Little, Brown and Company, 1964.

Hodara, M.: Ein Fall von Sporotrichose der Genital und Analgegend und der Mundschleimhaut. Dermat. Wchschr. *77*:1328, 1923.

Howell, A., Jr., Stephan, R. M., and Paul, F.: Prevalence of Actinomyces israelii, A. naeslundii, Bacterionema matruchotii and Candida albicans in selected areas of the oral cavity and saliva. J. Dent. Res. *41*:1050, 1962.

Hulse, W. F.: Laryngeal histoplasmosis. Report of a case. A.M.A. Arch. Otolaryng. *54*:65, 1951.

Jones, E. L.: Torula infection of the nasopharynx. South. Med. J., *20*:120–126, 1927.

Karcher, K. H.: Die europaische Blastomykose von Busse-Buschke in Hdb. Haut-Geschlkrh. IV/*4*:75–96. Berlin, Springer-Verlag, 1963.

Karunaratne, W. A. E.: Rhinosporidiosis in man. London, The Athlone Press, 1964.

King, H. C., and Cline, J. F. X.: Histoplasmosis involving the larynx. A.M.A. Arch. Otolaryng. *67*:649, 1958.

Kohlmeier, W.: Torulose der Nasennebenhoehlen. Zbl. Allg. Path. Anat. *93*:92 (1p), 1955.

Kressman-Debus, E.: Blastomykose des Ohres. Z. Laryng. Rhinol. *28*:338, 1949.

Kurung, J. M., and Yegian, D.: Medium for maintenance and conversion of H. capsulatum to yeastlike phase. Amer. J. Clin. Path. *24*:505–508, 1954.

LaTouche, C. J., Sutherland, T. W., and Telling, M.: Rhinocerebral mucormycosis. Lancet *2*:811, 1963.

Lyons, G. D.: Mycotic disease of the larynx. Ann. Otol. *75*:162–175, 1966.

McBride, R. A., Corson, J. M., and Dammin, G. J.: Mucormycosis: Two cases of disseminated disease with cultural identification of rhizopus; Review of literature. Amer. J. Med. *28*:832, 1960.

McLellan, M. S., Strong, J. P., Williams, P. M., and Baker, R. D.: Middle ear mycosis in a premature infant. Arch. Otolaryng. *82*:612–614, 1965.

Mumma, C. S.: Coccidioidomycosis of the epiglottis. Arch. Otolaryng. *58*:306–309, 1953.

Norris, J. C., and Armstrong, W. B.: Membraneous cryptococcic nasopharyngitis (Cryptococcus neoformans). Arch. Otolaryng. *60*:720–722, 1954.

Okudaira, M., and Schwarz, J.: Tracheobronchopulmonary mycoses caused by opportunistic fungi, with particular reference to aspergillosis. Lab. Invest. *11*:1053–1064, 1962.

Philipp, S.: Ein Fall von Sporotrichose der Mundhohle. Inaug. Diss. Koln, 1921.

Prockop, L. D., and Silva-Hutner, M.: Cephalic mucormycosis (phycomycosis). Arch. Neurol. *17*:379, 1967.

Savetsky, L., and Waltner, J.: Aspergillosis of the maxillary antrum. Report of a case and review of the available literature. Arch. Otolaryng. *74*:695–698, 1961.

Schwarz, J., and Baum, G. L.: Blastomycosis. Amer. J. Clin. Path. *21*:999–1029, 1951.

Schwarz, J., Baum, G. L., and Straub, M.: Cavitary histoplasmosis complicated by fungus ball. Amer. J. Med. *31*:692, 1961.

Sharp, W. B., John, M. B., and Robinson, J. M.: Etiology of otomycosis. Texas J. Med. *42*:380, 1946.

Smyth, G. D. L.: A preliminary report on fungal infections of mastoid and fenestration cavities. J. Laryng. *75*:703, 1961.

Sones, C. A., Rotkow, M. J., and Dunn, R. C.: Acute disseminated histoplasmosis. Report of a case in an adult. J. Iowa State Med. Soc. *45*:463, 1955.

Straatsma, B. R., Zimmerman, L. E., and Gass, J. D. M.: Phycomycosis: A clinicipathologic study of fifty-one cases. Lab. Invest. *11*:963, 1962.

Symmers, W. St. C.: Torulosis. Lancet *2*:1068, 1953.

Taschdjian, C. L., and Kozinn, P. J.: Laboratory and clinical studies on candidiasis in the newborn infant. J. Pediat. *50*:425, 1957.

Tedeschi, L. G., and Cheren, R. V.: Laryngeal hyperkeratosis due to primary monilial infection. Arch. Otolaryng. *87*:82, 1968.

Utz, J. P., Roberts, W. C., Cooper, T., Kravetz, H. M., and Andriole, V. T.: Candida endocarditis: An emerging peril in cardiovascular surgery. Ann. Intern Med. *54*:1058, 1961.

Vedder, J. S., and Schorr, W. F.: Primary disseminated pulmonary aspergillosis with metastatic skin nodules. J.A.M.A. *209*:1191, 1969.

Watjen, J.: Zur Kenntnis der Gewebsreaktionen bei Schimmelmykosen. Virchows Arch. Path. Anat. *268*:665, 1928.

Weed, L. A., and Anderson, H. A.: Etiology of broncholithiasis. Dis. Chest *37*:1, 1960.

Williams, A. O., von Lichtenberg, F., Smith, J. H., and Martinson, F. D.: Ultrastructure of phycomycosis due to Entomorphthora and Basidiobolus species. Arch. Path. *87*:459–468, 1969.

Winner, H. I., and Hurley, R.: Candida albicans. London, J. & A. Churchill, Ltd., 1964.

Zinneman, H. H., Hall, W. H., and Wallace, F. G.: Leishmaniasis of the larynx. Report of a case and its confusion with histoplasmosis. Amer. J. Med. *31*:654, 1961.

Section Five

PHARMACOLOGY

Chapter 16

TOPICAL DRUGS — BASIC AND APPLIED

by John D. Banovetz, M.D.

Before considering the practical and theoretical use of topical drugs in the ear, nose, and throat, the special features of the surfaces receiving the drugs must be emphasized. The normal ear canal is a short, dry, curved passage lined by cornified squamous epithelium resting without a subcutaneous layer directly on the underlying cartilage and bone. Epithelial debris follows a pattern of migration from the central drumhead to its periphery and out the canal. Only in the cartilaginous canal are found sebaceous and apocrine glands producing a unique secretion of protective value — cerumen. This cerumen contains a high percentage of fatty acids, and the best solution to dissolve and disperse it is water. The pH of the normal ear canal is slightly acid. Nasal mucosa is a highly specialized tissue consisting of epithelium and submucosa of varying thicknesses whose primary function is to expand or contract as a valve, allowing ingress and egress of air. Thickness varies with the impact of air currents; it is greater in the turbinates and septum and thinner in the sinuses. Typically the epithelium is ciliated and pseudostratified, but on exposed surfaces the cells approach a squamous appearance. Beneath the epithelium the turbinate and septal stroma contain cavernous venous sinuses which, by filling or emptying, adjust the nasal lumen. All this is richly supplied by cutaneous sympathetic and parasympathetic nerve fibers. Usually there is a cyclic rhythm in which the two sides of the nose are alternately congested or patent. Blanket pH is very close to 7.0 but may fluctuate a few tenths in normal noses. Cycling of nasal pH occurs with the menstrual cycle, an alkaline shift coinciding with the onset of menses. Lysozyme is considered to be a nasal defense in the mucous blanket and may be less active with an alkaline shift. However, menstruating women do not seem to be more susceptible to infection.

Ciliary action can be impaired to some degree at least by almost all drugs, and this impairment increases with concentration and time of exposure. Surface active agents, temperature variations, drying cigarette smoke, and toxic fumes like ammonia depress the cilia. Mineral oil preparations slow up the cilia and are cleared with great difficulty. Epinephrine in 1:1000 concentrations stops cilia but in very weak strengths has no effect. Weak solutions of phenylephrine do not harm cilia. Ephedrine up to 3 per cent is safe. Cilia can withstand some variation in tonicity (0.25 to 2.0 per cent), but limits are present and extremes stop the cilia; isotonic saline is the vehicle of choice for nasal medication. Tetracaine can stop ciliary activity at concentrations of 0.15 per cent or greater and should not be used for surface anesthesia. Dibucaine is also toxic at clinically used concentrations. Chlorprocaine, procaine, and lidocaine fail to produce permanent cell injury at clinically useful concentrations of 5 to 20 per cent. Cocaine appears to occupy a mid-position as regards ciliary toxicity, and the older studies show a 5 per cent concentration to be safe. Topical anesthetics like cocaine and pontocaine may also interfere with olfaction and may inhibit bacterial growth in nasal cultures.

In the mouth and pharynx is noncornifying epithelium with large submucosal lymphocyte aggregates. The nose, pharynx, and external ear have an indigenous bacterial and viral flora, but the middle ear, sinuses, and nasopharynx are sterile. It is into these environments that drugs are applied. Injury or inflammation will result in altered penetration and absorption of all drugs. One mechanism of drug reactions on epithelial surfaces is that the simple chemicals penetrate, combine with body proteins, and induce an immunological response to the conjugate, now an antigen. In some examples, degradation products of some drugs are supposed to combine more readily with body proteins than the drugs themselves. Immunocompetent lymphocytes accumulate in the area and are sensitized. After an incubation period of a week a delayed local tissue reaction can occur.

TOPICAL NASAL DECONGESTANTS

These sympathomimetic drugs include epinephrine, ephedrine, phenylephrine (Neo-Synephrine), propylhexedrine (Benzedrex), and the imidazolines: naphazoline (Privine), oxymetazoline (Afrin), tetrahydrozoline (Tyzine), and xylometazoline (Otrivin). By constricting the small arterioles the flow of blood into engorged edematous tissue is reduced, and the periarterial venous channels are allowed to empty, with resulting decongestion. Vasoconstriction results from a direct action of the drug on the alpha receptors of the vascular smooth muscle. Opening the airway allows blocked secretions to drain from the sinuses and meatus, with relief of subjective symptoms. Topical decongestants provide symptomatic relief regardless of whether the edema is caused by allergy, infection, or trauma. These agents play an important part in rhinologic diagnosis by facilitating visual examination. It is believed that they aid otitis media by opening the pharyngeal end of the eustachian tube, but this is a theory.

The topical application of nasal decongestants sometimes causes transient burning or a dry feeling in the nose. Prolonged use of vasoconstrictors in excessive amounts can lead to a chronic reactive hyperemia termed "rebound." Typically the patient first used the vasoconstrictor once or twice a day and now finds continual use ineffective. Initial vasoconstriction is followed by a secondary vasodilation; mucous cells pour out excessive secretion, and ciliary action is impaired. Combined, all these factors produce severe obstruction; therefore these compounds must be used only for short periods of less than a week. Systemic effects may occur in infants and children given a large number of drops of decongestants, the excess running into the pharynx and being swallowed. Tachycardia has been observed in small children after administration of Neo-Synephrine nose drops. For this reason a child should lie on his side with the head lower than the rest of the body, and only 2 to 3 drops should be placed into the lower nostril. Sweating, drowsiness, coma, somnolence, and shocklike states have been reported in children after administration of naphazoline (Privine) and tetrahydrozoline (Tyzine). Decongestants, especially the imidazoline family, should be used carefully in infants. Systemic effects are less likely to occur in adults. Vasoconstriction and tachycardia are undesirable in patients with hypertension, severe arterial disease (especially coronary or peripheral), and hyperthyroidism. Sympathomimetics have a glycogenolytic effect and may aggravate diabetes. Vasoconstrictors should not be given to patients receiving monoamine oxidase inhibitors (for example, Marplan, Niamid, Nardil, or Parnate) for fear of a severe hypertensive reaction.

Solutions of nasal decongestants are sterile when dispersed but can quickly become contaminated, acting as culture media and, there-

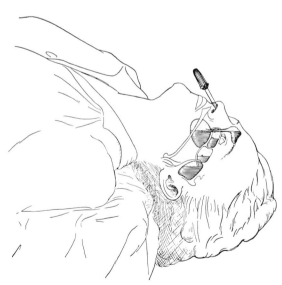

Figure 1 The "head low" position for the instillation of nose drops. In this procedure, only a small amount of medication is used (usually 5 to 10 drops), which would not be enough to produce a fluid level in the sinuses to the point shown in this illustration. In fact, the simple instillation of nose drops does not allow medication to enter the sinuses to any degree. In "displacement irrigation," however, several cubic centimenters of medication are used to produce a fluid level in the sinuses. (Boies, L. R., et al.: Fundamentals of Otolaryngology.)

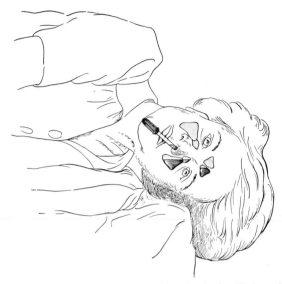

Figure 2 The Parkinson position for the instillation of nose drops. This represents the most desirable position with the patient on a side with her head lower than her shoulders. The nose drops are then introduced into the dependent nostril. Again, no medication actually forms this much of a level within the sinuses, but the aim of the procedure is to introduce a medication to produce vasoconstriction of the mucosa of the nasal space including the sinus ostia. (Boies, L. R., et al.: Fundamentals of Otolaryngology.)

alcohol 0.6 ml. and glycerin 0.6 ml. in normal saline 120 ml. The saline and glycerin lubricate and coat the mucosa, while the alcohol irritates the mucosa to stimulate mucous flow. Premarin has also been useful in this condition. Twenty milligrams are dissolved in 30 ml. normal saline and sprayed three times a day; its effects last as long as the medication is used, and the tissues revert back to the atrophic state on cessation of therapy. Biopsy of the mucosa shows thickening and regeneration.

In 1930 Dowling recommended packs of 10 per cent nitrate in glycerin and water inserted into the nose and left for 20 to 30 minutes. These were irritative, producing vasoconstriction and an outpouring of mucus. When the pack is removed, the patient blows out considerable secretion and feels relieved. Usually this treatment is repeated daily for five to seven days and a cumulative effect is noted. Unfortunately the place of this pack in rhinologic therapy has been lost because it has been used as a substitute for thoughtful diagnosis and because it was wrongly assumed to be antiseptic.

fore, reservoirs of reinfection. Patients should discard the bottle when the need for medication has passed, not be allowed to use the bottle with another person, and not present a previously used bottle to the pharmacist for refill. Between times of use the dropper should be dried and not allowed to stand in the bottle.

OLDER NASAL MEDICATIONS

Displacement irrigation is useful technique for treatment of ethmoiditis (Fig. 4). A nasal decongestant such as 0.5 per cent ephedrine in normal saline is used. Because of alternating suction several milliliters of solution may enter the sinus. Mucolytic agents like the enzymes trypsin and pancreatic desoxyribonuclease or acetylcysteine can be used. Clinical reports state their value, but controlled double-blind studies are few.

With advancing age there is drying and atrophy of the nasal mucosa. This atrophy is senile and not to be confused with idiopathic atrophic rhinitis. Sniffing of saline intranasally and the use of home humidifiers helps humidify the aging tissues. A symptomatic mildly irritating application is a nose drop of ethyl

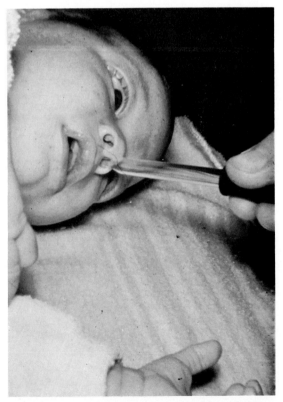

Figure 3 Inadvertent drug ingestion with resultant toxicity can be avoided by inserting nasal medications with infants in a side position. The excess will run out of the nose.

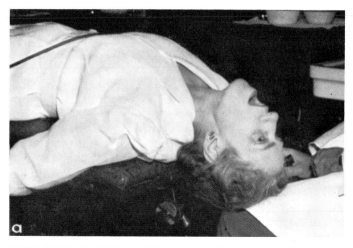

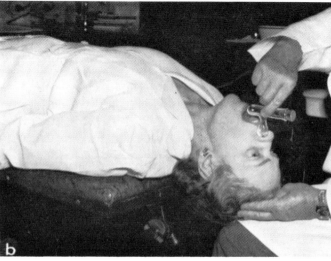

Figure 4 *(a)* The position of the patient for displacement irrigation. The patient is requested to breathe entirely by mouth, the medication is instilled into the side to be treated and tip of the suction bulb is inserted *(b)*, and alternate action and release of negative pressure is produced by holding a finger on and off the vent in the suction bulb while the opposite nostril is occluded by compression by the thumb of the operator's free hand. (Boies, L. R., et al.: Fundamentals of Otolaryngology.)

TOPICAL USE OF STEROIDS

Corticosteroids are normally poorly absorbed through intact skin, but inflamed or denuded skin can absorb large amounts as evidenced by studies with radioactive labeling and changes in serum and urinary 17-hydroxycorticosteroids. The amount absorbed varies with concentration, potency, vehicle, duration of treatment, size of area treated, use of occlusive dressings, and metabolism of the drug, as well as the epidermal barrier. As with systemic steroids, the effect of absorbed locally applied steroids depends upon the daily steroid fluctuations. To exert their effects, topical steroids must reach the vascular layer of the dermis. Edema has resulted from local use of a 9-α-fluorohydrocortisone, but clinical hypercorticism is rare from topical use. Adrenal suppression is a hazard, and precautions should be taken to minimize the amount absorbed. Stress may aggravate an otherwise unnoticed adrenal suppression. Topical agents of equivalent activity are 1 per cent hydrocortisone, 0.5 per cent prednisone, 0.1 per cent triamcinolone acetonide, 0.05 per cent urandrenolone, 0.025 per cent fluocinolone acetonide, 0.1 per cent dexamethazone 21-phosphate, and 0.25 per cent methylprednisolone acetate.

As early as 1951 Dill reported empirically that cortisone applied topically to the nose had a beneficial effect. Edema and secretions lessened and polyps became smaller. Topical corticosteroids should not be used on infections unless concomitant systemic therapy is given; rarely, pharyngeal fungal infections have occurred with topical steroids. Nasal polyps tend to recur when the steroids are stopped.

TOPICAL ANTIBACTERIAL THERAPY

Antiseptics

Ammoniated mercury ointment is an excellent older drug for limited use in the ear or nose. The mercury salts are safe for small areas because absorption is limited; however, since sensitivity may result, they have been largely replaced by antibiotic ointments. Hydrogen peroxide is a weak germicide whose chief benefit is its cleansing action. Boric acid is widely used as an ear dusting powder but has low antiseptic effectiveness and can cause fatal poisoning in infants if ingested or inhaled excessively. A commonly used prescription is:

> Boric acid) equal ⎫
> Neomycin) parts ⎬ to 2.5 gm.
> Hydrocortisone 25 mg.

Sig.: Insufflate three times daily from DeVilbiss 119 Powder Blower. Other antibiotics such as chloramphenicol may be substituted for neomycin.

Zinc stearate or absorbable dusting powder may be substituted. Boric acid is also used as a saturated solution in 70 or 95 per cent ethyl alcohol. This tincture owes its merit to the alcohol and not to the boric acid; it is mildly antiseptic and hydroscopic.

Antibiotics

The early use of sulfonamides and penicillins on the skin showed that hypersensitivity reactions could develop, which would preclude the patient's using the drug for a serious infection. To avoid sensitization, topical application of antibiotics should be limited to a short period, with use of a drug not likely to be needed systemically. Steroids are often combined with antibiotics to suppress inflammation; they usually do not prevent a hypersensitivity response to the antimicrobial. Penicillin, sulfonamides, tetracycline, and chloramphenicol are likely to cause reactions; neomycin, bacitracin, polymyxin, and colistin are examples of antibiotics that are of low toxicity topically but must be used with caution systemically. Bacitracin has a spectrum similar to that of penicillin, affecting gram-positive organisms including some staphylococci. Neomycin has a broad spectrum, being active against both gram-positive and gram-negative organisms. Polymyxin and colistin affect gram-negative organisms but are particularly effective against Pseudomonas.

Combinations of antibiotics may be used to widen the coverage. Topically they are quite safe, with the exception of neomycin which, if applied to a noninflamed ear, may be absorbed, with resulting ototoxicity. In ears containing hyperplastic mucosa there is still a lessened but real danger of absorption. Neomycin has been used as an irrigating solution for sinus tracts, for bowel preparation, and for long-term topical application. From these uses occasional examples of absorption with resulting nephrotoxicity and ototoxicity have been observed. Usually systemic penetration is poor. Applied to the normal middle ear chloramphenicol has been shown to be ototoxic also. Recently neomycin has been blamed increasingly for skin sensitization reactions, although the incidence is still low. This may explain instances in which external otitis improved and then worsened again. To avoid such sensitivity reactions, use of topical neomycin should be limited to a week at most.

In addition to topical antibiotics a variety of other agents are combined for local use in the ear. Normally the pH of the ear canal skin is slightly acid, but infected canal skin becomes alkaline. Ear drops are frequently acidified with acetic acid for this reason. Acetic acid also has mild bactericidal and fungicidal properties. Alcohol or propylene glycol are added for hydroscopic effect, preventing water maceration of the canal skin. Detergents may be added for surface wetting and spreading effect. Cresatin, metacresyl acetate, a phenol derivative, and 2 per cent salicylic acid in alcohol are fungicidal.

Severe external otitis, like any severe dermatitis, requires mild treatment. Burow's solution 1:20 (aluminum subacetate and glacial acetic acid) is nonsensitizing and nontoxic. Dressings wet with the solution mechanically debride crusts and are mildly antiseptic.

Ear drops are commonly prescribed for pain accompanying otitis media. Ten grains of phenol dissolved in one ounce of glycerin were formerly used, but this preparation has been discarded; the phenol caused desquamation of the drumhead and ear canal. Auralgan, a proprietary containing antipyrine and benzocaine in glycerin, can be used. Five to ten drops are instilled warm every two hours. Pain relief, as a rule, is better accomplished by systemic than by topical medication.

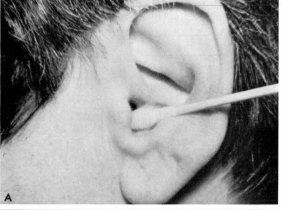
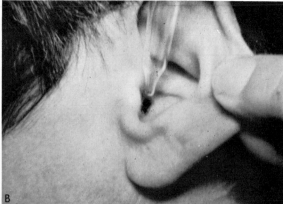
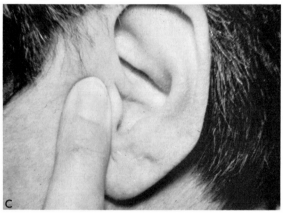

Figure 5 Technique of inserting ear drops. The ear to be treated should be upright so the ear canal is vertical. *A,* Excessive debris is removed from the outer part of the canal. No attempt is made to wipe the drumhead. *B,* At least 3 to 4 drops of medication is used. *C,* To and fro pressure on the tragus helps ballot the medication inward. After a 30 second wait, the patient may arise and the excess be allowed to run from the ear canal.

PREOPERATIVE SURFACE PREPARATION

It is impossible to sterilize the skin because most of its bacterial flora are too deeply imbedded to be removed without injury to the tissue. For the most part these are nonpathogenic flora. There are many superficial organisms that can be removed by skin preparations. Preliminary scrubbing of the skin before surgery is an established adjunct for removing bacteria or rendering them noninfective. Iodine is one of the most effective bactericides known and is used as a 2 per cent aqueous or alcoholic solution; alcohol is not essential for its use. Less irritating to the tissue and hopefully, but not positively, as effective as simple iodine are the iodophors like Betadine or Virac. These are complexes of iodine in a carrier from which it is slowly released.

Several quaternary ammonium compounds like benzalkonium (Zephiran) and cetylpyridinium (Ceepryn) are used for skin preparation. They are cationic detergents and their action is decreased by soap (anionic detergent); hence, their use must be preceded by rinsing away of soap with water and 70 per cent alcohol. *Pseudomonas aeruginosa* and *Mycobacterium tuberculosis* are resistant to quaternary ammonium compounds; *Staphylococcus aureus* is usually susceptible to concentrations of 1:1000. Hexachlorophene is a chlorinated phenol more effective against gram-positive than gram-negative organisms. It has no action on the tubercle bacillus or spores and should be used repeatedly for best effect. Daily scrubbing keeps the bacterial count low but may cause skin dryness. Tamed iodine, hexachlorophene followed by detergent, and hexachlorophene with soap all provide excellent skin preparation and a low rebound bacterial growth. Scrubbing must also be mechanically thorough, being done by a counted stroke method or for a timed period. The longer the scrubbing is done, the more thorough the removal of bacteria. Shaving of the skin should be done just before surgery rather than on the preceding night. Micro injury and tiny razor lacerations provide entry for bacteria and possible infection.

Other measures must be utilized with local anti-infectives. For example, mechanical measures for removing foreign material and assuring drainage are more important than the topical application of an antiseptic to a wound. Meticulous cleanliness must always accompany the use of local anti-infectives.

Preparation of the ear canal before elective surgery concerns the otologist. Normal ear canals usually contain only bacteria of low pathogenicity (diphtheroids and coagulase-negative staphylococci). *Staphylococcus aureus,* coagulase positive, is rare but is the most commonly recovered pathogen. A variety of local anti-infectious agents have been used in various studies, all of them successfully. Although no one has proved a correlation between sensorineural hearing loss after surgery and the presence of pathogenic bacteria preoperatively, such is suspected. Of greatest importance is the examination of the ear canals preoperatively, with postponement of elective surgery in the presence of a treatable infection. For example, stapedectomy when there is a mild external otitis should be preceded by a thorough mechanical cleaning of the canal for removal of debris and cerumen. Of less importance is the type of preparation used, provided it is not caustic; the total time spent cleaning is more important.

TOPICAL MEDICATION FOR THE THROAT

Definitive topical treatment of pharyngeal disease is not possible except in monilial infections, for which nystatin is used. For the most part treatment is symptomatic. Patients, feeling better after use of these adjuncts, will continue treatment, but the critical physician must regard them as art, not science. Painting of sore throats with 2 per cent silver nitrate or Mandel's solution is comforting but certainly not antibacterial. The formula is:

Iodine	0.3 mg.
Potassium iodide	0.3 mg.
Glycerin	30.0 ml.
Oil of gaultheria	0.3 mg.

Medicated troches do not deliver drugs below the epithelial surface but may have some surface cleansing action. They should always carry a low risk of sensitization.

Gargles and throat irrigations are best done with normal saline as warm as can be tolerated. Useful solutions include (1) isotonic saline solution made by dissolving 1/2 teaspoonful of table salt in one full glass of hot water; and (2) one teaspoonful sodium perborate powder dissolved in a glass of hot water. The old Dobell's solution is:

Sodium borate	15.0 cc.
Sodium bicarbonate	15.0 cc.
Liquefied phenol	3.0 cc.
Glycerin	35.0 cc.
Water	1000.0 cc.

One part of this is used in one or two parts of hot water. Throat irrigations are more effective in delivering solution to the pharynx than gargles. Gargling closes the anterior tonsillar pillars.

TOPICAL USE OF DRUGS IN THE MIDDLE EAR AND MASTOID

Since the infancy of otology, topical drugs have been inserted into chronically infected ears. The key question is whether they may adversely affect the hearing, balance, or epithelium while performing their main purpose. With the advent of stapes surgery and tympanoplasty, new emphasis has been placed on drugs because they are now used in surgery for noninfectious conditions.

In the 1930's a number of studies were done in which crystals were placed on the round window and the hearing measured. Cocaine, quinine, procaine, sodium chloride, and calcium chloride all depressed the cochlea. Saline solution did not adversely affect the hearing, and Fowler noted boric acid had little effect.

It is well known that the antibiotics neomycin, streptomycin, and kanamycin applied to a clean noninfected middle ear can cause toxicity. Streptomycin has been used in this way to destroy the ear in Meniere's disease. This danger is less acute in a chronically inflamed ear or mastoid bowl with thick hyperplastic mucosa. In this situation the risk seems more hypothetical than real.

Other antibiotics have also been implicated. The topical use of chloramphenicol has been followed by cochlear damage in man, and in guinea pigs decreased electrical potentials have been measured. Polymyxin, too, has proved toxic in animals, primarily to the vestibular system. What of the drugs used in elective surgery? Epinephrine 1:1000 applied to the round window has no deleterious effect on the electrical potentials. Even when introduced into the scala tympani, epinephrine had no

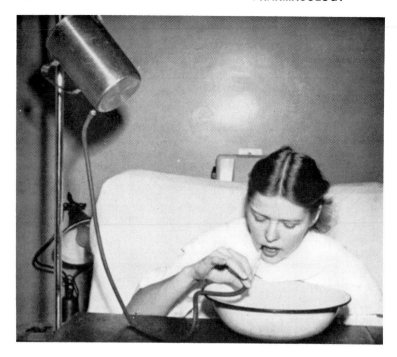

Figure 6 The equipment for and the position of the patient taking a hot throat irrigation. (Boies, L. R., et al.: Fundamentals of Otolaryngology.)

adverse effects; therefore, it can be used in stapes surgery even with an open oval window. Cocaine 10 per cent, tetracaine 2 per cent, and hexylcaine 5 per cent caused severe depression of the cochlea. Procaine 2 per cent, lidocaine 1 per cent, and hexylcaine 1 per cent allowed full recovery of the cochlear potentials and seem a good choice for surgery.

MISCELLANEOUS TOPICAL DRUGS

Hemostatic Agents

Thrombin is prepared from bovine prothrombin for topical use to control small vessel and capillary bleeding. Gelfoam is a gelatin base sponge that is completely absorbed and is used to stem capillary bleeding. It has no hemostatic property beyond providing a large surface area. Oxycel (oxidized cellulose) is a treated surgical gauze that promotes clotting by a reaction between hemoglobin and cellulose acid. It inhibits epithelialization and usually absorbs in a week.

Enzymes

The use of several enzymes has been proposed for lessening surgical and traumatic edema, such as plant protease concentrate, chymotrypsin, streptokinase-streptodornase, amylase, and proteolytic enzymes from carica papaya. The rationale is that these enzymes break down fibrin, preventing it from occluding the capillary and lymph vessels of edematous tissue. Chymotrypsin has been used topically to dissolve viscous middle ear fluid, facilitating its removal. Carica papaya enzymes have been used when the esophagus is plugged by a meat bolus without bone in it. When the meat is softened the bolus can pass into the stomach. Streptokinase-streptodornase has been used topically as a debriding agent. Whether given orally or intramuscularly, these drugs have not been universally accepted. In edema of traumatic or inflammatory origin patients are difficult to compare objectively and to watch for study purposes. Some physicians feel these drugs are not of value. Side effects from topical or oral use have been few. Intramuscularly, chymotrypsin, being an antigen, can cause anaphylactic reactions. Plant protease concentrate and enzymes from carica papaya may augment anticoagulants and are contraindicated in such patients.

Antihistamines

Topical use of antihistamines is likely to give rise to skin or mucosal sensitivity reactions; therefore, the systemic route is preferred.

WATER VAPOR THERAPY

Water is a major therapeutic agent used in respiratory tract disease. One must understand the physics and biology of vapor and aerosol treatment. Water vapor and humidity refer to gaseous water, sometimes termed "molecular water." Relative humidity is the ratio of the actual amount of water vapor present in air to the total amount of water vapor the air could hold; it always pertains to a specific temperature. Aerosol, by definition, is the suspension of minute particles of liquid in a gas. These particles are visible; hence, the term "mist" or "fog." Aerosols are classified on the basis of particle size and on the volume of vehicle aerosolized per minute. Usually this is milliliters of water per minute. Particle size may vary from 100 to 0.005 μ, but commonly aerosols are in the 10 to 0.1 μ range.

The machines used to produce water therapy are humidifiers and aerosol generators, although they overlap in both function and application; some machines produce more water vapor and are primarily humidifiers and others produce more particulate water and are aerosol generators. The jet type machines employ the Venturi principle and are commonly used heated and unheated both for humidifiers and generators. A pass-over humidifier blows air across a heated reservoir. Impellor machines use rotating fins or spinning discs for breaking water into particles and throwing it into the air. In ultrasonic generators high frequency sound waves break up the water into the very small particles able to penetrate the lower respiratory tract.

There is a definite relationship between particle size in aerosols and depth of deposition in the respiratory tree. Because of their inertia when suspended in the air stream, larger particles tend to deposit on the walls of the upper airway, trachea, and major bronchi. For example, large particles of 50 to 100 μ are deposited in the nose and larynx. Few particles over 10 μ penetrate beyond the larynx; to reach the alveoli, particles must be in the range of 1 to 5 μ. Here inertial impaction is no longer the mechanism of deposition, but sedimentation occurs in the smaller bronchioles. In the smallest alveoli brownian movement causes particle deposition. For therapy the nebulizer should provide particle size that will deposit in the area being treated; for example, in treatment of croup a large particle is necessary. Other factors also affect the deposition of particles in the respiratory tract. The smaller the bronchial tree, the greater the deposition at any particular size, and the smaller the particle needed to reach the bronchiole. The slower the respiratory rate and the deeper the breath, the greater the deposition.

Humidifiers are used to aid the respiratory tree in supplying water vapor to inspired gases. The nose, pharynx, and upper trachea guarantee that each cubic meter of inspired air contains 44 gm. of water vapor. If they are unable to do so, water moves from the lower respiratory tract mucosa to the gas. Breathing dry gas from a tank, or the presence of impervious mucosal crusts on airway surfaces, may produce a "humidity deficit." Temporary loss of nasal function after nasal surgery or after laryngectomy can ordinarily be compensated, but when combined with dry winter air as in the Northern states, pathologic dryness can occur.

Aerosols deliver water to the respiratory tree to dilute secretions and to moisten crusts, making easier their removal by cough or by ciliary action. Aerosol water may also evaporate, adding to a gas's water vapor level.

In spite of its many benefits, there are hazards to clinical use of water vapor. Hoffman and Finberg (1955) noted a rise in Pseudomonas infections coincident with the increased use of high humidity atmospheres in newborn nurseries. It is for practical purposes almost impossible to prevent bacterial contamination of water used for vapor therapy and, hence, contamination of patients. Nevertheless, strict housekeeping and sterilization techniques must be used. Aseptic techniques must be used in changing tracheostomy tubes and in performing tracheal suction. Only in this way can contamination be minimized.

Concern has been expressed that aerosol water may be retained, leading to water intoxication. Ordinarily this is not an important aspect of total body fluid maintenance, but it may become important in a uremic patient or a newborn.

If a patient is in a high environmental temperature, the respiratory tree must play a role in heat dissipation. Ordinarily most heat loss occurs through the skin, but this loss can be negated by high environmental temperature. Should the respiratory avenue also be blocked by breathing a hot, humid mist, heat retention hyperpyrexia may occur, with heavy cardiovascular strain. There is no evidence that the lung is damaged by high density mist. Shakoor et al. (1968) were unable to demonstrate changes in surfactant activity, pulmonary mechanics, or histological appearance of lung exposed to ultrasonically suspended mist inhaled directly into the trachea.

Patients with upper respiratory infections are more comfortable breathing well humidified air, but there is no good evidence that mist therapy favorably alters the disease. Unheated jet or spinning disc machines together with tents are sufficient and are well tolerated, even for long periods.

Following tracheostomy at least 70 per cent of the water normally supplied by the proximal airway should be provided for the patient. Thirty grams per cubic meter is the minimal acceptable water content. Heated vapor or jet nebulizers and ultrasonic nebulizers can supply this level, but unheated nebulizers and bubble humidifiers cannot.

To propel inhaled mist beyond the carina, there must be a water content over 44 gm./cu. m., and there must be minimal baffling in the upper airways. Nasal breathing offers too much baffling effect and oral breathing requires a maximum effort to retract the palate and soft tissues. Tracheostomy or endotracheal tube are necessary, together with an ultrasonic or highly efficient jet nebulizer for maximal deposition in the distal bronchi. Baffling as well as particle size is important for pulmonary water deposition.

REFERENCES

Boies, L. R., Hilger, J. A., and Priest, R. E.: Fundamentals of Otolaryngology. Philadelphia, W. B. Saunders Company, 1964.

Corssean, G., and Allen, C. R.: Cultured human respiratory epithelium: Its use in comparison of the cytotoxic properties of local anesthetics. Anesthesiology 21:237, 1960.

Dowling, J. I.: Non-surgical treatment of ethmoiditis. Laryngoscope 40:633, 1930.

Egan, D. F.: Humidity and water aerosol therapy. Conn. Med. 31:353, 1967.

Graff, T. D., and Benson, D. W.: Systemic and pulmonary changes with inhaled humid atmospheres. Anesthesiology 30:199, 1969.

Gulick, W. L., and Cutt, R. A.: The effect of epinephrine upon the ear. Ann. Otol. 71:105, 1962.

Hoffman, M. A., and Finberg, L.: Pseudomonas infections in infants associated with humidity environments. J. Pediat. 46:625, 1955.

Seudi, J. V., Kimura, R. T., and Reinhard, J. F.: Study of drug action on mammalian ciliated epithelium. J. Pharmacol. Exp. Ther. 102:132, 1951.

Shakoor, M., Sabean, J., Wilson, K., Hurt, H., and Graff, T.: High density water environment by ultrasonic humidification: Pulmonary and systemic effects. Anesth. Analg. (Cleveland) 47:638, 1968.

Stother, W. F., Parker, D. E., Rahm, W. E., and Crump, J. F.: The effects of anesthetics upon the ear. Ann. Otol. 69:969, 1960; 70:403, 1961; 71:116, 1962; 73:141, 1964.

Chapter 17

SYSTEMIC DRUGS

by Donald B. Hunninghake, M.D., and John D. Banovetz, M.D.

Rather than try to cover all systemic drugs and, in effect, cover none, this chapter deals with those most frequently prescribed by otolaryngologists. Antibiotics, corticosteroids, antivertiginous agents, antihistamines and antitussives are reviewed, with a statement of the broad principles of their use. Since deafness and vertigo can result from administration of many drugs, ototoxic medication must be discussed. For more complete pharmacological experience, the reader should consult the classic texts.

OTOTOXIC DRUGS

Inner ear damage is an infrequent but serious sequela of drug use. At present, most labyrinthine injury results from salicylates and a group of streptomyces-derived antibiotics. Quinine, nitrogen mustard, chloroquine, and ethacrynic acid are also ototoxic.

Suspended in a fluid-filled labyrinth of the temporal bone is the inner ear with its cochlear and vestibular divisions. Sound waves or head motion cause waves in this fluid, distorting the sensory hair-containing cells. This distortion of the hair cell is the mechanism for transfer of mechanical wave energy to neuroelectrical energy. There are an abundance of mitochondria and a rich supply of enzymes in the hair cells and the adjacent striae vascularis and nerve endings. Glucose is probably the principal source of energy for the inner ear. The primary site of action of ototoxic drugs in the ear is not known but is probably in the enzymes of the hair cell.

Evidence indicates that ototoxic drugs have an affinity for the cochlea, accumulating selectively and interfering with energy supply. Although studies have shown equivocal central nervous system effects of these drugs, they have shown destroyed otic labyrinths in both experimental animals and human temporal bones. These otic findings can well explain the vertigo and deafness observed clinically. After ingestion of the drugs, the first finding is degeneration of the hair cells of the cochlea, cristae of the semicircular canals and maculae of the saccule and utricle. As the dosage increases, destruction spreads until the whole end-organ is destroyed (Meuwissen and Robinson, 1967; El-Mofty and El-Serafy, 1966).

Salicylates

Salicylate ototoxicity is unique in that it is reversible. No histologic changes have ever been observed following high doses of salicylates. Salicylates are known to inhibit at least three groups of cellular enzymes in intermediary metabolism, and this enzyme inhibition may produce the otologic effect. Salicylates have been demonstrated in the striae vascularis and spiral ligament. The sodium, potassium, and protein levels of inner ear fluids are unchanged after salicylate ingestion. Salicylates are rapidly metabolized and excreted by the kidney.

Acute ingestion of large doses of salicylates, as in suicide attempts, produces a characteristic picture. Tinnitus and a bilateral sensorineural flat hearing loss develop (Meyers and Bernstein, 1965). Discrimination for speech stays good. The salicylate level usually produces hearing loss at about 20 mg. per 100 ml. and roughly rises with worsening hearing loss. Hearing loss reaches about 40 decibels when the blood level reaches 40 mg. per 100 ml.; it stays at this level even if the blood level rises.

Vestibular reaction measured by Halpike calorics and electronystagmoidography shows depressed function. Silverstein et al. (1967) have shown depression of the cochlear microphonic.

Falbe-Hansen in the 1940's stated that small doses of salicylates would in time accumulate and affect the ear. McCabe and Dey (1965) studied young women taking 15 five-grain tablets per day for four days and noted hearing reduced as a function of time. These patients all had serum salicylate level of 20 mg. per 100 ml. or higher. The salicylate level seems to be the key to the development of toxic effects, since many patients have taken salicylates daily for years without harm.

Antibiotics

Streptomycin, kanamycin, neomycin and gentamycin are the principal ototoxic antibiotics in clinical use. Dihydrostreptomycin has been removed from the market because of its severe erratic ototoxicity and lack of unique antimicrobial advantage.

These drugs must be given parenterally because of poor gastrointestinal absorption. However, in inflamed or obstructed bowel, absorption may be much greater. Healthy bowel absorbs 3 per cent of neomycin, but severe toxicity has resulted from giving neomycin in the presence of inflamed bowel mucosa, in hepatic disease, in repeated colon irrigations or in chronic skin ulcers. Normal skin does not absorb these drugs, but burned or damaged skin may.

After intramuscular injection these drugs are rapidly distributed, and peak concentrations result in the blood within a few hours. Streptomycin, kanamycin and neomycin penetrate the ear more slowly, reaching a peak concentration later. They are also eliminated more slowly, so that repeated doses can lead to accumulation. Interestingly, neomycin, the most ototoxic, is the slowest to leave the inner ear fluids. It should be emphasized that the levels in the blood are not equal to or even necessarily related to the inner ear levels (Table 1). The slow release may also explain why ototoxic effects persist or even get worse after the drug has been discontinued. Penetration of the inner ear is enhanced by the presence of a concurrent otitis media.

If renal function is normal, these antibiotics are eliminated largely unchanged. Renal concentrations may become very high; hence, they are effective renal antibiotics. All these drugs penetrate the central nervous system, with the possible exceptions of kanamycin and gentamycin. Kanamycin probably penetrates, but there is some disagreement on this point. Gentamycin penetrates poorly; adequate cerebrospinal fluid levels usually cannot be achieved by intramuscular injection alone but require intraventricular injection (Newman and Holt, 1967).

Since removal of these drugs depends almost entirely on the kidney, in renal failure a single dose may require days for excretion. Even regular doses will give excessive plasma levels which will add to the renal tubular damage and augment ototoxicity. Renal excretion depends upon the glomerular filtration rate, and newborns with their immature filtration mechanisms will retain these drugs. In one study the plasma half-life of kanamycin in infants less than 18 hours old averaged 18 hours in comparison with two hours for adults (Eichenwald, 1967).

Clinically the main factors that determine ototoxicity are the plasma concentration and the duration of the drug therapy. The cause of excessive plasma concentration is usually poor renal function. Pre-existing renal disease, renal newborn immaturity, increasing age, pre-existing hearing loss, and the use of two or more ototoxic drugs predispose to ototoxicity.

In the presence of renal disease patients should be treated according to Kunin's (1967) routines. These reduce the dose with *compromised* renal function on a scheduled basis.

Hearing loss usually affects the high tones first but can progress to all frequencies. There

TABLE 1. Relative Effects of Ototoxic Antibiotics

DRUG	VESTIBULE	COCHLEA	KIDNEY
Streptomycin	4+	+	+
Dihydrostreptomycin	+	4+	+
Neomycin	+	4+	3+
Kanamycin	+	3+	3+
Gentamycin	4+	+	+

may or may not be a latent period. Tinnitus or aural pressure may or may not accompany the hearing loss. It is not safe to expect tinnitus to precede the loss or to wait for audiometric changes before stopping the drug. The loss may progress to total deafness even if the drug is stopped. Hearing loss may even begin after the drug has been stopped. There is no effective treatment for the loss, and no drug can be concurrently administered to block ototoxicity. The panthoxenate salts of streptomycin and kanamycin have been tried but they have not been less ototoxic. Vertigo may accompany the hearing loss also; streptomycin is unique in that it usually causes vertigo before hearing loss. Ototoxic hearing loss is always permanent.

Vertigo can also progress to severe ataxia, but with time some compensation occurs.

The following are precautions to observe to aid in the prevention of ototoxicity: Minimum effective doses should be employed for as short a duration as feasible. Avoid sequential or concurrent use with other ototoxic drugs. Extreme caution must be employed when these drugs are used in a patient with renal failure. Question the patient about aural pressure and tinnitus and stop therapy when they appear. Auditory and renal function should be evaluated at least weekly. Special care must be used if the patient has pre-existing hearing loss. Lastly, the patient should be kept well hydrated.

Streptomycin. Streptomycin is one of the safer ototoxic drugs because it usually causes vertigo first and only later tinnitus and hearing loss. It has greater affinity for the vestibular system than the auditory.

The risk of developing vertigo from a total dose of 1 gm. per day is slight for treatment periods up to one month. If the dose is 2 gm. per day, vertigo is likely to develop during the second week. Barr et al. (1949) noted that the vestibular risk was small in daily doses of 0.5 to 1.0 gm., provided the total dose did not exceed 60 grams.

In another study Tompsett (1948) noted that less than 20 per cent of patients developed vestibular dysfunction if given 1 gm. a day for as long as four months. Intermittent therapy is less likely to cause toxic symptoms than daily therapy. Recommended doses for children are 15-30 mg./kg./day, with the lower dose chosen for prematures and newborns. Loss of hearing from streptomycin therapy administered with these precautions is unusual. If streptomycin is used intrathecally, severe deafness results.

Use of streptomycin has been studied in pregnant women for its effects on the fetal ear. Robinson (1964) has reported complete infant deafness and loss of caloric response after administration of 16 and 26 gm. of streptomycin. He cites this as a rare occurrence. Conway (1965) studied 17 children whose mothers received streptomycin during pregnancy and found real but mild defects in balance and audition.

Dihydrostreptomycin, in contrast to streptomycin, is a real villain, because it can cause severe permanent hearing loss even after it has been stopped. It is erratic and unpredictable; fortunately dihydrostreptomycin is no longer medically available in the United States (Shambaugh et al., 1959).

Kanamycin. Kanamycin is not so toxic as neomycin if used with strict precautions. In adults 1 or 2 gm. per day can be used for seven to ten days. Finegold (1966) reports only mild ototoxicity if the dose is 15 mg./kg./day or less in adults. In young patients with good kidney function at least 32 gm. were required to produce hearing loss; some patients tolerated 134 gm. before hearing loss ensued. In patients with renal insufficiency, as little as 5 gm. has caused deafness. Long-term studies of newborns treated with kanamycin for neonatal sepsis with 12-15 mg./kg./day failed to show any hearing loss.

In contrast to streptomycin, kanamycin can be removed by peritoneal dialysis. Kanamycin probably does not pass the placenta to any appreciable extent (Finegold, 1966).

Neomycin. When first introduced, neomycin was used parenterally, but as little as 8 gm. in four days was found to cause deafness. Now it has been largely restricted to topical or oral use. Kanamycin has the same wide antibacterial spectrum and is less toxic. Only 3 per cent of the ingested dose is absorbed from the gastrointestinal tract, but in the presence of diseased bowel or repeated use, toxic blood levels may be reached. Deafness has occurred following the treatment of prolonged diarrhea with neomycin in Kaopectate and following repeated use for irrigating sinus tracts. Neomycin's effects have been primarily cochlear, but in severe poisoning vestibular damage may occur as well.

Like the other ototoxic drugs, neomycin attacks the cochlear hair cells, resulting in permanent sensorineural hearing loss (Greenwood, 1959).

Gentamycin. Gentamycin may be effective when bacteria are resistant to neomycin and kanamycin and is an excellent choice for gram-negative infections caused by Pseudomonas, Proteus, *Escherichia coli* and Klebsiella-Aerobacter. Its most serious side effect is vestibular damage. This usually occurs with excessive plasma levels or in patients with renal failure; serum levels of 10–12 μg./ml. are recommended to reduce the level of ototoxicity. Hearing loss and renal damage are less likely to occur (Jao and Jackson, 1964).

Other Ototoxic Drugs

Polymyxin B. Fortunately the ototoxic effects of polymyxin were discovered when the drug was given to guinea pigs parenterally, and its human use has been restricted to severe gram-negative infections. In guinea pigs it affected the vestibular system to a greater degree than the hearing.

Colistin. This may cause ataxia and deafness if plasma levels are high. It is principally used in Pseudomonas infection at doses of 2–10 mg./kg./day.

Viomycin. This antituberculosis drug has produced vertigo and hearing loss following long-term use. It should never be given concomitantly with streptomycin.

Vancomycin (Vancocin). When given intravenously in high serum concentrations (over 80–95 μg./ml.), hearing loss has resulted. Its use in renal insufficiency may produce hearing loss at lower serum concentrations.

Nitrogen Mustard. This anticancer drug given in high but sublethal doses can produce clinical tinnitus, vertigo, and hearing loss. Cummings has reported typical ototoxic findings in temporal bones of treated patients.

Chloroquine Phosphate. Chloroquine has been used in lupus erythematosus, rheumatoid arthritis, malaria, and scleroderma. It may produce ototoxic symptoms and the typical temporal bone findings. When given to pregnant women, it can cross the placenta, affecting the fetal ear. The fetal ear seems most susceptible during the first trimester (Hart and Naunton, 1964).

Ethacrynic Acid (Edecrin). Ethacrynic acid is a recently developed diuretic that has been implicated as causing hearing loss. This may be transient and usually occurs only in patients with poor renal function. Matz and Naunton demonstrated that an initial reversible hearing loss may become permanent in experimental animals (Schneider and Becker 1966; Matz and Naunton, 1968).

ANTIBACTERIAL AGENTS

The specific diagnosis and treatment of various infectious diseases are discussed in other portions of the text. For each pathogenic organism there is generally one drug, or occasionally a combination of drugs, that is likely to be a better choice—in terms of both effectiveness and safety—than other drugs and combinations. When the patient does not respond to a first-choice drug or cannot tolerate it, there is usually a preferred order of choice among alternative drugs. A recent consensus on the choice of systemic antimicrobial drugs is recommended. Some of the causes of failure are unavoidable, but many are iatrogenic. Causes of failure include incorrect clinical or bacteriological diagnosis; improper selection, method of administration or dosage of drugs; futile prophylaxis; inaccessible lesion; drug resistance; deficiency in host defenses; alteration in bacterial flora and superinfection; and drug toxicity and hypersensitivity (The choice of systemic antimicrobial drugs. Med. Lett. Drugs Ther. *10*:77, 1968).

Penicillin

Penicillin is still the most effective antibiotic for treating a number of infections. It is used primarily to treat infections due to gram-positive cocci in otorhinolaryngology. It is bactericidal in action and appears to interfere with bacterial cell wall formation by interfering with the synthesis of an unique mucopeptide essential to bacterial wall structure. Excretion is primarily by the kidney. The incidence of hypersensitivity reactions has increased and death from anaphylactic shock occurs often enough to cause concern and to re-emphasize that it should not be used indiscriminately. A patient who is allergic to one preparation is very likely allergic to the others. It is true that some of the allergic responses may not be due to penicillin per se but rather to macromolecular components, degradation products, and polymers in the injected material (Stewart, 1970). Skin testing with whole drug, penicilloyl-polylysine, and the rabbit basophil cell degranulation test have been helpful in determining allergic individuals, but are not uniformly reliable.

Penicillin G has two important features that may limit its use. They are destruction in an acid media, which means poor absorption because of rapid destruction in the stomach. Also, many bacteria, primarily staphylococci and a number of gram-negative organisms, secrete penicillinase, which attacks the B-lactam ring of penicillin and inactivates the drug. Newer penicillins have been developed which have varying degrees of resistance to gastric acid or are effective in the presence of penicillinase-producing organisms. Some of the more commonly utilized penicillin preparations are listed here (Friend, 1966 a and b).

Penicillin G. This is administered both orally and parenterally. Absorption after an oral dose is only about 20 per cent, but oral administration may still be satisfactory for treating susceptible organisms. It is less costly than the newer penicillins. Procaine penicillin and benzathine penicillin G (Bicillin) with progressively longer durations of action are the two repository preparations generally used.

Phenoxymethyl penicillin (Pen-Vee K, Compocillin V-K and V-Cillin K). This was the first of the acid-stable penicillins and is very popular for oral administration. It is not penicillinase resistant.

Phenoxyethyl methyl penicillin (Chemipen, Darcil, Dramcillin, Maxipen, Semopen and Syncillin). This drug is also acid resistant and can be given orally, but is not penicillinase resistant.

Methicillin (Staphcillin, Dimocillin R-T). This agent was the first of the penicillinase-resistant penicillins and was a major advance in the treatment of penicillinase-producing staphylococci. It is not acid stable and must be given parenterally. It is unstable in aqueous solutions and rapidly deteriorates in acid solutions. It induces penicillinase activity in staphylococci and resistance may develop. Some feel that it is less potent than other penicillins of this series, but many treatment failures probably occurred because inadequate doses were used.

Oxacillin (Prostaphlin, Resistopen). This drug is both relatively acid resistant and penicillinase resistant. Approximately 60 per cent is absorbed upon oral administration, although absorption tends to be somewhat erratic. It is available only for oral administration and is better absorbed on an empty stomach. It was the first orally effective drug in this series for penicillinase-producing staphylococci and is primarily excreted by the kidney.

Cloxacillin (Tegopen). It is both penicillinase resistant and relatively acid stable; it is available only for oral administration. It differs from oxacillin by having a chlorine in the side chain. It may be better absorbed, absorption is less impaired by food and a significant amount is metabolized by the liver.

Dicloxacillin (Dynapen). This is both acid resistant and penicillinase resistant. It is partially metabolized by the liver and partially excreted by the kidney. It is used only orally.

Nafcillin (Unipen). This drug is relatively acid resistant and penicillinase resistant. Its absorption from the gastrointestinal tract is somewhat erratic and it is partially inactivated by acid. As the soluble sodium salt, it can also be given intramuscularly or intravenously. Thrombophlebitis has occurred following intravenous administration. Approximately 90 per cent is excreted in the bile and 10 per cent in the urine. It is also more stable in solution than methicillin.

Several comments must be made about the five preceding penicillinase-resistant penicillins. There is much discussion about variances in their activity against many gram-positive cocci such as hemolytic streptococci and pneumococci. Depending upon the severity of the infection, penicillin G (parenteral or oral) or penicillin V (oral) is the drug of choice. They are more effective and less expensive. Only if the etiology of the infection is unknown and penicillinase-producing staphylococci are suspected to be involved does this become pertinent. There is also no uniform agreement on the most effective drug in this series for penicillinase-producing staphylococci (Friend, 1966a; Kunin, 1969). Much attention also has been paid to serum levels of these drugs. The pharmacological activity of a drug at any given time is dependent upon the portion of the drug which is not bound to protein. Kunin (1966) has demonstrated that there is considerable variation in the protein binding of these drugs and this must be taken into account.

Ampicillin (Omnipen, Penbritin, Polycillin). It is acid stable and can be given orally and is also available for parenteral administration. It is not penicillinase resistant. It differs from other penicillins in that it has a wider spectrum of action, including many gram-negative organisms. Although extensively used in both adults and children it has been popular in pediatric practice where ears and meninges may be infected with pneumococcus, group A streptococcus, *Haemophilus influenzae*, or meningococcus. There is almost a uniform development of a rash when this drug is administered to patients with pharyngeal lesions associated with infectious mononucleosis. The same side effects occur as are seen with penicillin, but disturbances in liver function and diarrhea appear to be more common. The drug is primarily excreted in the urine, but is also concentrated in the bile.

Cephalosporins

The cephalosporins, which have recently been introduced into therapy, are a group of semisynthetic antibiotics developed from a cephalosporin fungus (Weinstein and Kaplan, 1970). They are active against gram-positive cocci, though less active than penicillin, and are active against certain gram-negative organisms including *Proteus mirabilis*, *E. coli*, *H. influenzae*, and Klebsiella. They inhibit cell wall synthesis. They are primarily excreted by the kidney, so the dose must be reduced in the presence of severe renal disease. They are indicated primarily as an alternative to penicillin in patients who are allergic to penicillin or for treating susceptible gram-negative bacilli infections. They are also active against penicillinase-producing staphylococci, with cephalothin being more active than cephaloridine. Fever, eosinophilia, anaphylaxis, serum sickness, and various skin rashes occur in about 5 per cent of treated patients. A small number of patients who are allergic to penicillin have had anaphylactic reactions when cephalosporins were administered, but there is still disagreement over whether this represents a true cross-sensitization with penicillin (Stewart, 1967). Renal tubular necrosis, primarily following large doses of cephaloridine, has been reported, as have occasional Coombs' positive reactions with cephalothin. The compounds listed here are currently available for clinical use.

Cephalothin (Keflin). This must be administered parenterally and is felt to be more effective than cephaloridine in penicillinase-producing staphylococcal infections and safer in patients with impaired renal function. Intramuscular injection is painful. The most clinical experience is available with this compound.

Cephaloridine (Loridine). It must also be administered parenterally, but is less painful on intramuscular injection than cephalothin.

Cephaloglycine (Kafocin). This drug is fairly well absorbed from the gastrointestinal tract and is administered orally. Administration after meals decreases absorption. This drug has only recently been marketed, and the greatest experience is in management of urinary tract infections.

Erythromycin

Erythromycin is a bacteriostatic drug clinically effective against certain infections caused by gram-positive bacteria, especially beta-hemolytic streptococci, pneumococci and staphylococci. Its spectrum of activity is similar to penicillin, but it is not considered to be so potent as penicillin. For this reason it is not considered a drug of first choice and penicillin is preferred. It is used to treat susceptible infections in patients who are allergic to penicillin, especially in cases of streptococcal pharyngitis. Some physicians wish to avoid the use of penicillin in simple types of gram-positive infections and utilize erythromycin. Penicillinase-resistant penicillins are also the drugs of choice in treating penicillinase-producing staphylococcal infections. Intramuscular administration is painful and irritating. There are many different erythromycin preparations. With the exception of erythromycin estolate (Ilosone), they are all liable to destruction by gastric acid and should preferably be administered when the stomach is empty. Ilosone is acid stable, and higher blood levels have been reported. However, Ilosone produces a hypersensitivity reaction manifested by intrahepatic cholestasis and jaundice.

Lincomycin (Lincocin)

Lincomycin is a bacteriostatic drug with an antibacterial spectrum similar to erythromycin and penicillin G. Its potency, indications for use, as well as the preferences for penicillin are similar to those described for erythromycin. It is generally used interchangeably with erythromycin, but there are two significant differences: One is that lincomycin can be given intramuscularly. Also, the development of resistance by staphylococci appears to be less marked than with erythromycin. Hence, it has been used more for treating staphylococcal infections, but again in severe infections caused by penicillinase-producing staphylococci a penicillinase-resistant penicillin is preferred. The oral form of the drug is absorbed erratically, and gastrointestinal symptoms, especially diarrhea, are common. The hepatotoxicity reported with erythromycin estolate has not been a problem with lincomycin. A chlorinated derivative of lincomycin (Cleocin) has replaced the parent compound for oral administration.

Tetracyclines

The tetracyclines are primarily bacteriostatic in action and act by inhibiting protein synthesis. Generally they are not the drugs of first choice in infections seen by otolaryngologists. Although oral administration with few side effects and their broad spectrum of activity have made them popular, more effective antibiotics for specific infections are available. The older tetracyclines, chlortetracycline (Aureomycin), oxytetracycline (Terramycin) and tetracycline itself are well known. The newer ones include declocycline (Declomycin), methacycline (Rondomycin) and doxycycline (Vibramycin). The primary differences among these drugs are in the rapidity and mode of excretion from the body. The newer tetracyclines have longer durations of action and are administered less frequently, but it does not appear that the antibacterial spectrum of any of the tetracyclines is significantly different. Photosensitization reactions are more frequent with the longer acting tetracyclines. The absorption of all tetracyclines is impaired when they are taken with milk products or drugs containing calcium, magnesium, or aluminum; doxycycline's absorption is least impaired. Hepatic damage is especially likely in pregnant women or in patients with impaired renal function. Adverse effects on the fetus and children up to about 12 years of age include changes in bones and teeth. The various complications related to tetracycline administration, including the Fanconi syndrome from degradation products of outdated tetracycline, have been summarized (Clendenning, 1965).

Chloramphenicol

Despite warnings from the manufacturers and many other sources that chloramphenicol can cause fatal bone marrow injury, misuse of the drug has continued. Because of the possibility of serious adverse effects, especially blood dyscrasias, most Medical Letter consultants believe that chloramphenicol should be used systemically only for the treatment of severe life-threatening infections, and then only when clinical experience indicates that the drug is likely to be more effective than any other agent; or when other effective agents may be more hazardous. In vitro susceptibility tests showing that chloramphenicol is more active than other agents against the infecting organism should never be accepted as the sole indication for chloramphenicol. The use of these guidelines is strongly recommended (Chloramphenicol. Med. Lett. Drugs Ther. *10*:33, 1968).

Sulfonamides

The sulfonamides were the first effective antibacterial agents that could be administered in safe therapeutic dose ranges. As newer, more effective antibiotics have been developed, their place in the therapeutic armamentarium has been narrowed. The sulfonamides are effective against many gram-positive organisms, some gram-negative diplococci and bacilli. Sulfonamides should not be used indiscriminately for upper respiratory infections, and they are not first choice for acute sinusitis, acute otitis media, or β-streptococcal tonsillitis. Sulfonamides remain valuable in some forms of meningitis and for patients with allergies to many antibiotics, renal infections, nocardiosis, or trachoma.

The sulfonamides act by competitive inhibition of para-aminobenzoic acid, an essential growth factor for many bacteria. The individual pharmacological differences of many of the available preparations have been reviewed (Weinstein et al., 1960). Recently several long-acting sulfa preparations became available, but the extended duration of high concentrations of sulfonamides increases the frequency, severity, and persistence of adverse effects. The long-acting preparations have also been associated with the Stevens-Johnson syndrome, although a cause and effect relationship has been questioned (Bianchini, 1968). The use of the shorter acting preparations is recommended.

Corticosteroids

The corticosteroids are used clinically as replacement therapy in Addison's disease, to suppress pituitary ACTH secretion, to suppress undesirable inflammatory responses, and in certain hypersensitivity states. ACTH and cortisol and its synthetic analogs suppress or prevent the inflammatory response, whether the inciting agent is chemical, immunological, or mechanical. They suppress or prevent the gross changes of inflammation, including redness, heat, swelling, and tenderness. Microscopically edema formation, fibrin deposition, capillary dilatation, phagocytic migration, capillary and fibroblast proliferation, collagen deposition, and cicatrization are suppressed or prevented. The biochemical pathways by which steroids inhibit the inflammatory response are unknown, The theories of inflammation and the effect of anti-inflammatory agents have been extensively reviewed (Zweifach et al., 1965; Bondy, 1969). Stabilization of the lysosomes of white blood cells and prevention of release of hydrolytic enzymes has been suggested. Depression of respiration and of mucopolysaccharide synthesis required for wound healing has also been suggested. The major effect of corticosteroids on allergic reactions appears to be due to the inhibition of the inflammatory response initiated by the antigen-antibody interaction. The level of circulating antibody is not significantly altered in man except for the titer of certain auto-antibodies, but the rapid release of antibodies resulting from amnestic response may be decreased. Combination of antigen with antibody is not altered by steroids, but large doses of steroids may influence components of the complement system. Although the mechanism is unknown, the injury to cells that results from union of antigen with antibody is prevented.

Cortisol (hydrocortisone) is the main anti-inflammatory corticosteroid hormone secreted by the adrenal cortex. A normal adult human secretes about 25 mg. daily in nonstressful periods. Hence, in replacement therapy in hypoadrenalism or hypopituitarism, physiological replacement doses approximating this level are utilized. Much larger or pharmacological doses are frequently needed to suppress inflammation.

There is a circadian rhythm in cortisol secretion that is reflected in both the plasma concentration and the urinary excretion of 17-hydroxycorticosteroids (17-OHCS) (Liddle, 1966). In normal subjects with a pattern of daytime activity and nocturnal sleep the plasma 17-OHCS reach a peak about 8 A.M. and decline throughout the day to a low between 8 P.M. and midnight, then begin to rise again about 4 A.M. The plasma adrenocorticotrophin (ACTH) levels are parallel. Centers in the hypothalamus which are responsive to neural and humoral mediators govern the secretion of peptide substances (corticotrophin-releasing factor) which regulate pituitary-adrenal function. They stimulate the secretion and release of ACTH by the anterior pituitary. It appears that these hypothalamic centers are suppressed by high levels of circulating corticosteroids.

The long-term administration of corticosteroids is frequently associated with adrenal suppression and signs of hypercorticism. Diabetes mellitus, peptic ulcer, tuberculosis, or other chronic infections, hypertension and cardiovascular disease, osteoporosis, electrolyte disturbances, and psychological difficulties may be unmasked or aggravated. Impairment of growth occurs in children. Current information suggests that if one administers corticosteroids in a manner less likely to disturb the above cycle, such as avoiding high steroid levels during the evening, or enables the body to escape from elevated steroid levels for periods of time, there is less disturbance of homeostatic mechanisms and fewer side effects. Application of this knowledge has led to better tolerated programs for corticosteroid administration. Thorn (1966) has summarized many of the important clinical considerations in the clinical use of corticosteroids.

An alternate day program of steroid administration with a 48 hour single morning dosage regimen has been found useful in minimizing the toxic side effects of corticosteroids while maintaining their desirable anti-inflammatory and immunosuppressive effects. Early reports of the use of this regimen included dermatologic disorders (Reichling and Kligman, 1961), asthma, various dermatoses, and other allergic disorders (Harter et al., 1963). These studies have subsequently been confirmed and extended to nephrosis (Soyka, 1967), rheumatoid arthritis, and other collagen diseases, and a variety of other disease states. The consensus is that effectiveness of the alternate day approach in many disease states is either equal to or slightly less than conventional multiple dose administration; pituitary-adrenal reserve function is maintained (Adams et al., 1966; Ackerman and Nolan, 1968); and there are fewer undesirable effects on bone, skin, and connective tissues. Dougherty et al. (1958) demonstrated that cortisol need not be present in inflamed tissue for a prolonged period in order to inhibit inflammation, and clinically the duration of the anti-inflammatory effect of the corticosteroids exceeds the duration of their presence in the body. Although certain patients may require more frequent administration of the corticosteroids to achieve the desired pharmacological effect either initially or chronically, the generally favorable therapeutic response and diminished side effects of this regimen suggest that it could be more widely employed.

The use of an intermittent schedule of corticosteroid administration (Lange et al., 1958; Adams et al., 1964), that is, on 3 to 5 consecutive days of each week, has also been reported to produce beneficial therapeutic effects with fewer side effects and is generally not associated with pituitary-adrenal hypofunction (Danowski et al., 1964). This method has not been extensively investigated and does not appear to be so popular as the alternate day approach. Single dose steroid administration daily in the morning has also been studied (Dubois and Adler, 1963; Matthews, 1964; Demos et al., 1964). Diminished toxicity and less pituitary-adrenal hypofunction have been reported. Others have reported that the incidence of side effects is unchanged from the multiple dose per day regimen (Demos et al., 1964). The synthetic corticosteroids have longer plasma half-lives than cortisol (Melby, 1961), and if one utilized a steroid with a long half-life, the incidence of side effects might be greater. If large doses of corticosteroids are administered, the multiple dose per day schedule appears to be associated with the greatest incidence of side effects and pituitary-adrenal suppression. In lieu of the favorable results reported with schedules such as the alternate day approach, the use of depot and sustained-release steroid preparations has been questioned (Reichling and Kligman, 1961).

There is individual variation in the incidence of side effects and pituitary-adrenal suppression with corticosteroid administration in patients, and some patients may be able to tolerate large doses over prolonged periods with sequelae. The incidence of untoward effects increases with increasing steroid dosage, but the mode of administration of steroids is also important.

ACTH has been used for many steroid-responsive conditions but is rarely used for prolonged periods of time. The disadvantages of ACTH include salt and water retention, necessity for parenteral administration, and difficulty in obtaining uniform daily steroid responses. The symptoms and signs of hypercorticism may also develop. The most important use is in diagnosing disorders of the adenohypophysis and adrenal cortex. Chronic administration does not appear to inhibit growth in children and it has sometimes been recommended in female patients to provide natural androgens since corticosteroid administration may inhibit their secretion by the adrenal. Chronic administration of ACTH suppresses hypothalamic and pituitary activity, while the adrenal glands remain functional. Adrenal steroids suppress all three. ACTH has also been recommended for use in patients with pituitary-adrenal suppression resulting from prolonged corticosteroid therapy during the period of withdrawal of adrenal hormone therapy. Graber et al. (1965) found that recovery of pituitary function (plasma ACTH leveis) preceded recovery of adrenal function (plasma

cortical levels). If correction of pituitary function is necessary before adrenal recovery, the rationale for the use of ACTH to stimulate the adrenal cortex during corticosteroid withdrawal is unclear (Med. Lett. Drugs Ther. *10*:62, 1968).

There does not appear to be any qualitative difference in the anti-inflammatory effect produced by the various commercially available corticosteroid preparations. They do differ in their potency on a milligram basis and in degradation rates in the body. The salt-retaining properties may vary, and this effect of the synthetic analogs is considerably less than cortisol or cortisone. Anti-inflammatory effect is directly related to glucogenic activity, while salt-retaining activity is inversely proportional. Characteristic features of some of the oral corticosteroid preparations are presented in Table 2.

All the steroids listed in Table 2 may be administered orally. Many corticosteroids are also available for parenteral administration. The succinate or phosphate derivatives of hydrocortisone, prednisolone, methylprednisolone, and dexamethasone are highly soluble, have a rapid onset of action, and are rapidly excreted. Others such as cortisone acetate, methylprednisolone acetate, and triamcinolone acetonide are more insoluble and are slowly absorbed and excreted, and the onset of action is delayed. Various preparations are also available for injection into confined spaces, such as intrabursal and intra-articular. Corticosteroids have also been incorporated into various vehicles for local application to the skin, eyes, or mucous membranes. Several agents with potent topical activity include triamcinolone acetonide, betamethasone valerate, fluocinolone acetonide, flurandrenolone acetonide and fluorometholone.

TABLE 2. *Characteristics of Oral Corticosteroids*

USP NAME	ANTI-INFLAMMATORY (RELATIVE POTENCY)	MINERALO-CORTICO-STEROID (RELATIVE POTENCY)
Hydrocortisone	1.0	0.03
Cortisone	0.8	0.03
Prednisone	4.0	0.04
Methylprednisone	6.0	0.02
Triamcinolone	5.0	0
Betamethasone	30.0	0
Dexamethasone	30.0	0
Fludrocortisone	10.0	4.2
Desoxycorticosterone	0.0	1.0
Aldosterone	0.1	20

Corticosteroids have been used for a wide variety of ENT disorders. Frequently they are used only on a short-term basis or in small dosages, and the severe side effects previously discussed are not encountered. They have frequently been employed empirically in a variety of disorders, and uniform agreement on the utility or best means of administration (i.e., topically vs. systemic) is not present. Their value in specific disease states is discussed in other sections of this text. In general, they have been more extensively employed in the treatment of bronchial asthma, esophageal caustic burns, acute laryngotracheobronchitis, Bell's palsy, allergic and vasomotor rhinitis, and nasal polyps.

DRUGS FOR VERTIGO

Disturbances in equilibrium with or without nausea and vomiting occur in a variety of unrelated disease states. A disturbance in the spatial orientation of the body develops when inconsistent information from the peripheral receptors is fed into the central nervous system. A sense of turning or falling of the body in relation to the environment develops. Vertigo is a staggering motion or falling accompanied by nystagmus, past pointing, tachycardia, nausea, vomiting, diaphoresis and hypertension. A variety of mechanisms produce vertigo. These include: (1) irritation or destruction of the labyrinth, vestibular nerve, or vestibular pathways in the brain stem, cerebellum, or cortex; (2) visual disturbances; (3) loss of proprioceptive reception from the neck, trunk, or extremities; (4) direct toxic action on the central nervous system as in alcoholism; (5) decreased cardiac output or decreased red cell volume as in cardiac arrhythmias of anemia; and (6) psychogenic disease.

Unfortunately the exact physiologic mechanisms of equilibrium disturbances are unknown. Labyrinthine stimulation of both semicircular canals and otoliths produces vertigo but not necessarily in identical ways. Meniere's disease affects the entire labyrinth; Berg's positional vertigo appears to be a disorder of the otolith, particularly the utricle, but this is not absolutely proved. It is generally agreed that the labyrinths play an important role in motion sickness, but it has not been proved which part of the labyrinth is responsible. It was noted in the last century that many deaf mutes and other subjects with acquired damage to the inner ear were immune to motion sickness. At least two central nervous system (CNS) areas are related to vomiting; they are the chemoreceptive trigger zone which can be stimulated by drugs such as apomorphine and the vomiting center itself. The central mechanisms for vomiting are related to those for equilibrium, but they are not identical. Most drugs used for motion sickness have one or more of the following actions: antivertigo, antiemesis, or vasodilatation. These actions are often distinct and unrelated; for example, a potent antiemetic agent like chlorpromazine has practically no antivertigo properties.

Drug Evaluation

A number of methods have been used to evaluate the effect of drugs on motion sickness in man. Many large scale field trials were conducted during World War II on personnel involved in various sea and air maneuvers, and simulated controlled maneuvers were also utilized. These studies eliminated many inactive drugs and those producing significant side effects, but conflicting and confusing data were obtained with the clearly active drugs. Many of these discrepancies were probably the result of variations in the duration and type of motion; variations in the interval between medication and exposure to motion, mode of administration, and dosage level of drug; and variations in the previous exposure and tolerance of subjects. The expense and difficulties encountered in the field trials led to attempts to develop a reliable laboratory test for screening and evaluation of drugs for motion sickness, but no single test that is uniformly and exclusively predictive has yet been devised. Efforts to design such a test are hampered by lack of specific knowledge of both the physiology of the disorder itself and the mechanism of action of the effective drugs.

Studies in man and animals have involved measurements of nystagmus after stimulation of the semicircular canal by rotation or caloric tests. The evidence suggests that drugs effective in motion sickness modify this response, and nystagmus is either depressed or abolished. Incompletely answered is the question of whether the depression of nystagmus is limited to this group of drugs and if this is an end-organ effect or a nonspecific depression of cortical activity resulting from the sedative properties of these drugs. Nystagmus response does depend somewhat upon the state of mental alertness and can be heightened with amphetamine.

Tilting chairs or parallel swings have been used to stimulate the otoliths, and some of the effective drugs depress this response. Another test employed is the ability of these drugs to block apomorphine-induced vomiting. Hyoscine and promethazine, which are effective in treating vertigo, depressed vomiting in this test, but chlorpromazine, an ineffective agent for treating vertigo, was even more effective in depressing vomiting. Graybiel et al. (1967) have had extensive experience with the production of canal sickness by use of a slow rotation room where the stressful Coriolis accelerations could be quantitated and a specific level of motion sickness can be attained. Their studies indicate a positive correlation between production of canal sickness and observed air sickness and caloric sensitivity. They were also able to rank 16 antimotion sickness drugs in terms of effectiveness by this method. Although use of the slow rotation room may be the best laboratory test currently available, there are also limitations to the validity of the results when applied to actual operational conditions.

Antimotion sickness drugs have also been studied in vitro for their ability to antagonize histamine and acetylcholine. Most of the effective drugs have either antihistaminic activity or anticholinergic activity, but these parameters cannot be used as the sole criterion for efficacy. Several drugs effective in motion sickness can control the adverse syndrome produced by intracarotid injection of diisopropyl fluorophosphate in animals and this is another study tool. Its exact importance and clinical correlation are yet unclear. In summary, carefully designed field trials are still essential for defining efficacy of antimotion sickness drugs, but these trials are complicated by many variables, including the diverse etiologies of the syndromes being treated. There is a difference between prolonged sea travel and short exposure to severe motion. Meniere's disease with its spontaneous remissions is different from poststapedectomy vertigo.

Specific Drugs

A careful review of the results of the previously described experiments and clinical trials revealed that five drugs were unquestionably of value in the treatment of motion sickness; these are L-hyoscine, diphenhydramine, cyclizine, meclizine, and promethazine (Brand and Perry, 1966). Other drugs may be helpful in certain situations, but evidence for their efficacy is less convincing.

These drugs are more effective when given prophylactically, and some general guidelines to onset and duration of action are given in Table 3. Hyoscine has a more rapid onset, a short duration of action and appears to be the preferred form of therapy when the goal is quick-acting, short-term protection against severe motion sickness. Cyclizine, diphenhydramine, meclizine, and promethazine have progessively longer durations of action and would be preferred for longer exposures to motion. The protection offered by cyclizine and meclizine appears to be equal to the others, but their side effects, especially sedation, may be less and might be preferred if mental alertness were important. Diphenhydramine and promethazine are more likely to produce sedation, which could be an advantage in apprehensive individuals. The reported efficacy of these drugs in motion sickness varies widely, but most trials report that 70 or more per cent of those who would otherwise become ill are protected. Some of the important features of these drugs are summarized in Table 3.

A variety of drugs have been used to treat disturbances in equilibrium. As previously indicated, the use of certain drugs in motion sickness has been shown to be beneficial. The use of drugs for treating other types of equilibrium

---

TABLE 3.   *A Comparison of Drugs for Motion Sickness*

NAME	TRADE NAME	SPEED OF ONSET (hrs.)	DURATION (hrs.)	DOSE (mg.)
Cyclizine	Marezine	1	4	50
Diphenhydramine	Dramamine	1	6	50
Hyoscine	Scopolamine	$\frac{1}{2}$–1	4	0.6–1.0
Meclizine	Bonine, Bonamine	1	12	50
Promethazine	Phenergan	$1\frac{1}{2}$	12	25–50

disturbances is more empirical, and controlled clinical studies demonstrating efficacy are generally lacking. These drugs include antihistamines, anticholinergics, vasodilators, tranquilizers, and other central nervous system depressants. A survey of the structural formulas of these drugs indicates that it would be hard to define a structure-function relationship.

Antihistamines. Some of the more effective drugs for treating motion sickness and other disturbances of equilibrium are found in this group of drugs. Efficacy of treating vertigo is not directly related to antihistaminic activity. Dimenhydrinate has been shown to be of value in treating motion sickness. It is also used in Meniere's disease, acute labyrinthitis, and nonspecific vertigo, but controlled clinical studies are rare. Gutner et al. (1951) showed that dimenhydrinate depressed vestibular function when stimulated by galvanic current or caloric testing. Dimenhydrinate also modifies those postural reflexes which are believed to be medicated through the otoliths in the rabbit (Fermin et al., 1950). Promethazine is also an effective antivertiginous drug, but its marked sedative effect may limit its usefulness. It also decreases the incidence of apomorphine-induced vomiting in man (Isaacs and MacArthur, 1954).

Meclizine and cyclizine are effective in motion sickness and are frequently employed in other types of vertigo. Dimenhydrinate, cyclizine, promethazine, and meclizine have all been shown to be capable of depressing calorically induced nystagmus in guinea pigs (Richards et al., 1963). In one special preparation cyclizine failed to modify action potentials picked up from the eighth nerve response to electrical stimulation of the lateral semicircular canal. The authors concluded that cyclizine has no influence on the vestibular nerve or primary vestibular nuclei and suggested that its locus of action was in the cerebellum or cerebrum (Cramer and Dowd, 1961). Meclizine and cyclizine have produced birth defects in experimental animals, and these drugs should not be prescribed in pregnancy. Drowsiness may be a prominent side effect of antihistamines and impairment of motor function may occur. They must be prescribed with caution to motor vehicle operators and patients with other occupations in which mental alertness is essential.

Anticholinergics. Hyoscine (scopolamine) and atropine are examples of this group; the former is highly recommended for short-term motion sickness prevention. Side effects, including dry mouth, drowsiness, vertigo, and blurred vision, are frequent. Prolonged use can cause headache, cardiac acceleration and, occasionally, hallucinations. The therapeutic ratio of antivertiginous drugs must also be considered. One study of hyoscine in motion sickness at dosage levels of 0.5 and 1.0 mg. revealed that the higher dosage level offered only 3 per cent greater protection, while the incidence of visual disturbances was increased by 25 per cent. Some of the newer synthetic belladonna drugs which are effective in parkinsonism have been investigated for treatment of vertigo. Benztropine mesylate (Cogentin) and trihexyphenidyl HCl (Artane) appear to be less effective than hyoscine.

CNS Depressants. Sedatives were the first drugs to be used to treat vertigo and, while having no specific effect on vestibular function, do relieve fear and anxiety. They are useful in conjunction with other antivertigo preparations.

Tranquilizers. Emotional factors are certainly part of any vertiginous episode, and the reported effectiveness of this group may be partially the result of relief of anxiety. These drugs also act on the chemoreceptor trigger zone to depress vomiting. Promethazine, which falls into both the antihistamine and tranquilizer group, is more effective in motion sickness; its disadvantage is its sedation. Prochorperazine (Compazine) and trifluoperazine (Stelazine) have had favorable reports.

Miscellaneous Agents. Trimethobenzamide (Tigan), 250 mg. orally or 200 mg. intramuscularly, tends to block vomiting primarily by acting on the chemoreceptor trigger zone. It has been used alone or in combination with nicotinic acid, a vasodilator. There is little evidence that it is effective in motion sickness or vertigo.

Nicotinic acid and nicotinyl alcohol tartrate (Roniacol) are used empirically in ear disease. They cause vasodilatation of small blood vessels by a direct action, but there is no evidence that cerebral blood flow is increased (Scheinberg, 1950). Rather the best evidence is that there is no change in cerebral blood flow, vascular resistance, or oxygen and glucose consumption. Vertigo, nausea, and vomiting in geriatric patients frequently respond better to a vasodilator and antivertiginous drugs than to an antivertiginous drug alone. The efficacy of nicotinic acid is questionable; its use is probably more traditional than objective.

Histamine is a potent vasodilator causing arteriolar dilatation and increased capillary permeability when injected. It has been used (2.75 mg. in 250 ml. 5 per cent dextrose/water) intravenously for Meniere's syndrome. Dilute histamine hyposensitization is also advocated (Shambaugh, 1950). One postulate states that Meniere's disease is due to the local accumulation of histamine in nonphysiologic toxic concentration. This causes arteriolar dilatation and loss of capillary solids and fluids with resultant endolymph accumulation and cochlear duct dilatation. Based on this hypothesis, a histamine analog, betahistine dihydrochloride (Serc), has been advocated to decrease the frequency of vertiginous episodes in Meniere's disease. The evidence for its efficacy is currently being seriously questioned.

Evaluation of drugs in Meniere's disease is very difficult because the natural course may be unpredictable, with spontaneous remissions and exacerbations of varying lengths. Eriodictyon glycoside (lemon bioflavinoid complex) has been noted by Williams to improve vertigo in Meniere's disease. Its physiologic mechanism is unknown. The effect was judged solely on improvement of hearing in an attempt to be objective. Because of the pathologic observation of endolymphatic hydrops, diuretics of all kinds, from ammonium chloride to chlorothiazide, have been used without consistent results. Severe diets, usually salt poor, have also been ineffective. Droperidol and fentanyl citrate (Innovar), a neuroleptanalgesic, has been noted to depress the vestibular system. A dose of 2 cc./70 kg. has been recommended intravenously for acute attacks of Meniere's syndrome (Dirk et al., 1969). It is yet too early for this to have received extensive trial.

Amphetamine alone has been reported to have antimotion sickness properties; it has been combined with other antimotion sickness drugs to counteract their depressant action. Empirically it has been given to abort attacks of Meniere's disease, but objective evidence of improvement is lacking. In general, combinations of antivertiginous drugs appear to be only as effective as a full strength dose of their most effective component. There is no evidence that nicotinic acid combined with meclizine (Antivert) is superior to meclizine alone.

ANTITUSSIVE AGENTS

Cough is a protective physiologic reflex and, to repeat an old truism, more people have died from an inability to cough than from the act of coughing itself. Yet there are instances when continued or severe paroxysms of coughing may be harmful. Further debilitation may occur from loss of sleep, decreased food intake, and nausea and vomiting. Severe paroxysms of cough may lead to undesired effects on the cardiopulmonary system. Urinary incontinence in women with pelvic relaxation can also be precipitated, and chronic cough has been implicated in hernia production. Coughing is also an excellent method of droplet dissemination of infected material. The causes of cough are legion, including many diseases of the lung and upper airway as well as some cardiovascular and gastrointestinal disorders.

A cough, whether reflex or voluntary, has three distinct phases: A rapid, deep inspiratory phase ends with closure of the glottis. The compressive phase is due to contraction of thoracic and abdominal muscles and results in an increase in intrathoracic pressure. Finally, the glottis opens and air is expelled at speeds up to 500 miles per hour. Cough is a reflex which is partly under voluntary control, but little is known about cortical regulation of cough. A central cough-regulating center appears to exist in the medulla. Afferent impulses arising from the external ear, pharynx, larynx, trachea, bronchi, pleura, diaphragm, or pericardium ascend via the glossopharyngeal, vagus, or phrenic nerves to this center. Cleaning the ear with a curette may produce coughing through the auricular branch of the vagus (Arnold's nerve). Enlargement of the left auricle in mitral stenosis may stimulate cough through the cardiac branches of the vagus nerve.

The existence of two types of receptors in the tracheobronchial tract which appear to be specific for mechanical or chemical stimulation was demonstrated by Widdicombe (1954). The receptors for mechanical stimuli are located primarily in the mucosa of the larynx and trachea, particularly the lower third including the carina. The receptors sensitive to chemical irritants are widely distributed throughout the respiratory tract. Bronchoconstriction may precipitate or accentuate cough. Pulmonary stretch receptors located in the smooth muscle surrounding the bronchioles are stimulated by inflation of the lung. The above mechanisms are noteworthy because drugs may raise the threshold for cough production by either a central or peripheral effect. In the bronchi, drugs may relieve bronchospasm, modify mucus, or produce local anesthetic effects.

Centrally Acting Antitussive Agents

Narcotics. The narcotics are the best known centrally acting antitussive agents.

They act principally by direct suppression of the cough center and by a nonspecific effect on the central nervous system to dull perception of cough stimuli. These agents also suppress respiration, cause bronchoconstriction, and reduce mucus production and ciliary activity of the bronchi. These latter effects may lead to impairment of adequate bronchial drainage in patients with bronchiectasis or asthma. The chronic use of cough mixtures containing narcotics poses the threat of addiction. Contrary to popular opinion, codeine addiction is not rare and may start with extended use of a cough mixture (Bickerman, 1968–69).

Codeine is still one of the most effective and popular antitussive agents, and experience has shown that it suppresses cough of many etiologies. In usual therapeutic doses codeine is approximately one fourth as depressant to respiration as is morphine. As the dose is increased there may be no commensurate increase in respiratory depression; toxic doses may tend to cause stimulation of the central nervous system. Codeine produces less drying effect and less constriction of bronchial smooth muscle than morphine.

The average oral adult dose of various narcotics required for cough suppression is listed in Table 4. Codeine and dihydrocodeinone, similar to codeine, are used more extensively for chronic suppression of cough. The other narcotics are also good cough suppressants, but may be associated with more prominent side effects than codeine if used chronically. They are generally used in specific situations such as acute pulmonary edema, or cough associated with intractable pain occurring with rib fractures or neoplasms, or for intractable paroxysms of cough. The use of narcotics in pa-

tients with chronic lung diseases may precipitate or accentuate pulmonary insufficiency.

Non-narcotics. A number of compounds have been developed which centrally depress the cough center and are devoid of addiction and the other undesirable side effects of the narcotics. Dextromethorphan and noscapine are representative of this group. A discussion of other non-narcotic antitussives which act centrally may be found in the review of Bickerman (1962). Benson et al. demonstrated in 1952 that dextromethorphan could inhibit cough induced by electrical stimulation of the tracheal mucosa in dogs. Studies employing citric acid-induced cough and clinical trials in patients have demonstrated significant cough depression, approximately equal to codeine. In clinical trials the incidence of side effects is low, considerably less than with codeine. Bronchoconstriction has been observed in animals. Dextromethorphan does not produce respiratory depression or addiction, and there is no evidence that tolerance develops. At dose levels below 5mg./kg. in animals there was no depression of ciliary activity. Dextromethorphan has enjoyed popularity for cough in the common cold syndrome, but Bickerman (1962) has not found it effective in cough associated with bronchiectasis or asthma.

Noscapine, a naturally occurring alkaloid in opium, is not a narcotic and has no addiction liability. It is about equal to codeine in antitussive action on a weight basis. The recommended adult dose for noscapine is 15 to 30 mg. three or four times a day; its wide margin of safety permits a single dose of 60 mg. for paroxysms of coughing. Noscapine has little effect on respiration and may be a bronchodilator, although evidence on this point is conflicting.

TABLE 4. Drugs Used for Cough Suppression

GENERIC AND TRADE NAME	AVERAGE ADULT DOSE (mg.)
Narcotics	
Morphine	2.0– 3.0
Codeine	8.0–15.0
Dihydrocodeinone (Hycodan)	5.0–10.0
Meperidine (Demerol)	25 –50
Dihydromorphinone (Dilaudid)	0.5– 1.0
Methadone (Dolophine)	1.5– 2.0
Non-narcotics	
Dextromethorphan (Romilar)	15 –30
Noscapine (Nectadon)	10 –30

Peripherally Acting Antitussive Agents

A variety of preparations are available which act nonspecifically to decrease irritation within the respiratory tract or facilitate the evacuation of retained secretions. The precise mode of action of some of the following substances is unknown. Antihistamines, antipyretics, decongestants, demulcents, expectorants, and local anesthetics are frequently employed in cough mixtures. Many preparations contain some or all of the preceding in addition to the previously described centrally acting drugs, and it is difficult to assess the value of individual ingredients.

Demulcents are bland substances like glycerin, honey, or cherry syrup which protectively coat the pharyngeal mucosa. This soothes the mucosa topically and may prevent drying and crusting. These compounds are often used as vehicles for other antitussive agents. The candy cough drops act similarly to lessen pharyngeal irritation.

Benzonatate is chemically related to the local anesthetic tetracaine and it acts locally on the stretch receptors and appears to depress polysynaptic spinal reflexes, thus inhibiting the transmission of cough impulses. In adults the optimal dose appears to be 100 mg. three or four times a day. The antitussive effect of 100 mg. of benzonatate is comparable to that produced with 15 mg. of codeine (Benson et al., 1952). There is no apparent effect on respiration.

Antihistamines are indicated primarily in the treatment of allergic cough, but they are widely used in cough medications. Other actions of antihistamines that may be helpful in suppressing cough include a central depressive action and drying effect. Drying of secretions is a mixed benefit; if it makes the secretions more viscous, the retention is enhanced. Oral decongestants may be added to cough syrups for their ability to constrict blood vessels and their bronchodilating action. The dose of both the antihistamine and the oral decongestant is often below that expected to produce an adequate therapeutic response.

Expectorants are drugs that aid in the removal of secretions from the respiratory tract; this may be done by different mechanisms. Glycerol guaiacolate is an expectorant that increases respiratory tract fluid, tending to lower its viscosity and facilitate its removal, virtually without side effects. Organic and inorganic salts like citrates, acetates, ammonium salts, and iodides are used to increase mucus.

The iodides and syrup of ipecac are gastric irritants which at subemetic doses produce a reflex increase in respiratory secretions. In comparison to glycerol guaiacolate, the iodides are probably more effective. Iodides may increase the protein bound iodine level and cause a variety of minor toxic effects like skin rash or salivary gland swelling. Substances like guaicol, chloroform, and terpin hydrate act to decrease respiratory secretions.

In summary, there is no single ideal medication for treatment of cough. Synthetic non-narcotic agents should receive first choice for nuisance coughs and those of short duration. In general, the antitussive effect is enhanced by giving the dose more frequently rather than by increasing individual doses. Humidification, although not within the scope of this chapter, is a valuable adjunct to cough control; using a humidifier in the room of a coughing child can be of great benefit.

ANTIHISTAMINES

The pharmacological properties of the various antihistamines are similar and can be divided into two major categories: histamine antagonism and direct effects of the drug on effector cells (Goodman and Gilman, 1965). A common structural feature of most antihistamines is a substituted ethylamine — CH_2CH_2N — which is also present in histamine. It is presumed that this portion of the molecule competes with histamine for receptor sites on the effector cells, (Wilhelm, 1962); most antihistamines are competitive antagonists of histamine (Marshall, 1955) and do not prevent the release of histamine. The antihistamines antagonize the majority of the pharmacological actions of histamine, with the gastric secretory effect of histamine being a notable exception.

Antihistamines can reduce the intensity of allergic and anaphylactic reactions, and this property plus their use in the prophylaxis and treatment of motion sickness constitute the major therapeutic indications for their use in ENT practice. These drugs are more effective in preventing the effects of histamine than in reversing them once they occur, and are used primarily for palliative or symptomatic relief only. The antihistamines block the bronchoconstrictor effects of histamine but are only feeble antagonists of bronchospasm induced by antigen-antibody reactions (Schild et al., 1951) and other bronchoconstricting agents like the kinins. These drugs are of limited value in treating anaphylaxis in man.

The antihistamines are readily absorbed from the gastrointestinal tract. Maximal effect from a single oral dose is obtained within one hour and the duration of action generally varies from three to six hours. Recently, timed release preparations have been developed and permit twice-a-day dosage. The metabolic fate of the antihistamines which have been studied, such as diphenhydramine, tripelennamine, and cyclizine, reveal that these compounds are primarily metabolized by the liver, with excretion of the metabolites in the urine. Many studies in animals have shown that a number of antihistamines are capable of stimulating the drug-metabolizing system in the liver (Conney and Burns, 1962). They have stimulated their own metabolism as well as the metabolism of many other drugs and endogenous substrates like estrogens and glucocorticoids. Unfortunately the significance of this in man has not been evaluated to determine the frequency of this interaction with other drugs or whether the decreased therapeutic effect sometimes seen with prolonged administration of an antihistamine is related to enhanced metabolism.

All the antihistamines elicit side effects, with certain side effects being more common with particular antihistamines, but there is also marked variation in individual patient responses to these drugs. The most common side effect of the antihistamines is sedation, although certain drugs like diphenhydramine are more likely to produce this effect. This CNS depressant effect is not related to the antihistamine effect, and the depression may be potentiated by alcohol and barbiturates. CNS stimulation may also be seen, but it is more likely to occur in poisoning, especially in children. Most antihistamines also have varying degrees of anticholinergic, local anesthetic, and quinidine-like effects, as well as direct stimulating effects on smooth muscle such as bowel, uterus, and bladder. Again the extent of these effects varies with individual compounds and is rarely great enough to be therapeutically beneficial but may be related to side effects. Complaints of blurred vision, dizziness, tinnitus, inability to concentrate, and dryness of the oropharynx may occur.

The antihistamines are widely used for symptomatic relief of upper respiratory infections caused by viruses. It is well established that these agents have no antiviral effect and do not shorten the duration of the common cold (Feller, 1950). Symptoms of allergic rhinitis may be relieved to some extent with antihistamines; they are more effective in relieving symptoms of acute allergic rhinitis than those due to chronic conditions. In seasonal hay fever, better results are obtained at the beginning of the season when pollen counts are lower. They have long been considered to be ineffective and contraindicated in the treatment of acute and chronic bronchial asthma which is not complicated by allergic rhinitis (Rapp, 1969). The intravenous use of antihistamines is valuable in acute allergic states, acute urticaria, acute pruritic states, and anaphylactic and anaphylactoid reactions to drugs, radiopaque dyes, and allergenic extracts. Many acute allergic dermatoses respond favorably to the use of antihistamines, and they are widely used for preventing motion sickness. They also appear to be of value in preventing allergic transfusion reactions (Wilhelm, 1955).

There are many antihistaminic preparations available. Some of these are derivatives of the same basic molecule and differ only in the salt form. Others are either racemic mixtures or the dextro-isomer. The antihistaminic effect is believed to reside primarily in the d-form; consequently, the d-forms of a number of antihistamines were developed in an attempt to decrease the incidence of side effects. Many preparations are also available which contain other antihistamines, sympathomimetics, anticholinergics, antitussives, analgesics, antibiotics, and other agents. Some of these combinations are useful, while others have not been proved and will undoubtedly be removed from the market in the future. Some representative drugs from the various chemical classes of antihistamines include the following.

Ethanolamines. Diphenhydramine (Benadryl) and dimenhydrinate (Dramamine) are the most widely used. They have prominent sedative and atropinelike effects. Diphenhydramine is also frequently used orally as a sedative and intravenously for acute allergic reactions. Dimenhydrinate is used most frequently in motion sickness.

Ethylenediamines. Tripelennamine (Pyribenzamine) is an effective antihistaminic, but is noted for its sedative properties.

Alkylamines. These include pheniramine (Trimeton), chlorpheniramine (racemic mixture—Chlortrimeton, Teldrin; d-isomer—Polaramine) and brompheniramine (racemic mixture—Dimetaine; d-isomer—Disomer). Because of the lower incidence of drowsiness, these compounds have enjoyed widespread popularity for daytime use; many varied dosage forms are available.

Cyclizine. Cyclizine (Marezine and meclizine (Bonine) are widely prescribed for motion sickness.

There is no single outstanding antihistamine. The best results will be obtained if one utilizes a very limited number of antihistamines, selecting compounds from the various groups outlined, and learns the pharmacological variations of individual compounds. Considerable variation in response occurs among patients. Titration of dose in individual patients is also important.

REFERENCES

Ototoxic Drugs

Barr, B., Floberg, L. E., Hamberger, C. A., and Koch, H.: Otologic aspects of streptomycin. Acta Otolaryng. (Suppl.) *75*:5, 1949.

Conway, N.: Streptomycin in pregnancy—effect on the fetal ear. Brit. Med. J. *1*:260, 1965.

Cummings, C.: Experimental observations on the ototoxicity of nitrogen mustard. Laryngoscope *78*:530, 1968.

Eichenwald, H. F.: Antibiotics and the newborn. Hosp. Prac. *2*:51, 1967.

El-Mofty, A., and El-Serafy, S.: The effect of ototoxic antibiotics on the oxygen uptake of the membranous cochlea, Ann. Otol. *75*:216, 1966.

Falbe-Hansen, J.: Clinical studies on the effect of salicylic acid and quinine on the human ear. Acta Otol. (Suppl.) *44*:50–74, 1941.

Finegold, S. M.: Toxicity of kanamycin in adults. Ann. N.Y. Acad. Sci. *132*:942, 1966.

Greenwood, G. J.: Neomycin ototoxicity. Arch. Otol. *69*:390, 1959.

Hart, C., and Naunton, R. F.: The ototoxicity of chloroquine phosphate. Arch. Otol. *80*:407, 1964.

Jao, R. L., and Jackson, G. G.: Gentamycin sulfate, new antibiotic against gram negative bacilli. J.A.M.A. *189*:817, 1964.

Kunin, C. M.: A guide to use of antibiotics in patients with renal disease, a table of recommended doses and factors governing serum levels. Ann. Intern. Med. *67*:151, 1967.

Matz, G. J., and Naunton, R. F.: Ototoxic drugs and poor renal function. J.A.M.A. *206*:2119, 1968.

McCabe, P. A., and Dey, F.: The effect of aspirin upon auditory sensitivity. Ann. Otol. *74*:312, 1965.

Meuwissen, H. J., and Robinson, G. C.: The ototoxic antibiotics, a survey of current knowledge. Clin. Pediat. *6*:262, 1967.

Meyers, E. N., and Bernstein, J. M.: Salicylate ototoxicity. New Eng. J. Med. *273*:587, 1965.

Newman, R. L., and Holt, R. J.: Intrathecal gentamicin in treatment of ventriculitis in children. Brit. Med. J. *2*:539, 1967.

Robinson, G.: Hearing loss in infants of tuberculous mothers with streptomycin therapy during pregnancy. New Eng. J. Med. *271*:949, 1964.

Schneider, W. J., and Becker, E. L.: Acute transient hearing loss after ethacrynic acid therapy. Arch. Intern. Med. *117*:715, 1966.

Shambaugh, G. E., et al.: Dihydrostreptomycin deafness. J.A.M.A. *170*:1657, 1959.

Silverstein, H., Bernstein, J. M., and Davies, D. G.: Salicylate ototoxicity—a biochemical and electrophysiological study. Ann. Otol. *76*:118, 1967.

Tompsett, R.: Relation of dosage to streptomycin toxicity. Ann. Otol. *57*:181, 1948.

Antibacterial Agents

Bianchini, J. R. et. al.: Drugs as etiologic factors in the Stevens-Johnson syndrome. Amer. J. Med. *44*:390, 1968.

Chloramphenicol. Med. Lett. Drugs Ther. *10*:33, 1968.

Clendenning, W. E.: Complications of tetracycline therapy. Arch. Dermat. *91*:628, 1965.

Friend, D. G.: Penicillin G. Clin. Pharmacol Ther. *7*:421 1966a.

Friend, D. G.: Penicillin therapy—newer semisynthetic penicillins. Clin. Pharmacol. Ther. *7*:706, 1966b.

Kunin, C. M.: Clinical pharmacology of the new penicillins. The importance of serum protein binding in determining antimicrobial activity and concentration in the serum. Clin. Pharmacol. Ther. *7*:166, 1966.

Kunin, C. M.: Current status of the new antibiotics. Virginia Med. Monthly *96*:29, 1969.

Stewart, G. T.: Hypersensitivity and toxicity of the B-lactam antibiotics. Postgrad. Med. J. (suppl.) *430*:31, 1967.

Stewart, G. T.: Penicillin allergy. Clin. Pharmacol. Ther. *11*:307, 1970.

The choice of systemic antimicrobial drugs. Med. Lett. Drugs Ther. *10*:77, 1968.

Weinstein, L., and Kaplan, K. The cephalosporins: Microbiological, chemical and pharmacological properties and use in chemotherapy of infections. Ann. Intern. Med. *72*:729, 1970.

Weinstein, L., Madoff, M. A., and Samet, C. M.: The sulfonamides. New Eng. J. Med. *263*:793; 842, 1960.

Corticosteroids

Ackerman, G. L, and Nolan, C. M.: Adrenocortical responsiveness after alternate day corticosteroid therapy. New. Eng. J. Med. *278*:405, 1968.

Adams, D. A., Gold, E. M., Gonick, H. C., and Maxwell, M. H.: Adrenocortical functions during intermittent corticosteroid therapy. Ann. Intern. Med. *64*:542, 1966.

Adams, D. A., Maxwell, M. H., and Gold, E. M.: Initial intermittent corticosteroid therapy of nephroses and its effect on adrenal reserve. Clin. Res. *12*:247, 1964.

Bondy, P. K.: Duncan's Diseases of Metabolism. 6th ed. Philadelphia, W. B. Saunders Company, 1969, pp. 827–885.

Danowski, T. S., Bonessi, J. V., Sabeh, G., Sutton, R. D., Webster, M. W., and Sarver, M. E.: Probabilities of pituitary-adrenal responsiveness after steroid therapy. Ann. Intern. Med. *61*:11, 1964.

Demos, C. H., Krasner, F., and Groel, J. T.: A modified (once a day) corticosteroid dosage regimen. Clin. Pharmacol. Ther. *5*:721, 1964.

Dougherty, T. F., Brown, H. E., and Berliner, O. L.: Metabolism of hydrocortisone during inflammation. Endocrinology *62*:455, 1968.

Dubois, E. L., and Adler, D. C.: Single daily dose oral administration of corticosteroids in rheumatic disorders: An analysis of its advantages, efficacy and side effects. Curr. Ther. Res. *5*:43, 1963.

Graber, A. L., Ney, R. L., Nicholson, W. E., Island, D. P., and Liddle, G. W.: Natural history of pituitary-adrenal recovery following long-term suppression with corticosteroids. J. Clin. Endocr. *25*:11, 1965.

Harter, J. G., Reddy, W. J., and Thorn, G. W.: Studies on an intermittent corticosteroid dosage regimen. New Eng. J. Med. *269*:591, 1963.

Lange, K., Wasserman, E., and Slobody, L. B.: Prolonged intermittent steroid therapy for nephrosis in children and adults. J.A.M.A. *168*:377, 1958.

Liddle, G. W.: Analyses of circadian rhythms in human adrenocorticol secretory activity. Arch. Intern. Med. *117*:739, 1966.

Matthews, H. A.: Preliminary report on single daily dose corticosteroid therapy. Med. Times *90*:934, 1962.

Medical Letter: ACTH versus corticosteroids. *10*:62, 1968.

Melby, J. C.: Adrenocorticosteroids in medical emergencies. Med. Clin. N. Amer. *45*:875, 1961.

Reichling, A. H., and Kligman, A. M.: Alternate day corticosteroid therapy. Arch. Dermat. *83*:980, 1961.

Soyka, L. F.: The nephrotic syndrome: Current concepts in diagnosis and therapy advantages of alternate day steroid regimen. Clin. Pediat. *6*:77, 1967.

Thorn, G. W.: Clinical considerations in the use of corticosteroids. New Eng. J. Med. *274*:775,1966.

Zweifach, B. W., Grant, L., and McCluskey, R. T. (ed.) The Inflammatory Process. New York, Academic Press, 1965.

Drugs for Vertigo

Boedts, D. A., and Vandenhove, P. T.: Droperidol-fentanyl citrate in equilibratory disturbances. Arch. Otolaryng. (Chicago) *89*:715, 1969.

Brand, J. J., and Perry, W. L. M.: Drugs used in motion sickness—A critical review of the methods available for the study of drugs of potential value in its treatment and of the information which has been derived by these methods. Pharmacol. Rev. *18*:895, 1966.

Cramer, R. L., and Dowd, P. J.: Some new neurophysiologic studies on motion sickness and its therapy. U.S. School Aerospace Medicine 62–69, November, 1961.

Deane, F. R., Wood, C. D., and Graybiel, A.: Effect of drugs in altering susceptibility to motion sickness in aerobatics and the slow rotation room. Aerospace Med. *38*:842, 1967.

Fermin, H., Van Deinse, J. B., and Hammelburg, E.: The effect of dimenhydrinate upon the labyrinth. Acta Otolaryng. *38*:543, 1950.

Gutner, L. B., Gould, W. J., and Batterman, R. C.: Action of dimenhydrinate (Dramamine) and other drugs on vestibular function. Arch. Otolaryng. *53*:308, 1951.

Isaacs, B., and MacArthur, J. G.: The influence of chlorpromazine and promethazine on vomiting induced by apomorphine in man. Lancet *2*:570, 1954.

Richards, A. B., Hughes, F. W., and Forney, R. G.: Evaluation of anti-motion sickness drugs by component measurements of nystagmus in guinea pigs. Curr. Therap. Res. *5*:587, 1963.

Scheinberg, P.: Effect of nicotinic acid on cerebral circulation, with observations on extracerebral contamination of cerebral venous blood in nitrous oxide procedure for cerebral blood flow circulation. *1*:1148, 1950.

Shambaugh, G. E., Jr.: Histamine in treatment of certain types of headache and vertigo following fenestration operation. Arch. Otolaryng. *51*:781, 1950.

Williams, H. L., Maher, F. T., Corbin, K. B., Brown, J. R., Brown, H. A., Hedgecock, L. D.: Eriodictyol glycoside in the treatment of Meniere's disease. Ann. Otol. *72*:1082–1101, 1963.

Antitussive Agents

Benson, W. M., Stefko, P. L., and Randall, L. O.: Comparative pharmacology of D-DL-L-dromoran and related ether derivatives. Fed. Proc. *11*:322, 1952.

Bickerman, H. A.: Clinical pharmacology of antitussive agents. Clin. Pharmacol. Ther. *3*:353, Bickerman, H. A.: Antitussive agents. *In* Drugs of Choice, 1968–69. St. Louis, The C. V. Mosby Company.

Widdicombe, J. G.: Receptors in the trachea and bronchi of the cat. J. Physiol. *123*:71, 1954.

Antihistamines

Conney, A. H., and Burns, J. J.: Factors influencing drug metabolism. Advances Pharmacol. *1*:31, 1962.

Feller, A. E., Badger, G. F., Hodges, R. G., Jordan, W. S., Rammelkamp, C. H., and Dingle, J. A.: The failure of antihistaminic drugs to prevent or cure the common cold and undifferentiated respiratory diseases. New Eng. J. Med. *242*:737, 1950.

Goodman, L. S., and Gilman, A. (eds.): The Pharmacological Basis of Therapeutics. New York, The Macmillan Co., 1965, pp. 614-643.

Marshall, P. B.: Some chemical and physical properties associated with histamine antagonism. Brit. J. Pharmacol. *124*:547, 1955.

Rapp, D. J.: Management of the child with allergic asthma and rhinitis. Pediat. Clin. N. Amer. *16*:257, 1969.

Schild, H. O., Hawkins, D. F., Mongar, J. L., and Herxheimer, H.: Reaction of isolated human asthmatic lung and bronchial tissue to specific antigen. Histamine release and muscular contraction. Lancet *2*:376, 1951.

Wilhelm, R. E.: The newer anti-allergic agents. Pediat. Clin. N. Amer. *45*:887, 1961.

Wilhelm, R. E., Nutting, H. M., Jennings, E. R., and Brines, O. A.: Antihistamines for allergic and pyrogenic transfusion reactions. J.A.M.A. *158*:529, 1955.

HISTOLOGY AND PATHOLOGY

Chapter 18

HISTOLOGY AND PATHOLOGY OF THE EAR

TEMPORAL BONE REMOVAL FOR DISSECTION AND HISTOLOGICAL EXAMINATION

by

Michael M. Paparella, M.D.

Human temporal bones are useful for the study of anatomy, histology and pathology and for practice microscopic surgical dissection. The temporal bone must be removed from the skull for adequate study. The specimen contains the external auditory canal, middle ear, mastoid, inner ear structures and surrounding petrous pyramid.

REMOVAL OF TEMPORAL BONE

When a complete autopsy permit has been obtained, the temporal bones should be removed as quickly as possible after death to retard postmortem degenerative changes. No external disfigurement or other complication to the cadaver should result.

The calvarium is removed in the usual way. The brain is then removed, with care being taken to cut the seventh and eighth cranial nerves sharply at the surface of the internal auditory meati (Fig. 1). Thus, the nerve trunks will remain with the temporal bone specimens. The brain may be preserved and studied for central auditory and vestibular lesions when desired.

The two recommended techniques of removal are: (1) the block method and (2) the bone plug method.

Block Method

A motor-driven saw or, preferably, the commonly available Stryker saw* (rocker-

type oscillating saw) may be used. With the block method four saw cuts are made as outlined in Figure 2.

The *first cut* is made at a right angle as close to the apex of the petrous bone as regional anatomy will allow. With this method the eustachian tube can be removed for study if this cut is made farther forward.

The *second cut* is made parallel to the first cut through the mastoid process as close to the lateral wall as possible. More of the mastoid process is helpful for temporal bone dissection and less is necessary for histological study.

The *third cut* joins cuts 1 and 2 and is made approximately 1 inch anterior and parallel to

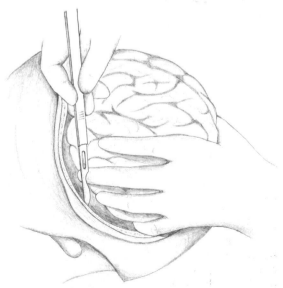

Figure 1. Removing brain, and transection of seventh and eighth cranial nerves.

---

*The Stryker saw can be obtained from the Orthopedic Frame Company, Kalamazoo, Michigan.

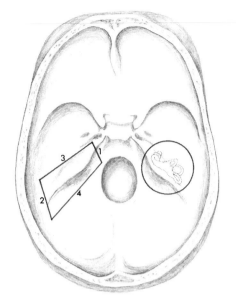

Figure 2. Outlining block and bone plug method of removal.

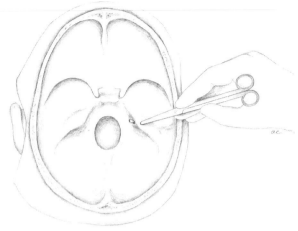

Figure 3. Arcuate eminence.

the petrous ridge in the floor of the middle cranial fossa. This cut includes the bony external canal.

The *fourth and final cut* is made in the horizontal plane close to the floor of the posterior cranial fossa. This undermining cut severs the bone from its inferior attachments. The temporal bone is still not loose, and great care must be taken to avoid crushing it. A "lion-jawed" forceps is used to grasp the specimen, and the remaining bony connections are loosened by a gentle rocking motion, which will free the specimen for further dissection. A sharp chisel, knife or scissors are used to cut remaining ligamentous fibrous and bony attachments.

Whether the temporal bone is removed by the bone plug method or the block method, the carotid artery should then be grasped and a ligature placed around this vessel. In addition, a suture may be placed in the external auditory canal to prevent any leakage of fluid (Fig. 6).

Bone Plug Method

This method was introduced and described by Schuknecht (1968) (Fig. 2). The saw should be centered over the arcuate eminence (superior semicircular canal prominence on the superior surface) and directed to the floor of the middle cranial fossa (Fig. 3). This technique requires the use of a specially designed oscillating bone plug saw attached to the conventional Stryker apparatus; the procedure is simple

and provides adequate tissue for study. For the adult skull a 1.5 inch diameter saw adjusted to a depth of 1.5 inch is used, whereas a 1 inch diameter saw adjusted to a depth of 1 inch is used for smaller skulls.

The head is steadied by an assistant and a stream of water is directed at the blade for lubrication (Fig. 4). Cutting is completed when a loss of resistance is felt, suggesting penetration through the base of the skull. An improved cutting action is acquired by slight rotation of the saw. The plug is then grasped with the "lion-jawed" forceps (Fig. 5) and the bone is rotated, permitting visualization of the intern-

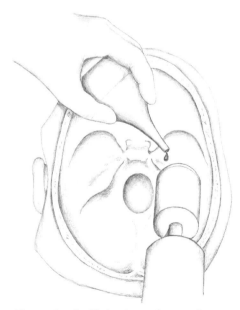

Figure 4. Oscillating bone plug saw in use.

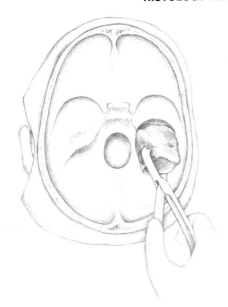

Figure 5. "Lion-jawed" forceps grasping specimen.

al carotid artery on its inferior surface; this is grasped with a curved hemostat and ligated (Fig. 6). Additional attachments are cut with a knife, scissors or osteotome.

TEMPORAL BONE DISSECTION

Surgical dissection of the temporal bone is an essential prerequisite for otology training in

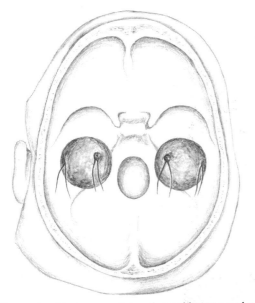

Figure 6. Ligatures on internal carotid artery and external auditory canal.

residency programs or for otolaryngologists who wish to practice certain techniques. Fresh temporal bones can be wrapped in water-soaked cotton or they may be placed in Teflon bags, all the air expelled, and the bones frozen, which helps to preserve the soft tissues for later use.

A temporal bone dissection station should be arranged to simulate actual operating room conditions as closely as possible. Essential items of equipment include a proper table and comfortable chair, an operating microscope, a motor-driven drill or other otological drill, suction, a complete assortment of otological instruments and a temporal bone holder. In general, two types of temporal bone holders can be used: one which imbeds and fixes the temporal bone in a medium such as plaster of paris, or another which secures the temporal bone specimen, allowing for study of all surfaces and relationships of the bone during dissection (Fig. 7).

It is not within the scope of this chapter to provide a guide for surgical or anatomical dissection. In teaching or learning otological surgery, however, it is possible to use an illustrated step-by-step guide which allows the resident or otolaryngologist to practice most of the surgical techniques in a single temporal bone specimen (Saunders and Paparella, 1968).

Many normal temporal bones should be used for practice dissection before any procedures are attempted in a living human being. The tympanic membrane with the attached malleus or the incus may be removed from temporal bones of healthy patients, preserved and saved for later use as a homologous transplant in tympanoplasty surgery.

HISTOLOGICAL PREPARATION OF THE TEMPORAL BONE

If the patient has had otological difficulties, including hearing and vestibular disorders, the temporal bone should be preserved for histological study. All pertinent clinical data, especially the results of auditory or vestibular function tests, should be recorded. Such patients may be persuaded to bequeath their temporal bones to science at the time of death through the Deafness Research Foundation.

Autolysis can be retarded and more rapid fixation achieved by injecting formalin solution through the tympanic membrane to fill the middle ear promptly after death. When delay in removal of the specimen is unavoidable, the

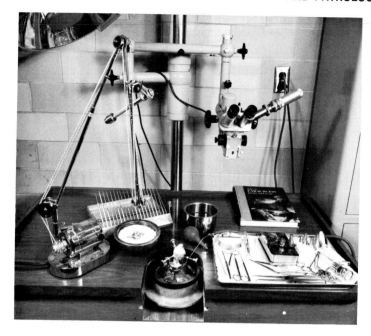

Figure 7. Typical temporal bone dissection table and set-up. Two types of temporal bone holders are demonstrated.

body should be refrigerated to reduce autolytic changes; the temporal bones should be removed within 24 hours.

Excess soft tissues and bone are trimmed from temporal bone block specimens by use of scissors and rongeur. The specimen removed by the bone plug method is smaller and can usually be placed in the fixative solution with little or no trimming.

After the bones have been removed they should immediately be placed in 400 ml. of 10 per cent formalin (one part commercial formalin to four parts distilled water) or in Heidenhain's Susa fixative solution. The jar containing the fixative and the specimen is placed in the refrigerator for a period of 48 hours. It is desirable to shake the jar once or twice a day to improve penetration of the fixative. After the bones have remained in the fixative for two to three days or more they may be shipped to a laboratory properly equipped to examine temporal bones. They should be placed in a plastic or glass jar which has been filled to the top with the fixative (formalin or Heidenhain's Susa) and properly sealed with tape or paraffin. The jar is packed in a carton with sufficient padding

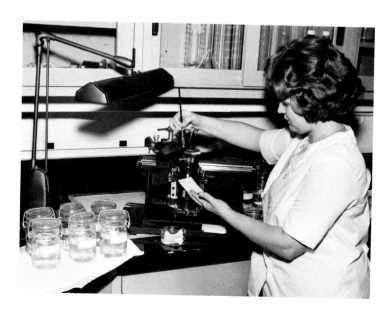

Figure 8. Technician cutting temporal bone specimen on sliding microtome.

to protect it from breakage and mailed by either first class or air mail.

The preparation of temporal bones for light microscopic study is a somewhat complex and expensive process requiring an average of seven to nine months for human specimens and a shorter time for animal temporal bone specimens. The trick is to decalcify one of the hardest bones of the body (petrous bone) while at the same time preserving all the detailed and delicate structures of the membranous labyrinth. Proper histological slides for interpretation are dependent upon: (1) reduction of post-mortem autolysis as suggested previously, and (2) elimination of preparation artifacts. Specially trained technical personnel working in a properly equipped temporal bone laboratory are necessary (Fig. 8). It is desirable for the temporal bone laboratory to function in conjunction with the general pathology laboratory of a hospital, which will help to ensure the cooperative interest of the pathologist.

Table 1 provides an outline for the procedures in histological preparation. More detailed instructions should be obtained from the literature (Schuknecht, 1968).

TABLE 1. Histological Preparation of Temporal Bone Specimens

STEP	TIME	SOLUTION	TECHNIQUE
Fixation	1st & 2nd weeks or 48 hours	10% Buffered formalin or Heidenhain Susa	Fixation in refrigerator 1st week, at room temp. 2nd week or Fixation in refrigerator
Decalcification	3rd to 9th week	5% Trichloroacetic acid	Solution is changed every day for the first week, three times weekly after that. Test for calcium with 5% ammonium oxalate in the fourth week. Test every other day until three negative reactions are recorded.
Neutralization	One day	5% Sodium sulfate	Place in solution.
Rinse	One day	Water	Rinse in running tap water.
Dehydration	10th & 11th weeks	Concentrations of alcohol	Change daily through concentrations of: 35%, 50%, 70%, 80%; two changes of 95%; three changes of absolute alcohol.
Clearing	Two days	½ Ether, ½ absolute alcohol	Change daily.
Embedding	12th thru 25th weeks	Concentrations of celloidin	Place in 1% celloidin for two weeks, then place in 3% celloidin for three weeks, then place in 6% celloidin for four weeks, then place in 12% celloidin for four weeks.
Hardening	26th thru 30th weeks	12% Celloidin	Ether and alcohol permitted to evaporate slowly to prevent formation of air bubbles.
Mounting	After hardening (1 to 2 hours)		The surface of the block is softened with ether-alcohol solution, pressed on a mounting block layered with 12% celloidin, and hardened in chloroform. The blocked specimen may be stored in 80% alcohol until time for sectioning.
Cutting	After mounting (2 to 3 hours)		Block is sectioned on a sliding microtome. Sections are cut in a horizontal plane with the modiolus of the cochlea at a thickness of 20μ. Sections can also be cut in a vertical plane parallel to the axis of the bony modiolus.
Staining	After cutting (6 to 8 hours)		Routine hematoxylin and eosin staining. Other histological stains can also be used.

Normal Histology of the Human Temporal Bone

The following temporal bone sections are selected to demonstrate anatomical relationships: Normally every fifth section is stained with hemotoxylin and eosin for study. Each section is 20μ thick, so that the distance between each stained section is five times 20μ, or 100μ (0.1 mm.). The first temporal bone seen in Figures 9 through 19 is No. 22 and the second is No. 62, so the distance between these two sections is 800μ or 0.8 mm.

Examples of Pathology

Comprehensively it is not possible in this chapter to describe the pathology of the temporal bone. Further discussion of otological pathology will be found in the appropriate chapters of Volume II. Figures 20 to 22 illustrate examples of the disease processes which may be encountered.

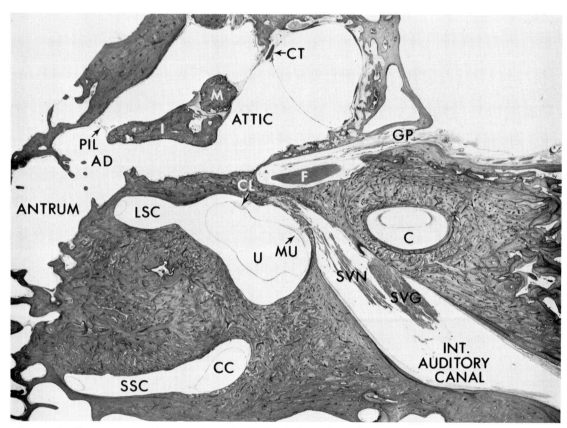

Figure 9. Normal temporal bone specimen No. 22, left. I, Incus; M, malleus (head); C, cochlea; CT, chorda tympani nerve; F, facial nerve; GP, greater superficial petrosal nerve; AD, aditus ad antrum; PIL, posterior incudal ligament; LSC, lateral semicircular canal; CL, crista of lateral semicircular canal; MU, macula of utricle; U, utricle; CC, crus commune; SSC, superior semicircular canal; SVN, superior vestibular nerve (VIII); SVG, superior vestibular ganglion (scarpas).

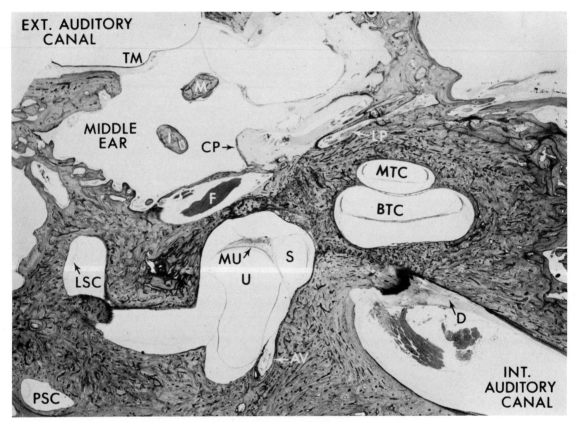

Figure 10. Normal temporal bone, specimen No. 62, left. MTC, Middle turn of cochlea; BTC, basal turn of cochlea; M, malleus (handle); I, incus (long process); TM, tympanic membrane; CP, cochleariform process; LP, lesser superficial petrosal nerve; PSC, posterior semicircular canal; LSC, lateral semicircular canal (membranous); MU, macula of utricle; U, utricle; S, saccule; AV, aqueduct of vestibule (endolymphatic duct); D, dura; F, facial nerve.

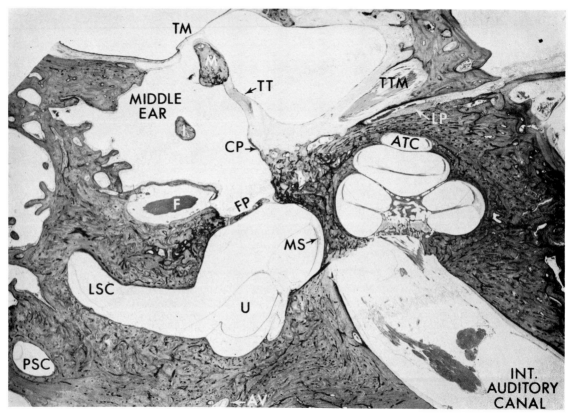

Figure 11. Normal temporal bone, specimen No. 77, left. LP, Lesser superficial petrosal nerve; TM, tympanic membrane; M, malleus (short process); TT, tensor tympani tendon; TTM, tensor tympani muscle; CP, cochleariform process; I, incus (long process); F, facial nerve; FP, footplate (stapes); MS, macula of saccule; U, utricle; AV, aqueduct of vestibule; PSC, posterior semicircular canal; LSC, lateral semicircular canal; ATC, apical turn of cochlea.

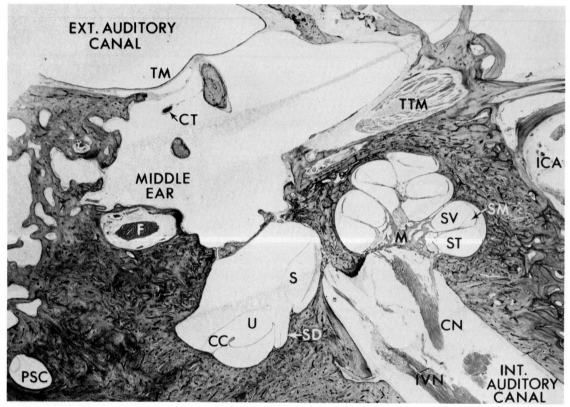

Figure 12.   Normal temporal bone, specimen No. 106, left. SV, Scala vestibuli; SM, scala media; ST, scala tympani; M, modiolus; CN, cochlear nerve; IVN, interior vestibular nerve; ICA, internal carotid artery; F, facial nerve; CT, chorda tympani nerve; Tm, tympanic membrane; U, utricle; S, saccule; SD, saccular duct; PSC, posterior semicircular canal; CC, crus commune; TTM, tensor tympani muscle.

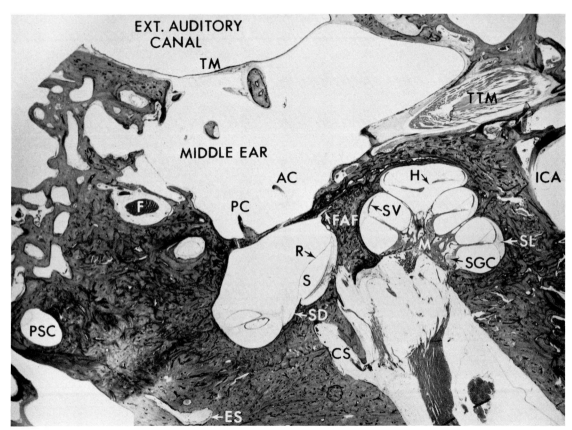

Figure 13. Normal temporal bone, specimen No. 124, left, FAF, Fissula antefenestram; SL, spiral ligament; SV, stria vascularis; H, helicotrema; M, midmodiolar view of cochlea; SGC, spiral ganglion canal (Roesenthal's); CS, canalis singulare (for nerve to posterior semicircular canal ampulla); ES, endolymphatic sac (bony portion); S, saccule; SD, saccular duct; R, reinforced part of saccular wall; PC, posterior crus of stapes; AC, anterior crus of stapes; TM, tympanic membrane; TTM, tensor tympani muscle; ICA, internal carotid artery; F, facial nerve; PSC, posterior semicircular canal.

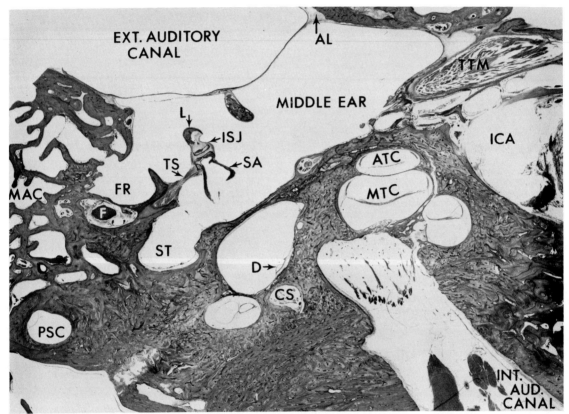

Figure 14. Normal temporal bone, specimen No. 152, left. TS, Stapedius tendon; ISJ, icudostapedial joint; L, lenticular process of incus; AL, annular ligament; F, facial nerve; SA, arch of stapes; PSC, posterior semicircular canal; D, ductus reuniens; ATC, apical turn of cochlea; MTC, middle turn of cochlea; ICA, internal carotid artery; TTM, tensor tympani muscle; ST, sinus tympani (infrapyramidal recess); FR, facial recess (suprapyramidal recess); MAC, mastoid air cells; CS, canalis singulare.

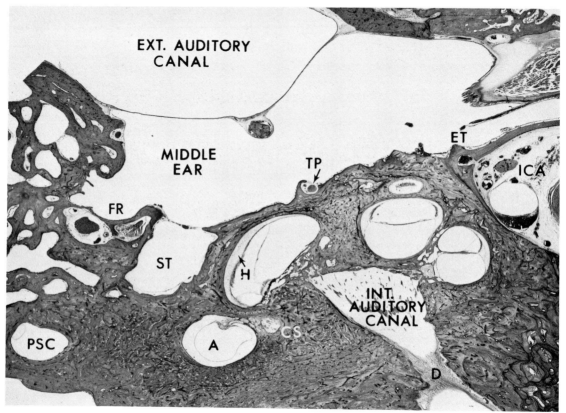

Figure 15. Normal temporal bone, specimen No. 171, left. H, Hook portion of cochlea (spiral ligament); CS, canalis singulare; A, posterior semicircular canal ampulla; PSC, posterior semicircular canal (limb); ST, sinus tympani; FR, facial recess; TP, tympanic plexus (Jacobson's nerve); ET, eustachian tube (protympanum); ICA, internal carotid artery; D, dura.

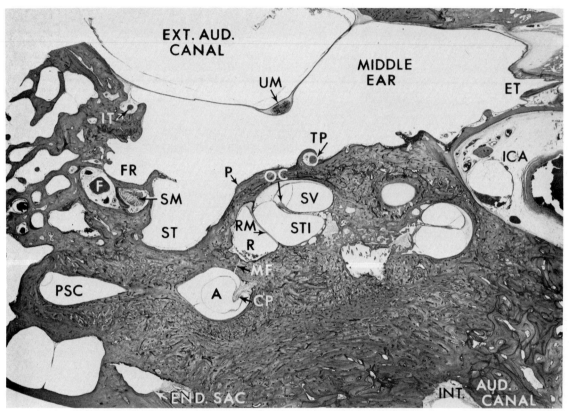

Figure 16. Normal temporal bone, specimen No. 192, left. ET, Eustachian tube; IT, iter chordae posticus (chorda tympani nerve); UM, umbo; TP, tympanic plexus (Jacobson's nerve); P, promontory; A, ampullated end of posterior semicircular canal; CP, crista ampularis; PSC, posterior semicircular canal; ICA, internal carotid artery; F, facial nerve (vertical portion); ST, sinus tympani; FR, facial recess; SM, stapedial muscle (in pyramidal process); MF, microfracture between ampullated end of posterior semicircular canal and round window niche (common finding in adults); R, round window niche; RM, round window membrane; OC, organ of Corti; STI, scala tympani; SV, scala vestibuli; END. SAC, endolymphatic sac. (Dural portion not shown.)

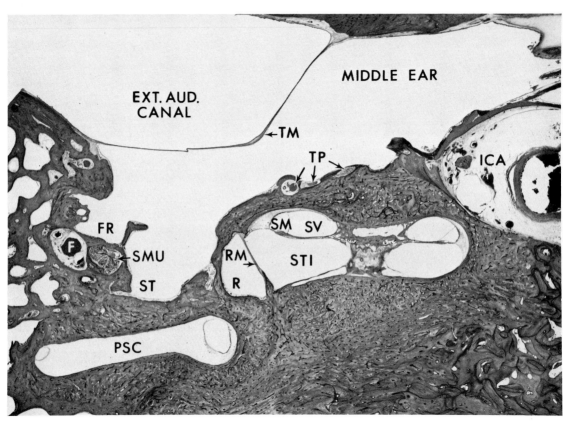

Figure 17. Normal temporal bone, specimen No. 210, left. R, round window niche; RM, round window membrane; PSC, posterior semicircular canal (lower turn); FR, facial recess; SMU, stapedial muscle; ST, sinus tympani; F, facial nerve (vertical portion); TP, tympanic plexus (arrows); STI, scala tympani; SM, scala media; SV, scala vestibuli; ICA, internal carotid artery; TM, tympanic membrane.

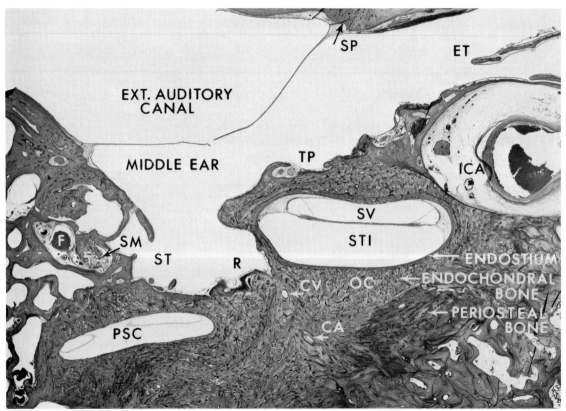

Figure 18. Normal temporal bone, specimen No. 240, left. CA, Cochlear aqueduct; CV, cochlear vein (canal of cotunnius); PSC, posterior semicircular canal; R, round window niche; ST, sinus tympani; SM, stapedius muscle; F, facial nerve; TP, tympanic plexus; OC, otic capsule (showing endostium, endochondral and periosteal bone); ET, eustachian tube; ICA, internal carotid artery; SV, scala vestibuli; STI, scala tympani; SP, sulcus tympanicus.

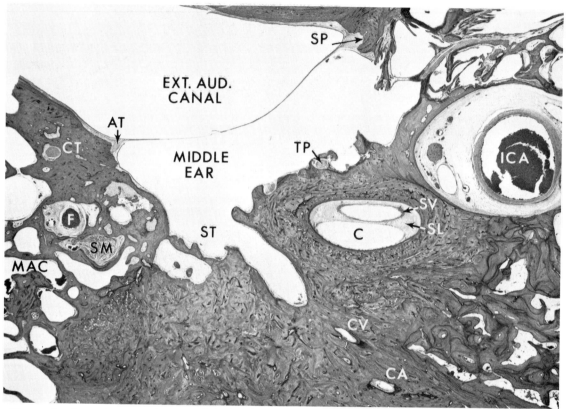

Figure 19. Normal temporal bone, specimen No. 281, left. SM, Stapedius muscle; F, facial nerve; MAC, mastoid air cells; TP, tympanic plexus; SP, sulcus tympanicus; AT, annulus tympanicus; CV, cochlear vein; CA, cochlear aqueduct; ICA, internal carotid artery; ST, sinus tympani; C, cochlea; SV, stria vascularis; SL, spiral ligament; CT, chorda tympani.

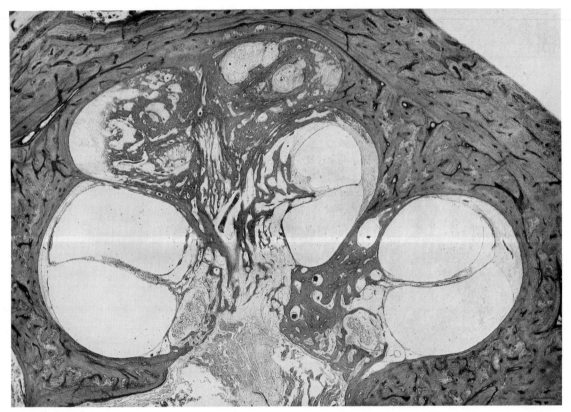

Figure 20. Cochlea of patient with embolic obstruction of arterial supply to apex resulting in fibrosis and pathological bone formation.

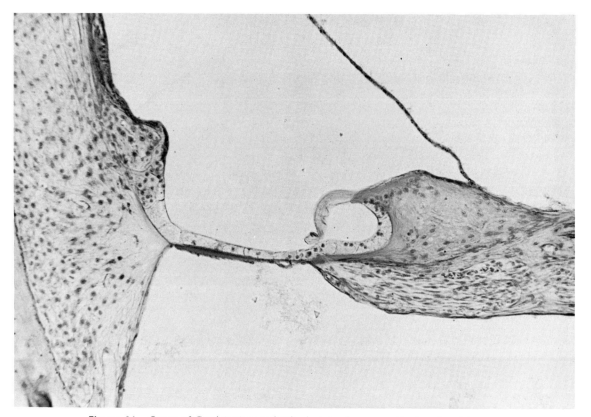

Figure 21. Organ of Corti (cat) completely destroyed as a result of profound trauma.

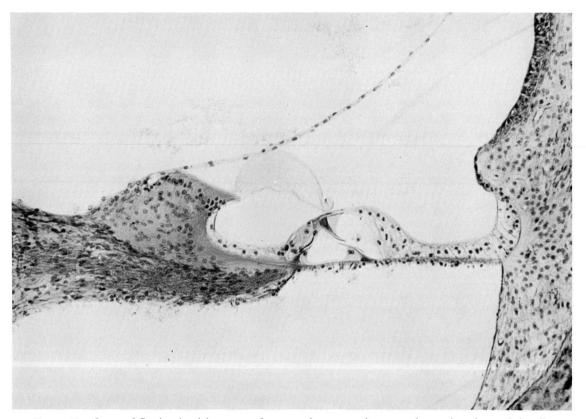

Figure 22. Organ of Corti as it might appear after ototoxic or acoustic trauma destruction of outer hair cells.

REFERENCES

Bast, T. H., and Anson, B. J.: The Temporal Bone and the Ear. Springfield, Ill., Charles C Thomas, 1949.

Gallagher, J. C.: Histology of the Human Temporal Bone (syllabus). Washington, D. C., American Registry of Pathology, 1967.

Saunders, W. H., and Paparella, M. M.: Atlas of Ear Surgery. St. Louis, The C. V. Mosby Co., 1968.

Schuknecht, H.: Temporal bone removal at autopsy. Arch. Otolaryng. 87:33-41, 1968.

Wolf, D., Bellucci, R. J., and Eggston, A. A.: Microscopic Anatomy of the Temporal Bone. Baltimore, The Williams & Wilkins Co., 1957.

The Temporal Bone Banks Program for Ear Research. I. Technique for acquiring and preparing the human temporal bone for the study of middle and inner ear pathology. II. Directory of temporal bone banks. Trans. Amer. Acad. Ophthal. Otolaryng. 70:871, 1966.

THE ULTRASTRUCTURE OF THE COCHLEAR DUCT*

by

Arndt J. Duvall, III, M.D.

and

Cedric A. Quick, M.D.

Microscopic examination of histological specimens is one of the most valuable methods of obtaining biological information. The development of phase microscopy attained the limit of resolution of the light microscope. This resolution approximates 0.2μ, a limit imposed by the wavelength of light, precluding adequate resolution at magnifications over 1100 times. With increasing knowledge it became evident that there were definitive structures smaller than those visualized by light microscopy. If better resolution and higher magnification could be obtained, the detailed form of these structures could be further studied. This has been achieved by the electron microscope, which utilizes a beam of electrons instead of light waves.

The first practical electron microscope was invented over 30 years ago. It soon came into use in metallurgy and the related industries, but a lack of techniques for producing sufficiently thin tissue sections prevented its use as a practical tool in biology until the 1950's. The electron microscope allows resolution in the order of 1 to 2Å. (Å. = 10^{-8} cm.) and consequently magnifications of over a million times (Sjostrand, 1967). Electrons pass through thin sections of a specimen and through systems of magnetic lenses and are finally made to impinge upon a fluorescent screen or a photographic plate. This electron beam is influenced to such an extent by its environment that it must be produced in a near vacuum. The sections must be extremely thin to allow "clean" penetration without scattering of the electrons. Producing sufficiently thin sections (250 Å.) without chatter or folds is the chief technical stumbling block of biological electron microscopy.

Electron microscopy has made new demands on fixation and preparation of specimens. At high magnification postmortem changes are easily visualized, necessitating

standards of specimen collection more rigorous than those of light microscopy. For ethical and anatomical reasons biopsy of the normal human cochlea is not feasible, and postmortem material is rarely obtained within the necessary time limit. Therefore, experimental animals have provided the major material for study.

The final electron image thrown onto the fluorescent screen or photographic plate is similar to a radiograph—it is one of lines, spaces, and shadows. There are few fixed parameters which will help to distinguish the normal from the abnormal. Only by many hours of patient scanning with the electron microscope will this ability be acquired.

Throughout this chapter only an outline of electron microscopy of the cochlea will be attempted. For the sake of brevity, descriptions will be confined to structures that can be delineated only with the electron microscope and are of particular interest. The reader is referred to individual publications and to the electron microscopic texts on the inner ear for more detailed descriptions (Engstrom et al., 1966; Spoendlin, 1966; Iurato, 1967).

GENERAL CONSIDERATIONS

Throughout the cochlea the epithelium enclosing the endolymph is surrounded by a basal lamina (basement membrane) (Fig. 40) which is continuous except where the nerves penetrate the basilar membrane (Fig. 32) and behind the *stria vascularis* (Fig. 39). The endolymphatic surface of this lining epithelium is a three-layered plasma membrane which is thicker than usual (130 Å. as opposed to 90Å.) and is thrown into folds called microvilli. Each cell is attached to its neighbor by a so-called "tight junctional complex" (*zonula occludens, zonula adherens,* and *macula adherens* or desmosome) (Fig. 40 insert) (Farquahr and Palade, 1963). Neural elements are found only in association with hair cells, and nowhere else in the cochlear duct.

*This work was supported by the National Institute of Neurological Diseases and Stroke, grants #NB04615, #NB05349, and #NB04403.

Every cochlear cell has the usual cytoplasmic organelles commonly described by electron microscopists. Only when their arrangements are significant will attention be drawn to them in the following text.

Limbus Spiralis

The limbus (Fig. 23) is a platform composed mainly of connective tissue continuous with that of the basilar membrane. Its flat, superior

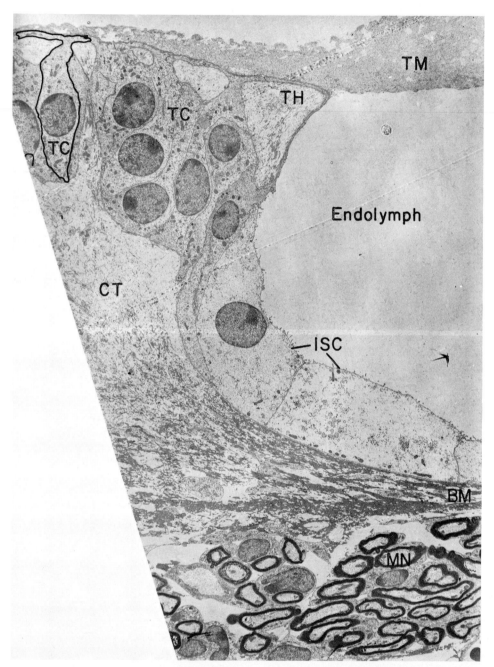

Figure 23. Limbus and inner sulcus of the guinea pig cochlea. The T-shaped cells (TC) line the superior surface of the elevated platform, the limbus. The tectorial membrane (TM) is seen as a filamentous, acellular structure projecting out from the "tooth of Huschke" (TH). Inner sulcus cells (ISC) line the endolymphatic space running down the limbus onto the basilar membrane (BM). Beneath the basilar membrane are myelinated nerves (MN). These afferent and efferent nerves gain or lose, respectively, their myelin sheaths as they penetrate the basilar membrane. The filaments of the limbus connective tissue (CT) are continuous with those of the basilar membrane. (Approx. 2300×.)

surface is covered by T-shaped cells on which sits the acellular tectorial membrane. The T cells are seen very early in embryological development, as is the tectorial membrane. If one accepts the hypothesis that the tectorial membrane is secreted, then the T cells are probably responsible for this function.

Inner sulcus cells line the limbus along its vertical surface, running from the auditory tooth of Huschke along the basilar membrane to the inner supporting cells. The inner sulcus cells are similar in appearance to Claudius cells (Fig. 35).

Basilar Membrane

The basilar membrane is composed primarily of extracellular amorphous substance and radial filaments (Figs. 23, 25 *b* and 32). It is traditionally divided into an inner *pars tecta* and an outer *pars pectinata*. In the pars tecta the filaments lie side by side, whereas in the pars pectinata they are grouped into fibers ranging from 0.5 to 1.5μ in diameter (Iurato, 1962). The filaments of the basilar membrane are continuous with those of the limbus (Fig. 23) and spiral ligament. Lining the tympanic surface of the basilar membrane is a layer of connective tissue that is continuous with the rest of the *scala tympani* and contains loops of capillaries.

The Organ of Corti

The organ of Corti consists of a row of inner hair cells and three rows of outer hair cells, associated neural elements, and different types of supporting cells. Occasionally there are "extra" outer hair cells, resulting in a fourth row.

The inner hair cell (Fig. 24) appears less differentiated than the outer hair cell. It resembles an obliquely placed Type I vestibular hair cell (Fig. 25 *a*). Interestingly, during embryonic development the outer hair cells also have this flasklike shape (Fig. 25 *b*). The more elaborate ultrastructure of the adult outer hair cell may indicate a higher order of function. It has been suggested that it performs a greater degree of frequency analysis.

The cylindrical outer hair cells are longer in the apical turns than in the basal turns (Fig. 26). Lining their vertical walls are layers of flattened cisternae. Mitochondria are collected in the subcuticular region and at the infranuclear pole, and dispersed along the vertical walls.

At the surface of the hair cell (Figs. 27 and 28) is a cuticular plate from which project stiff stereocilia that are superficially embedded into the overhanging tectorial membrane (Fig. 26). These stereocilia are arranged in rows and form a characteristic pattern. Those of the outer hair cell are "W" in shape (Fig. 27 *a*), with the limbs facing away from the *stria vascularis*. Toward the stria vascularis and at the apex of the formation, a basal body (Fig. 28) lies in a small hole in the cuticular plate (Engstrom et al., 1962; Flock et al., 1962). On the inner hair cell, the stereocilia form a flattened "M" (Fig. 27 *b*), like the wings of a bird in flight. The basal body or centriole sits in front of the pattern, again toward the stria (Duvall et al., 1966). This arrangement is similar to that of the vestibular system (Flock, 1964), in which the basal bodies have associated kinocilia like those found in respiratory ciliated cells. Kinocilia extend from the basal bodies of the embryonic cochlea (Fig. 26 insert) but are absent in the mature hair cell. The significance of this anatomical polarization in the cochlea is not understood, whereas the arrangement in the vestibular system coincides with the physiological polarization. Serial sectioning has failed to identify more than one centriole, apart from the basal body, in any one hair cell (Fig. 28) (Duvall et al., 1966).

The major mechanical support of the organ of Corti is derived from the pillar cells and the reticular lamina (Engström and Wersäll, 1953). The latter is formed primarily by coalescence of tonofibrils of Deiters' cells (Figs. 26 and 27 *a*).

A firm knowledge of the normal appearance of the hair cell has borne fruit in research, because it has been seen that the first effects of damage are often reflected in the intracellular organelles of hair cells (Figs. 29 and 30) (Duvall and Wersall, 1964; Hawkins and Engstrom, 1964; Lundquist and Wersall, 1966).

Innervation of the Organ of Corti. Electron microscopy has resulted in an increase in our knowledge of organ of Corti innervation (Spoendlin and Gacek, 1963; Smith and Rasmussen, 1965; Spoendlin, 1966, 1969). Ultramicroscopically, efferent nerve *endings* can be distinguished from afferent *endings*. Unfortunately the afferent and efferent nerve *fibers* cannot be easily distinguished morphologically. The following discussion outlines the innervation as it is presently understood.

All nerves enter from the modiolus and are composed of afferent and efferent fibers. Where these nerves lie in the osseous spiral lamina or beneath the basilar membrane, they

(Text continued on page 516)

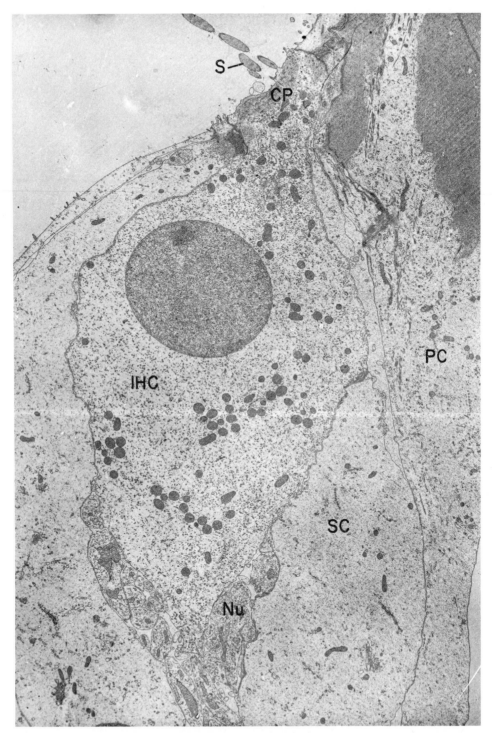

Figure 24. The inner hair cell (IHC) is obliquely placed and flask-shaped. The nucleus is central. Neural elements (Nu) cup the lower pole. Stereocilia (S) emerge from the cuticular plate (CP). Inner supporting cells (SC) surround the hair cell. Inner pillar cell (PC). (Approx. 5300×.)

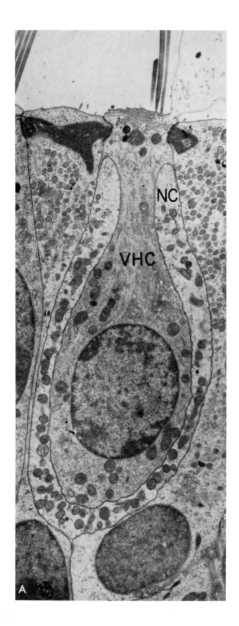

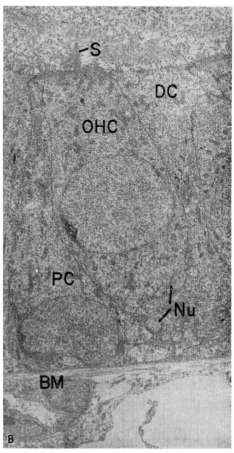

Figure 25. Comparative electron micrographs showing similarities to inner hair cell (Figure 24). *A*, A Type I vestibular hair cell (VHC) of guinea pig ampulla with its centrally placed nucleus and flask shape. The nerve chalice (NC) almost completely surrounds the hair cell. (Approx. 4800×.) *B*, The first outer hair cell (OHC) of a 40-day guinea pig embryo (length of gestation = 70 days). Nu, neural elements; S, stereocilia; BM, basilar membrane; DC, Deiters' cells; PC, outer pillar cells. (Approx. 2700×.)

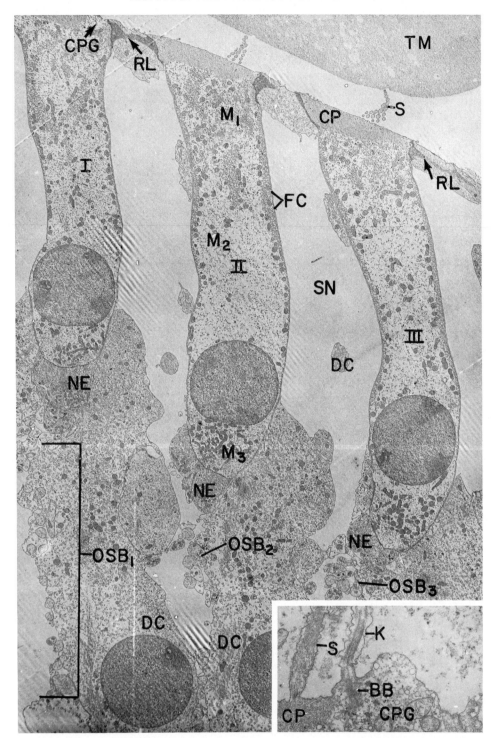

Figure 26. Outer hair cells (I, II, III) in basal turn of guinea pig at birth. Note the regular cylindrical shape and inferiorly placed nucleus. Mitochondria are dispersed in the subcuticular region (M_1) and along the vertical walls (M_2). There is also an abundance at the lower pole (M_3). Lining the vertical surfaces are well defined flattened vesicles or cisternae (FC). Except for a small gap (CPG), the cuticular plate (CP) occupies the endolymphatic surface of hair cells. Stereocilia (S) emerge from the cuticular plate and are embedded in the tectorial membrane (TM). Deiters' cells (DC) surround the lower poles of the hair cells, nerve ending "tulips" (NE), and outer spiral bundles (OSB). RL, reticular lamina; SN, spaces of Nuel. (Approx. 3100×.)

Insert: endolymphatic surface of an embryo outer hair cell (40 days) showing details of a cuticular plate gap (CPG). A kinocilium (K) extends from the basal body (BB). In the adult, only the basal body remains. (Approx. 17,000×.)

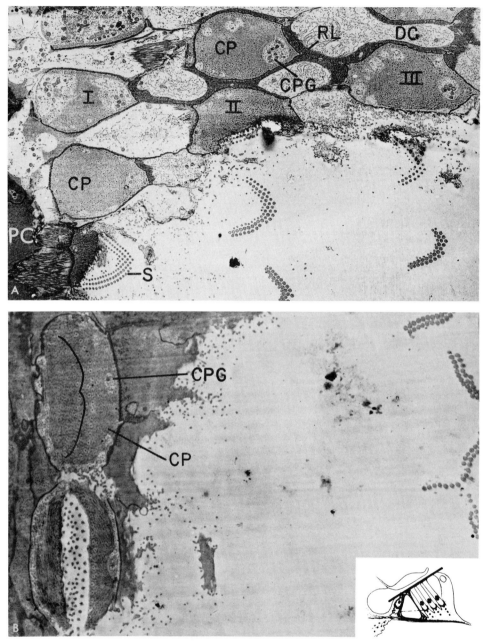

Figure 27. Transverse sections at the level of the tops of the hair cells (see line drawing). *A,* Outer hair cell (I, II, III) tops are surrounded by the reticular lamina (RL). Note the cuticular plate gap (CPG) in the cuticular plate (CP). The stereocilia (S) form a "W" pattern. PC, outer pillar cell; DC, Deiters' cell. (Approx. 2800×.) *B,* Inner hair cell tops showing cuticular plate (CP), cuticular plate gap (CPG) and characteristic "m" stereocilia pattern. (Approx. 4500×.)

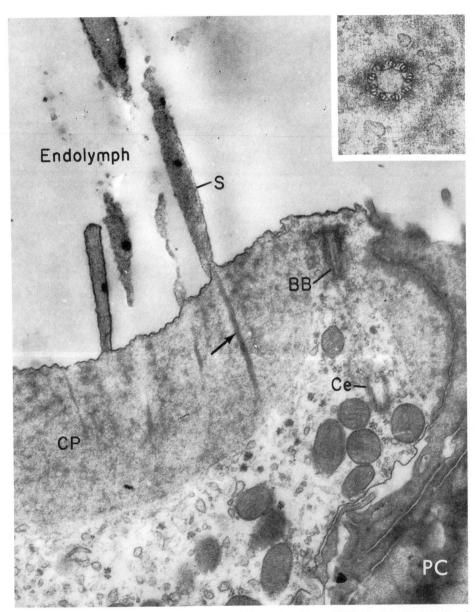

Figure 28. Top of adult inner hair cell with longitudinally cut basal body (BB) lying in the cuticular plate gap. An obliquely cut centriole (Ce) lies beneath. The fibrous core (→) of a stereocilium (S) is seen entering into the cuticular plate (CP). PC, inner pillar. (Approx. 30,000×.) Insert: Cross section of a basal body. It shows nine longitudinally oriented triplet fibers characteristic of both basal body and centriole. (Approx. 60,000×.)

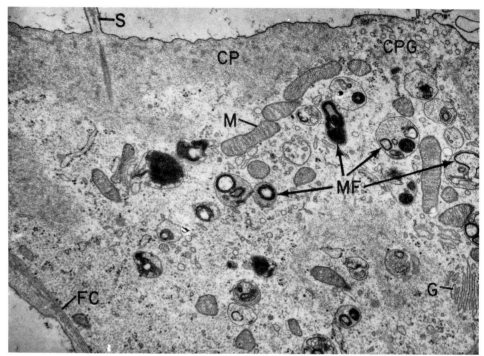

Figure 29. Subcuticular cytoplasmic pathology in outer hair cell following intramuscular kanamycin (300 mg/kg times 16 days). Earliest pathology is myelin-like figure formation in what are probably degenerating mitochondria (MF). These changes are not visible with the light microscope. CP, cuticular plate; CPG, cuticular plate gap; M, mitochondria; G, Golgi apparatus; S, stereocilium; FC, flattened cisternae. (Approx. 21,000×.)

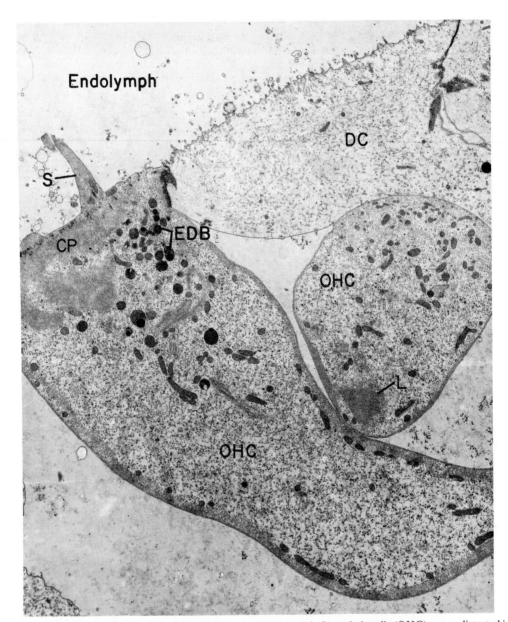

Figure 30.   Young chinchilla cochlea after exposure to intense sound. Outer hair cells (OHC) are so distorted in shape that one is cut in cross-section. Stereocilium (S) is enlarged, and there are abnormal groupings of laminated cisternae (L). Many electron-dense bodies (EDB) are concentrated below the cuticular plate (CP). Morphologically similar bodies are present in hair cells of elderly humans. (Kimura et al., 1964.) DC, Deiters' cell. (Approx. 3600×.)

are wrapped in myelin sheaths. Above the basilar membrane the myelin is absent, and nerves are covered by sarcolemmal sheaths only. Most of these fibers are collected into bundles which run spirally or radially (Fig. 31).

Both the inner and outer hair cells have afferent innervation. The efferent innervation appears to be predominant to the outer hair cells. The question of the extent of nerve-to-nerve synapse is unsolved.

Beneath the inner hair cells are inner spiral bundles (Fig. 32) composed mainly of efferent fibers which spiral in both directions along the cochlea. Some fibers cross between the inner pillar cells and form the tunnel spiral bundle. Transection of the olivocochlear bundle results in degeneration of the tunnel spiral bundle, indicating its efferent nature. Intermittently fibers of the tunnel spiral bundle turn at right angles, cross the tunnel, and innervate outer

hair cells. Some of these fibers spiral a short distance in an outer spiral bundle (Fig. 26) before innervating outer hair cells.

Most of the afferent fibers to the organ of Corti synapse directly with the inner hair cells (Figs. 24 and 32). Some take a short spiral course in inner spiral bundles and then pass obliquely to the outer hair cells between the inner pillar cells below the tunnel spiral bundle. Cross-sections show that an average of one fiber passes between each pillar cell (Spoendlin, 1969) and then lies on the floor of the tunnel, often encased in tunnel cells (Fig. 32 insert). These afferent fibers join the three outer spiral bundles (Fig. 24), which are thought to run toward the base. The small number of afferent fibers on the tunnel floor, compared with the large number of afferent nerve endings on the outer hair cells, indicates extensive nerve branching.

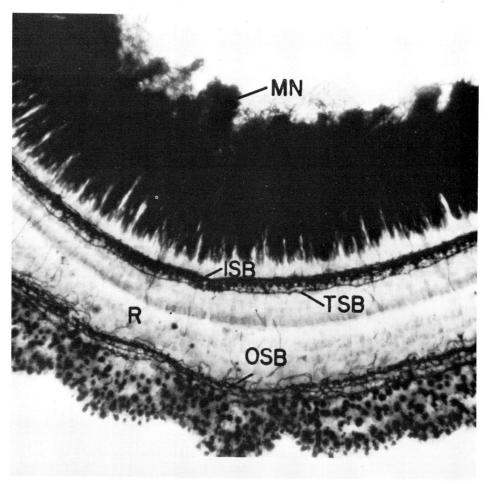

Figure 31. Surface preparation of the fourth turn of a guinea pig cochlea (osmium tetroxide-zinc oxide stain). Note the relative position of the myelinated nerves (MN) in the spiral osseous lamina, inner spiral bundles (ISB), tunnel spiral bundle (TSB) and three outer spiral bundles (OSB). Radial nerves (R) are seen crossing the tunnel. The myelinated intraganglionic spiral bundle cannot be seen because of the dark staining of the radial myelinated fibers in the spiral osseous lamina.

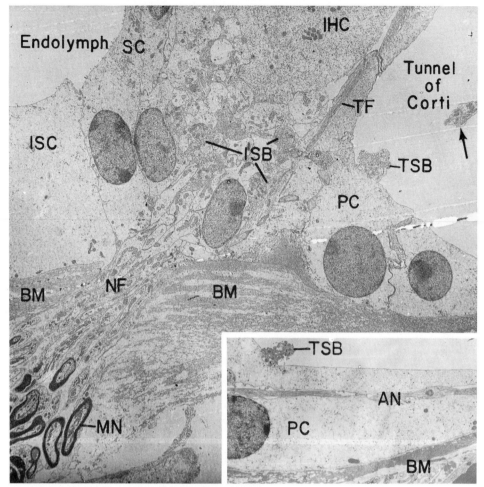

Figure 32. Beneath the inner hair cell (IHC), inner spiral bundles (ISB) are encased in inner supporting cells (SC). Tunnel spiral bundle (TSB) lies adjacent to the inner pillar (PC) in tunnel of Corti. Note efferent fibers (→) from tunnel spiral bundle crossing tunnel of Corti. Nerve fibers (NF) are myelinated (MN) only below the basilar membrane (BM). TF, tonofibrils; ISC, inner sulcus cells. (Approx. 2000×.)
Insert: Afferent nerves (AN) crossing floor of tunnel encased in pillar cell. (Approx. 3000×.)

Afferent and efferent nerve endings are grouped at the lower pole of hair cells and differ ultrastructurally (Rodriquez-Echandia, 1967). The efferent are more prevalent on the outer hair cells in the basal turns, particularly the innermost rows. These endings are also more numerous than the number of efferent fibers crossing the tunnel, indicating extensive efferent fiber branching. Nerve fibers of afferent or efferent variety supply more than one outer hair cell, and any one hair cell will therefore be supplied by more than one nerve fiber.

The efferent ending is large, and the flattened adjacent surfaces of the nerve ending and outer hair cell are called synaptic membranes. These synaptic membranes are separated by a synaptic gap of about 200 Å. in the guinea pig. Above the synaptic membrane of the hair cell lies a flattened vesicle called the postsynaptic cisterna (Fig. 33 b). The nerve ending cytoplasm is characterized by many large mitochondria and numerous synaptic vesicles, most of which are uniform in size. A few have dense cores and are larger.

The afferent ending is smaller than the efferent (Fig. 33 a). It has a thickened postsynaptic membrane and contains smaller mitochondria. The synaptic vesicles are irregular in size. Attached to the thickened presynaptic membrane of the hair cell are small electron-dense rods which protrude into the cytoplasm of the hair cell (Fig. 33 c). These synaptic bars are surrounded by vesicles. The synaptic gap varies between 150 and 175 Å. and may con-

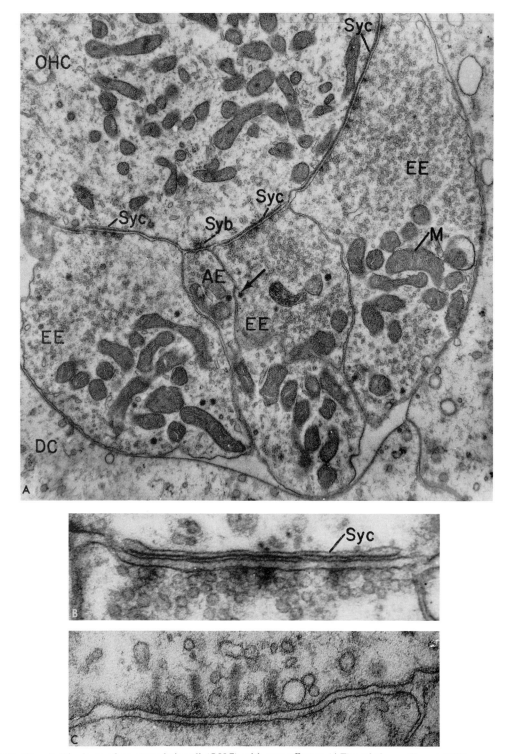

Figure 33. *A*, The base of an outer hair cell (OHC) with one afferent (AE) and three efferent (EE) nerve endings. The larger efferent endings are characterized by synaptic cisternae (Syc) which are located within the hair cell above its synaptic membrane. The cytoplasm of these endings contain numerous uniform-sized synaptic vesicles and large mitochondria (M). Within the hair cell above the afferent ending (AE) are synaptic bars (Syb). The afferent ending contains vesicles of varying sizes. Both types of endings contain some vesicles with electron-dense cores (→). (Approx. 22,000×.) *B*, Efferent synaptic area. Note vesicle condensations on presynaptic membrane and electron-dense material in the adjacent synaptic gap. (Approx. 73,000×.) *C*, Afferent synaptic area with a synaptic ribbon composed of four synaptic bars and surrounding vesicles. The bars are attached to the presynaptic membrane of the hair cell. Note the electron-dense line in the synaptic gap. (Approx. 66,000×.)

tain filamentous material which is often distinguishable as an electron-dense line.

The majority of endings innervating the inner hair cells are afferent. The endings are small and characterized by synaptic bars and thickened pre- and postsynaptic membranes. There are no endings on the inner hair cell with the arrangement of organelles characteristic of the efferent endings of the outer hair cells.

Hensen's Cells

At the lateral border of the organ of Corti, the cells of Hensen are collected together in a characteristic rosette, especially in the apical turns (Fig. 34). On the endolymphatic surface microvilli are more numerous and longer than those of any other cell type within the cochlear duct. The nucleus is centrally placed in the cell and lies along the radial axis of the rosette.

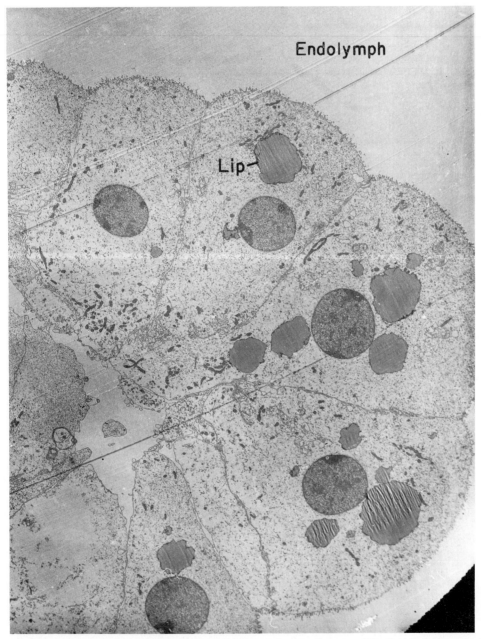

Figure 34. Hensen's cells of fourth turn in their characteristic "rosette" pattern. The lipid inclusions (Lip) are well shown, as are the long numerous microvilli on the endolymphatic surface. (Approx. 2800×.)

Cytoplasmic lipid inclusions are found mainly in the cells of the apical turns. In the embryo similar lipid inclusions are found in the inner supporting cells.

Claudius' Cells

The cuboidal Claudius' cells line the floor of the external sulcus from Hensen's cells to the external sulcus cells. Their function has long eluded investigators. The insipid appearance of the cell cytoplasm gives no clue to their function. It has been suggested (Duvall and Quick, 1969) that Claudius' cells may be one of the repositories of particulate matter, as is evidenced by the increase in lysosomes seen in these cells in experiments in which endogenous debris was created within, or exogenous tracers were introduced to, *scala media* (Fig. 35).

The External Sulcus Cells

The external sulcus cells form a continuous band throughout the cochlear duct and are situated behind the spiral prominence epithelium and Claudius' cells (Figs. 36 and 37) (Duvall, 1969). In the apical turns the external sulcus cells partly emerge from between these cell groups, exposing a surface to the endolymph. From the deep surface of the band, multicellular projections or pegs extend into the spiral ligament. The number and size of these pegs decrease toward the apex. Contrary to the popular belief, cells of the pegs are not arranged in a rosette and no extracellular lumen is present. A capillary network intertwines through the spiral ligament connective tissue around the pegs (Fig. 37).

Microfilaments are a distinguishing cytoplasmic feature of the external sulcus cells (Fig. 36 insert). These are also found in the epithelium of the endolymphatic sac. The plasma membranes of external sulcus cells interdigitate extensively with each other (Fig. 38 *a*).

The external sulcus cells contain frequent large, ovoid bodies which are surrounded by a unit membrane and are devoid of any outstanding organelles (Fig. 38 *a*). These membrane-enclosed bodies (MEB) are also found nearby in perivascular spaces, in the cytoplasm of peri-

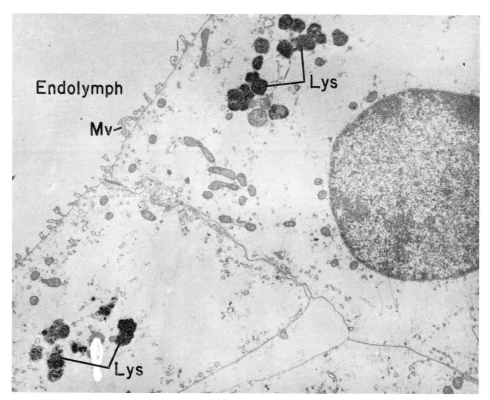

Figure 35. Claudius cells. Following placement of Ferritin into scala vestibuli, lysosomes (Lys) become prevalent in Claudius cells. Lysosomes are organelles that break down cell constituents and foreign material. Mv, microvilli. (Approx. 11,000×.)

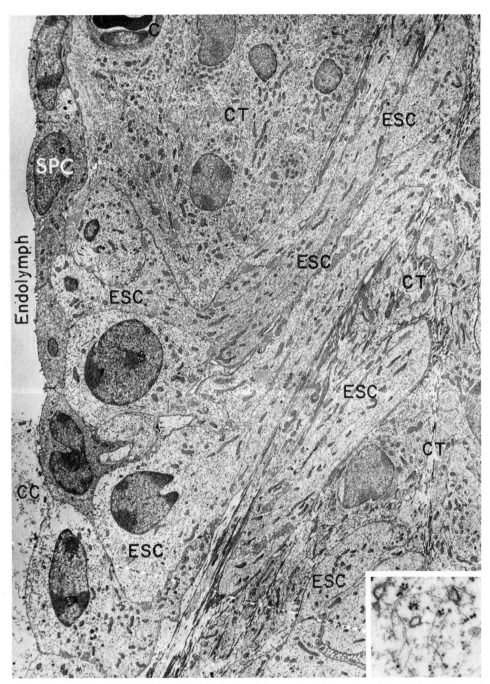

Figure 36. External sulcus cell complex (ESC) in the second turn of a guinea pig cochlea. Multicellular projections or pegs extend into the spiral ligament connective tissue (CT). In the basal turns the external sulcus cells are not directly exposed to the endolymph because the spiral prominence epithelium (SPC) and Claudius cells (CC) line the surface. C, spiral prominence capillary. (Approx. 2300×.)

Insert: Microfilaments of external sulcus cell cytoplasm. (Approx. 31,000×.)

cytes and endothelial cells, and within the capillary lumen (Fig. 38 *b*). This anatomical evidence would tend to support Saxen's (1951) original hypothesis that the external sulcus cells perform a removal function. In recent studies with electron-opaque tracers in the endolymph, no evidence of these tracers was found in the membrane-enclosed bodies or even within the external sulcus cells (Duvall and Quick, 1969). This paradoxical situation has yet to be resolved.

Spiral Prominence

The spiral prominence is a rounded bulge in the lower portion of the lateral cochlear wall below the stria vascularis (Fig. 36). It is covered by a single layer of flattened cuboidal cells. The nuclei occupy a large portion of the cells and are usually bilobed. This cell layer resembles the light cells of the vestibular *planum semilunatum*. Subepithelial connective tissue composes the bulk of the prominence and is similar to that of the spiral ligament, but

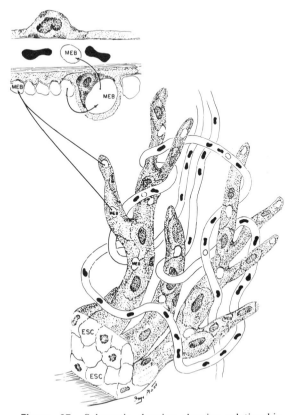

Figure 37. Schematic drawing showing relationship between external sulcus cell complex and spiral ligament capillaries. MEB, membrane-enclosed bodies.

has a greater cell density. One or more capillaries are always situated near the center of the spiral prominence.

Stria Vascularis

The stria vascularis is considered a vascular epithelium (Fig. 39) (Rodriquez-Echandia and Burgos, 1965). It extends from the spiral prominence to the attachment of Reissner's membrane, thus forming the major portion of the lateral cochlear wall. Prior to the advent of electron microscopy, its complicated morphology was not adequately delineated. It is composed of three types of cells—the marginal or chromophil (dark) cells, the intermediate or chromophobe (light) cells, and the basal cells. The capillary network within the stria is separated from the stria by a double basal lamina.

The marginal cells line the endolymphatic surface and are thought to be the only cell type derived from the otocyst (Kikuchi and Hilding, 1966). In a state of partial atrophy they can resemble the dark cells of the vestibular labyrinth (Kimura, 1969). The scala media surface has a few short microvilli. The deep portions of the cell are thrown into long, thin, tentacle-like projections, giving the cell a large surface area in relation to its volume. They interdigitate with similar, but somewhat thicker, processes of the intermediate cells. Processes from both types of cells frequently lie adjacent to the basement membrane of the capillaries. The marginal cell cytoplasm contains dense ground substance and numerous large mitochondria in their processes. Near the endolymphatic surface are a large number of rough-surfaced microvesicles of various sizes.

The intermediate cells lie behind the marginal cells. They have a pale cytoplasm with fewer mitochondria, and they are irregularly stellate in form. Projections of the intermediate cells extend toward the endolymphatic surface to interdigitate with those of the marginal cells.

The basal cells are long flat cells connected by frequent desmosomes. Their cytoplasm is pale. They may lie adjacent to capillaries and often completely surround them. Groups of basal cells intermittently project toward the endolymphatic surface but reach that surface only at the upper and lower ends of the stria vascularis. There is no basement membrane separating the stria from the spiral ligament. In guinea pigs the intermediate and basal cell layers contain melanin granules. Melanocytes may be dispersed within the stria.

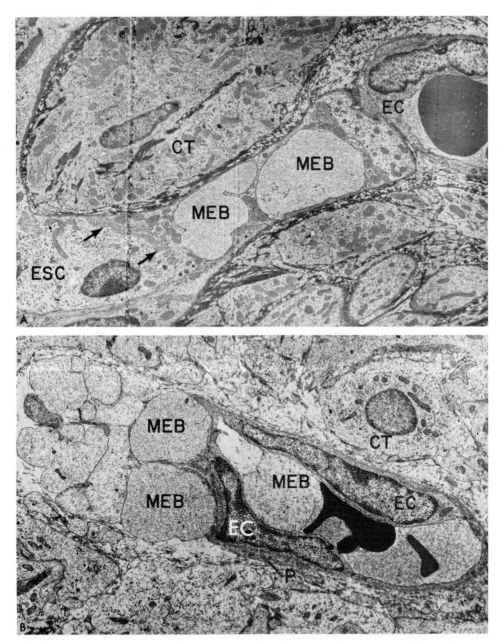

Figure 38. *A,* Membrane-enclosed bodies (MEB) are seen within external sulcus cell pegs (ESC) adjacent to an endothelial cell (EC) of a spiral ligament capillary. The characteristic interdigitation of external sulcus cell plasma membranes is arrowed ($\rightarrow$) CT, spiral ligament connective tissue. (Approx. 5000×.) *B,* Membrane-enclosed bodies (MEB) are shown within the capillary lumen and in the perivascular space. P, pericyte. (Approx. 4000×.)

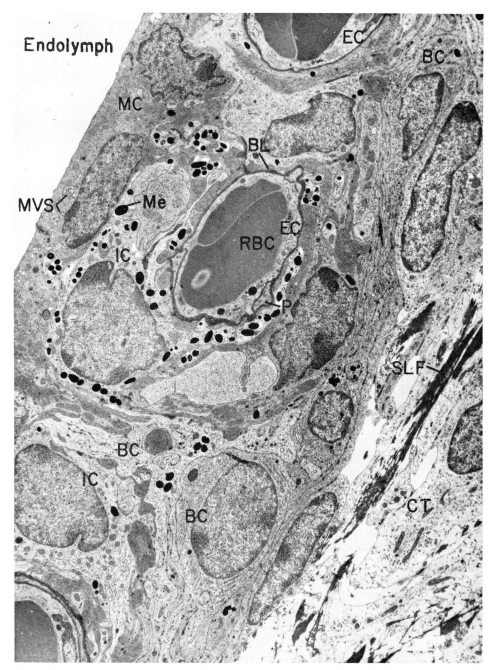

Figure 39. Stria vascularis. The marginal (dark) cell (MC) cytoplasm contains an electron-dense ground substance, many microvesicles (MVS) but few microvilli. The intermediate (light) cells (IC) have a less dense ground substance. Long cytoplasmic projections of the marginal and intermediate cells intertwine with each other and lie adjacent to the basal lamina (BL) of capillaries. Beneath these two cell types is a layer of basal cells (BC) characterized by numerous interconnecting desmosomes. Melanin granules (ME) are found in the cytoplasm of basal and intermediate cells. EC, endothelial cell; P, pericyte; CT, spiral ligament connective tissue; SLF, spiral ligament fibers. (Approx. 4900×.)

Certain morphological features suggest possible functions: The anatomical appearance of the stria is consistent with secretion or absorption. The rich endowment of mitochondria indicates high metabolic activity within the stria. Elaboration of the cell margins, greatly increasing surface in relation to volume, suggests ionic transport (Fawcett, 1962).

Reissner's Membrane

In the guinea pig Reissner's membrane has two cell layers. The scala vestibuli layer is thin and composed of elongated, flattened cells which are continuous with identical cells that line the whole scala vestibuli. Frequent pores are seen between adjacent cells (Fig. 40) (Duvall and Rhodes, 1967).

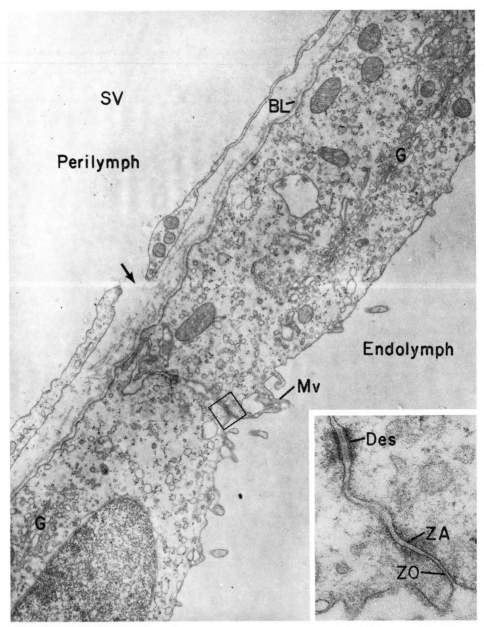

Figure 40. Reissner's membrane. The upper, thin scala vestibuli layer contains a pore (→). The more substantial scala media layer has a basal lamina (BL). All cells lining the endolymph are connected by "tight junctions," details of which are shown in the insert. G, Golgi apparatus. (Approx. 14,000×.)

Insert: Des, desmosome; ZA, zonula adherens; ZO, zonula occludens. (Approx. 86,000×.)

The flattened cuboidal cells of the scala media layer appear to have no formed connections with the scala vestibuli layer. However, between the layers, but always adjacent to the scala media layer, is a basal lamina.

From its structure the scala vestibuli layer would seem to offer little resistance to the passage of fluid, electrolytes, and particulate matter. Farquhar and Palade (1963) feel that the basal lamina might play a significant role in selectivity. The microvesicles of the scala media layer suggest proteinaceous transfer; and, in fact, micropinocytotic transfer has been observed within these cells experimentally. Passage between cells connected by "tight junctions" (Fig. 40 insert) is a matter of heated debate (Luft, 1966; Karnovsky, 1967; Revel and Karnovsky, 1967). Tracer experiments performed by the authors (1969) have shown passage through the scala media layer by both micropinocytosis and transfer through their "tight junctions." Electron-dense debris created within the scala media fails to pass further out than lysosomes within the scala media layer. It has been postulated, therefore, that Reissner's membrane offers a one-way barrier to particulate matter. More work is needed both to substantiate this hypothesis and to explore the movement of electrolytes and fluids in this region.

SUMMARY

A brief review of the ultrastructure of the cochlear duct has been presented. Electron microscopy has contributed significantly to our knowledge of this important organ. However, the electron microscope may have raised as many questions as it has answered. Morphology alone cannot delineate function but can only suggest it. The combination of electron microscopy with the tools of histochemistry, biochemistry, and electrophysiology will further advance our knowledge of the cochlea. The future offers rich opportunities to inquiring minds willing to utilize all these tools.

REFERENCES

Duvall, A. J.: The ultrastructure of the external sulcus in the guinea pig cochlear duct. Laryngoscope 79:1–29, 1969.

Duvall, A. J., Flock, A., and Wersall, J.: The ultrastructure of the sensory hairs and associated organelles of the cochlear inner hair cell with reference to directional sensitivity. J. Cell Biol. 29:497–505, 1966.

Duvall, A. J., and Quick, C. A.: Tracers and endogenous debris in delineating cochlear barriers and pathways— An experimental study. Ann. Otol. 78:1041–1057, 1969.

Duvall, A. J., and Rhodes, V. T.: Reissner's membrane, an ultrastructural study. Arch. Otolaryng. 86:143–151 1967.

Duvall, A. J., and Wersall, J.: Site of action of streptomycin upon inner ear sensory cells. Acta Otolaryng. 57:581–598, 1964.

Engstrom, H., Ades, H. W., and Anderson, A.: Structural Pattern of the Organ of Corti. Baltimore, The Williams & Wilkins Co., 1966.

Engstrom, H., Ades, H. W., and Hawkins, J. E.: Structure and functions of the sensory hairs of the inner ear. J. Acoust. Soc. Amer. 34:1356–1363, 1962.

Engstrom, H., and Wersall, J.: Structure of the organ of Corti—II. Supporting structures and their relations to sensory cells and nerve endings. Acta Otolaryng. 43:323–334, 1953.

Farquhar, M. G., and Palade, G. E.: Junctional complexes in various epithelia. J. Cell Biol. 17:375–412, 1963.

Fawcell, D. W.: Physiologically significant specializations of the cell surface. Circulation 26:1105–1132 1962.

Flock, A.: Electron microscopic and electrophysiological studies on the lateral line canal organ. Acta Otolaryng. 199(Suppl.):1–90, 1964.

Flock, A., Kimura, R., Lundquist, P.-G., and Wersall, J.: Morphological basis of directional sensitivity of the outer hair cells in the organ of Corti. J. Acoust. Soc. Amer. 34:1351–1355, 1962.

Hawkins, J. E., and Engstrom, H.: Effect of kanamycin on cochlear cytoarchitecture. Acta Otolaryng. 188(Suppl.):100–107, 1964.

Iurato, S.: Submicroscopic structure of the membraneous labyrinth—III. The supporting structure of Corti's organ. Z. Zellforsch. 56:40–96, 1962.

Iurato, S.: Submicroscopic Structure of the Inner Ear. New York, Pergamon Press, 1967.

Karnovsky, M. J.: The ultrastructural basis of capillary permeability studied with peroxidase as a tracer. J. Cell Biol. 35:213–236, 1967.

Kikuchi, K., and Hilding, D. A.: The development of the stria vascularis in the mouse. Acta Otolaryng. 62:277–291, 1966.

Kimura R. S.: Distribution, structure, and function of dark cells in the vestibular labyrinth. Ann. Otol. 78:542–561 1969.

Kimura, R. S., Schuknecht, H. F., and Sando, I.: Fine morphology of the sensory cells in the organ of Corti of man. Acta Otolaryng. 58:390–408, 1964.

Luft, J. H.: Fine structure of capillary and endocapillary layer as revealed by ruthenium red. Fed. Proc. 25:1773–1783, 1966.

Lundquist, P.-G., and Wersall, J.: Kanamycin induced changes in cochlear hair cells of the guinea pig. Z. Zellforsch. 72:543–561, 1966.

Revel, J. P., and Karnovsky, M. J.: Hexagonal array of subunits in intercellular junctions of the mouse heart and liver. J. Cell Biol. 33:C7–C12, 1967.

Rodriguez-Echandia, E. L.: An electron microscopic study on the cochlear innervation, I. The recepto-neural junctions at the outer hair cells. Z. Zellforsch. 78:30–46, 1967.

Rodriguez-Echandia, E. L., and Burgos, M. H.: The fine structure of the stria vascularis of the guinea pig inner ear. Z. Zellforsch. 67:600–619, 1965.

Saxen, A.: Histological studies of endolymph secretion and resorption in the inner ear. Acta Otolaryng. 40:23–31, 1951.

Smith, C. A., and Rasmussen, G. L.: Degeneration in the efferent nerve endings in the cochlea after axonal section. J. Cell Biol. 26:63–77, 1965.

Sjostrand, F. S.: Electron Microscopy of Cells and Tissues. New York, Academic Press, 1967.

Spoendlin, H. H., and Gacek, R. R.: Electron microscopic study of the efferent and afferent innervation of the organ of Corti in the cat. Ann. Otol. 72:660–686, 1963.

Spoendlin, H.: The organization of the cochlear receptor. In Bibliotheca oto-Rhino-laryngologie. Vol. 13. Switzerland, Karger, 1966.

Spoendlin, H.: Innervation patterns in the organ of Corti of the cat. Acta Otolaryng. 67:239–254, 1969.

SCANNING ELECTRON MICROSCOPIC MORPHOLOGY OF THE EAR

by

David J. Lim, M.D.

Since the introduction of the scanning electron microscope (SEM) to the field of biology in the mid 60's, substantial progress has been made in its application to the study of the ear. Three-dimensional views of the ear on an ultrastructural level obtained with the SEM have added a new dimension to the understanding of this complex organ. These new views bridge the gap between the understanding of the ear provided by light microscopy and that provided by transmission electron microscopy (TEM). This section is intended to provide otolaryngologists with a better concept of the morphology of the ear through the use of scanning electron microscopy. It is not an exhaustive description of all the anatomic structures in the ear; some important structures are not discussed since the SEM has not provided new insight into them.

How the SEM Differs from the TEM

Unlike the conventional TEM, which uses thin sectioned tissue, the SEM can examine most biological tissue without sectioning, thereby providing a surface view of the cells. In the SEM a narrow, constantly scanning electron beam, about 200 Å in diameter, is focused on cell surfaces which have been coated with a thin layer of conductive metal. As the electrons bombard the surface of the metal-coated tissue in a vacuum tube, they cause the emission of secondary electrons, which are collected, electronically amplified, and projected on a cathode ray tube (CRT) (Fig. 41). The SEM, therefore, consists of a column (vacuum tube), a vacuum system, and an electronic signal amplifier and displayer (CRT) (Fig. 42).

In contrast to the complex image processing in the SEM, the image in the TEM, as in the light microscope, is a result of heavy metal staining of the tissue, which provides electron contrast for a fluorescent screen. In the TEM, sectioned and stained specimens are placed in the pathway of the electron beam, but in the SEM, the bulky sepecimens are placed at terminals of the primary electron projection. This latter arrangement allows greater maneuverability of the specimen in the SEM than is possible in the TEM.

MIDDLE EAR

Tympanic Membrane

The tympanic membrane is formed by the pars flaccida and the pars tensa. The *pars flaccida,* also known as Shrapnell's membrane, consists of the epidermal, middle lamina propria, and inner mucosal layers. The middle lamina propria is made up of loose connective tissues with elastic and collagen fibers (Fig. 44A). The abundance of elastic fibers accounts for the elasticity of this part of the membrane, although the pars flaccida is generally thicker than the pars tensa in man. The pars flaccida is of particular clinical importance in relation to cholesteatoma development. The *pars tensa* also consists of three layers (Fig. 43). However, the lamina propria in the tensa consists of outer radial and inner circular fibers (Fig. 44). These fibers have been considered collagen, but recent electron microscopic and biochemical studies have shown that they are fine fibrils of an unidentified nature, possibly keratin or reticulin. The outer radial fibers are generally well developed near the umbo, while the circular fibers are better developed in the periphery of the membrane. Besides these two distinct fiber layers, there are a few parabolic, transverse, and

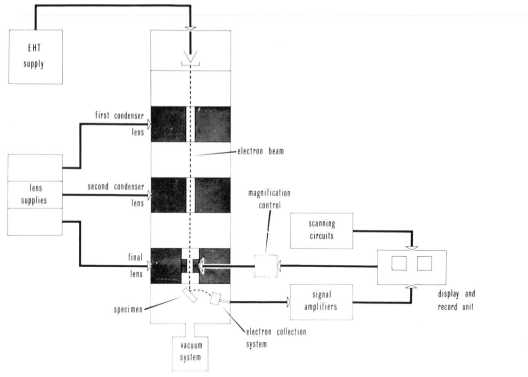

Figure 41. A diagram of the scanning electron microscope. (Courtesy of the Kent-Cambridge Instrument Co.)

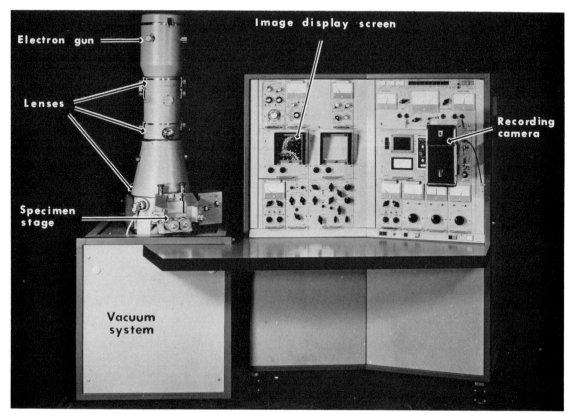

Figure 42. Front view of the scanning electron microscope. (Courtesy of the Kent-Cambridge Instrument Co.)

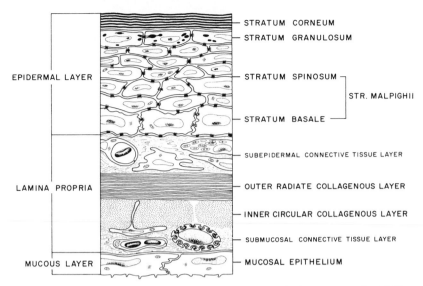

EPIDERMAL LAYER
— STRATUM CORNEUM
— STRATUM GRANULOSUM
— STRATUM SPINOSUM
STR. MALPIGHII
— STRATUM BASALE

LAMINA PROPRIA
— SUBEPIDERMAL CONNECTIVE TISSUE LAYER
— OUTER RADIATE COLLAGENOUS LAYER
— INNER CIRCULAR COLLAGENOUS LAYER
— SUBMUCOSAL CONNECTIVE TISSUE LAYER

MUCOUS LAYER
— MUCOSAL EPITHELIUM

Figure 43.   Schematic diagram of the pars tensa (Acta Otolaryng. *66:* 181, 1968).

crescentic fibers which are also a part of the total tympanic membrane fiber arrangement.

Lining Epithelium of the Eustachian Tube and the Middle Ear Mucosa Cavity

The lining epithelium of the eustachian tube is formed by ciliated cells (80 per cent in humans) and secretory cells (goblet cells) (Fig. 45*A*). The side near the pharyngeal opening contains seromucous glands which open to the epithelial surface. On the other hand, the lining of the middle ear cavity is generally described as a simple mesothelial-like squamous epithelium. Recent electron microscopic studies have provided us with evidence that the lining of the middle ear cavity is formed by numerous ciliated as well as secretory cells. About 10 per cent of the epithelial cells are ciliated on the promontory of the normal adult. A typical mucous blanket can be seen on the promontory and in the antrum (Fig. 45*B*). This information suggests that the middle ear cavity and the eustachian tube are provided with a mucociliary transportation system which could be considered part of the defense system of the middle ear. In addition to this mechanical defense system, the possible presence of an enzymatic defense system has been postulated; however, further definitive data are needed.

COCHLEA

Surface View of the Organ of Corti

There are altogether about 12,000 outer hair cells and 3500 inner hair cells in humans. The outer hair cells are arranged in three or four rows. Each outer hair cell has about 100 to 300 sensory hairs arranged in a "V" or "W" formation projecting from the cuticular plate (Figs. 46 and 47). The inner hair cells appear in a single row across the pillar cell phalanx. Each inner hair cell has about 50 to 70 sensory hairs; they are not arranged in so pronounced a "V" formation (Fig. 46*B*). The hairs of both inner and outer hair cells are arranged in a steplike pattern in which the outer row is the tallest (Fig. 47). Only the tallest hairs are firmly attached to the tectorial membrane (see Tectorial Membrane).

Although it has been well established that hearing depends on the hair cells, little is known of the exact process of sensory cell excitation. The current belief is that the shearing motion of the organ of Corti in relation to the tectorial membrane leads to excitation of the sensory cell. There is general agreement that the initial event of sensory cell excitation is physical—the bending of hairs (Békésy). However, how this bending of the hairs triggers cell excitation is not known. Vinnikov and Titova (1964) have suggested that an enzymatic ion pump, located on the surface of the hair-bearing side of the

(Text continued on page 533)

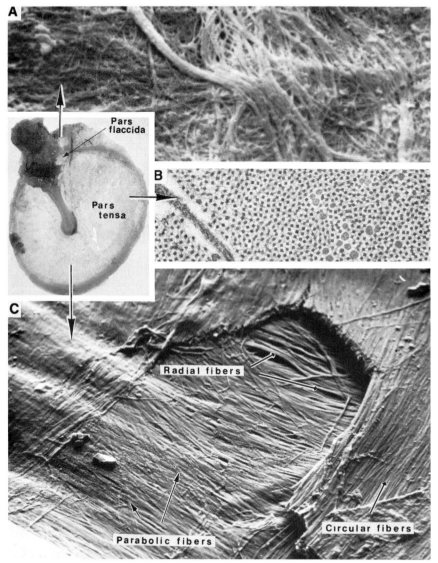

Figure 44. *A*, Irregularly arranged elastic and collagen fibers in the pars flaccida. *B*, Major components of the pars tensa fibers are formed by square fibrils; the round ones are collagen. *C*, Fiber arrangement of the pars tensa. Insert is a dissected human tympanic membrane. (Photo by T. Shimada.)

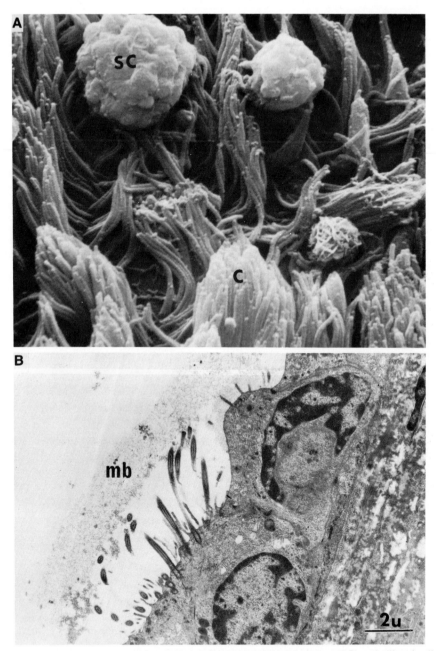

Figure 45. *A*, The lining epithelium of the bony eustachian tube shows secretory (SC) and ciliated cells (C). *B*, TEM micrograph of a ciliated cell from the human promontory with mucous blanket (MB) shows evidence of metachronal motion of the cilia. (With permission of Ann. Otol.).

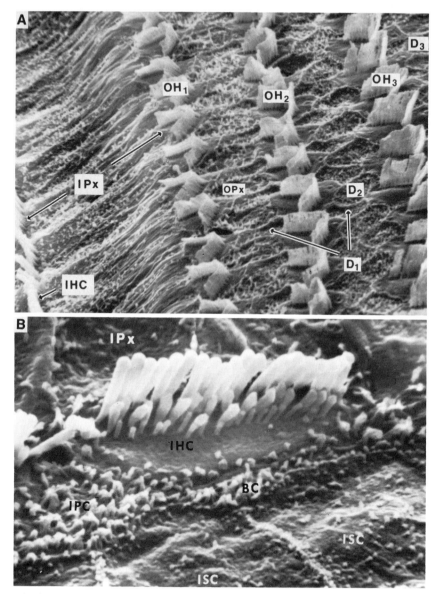

Figure 46. *A*, Surface view of the organ of Corti shows inner hair cells (IHC), head plates of the inner pillar cells (IPX), three rows of the outer hair cells (OH$_1$, OH$_2$, OH$_3$), phalanges of the outer pillar cells, and phalanges of first (D$_1$), second (D$_2$) and third (D$_3$) rows of the Deiter cells. *B*, Close-up view of the inner hair cell (IHC) shows step-like arrangement of the sensory hairs (stereocilia). Small phalanx of the inner phalangeal cell (IPC) possesses numerous microvilli. BC = border cells; IPX = head plate of the inner pillar cells; ISC = inner sulcus cells. (With permission of Arch. Otolaryng.)

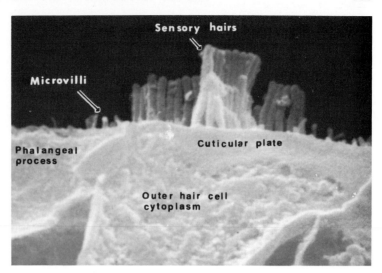

Figure 47. Fractured outer sensory cell shows step-like arrangement of the sensory hairs.

sensory cell, causes the end-organ excitation. Vilstrup et al. (1960) have suggested the possibility that the electric potential ("displacement potential") caused by displacement of the hyaluronic acid in the endolymph is responsible for the sensory cell excitation. On the other hand, Engström and his co-workers (1962) suggested that the hairs act as *levers,* transmitting mechanical energy from the tectorial membrane to the basal body, which is the essential excitable structure of the sensory cell. Still another view was put forth by Davis (1958), who suggested that the batterylike endolymph potential in the cochlea flows from the endolymph in the scala media to the neuron through the sensory cells. At the interface of the endolymph and the sensory cell, a *variable resistor,* presumably sensory hairs, should be able to raise or lower the resistance through the bending of the hairs. Lawrence (1967) modified Davis' hypothesis by suggesting that the tectorial membrane has zero electric potential and serves as a *semiconductor* between the positive resting potential of the endolymph and the negative resting potential of the organ of Corti.

Nerve Supply of the Organ of Corti

The cochlear nerve, which is derived from the cochlear ganglion in Rosenthal's canal, travels through thin bony plates (osseous spiral lamina) as bundles of myelinated nerve fibers. These bundles lose their myelin coating at the level of the basilar membrane beneath the inner hair cells. The perforations in the basilar membrane are called the *habenulae perforatae.*

These nerve bundles are formed by both afferent and efferent (olivocochlear) fibers. Both afferent and efferent nerves are supplied to the inner and outer hair cells.

As the nerve fibers enter the cochlea, they form the following bundles: (1) inner spiral bundles, (2) radial tunnel bundles, (3) spiral tunnel bundles, (4) outer spiral bundles, and (5) short radial fibers (Fig. 48). The exact pattern of nerve distribution in the cochlea is not yet clearly understood because of the tortuous course of the nerve fibers. It is believed that each of the nerve fibers supplies more than one outer sensory cell and that they travel considerable distances either in the tunnel bundles or in the external spiral bundles. The population of the afferent and efferent nerve endings and their distribution in the guinea pig and the chinchilla are mapped out by Smith and her coworkers. According to them, the number of cochlear nerve terminals per cell seems to be greater in the apical part of the cochlea. In the chinchilla, 30 small endings (afferent) were counted on a single cell. It was further concluded that the afferent and efferent endings were approximately equal in number in the entire basal turn and on the first row of hair cells in all turns. But in the upper turns, the afferent nerve endings greatly outnumbered the efferent terminals.

Tectorial Membrane

The tectorial membrane is made up of gelatinous materials containing keratinlike fibrils and sulfated mucopolysaccharide ground sub-

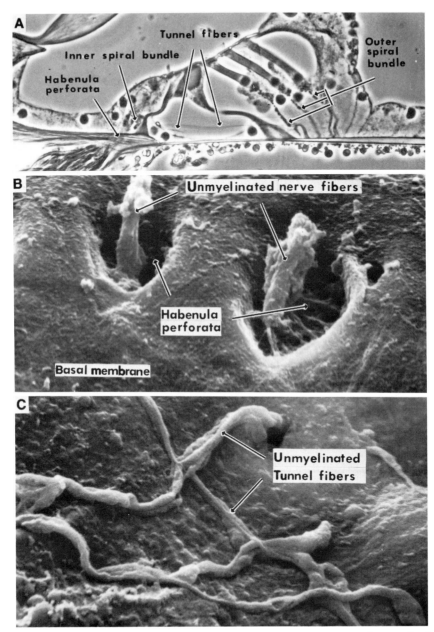

Figure 48. Light (*A*) and SEM (*B,C*) micrographs show various unmyelinated nerve bundles traveling inside the guinea pig organ of Corti.

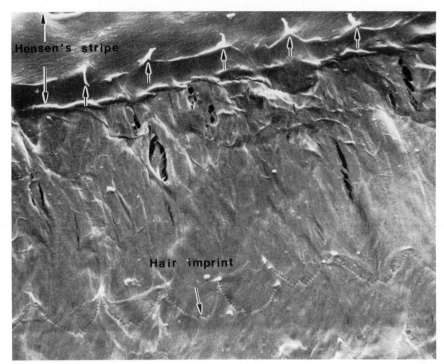

Figure 49. Undersurface of the squirrel monkey tectorial membrane shows regularly arranged trabeculae-like structures along the Hensen's stripe and first and second rows of the outer hair cells' hair imprints. Only the tallest row of the hairs left an imprint.

stances (Iurato, 1967). It can be roughly divided into three parts: (1) the limbal portion in contact with the interdental cell phalanx; (2) the midportion covering the inner sulcus, including the organ of Corti; and (3) the marginal network ("Randfasernetz"). The marginal network is believed to be attached to the third row of the Deiters' cell phalanx and/or Hensen's cell, either by fingerlike projections or by ladderlike structures. The outer surface of the membrane is loosely covered with a network of fibers similar to the material found in the marginal network. A linear band runs along the entire length of the tectorial membrane. This band, called "Hensen's stripe," has trabeculaelike structures arranged in intervals the width of one inner hair cell. These structures are believed to anchor the tectorial membrane to the inner phalangeal cells and/or inner border cells (Fig. 49). Whether or not the sensory hairs of the inner hair cells are firmly embedded in the membrane has been the subject of debate. Recent electron microscopic evidence suggests that the tall hairs of the outer hair cells are partially embedded in the tectorial membrane. The undersurface of the tectorial membrane, when seen by SEM, always shows three or four rows of imprints of the outer sensory cell hairs. On the other hand, there is no trace of any such imprints left by the inner hair cells.

Outer and Inner Pillar Cells

In cross-sectioned views the outer and inner pillars can be seen to form a triangle and to support the sensory cells. The reticular laminae between the inner and outer hair cells are formed by the head plate of the inner pillar cells (Fig. 46). The upper portion of the outer pillar cell gives firm support directly beneath the head plate of the inner pillar, but its phalanx forms a portion of the reticular lamina between the first and second rows of the outer hair cells (Fig. 46). The pillars are arranged at regular intervals, allowing the "cortilymph (Engström, 1960; Rauch, 1964) to flow freely in the tunnel, and the radial tunnel fibers to pass freely between the pillars. The bases of the pillars are firmly attached to the surface of the basilar membrane by broad footings.

Inner Phalangeal Cells

The inner phalangeal cells support the inner hair cells. Their phalanges form a portion of the reticular lamina between the inner hair cells and border the pillars of the inner pillar cells and the border cells (Fig. 46B). Cytologically, inner phalangeal cells are similar to border cells. The presence of numerous long microvilli on

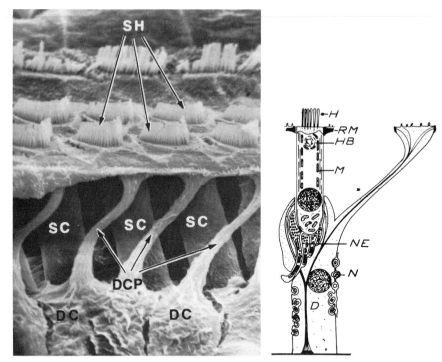

Figure 50.   The relationship between the third row of outer hair cells and the Deiters' cell (DC) is shown. Observe the slanted position of the Deiters' cell processes (DCP). SH = sensory hairs, SC = sensory cells. Insert is a diagrammatic representation of these cells by Engström and Wersäll. D = Deiters' cell, H = sensory hairs, RM = reticular membrane, HB = Hensen's body, M = mitochondria, NE = nerve endings, N = nerve. (Reproduced from Bourne, G., and Danielli, J. (eds.): International Review of Cytology, Vol. VII, p. 548. New York, Academic Press, 1958.)

the surface of the inner phalangeal cells suggests the possibility that these cells serve as anchoring points for the trabeculae of Hensen's stripe.

Deiters' Cell (Outer Phalangeal Cell)

The Deiters' cell consists of a tubular cell body, slender cell processes, and an umbrella-like phalanx. The upper part of the cell body embraces the lower part of the hair cell; therefore, this part of the cell is sometimes referred to as the Deiters' cell cup. The positions of the cell body and its cell phalanx are exactly one cell apart. In other words, a Deiters' cell embraces an outer hair cell (A), but its phalangeal process is attached between hair cells B and C, located toward the apex (Fig. 50). The function of the Deiters' cell is to support the outer hair cells. In the event of outer hair cell degeneration due to acoustic trauma, the phalanx closes the gap left by degenerated outer hair cells. There is evidence that the phalanges of the third row of Deiters' cells might serve as anchoring points for the marginal network of the tectorial membrane (Kimura).

Spiral Ligament

When examined with the SEM, the sponge-like spiral ligament appears as a meshwork of fibrils. According to Iurato (1967), these fibrils are chemically similar to keratin rather than to collagen. The spiral ligament extends to the scala vestibuli as well as to the tympani and is thereby soaked with the perilymph. Some areas of the spiral ligament facing the scala vestibuli and the scala tympani are not completely covered with cells, thus allowing free flow of perilymph. The exact function of the spiral ligament is not known; however, it is believed that this ligament acts as an anchor for the basilar membrane and houses the stria vascularis.

Limbus Spiralis

The limbus spiralis is formed by loose connective tissue similar to the spiral ligament and contains large numbers of blood vessels. The basilar membrane also anchors to the limbus as it did in the spiral ligament. Its surface faces the

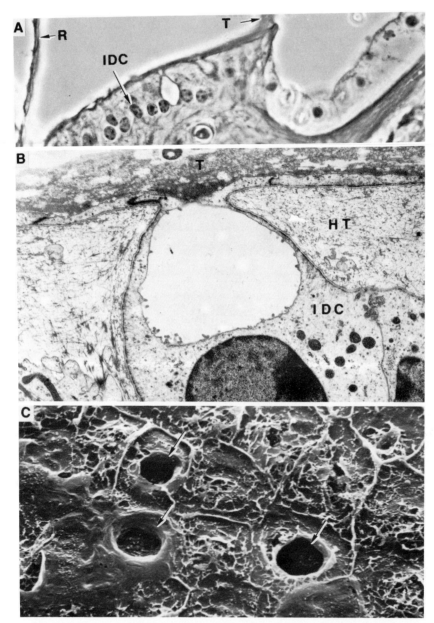

Figure 51. *A*, Light micrograph shows Reissner's membrane (R), tectorial membrane (T), and interdental cell (IDC). Observe the clear space in the limbus which is interpreted as "cytoplasmic ductule" in the interdental cells. *B*, A large invaginated cytoplasmic membrane of the interdental cell (IDC) is seen with the TEM. T=tectorial membrane; HT= Huschke's teeth. *C*, Surface view of the interdental cells is provided by removing the tectorial membrane attachment from the limbus. Arrows point to the invaginated ("ductule") interdental cells.

scala media as well as the scala vestibuli. Borghesan postulated that the vascular zone of the limbus spiralis facing the scala vestibuli contributes to the formation of the perilymph.

The part that faces the scala media is covered mainly with Huschke's teeth cells (interdental cells). In cross-section these cells appear to have the shape of the letter "T"; therefore, they are also referred to as the "T" cells. Iurato (1967) and other investigators believe that, in addition to their obvious function as anchors for the tectorial membrane to the limbus, the interdental cells also secrete tectorial membrane ground substances. Another less widely accepted function of the "T" cells is secretion of endolymph (Voldrich). Occasionally indentation of the center portion of the phalanx of this cell is observed, but the functional meaning of this observation is unclear (Fig. 51).

Reissner's Membrane

Reissner's membrane is formed by two layers of different types of cells (Fig. 52). The epithelial cells facing the endolymph have junctions that tightly bridge the cell. When they are viewed from the surface, these epithelial cells reveal a regular hexagonal arrangement. The surface in contact with the endolymph is covered with numerous microvilli, whereas the cells facing the scala vestibuli resemble endothelial cells in that their cell margins loosely overlap and they do not have a well developed tight junction. According to the "radial flow" theory of endolymph production proposed by Naftalin and Harrison, Reissner's membrane presumably serves as a filter, allowing certain ions to pass through, while it acts as a barrier to others.

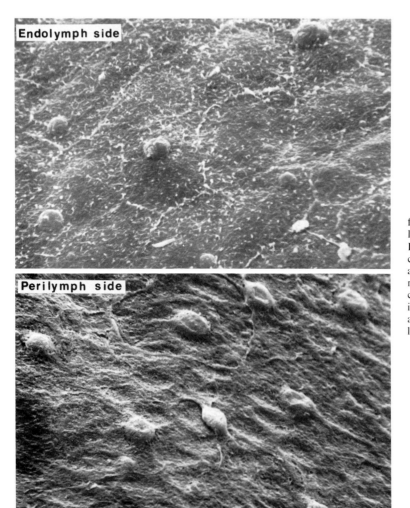

Endolymph side

Perilymph side

Figure 52. Reissner's membrane facing the endolymph side and perilymph side is shown. (Lim, D.: J. Laryng. *84*:422, 1970). The cells covering the endolymph side are well arranged hexagons with numerous microvilli on their surfaces, but the cells covering the perilymph side are irregular in shape and overlap one another. The latter cells are much larger than the former.

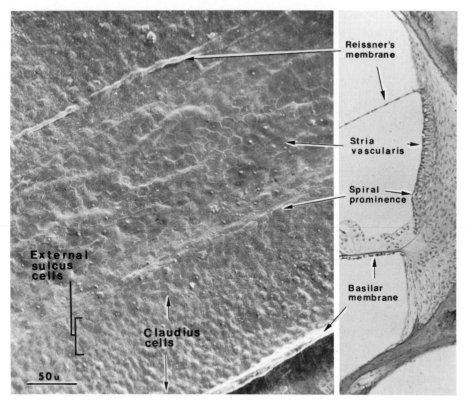

Figure 53. Surface view of the stria vascularis, spiral prominence, external sulcus cells, and Claudius cells is shown. (Lim, D. J., and Lane, W. C.: Trans. Amer. Acad. Ophthal. Otolaryng. *73*:845, 1969). Insert is a light micrograph of same area.

Spiral Prominence and External Sulcus Cells

The epithelial cells covering the spiral prominence are elongated hexagons whose long axis parallels the plane of the basilar membrane (Fig. 53), whereas the external sulcus cells are strictly hexagonal. When the external sulcus cells are covered by bordering Claudius cells, their margins become indistinct. The function of these two cell groups is not clearly understood. Although Shambaugh hypothesized that the external sulcus cell has a secretory function, morphological evidence in support of this concept is weak. Recent electron microscopic studies have revealed that the external sulcus cell possesses treelike cytoplasmic processes with numerous vessels wrapped around them. Saxen postulated that the external sulcus cells participate in phagocytosis and absorption of the inner ear fluid.

Stria Vascularis

When the stria vascularis is sectioned, it can be seen that it is formed by three different types of cells: outer marginal cells, middle intermediary cells, and basal cells. The outer marginal cells are hexagonal on the surface and are covered with a small number of microvilli and numerous pinocytotic vesicles (Fig. 53). The base of this cell interdigitates in a complex pattern with the intermediary cells. The outer marginal or epithelial cells possess large numbers of mitochondria. The stria vascularis is provided with a rich vascular network which forms a loop at the level of the spiral prominence. The function of the stria is still a source of controversy: some argue that it is absorptive, whereas others argue that it is secretory. In either case, the implication is that the stria contributes to the makeup of the endolymph.

VESTIBULE

The sensory organs of the vestibule or labyrinth in mammals are formed by three cristae ampullares and two maculae, utricle and saccule. They are the proprioceptors of rotatory and gravitational sensations. Besides these organs, the vestibule has an endolymphatic sac which extends from the otolithic organs and terminates as a blind pouch intradurally. This sac is believed to perform absorptive and phagocytic functions.

Otolithic Organs

The *saccule* is the only vestibular organ that is directly connected to the cochlea by way of the *ductus reuniens* and embryologically belongs to the pars inferior, as does the cochlea. The saccule is in the shape of an inverted L, and its "knee" points toward the cochlea. The saccule is securely fixed in a bony depression, the spherical recess of the temporal bone. The *utricle* is in the shape of an open shell with its plane approximately at right angles to the saccule and partially secured to a bony depression, the elliptical recess of the temporal bone.

Otolithic Membrane

Both saccule and utricle are termed otolithic organs because of their otolithic membranes. This membrane is formed by two parts: a gelatin layer and statoconia. When the surface of the membrane is examined, the "snowdrift lines" of Engström can be seen (Fig. 54). In the utricle this snowdrift line is in the shape of a U and appears to be a depression. In the saccule it is L-shaped and elevated like a snow-covered mountain ridge. These lines correspond to the "striola" of Werner, which is visible in a surface preparation as a light area on the sensory epithelium.

Only recently clusters of small holes in the otolithic membrane along the striola were observed with microradiography (Lindeman, 1969) and SEM (Lim, 1969). Why these holes are present is not clearly understood. However, the presence of holes along the snowdrift lines suggests the possibility that the endolymph can flow freely into the subcupular space in this region. In a test tube experiment with gel-grown calcite crystals, the smaller crystals are found, as a rule, along the gel interface. It is interesting to note that the smaller otoconia are found on the outer surface of the membrane and also along the snowdrift lines (Fig. 54).

In mammals the *statoconia* are believed to consist of calcium carbonate in calcite form. The statoconium has a smooth, barrel-shaped body with two pointed tips (Fig. 55). The pointed end is formed by three surfaces. The size of a statoconium varies considerably, ranging between 0.5 and 10μ.

The exact mechanism and origin of otolithic formation are not clearly understood; however, when isotope-labeled calcium was given to laboratory animals, some of the otoliths became labeled. This finding, according to Belanger, indicates that new calcium is incorporated into the otoconia. Regarding the origin of otoconia, Vilstrup has suggested that these crystals are formed in the endolymphatic sac in the embryonic stage and transported to the otolithic organs (transportation theory). On the other hand, some believe that these crystals are formed in the gelatin membrane (in situ formation theory). In the latter theory the calcium carbonate crystallizes in the gelatin, using the gel molecules as "critical nuclei." The importance of gelatin (mucopolysaccharide) in otoconia formation has been given further emphasis by observations made by Erway and his coworkers (1970). They were able to effect the absence or malformation of otoconia by eliminating manganese from the diet administered to pregnant mice in the early stages of their pregnancy. These investigators reasoned that the manganese is essential for the normal biosynthesis of the mucopolysaccharide and that deficient mucoprotein is the underlying cause of otolith malformation. Further, when the otoconia are decalcified, they leave protein residues.

The *relationship between the sensory epithelium* and the *gelatin membrane* has been the subject of considerable interest among morphologists and physiologists. Whether the gelatin substance completely covers the hairs remains a subject of dispute. Recent electron microscopic observations suggest that only the tall stereocilia and kinocilia are partially embedded in the gelatin layer, whereas the remainder of the sterocilia can float freely in the subcupular space (Fig. 56). Whole bundles of sensory hairs are surrounded by anchoring fibrils of the gelatinous substances (Dohlman, 1971). The supporting cells which surround the sensory cells contain numerous granules which are believed to be secretory in nature. Exactly what they secrete is still unknown; however, it is postulated that the "veil"-like anchoring fibrils are secreted by these supporting cells.

Sensory Epithelia

According to Wersäll, the sensory epithelia of the vestibule are formed by two types of sensory cells (Fig. 57). The Type I sensory cell is goblet-shaped and has a cuplike nerve ending (nerve calyx) which is believed to be an afferent nerve ending. Occasionally an efferent nerve

(Text continued on page 545)

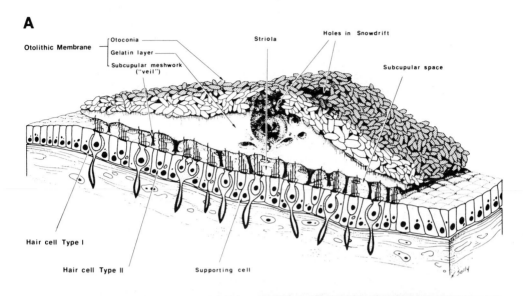

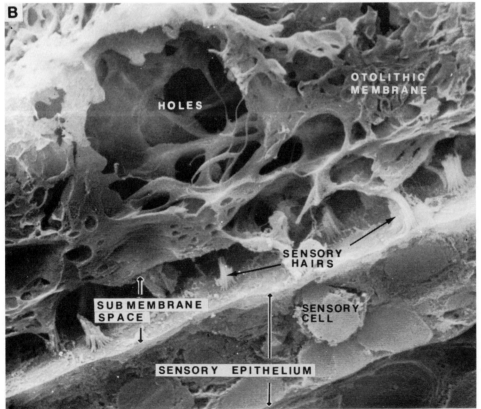

Figure 54. *A,* An artist's concept of the saccule illustrates the relationship between the otolithic membrane and the sensory epithelium. *B,* Fractured saccule shows side view of the sensory epithelium and the gelatin membrane. Numerous holes connected to the surface of the membrane are seen in the striola region. Reticular fiber arrangement of the gelatin membrane in the "otolithic striola" is depicted. (Lim, D. J.: Arch. Otolaryng. *94:*69–76, 1971).

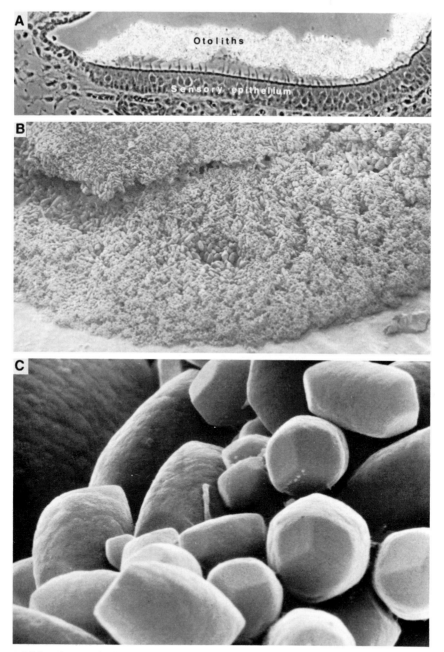

Figure 55. *A*, Light microscopic view of the otolithic membrane of the utricle. *B*, Surface view of the guinea pig otoliths in the utricle. (Lim, D. J., and Lane, W. C.: Trans. Amer. Acad. Ophthal. Otolaryng. *73*:866, 1969). *C*, Close-up view of the human otoliths.

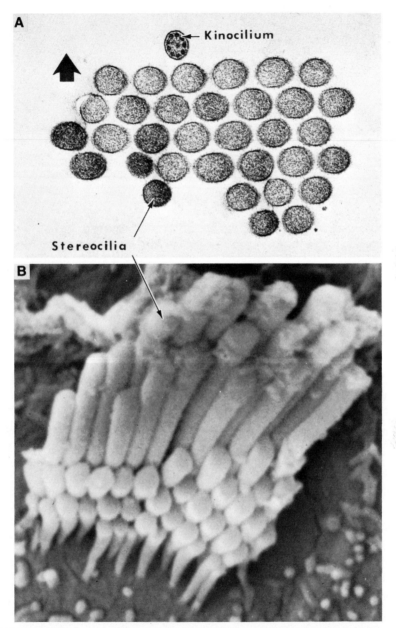

Figure 56. *A*, TEM micrograph of vestibular sensory hairs shows a kinocilium and numerous stereocilia. An arrow indicates the direction of sensory hair polarization. *B*, An SEM view of the same. Only tall stereocilia are covered with gelatinous substances. Observe the gradation in height of the sensory hairs.

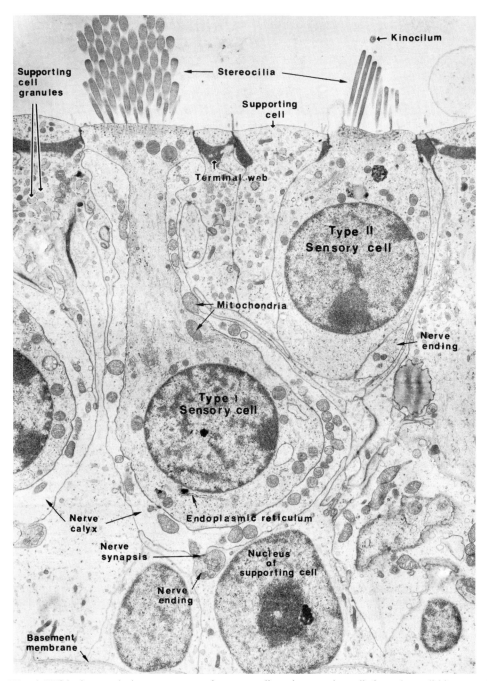

Figure 57.   A TEM micrograph shows two types of sensory cells and supporting cells from the otolithic organ. (Lim, D. J.: Arch. Otolaryng. *94*:69–76, 1971.)

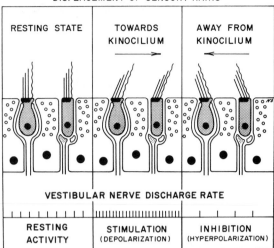

DISPLACEMENT OF SENSORY HAIRS

| RESTING STATE | TOWARDS KINOCILIUM | AWAY FROM KINOCILIUM |

VESTIBULAR NERVE DISCHARGE RATE

| RESTING ACTIVITY | STIMULATION (DEPOLARIZATION) | INHIBITION (HYPERPOLARIZATION) |

Figure 58. Artist's conception of vestibular sensory cell excitation by shearing force. (Redrawn from Wersäll, J., Gleisner, L., and Lundquist, P.-G.: *In* DeReuck, A., and Knight, J. (eds): Myotatic, Kinesthetic and Vestibular Mechanisms. Boston, Little, Brown and Company, 1967.)

ending is attached to the surface of the nerve calyx. At times the nerve calyx embraces more than one sensory cell and forms double calyces. The Type II sensory cell is cylindrical and is provided with buttonlike nerve endings, both afferent (agranular) and efferent (granular).

There are about 10,000 sensory hair cells in the utricle and about 7500 sensory cells in the saccule of the guinea pig (Lindeman, 1969). Each hair of the sensory cells consists of one kinocilium and about 80 to 90 stereocilia. The kinocilium has 2+9 internal filaments similar to those of the motile cilia, but two central filaments are frequently interrupted in sensory cilia, whereas the stereocilia are formed by an amorphous matrix without internal filaments. The kinocilium is present near the largest stereocilia, which are arranged in church pipe organ patterns (Fig. 56). The shearing motion toward the kinocilium from the stereocilia side presumably excites the sensory cells, and stimulation in the reverse direction inhibits the neural discharge (Fig. 58).

This kinocilium-stereocilia arrangement is also referred to as the direction of sensory hairs, with the kinocilium at the head and the stereocilia behind. An arrow is generally used in a diagram to indicate this arrangement in a single sensory cell. This arrangement is polarized along the striola. In the saccule, the hairs on either side of the striola are turned away from one another, while in the utricle they face one another (Fig. 59). In the ampulla of the semicircular canal, the direction of sensory hair arrangement is the same on each crista. In the horizontal crista, the direction of hair arrangement is toward the utricle, whereas it is opposite in the vertical cristae.

Semicircular Canals and Cristae Ampullares

There are three semicircular canals connecting the three cristae ampullares and the utricle. The superior and posterior canals form the common duct. These three canals are arranged at right angles to one another. Because of this arrangement, these organs are considered to be sensing devices for angular motion in each respective plane. The walls of the ampulla and the semicircular canals are formed by two layers of cells: inner epithelial and outer mesothelial-like cells. The *crista ampullaris* forms a saddlelike mound of tissue which is richly supplied with myelinated nerve fibers and capillaries embedded in connective tissue. Its surface is covered with sensory epithelium formed by two types of sensory cells and supporting cells identical to those of the macula. The only difference is that the sensory cells are much taller in the crista than in the macula, and their gradations in height are greater in the crista (Fig. 60). The long kinocilium is extremely wavy in appearance. The stereocilium takes the shape of a baseball bat. It has a narrow point inserted into the cuticular plate of the sensory cells and a dilated tip. The kinocilium, on the other hand, is usually uniform in thickness along its entire length. On top of these hairs is the cupula, which is formed by a mound of gelatin. The cupula has a definite texture in a fixed specimen. It contains numerous tubular structures and resembles a honeycomb. In the natural state, the cupula presumably is in contact with the dome of the ampulla (Steinhausen).

Whether the sensory hairs are fully embedded in the cupula has been the subject of the same kind of discussion which has focused

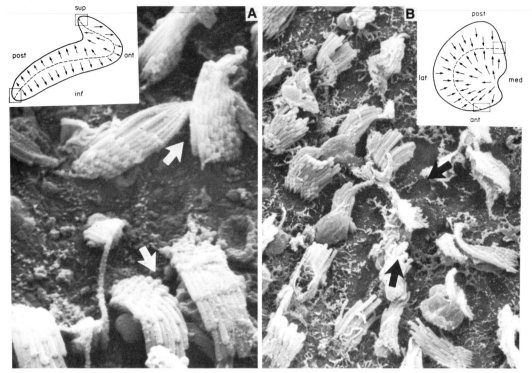

Figure 59.   *A,* Polarized sensory hair arrangement in the saccule is indicated by arrows. *B,* Arrows indicate polarized sensory hair arrangement in the utricle. (*A* and *B* from Lim, D. J.: Arch. Otolaryng. *94*:69–76, 1971.) Inserts are artist's conception of the sensory hair polarization along the striola in the saccule (left) and the utricle (right). (Reproduced from Lindeman, H.: Studies on the Morphology of the Sensory Regions of the Vestibular Apparatus. Berlin, Springer-Verlag, 1969.)

upon the gelatin membrane of the otolith organs. Electron microscopic findings seem to support the notion that there is a subcupular space. These findings suggest that the entire length of the sensory hair is not embedded in the cupula. The cupula is thought to be formed from a protein-mucopolysaccharide complex which is sulfated (Dohlman, 1960).

Planum Semilunatum

The half-moon-shaped areas on both sides of the lateral walls of the ampulla are designated as the plana semilunata (Fig. 61). The function of the planum in mammals is not yet clearly understood. Dohlman (1960) demonstrated that when ^{35}S is given to the pigeon, it is immediately incorporated into the planum cells and soon moved to the cupula. Therefore, in birds, the planum is considered to be secretory epithelium. Whether the secreta are endolymph components or part of the cupula is still open to question.

Dark Cells of the Vestibule

It is worth mentioning that the dark cells, so called because of their osmiophilic nature, have a distinct pattern of distribution in the vestibule (Kimura). The dark cells are present only in the slope of the crista. Among all the vestibular organs, the saccule is the only organ which does not possess these cells. Melanocytes have been observed lining the portion of the wall below the dark cells. The function of these cells is not yet clearly understood. Kimura and others have postulated that the dark cells might be responsible for contributing to the vestibular endolymph formation. These cells are morphologically similar to the marginal cells of the stria vascularis of the cochlea in that they have numerous vesicles and enormous interdigitations of the cytoplasmic membrane. Because of these morphological characteristics, it has been suggested that the dark cells have an absorptive function (Dohlman, 1960). It is also interesting to note that the dark cells appear to produce a mass of cytoplasmic debris on the cell surface, easily recognized with the SEM (Fig. 62).

The function of the melanocytes in the vestibule is not clearly understood. Recently, Erway and others (1970) have hypothesized that the melanocytes in the vestibule contribute to the normal metabolism of manganese, which is considered essential for the biosynthesis of mucopolysaccharides.

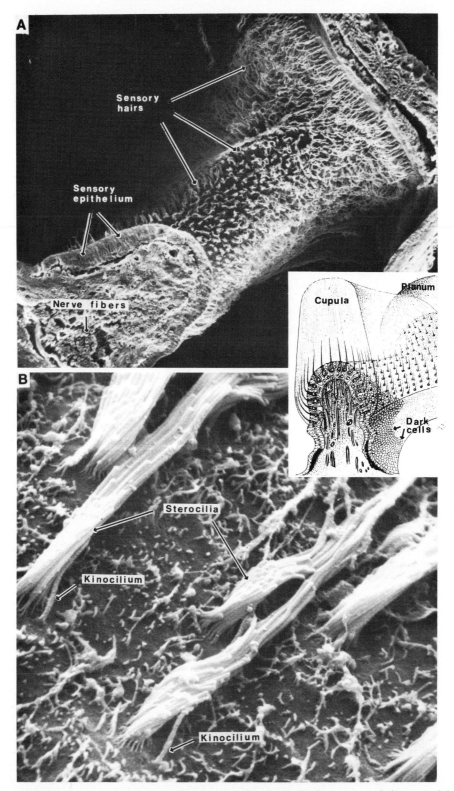

Figure 60. *A*, Bird's-eye view of the guinea pig crista ampulla shows that long sensory hairs are mainly distributed along the periphery of the sensory area and short ones in the center. *B*, Close-up view of the long sensory hairs of the crista as seen with the SEM. Observe the well-developed microvilli on the supporting cell surface. (*A* and *B* from Lim, D. J.: Arch. Otolaryng. *94*:69–76, 1971.) *C*, Insert is artist's conception of the crista showing cupula, planum semilunatum, and dark cells. (Engström, H., and Wersäll, J.: *In* Bourne, G., and Danielli, J. (eds.): International Review of Cytology, Vol. VII. New York, Academic Press, 1958.

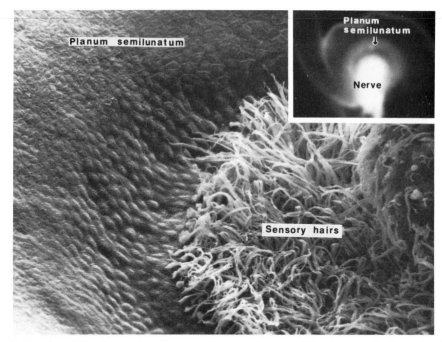

Figure 61. Inside view of the planum shows numerous hexagonal arrays of the planum cells. Insert is a lateral view of the ampulla with the surgical microscope.

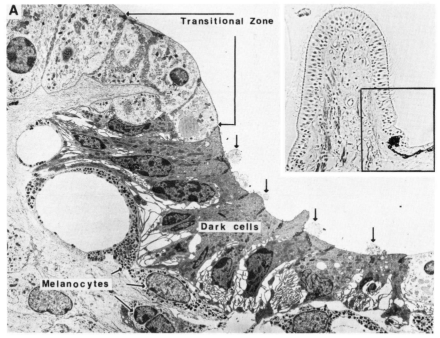

Figure 62. *A*, TEM micrograph of the dark cells whose surfaces are covered with cytoplasmic debris (arrows) is shown. The vacuolization and cytoplasmic interdigitation are characteristic of this cell. The melanocytes are generally found directly beneath the dark cells. An insert shows the area examined in A and B.

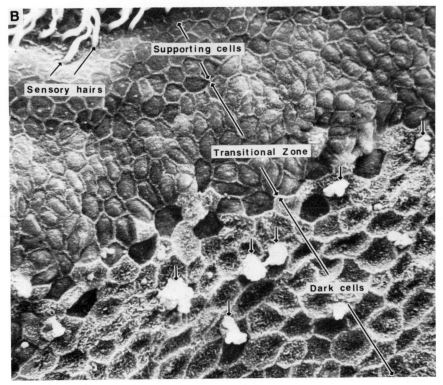

Figure 62. *Continued. B,* Same area as in the insert observed with the SEM shows dark cells with numerous cellular debris (arrows). (With permission of Ann. Otol.)

REFERENCES

Middle Ear

Hentzer, E.: Ultrastructure of the normal mucosa in the human middle ear, mastoid cavities and the Eustachian tube. Ann. Otol. *79*:1143–1157, 1970.

Johnson, F. R., McMinn, R. M., and Atfield, G. N.: Ultrastructural and biochemical observations on the tympanic membrane. J. Anat. *103*(2):297–310, 1968.

Kawabata, I., and Paparella, M. M.: Ultrastructure of the normal human middle ear mucosa. Ann. Otol. *78*:125, 1969.

Lim, D. J.: Human tympanic membrane, an ultrastructural observation. Acta Otolaryng. *70*:176–186, 1970.

Lim, D. J., and Shimada, T.: Secretory activity of normal middle ear epithelium, scanning and transmission electron microscopic observations. Ann. Otol. *80*:319–329, 1971.

Lim, D. J., Paparella, M. M., and Kimura, R.: Ultrastructure of the Eustachian tube and middle ear mucosa in the guinea pig. Acta Otolaryng. *63*:425–444, 1967.

Sade, J.: Middle ear mucosa. Arch. Otolaryng. *84*:137–143, 1966.

Shimada, T., and Lim, D. J.: Distribution of ciliated cells in the human middle ear. Ann. Otol. *81*:203–211, 1972.

Inner Ear

Békésy, von G.: Experiments in Hearing. New York, McGraw-Hill Book Co., Inc., 1960.

Belanger, L. F.: Observation on the development, structure and composition of the cochlea of the rat. Ann. Otol. *65*:1060–1073, 1956.

Bloom, W., and Fawcett, D. W.: Ear. *In* A Textbook of Histology. 9th ed. Philadelphia, W. B. Saunders Company, 1968, p. 812.

Borghesan, E.: Modality of the cochlear humoral circulation. Laryngoscope *67*:1266–1285, 1957.

Davis, H.: A mechano-electrical theory of cochlear action. Ann. Otol. *67*:789–801, 1958.

Dohlman, G. F.: Histochemical studies of vestibular sensory areas: Efferent innervation of vestibular sensory areas. *In* Rasmussen, G. L., and Windle, W. F. (eds.): Neural Mechanisms of the Auditory and Vestibular Systems. Springfield, Illinois, Charles C Thomas, 1960, pp. 258–275.

Dohlman, G. F.: The attachment of the cupulae, otolith and tectorial membranes to the sensory cell areas. Acta Otolaryng. *71*:89–105, 1971.

Engström, H.: The cortilymph, the third lymph of the inner ear. Acta. Morph. Neerl. Scand. *3*:195–204, 1960.

Engström, H., Ades, H. W., and Andersson, A.: Structural Pattern of the Organ of Corti: A Systematic Mapping of Sensory Cells and Neural Elements. Baltimore, The Williams & Wilkins Company, 1966.

Engström, H., Ades, H., and Bredberg, G.: Normal structure of the organ of Corti and the effect of noise-induced cochlear damage. *In* Wolstenholme, G., and Knight, J. (eds.): Sensorineural Hearing Loss. CIBA Foundation Symposium. London, J & A Churchill, Ltd., 1970, pp. 127–152.

Engström, H., Ades, H. W., and Hawkins, J. E.: Structure and functions of the sensory hairs of the inner ear. J. Acoust. Soc. Amer. *34*:1356–1363, 1962.

Engström, H., and Wersäll, J.: Structure and innervation of the inner ear sensory epithelia. *In* Bourne, G. H., and Danielli, J. F. (eds.): International Review of Cytology. New York, Academic Press, 1958, p. 535.

Erway, L., Hurley, L. S., and Fraser, A. S.: Congenital ataxia and otolith defect due to manganese deficiency in mice. J. Nutr. *100*:643–654, 1970.

Flock, Å., Kimura, R. S., Lundqvist, P.-G., and Wersäll, J.: Morphological basis of directional sensitivity of the outer hair cells in the organ of Corti. J. Acoust. Soc. Amer. *34*:1351–1355, 1962.

Hilding, A. C.: Studies on the otic labyrinth: On the origin and insertion of the tectorial membrane. Ann. Otol. *61*:757–769, 1952.

Igarashi, M., and Kanda, T.: Fine structure of the otolithic membranes in the squirrel monkey. Acta Otolaryng. *68*:43–52, 1969.

Iurato, S.: Submicroscopic Structure of the Inner Ear. New York, Pergamon Press, 1967.

Kikuchi, K., and Hilding, D.: The development of the organ of Corti in the mouse. Acta Otolaryng. *60*:207–222, 1965.

Kimura, R. S.: Hairs of the cochlear sensory cells and their attachment to the tectorial membrane. Acta Otolaryng. *61*:55–72, 1966.

Kimura, R. S.: Distribution, structure, and function of dark cells in the vestibular labyrinth. Ann. Otol. *78*:542–561, 1969.

Kimura, R. S., Schuknecht, H. F., and Sando, I.: Fine morphology of the sensory cells in the organ of Corti of man. Acta Otolaryng. *58*:390–408, 1964.

Lawrence, M.: Electric polarization of the tectorial membrane. Ann. Otol. *76*:287–312, 1967.

Lim, D. J.: Three dimensional observation of the inner ear with the scanning electron microscope. Acta Otolaryng. Suppl. 255, 1969.

Lim, D. J.: Vestibular sensory organs, a scanning electron microscopic investigation. Arch. Otolaryng. *94*:69–76, 1971.

Lindeman, H. H.: Studies on the morphology of the sensory regions of the vestibular apparatus. *In* Advances in Anatomy, Embryology and Cell Biology. Vol. 42. Berlin, Springer-Verlag, 1969.

Marovitz, W., Thalmann, R., and Arenberg, I.: Specialized extracellular structures of the inner ear. *In* Johari, O.

(ed.): Proc. 4th Ann. IITRI SEM Symposium, Chicago, 1971, pp. 315–320.

Naftalin, L., and Harrison, M.: Circulation of labyrinthine fluids. J. Laryng. *72*:118–136, 1958.

Paparella, M. M.: Biochemical Mechanisms in Hearing and Deafness. Springfield, Illinois, Charles C Thomas, 1970.

Rasmussen, G. L.: Neural Mechanisms of the Auditory and Vestibular Systems. Springfield, Illinois, Charles C Thomas, 1960.

Rauch, S.: Biochemie des Hörorgans. Stuttgart, Georg Thieme Verlag, 1964.

Saxen, A.: Histological studies of endolymph secretion and resorption in the inner ear. Acta Otolaryng. *40*:23–31, 1951.

Shambaugh, G. E.: On the structure and function of the epithelium in the sulcus spiralis externus. Arch. Otolaryng. *37*:538–546, 1908.

Spoendlin, H.: The organization of the cochlear receptor. *In* Rüedi, L. (ed.): Advances in Oto-Rhino-Laryngology. Vol. 13. Basel, S. Karger, 1966.

Spoendlin, H.: Auditory, vestibular, olfactory and gustatory organs, *In* Bischoff, A. (ed.): Ultrastructure of the Peripheral Nervous System and Sense Organs. St. Louis, The C. V. Mosby Co., 1970, p. 173.

Steinhausen, W.: Über die Beobachtung der Cupula in den Bogengangsampullen des Labyrinths des lebenden Hechts. Arch. Ges. Physiol. *232*:500–512, 1933.

Vilstrup, T.: On the formation of the otoliths. Ann. Otol. *60*:974–981, 1951.

Vilstrup, T., et al.: (Cited by Dohlman, G. F.) Histochemical studies of vestibular mechanisms. *In* Rasmussen, G. L., and Windle, W. F. (eds.): Neural Mechanisms of the Auditory and Vestibular Systems. Springfield, Illinois, Charles C Thomas, 1960, p. 270.

Vinnikov, J. A., and Titova, L. K.: The Organ of Corti, Its Histophysiology and Histochemistry. New York. Consultants Bureau, Inc., 1964.

Voldrich, L.: Morphology and function of the epithelium of the limbus spiralis cochlea. Acta Otolaryng. *63*:505–514, 1967.

Wersäll, J.: The minute structure of the crista ampullaris in the guinea pig as revealed by the electron microscope. Acta Otolaryng. *44*:359–369, 1954.

Chapter 19

HISTOLOGY AND PATHOLOGY OF THE NOSE AND SINUSES

by Paul Lober, M.D.

NASAL CAVITY AND PARANASAL SINUSES

Histology

The nasal cavities and paranasal sinuses form a continuous interconnecting structure. They represent a conducting portion of the respiratory tract modified for contact with environmental air. Because of their similarity, the histological features of the entire space may be covered in a single discussion. The paranasal sinuses do not directly conduct air, and their function, if any, is still obscure (Blantar and Biggs, 1969).

The skin of the nose continues through the external nares into the first portion of the nasal cavities, the vestibule. Hairs are enlarged and thickened in this area. The pilosebaceous apparatus is similar to that of the skin. Inside the vestibule, at a variable distance from the exterior, there is an abrupt transition of the stratified squamous epithelium into mucus-secreting, pseudostratified, ciliated, columnar epithelium, which lines the remainder of the space. This is sometimes modified at a few points into stratified squamous type epithelium where the exterior air strikes an exposed surface, as at the lower extremities of the turbinates. Goblet cells are frequent in the respiratory epithelium. An integral part of the mucosa is the continuous sheet of mucus on the surface, propelled by beating cilia.

A distinct basement lamina divides the mucosa and submucosa. The submucosa of the nasal cavities is relatively thick. It contains many large venous channels, particularly over the conchae. Although these bear some similarity to erectile tissue, they lack smooth muscle in their septa. There are mixed mucous and serous glands in the submucosa, which open directly on the surface (Bloom and Fawcett, 1968).

The posterior portion of the nasal spaces frequently shows aggregates of lymphatic tissue in the submucosa. These may contain well-formed lymphoid follicles. In these areas, lymphocytes and other inflammatory cells may be seen within the mucosa itself, having apparently migrated from deeper germinal centers or vessels. There may be a very intimate blending of lymphocytes with epithelium (Fig. 1).

The accessory sinuses show a similar respiratory epithelial lining. The mucous glands of the submucosa are fewer and smaller and blood vessels less prominent. There are only scattered lymphocytes. The entire submucosa is thinner, somewhat more fibrous and tightly adherent and continuous with the periosteum of the underlying bone. The cilia beat toward the orifice into the nasal cavity.

At the apex of the nasal cavities the surface epithelium is modified for olfaction. The mucosa in this olfactory area is yellowish brown rather than pink. It extends from the roof 8 or 10 mm. on each side of the nasal septum and covers the supreme nasal concha. It amounts to about 5 sq. cm. of mucosa altogether. The

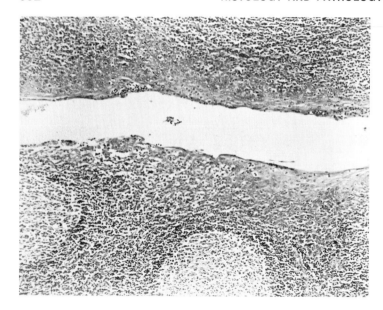

Figure 1. Photomicrograph of tonsillar crypt showing the intimate blending of lymphoid tissue and epithelium as "lymphoepithelium." (Hematoxylin and eosin, × 100.)

olfactory sensory organ is primitive as compared to the ear or eye.

The pseudostratified epithelium is about 60 micra thick in this area. There are tall narrow supporting cells showing long microvilli on the surface and axial fibrils. Conical basal cells form a layer between the attachments of the supporting cells to the basement membrane. They show branching processes.

The olfactory sensory cells in the mucosa are modified bipolar nerve cells. The nuclei are below those of the supporting cells. The dendrite projects to the surface where it extends as an olfactory vesicle. Long nonmotile cilia attached to the vesicle lie within the surface layer of mucus. At the base of the olfactory cell is the axon, which continues into the lamina propria as a fiber of the olfactory nerve. These fibers are gathered into about 20 bundles which pass through the cribriform plate of the ethmoid (Bloom and Fawcett, 1968; Schneider, 1967).

Deep to the olfactory epithelium is a thin lamina propria continuous with periosteum. Blood vessels and lymphatics here communicate with those of the arachnoid through the olfactory nerve sheaths. The glands are of branched tubuloalveolar type (Bowman's glands). There are no lymphoid aggregates.

Pathology

Developmental Abnormalities

Gross anatomical deficiencies in structure of the nose are not uncommon. These range from complete atresia of the nasal cavity to deviations of the nasal septum (Unger, 1965). Atresia of the choanae may be produced by a bony or sometimes only membranous septum (Flake and Ferguson, 1965), possibly representing a persistent buccopharyngeal membrane (Boyd, 1945; Peebles et al., 1965). About half are bilateral (Flake and Ferguson, 1965). In the newborn, and especially in the premature infant, death by asphyxiation frequently occurs if the diagnosis is not made at once, since mouth breathing has not yet been learned by the infant (Bales, 1966; Fearon and Dickson, 1968).

Deficient or absent pneumatization of sinuses may accompany bony facial deformity (Kietzer and Paparella, 1969). This appears to be the result of a failure in remodeling of the bone rather than of a primarily abnormal structure.

Inclusions of aberrant tissue in the nasal walls may give rise to cysts or tumors. Embryonic tissue may be retained at points of junction of primitive segments during formation of the facial skeleton. Most commonly these are manifest as midline cysts lined by skin containing pilosebaceous structures (dermoid cysts) (Pratt, 1965). Other tissues may be included. Central nervous system tissue may occur outside the cranium in about 1 in 4000 births (Blumenfeld and Skolnick, 1965). Cystic structures lined by glial tissue may project into the nasal cavity (encephalocele) or solid tumors may result (glioma) (Fig. 2). These are most commonly seen around the dorsum of the nose (sincipital) as a nasal mass superior to the middle meatus. They also occur at nasofrontal,

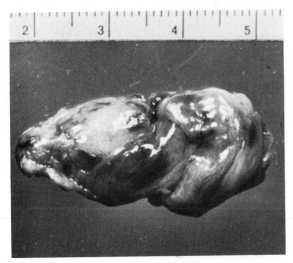

Figure 2. Nasal glioma from male infant, 5 months old. It projected into the left nasal space and consisted of mature neuroglial tissue.

naso-ethmoidal and naso-orbital junctions. The tissue is well differentiated, is composed of glial cells and fibers and does not represent a neoplasm. There may be a connection of the cavity of the cyst with the cerebral ventricular system.

Localized dilatations of blood vessels of small size may occur on a hereditary basis (hereditary hemorrhagic telangiectasia) (Fox, 1959). In the nasal cavity these may become manifest by episodic bleeding. Although the hemorrhages may be severe, death from this cause is rare (Stecker and Lake, 1965). The lesion is usually on the nasal septum. Other parts of the mouth or face may be involved, and there may be pulmonary arteriovenous fistulas (Hodgson et al., 1959). The lesion does not appear to progress with age (Stecker and Lake, 1965).

Concha bullosa is an enlarged pneumatized middle turbinate which extends into the nasal cavity (Ash and Raum, 1956).

Congenital perforations or incomplete closures of the nasal septum occur. They are uncommon as compared with acquired lesions off the septum (Unger, 1965).

Inflammatory Processes

The nasal cavities are exposed directly to all the gaseous and particulate pollutants of environmental air. Nearly all are removed by solution or by trapping in the mucus layer covering the epithelium. Irritants held to the epithelial cells in this way may lead to hyperemia, congestion, edema, and cellular infiltration of the tissue, the changes of an acute rhinitis. A sensitized mucosa may react to otherwise innocuous materials. Microorganisms may produce a similar response.

Symptoms of the common cold may be produced by identifiable viruses (Snow, 1969), some in epidemic form. Similar acute rhinitis may be related to systemic factors not yet elucidated. It is difficult to establish a demonstrable relation of acute rhinitis to simple exposure to a cold environment (Douglas et al., 1968). It has been shown clinically, however (Fowler, 1943), and it is common experience that vasomotor mechanisms may produce an acute rhinitis with hyperemia and exudation of fluid and mucus. This reaction may be triggered by allergic hypersensitivity. Liberation of histamine in the affected tissues can explain the phenomenon. It is nearly impossible to separate the allergic reactions from a secondary infectious component.

Hemorrhagic rhinitis may be associated with contact with environmental chemicals (apple-packer's epistaxis) (Garland, 1967).

Acute rhinitis is characterized by congestion and edema of the submucosa, which leads to thickening of tissues and obstruction to the airway. Hypersecretion of mucus from both glands and mucosal cells occurs, as well as transudation of fluid. Later, purulent rhinitis may be imposed, with migration of polymorphonuclear leukocytes. Eosinophilic leukocytes are nearly always present but may predominate in allergic states. Fibrinopurulent exudate may form on mucous surfaces.

Chronic rhinitis involves additional changes. Hyperplasia of fibrous tissue may lead to more or less permanent thickening of submucosa, and there may be aggregation of lymphoid and plasma cells. If there has been destruction of tissue with ulceration, or with contraction of fibrous tissue, an atrophy is produced, with thinning of mucosa and loss of mucous glands. Ozena is the condition of enlarged nasal spaces lined by flattened, dry atrophic mucosa which may be crusted and foul-smelling. Some cases appear to occur without a preceding chronic sinusitis. Removal of turbinates surgically may have a similar result.

The causative organism of chronic rhinitis is generally not clear, since there may be a mixed bacterial population.

Probably protective antibodies are present in nasal secretion which may neutralize entrant viruses at the mucous membrane surface and prevent clinical infections (Rossen et al., 1970). Ciliary action is also important in preventing infection (Dolowitz and Dougherty, 1966).

Acute sinusitis may be painful from pressure of fluid within the sinus if the orifice is blocked by edema or exudate. The mucosal changes are similar to those in rhinitis. Chronic sinusitis may lead to proliferation with permanent closure of the orifice. In purulent sinusitis the sinus may be ulcerated and filled with fibrino-purulent exudate, converting it to an abscess. Many forms are described, depending on the preponderance of the type of chronic tissue reaction (Ash, 1939).

The bony walls surrounding the sinuses are thin, and increased pressure may lead to ische-mic necrosis with local spread of the infective agent. The most serious complication is a men-ingitis. The orbital cavity may be invaded from maxillary or ethmoidal sinuses. Cavern-ous sinus thrombosis may follow sphenoidal sinusitis (Wasserman, 1967). The anterior cra-nial cavity may be involved through the fron-tal, sphenoidal, or ethmoidal sinuses. Osteo-myelitis of the frontal bone from a frontal sinu-sitis may involve large portions of the bone.

Specific infectious rhinitis may occur with streptococci, staphylococci, pneumococci, or even with Vincent's organisms. A pseudomem-branous inflammation may be produced by diphtheria bacilli and by streptococci.

Congenital syphilis may involve the vomer, leading to a flattened nasal bridge. A specific ulcerating rhinitis occurs in the secondary stage. Fungi may involve the nasal structures primarily (Hora, 1965). Mucormycosis may extend from nasal cavity to brain (rhinocerebral type) (Castleman and McNeely, 1968; De-Weese et al., 1965).

Nasal polyps are localized, pedunculated hy-perplasias of mucosa and submucosa. They are related to chronic inflammation and, in particu-lar, to allergic states. Probably there is interfer-ence with vascular outflow. Eosinophils are nearly always present whether or not an aller-gic history can be elicited. Polyps show a cov-ering of generally normal-appearing respira-tory epithelium. The basement lamina frequent-ly appears thickened or prominent. The core of the polyp shows some dilated capillary or venous channels and abundant, loose, fibrous stroma poor in cells, which are separated by a small amount of intercellular material. There are usually nests of eosinophilic leukocytes just beneath the mucosa, with more scattered plasma cells. There are generally few lympho-cytes or neutrophils. The surface epithelium may be ulcerated or may undergo squamous metaplasia where it is exposed to the air stream. Polyps are generally bilateral, espe-cially when related to allergy.

Nasal polyps are found in about 6 per cent of children with cystic pancreatic fibrosis (mu-coviscidosis) (Despons and Stoller, 1965; Ma-gid et al., 1967). This may not be significant (Blumstein, 1966). The glands are reported to show the cystic changes with dilated ducts seen in other sites. Ciliary action is normal (Magid et al., 1967).

Tuberculosis and sarcoidosis of the nasal cavity occur with characteristic granulomas.

Rhinosporidiosis is a specific granulomatous disease, usually starting in the nose, which has now been reported from many parts of the world but is most widely seen in India. It is due to a fungus, *Rhinosporidium seeberi* (Gupta 1966; Karunaratne, 1936).

Rhinoscleroma is somewhat more common. *Klebsiella rhinoscleromatis* is found in the early stages of the disease and is generally intracytoplasmic. In the early stages there is exuberant proliferation within the nasal cavity of fibroblasts and large foamy Mikulicz's cells. The late stage shows scarring. The disease may go undiagnosed for many years (Furnas, 1968; Klassen, 1965; Shaw and Martin, 1961; Winborn, 1967).

Obscure chronic inflammatory processes ap-parently beginning in or around the nasal cav-ities and sinuses which go on to extensive de-struction of tissue and often the death of the individual have been termed lethal midline granuloma (Bryce and Crysdale, 1969; Singh et al., 1958; Stewart, 1933). It is clear that not all these cases represent a single entity, and such an entity may not even exist (Eichel and Ma-berg, 1968).

The inflammatory process is proliferative, with mixtures of fibroblasts, capillaries, histio-cytes, lymphocytes, plasma cells, and polymor-phonuclear leukocytes in various proportions. Ulceration and tissue destruction ensue. It is not always located in the midline. True granu-lomas in the histological sense of epithelioid cell nodules with multinucleated giant cells are not seen.

In these cases of lethal midline granuloma, organisms are not identified, nor is recogniz-able lymphoma or other malignancy found at autopsy. The usual involvement of lower respi-ratory and urinary tracts and of vessels charac-teristic of Wegener's granulomatosis is not found at the onset (Spear and Walker, 1956), although more widespread involvement even-tually may occur. Many cases appear to have polyarteritis nodosa lesions at autopsy (Astrom and Lidholm, 1963; Brown and Woolner, 1960). Some authorities think that it is indistinguishable from Wegener's granulomatosis (Castleman and McNeely, 1965; Friedman, 1964; Yarington et al., 1965). The process may be called more properly "polymorphic reticulosis" (Eichel and Mabery, 1968). It must be distinguished from cases of reticulum cell sarcoma with secondary infection (Brown and Woolner, 1960).

Systemic lupus erythematosus may produce ulcerating lesions of nasal mucosa. During acute episodes these lesions have been known to perforate the nasal septum (Alcala and Alarcon, 1969).

Rhinoliths start as foreign bodies in the nasal space which become calcified over the years. They have been reported up to 7 cm. in size (Carder and Hill, 1966). A rare complication of the nostril is rhinitis caseosa or cholesteatoma of the nose (Ash and Raum, 1956). The cavity becomes filled with desquamated epithelial debris following squamous metaplasia of the lining epithelium. A similar process produces cholesteatoma of the maxillary sinus (Pogorel and Budd, 1965). Congenital cholesteatoma of the temporal bone may extend into a sinus (Cole and McCoy, 1968).

Tumors

There is no one predominant tumor of the nasal cavities. About half of the neoplasms which occur are malignant. About one fourth of the tumors of the paranasal sinuses originate in the bone (Ash et al., 1964). Thinness of bony partitions facilitates spread of malignant tumors to adjacent structures. Symptoms of obstruction to the airway may be late, even in the nasal cavity proper, and lesions in the sinuses may be completely silent clinically.

The surface epithelium lining the nasal cavity and sinuses produces the greatest number of tumors. The epidermis and dermis lining the vestibule may produce basal or squamous cell carcinomas or skin gland neoplasms. Verrucas and keratoses may occur just inside the nares.

The respiratory epithelium produces some unique papillary lesions. Exophytic squamous papillomas (Norris, 1962) may arise anywhere but are most common on the septum. About one fourth of the cases seem to have multiple sites of origin. These growths show orderly elongated fronds of vascular fibrous tissue, continuous with the submucosa, which support

layers of regular stratified epithelium. This appears thickened and multilayered. Cells tend to undergo surface flattening and show maturation. Rarely is there any keratinization or formation of a granular layer. Mitoses are uncommon. There is no tendency to fusion of processes in the benign lesions and no downward growth. Bone erosion is not seen (Kramer and Som, 1935). These tumors may cover a wide area of the upper nasal cavity before being discovered. They are twice as frequent in men as in women.

Although exophytic papillomas may recur in about one fourth of patients (Norris, 1963), frank invasive epidermoid carcinoma arising from this growth is uncommon. No relationship to a virus has been demonstrated (Gaito et al., 1965). Some papillary tumors are formed in part or entirely by columnar rather than squamous epithelium (Fig. 3). It is generally tall, with basal nuclei and pale, mucus-secreting cytoplasm and is frequently ciliated. Although sometimes the cells are crowded, they are uniform and lie upon an intact basement lamina (Cody, 1967; Kramer and Som, 1935). This can be interpreted as glandular metaplasia of the respiratory mucosa (schneiderian), although columnar cells normally form the superficial layer.

A considerable degree of pleomorphism can be accepted in papillomas without considering them histologically malignant. This can appear as a high degree of dyskeratosis. Similar changes in glandular papillary or solid tumors (adenoma) are less common and may be more significant. Recurring glandular tumors have been called adenoma malignum (Ash et al., 1964).

Another variety of papillary tumor exhibits a more solid type of growth. This has been called an inverting papilloma (papillary sinusitis, polyp with metaplasia) (Fig. 4). In these, there is an edematous stroma like that of the inflammatory nasal polyp, into which thickened folds of multilayered epithelium have grown. The epithelial cells are uniform, show some maturation on the surface, but are generally less flattened than those in the squamous papilloma. There is little mitotic activity and no real invasion. They do not cornify. The gross appearance is that of a smooth polypoid mass rather than a papillary surface. Question has arisen as to whether these should be regarded as true neoplasms rather than metaplasias in a polyp. At times, however, they are quite extensive.

The two types of papilloma seem to be unrelated. Sinuses are more often involved with

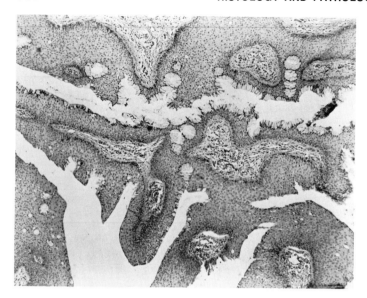

Figure 3. Photomicrograph of recurrent papilloma from left nasal septum of a woman, 54. Note the mucous cells interspersed in the stratified squamous epithelium. (Hematoxylin and eosin, × 40.)

inverting papillomas, perhaps because bone destruction may occur even though the tumor is histologically benign (Skolnik et al., 1966). An associated squamous cell carcinoma arises in from 2 to 15 per cent of patients (Fechner and Alford, 1968; Osborn, 1970; Skolnik et al., 1966). Men develop inverting tumors three times more often than women. The average age at onset is 49 as compared to 44 for exophytic lesions (Norris, 1963). There appears to be a greater tendency for inverting papillomas to recur. A diffuse squamous metaplasia of the nasal mucosa elsewhere may explain the high recurrence rate (Cummings and Goodman, 1969). Radiation may account for a few malignant transformations (Mabery et al., 1965).

Only about 10 per cent of each type of papilloma appears to originate in the sinus rather than in the nasal cavity proper (Norris, 1962).

Primary squamous cell carcinoma of the nasal cavity may be associated with a papilloma (Osborn, 1970), but more frequently it is without an antecedent lesion. These generally are not cornifying and are sometimes referred to as transitional cell carcinoma or schneiderian carcinoma.

Use of the term "transitional" to denote either tumors or epithelium of the upper respiratory tract is unfortunate (Osborn, 1970). It does not appear that a particular type of epithelium occurs here (Schneider, 1967). The minor differences described in the lining of upper

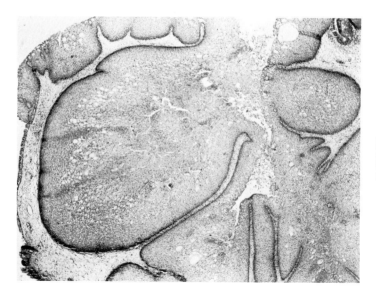

Figure 4. Photomicrograph of inverting papilloma of nasal cavity in a man of 65. Broad columns of stratified epithelium are invaginated into fibrous stroma. (Hematoxylin and eosin, × 25.)

air passages may represent lymphoid infiltration.

About 2 per cent of all carcinomas develop in the nose or sinuses. They do not seem to metastasize so readily as similar tumors in other areas (Ash et al., 1964). In the nasal cavity the tumor usually arises on the middle or inferior turbinate, rarely on the septum or in the ethmoidal area (Ackerman and Del Regato, 1962). It is composed of solid sheets or columns of moderately large epithelial cells in a pavementlike pattern. Cell boundaries are usually distinct. The nests of epithelium are sharply bounded, but there may be a variable amount of lymphocytic infiltration which obscures it. This may be of a quantity to suggest the type of tumor known as lymphoepithelioma (Fig. 5). A gradual transition between tumor types is seen.

A special type of squamous cell carcinoma arises as an ulceration of the septum at the mucocutaneous junction (Lyons, 1969). Adenocarcinomas arise more commonly in the upper portions of the nasal cavities (Fig. 6). They are commonly pseudopapillary. A type composed of cylindrical clear cells is sometimes called a colloid carcinoma (Worsoe-Peterson, 1965). Others produce more abundant mucus and a third type is made up of more opaque eosinophilic cells like the oxyphilic cells of salivary type glands (oncocytes). They may be mixed with lymphocytes (Ash et al., 1964). There are repeated recurrences before any more distant metastases appear.

A special type of adenocarcinoma is the adenoid cystic carcinoma, derived from submucosal glands rather than from the surface epithelium. This is composed of large nests or sheets of relatively small, dark-staining cells of indifferent shape which contain rounded glandlike spaces. The spaces may contain granular or mucoid material. The epithelial cells are not columnar, but those at the periphery of the nest may be cuboidal in shape. The tubular character of the secretion expressed from the "Swiss-cheese"-like spaces was responsible for the name "cylindroma," given to these tumors in early descriptions. They are unusual but ubiquitous in the respiratory system. Adenoid cystic carcinoma has an ominous prognosis for long-term survival (McDonald and Havens, 1948), in spite of very slow progression.

A rapidly growing variant of gland ductal carcinoma which shows areas of both squamous and adenocarcinoma has been described as adenosquamous carcinoma in two cases in the nasal cavity (Gerughty et al., 1968) as well as elsewhere in the mouth and larynx.

Carcinoma of the nasal cavity may spread by lymphatics to the retropharyngeal nodes from posterior in the cavity, to the deep internal jugular nodes from the midportion, and to tonsillar and anterior jugular nodes from the nasal floor and septum (Ackerman and Del Regato, 1962).

Paranasal sinus carcinoma amounts to about 5 per cent of upper respiratory tract malignancies (Baker et al., 1966). About 85 per cent are in males (Salinger, 1966). Carcinoma of the maxillary sinus generally arises in the lower portion of the sinus and may not give rise to symptoms before it is far advanced and presents as an enlargement of the cheek (Tabb,

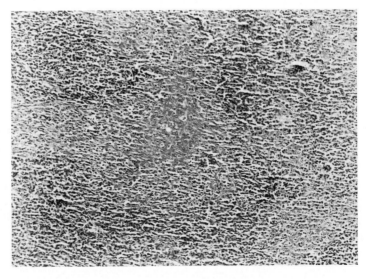

Figure 5. Photomicrograph of recurrent squamous cell carcinoma of lymphoepithelioma type from nasopharynx of woman of 45. Note the blending of epithelial cells in center with darker lymphoid cells. (Hematoxylin and eosin, × 100.)

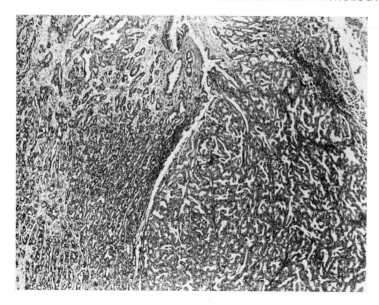

Figure 6. Photomicrograph of polypoid adenocarcinoma from left ethmoid region in a man 60 years old. It is made up of well formed, branching glands lined by columnar eosinophilic epithelium. (Hematoxylin and eosin, × 40.)

1957). Types of tumors seen are the same as in the nasal cavity (Takashi, 1956). Papillary tumors come to be compressed and solid. Two thirds of sinus tumors are malignant (Ash et al., 1964). About 80 per cent are squamous cell carcinomas (Badib et al., 1969). Adenocarcinoma is more frequent in the ethmoid sinuses (Ash et al., 1964).

Those tumors arising in the upper half of the maxillary sinus tend to involve the orbit. Chronic sinusitis does not seem to predispose to carcinoma (Ackerman and Del Regato, 1962). Patients exposed to Thorotrast have developed carcinoma years later (Ackerman and Del Regato, 1962; Poushter and Perl, 1965). Metastases from carcinoma of the antrum appear late in the course of the disease and are found in submaxillary and cervical nodes. Adenoid cystic carcinoma has a particularly poor outlook (Bassilios et al., 1967; Rofla 1969; Tauxe et al., 1962; Taylor et al., 1965).

Metastatic carcinoma of the maxilla nearly always involves the antrum. Renal cell carcinoma is particularly apt to appear as a solitary metastasis in this location. Metastases to other sinuses are rare (Bernstein et al., 1966; Morgenstein, 1968; Toomey and Frazer, 1967).

The ethmoid, frontal, and sphenoidal sinuses are far less likely to give rise to a neoplasm. They are involved in about that order (Badib et al., 1969).

Tissues other than the surface epithelium may give rise to tumors. Tumors of salivary gland type can be found in the submucosa of the nasal cavity and antrum. Most commonly this is a benign mixed tumor (Fig. 7).

Malignant lymphoma is the second most common malignant tumor of the nasal cavities. These tend to develop posteriorly. Most are of lymphoblastic type (lymphosarcoma), although lymphocytic forms (lymphatic leukemia) (Sanford and Becker, 1967) and reticulum cell sarcoma occur (Silver et al., 1968).

Extramedullary plasmacytoma is peculiar to the upper respiratory tract (Figi et al., 1945). It amounts to nearly 1 per cent of malignancies of the upper tract. The tumor is composed of sheets of recognizable plasma cells. They may show some enlargement and pleomorphism. Histological changes are not helpful in predicting the likelihood of dissemination. Bone involvement indicates a poor prognosis (Poole and Marchetta, 1968). It occurs chiefly in men aged 40 to 70. There may be an interval of a decade before dissemination is discovered. Multiple growths may occur in the respiratory tract without other evidence of disease, either concurrently or as recurrences. An inflammatory mass may contain many small uniform plasma cells, but they are accompanied by a variety of other inflammatory cells.

Malignant melanoma may arise from melanocytes in the respiratory epithelium or from the epidermis lining the vestibule (Ravid and Estenes, 1960). They amount to about 4 per cent of malignant tumors of the nasal cavity. Four cases are reported from the maxillary sinus (Crone, 1966), although some of these are doubtful (Ravid and Estenes, 1960). Most are seen on the septum, where areas of pigmentation are found (Lewis and Martin, 1967). There is nearly always stratified squamous

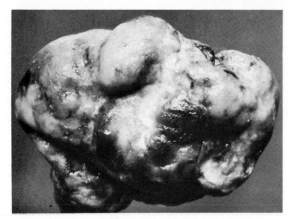

Figure 7. Benign fibrous tumor from nasal cavity of a girl, 12, diagnosed as fibroma. It lacked the vascularity of angiofibromas.

epithelium on the surface (Ravid and Estenes, 1960).

Hemangioma of the nasal septum is described as a source of epistaxis. These usually appear to be telangiectases or pyogenic granulomas (Ash and Old, 1950). Other vascular neoplasms are rare; five hemangiopericytomas and a glomangioma are described (Lenczyk, 1968; Pantazopoulos, 1965).

Neurogenic tumors of the nasal cavity are of great interest. They amount to about 3 per cent of true nasal tumors (Lewis et al., 1965). The olfactory neuroblastoma (neuroepithelioma, esthesioneuroma) (Silcox, 1966) arises above the line of the free border of the middle turbinate. It appears to originate in neural elements of the olfactory epithelium. It is composed of a feltwork of fine neurofibrils containing nests of small, dark-staining, angular cells. These nests may occasionally show rosette formations in which the nuclei form a glandlike circle of epithelial appearance. These may be termed neuroepitheliomas (Gerard-Marchant and Micheau, 1965). There may be calcified laminated psammoma bodies (Caballes, 1965). Some show scattered tumor nests in fibrous tissue. The appearance is similar to that of neuroblastoma arising in sympathetic tissue. The histological structure is not helpful for prognosis. All invade the surrounding tissues locally. Distant metastases to cervical nodes and lungs occur in about 20 per cent of patients (Lewis et al., 1965; Skolnik et al., 1966). There is about a 50 per cent five-year survival after treatment (Hutter et al., 1963; Lewis et al., 1965; Skolnik et al., 1966). Metastases are said to be less frequent in adults (FitzHugh et al., 1965). Those tumors showing true rosettes are reported not to have

metastasized (Hutter et al., 1963), but some consider them more liable to recurrence (Gerard-Marchant and Micheau, 1965). Olfactory neuroblastomas occur most commonly in males aged 11 to 20 and 31 to 40. Cases are reported from nine to 79 years (Skolnik et al., 1966). They can be produced experimentally in Syrian hamsters (Herrold, 1964).

In addition to the neuroblastoma, which is a true neoplasm, some tumors of neurogenic origin in the olfactory area represent nests or extensions of normal central nervous system tissue (Smith et al., 1963). It may be extranasal at the root of the nose. These nasal gliomas lack the undifferentiated neuroblastic cells and are composed of mature astrocytic cells and even neurons in a fine glial stroma. There may be a stalk connecting this tissue with the brain (Ross, 1966). It may project as a polyp into the nasal cavity. If there is a lumen which communicates with the subarachnoid space or cerebral ventricle, this is an encephalocele (Smith et al., 1963). Neurilemmomas also occur (Ackerman and Del Regato, 1962).

Chromophobe adenomas of the pituitary gland may erode into the nasal cavity and form a polypoid tumor (Kay et al., 1950). A meningioma may arise as a primary tumor in a sinus (Ash et al., 1964). Chordoma derived from notochord tissue has been reported (Adams, 1948; Pastore et al., 1949). Angiofibroma may develop in the sinus as well as in the nasopharynx (Maniglia et al., 1969).

Developmental tumors might be expected in the complex area of the junction of processes in the head, and teratoid tumors are reported in nasal cavities and sinuses (Patchefsky et al., 1968). The first retinal anlage tumor was reported in the maxilla (Halpert and Patzer, 1947). Chordoma from the region of the basiocciput may invade the sphenoid sinus and obstruct the nasal cavity (Dahlin and MacCarty, 1952).

Tumors and masses within the facial bones necessarily will encroach on sinuses or the nasal cavity. Examples of this are ameloblastomas, odontomas, and dentigerous cysts of the maxillary alveolar ridge (Ackerman and Del Regato, 1962; Dodge, 1965). Osteomas or fibro-osteomas of frontal or ethmoidal regions may obliterate the sinuses (Soboroff and Nykiel, 1966). Fibrous dysplasia of the maxilla may be bilateral (cherubism) and involve the sinuses (Ward et al., 1969); Pantzopoulos, 1965). Giant cell lesions of the maxilla, whether reparative granulomas or true giant cell tumors, may involve the maxillary or ethmoid sinuses (Friedberg et al., 1969; Griffey and Tedeschi, 1968).

Paget's disease of bone may be followed by osteosarcoma of facial bones (Ackerman and Del Regato, 1962). Ewing's sarcoma of bone is reported. Chondroma and chondrosarcoma of ethmoid or nasal septum have occurred. A mucoid tumor of connective tissue origin, myxoma, has been described in the ethmoid region (Ackerman and Del Regato, 1962). Deposits of amyloid in primary amyloidosis may simulate a neoplasm in the nasal septum (Garrett, 1968).

REFERENCES

Ackerman, L. V., and Del Regato, J. A.: Cancer of the respiratory system and upper digestive tract. *In* Cancer, Diagnosis, Treatment and Prognosis. St. Louis, The C. V. Mosby Co., 1962.

Adams, W. S.: A case of chordoma of the right frontal sinus. J. Laryng. *62*:93-95, 1948.

Alcala, H., and Alarcon, S. D.: Ulceration and perforation of the nasal septum in systemic lupus erythematosus. New Eng. J. Med. *281*:722-723, 1969.

Ash, J. E.: Sinusitis from the viewpoint of the general pathologist. Trans. Amer. Acad. Ophthal. Otolaryng. *44*:304-320, 1939.

Ash, J. E., Beck, M. R., and Wilkes, J. D.: Tumors of the upper respiratory tract and ear. AFIP Atlas of Tumor Pathology, Section IV, Fascicles 12 and 13, 1964.

Ash, J. E., and Old, J. W.: Hemangioma of septum. Trans. Amer. Acad. Ophthal. Otolaryng. *54*:350-356, 1950.

Ash, J. E., and Raum, M.: An Atlas of Otolaryngic Pathology. Amer. Acad. Ophthal. Otolaryng., Washington, D.C., A.F.I.P., 1956.

Astrom, K. E., and Lidholm, S. D.: Extensive intracranial lesions in a case of orbital nonspecific granuloma combined with polyarteritis nodosa. J. Clin. Path. *16*:137-143, 1963.

Badid, A. O., Kurobara, S. S., Webster, J. H., and Shedd, D. P.: Treatment of cancer of paranasal sinuses. Cancer *23*:533-537, 1969.

Baker, R., Cherry, J., Lott, S., and Bischofberger, W. B.: Carcinoma of maxillary sinus. Arch. Otolaryng. *84*:201-204, 1966.

Bales, G. A.: Choanal atresia in the premature infant. Laryngoscope *76*:122-126, 1966.

Bassilios, M. I., Raum, C., Jarmolych, J., and Goffin, F.: Cylindroma of right maxillary antrum. Laryngoscope *77*:365-371, 1967.

Bernstein, J. M., Montgomery, W. W. and Balogh, K.: Metastatic Tumors to the Maxilla, Nose and Paranasal Sinuses. Laryngoscope *76*:621-650, 1966.

Blantar, P. L., and Biggs, N. C.: Eighteen hundred years of controversy: The paranasal sinuses. Amer. J. Anat. *124*:135-147, 1969.

Bloom, W., and Fawcett, D. W.: A Textbook of Histology. Philadelphia, W. B. Saunders Company, 9th ed., 1968, pp. 629-651.

Blumenfeld, R., and Skolnick, E. M.: Intranasal encephaloceles. Arch. Otolaryng. *82*:527-531, 1965.

Blumstein, G. I.: Nasal polyps. Arch Otolaryng. *83*:266-269, 1966.

Boyd, M. E.: Congenital atresia of posterior nares. Arch Otolaryng. *41*:261-271, 1945.

Brown, H. A., and Woolner, L. B.: Findings referable to the upper part of the respiratory tract in Wegener's granulomatosis. Ann. Otol. *69*:810-829, 1960.

Bryce, D. P., and Crysdale, W. S.: Non-healing granuloma: A diagnostic problem. Laryngoscope *79*:794-805, 1969.

Caballes, R. L.: Psammoma bodies in olfactory neuroblastoma. Laryngoscope *75*:1749-1755, 1965.

Carder, H. M., and Hill, J. T.: Asymptomatic rhinolith. Laryngoscope *76*:524-530, 1966.

Castleman, B., and McNeely, B. U.: Wegener's granulomatosis involving sinuses, lungs, tongue, larynx, trachea, bronchi. New Eng. J. Med. *273*:652-659, 1965.

Castleman, B., and McNeely, B. U.: Mucormycosis, rhinocerebral type, involving paranasal sinuses and right internal carotid and middle cerebral arteries. New Eng. J. Med. *279*:1220-1229, 1968.

Cody, C. C.: Inverting papillomata of the nose and sinuses. Laryngoscope *77*:584-598, 1967.

Cole, T. B., and McCoy, G.: Congenital cholesteatoma of temporal bone and sphenoid sinus. Arch. Otolaryng. *89*:576-579, 1968.

Crone, R. P.: Malignant amelanotic melanomas of the nasal septum and maxillary sinus. Laryngoscope *76*:1826-1833, 1966.

Cummings, C. W., and Goodman, M. L.: Inverted papilloma of the nose and paranasal sinuses. Amer. J. Clin. Path. *52*:766 (Abstract), 1969.

Dahlin, D. C., and MacCarty, C. S.: Chordoma: A study of 59 cases. Cancer *5*:1170-1178, 1952.

Despons, J., and Stoller, F. M.: Nasal polyposis in mucoviscidosis. Laryngoscope *75*:475-483, 1965.

DeWeese, D. D., Schlenning, A. J., and Robinson, L. B.: Mucormycosis of the nose and paranasal sinuses. Laryngoscope *75*:1398-1407, 1965.

Dodge, O. G.: Tumors of the jaw, odontogenic tissues and maxillary antrum (excluding Burkett's lymphoma) in Uganda Africans. Cancer *18*:205-215, 1965.

Dolowitz, D. A., and Dougherty, T. F.: Study of cilia and connective tissue in normal and hyperplastic nasal mucous membrane. Laryngoscope *76*:1380-1388, 1966.

Douglas, R. G., Lindgren, K. M., and Couch, R. B.: Rhinovirus and the common cold. Exposure to cold environment. New Eng. J. Med. *279*:776-777, 1968.

Eichel, B. S., and Mabery, T. E.: The enigma of lethal midline granuloma. Laryngoscope *78*:1367-1386, 1968.

Fearon, B., and Dickson, J.: Bilateral choanal atresia in newborn. Plan of action. Laryngoscope *78*:1487-1499, 1968.

Fechner, R. E., and Alford, D. O.: Inverted papilloma and squamous cell carcinoma. Arch Otolaryng. *88*:507-512, 1968.

Figi, F. A., Broders, A. C., and Havens, F. Z.: Plasma cell tumors of the upper part of the respiratory tract. Ann. Otol. *54*:283-297, 1945.

FitzHugh, G. S., Allen, M. S., Reicker, T. N., and Sprenkle, P. M.: Olfactory neuroblastoma (esthesioneuroepithelioma). Arch. Otolaryng. *81*:161-168, 1965.

Flake, C. G., and Ferguson, C. F.: Congenital choanal atresia in infants and children. Arch. Otolaryng. *81*:425-426, 1965.

Fowler, E. P., Jr.: Unilateral vasomotor rhinitis due to interference with the cervical sympathetic system. Arch. Otolaryng. *37*:710-712, 1943.

Fox, M. I.: Hereditary hemorrhagic telangiectasia. Conn. Med. 23:224–230, 1959.

Friedberg, S. A., Eisenstein, R., and Wallner, L. J. Giant cell lesions involving the nasal accessory sinuses. Laryngoscope 79:763–776, 1969.

Friedman, I.: The clinical diagnosis of malignant granuloma and Wegener's granulomatosis. Proc. Roy. Soc. Med. 57:280–297, 1964.

Furnas, D. W.: Recognition of scleroma (rhinoscleroma). Laryngoscope 78:1948–1952, 1968.

Gaito, R. A., Gaylord, W. H., and Hilding, D. A.: Ultrastructure of human nasal papilloma. Laryngoscope 75:144–152, 1965.

Garland, J.: Apple-packer's epistaxis. New Eng. J. Med. 276:413–414, 1967.

Garrett, J. A.: Amyloid deposits in the nose and maxillary sinuses. Arch. Otolaryng. 87:411–412, 1968.

Gerard-Marchant, R., and Micheau, C.: Microscopical diagnosis of olfactory esthesioneuromas. J. Nat. Canc. Inst. 35:75–82, 1965.

Gerughty, R. M., Hennigar, G. R., and Brown, F. M.: Adenosquamous carcinoma of the nasal, oral and laryngeal cavities. Cancer 22:1140–1155, 1968.

Griffey, L. E., and Tedeschi, L. G.: Giant cell tumors of ethmoid. Arch. Otolaryng. 87:615–617, 1968.

Gupta, O. P.: Rhinosporidiosis. unusual extranasal manifestation. Laryngoscope 76:1842–1849, 1966.

Halpert, B., and Patzer, R.: Maxillary tumor of retinal anlage. Surgery 22:837–841, 1947.

Herrold, K. M.: Introduction of olfactory neuroepithelial tumors in Syrian hamsters by diethylnitrosamine. Cancer 17:114–121, 1964.

Hodgson, C. H., Burchell, H. B., Good, C. A., and Clagett, O. T.: Hereditary hemorrhagic telangiectasia and pulmonary arteriovenous fistula. Survey of a large family. New Eng. J. Med. 261:625–636, 1959.

Hora, J. F.: Primary aspergillosis of paranasal sinuses and associated areas. Laryngoscope 75:768–773, 1965.

Hutter, R. V. P., Lewis, J. S., Foote, F. W., Jr., and Tollefsen, H. R.: Esthesioneuroblastoma Amer. J. Surg. 106:748–753, 1963.

Karunaratne, W. A. E.: The pathology of rhinosporidiosis. J. Path. Bact. 42:193–202, 1936.

Kay, S., Leer, J. K., and Stout, A. P.: Pituitary chromophobe tumors of the nasal cavity. Cancer 3:695–704, 1950.

Kietzer, G., and Paparella M. M.: Otolaryngological disorders in craniometaphyseal dysplasia (leontiasis ossea). Laryngoscope 79:921–941, 1969.

Klassen, J.: Rhinoscleroma treated with Streptomycin and Dexamethason. Arch. Otolaryng. 82:74–77, 1965.

Kramer, R., and Som, M. L.: True papilloma of nasal cavity. Arch. Otolaryng. 22:22–43, 1935.

Lenczyk, J. M.: Nasal hemangiopericytoma. Arch. Otolaryng. 87:536–539, 1968.

Lewis, J. S., Hutter, R. V. P., Tollefson, H. R., and Foote, F. W.: Nasal tumors of olfactory origin. Arch. Otolaryng. 81:169–174, 1965.

Lewis, M. G., and Martin, J. A. M.: Malignant melanoma of nasal cavity in Ugandan Africans. Cancer 20:1699–1705, 1967.

Lyons, G. D.: Squamous cell carcinoma of the nasal septum. Arch. Otolaryng. 89:585–587, 1969.

Magid, S. L., Smith, C. C., and Dolowitz, D. A.: Nasal mucosa in pancreatic cystic fibrosis. Arch. Otolaryng. 86:212–216, 1967.

Maniglia, A. J., Mozzarella, L. A., Minkowitz, S., and Moskowitz, H.: Maxillary sinus angiofibroma treated with cryosurgery. Arch. Otolaryng. 89:527–532, 1969.

Mabery, T. E., Devine, K. D., and Harrison, E. G.: The problem of malignant transformation in nasal papilloma. Arch. Otolaryng. 82:296–300, 1965.

McDonald, J. R., and Havens, F. Z.: Study of malignant tumors of glandular nature found in nose, throat and mouth. Surg. Clin. N. Amer. 28:1087–1106, 1948.

Morgenstein, K. M.: Bronchogenic carcinoma metastatic to maxillary sinus. Laryngoscope 78:262–269, 1968.

Norris, H. J.: Papillary lesions of nasal cavity and paranasal sinuses. Laryngoscope 72:1784–1797, 1962.

Norris, H. J.: Inverting papillomas: A study of 29 cases. Laryngoscope 73:1–171, 1963.

Osborn, D. A.: Nature and behavior of transitional tumors in the upper respiratory tract. Cancer 25:50–60, 1970.

Pantzopoulos, P. E.: Glomangioma of nasal cavity—case study. Arch. Otolaryng. 81:83–86, 1965.

Pantzopoulos, P. E.: Monostotic fibrous dysplasia of paranasal sinuses. Laryngoscope 75:335–344, 1965.

Pastore, P. N., Sabyoun, P. F., and Mandeville, F. B.: Chordoma of the maxillary antrum and nares. Arch. Otolaryng. 50:647–658, 1949.

Patchefsky, A., Sundureker, W., and Warden, P. A.: Malignant teratoma of the ethmoid sinus. Cancer 21:714–721, 1968.

Peebles, E. M., Dent, J. H., and Rutledge, L. J.: Choanal atresia in the newborn infant: Report of 2 cases with detailed anatomic studies. Laryngoscope 75:783–792, 1965.

Pogorel, B. S., and Budd, E. G.: Cholesteatoma of maxillary sinus. Arch. Otolaryng. 82:532–534, 1965.

Poole, A. G., and Marchetta F. C.: Extramedullary plasmacytoma of the head and neck. Cancer 22:14–21, 1968.

Poushter, D., and Perl, T.: Carcinoma of the maxillary sinus with residual Thorotrast. Laryngoscope 75:74–83, 1965.

Pratt, L. W.: Midline cysts of nasal dorsum, embryologic origin and treatment. Laryngoscope 75:968–980, 1965.

Ravid, J. M., and Estenes, J. A.: Malignant melanoma of nose and paranasal sinuses and juvenile melanoma of the nose. Arch. Otolaryng. 72:431–444, 1960.

Rofla, S.: Mucous gland tumors of paranasal sinuses. Cancer 24:683–691, 1969.

Ross, D. E.: Nasal glioma. Laryngoscope 76:1602–1611, 1966.

Rossen, R. D., Butler, W. T., Waldenon, R. H., Alford, R. H., Hornick, R. B., Togo, Y., and Kasel, J. A.: The proteins in nasal secretion. J.A.M.A. 211:1157–1161, 1970.

Salinger, S.: The paranasal sinuses: neoplasms and other growths, Part II. Laryngoscope 76:127–160, 1966.

Sanford, D. M., and Becker, G. D.: Acute leukemia presenting as nasal obstruction. Arch. Otolaryng. 85:102–104, 1967.

Schneider, R. A.: The sense of smell in man. Its physiologic basis. New Eng. J. Med. 277:299–303, 1967.

Shaw, H. J., and Martin, H.: Rhinoscleroma—A clinical perspective. J. Laryng. 75:1011–1039, 1961.

Silcox, L. E.: Olfactory neuroblastoma. Laryngoscope 76:665–673, 1966.

Silver, W. E., Daly, J. F., and Friedman, M.: Reticulum cell sarcoma of nose and nasal sinuses. Arch. Otolaryng 87:532–535, 1968.

Singh, M. M., Stokes, J. F., Drury, R. A. B., and Walshe, J. M.: The natural history of malignant granuloma of the nose. Lancet 1:401–403, 1958.

Skolnik, E. M., Lowry, A., and Friedman, J. E.: Inverted papilloma of the nasal cavity. Arch. Otolaryng. 84:644–653, 1966.

Skolnik, E. M., Mossari, F. S., and Teuta, L. T.: Olfactory neuroepithelioma. Arch. Otolaryng. *84*:644–653, 1966.

Smith, K., Schwartz, H., Luse, S., and Ogura, J.: Nasal gliomas, a report of 5 cases with electron microscopy of 1. J. Neurosurg. *20*:968–981, 1963.

Snow, J. B.: Classification of respiratory viruses and their clinical manifestations. Laryngoscope *79*:1485–1493, 1969.

Soboroff, B. J., and Nykiel, F.: Surgical treatment of large osteomas of ethmo-frontal region. Laryngoscope *76*:1068–1081, 1966.

Spear, G. S., and Walker, W. G.: Lethal midline granuloma (granuloma gangraenescens) at autopsy. Bull. Johns Hopkins Hosp. *99*:313–332, 1956.

Stecker, R. H., and Lake, C. F.: Hereditary hemorrhagic telangiectases. Arch. Otolaryng. *82*:522–526, 1965.

Stewart, J. P.: Progressive lethal granulomatous ulceration of the nose. J. Laryng. *48*:657, 1933.

Tabb, H. G.: Carcinoma of the antrum. Laryngoscope *67*:269–341, 1957.

Takashi, M.: Carcinoma of paranasal sinuses. Amer. J. Path. *32*:501–519, 1956.

Tauxe, W. N., McDonald, J. R., and Devine, K. D.: A century of cylindromas. Arch. Otolaryng. *75*:364–376, 1962.

Taylor, J. S., Cooley, H. N., and Hicks, J. J.: Cylindroma of maxillary antrum. Laryngoscope *75*:1727–1736, 1965.

Toomey, J. M., and Frazer, J. P.: Metastatic adenocarcinoma of frontal sinus. Arch. Otolaryng. *85*:407–409, 1967.

Unger, Max: Architecture of the nasal septum—how deviations are formed. Laryngoscope *75*:322–332, 1965.

Ward, P. H., Allen, C., and Owen, R.: Monostotic fibrous dysplasia of maxilla. Laryngoscope *79*:1295–1306, 1969.

Wassermann, D.: Acute paranasal sinusitis and cavernous sinus thrombosis. Arch. Otolaryng. *86*:205–209, 1967.

Winborn, C. D.: Rhinoscleroma. Arch. Otolaryng. *85*:223–225, 1967.

Worsoe-Peterson, J.: Colloid carcinoma of the nasal cavity and sinuses. Arch. Otolaryng. *82*:181–185, 1965.

Yarington, C. T., Abbott, J., and Raines, D.: Wegener's granulomatosis. Laryngoscope *75*:259–269, 1965.

Chapter 20

HISTOLOGY AND PATHOLOGY OF THE THROAT, LARYNX, ESOPHAGUS, AND TRACHEOBRONCHIAL TREE

by Paul Lober, M.D.

PHARYNX

Histology

The pharynx is structurally and functionally divided into three distinct parts. The nasal pharynx is the upper portion, continuous with the nasal cavities through the choanae, which is adapted for conduction of air. It extends to the posterior margin of the soft palate. It is held open by bony walls. The roof is close to the body of the occipital bone and sphenoid, and the foramen lacerum and foramen ovale are close by. Closely related structures are the gasserian ganglion, the cavernous sinus, the third and fourth cranial nerves, and the optic nerve. A lateral recess surrounded by lymphoid tissue extends laterally along the posterior wall of the eustachian tube on each side as deep as 1.5 cm. in the adult (fossa of Rosenmüller) (Ash and Raum, 1956).

The mucous membrane, as in the nasal cavities, is formed of pseudostratified, columnar, ciliated epithelium. The cilia beat downward toward the mouth. The epithelium lies on a thin basement lamina which covers a thin fibrous lamina propria. There is a thick elastic layer beneath this which separates the mucosa from the underlying wall of skeletal muscle. The elastic fibers penetrate between bundles or

fuse with the periosteum of the skull at the fornices. At the lateral wall of the nasal pharynx there is a small amount of submucosal fibrous tissue.

The posterior and lateral walls show a transition of respiratory epithelium into stratified epithelium, which at first is columnar and then becomes squamous with small papillae. The level of this transition rises with increasing age.

Mixed mucous and serous glands are seen under the respiratory mucosa and mucous glands alone are seen under the stratified squamous. They lie in the muscle and open through ducts which pass through the elastic layer.

Aggregates of lymphoid tissue occur characteristically in the mucosa of the nasopharynx. These are particularly large in the roof (tonsil of Luschka) and posterior wall (pharyngeal tonsil or adenoid tissue). This area opposite to the choanae is strategically located for trapping of particles from inspired air. Other large collections may be found in the lateral walls around the eustachian tube orifices and on the palate. The lymphoid tissue shows well formed follicles and lies in the lamina propria with a thin capsule. There is a close relationship of lymphoid cells with overlying epithelium over broad areas. Lymphocytes infiltrate the epithelium and obscure the basement lamina. This is

563

so characteristic that the combination is frequently referred to as lymphoepithelium (Ash, 1966).

Epithelial clefts or folds occur between nodules of lymphoid cells, but these are not so deep as the true crypts of the palatine tonsil. Septa of fibrous and elastic tissue containing some seromucinous glands divide the tonsil. Glands also lie outside the capsule, which may empty into the folds. The lymphatic tissue contains no sinuses, and blind-ending lymphatic channels surround the tonsil. Atrophy begins at puberty, and the adult shows only a little lymphatic tissue, usually covered by stratified squamous epithelium.

The oral pharynx extends from the soft palate to the hyoid bone. It serves for passage of both air and solids. Structures included are the palatine tonsils and palatine folds, base of the tongue, glosso-epiglottic space and, in some descriptions, the epiglottis (Ackerman and Del Regato, 1962).

The entire space is lined with relatively thin, stratified, squamous epithelium, noncornifying. Lymphoid aggregates are found in the base of the tongue and soft palate, and in the palatine tonsil, completing "Waldeyer's ring." The lymphoid tissue seems designed to intercept materials entering the body by mouth. As in the nasal pharynx, the epithelium lies upon a thin layer of dense fibrous lamina propria which shows small papillae. There is an elastic layer in place of the muscularis mucosae which blends with septa of the underlying skeletal muscle. This layer has an inner longitudinal and an outer oblique layer. There is no submucosa. Mucous glands lie deep to the elastic layer, in the muscle.

The palatine or faucial tonsil is a bilateral organ lying between the faucial pillars. It is likewise covered with stratified squamous epithelium. This forms 10 to 20 deep crypts and, in the crypts and on the surface, becomes intimately blended with lymphocytes (pseudoreticular). They appear to migrate into and through the epithelium. The lamina propria is a thin fibrous layer with small papillae. The deeper tissue is formed by a thick layer of dense lymphatic tissue which completely obliterates the lamina propria around the crypts. Lymphoid follicles with secondary centers are ranged about the crypts, generally in a single layer. Partitions of fibrous tissue extend between the crypts and their lymphatic envelopes. In addition to lymphocytes, there are a few polymorphonuclear leukocytes and frequent plasma cells within the tissue. A dense fibrous

capsule underlies the tonsils and is continuous with the elastic layer. Glands lie outside the capsule and open on the free surface, not in the crypts. A decreased number of cells and follicles are seen with advancing age, but the tonsil is not less active (Kelemen, 1943). Fibrosis is the result of preceding infection, not of atrophy.

The hypopharynx or laryngeal portion of the pharynx is the continuation of the pharynx inferiorly. The upper boundaries are arbitrary, but are usually taken to be at the orifice of the larynx. It includes the piriform sinuses and aryepiglottic folds down to the lower border of the cricoid cartilage. This is at the level of the sixth cervical vertebra where the pharynx blends into the structure of the esophagus. The hypopharynx, being U-shaped, shows medial walls against the larynx, as well as lateral and posterior walls.

The histological structure of the oral pharynx is continued. At the lateral walls inferiorly, a loose fibrous submucosa appears between the muscle layers and the elastic layer. The epithelium throughout is of stratified squamous type, with a thin, dense lamina propria and small papillae. There are increased numbers of mucous glands deep to the elastic layer. The muscularis mucosae does not appear until the esophagus is reached. Lymphoid tissue is nearly absent.

Pathology of Nasal Pharynx

Developmental Abnormalities

The roof of the nasopharynx shows an anteroposterior fissure which ends in a pocket posteriorly. This is the pharyngeal pouch or bursa pharyngea. It appears to be related to the degenerating notochord rather than Rathke's pouch (Guggenheim, 1953; Huber, 1912; Snook, 1934). This is rarely the site of a true embryonal bursa in the adult which may extend above the pharyngeal constrictor muscles to the occipital bone. Retention cysts may develop. The true bursa is deep to fascia and not removed by adenoidectomy (Guggenheim, 1953). A pharyngeal recess or crypt at the site of the pharyngeal tonsil may be sealed off and form a superficial abscess or cyst, which is removed with the tonsil. The term Tornwaldt's disease may refer to any of these cystic swellings in the posterior nasopharynx. A rare dermoid or teratoma is seen at this location (Boies and Harris, 1965). Within the mucosa of the roof in the midline may be found nests of anterior pituitary lobe tissue, representing the site of Rathke's pouch.

Other congenital defects of the nasopharynx are rare. Nasopharyngeal stenosis or occlusion is usually due to inflammatory adhesions following surgery or, formerly, to syphilis (Lehmann et al., 1968).

Inflammatory Processes

Inflammation of the nasopharyngeal walls may be serious because of the proximity of important structures. Swelling of lymphoid tissue is likely to block the orifices of the eustachian tubes, at least periodically, and larger masses of hyperplastic pharyngeal tonsillar (adenoid) tissue may obstruct the airway in children who have a shallow nasopharynx by impinging on the soft palate. Rarely this has led to pulmonary hypertension and heart failure (Levy et al., 1967).

The tonsillar tissue may show an infiltration of phagocytes and plasma cells in chronic infections, with increased numbers of polymorphonuclear leukocytes, including eosinophils, in more acute inflammations. Acute pharyngitis is generally accompanied by rhinitis. There is edema and vascular congestion, with increased mucus secretion and fluid transudation. Edema extends into palate and uvula. Collections of exudate with necrotic mucosa may form patches of pseudomembrane. The exudate is principally made up of polymorphonuclear leukocytes. The inflammation is most visible over the tonsil and posterior wall but generally involves the entire lining. A similar reaction appears to be produced by a variety of microorganisms, but streptococci appear to excite the most severe inflammation (Ash and Raum, 1956).

More chronic changes include hyperplasia of lymphoid tissue and an interstitial exudate of lymphocytes, plasma cells, and macrophages. There may be a mild increase in the number of reticular and collagen fibers, but dense scar is unusual. The exudate may interfere with drainage of crypts and gland ducts.

Hyperplasia of pharyngeal tonsillar tissue is produced by an increase in number and size of lymphoid follicles. It may follow allergic states rather than true infections. The adenoid tissue may enlarge if the palatine tonsils are removed.

With immunosuppression therapy, uncommon pathogenic organisms may gain a foothold (Castleman and McNeely, 1968). Lethal midline granuloma may begin in the nasopharynx. Infections with *Corynebacterium diphtheri-*

ae are apt to produce a pseudomembrane consisting of tough adherent fibrin and necrotic epithelium. The bacteria may persist in the carrier state.

A complication of severe nasopharyngitis may be a retropharyngeal abscess. Most often this starts in a peripharyngeal space where nodes draining the infection may break down. It is uncommon in adults. A single postvisceral space lies behind the peripharyngeal spaces and extends into the mediastinum. Both also extend laterally to the carotid sheath. About 15 per cent of abscesses develop mediastinitis or massive hemorrhage if untreated. A prevertebral space lies behind the prevertebral fascia. It may be the site of an abscess arising from vertebral disease (Davidson, 1949). Middle-ear infection may be the source of retropharyngeal abscess by direct extension through the bone. The abscess commonly drains through the mucosa and not laterally into parapharyngeal tissues.

Tuberculosis has been found at autopsy in the nasopharynx in as many as 75 per cent of patients having pulmonary tuberculosis (Szanto and Hollender, 1944). This would be higher than the incidence of laryngeal tuberculosis. The diagnosis may require histological examination of unbroken mucosa. An ulcerating lesion in the nasopharynx might be a source of bacilli when sputum is positive and in reinfection. Usually it is located posteriorly or in the roof of the nasopharynx, where sputum strikes.

Syphilitic lesions of the second stage, mucous patches, are seen in the nasopharynx. An extension of syphilitic rhinitis and diffuse interstitial inflammation may produce structural deformity in the third stage.

Tumors

Because of peculiaritis of structure and location, neoplasms of the nasopharynx tend to bring about distinct clinical entities. Benign tumors in the nasopharynx are outnumbered four to one by malignant ones (Ash and Raum, 1956). Most interesting of the benign tumors is the juvenile nasopharyngeal angiofibroma. There is some doubt about its true identity as a neoplasm (Evans, 1966). It is made up of an intertwining mass of fibroblastic tissue containing thin-walled blood vessels of capillary size or somewhat larger. It probably represents an angioma with a prominent and characteristic stroma. The fibroblastic cells may be stellate in shape. They are sometimes irregular in size and staining reaction, much like their appearance in some breast tumors (cystosarcoma) or in neurofibromas (Sternberg, 1954). The vessels are occasionally muscular (Balogh and Caulfield, 1967). There is a tendency for increased fibrous tissue in older lesions (Evans, 1966). The vessels appear to be an integral part of the neoplasm. Although they are said to regress in size in later years, this appears actually to be uncommon (Evans, 1966; Sternberg, 1954). They are difficult to eradicate and may cause severe deformities of the facial skeleton (Martin et al., 1948; Patterson, 1965). They occur in boys 10 to 17 years of age (Rodriguez, 1966). Although cases have been reported in females (Osborn and Sokolovski, 1965; Rominger and Santore, 1968), these may be examples of simple fibromas (Harma, 1958). Testosterone treatment does not cause regression (Apostal and Frazell, 1965). Metastases have been reported, but the tumor may not have been correctly identified in these cases (Hormia and Koskinen, 1969). Growth is limited but deformity requires removal.

Carcinoma is the most important malignant tumor of the nasopharynx. It amounts to 0.5 to 1.0 per cent of all cancers. Two thirds occur in men. The tumor tends to appear in younger ages, the peak incidence occurring at ages 40 to 45 years (Ackerman and Del Regato, 1962). Much confusion has arisen from the nomenclature of carcinomas of the nasopharynx. Probably all but a few glandular tumors arise from the surface epithelium. The term transitional, referring to their origin in the epithelium that lines the excretory gland ducts, is inappropriate for these tumors. A variable amount of lymphoid tissue is frequently incorporated into the tumor, as it is into the normal mucosa of the nasopharynx. The lymphoid tissue is not malignant, and the term lymphoepithelioma is misleading (Cappell, 1934). It should be used sparingly and only to indicate a variety of squamous cell carcinoma which carries large amounts of lymphoid stroma. There is a gradual transition from more conventional types of squamous cell carcinoma (Perez et al., 1969; Teoh, 1957; Yeh, 1962). Frankly cornifying or well differentiated squamous cell carcinoma is unusual in the nasopharynx (Ackerman and Del Regato, 1962). A predilection for Chinese individuals, even after emigration, is well documented (Lin et al., 1969; Martin and Quan, 1951; Pang, 1965; Sturton et al., 1966; Teoh, 1952; Yeh, 1962). It is not clear that environmental factors such as incense have been eliminated (Sturton et al., 1966), and the predilection may not be genetic.

The primary lesion of carcinoma may be an exophytic or lobulated mass in the lateral fornices or where space permits, or, less commonly, it may be a deep fissure or ulcer surrounded by infiltrating tumor. Some are pedunculated even though undifferentiated histologically. A few carcinomas show areas of frank squamatization with keratin pearls. Most are formed of solid sheets of indifferent epithelial cells, usually in a pavement arrangement, separated by collections of lymphoid tissue or fibrous stroma. Nuclei are usually large and somewhat variable in size and outline, and nucleoli may be distinct. There may be large number of mitoses, with relatively little pleomorphism. Cytoplasm is often indistinct, as are cell boundaries, and these cells may be confused with reticular cells. There may be uniform, closely packed cells without lymphoid stroma (transitional cell type) (Evans, 1966).

Lymphatic spread occurs early in the course of the disease, often before the primary lesion is discovered. Those tumors on the roof and posterior wall may go to retropharyngeal nodes, some to the highest nodes along the internal jugular vein. Those tumors on the lateral wall may spread first to the retropharyngeal and jugular nodes but may also invade the base of the skull and important parapharyngeal structures (Ackerman and Del Regato, 1962).

Distant metastases occur more commonly than in nearly any other carcinoma of head and neck origin. Lungs and bones and liver are most commonly involved (Kaplan et al., 1969; Papavasilion, 1968; Rubenfeld et al., 1962; Teoh, 1957). When the internal jugular vein is invaded, all these sites show distant metastases (Teoh, 1957). Invasion of the skull bone is nearly as common as node metastases in late cases (Teoh, 1957) and about half of these have intracranial extension. Pulmonary spread by direct extension from the mediastinum has been suggested (Sasaki, 1968). Distant metastases from well differentiated keratinizing tumors are rare.

The prognosis of carcinoma of the nasopharynx must be based upon accurate classification of tumors. Reports of large groups of treated "cancer" are not helpful if they include lymphomas, adenoid cystic carcinomas, and other malignant tumors. About one third survival at five years may be the best that can be expected, if most are detected early (Perez et al., 1969; Shedd et al., 1967; Wang et al., 1962). Radiation is the treatment of first choice, since the usually poorly differentiated carcinoma is radiosensitive. Radical neck dissection adds nothing to treatment (Perez et al.,

1969). Hydroxyurea has been used for chemotherapy (Lucas and Lehrnbecker, 1969).

Malignant lymphoma of the nasopharynx tends to occur in age groups older than those subject to carcinoma and in children (Ackerman and Del Regato, 1962). One would expect a higher incidence in the respiratory tract than elsewhere because of the abundant lymphoid tissue normally present. Some have considered reticulum cell sarcoma to be the commonest malignant lesion of the nasopharynx (Ash, 1966), but this appears to be due to misinterpretation of undifferentiated carcinomas. In most series of malignant tumors (Perez et al., 1969; Matz and Conner, 1968; Vaeth, 1960), malignant lymphomas form a small minority. The large celled type or reticulum cell sarcoma is composed of broad sheets of fairly uniform cells, with large nuclei and prominent nucleoli. There may be frequent mitoses. The resemblance to epithelium may be close. There may be variable members of lymphocytes. Lymphocytic or lymphoblastic lymphoma (lymphosarcoma) is composed of more readily identified smaller cells of definitely lymphoid differentiation. Reticulum cell sarcoma appears to be more common in male children (Borella, 1964). Lymphoma is more radiosensitive than carcinoma. Peripheral nodes may be involved simultaneously or apparently by spread (Castleman and McNeely, 1968). The tumor may be pedunculated or present as an ulcerated mass. Hodgkin's disease has been reported (Ash and Raum, 1956; Ghossein and Najjar, 1967).

Less common tumors of the nasopharynx are seen in considerable variety. In children and adolescents the embryonal rhabdomyosarcoma may arise in the walls of the nasopharynx (Cappell, 1938; Prior and Stoner, 1957; Stobbe and Dargeon, 1950). It may grow as a polypoid translucent soft grapelike mass (sarcoma botryoides), as it is seen in the urogenital tract. It is composed of small, dark cells, with little cytoplasm and occasional wisps of dense eosinophilic fibers, rarely cross-striated. It may be mistaken for a lymphoma histologically because of the small, dark, uniform cells. Tumors of the nasopharynx in children are rare (less than 1 per cent of adults) (Martin, 1940), but many are carcinomas. Teratomas have been reported (Sollee, 1965). A sessile chondroma arising around the eustachian tube or base of the sphenoid bone occurs primarily in young men before age 18. Chondrosarcoma has occurred in this location in an older individual (Timmis, 1959). A schwannoma may present in the wall of the pharynx (Guggenheim, 1953). More often these are attached to the vagus or another upper cervical nerve (Slaughter and de Peyser, 1949).

Adenoid cystic carcinoma (cylindroma) is present in small numbers in the nasopharynx as elsewhere throughout the respiratory tract (Kramer and Som, 1939) (Fig. 1). It is apt to occur in the fossa of Rosenmüller, but may occur anywhere, apparently arising from mucosal glands. It usually has a very distinctive pattern, being formed of nests of relatively small, moderately dark-staining, uniform epithelial cells. The nests show circular glandlike spaces, making a cribriform or netlike structure. The glands are lined by cells identical to those in the more solid areas. Mitoses are uncommon. The tumor exhibits the same inexorable, slow, diffusely invasive course seen in other sites.

Extramedullary plasmacytoma is more common in the nasopharynx than elsewhere in the mouth and upper air passages (Dolin and Dewar, 1956). It may be ablated without recurrence during the subsequent life span of the patient, but most often is followed or accompanied by multiple foci (multiple myeloma) and generalized disease. The histological appearance does not aid in foretelling the outcome.

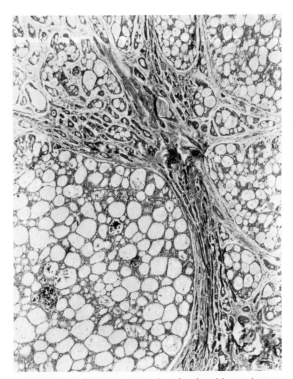

Figure 1. Photomicrograph of adenoid cystic carcinoma (cylindroma) in an 87 year old man. It arose from submucosal glands and invaded the maxilla. Large nodules of tumor show a netlike arrangement of epithelial cells surrounding small rounded spaces. (Hematoxylin and eosin, × 40.)

It is composed of relatively large and slightly irregular plasma cells, often resembling lymphoma under a low-power microscope, except that the nuclei appear more widely separated.

Among the rarest tumors of the nasopharynx are chordoma and synovial sarcoma. The origin of chordoma from remnants of notochord in the posterior pharyngeal wall is clear. The large vacuolated cells in a mucoid matrix are characteristic (Wang and James, 1968). Growth is slow and metastasis unusual, but it is nearly impossible to extirpate the tumor in this location. Synovial sarcoma is generally easily recognized histologically by the combination of fibrosarcomatous stroma and glandlike spaces containing mucin and lined with tall columnar cells. It arises from obscure origins in the soft tissue of the neck (Jernstrom, 1954).

Pathology of the Oral Pharynx

Developmental Abnormalities

The walls of the oropharynx are rarely the site of ectopic central nervous system tissue (Shapiro and Mix, 1968; Walker et al., 1963) or of congenital cysts, presumably of branchial cleft origin (Petersen, 1962). Rare teratoid tumors appear in the tonsil (Blair and Sanchez, 1969).

Inflammatory Processes

Inflammatory lesions of the oral pharynx often parallel those in the nasal portion. It is clear that some infections of the pharynx, and particularly of the tonsil, however, are foodborne (Hill et al., 1969). The bacterial flora may even be related to the lower intestinal tract (Johanson et al., 1969). Exudate in the oral pharynx may be more readily dislodged from the surface, but pseudomembranes may form. Ulcerative pharyngitis may lead to scarring and deformity (Bosma et al., 1968). Histoplasma can be isolated (Weed and Parkhill, 1948).

Tonsillitis frequently is suppurative in character, with collections of purulent exudate within sealed-off crypts. Deep foci may be surrounded by fibrous tissue. The capsule is resistant to infection, but peritonsillar spread of infective material may lead to abscess within the parapharyngeal space.

The oral pharynx is exposed to direct trauma and laceration, as with objects held in the mouth while being struck or during a fall. A finger in the mouth of the newborn infant during delivery may lead to a traumatic or pseudodiverticulum (Girdany et al., 1969). Breaks in the surface epithelium may be filled by exuberant overgrowth of fibroblasts and capillaries, with leukocytic infiltrate (pyogenic granuloma) (Kerr, 1951). True diverticula of the oropharynx are not reported.

The tonsil, like the nasal pharynx, is a frequent site of tuberculosis in patients with pulmonary infection; however, this is rarely the site of the presenting lesion (Sanford and Becker, 1966). Sarcoidosis is a rare incidental finding in tonsils that have been removed (Yarington et al., 1967). Ectopic tissues are found in palatine tonsils, notably cartilage and bone, with a rare teratoma (Friend, 1926; Rosenberg, 1935; Wilkinson, 1929). Tonsillectomy in early life does not appear to predispose to later malignancy (Gross, 1966). A punched-out ulceration of the tonsil may be syphilitic in origin.

Tumors

Thickening and cornification of the surface epithelium (leukoplakia) is much less common than in the oral cavity. Only if this is accompanied by the cellular changes of dysplasia is there any relationship to malignancy (Soule, 1968). These changes are enlargement and irregularity of nuclei; failure of maturation of nuclei toward the surface; mitoses, particularly abnormal mitoses in the upper layers; and, generally, hyperchromicity and disorganization.

Carcinoma of the oral pharynx occurs generally in the sixth and seventh decades. About 90 per cent occur in men (Ackerman and Del Regato, 1962; Soule, 1968). This is apt to occur as a diffuse infiltration or as a shallow ulcer over the anterior pillar above the tonsil and soft palate. They are squamous cell carcinomas, which are relatively better differentiated than those of the nasal pharynx. A few are papillary in character.

Those carcinomas arising in the posterior wall are less well differentiated and tend to grow outward toward the lumen. The lateral wall tumors extend downward. Squamous cell carcinomas arising in and around the epiglottis occur somewhat earlier in life (fifth and sixth decades) (Ackerman and Del Regato, 1962). A large polypoid mass may develop on the epiglottis, whereas those arising in the valleculae are ulcerating (Woolner, 1968). They account for about 25 per cent of "extrinsic" laryngeal tumors (Shaw and Epstein, 1959) and 8 to 15 per cent of all perilaryngeal cancers (Shahrokh et al., 1961; Withalm, 1953). More than half have positive nodes when first seen (McCall et al., 1957; Shaw and Epstein, 1959). Carcinoma of the base of the tongue is much less common (one fourth to one sixth) than that of the anterior portion. It is deeply infiltrating, with penetrating fissures, but in general it is relatively well differentiated (Ackerman and Del Regato, 1962). The prognosis is poor (Seda and Snow, 1969).

Some etiological factors in carcinoma of the pharynx are thought to be extrinsic. There appears to be a relationship of increased incidence to hepatic cirrhosis, heavy alcohol consumption, and heavy smoking (Keller, 1967). The high incidence in India has been related to peculiarities of cigarette smokers' habits (Paymaster, 1962 and 1964). Multiple malignancies occurring in the respiratory and alimentary tract, however, suggest an inherent capability of the epithelium to produce malignancy (Epstein et al., 1960; Marchetta et al., 1965; Wynder et al., 1969).

Carcinoma of the palatine tonsil is usually a noncornifying squamous cell carcinoma (Evans, 1966). It may be superficial for long periods while spreading over the surface. This may have the appearance of thickened mucosa or of a superficial ulcer, generally at the upper pole. Leukoplakia is not a precursor (Ash, 1966; Parkhill, 1968). This carcinoma is second in frequency in the upper air passages to carcinoma of the larynx (Ackerman and Del Regato, 1962). These amount to 1.5 to 3.0 per cent of all cancers (Daly and Friedman, 1960). Males in sixth to seventh decades are predominantly affected. It is rarely bilateral (Holden and Howard, 1966).

Carcinomas of the tonsil, soft palate, and anterior pillar spread first to subdigastric nodes anterior to the jugular chain (Ackerman and Del Regato, 1962; Martin and Sugarbaker, 1941). About 11 per cent have shown bilateral spread (Teloh, 1952). Those of the base of the tongue commonly spread bilaterally to cervical nodes. The outlook for survival is probably best for carcinoma of the tonsil, amounting to 32 to 43 per cent for five years (Scanlon et al., 1958). In reporting statistics, only tumors of the same type and location should be compared.

Malignant lymphoma is a less common tumor of the palatine tonsil (Johnson, 1960; Parkhill, 1968). It is likely to appear as a polypoid lobulated soft growth, possibly pedunculated, which is covered for the most part by intact mucosa. It is composed of sheets of lymphocytic cells, usually of fairly uniform size, sometimes of large reticulum cells. Terminology and classification will depend on estimations of cell size and degree of differentiation into lymphocytes. It is more common than carcinoma in the third and fourth decades. A few lymphomas are seen in the pharyngeal walls or epiglottis.

Other benign or malignant tumors of the oral pharynx are uncommon. Adenocarcinomas, usually adenoid cystic type, can be encountered usually from the soft palate laterally (Smant and French, 1961); a rare example is an adenocarcinoma of the epiglottis (Ahned, 1956). These tumors produce a submucosal mass. Solitary plasma cell myeloma may occur on the tonsil or elsewhere (Webb et al., 1962).

Any soft tissue sarcoma in the neck may impinge on the pharyngeal wall, such as liposarcoma, fibrosarcoma, or rhabdomyosarcoma. Other malignant tumors are represented usually by single case reports as hemangiopericytoma (Stout and Murray, 1942) and mucoepidermoid carcinoma (Fig. 2). Melanoma of the tonsil is less common than melanoma in the oral cavity (Moore and Martin, 1955). Synovial sarcoma may arise in the soft parts of the neck and involve the pharynx (Martens, 1958). They need not be associated with a joint. Acinic cell carcinoma (Wendling, 1968) and rare salivary gland neoplasms may arise from mucous glands.

Benign tumors of the oropharynx are considerably less common than malignant. Neurilemmoma appears to be the most common. They are attached to adjacent nerves, sometimes the vagus or hypoglossal (Figi, 1933; Iliades and Watson, 1967; Kragh et al., 1960; Obermann and Sullenger, 1967). Lipomas occur in the posterior wall (Glyn-Jones, 1952; Harper, 1959). Squamous papilloma is the only benign tumor of consequence which appears on the tonsil (Fig. 3). It has no malignant propensities but must be distinguished from papillary forms of carcinoma (Parkhill, 1968).

Polypoid structures of loose fibrous tissue, sometimes containing fat, may be inflammatory in origin (Laskiewicz, 1962; Soule, 1968; Sohn and Feverstein, 1967). A fibroma which lacks the vessels of the nasopharyngeal angiofibroma has been described (Vaheri and Narma, 1957).

Hemangiomas and lymphangiomas are uncommon (Cocke, 1961). Benign mixed tumors

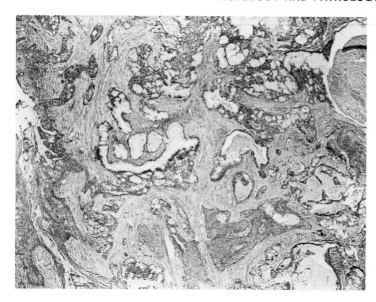

Figure 2. Photomicrograph of muco-epidermoid carcinoma arising in sub-mucosal glands of palate in a woman 26 years old. Cystic spaces are lined by tall mucus-secreting cells and by stratified squamous epithelium. (Hematoxylin and eosin, × 40.)

may become very large (Soule, 1968), but there is rarely a malignant change (Havens and Butler, 1955). Myxoma and xanthoma are described in relation to the oral pharynx (Dutz and Stout, 1961; New, 1935). Leiomyoma is rare (Seymour-Jones, 1959), and leiomyosarcoma has been reported (Fuller et al., 1966). Chordoma may present in the oral pharynx as well as in the nasal pharynx (Schindel and Markowicz, 1966). A chemodectoma of glomus jugulare or vagal body may bulge into the pharynx (Johnson et al., 1962; Schermer et al., 1966) (Fig. 4). Granular cell myoblastomas are rare beyond the

tongue (Frenckner, 1938). A cystic papillary benign tumor of palate (cystadenoma) appears to arise from mucous glands (Goldman, 1967; Soule, 1968). Osteoma of the mandible is reported in the tonsillar area (Jordan, 1958).

Other benign cystic tumors do not appear to be neoplastic. Some in the epiglottis and valleculae appear to be retention cysts and contain thick mucus (Woolner, 1968). Amyloid deposits in the lamina propria of the pharyngeal wall may produce a polypoid tumor (Bauer and Kuzma, 1949; Kyle and Bayrd, 1961; Soule, 1968).

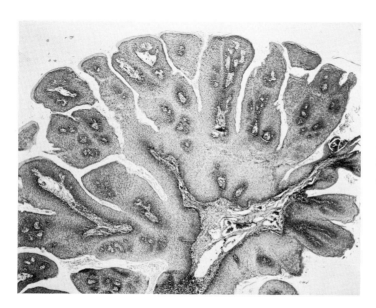

Figure 3. Photomicrograph of squamous papilloma of left tonsillar area in a man of 24. Fibrovascular fronds are covered by uniform stratified squamous epithelium. (Hematoxylin and eosin, × 40.)

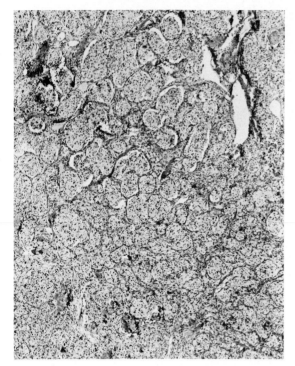

Figure 4. Photomicrograph of a chemodectoma from a woman, 45. The ball-like nests of tumor cells are surrounded by strands of vascular stroma. (Hematoxylin and eosin, × 40.)

Pathology of the Hypopharynx

Congenital Abnormalities

At the junction with the esophagus, congenital abnormalities in the development of the hypopharynx may lead to constrictions or defects in the wall (Keith, 1910).

Pharyngoesophageal diverticulum arises between the inferior constrictor muscle and the cricopharyngeus, where there appears to be a deficiency in the muscle coat. Periodically increased intraluminal pressure during swallowing eventually leads to formation of a pocket of mucosa, lamina propria, and a few muscle fibers, which penetrates between muscle bundles to expand into the more yielding tissues of the parapharyngeal space. The majority do not appear before the age of 50, although the muscle defect may be congenital. Most are on the left side. The aperture into the pharynx is generally wide and loosely open when the muscle is not contracted. Ulceration is common, but squamous cell carcinoma arising in the diverticulum is uncommon (Lahey, 1946; Liberson and Riese, 1960; Pierce and Johnson, 1969).

Inflammatory Processes

The hypopharynx is less exposed to external infection, and inflammatory lesions are less common than in nasal or oral portions.

Tumors

Neoplasms of the hypopharynx are similar to but generally less common than those of the other portions of the pharynx. Nearly all are squamous cell carcinomas, usually moderately to completely undifferentiated (Evans, 1966). They occur chiefly in males, although postcricoid carcinoma occurs more frequently in women. Most arise on the posterior wall, pyriform sinus, or retrocricoid areas (Ackerman and Del Regato, 1962). Those of the posterior wall appear to be limited to superficial spread for long periods, whereas those of the lateral wall tend to involve the adjacent deeper structures more readily. These include the thyroid cartilage, internal jugular vein, and internal carotid artery. Those arising on the medial walls involve the laryngeal ventricle and true and false cords. They may be called extrinsic carcinomas of the larynx (Fig. 5). The tumors of the aryepiglottic folds resemble those of the epiglottis in being exophytic, papillary, or polypoid. These may be classified as supraglottic carcinomas of the larynx. Retrocricoid carcinomas tend to be annular and to extend into the esophagus. They are associated with the Paterson-Plummer-Vinson syndrome (Ahlborn, 1936; Coleman, 1957; Wynder et al., 1957) in one half to two thirds of patients. It has been estimated that one out of 75 patients with the syndrome will develop this tumor (Jones, 1961). A few carcinomas seem to have been related to therapeutic radiation many years before (McGraw, 1965; Sonn and Peimer, 1955; Tsukamoto and Tazaki, 1954). No other etiological factors have been suggested. Those of the posterior wall and aryepiglottic fold appear to have the best prognosis. Pyriform sinus tumors are the second most frequent source (to the nasopharynx) of metastatic carcinoma in cervical nodes with a previously undiscovered primary lesion (Brown and Devine, 1960).

Lymphatic drainage is through the thyrohyoid membrane to the internal jugular nodes. Bilaterally involved nodes have been reported in 67 per cent when the tumor crosses the midline and contralaterally involved nodes in 19 per cent when the tumor is confined to one side (Hamilton and Oppenheim, 1955). Medial wall tumors tend to spread toward the medias-

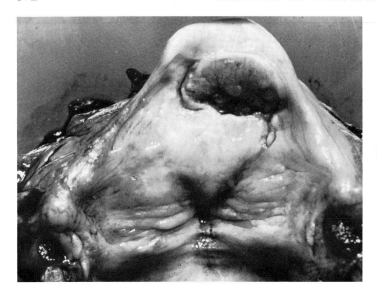

Figure 5. Squamous cell carcinoma of the epiglottis in a 51 year old man. The laryngeal surface shows an indurated ulcerated plaque measuring 2.0 × 1.5 cm.

tinum. Surgical treatment appears to be preferred (Ballantyne, 1967; Brown and Devine, 1960; Cunningham and Catlin, 1967; Raven, 1952).

THE LARYNX

Histology

The larynx is that portion of the respiratory tract conducting air from the common oral pharynx into the trachea and lower respiratory tract and includes the sphincter or glottis. It is held open, as in the nasal cavity, by cartilages. The thyroid and cricoid cartilages are unpaired and composed of hyaline cartilage. The paired cartilages are of fibroelastic structure except for the lower part of the arytenoids. Intrinsic skeletal muscles connect the cartilages.

Within this framework is a tubular lumen lined by epithelium. There is a transition in the lower half of the posterior surface of the epiglottis and just inside the aryepiglottic folds, from the stratified squamous epithelium of the pharynx into the pseudostratified ciliated columnar epithelium of the entire lower tract. The cilia are 3.5 to 5.0 μ in length and beat toward the mouth (Bloom and Fawcett, 1968).

Goblet cells in variable numbers are scattered among the ciliated cells. There is a distinct basement lamina, which lies on a thin fibrous lamina propria. This stroma is variable in thickness, being more abundant over the epiglottis and aryepiglottic folds and fairly thick over the cords, whereas in the lower portion it is relatively scarce. There are mixed

mucous and serous glands of tubulo-acinous structure throughout, except for the areas of the true cords. The ducts open on the surface, and there are some mucous cells in the duct lining. The anterior surface of the epiglottis may contain a few taste buds. Rete pegs are practically absent in the stratified squamous epithelium of this area. The vocal cords are covered by thin, stratified squamous epithelium.

The lamina propria throughout the larynx contains elastic fibers. These are accentuated over the true cord. Each cord is really a band of elastic tissue extending from the thyroarytenoid muscle to the rim of the glottis. A layer of elastic fibers is condensed just under the epithelium with a second layer just above the muscle (thyroarytenoid ligament). The intervening looser layer of the lamina propria has been called Reinke's space. It extends no more than 2 mm. from the margins of the cords.

The ventricles of the larynx are deep pockets lined by respiratory epithelium which invaginates between true and false cords and extends upward just superficial to the cartilage. The lamina propria here is closely attached to perichondrium. There may be a slight fold at the base containing lymphoid aggregates (laryngeal tonsil). The lamina propria around the ventricle contains many mucous glands.

Below the glottis, the laryngeal mucosa shows a thin lamina propria. There are fewer glands and goblet cells. A dense elastic layer continues below this (elastic cone), and the transition into trachea is arbitrarily taken to be at the lower border of the cricoid cartilage.

Lymphatic channels drain to upper cervical nodes and to nodes along the trachea but they are sparse over the cords. Elsewhere they are found in the lamina propria.

Pathology

Congenital Abnormalities

Complete stenoses of the larynx are incompatible with extrauterine life. Partial atresia may be present and may persist into adult life (Baker and Savetzky, 1966). Webs between vocal cords and supraglottic and infraglottic structures have been described. "Hard" subglottic types contain cartilage, whereas "soft" types are of fibrous tissue. They have been thought to represent failure of recanalization (McMillan and Duvall, 1968) but may also be the result of the arrest of epithelial development at different stages (Smith and Bain, 1965).

Cysts of the larynx may be congenital and represent pinching off of the ventricle (Suehs and Powell, 1967). Embryonic inclusion cysts may be of branchial cleft origin and show ciliated columnar epithelium, with some lymphoid tissue (Ash and Raum, 1956). Most cysts are of retention type, however (Leonard et al., 1967). An abnormal cry at birth has been associated with mental retardation, microcephaly, hypotonia, and laryngomalacia (cri du chat syndrome). There are a relaxed epiglottis and diamond-shaped vocal cords (Ward et al., 1968).

Laryngocele may be congenital or acquired. An internal type dissects upward into the aryepiglottic fold. The external type may protrude above or even through the thyroid cartilage through the hyothyroid membrane to be apparent in the neck in the lateral submandibular space (Ferguson, 1967). There appears to be a relatively thin layer of fibrous tissue separating the ventricle from the supraglottic space (Putney, 1968). Increased incidence is reported in musicians who play wind instruments (Macfie, 1966).

Ventricular hernia is a bulging of the mucosa of the ventricle into the lumen as a polypoid smooth mass, and inflammatory changes may occur (Ash and Raum, 1956).

Inflammatory Processes

Laryngitis may be threatening to life because of the narrow airway and rigid walls. This is particularly true in young children. Acute inflammatory processes in epiglottis and aryepiglottic folds in children under five years of age are often caused by *Haemophilus influenzae* Type B and may be a cause of sudden illness and death (Baxter, 1967; Cole, 1967). Edema of the lamina propria may be particularly severe where it has a loose structure over the epiglottis, aryepiglottic folds, and vocal cords. The edema in acute supraglottis is accompanied by congestion of vessels and some mononuclear infiltrate. There is often adherent fibrinous exudate on the mucosal surface. A similar sudden edema is produced by an allergic urticarial reaction. There is little cellular infiltrate and superficial exudate. Localization is the same and is dictated by the structure of the tissue.

Acute laryngotracheal bronchitis is a similar process in children which, in addition, involves the lower tract. Thick exudate in bronchi and trachea rather than the edema of the laryngeal structures may produce distress, although edema of the subglottic mucosa may be a contributing factor (Neffson, 1944; Ross, 1969). Pseudomembranous laryngitis may be produced by streptococci, although diphtheria is still endemic in the United States (Lang, 1965). The membrane in either case is composed of adherent fibrinous exudate and necrotic mucosa, leaving vascular lamina propria exposed when it is removed. The pseudomembrane of diphtheria is said to be grayer and more adherent than that produced by streptococci (Ash and Raum, 1956). Destruction of tissue or hemorrhage may occur in acute laryngitis without membrane formation. Most acute laryngitis represents an inflammation descending from the pharynx during an acute upper respiratory infection.

Ulcerations of both cords where they are in contact (contact ulcers) apparently are related to injury. This is usually seen posteriorly over the vocal processes of the arytenoids. It may be related to reflux of gastric juice (Cherry and Margulies, 1968; Delahunty and Cherry, 1968).

Chronic laryngitis is characterized by thickened mucosa, with aggregates of lymphocytes and polymorphonuclear leukocytes in the lamina propria. There is glandular hypertrophy and increased vascularity. The thickening may be localized to produce a polyplike area. Such changes may be produced by trauma, by chronic irritation by fumes, or by chronic upper respiratory infections. Atrophic laryngitis (sicca) shows reduced numbers of glands and vessels. There may be squamous metaplasia over large areas (Ash and Raum, 1956).

Tuberculosis of the larynx is common in patients with pulmonary tuberculosis and positive sputum. The lesions are usually located posteriorly, over the arytenoids, in the interarytenoid space, and over the vocal cords and posterior surface of the epiglottis. Long-standing lesions may penetrate deeply and deform the cartilages. The lesions are characteristic necrotizing epithelioid granulomas. A less specific chronic inflammatory infiltration may precede the granuloma stage. Organisms should be demonstrated (Castleman and McNeely, 1968).

Syphilis most commonly produces mucous patches in the larynx in the secondary stage. Condylomas and gummas of the third stage are rare. Congenital infection may cause diffuse hyperplasia of the mucosa. Blastomycosis may involve the larynx. Suffocation by nodular lesions in the larynx may be a cause of death in leprosy. The tuberculoid lesion is uncommon, but tuberculosis is a frequent complication of leprosy (Ash and Raum, 1956), and granulomas may therefore be present. Monilia infection may be related to hyperkeratosis (Tedeschi and Cheren, 1968).

Sarcoidosis may involve the larynx in as many as 5 per cent of patients (Devine, 1965). Although the true cords are uncommonly involved, there may be diffuse thickening of supraglottic structures. Lupus erythematosus and mucous membrane pemphigoid are reported to involve the larynx (Polliack, 1968; Scarpelli et al., 1959). Thickening of vocal cord mucosa with material resembling that in myxedema may be found in hypothyroidism (Ritter, 1965). Rheumatoid arthritis affecting the cricoarytenoid joint may lead to laryngeal symptoms (Bienenstock et al., 1963). Myositis ossificans of laryngeal musculature may cause stridor (Pappas and Johnson, 1965), and trichinosis of the muscle may produce hoarseness (Kean, 1966).

A peculiar polychondritis involving the laryngeal and tracheal cartilages causes eventual replacement of cartilage by fibrous tissue. Some cases resemble Wegener's granulomatosis (Daly, 1966; Pearson et al., 1960).

Trauma to the larynx in the form of a blunt blow may displace cartilages without much damage to the soft tissues of the neck. This may happen to the front seat passenger thrown against a padded dashboard (padded dash syndrome) (Butler and Moser, 1968).

Endotracheal intubation, especially over long periods, may result in ulceration and later production of pyogenic granuloma (Barton, 1953) (Fig. 6). The lesions may be in the subglottic space against the cricoid (Bergstrom et al., 1962) or on the tip of the vocal process of one or both arytenoids (Jackson, 1953). Even a brief exposure may produce ulceration (Way and Sooy, 1965). Temporary difficulty is common after 48 hours of intubation (Hedden et al., 1969; Tonkin and Harrison, 1966), and permanent hoarseness may occur (Donnelly, 1969). Local lesions are present in a high percentage of autopsied patients (Stein et al., 1960). Granulation tissue at the site of injury may produce recurrent polypoid lesions much later. These are composed of proliferating fibroblasts and capillaries growing into a superfi-

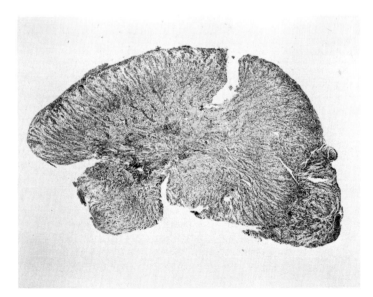

Figure 6. Photomicrograph of pyogenic granuloma of larynx from a man of 38. Note the proliferating capillaries and fibrous tissue strands radiating outward toward the ulcerated surface. (Hematoxylin and eosin, × 40.)

cial layer of fibrinous exudate. Eventual overgrowth of the epithelium from the margins may occur, leaving a vascular fibrous polyp. Radiation has been used to prevent recurrence (Smith et al., 1969).

Tumors

The vocal cord polyp or nodule is a common but poorly understood lesion resembling the pyogenic granuloma (Fig. 7). It usually appears as a single lesion on the anterior third of the vocal cord. It has been related to misuse of the voice, but many cases appear to be spontaneous. Although it would be impossible to follow a single lesion serially, several stages of development have been described (Ash and Schwartz, 1944). The smaller lesions, thought to be at an early stage, show fibroblastic proliferation in the lamina propria and present as firm, flattened plaques. A polypoid stage, most frequently seen by pathologists, consists chiefly of greatly thickened lamina propria of loose edematous structure. There is generally no alteration of the surface epithelium and little inflammatory cellular infiltrate. A promi-

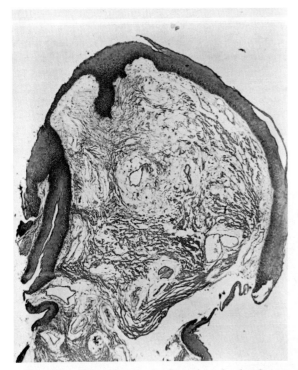

Figure 7. Photomicrograph of vocal cord polyp from a man 31 years old. Note the loosely arranged edematous fibrous stalk with large vascular channels covered by well differentiated epithelium. (Hematoxylin and eosin, × 40.)

nent and perhaps thickened epithelial basement lamina is easily seen. There are variable numbers of thin-walled vessels, apparently large capillaries, or venules in this stroma. A varix stage is described when these are unusually prominent and large. There is rarely any external bleeding, however. Deposit of fibrinous or thrombotic material in the vessels and surrounding tissue leads to a so-called amyloid stage or amyloid tumor. It appears unlikely that all such polyps pass through all these stages. The term vocal cord polyps appears most appropriate for the majority. No relationship to allergic conditions has been demonstrated.

True amyloid may be deposited in the larynx in a more diffuse manner. This is the most frequent site in the respiratory tract in primary systemic amyloidosis but is rare in secondary amyloidosis (Heiner, 1968). It involves the vestibule, false cord, aryepiglottic fold, or subglottic area, with diffuse thickening of mucosa and deposits of smooth hyaline material around vessels and in the fibrous lamina propria.

Thickening and hyperkeratosis of the epithelium over the vocal cords is seen frequently, either in the presence of underlying inflammation or as an apparently primary process. Rete pegs are accentuated and a granular layer appears in the epithelium, with the accumulation of a thick keratinizing layer above.

The surface may become verrucous or papillary, suggesting lateral growth of epithelium as well. There may be an abrupt transition to normal-appearing stratified squamous or respiratory epithelium. If the cells are uniform and show normal stages of maturation toward the surface, it may be regarded as a benign process. There is generally little inflammatory infiltrate in the lamina propria. The relationship to chronic inflammation, infection, irritation, or trauma is obscure. This may be termed pachydermia laryngis, but "hyperkeratosis" appears sufficient. The term leukoplakia may be employed, since it indicates literally only a thickened opaque white area on the mucosa. More commonly, leukoplakia is used in the sense of a dyskeratosis or premalignant lesion and, hence, probably should be avoided without a clear understanding of the character of the lesion concerned.

Without microscopic examination, simple hyperkeratosis cannot be distinguished from those thickenings which exhibit growth activity in the direction of malignancy. Dysplasia, or atypical epithelial hyperplasia, is characterized by cellular irregularity in size and staining reaction, loss of normal maturation toward the surface, increasingly frequent mitoses, and general hyperchromicity. Malignant changes include complete loss of polarity and maturation, presence of abnormal mitoses, and disruption of the basal layers. Malignant change may be confined to the surface epithelium (in situ carcinoma) or there may be penetration of the basement lamina by epithelial cells, with downward invasion into the lamina propria. A continuum of changes may be observed from normal through hyperplasia and dysplasia to frank carcinoma. Unfortunately, the point of separation must sometimes be arbitrary (Holinger, 1966). Without invasion, however, metastasis does not occur (Kuhn et al., 1957).

Carcinomas of the larynx amount to about 20 per cent of malignant lesions of the head and neck (Rogers et al., 1966). They arise primarily on the anterior portions of the vocal cords or in the ventricles and are almost all relatively well differentiated squamous cell carcinomas. About 90 per cent occur in men. Origin from a pre-existing dyskeratosis or papilloma may be demonstrable (Ash and Raum, 1956). They are generally slow-growing and tend to metastasize late, partly from lack of lymphatic channels in the cord. Carcinomas originating in the epiglottis, aryepiglottic folds, and pyriform fossae (extrinsic carcinoma) are more properly considered carcinomas of the hypopharynx. The location of the primary lesion is the determining factor in the frequency of spread to the pre-epiglottic space, through the thyroid cartilage, or to the anterior cervical nodes (Ogura, 1955).

The usual carcinoma of the vocal cord is composed of infiltrating columns and sheets of focally cornifying epithelial cells. They are somewhat irregular and there are variable numbers of mitoses. Usually there is considerable cytoplasm, particularly in the centers of large nests, and intercellular bridges may be apparent. The stroma usually shows some infiltration of lymphocytes and plasma cells. The carcinoma tends to be confined by the cartilages and elastic membranes for some time. Fixation of the vocal cord indicates that the lamina propria (Reinke's layer) has been penetrated (Ash and Raum, 1956). Some carcinomas show smaller cells with less cytoplasm and resemble basal cell carcinomas of the skin. They are less differentiated. Eventual lymphatic spread is to the anterior cervical and mediastinal nodes, reported in up to 31 per cent of infiltrating carcinomas (Kuhn et al., 1957). The prognosis is better in women, who are more likely to have types other than squamous cell carcinoma (Kirchner and Malkin, 1953).

A history of smoking is closely related to the incidence of squamous cell carcinoma of the larynx (Auerbach et al., 1970; Ellis and Liderman, 1960). Previous radiation therapy for papillomatosis has been implicated in subsequent development of carcinoma (Majoros et al., 1963; VerMeulen, 1966). However, carcinoma of the larynx in persons under age 20 may be unrelated to either papillomatosis or irradiation (Glyn-Jones and Gabriel, 1969). It has a good prognosis. Incidence of laryngeal carcinoma appears to be rising (Von Essen et al., 1968).

Clinical staging is necessary to compare results of treatment (Alexander and Cassady, 1966; Goldman et al., 1966; McNelis, 1965; Trible and Kahauer, 1969). Location and histologic degree of differentiation of the tumor are also important.

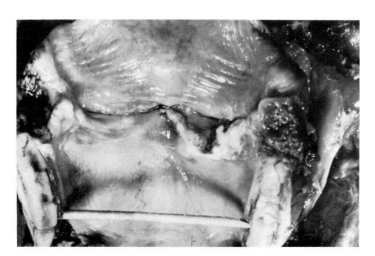

Figure 8. Squamous cell carcinoma of the larynx in a man, 51. The right vocal cord is replaced by ulcerating tumor, while the false cord is not involved.

Multiple primary carcinomas of the respiratory tract may frequently include the larynx (Titche, 1966). Radiation therapy may destroy the primary growth (Perez et al., 1968). Fibrous encapsulation of cervical nodes may prevent recurrence (Goldman et al., 1969). Disseminated nests may remain viable, however (Goldman et al., 1966).

Adenocarcinomas of the larynx are rare. Most can be classified as adenoid cystic carcinoma. They have the appearance and course of those seen elsewhere in the respiratory tract (Toomey, 1967).

A rare polypoid tumor shows a transition of squamous cell carcinoma of the surface epithelium into a spindle-celled, sarcomalike, deeper mass. These are probably all squamous cell carcinomas, although metastases sometimes resemble sarcoma. They have been classified as pseudosarcoma, carcinosarcoma, or fibroma with superficial carcinoma (Ash and Raum, 1956; Minckler et al., 1970). They appear to have a relatively favorable prognosis (Himalstein and Humphrey, 1968; Sherwin, 1963). Similar tumors are seen in the esophagus, tongue, and skin.

Papillomas of the larynx occur in young children and in adults. In each case they are composed of elongated vascular fibrous projections from the lamina propria which are covered with layers of well-differentiated stratified squamous epithelium. This may show hyperkeratosis but it is rarely dyskeratotic. These papillomas tend to develop on the anterior third of the cord or at the commissure. Those in children tend to recur but regress at adolescence. They are frequently multiple and may extend into the lower tract (Kirchner and Malkin, 1951). A viral etiology is not confirmed (Dekelbaum, 1965), but skin warts may be associated (Kaufman and Balogh, 1969). Adult papillomas are more often single than multiple (Dekelbaum, 1965). They may disappear with pregnancy (Holinger et al., 1968).

Many types of benign tumors have been found to originate in or around the larynx (New and Erich, 1938). A few glandular tumors arising from mucous glands are usually subglottic (Capo, 1956; Kroe et al., 1967; Sabri and Hajjar, 1967). Mixed tumors are most common. Neurofibromas and neurilemmomas may encroach on the larynx (Goethals and Lillie, 1961; Holinger and Cohen, 1950). Benign and malignant cartilaginous tumors most commonly arise in the cricoid cartilage. They tend to remain localized, even if histologically malignant (Brandenburg et al., 1967;

Goethals et al., 1963; Hora and Weller, 1961; Huizenga and Balogh, 1967; Putney and Moran, 1965). Chemodectomas arising from the inferior laryngeal glomus may impinge on the wall of the subglottic area (Baxter, 1965; Martinson, 1968). So-called granular cell myoblastoma arises from the vocal cords. The overlying epithelium may show pseudoepitheliomatous hyperplasia. These are probably neurogenic tumors and not related to muscle (Cracovaner and Opler, 1967; Iglauer, 1942; Pope, 1965; Schneider et al., 1969). A true rhabdomyoma may exist, however (Battifora et al., 1969).

Melanoma may be primary on the mucosa of the larynx (Pantazapoulos, 1964) Melanoblasts in the junctional area of the epithelium must be demonstrated, since metastatic tumors of the mucosa may also occur (Chamberlain, 1966). True osteogenic sarcoma may arise in the laryngeal cartilages (Sprinkle et al., 1966). Other soft-tissue sarcomas may involve the larynx (Pratt and Goodof, 1968). Metastatic carcinomas are rare in the larynx, as they are in spleen and skeletal muscle (Fields, 1966; Mazzarella et al., 1966). Leukemic infiltrates in laryngeal structures may be found in a large percentage of patients dying of leukemia, but they are seldom symptomatic (Shilling et al., 1967).

THE ESOPHAGUS

Histology

The esophagus is considered to commence at the level of the lower border of the cricoid cartilage and to extend to the junction with the cardia of the stomach. Both boundaries are arbitrary. There is a gradual transition in structure from the hypopharynx above. Below, the transition to the stomach is generally taken to be at the point where esophageal mucosa is replaced by gastric mucous membrane, but this may occur at a point somewhat higher than would be indicated by anatomical structure. The esophageal mucosa is not known to line any part of the stomach in man, as it may in rodents (Blount and Lachman, 1953).

The entire esophagus is lined with stratified squamous epithelium which may be from 500 to 800 μ in thickness and consists of 8 to 20 layers of cells. It does not normally show cornification at the surface, although small numbers of precursor keratohyaline granules may be seen (Bloom and Fawcett, 1968). It is indistinguishable from pharyngeal mucosa above, but undergoes an abrupt transition to simple columnar mucosa at the cardia of the stomach. This boundary is grossly visible, since the columnar epithelium transmits the color of the underlying blood, whereas the thicker esophageal mucosa tends to be pale. There is regeneration of the epithelium from the basal layer, which shows scattered mitoses. Normally there is an orderly progression of maturation changes in the cells approaching the surface, and nuclei are retained in surface cells, which are cast off intact. There is a thin basement membrane separating the epithelium from the underlying lamina propria This is composed of relatively thin collagen and elastic fibers with scattered fibrocytes and contains some lymphocytes. The lymphocytes may form distinct nodules adjacent to gland ducts. The lamina propria shows numerous papillae supporting the epithelium.

The submucosa is separated from the mucosa by the muscularis mucosae. This thin layer of smooth muscle shows longitudinal fibers and some elastic tissue. It becomes thicker and blends with that of the stomach below. Above, it replaces the elastic layer of the pharynx. It does not exceed 400 μ in thickness.

The submucosa is composed of denser collagen and elastic fibers than is the lamina propria. There are a few nests of fat cells. It provides the wall with some strength, and its thickness allows the mucosa to fold longitudinally when the esophagus is not distended. There are also networks of finer elastic fibers and some small infiltrates of lymphocytes, generally gathered about glands.

The bulk of the esophageal wall is formed by the muscularis propria. This is 0.5 to 2.2 mm. thick when relaxed. It is composed of both smooth and skeletal types of muscle fibers. These are not arranged in completely regular circular or longitudinal layers. There is, however, an inner layer containing many spiral or oblique bundles; it is continuous with the inferior constrictor of the pharynx. An outer layer is formed of more longitudinally oriented fibers.

The skeletal muscle of the pharynx continues in both inner and outer layers in the upper fourth of the esophagus. Gradual replacement of skeletal by smooth muscle occurs down through the upper half. In the lower third there is no remaining skeletal muscle. The muscle layers are continuous with those of the stomach below. The connection of esophageal muscle with the inferior constrictor of the pharynx is complex (Blount and Lachman, 1953.)

The tunica adventitia lies outside the muscle layer. It is a loose fibrous layer which joins the esophagus to neighboring structures. There is no serosa.

The submucosa contains the esophageal glands proper. They are distributed irregularly throughout the esophagus and can be seen grossly. They are branched tubuloalveolar structures lined by mucus-secreting cells. There are no serous elements. The glands are compound, and the smallest ducts fuse into a larger main duct which opens on the surface of the mucosa. The main duct shows a stratified squamous lining and the smaller ducts have low columnar epithelium.

The lamina propria shows a second type of gland, the esophageal cardiac glands. They are like those of the cardia of the stomach, formed of curled tubules lined by pale granular cuboidal cells. They appear to contain some mucin and are connected to the surface by a duct lined by mucus-secreting cells. This opens at the tip of a papilla in the lamina propria. These glands occur only in the upper part of the esophagus, between the cricoid and the level of the fifth tracheal ring, and at the lower end of the esophagus near the cardia itself.

The blood supply of the esophagus is derived from several vessels along its course (inferior thyroid, esophageal branches of the aorta, intercostals, inferior phrenic, and left gastric). The wall is pierced from the adventitia by small arteries, and a plexus of veins is found in the adventitia as well. The submucosa contains many longitudinal vessels, and there are thin-walled vessels extending into the papillae of the lamina propria.

Two autonomic nerve plexuses are found in the esophageal wall, supplied by the thoracolumbar division of the sympathetic system and by the vagus (parasympathetic). Groups of nerve cells with their filaments and bundles of nerve fibers are seen in the interval of the fibrous tissue separating the inner and outer layers of the muscularis propria. These are the elements of the myenteric plexus (of Auerbach). The axons supply the smooth muscle of the muscularis propria. Other less conspicuous groups of ganglion cells and fibers are seen in the submucosa. These are in smaller numbers. Their fibers appear to supply the muscularis mucosae. They form the submucous plexus (of Meissner).

The epithelium of the esophagus is derived from the endoderm, which at first is simple columnar in type. In the embryo this becomes two-layered and then ciliated. By the eleventh week, rounded cells appear between the layers, developing into a squamous epithelium that replaces the columnar cells, which are then forced to the surface and desquamated. In the adult, portions of the esophagus may continue to be lined by columnar epithelium. This may be grossly visible from its pink color. The distinct outline of these patches may suggest an erosion. These areas are usually in the parts of the esophagus which contain cardiac-type glands. The epithelium may be more complex in these areas, even forming tubular glands lined by zymogenic and parietal cells, as in the stomach (Bosher and Taylor, 1951; Mottet, 1968; Rector and Connerley, 1941; Schridde, 1904). Such areas of aberrant mucosa can be found in about 10 per cent of individuals. They should not be interpreted as misplaced gastric mucosa, although this mucosa may more or less closely resemble that of the stomach.

Pathology

Congenital Abnormalities

Aside from the presence of islands of aberrant mucosa the most common congenital abnormality is atresia (Plass, 1919). It occurs in from 0.01 to 0.04 per cent of live births. In about 88 per cent there is, in addition, a tracheoesophageal fistula tract (Tenta and Ford, 1967). A fistula without atresia is much less common and is seen in only 1 to 4 per cent. A familial occurrence is rare. About half of the individuals born with tracheoesophageal fistulas have other abnormalities. Evidently there is a failure of the tracheoesophageal tube of the embryo to become completely divided by the developing septum. The detailed explanations of this failure do not account for all the varieties of structure encountered, however (Rosenthal, 1931; Tenta and Ford, 1967).

A common form is for the upper esophageal segment to end in a blind sac, while the lower segment from the stomach opens into the posterior wall of the trachea above the bifurcation. The communication with the trachea may be a rounded opening or a small slit. Similar slits may join the esophagus and larynx. In this case, fusion of the cricoid cartilage posteriorly may be prevented (Blumberg et al., 1965; Imbrie and Doyle, 1969).

In cases in which the fistula is small, and the esophagus patent, the patient may survive untreated (Tenta and Ford, 1967). Surgical repair is frequently possible (Haight, 1944).

Other forms of tracheoesophageal fistula show a communication between proximal esophagus and trachea, or between both segments (or neither) and the trachea (MacGregor, 1960).

Congenital esophageal stenosis is about one tenth as common as tracheoesophageal fistula (Bluestone et al., 1969). It is difficult to distinguish congenital varieties of stenosis with or without webbing from acquired varieties or from cardiospasm (Shamma'a and Benedict, 1958). There may be submucosal thickening, most commonly at the junction of the middle and lower thirds. A lower esophageal ring deformity found on x-ray may be difficult to identify at postmortem examination (Schatzki and Gary, 1953). It is most often a congenital mucosal ring at the cardioesophageal junction (Goyal et al., 1970).

All degrees of duplication of the esophagus have been reported, from intramural cysts to complete double esophagus (Bishop and Koop, 1964; Bremer, 1944; Rosemak and Van Vactor, 1951). One common explanation, that at one stage of embryological development the esophagus is a solid epithelial tube, is not conclusively proved (Tenta and Ford, 1967). However, such a hypothesis would explain the fact that more than one lumen may recanalize by vacuolization of the solid epithelial tube.

These duplications are closely related to enterogenous cysts of the thorax These appear to arise from the foregut itself, since they have an independent musculature, generally lacking or incomplete in most frank duplications. They are also related to defects in the vertebrae, perhaps through adherence of the foregut to the neurenteric canal or through a relation to the regressing notochord (Rosenthal, 1931).

Cysts within the esophageal wall are nearly all of congenital origin, although a few may be derived from occluded glandular ducts. In the middle third, most cysts are of primitive foregut origin. Bronchial cysts should contain cartilage as well as be lined by ciliated epithelium. Cysts in the lower third are more often gastroenteric. The origin of many cannot be identified (Desforges and Streider, 1960; Stout and Lattes, 1957; Totten et al., 1953).

Diverticula

Diverticula of the esophagus are fairly common and often troublesome. Most often the diverticulum includes all the layers of the esophagus, including the muscle coats, and is produced by adherence of the outer layers to adjacent structures. Such a pocket is a "true" diverticulum structurally, since the muscle layers are intact. The adhesions may be congenital in origin, related to incomplete separation of trachea and esophagus, or they may be the result of contraction of an inflammatory fibrous proliferation. This sometimes has resulted from tuberculous adenitis or other lymph node inflammation. Scarring following radiation therapy or surgery may do likewise. The diverticulum produced in this way has a tentlike shape with broad aperture and rarely retains food or secretion or ulcerates. It is often located anteriorly near the tracheal bifurcation.

The more significant type of diverticulum in producing complications is that in which the muscle layers are interrupted. Pressure from inside the lumen, pulsion, causes the mucosa and portions of the submucosa to evaginate through the aperture in the muscle. This does not usually happen unless there is some preexisting defect in the structure of the muscle. Such anatomically defective areas occur most often in the upper one third where the fibers of the inferior constrictor muscle of the pharynx blend into the muscle layer of the esophagus proper. Those diverticula, which occur at the junction of esophagus and pharynx, are more properly considered to be in the pharynx. In the lower part of the esophagus increased pressure within the lumen may be more important in providing pulsion diverticula than a muscle defect. The pressure may be elevated above a congenital web, or within a hiatal hernia, or with cardiospasm. Such pulsion diverticula tend to have a relatively narrow aperture and may fill with food and secretion, which may be expelled by projectile vomiting or lead to choking spells. Ulceration and even perforation may occur within the diverticulum. It is rare to find diverticula in a person younger than age 15, and a secondary rather than congenital origin of the muscle defects has been postulated (James, 1946; King, 1947).

Varices

Abnormally dilated veins in the submucosa of the esophagus are dangerous to life, since they are exposed to frequent trauma and are inaccessible to direct treatment. These varices are generally produced when blood pressure in the portal venous system is elevated over long periods. There is little supporting tissue around these large thin-walled channels, and the overlying mucosa is thin and delicate. Rupture and hemorrhage may be produced during a peak elevation of blood pressure in these channels, as in straining, vomiting, or coughing. Peptic

erosion of the overlying mucosa is probably not necessary (Liebowitz, 1961). Ten or 15 per cent of patients may die from the first hemorrhage (Baker et al., 1959). Lowering of portal blood pressure by portacaval anastomosis may reduce the danger of hemorrhage but does not improve the ultimate survival of the patient (Conn and Lindenmuth, 1968).

Varices are found generally in the lower third, where the esophageal veins offer a connection between the coronary veins of the stomach, part of the portal system, and the azygos veins which drain into the superior vena cava. The normal direction of blood flow is reversed.

Varices are demonstrated pathologically with some difficulty unless the channels can be preserved in their distended condition. They follow the longitudinal folds of the esophagus. Chronic inflammatory changes seen in their walls may be secondary to agonal changes.

Inflammatory Processes

The esophagus may be the site of acute and chronic inflammatory processes. Most often these are associated with ulceration of the mucosa. However, the infection may spread from mediastinal nodes, pericardium, or pleura through the adventitia.

There is usually a mixed bacterial culture, although hematogenous spread of a specific organism may involve the esophagus. Uncommonly, a fungal disease or a granulomatous disease such as tuberculosis may localize apparently primarily in the esophagus. Fungal diseases have become more common with manipulation of the immune mechanisms and use of antibiotics. Esophagitis is seen in terminal uremia.

Erosions and ulcerations seen at postmortem examination are often the result of reflux of gastric juice just before or after death. The finding of a cellular inflammatory infiltrate in the surrounding tissue establishes the process as antemortem. During life, reflux of gastric juice may lead to persistent chronic inflammations. Actual peptic ulcers are discussed later.

All these processes may elicit an inflammatory reaction which is not specific histologically. First of all there is probably a dilatation of vessels, chiefly capillaries, with focal leukocytic infiltration beneath the mucosa. If ulceration occurs, the surface is covered with fibrinous exudate. The submucosa in chronic esophagitis shows large phagocytic cells derived from histiocytes or lymphocytes and nests of lymphocytes in the deeper layers. There is proliferation of fibroblasts and capillaries. The fibrinous exudate may organize. A longstanding process leads to fibrous scarring in the submucosa, or deeper if the muscle is destroyed. Granulomas of characteristic form are produced in tuberculosis and related fungal diseases.

Peptic ulceration owing to reflux of gastric acid peptic contents during life is common (Barrett, 1950) (Fig. 9). A defect in the diaphragm is the most important factor and may be associated with some type of hiatus hernia (Hagarty, 1960). The histological appearance is similar to that of gastric or duodenal wall in similar conditions. The stratified squamous epithelium erodes first, since it has little mucus protection against digestion. With loss of epithelium there is an acute infiltration of lamina propria and soon of submucosa by polymorphonuclear leukocytes, with dilatation of capillaries and edema of fibrous tissue. Mononuclear phagocytic cells and lymphocytes accumulate in deeper tissues. With the passage of time there is fibroblastic proliferation and eventual scarring of the submucosa. The muscle layers may be destroyed and replaced by scar. Perforation may occur before fibrosis takes place, with the severe complication of spillage of contents into the mediastinum. Hemorrhage is common. Most peptic ulcerations are in the lower esophagus. The term "peptic ulcer" does not necessarily mean the ulceration of aberrant "gastric" mucosa of the esophagus, although this may occur (Barrett's ulcer). The pink appearance of glandular mucosa

in contrast to the opaque white of stratified squamous epithelium should not be mistaken for patches of erosion. Few peptic ulcers can be accounted for by "ectopic" mucosa (Allison, 1948).

The gastroesophageal sphincter mechanism is complex. The tone or strength of the sphincter appears to be dependent on gastrin secretion rather than on the level of free acid in gastric juice (Castell and Harris, 1970).

Perforation of the esophagus by trauma can occur not only from instrumentation or foreign objects but also during severe vomiting or retching. The syndrome was described by Mallory and Weiss (1929, 1932). Massive bleeding may occur (Dobbins, 1963; Freeark et al., 1964). The tear usually occurs longitudinally just at the gastroesophageal junction. This appears to be related to the diaphragmatic attachments at that point. Such tears may be related to hiatal hernias. The esophagus may dilate abnormally without proper support in this area. It has also been proposed that waves of retrograde contraction may force open a contracted spastic terminal esophagus. The actual tear may be visualized with difficulty. A pre-existing chronic ulcer may perforate under the same circumstances. After a few days the original tear may resemble an inflammatory ulcer histologically.

The ingestion of caustics (chiefly sodium hydroxide) produces an acute esophagitis with necrosis. The most damage is produced at the points of slowing of the bolus or narrowing of the esophagus, that is, just above the cricoid, at the aortic arch, and just above the cardia. If the muscle is destroyed, proliferation and contraction of a collagenous scar soon produces stricture. Experimental re-epithelialization has been slow, and early dilatation (before 10 days) seems illogical (Bosher et al., 1951).

Bacterial invasion does not appear decisive in formation of a later stricture, but destruction of the muscle by the chemical is necessary. At least half the patients ingesting lye do not need active treatment (Bikhazi et al., 1969). The great majority of cases of lye ingestion are accidental and occur in children (60 per cent of patients are under 3 years of age). According to Kiviranta (1949–1950) it is not a popular form of suicide. The site of a previous lye stricture is said to be predisposed to the formation of carcinoma (Bigelow, 1953). This seems to be a rare and perhaps fortuitous occurrence.

A seldom recognized form of esophagitis is produced by herpesvirus. Intranuclear inclusions and giant cells are seen in the inflamma-

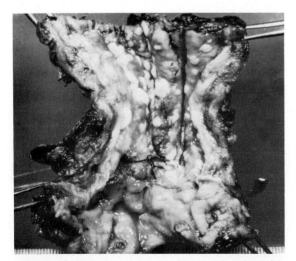

Figure 9. Chronic esophagitis with extensive ulceration related to reflux of gastric juice from a 19 year old girl. Islands of pale mucosa remain between the ulcers.

tory infiltrate, and it may be associated with ulceration (Moses and Cheatham, 1963).

Scleroderma (systemic sclerosis) produces extensive fibrosis in the esophageal wall, beginning in the submucosa and eventually replacing much of the smooth muscle. The fibrous tissue is relatively poor in cells. The overlying epithelium becomes atrophic and readily ulcerates.

As noted earlier, herniation of portions of the stomach through the esophageal hiatus in the diaphragm (hiatus hernia) is commonly associated with esophageal disease. The "bell" type, which is most common, shows a symmetrically dilated portion of stomach above the diaphragm attached to what appears to be a shortened esophagus. The hiatus is not much enlarged. A paraesophageal type of hernia shows a sac of stomach protruding through a defect in the diaphragm beside an esophagus of normal length. An unusual type is seen in which a large part of the stomach extends into the thorax through a large orifice (esophagogastric type) (Hagarty, 1960; Robbins, 1967).

Achalasia

Dysphagia is the symptom of difficult or painful swallowing (Stembien and Dogradi, 1967). It may be produced by any obstruction of the esophagus. Extrinsic masses or enlarged organs may infringe on the lumen. Even exostoses of the spine may cause pressure on the esophagus (Facer, 1967; Perrone, 1967). An esophagus without grossly visible obstruction may fail to transmit food properly. This is achalasia (or cardiospasm) and seems to result from a failure of coordination of muscle contraction. It has been related to a defect in innervation characterized by abnormalities in the intrinsic nerve plexus (Rake, 1927). In long-standing cases, the esophagus dilates and elongates through most of its extent. Only at the distal end, the so-called vestibule of the stomach, may there be a persistent ringlike contraction. The lesion thus resembles congenital megacolon (megaesophagus) (Hurst and Rake, 1930; Ingelfinger and Kramer, 1953; Schatzki and Gary, 1953).

Absence of ganglion cells in the distal segment of the esophagus may occur in some cases, but this is not so constant a finding as in Hirschsprung's disease (Rake, 1927). More commonly, ganglion cells appear degenerate or reduced in numbers (Cassella et al., 1964). Changes in the vagus nerve and atrophy of muscle are described (Cassetta et al., 1964).

At the time of study, these esophagi frequently show marked fibrosis, chronic inflammatory cell infiltrates, and thickened or ulcerated mucosa. It is difficult to determine whether the nerve changes are primary or secondary. Uncomplicated cases are seldom examined, biopsies of deep muscle layers cannot be obtained easily in clinical cases, and the myenteric plexus does not have the orderly distribution between muscle layers which is seen in the colon.

In early stages of cardiospasm, there may be a psychogenic factor which may be reversible (Wolf and Almy, 1949). This may represent a disease different from true achalasia.

Tumors

By far the most common malignancy of the esophagus is carcinoma. It produces about 2 per cent of deaths due to carcinoma. All but a small fraction (2 to 3 per cent) are of squamous cell type (Boyd et al., 1958). The incidence of carcinoma of the esophagus is much higher in some parts of the world than in the United States. The highest incidence appears to be in India (Desai et al., 1969). Puerto Rico has an elevated incidence of 11 per cent of all cancer deaths (Martinez, 1964). It is the commonest malignant tumor of the Alaskan Eskimo (Hurst, 1964). Etiological factors in the environment, particularly in ingested food, appear to be very important (Wynder and Bross, 1961). Heavy drinking of alcohol elevates the incidence up to 25 times. It is not clear, however, whether hot or spicy food is a significant factor.

The incidence in males predominates in a ratio usually of about 5 to 1, and the great majority of tumors occur in the over-50 age group.

It is likely that invasive squamous cell carcinoma is preceded by malignant changes in the surface epithelium, in situ carcinoma, which are inapparent clinically. Their duration prior to invasion is probably short. It is often possible to find some superficial changes at the margins of invasive tumors, sometimes over wide areas. Rarely, the carcinoma is confined completely to the mucosa (Ushigomi et al., 1967). Nevertheless, exfoliative cytology has not proved to be very useful as a screening procedure. Quite accurate results have been produced with special efforts, however, in patients suspected of tumor (Prolla et al., 1965). Leukoplakia or keratinizing thickening of the epithelium may follow prolonged stasis and chronic inflammation, as in megaesophagus or in diverticula. Rarely a squamous cell carcinoma may appear at this site.

Carcinoma of the esophagus is rarely induced by radiation in man. It is almost unknown in experimental animals, but may be induced by gamma radiation in mice (Gates and Warren, 1968).

The sites of predilection suggest that stasis or slowing of the luminal contents may be a factor in pathogenesis. Hiatal hernial sacs, diverticula and megaesophagi have been said to increase incidence. None of these conditions can be said to be premalignant, however. Carcinoma at the site of previous lye stricture is known to occur. About 50 per cent of carcinomas are in the lower third, and about 33 per cent are in the middle third, with the smallest number in the proximal third.

Initially the gross lesion is a smooth plaque which readily ulcerates and spreads both longitudinally and circumferentially. Although most lesions completely encircle the esophagus at the time of treatment, it is common to find a preserved band of normal mucosa extending longitudinally across the tumor, even in late stages (Fig. 10). The lesion is most commonly an oval, heaped-up tumor with central ulceration.

The malignant epithelium invades the submucosa and is exposed to lymphatic channels early in the course. These may carry the cells longitudinally or into deeper layers. Intramural spread is demonstrated in at least half the cases (Burgess et al., 1951).

The esophagus does not have a serosa, and there is no barrier to direct extension of the carcinoma into the contiguous structures. A fistula tract into trachea or bronchi or vessel may develop (Laubscher, 1970). Ordinarily the only symptom is a disturbance of swallowing which is gradual in progress. Complete obstruction is a very late event.

Lesions in the lower third and some in the midportion may spread to lymph nodes in the abdomen as well as to the mediastinum. A metastasis may be more prominent than the primary lesion (Talerman and WooMing, 1968). Those in the upper portion are more likely to spread into the neck; those in the upper third are said to be more likely to be confined to the wall, but this fact may be the result of earlier discovery of these lesions (Burgess et al., 1951). Because symptoms are late and spread is early, treatment has been largely ineffective (Boyd et al., 1954; Kay, 1963).

If one considers only the carcinomas occurring in women, about 56 per cent are in the upper third (Burgess et al., 1951). This may represent the effect of cases of Plummer-Vinson syndrome. The average age is about three years younger in women than in men (54 vs. 57 years). Carcinoma of the esophagus appears to be much more common in the Alaskan Eskimo women than in the men (Hurst, 1964).

Adenocarcinomas may arise in the esophagus proper. These could develop from esophageal or cardiac-type glands without involving the possibility of an origin from ectopic glandular mucosa. Most of these are in the lower third. An interval of normal esophagus must be demonstrated between the tumor and the stomach to allow these to be distinguished from adenocarcinomas arising in the cardia of the stomach, which are overwhelmingly more common. Probably not more than 3 per cent of

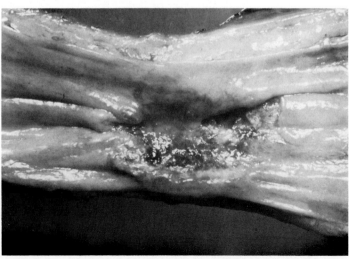

Figure 10. Squamous cell carcinoma of the esophagus in a man of 94. It measured 2.5 cm. in length and was not completely annular.

carcinomas of the esophagus are glandular. The prognosis does not appear to be any better than that for squamous cell carcinoma (Block and Lancaster; 1964; Boyd et al., 1958; Goldfarb, 1967; Turnbull and Goodner, 1968).

Several variants of squamous cell carcinoma occur. It may be verrucous, relatively well differentiated, and slow-growing (Minielly et al., 1967). Rarely, the malignant epithelium may be confined to the surface (Ushigomi et al., 1967). A special form is polypoid. This may produce a sarcomalike cellular structure which is recognized as squamous cell carcinoma only upon intensive study and in certain areas (Fraser and Kinley, 1968; Lane, 1957; Lichtiger et al., 1970; Scarpa, 1966; Stout et al., 1949). These latter (pseudosarcomas) appear to have a much better prognosis and appear to correspond somewhat to spindle-celled carcinomas of skin (Underwood et al., 1951).

Paget's change in the mucosa of the esophagus has been reported in the presence of squamous cell carcinoma (Yates and Koss, 1968).

Adenoid cystic carcinoma (cylindroma) (Marcial-Rojas and Vallecillo, 1959) is known as well as mucoepidermoid carcinoma (Kay, 1968; Weitzner, 1970). Both probably arise from esophageal mucous glands. Metastatic carcinoma, particularly from the breast, may manifest itself through dysphagia. (Polk et al., 1967; Toreson, 1944). Primary melanoma arises from melanocytes in esophageal mucosa. Junctional changes must be demonstrated to prove the primary nature of the tumor (Boyd et al., 1954). A case has been reported in a child (Basque et al., 1970).

Nearly all benign intramural tumors of the esophagus are leiomyomas derived from the muscle coats (Schmidt et al., 1961). Most occur in the mid or lower third. Palisading of nuclei is not so common as elsewhere, and some of these tumors are interpreted as neurofibromas or fibromas (Stout and Lattes, 1957). There are a few nodular deposits of fat interpreted as lipomas. Small cartilaginous masses in the upper esophagus appear to be malformations derived from the primitive foregut, although osteochondromas are reported (Mahour and Harrison, 1967). Solitary fibromas, neurilemmomas, adenomas, and angiomas are rarities and poorly documented. These tumors do not become deeply ulcerated.

A fibrovascular polyp, sometimes on a spectacularly long stalk, occurs in the upper third and is generally attached at the level of the cricoid cartilage (Moersch and Harrington, 1944). Granular cell myoblastoma has been

reported. Inflammatory lesions may show papillary hyperplasia of overlying epithelium, but a true papilloma of the esophagus does not seem to occur in man. A mass of primary amyloidosis may appear as a tumor (Heitzman et al., 1962).

THE TRACHEA AND BRONCHI

Histology

The trachea lies below the cricoid cartilage and is held rigidly open by a series of C-shaped cartilages in the wall. Their defects are bridged by transverse smooth-muscle bundles posteriorly. They have a sheath of dense collagenous and elastic tissue forming a continuous flexible elastic tube. To this the mucosa is attached by a loose fibrous submucosa. The trachea is lined by ciliated pseudostratified columnar epithelium, characteristic of the respiratory tract. Surface cells, intermediate cells, and basilar germinal cells can be distinguished. The basement lamina is prominent and measures about 5μ (Spencer, 1968). The epithelium shows many goblet cells. Beneath the epithelium is a lamina propria containing numerous elastic fibers. They tend to form a longitudinal sheet. Small mixed tubulo-acinous glands are generally beneath the elastic layer. Posteriorly they may be in the muscle. There may be small lymphatic foci in the lamina propria. Lymphatic channels begin in the lamina propria and extend through larger channels in the submucosa to the nodes outside the wall. The trachea is joined to surrounding structures by loose areolar tissue without a serosa. With age the tracheal cartilages do not tend to ossify, as do those of the larynx.

The bronchial structure undergoes progressive changes as the bronchi divide and become smaller. The major bronchi to right and left lungs continue the structure of the trachea. Just at the carina, the epithelium may be stratified and the surface cells may even be squamous in type. At the entrance to the lungs, the main stem bronchi divide into primary bronchi for each lobe. Cartilaginous plates of irregular shape rather than rings surround the entire circumference of the walls of these bronchi. Muscle becomes more prominent and completely surrounds the bronchus. As the bronchi continue to divide, the cartilages become smaller and, in bronchi of 1 mm. diameter, they completely disappear. These are secondary or segmental bronchi. Longitudinal folds of the submucosa and mucosa are produced by contraction of circular muscle fibers. The layer of smooth muscle under the mucosa is formed of interlacing oblique and circular elastic and muscle fibers which do not form a distinct circular layer. In smaller bronchi the fibers are farther apart but continue through the respiratory bronchioles.

The mucosa of the major bronchi continues to the respiratory bronchioles. Mucous and mixed glands are present in the submucosa, usually deep to the muscle layer, as far as the cartilages extend into smaller branches. Lymphatic aggregates are present in somewhat greater numbers than in the trachea in the lamina propria. Follicles may be present, especially near bifurcations.

The outer layers of the bronchial wall are formed of dense collagenous tissue with many elastic fibers. This surrounds the cartilage plates and extends into surrounding structures of the lung. There may be some lymphatic nodules. Many small blood vessels extend into the muscle layer and through it into the lamina propria.

With loss of the cartilage and glands, the wall of the bronchus becomes thinner and appears to be composed of a single fibromuscular layer lined by mucosa. Respiratory bronchioles are those which first show a few branching alveoli, which start at about 0.5 mm. diameter.

The respiratory bronchioles are lined with ciliated columnar epithelium without goblet cells. The epithelium becomes more cuboidal and eventually loses its cilia. Bundles of smooth muscle fibers persist into alveolar ducts. The cuboidal epithelium may continue into the alveolar duct wall.

Alveolar ducts, numbering from two to eleven, branch from each of the respiratory bronchioles. These are surrounded by openings into the alveoli or alveolar sacs. The duct wall between the relatively large openings is surrounded by elastic and collagenous fibers and occasional smooth muscle cells. Alveolar sacs may include two to four alveoli.

An understanding of the structure of pulmonary alveoli is necessary for comprehension of the respiratory process. The alveolus is a thin-walled sac, with an opening replacing one side. The wall is a dense plexus of capillaries in a network of reticular and elastic fibers. The capillaries bulge into the alveoli and are larger than the spaces between them. Adjacent alveoli have common walls. Connecting pores of 7 to 9 μ in diameter have been found between adjacent alveoli. The mouths of alveolar sacs

are surrounded by collagenous rather than just reticulin fibers.

There is a thin, continuous cellular lining of alveoli, almost impossible to visualize by light microscopy (Low, 1953). It is separated from the capillary endothelium by a continuous basement lamina. Cell bodies of these greatly flattened epithelial cells can rarely be found. Somewhat larger rounded septal cells (great alveolar cells) may bulge into the lumen (Karrer, 1956). They appear to be epithelial but may have some secretory activity. Phagocytes found in the lumen may migrate from vessels (Bloom and Fawcett, 1968; Low and Sampaio, 1957).

Lymphatic channels do not appear beyond alveolar ducts. Those in bronchi drain toward the hilus, while a separate network of channels drains the pleura.

Pathology

Congenital Abnormalities

Congenital abnormalities of the trachea frequently also involve the esophagus and these are discussed in the section entitled "The Esophagus." A diffuse enlargement of trachea and bronchi is rare and appears to be congenital (Zizmor et al., 1965). Bronchogenic cysts of the mediastinum appear to represent parts of the primitive foregut. They may be left behind in close relation to trachea, carina, main bronchus, or esophagus. Cartilage and glands identify it as bronchial or tracheal (Eraklis et al., 1969; Lumpkin, 1966).

Stenosis of the trachea may occur without esophageal fistula. The most common form is a funnel-shaped constriction just above the bifurcation (Sardana, 1966). Webs of mucosa, or vascular rings, may constrict. Softening or disappearance of cartilage may lead to collapse; this may be secondary (Zarocostas, 1966).

Anomalies of development of the bronchopulmonary segment of the foregut may lead to segments of lung which do not connect with the normal bronchial tree (pulmonary sequestration). These may be intralobar (Borrie et al., 1963) extralobar, or may even communicate with the gut (Gerle et al., 1968). Cystic changes within the lung may be of congenital bronchial origin (Belanger et al., 1964; Moffat, 1960; and Tyson, 1947). In the adult, congenital cysts are difficult to differentiate from cystic bronchiectasis or chronic pulmonary abscess with re-epithelialization (Robbins, 1967).

If no carbon pigment is present in the wall, it may be regarded as congenital and it has never been part of the functioning lung. Cysts of the lung may be associated with those of kidney, liver, and pancreas.

Trauma

Trauma to the trachea may result in suffocation at once or in the later development of a stenosis at the site of fractured and dislocated cartilages (Novick, 1967). Foreign bodies are a common cause of bronchial obstruction, usually in young children. Often the aspiration is not perceived and the object is found after pulmonary symptoms have developed (Levine, 1969). The foreign body may be of intrinsic origin (broncholithiasis) (Schmidt et al., 1950). Stenosis may develop at tracheostomy sites.

Inflammatory Processes

Tracheitis probably occurs frequently in connection with pharyngitis and laryngitis but is overlooked. Tracheitis is prominent in acute laryngotracheobronchitis, and the trachea may be the site of pseudomembranous inflammation in diphtheria and streptococcal infection. When subjected to the airstream by a tracheostomy, there may be chronic inflammatory changes in the mucosa, with hypertrophy and squamous metaplasia of the epithelium.

Chronic bronchitis is seldom diagnosed as an entity in the United States but is more fre-quently recognized in Britain (Fletcher, 1959; Garston, 1961). Hyperplasia of mucosa with hypertrophy of mucous glands is described. Unaccompanied by emphysema it may lead to serious disability or death, (Hentel et al., 1963), although hyperplasia and emphysema are commonly related (Bates, 1968; Reid, 1959).

Acute bronchitis is a common sequel to upper respiratory infection. Presumably the inflammatory changes are similar to those of the upper tract. Only if pulmonary parenchyma is affected (bronchopneumonia) are there x-ray changes.

Pulmonary tuberculosis regularly involves small bronchi, and necrosis and cavitation may involve larger ones. Sarcoidosis lesions are found in the walls of major bronchi as epithelioid non-necrotizing granulomas, generally in the lamina propria (Figs. 11 and 12). They are usually not grossly visible. Some cases are closely related to infection with *Mycobacterium tuberculosis* (Gregorie et al., 1962; Haroutuman et al., 1964; Scadding, 1960).

Fungi may invade the bronchial tree in unusual conditions. *Candida albicans* (monilia) may form focal granulomatous lesions in the lung. They and other fungi are often, however, only secondary invaders. *Histoplasma capsulatum* may invade the bronchial tree primarily. Blastomycosis, coccidioidomycosis, and, more rarely, cryptococcosis may produce pulmonary lesions nearly identical to those of tuberculosis. Actinomycosis and nocardiosis may arise from aspirated organisms. They produce a more suppurative inflammatory reaction, as does mucormycosis (Robbins, 1967). Pulmonary

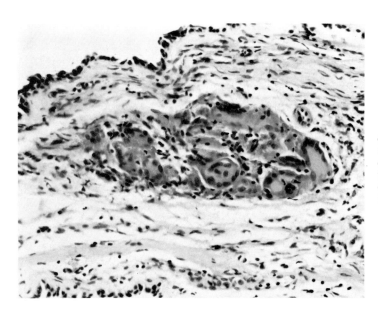

Figure 11. Photomicrograph of bronchial mucosa and submucosa containing a small granuloma thought to represent sarcoidosis in a man 30 years old. Tissue obtained by bronchoscopy. The granuloma contains several multinucleated giant cells. (Hematoxylin and eosin, × 250.)

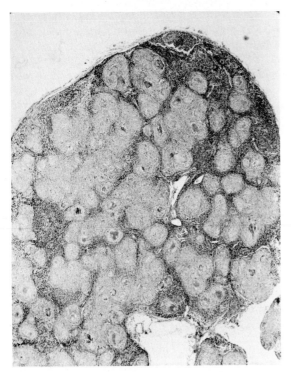

Figure 12. Photomicrograph of mediastinal lymph node containing numerous granulomas consistent with sarcoidosis, taken from a man of 28. Tissue obtained by mediastinoscopy. Some of the granulomas are becoming confluent. (Hematoxylin and eosin, × 25.)

sporotrichosis apparently is caused by aspiration of organisms (Baum et al., 1969).

A granulomatous disease of small bronchi and peribronchial tissues is caused by thermophilic actinomycetes and is known as farmer's lung (Wenzel et al., 1968). "Silo-filler's disease" is a necrotizing bronchiolitis related to exposure to fumes of nitric oxide.

Herpesvirus may cause lesions in the trachea and bronchi which demonstrate eosinophilic inclusions (Herout et al., 1966). Adenovirus also is known to cause necrotizing bronchial lesions (Wigger and Blanc, 1966). Cytomegalic inclusion disease of bronchi is seen in debilitated infants and adults (Fetterman et al., 1968).

Primary pulmonary (alveolar) disease inevitably involves at least smaller bronchi. Bronchial exudate or washings may reveal organisms in *Pneumocystis carinii* pneumonitis, or hyaline bodies in pulmonary alveolar proteinosis (Rosen et al., 1959).

Bronchiectasis is an abnormal enlargement and dilatation of bronchi and is always associated with a degree of chronic infection (Robbins, 1967). It may be produced by prolonged

bronchial stenosis (Ventura and Domaradski, 1967). Relief of the stenosis may reverse the changes if inflammation has not supervened (Drapanas et al., 1966). Atelectasis may also play a role (Anspach, 1934; Field, 1949; Mallory, 1947; Ogilvie, 1941). The bronchial wall becomes thickened and surrounded by increased amounts of collagenous tissue; it can no longer contract. The wall shows a diffuse infiltration of lymphocytes and plasma cells. Variable numbers of polymorphonuclear leukocytes are present, and the surrounding lung shows compression and evidence of chronic pneumonitis. Usually major bronchi are spared, except for apparently congenital varieties, but they may show chronic bronchitis.

Bronchiectasis is a common complication of mucoviscidosis (cystic fibrosis). Viscous mucous secretions of submucosal glands apparently lead to partial or complete obstruction of small bronchi, with secondary infection. Squamous metaplasia of bronchial epithelium is seen but it appears more likely to represent a secondary change rather than a primary cause of the bronchial disease. It has been related to vitamin-A deficiency owing to a lack of pancreatic enzymes (Robbins, 1967). Sinusitis is often associated with bronchiectasis. It is still not clear which of the two represents the earlier process.

Bronchial asthma is characterized by spasm of small bronchi and bronchioles frequently related to an allergic stimulus. The bronchi show plugs of mucous secretion and protein transudate. There is commonly edema of the mucosa and some hypertrophy of glands. An inflammatory infiltrate of lymphocytes, plasma cells, and eosinophilic leukocytes is seen. Hypertrophy of muscle is described, but thickening of the basement lamina of the mucosa is more striking (McCarter and Vazquez, 1966). Ciliary action appears to be inhibited (Dunnill, 1960). At autopsy secondary changes of the lung generally overshadow the primary asthmatic alterations (Cardell and Pearson, 1959; Gottlieb, 1964).

Emphysema is a disease of pulmonary overinflation, with enlargement of air spaces and tissue destruction (Robbins, 1967). It involves only the respiratory bronchioles (centrilobular) or all elements of the lobule distal to this (panlobular) (Thurlbeck, 1963). Larger bronchi are not affected. Eventual loss of respiratory capacity is caused by poor vascularization of thin-walled air spaces. Pathogenesis has been believed to be related to structural failure of the connective tissues of the lung (Ebert and

Pierce, 1963). Recent work shows a deficiency in alpha-1 antitrypsin, which is thought to allow destruction of elastin by proteases (Pierce et al., 1969). This deficiency is hereditary and explains familial incidence of some panlobular emphysema (Lieberman, 1969; Pierce et al., 1969; Talamo et al., 1966; Talbott, 1969).

Tumors

Tumors of the trachea are uncommon in relation to the size of the organ. About half are malignant (Miglets, 1965). Primary carcinoma is usually of squamous cell type (Hajdu et al., 1970). It amounts to less than 0.1 per cent of all malignancies. Incidence in males predominates five to one, and most patients are in the fourth to sixth decade. The prognosis is grave because of ease of spread and lateness of discovery; less than 25 per cent survive one year. Adenoid cystic carcinoma is even less common but shows its usual slower course (Markel et al., 1964; Zunker et al., 1969). Rare tumors arise from mucous glands, connective tissue, and cartilages (Ellman and Whittaker, 1947; Kay and Brooks, 1970).

Papillomas in the trachea and bronchi are associated with papillomatosis of the larynx and appear to represent multicentric origin (Buffmire et al., 1950). Most occur in children and eventually regress. Adult cases are more protracted, often solitary, and may involve a risk of malignancy (Al-Saleem et al., 1968; Kaufman and Klopstock, 1963; Laubscher, 1969). Rare papillary tumors show malignant cellular characteristics and spread extensively within the lumen but do not invade the wall (Smith and Dexter, 1963).

Primary chondroma or chondrosarcoma expands into the tracheal lumen (Daniels et al., 1967). More are seen in smaller bronchi. Fibrosarcoma has been described in the bronchus (Black, 1950). Malignant melanoma may arise in the tracheobronchial tree but is far more likely to be metastatic, even if a primary is unknown. Junctional changes must be demonstrated (Reid and Mehta, 1966). So-called granular cell myoblastomas are seen in the wall of trachea or bronchi. They may be multiple (Archer et al., 1963; Kramer, 1939; Rojer, 1965). Amyloid deposits in the mucosa may form a tumorlike mass (Duke, 1959; Karnberg et al., 1962).

Carcinoma arising in bronchial epithelium is one of the most common malignancies. Most are squamous cell carcinomas, and it is generally presumed that squamous metaplasia precedes the malignant change (Spain et al., 1970). This does not mean that squamous metaplasia is premalignant in character. It is not clear that superficial malignant change precedes invasive carcinoma by any appreciable period of time. However, atypical changes in the bronchial epithelium are more common in carcinomatous lungs and in smokers (Auerbach et al., 1962; Auerbach, Hammond et al., 1967). Multiple carcinomas occur clinically, but in only about 3 per cent of cases (Auerbach, Stout et al., 1967; Winter, 1966). Chromosomal abnormalities are reported (Falor et al., 1969). Squamous cell carcinomas are thought to occur more often in the larger central bronchi because of more frequent squamous metaplasia in this area (Ashley and Davies, 1967). The squamous cell carcinomas of the bronchus are more often poorly than well differentiated. They tend to encircle the bronchus, invade lung parenchyma and vessels directly, and spread readily to lymph nodes. Obstruction of the bronchus by exophytic growth leads to pulmonary symptoms. Although centrally located tumors are more accessible to diagnosis and may produce symptoms earlier, those located at the periphery have a better prognosis (Kern et al., 1968).

Classification of lung tumors is dependent upon interpretation of sometimes minor histological features and the criteria of individual pathologists; therefore, the percentages of tumors placed in various categories is quite variable in different centers. A standard classification has been published by the World Health Organization. It appears worthwhile to classify tumors as precisely as possible according to cell of origin, leaving the smallest number possible undifferentiated or unclassified.

Adenocarcinomas account for 11 to 28 per cent of primary lung tumors (Bennett et al., 1969; Guillan et al., 1967; Spencer, 1968). An association with smoking is reported (Guillan et al., 1967), although this factor is not generally considered so significant as in squamous cell tumors. Presumably these can arise directly from surface epithelium as well as from glands (Evans, 1966). The majority appear to be peripheral in origin. They frequently produce abundant mucin, but in poorly differentiated tumors a mucin stain may be necessary to detect it. There is a nearly equal sex incidence (Vincent et al., 1965). Peripheral adenocarcinomas must be carefully differentiated from metastatic carcinoma. Prognosis is no better than for squamous cell carcinoma (Bennett et al., 1969; Guillan et al., 1967). Degree of differentiation does not appear to be prognostic.

Undifferentiated carcinomas composed of small rounded or elongated hyperchromatic cells possessing very little cytoplasm have been called "oat cell" or small-celled carcinomas. They amount to about 10 per cent of bronchogenic carcinomas (Galofre et al., 1964; Kato et al., 1969). Some of these tumors show a transition into recognizable squamous cell carcinoma in some areas. They occur centrally in the lung and predominantly in men (19 to one). Probably they should be regarded as undifferentiated squamous cell carcinomas. A relationship to bronchial carcinoid tumor has been suggested, however (Bensch et al., 1968). The prognosis is grave, only asymptomatic patients being reported to survive five years (1.4 per cent) (Kato et al., 1969).

Terminal bronchiolar or "alveolar cell" carcinoma is a variant of adenocarcinoma which grows in a manner suggesting that the tumor cells line pre-existing alveoli (Fig. 13). This may be seen only at the growing edge, and the remainder of the tumor may be more irregularly glandular (Bennett and Sasser, 1969). It bears some resemblance to benign inflammatory lesions in which columnar epithelium comes to line immobilized alveoli (Decker, 1955). Probably it does not arise from a distinctive cell type. Most have a rapid malignant course (Watson and Farpour, 1966). It may be diffuse or multicentric in 30 per cent. Giant-cell carcinoma appears to represent poorly differentiated adenocarcinoma (Guillan and Zelman, 1966;

Herman et al., 1966); it has as poor a prognosis as the small-celled variety.

About half the adenocarcinomas appear to arise in pre-existing pulmonary scars (Bennett et al., 1969). The evidence for this is a focus of elastic and collagen fibers near the center of the tumor which shows abundant anthracotic pigment, trapped histiocytes, and cholesterol. Recognizable foreign-body reactions or tuberculous lesions are rarely found (Spencer, 1968). A few squamous cell carcinomas and small-celled tumors show a similar topography. It is known that metastatic tumor may also localize in a scar (Spencer, 1968). Many badly scarred lungs fail to show any evidence of malignant change, and the evidence for an etiological relationship is not complete.

A puzzling lesion is the tumorlet (Whitwell, 1955) of the peripheral lung (MacMahon et al., 1967). This is a small focus of dark cells resembling small-celled carcinoma or carcinoid in an area of scar or chronic inflammation. Rare metastases to local areas are reported, but there is no demonstrable relation to more common tumor types (Evans, 1966; Hausman and Weimann, 1967; Spencer, 1968). They must be distinguished from early carcinoma of peripheral lung (Berkheiser, 1966), from small carcinoid tumors (Spencer, 1968), and from pulmonary chemodectoma (Kohn et al., 1960). Rare, small clear-celled tumors also appear to be benign but of uncertain character (Liebow and Castleman, 1963). Rare carcinomas apparently of bronchial origin have been found to secrete gonadotropin (Cottrell, 1969) and parathormone (Turkington et al., 1966).

Cytological study of sputum is useful in

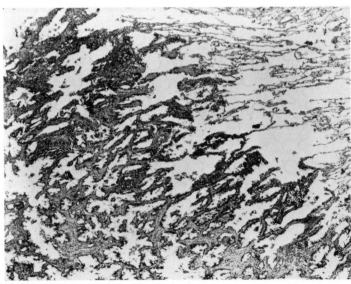

Figure 13. Photomicrograph of bronchiolar carcinoma of lung in a woman, 51. The advancing margin of the tumor appears to line pre-existing alveoli. It is forming more irregular glands in the left lower corner. (Hematoxylin and eosin, × 40.)

diagnosis of lung carcinoma, particularly those beyond reach of the bronchoscope (Koss et al., 1964; Melamed et al., 1963; Russell and Chang, 1967; Spjut et al., 1955). Induction of sputum or postbronchoscopy specimens may be necessary to demonstrate malignant cells (Fontana et al., 1962). Filter techniques may be an improvement (Russell and Chang, 1967).

Bronchial adenoma is the commonly accepted term for certain indolently malignant tumors apparently arising from bronchial glands (Fig. 14). Similar tumors are rarely found in the trachea. They have in common slow growth and late metastasis. Most often the lesion projects into one side of a major bronchus with an equal or larger growth within the wall or extending into adjacent lung. Only a few can be removed entirely by bronchoscope. They must be considered carcinomas but differ remarkably from other bronchogenic carcinomas and deserve a special category. The term "adenomatoid bronchial tumors" has been suggested (Weiss and Ingram, 1961).

The largest number are of carcinoid type and are composed of nests and small sheets of dark-staining cells, having little cytoplasm. They occasionally form small acinar structures. No connection with the overlying epithelium is seen, and this may be lifted up over the tumor. Invasion of peribronchial tissues is seen, although the tumor may remain within a fibrous capsule. About 10 per cent are found in bronchial nodes (Goodner et al., 1961; Markel et al., 1964). A relationship to argentaffinoma, as seen in the intestinal tract, is demonstrated by the presence of secretory granules in the cytoplasm (Toker, 1966). Serotonin production

has been demonstrated, and the carcinoid clinical syndrome can be produced by this tumor as well as by small-celled carcinoma (Fox, 1960; Frank and Lieberthal, 1963; Gowenlock et al., 1964; Williams and Azzopardi, 1960).

About 10 per cent of bronchial adenomas are of adenoid cystic (cylindroma) type (Soutter et al., 1954). These have the same structure as similar tumors throughout the respiratory tract. A fibrous stroma is infiltrated by columns and larger sheets of epithelial cells which contain rounded alveolar spaces, frequently containing mucoid material. These are the "cylinders" seen by Billroth. The epithelial cells are quite uniform, with little cytoplasm, and resemble basal cells of epidermis (McDonald, Moersch, and Tenney, 1945). They show an ability to infiltrate perineural spaces and metastasize more readily than carcinoid tumors.

A third type of bronchial adenoma is of mucoepidermoid type. This is much less common than either of the others. It is composed of epithelium frequently lining cystic spaces and exhibiting both mucus secretion and multilayered squamous-type patterns (Ozla et al., 1961).

In any of these tumors complete removal surgically is required for cure. Bronchial obstruction and suppuration may occur before metastasis (Payne et al., 1959). A "true" benign mucous gland adenoma occurs rarely in the bronchus (Kroe and Pitcock, 1967).

A hamartoma is a benign tumor composed of tissues normally present at the site but with an abnormal irregular arrangement. In the lung most hamartomas are primarily composed of

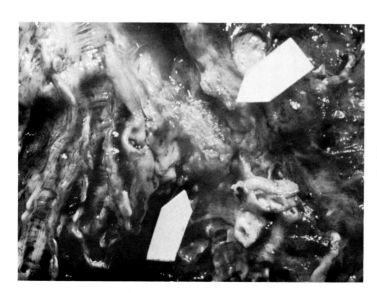

Figure 14. Bronchial adenoma of carcinoid type in the lateral basal bronchus of a 70 year old man. It projects into the bronchus as a polypoid mass 2 cm. in size.

masses of hyaline cartilage separated by fibrous tissue containing elongated ducts lined by columnar or respiratory epithelium. Some are endobronchial and may be mistaken for a chondroma of bronchial cartilage (Butler and Kleinerman, 1969; Hodges, 1958; McDonald, Harrington, and Claggett, 1945). The hamartoma may be composed of other tissues without cartilage (adenolipomyoma) (Karpas and Blackman, 1967). A lipoma of lung is rare (Plachta and Hershey, 1962).

Malignant lymphoma may appear as a primary lung tumor (Sternberg et al., 1959). Without involvement of lymph nodes or other organs, death is rare (Saltzstein, 1963), and most lymphoid masses in the lung are probably inflammatory pseudolymphomas. It is uncommon for generalized malignant lymphoma or leukemia to involve the lung (Green and Nichols, 1959; Robbins, 1953).

Plasmacytomas may apparently be primary in the lung (Romanoff and Milwidsky, 1962). Sarcoma arising in the connective tissue of the lung is uncommon (Agnos and Starkey, 1958). A true carcinosarcoma involving both epithelial and connective tissue elements has been described (Bergmann et al., 1951). However, these may be spindle-celled carcinomas similar to those in the esophagus and the larynx. A similar unusual tumor resembling fetal lung has been described in adults (pulmonary blastoma). It may be multicentric (Bauermeister et al., 1966; Minken, 1968) but appears to have a good prognosis.

Obscure granulomatous masses in the lung with some allergic manifestations may involve bronchi (Titus et al., 1962). Eosinophils may be prominent (eosinophilic granuloma) (Anderson and Forraker, 1959; Beckers et al., 1962). Histiocytomas (sclerosing angioma) are found in the lung (Liebow and Hubbell, 1956).

REFERENCES

Pharynx

Ackerman, L. V., and Del Regato, J. A.: Cancer. Diagnosis treatment and prognosis. 3rd ed. St. Louis, The C. V. Mosby Co., 1962, pp. 357–385.

Ahlborn, H. E.: Simple achlorhydric anemia, Plummer-Vinson syndrome, and cancer of the mouth, pharynx and esophagus. Brit. Med. J. 2:331–333, 1936.

Ahned, S.: Cylindroma of epiglottis. Arch. Otolaryng. 63:366–371, 1956.

Apostal, J. V., and Frazell, E. L.: Juvenile nasopharyngeal angiofibroma. Cancer 18:869–878, 1965.

Ash, J. E.: Organs of special senses. In Anderson, W. A. D.: Pathology. 5th ed. St. Louis, The C. V. Mosby Co., 1966, pp. 771–774.

Ash, J. E., and Raum, M.: An Atlas of Otolaryngic Pathol-

ogy. Amer. Acad. Ophthal. Otolaryng., Washington, D. C., A.F.I.P., 1956, pp. 212–215.

Ballantyne, A. J.: Principles of surgical management of cancer of the pharyngeal walls. Cancer 20:663–667, 1967.

Balogh, K., and Caulfield, J. B.: Ultrastructure and histochemistry of juvenile nasopharyngeal angiofibroma. Amer. J. Path. 50:22a, 1967.

Bauer, W. H., and Kuzma, J. F.: Solitary tumors of atypical amyloid (paramyloid). Amer. J. Clin. Path. 19:1097–1112, 1949.

Blair, O. M., and Sanchez, J. E.: Teratoid tumor of tonsil. Arch. Otolaryng. 89:745–747, 1969.

Boies, L. R. A., and Harris, D.: Nasopharyngeal dermoid of newborn. Laryngoscope 75:763–767, 1965.

Borella, L.: Reticulum cell sarcoma in children. Cancer 17:26–31, 1964.

Bosma, J. F., Graykowski, E. A., and Trygstad, C. W.: Chronic ulcerative pharyngitis. Arch. Otolaryng. 87:85–96, 1968.

Brown, P. M., and Devine, K. D.: Cancer of the pyriform sinuses. Arch. Otolaryng. 72:192–193, 1960.

Cappell, D. F.: On lymphoepithelioma of nasopharynx and tonsils. J. Path. Bact. 39:49–64, 1934.

Cappell, D. F.: Pathology of nasopharyngeal tumors. J. Laryng. 53:558–580, 1938.

Castleman, B., and McNeely, B. V.: Malignant lymphoma, lymphocytic type of nasopharynx and peripheral nodes (12 yr. duration) (case report). New Eng. J. Med. 279:33–41, 1968.

Cocke, E. W.: Cavernous hemangioma of the oral and hypopharynges. Amer. J. Surg. 102:798–802, 1961.

Coleman, F. B.: Post cricoid carcinoma following Paterson-Plummer-Vinson syndrome in a man. Guy Hosp. Rep. 106:75–79, 1957.

Cunningham, M. P., and Catlin, D.: Carcinoma of pharyngeal wall. Cancer 20:1859–1866, 1967.

Daly, J. F., and Friedman, M.: Carcinoma of the tonsil. Laryngoscope 70:595–615, 1960.

Davidson, M.: Abscesses of the retropharyngeal spaces in adults. Laryngoscope 59:1146–1170, 1949.

Dolin, S., and Dewar, J. P.: Extramedullary plasmacytoma. Amer. J. Path. 32:83–103, 1956.

Dutz, W., and Stout, A. P.: The myxoma in childhood. Cancer 14:629–635, 1961.

Epstein, S. S., Payne, P. M., and Shaw, H. J.: Multiple primary malignant neoplasms in the air and upper food passages. Cancer 13:137–145, 1960.

Evans, R. W.: Histological appearances of tumors. 2nd ed. Baltimore, The Williams & Wilkins Co., 1966.

Figi, F. A.: Solitary neurofibroma of pharynx. Arch. Otolaryng. 17:386–389, 1933.

Frenckner, P.: The occurrence of so-called myoblastomas in mouth and upper air passages. Acta Otolaryng. 26:689–701, 1938.

Friend, L. J.: Fibroadenolipoma of the tonsil. Arch. Otolaryng. 3:448–451, 1926.

Fuller, A. M., Van Vliet, P. D., Lillie, J. C., and Devine, K. D.: Pharyngeal leiomyosarcoma with fever of unknown origin. Arch. Otolaryng. 84:96–98, 1966.

Ghossein, N. A., and Najjar, M. Y.: Hodgkin's disease of the nasopharynx. Laryngoscope 77:247–251, 1967.

Girdany, B. R., Sieber, W. K., and Osman, M. Z.: Traumatic pseudodiverticulum of pharynx in newborn infants. New Eng. J. Med. 280:237–240, 1969.

Glyn-Jones, D.: Case of lipoma of pharynx. J. Laryng. 66:288–289, 1952.

Goldman, R. L.: Melanogenic papillary cystadenoma of soft palate. Amer. J. Clin. Path. 48:49–52, 1967.

Gross, L.: Incidence of appendectomies and tonsillectomies in cancer patients. Cancer 19:849–852, 1966.

Guggenheim, P.: Schwannoma of pharynx: Report of a case and review of the literature. Int. Coll. Surg. J. *19*:450–474, 1953.

Hamilton, J. E., and Oppenheim, H.: Carcinoma of extrinsic larynx – emphasizing metastatic disease. Amer. J. Surg. *90*:924–930, 1955.

Harma, R.: Nasopharyngeal angiofibroma. Acta Otolaryng. supplement 146, (Stockholm) 1958, pp. 1–74.

Harper, A. R.: Lipomata of upper air and food passages. J. Laryng. *73*:419–423, 1959.

Havens, F. Z., and Butler, L. C.: Mixed tumors of posterior pharyngeal wall. Ann. Otol. *64*:457–465, 1955.

Hill, H. R., Zimmerman, R. A., Reid, G. V., Wilson, E., and Kilton, R. M.: Food borne epidemic of streptococcal pharyngitis. New Eng. J. Med. *280*:917–921, 1969.

Holden, H., and Howard, N.: Bilateral lymphoepithelioma of tonsils. Arch. Otolaryng. *84*:433–435, 1966.

Hormia, M., and Koskinen, O.: Metastasizing nasopharyngeal angiofibroma. Arch. Otolaryng. *89*:523–526, 1969.

Huber, G. C.: On the relation of chorda dorsalis to the anlage of the pharyngeal bursa or median pharyngeal recess. Anat. Rec. *6*:373–404, 1912.

Iliades, C. E., and Watson, F.: Neurilemmoma of the pharynx. Laryngoscope *77*:1–7, 1967.

Jernstrom, P.: Synovial sarcoma of pharynx. Amer. J. Clin. Path. *24*:957–961, 1954.

Johanson, W. G., Pierce, A. K., and Sanford, J. P.: Changing pharyngeal bacterial flora of hospitalized patients. New Eng. J. Med. *281*:1137–1140, 1969.

Johnson, F.: Lymphosarcoma of tonsil. Laryngoscope *70*:846–852, 1960.

Johnson, W. S., Beahros, O. H., and Harrison, E. G.: Chemodectoma of glomus intravagale. Amer. J. Surg. *104*:812–820, 1962.

Jones, R. F. M.: Paterson-Brown Kelly syndrome (post cricoid carcinoma). J. Laryng. *75*:529–543, 1961.

Jordan, L. W.: Unusual tumors of tonsil area. Laryngoscope *68*:1044–1056, 1958.

Kaplan, G., Rubenfeld, S., and Gordon, R. B.: Unusual manifestations of carcinoma of the nasopharynx. Cancer *24*:781–785, 1969.

Keith, A.: Constrictions and occlusions of the alimentary tract of congenital or obscure origin. Brit. Med. J. *1*:301–305, 1910.

Kelemen, G.: The palatine tonsil in the 6th decade. Ann. Otol. *52*:419–443, 1943.

Keller, A. Z.: Cirrhosis, alcoholism and heavy smoking, associated with cancer of the mouth and pharynx. Cancer *20*:1015–1022, 1967.

Kerr, D. A.: Granuloma pyogenicum. Oral Surg. *4*:158–176, 1951.

Kragh, L. V., Soule, E. H., and Masson, J. K.: Benign and malignant neurilemmomas of head and neck. Surg. Gynec. Obstet. *111*:211–218, 1960.

Kramer, R., and Som, M. L.: Cylindroma of upper air passages. Arch. Otolaryng. *29*:356–370, 1939.

Kyle, R. A., and Bayrd, E. D.: Primary systemic amyloidosis and myeloma – 81 cases. Arch. Intern. Med. *107*:344–353, 1961.

Lahey, F. H.: Pharyngoesophageal diverticulum: Its management and complications. Ann. Surg. *124*:617–652, 1946.

Laskiewicz, A.: Pedunculated fibrolipomas of the pharynx. EENT Monthly *41*:369–373, 1962.

Lehmann, W. B., Pope, T. H., and Hudson, W. R.: Nasopharyngeal stenosis. Laryngoscope *78*:371–385, 1968.

Levy, A. M., Tabakin, B. S., Hanson, J. S., and Narkewicz, R. M.: Hypertrophied adenoids causing pulmonary hypertension and severe congestive heart failure. New Eng. J. Med. *277*:506–511, 1967.

Liberson, M., and Riese, K. T.: Carcinoma in a large pharyngoesophageal diverticulum. Gastroenterology *38*:817–820, 1960.

Lin, H. S., Lin, C., Yeh, S., and Tu, S.: Fine structure of nasopharyngeal carcinoma with special reference to anaplastic type. Cancer *23*:390–405, 1969.

Lucas, G. J., and Lehrnbecker, W.: Hydroxyurea in nasopharyngeal cancer. J.A.M.A. *210*:2397, 1969.

Marchetta, F. C., Sako, K., and Camp, F.: Multiple malignancies in patients with head and neck carcinoma. Amer. J. Surg. *110*:537–541, 1965.

Martens, V. E.: Unusual synovial tumors. J.A.M.A. *157*:888–890, 1955.

Martin, H. E.: Cancer of the head and neck in children. *In* Dargeon, H. W. (ed.): Cancer in childhood and a discussion of certain benign tumors. St. Louis, The C. V. Mosby Co., 1940, pp. 67–75.

Martin, H., and Quan, S.: Racial incidence of nasopharyngeal cancer. Ann. Otol. *60*:168–174, 1951.

Martin, H., Ehrlich, H. E., and Ahels, J. C.: Juvenile nasopharyngeal angiofibroma. Ann. Surg. *127*:513–536, 1948.

Martin, H., and Sugarbaker, E. L.: Cancer of the tonsil. Amer. J. Surg. *52*:158–196, 1941.

Matz, G. J., and Conner, G. H.: Nasopharyngeal cancer. Laryngoscope *78*:1763–1767, 1968.

McCall, J. W., Whitaker, C. W., and Karam, F. K.: Carcinoma of the epiglottis. Laryngoscope *67*:679–690, 1957.

McGraw, R. W., and McKenzie, A. D.: Carcinoma of the thyroid and laryngopharynx following irradiation. Cancer *18*:692–696, 1965.

Moore, E. S., and Martin, H.: Melanoma of upper respiratory tract and oral cavity. Cancer *8*:1167–1176, 1955.

New, G. B.: Xanthoma of pharynx and larynx. Arch. Otolaryng. *22*:449–453, 1935.

Oberman, H. A., and Sullenger, G.: Neurogenous tumors of head (pharynx) and neck. Cancer *20*:1992–2001, 1967.

Osborn, D. A., and Sokolovski, A.: Juvenile nasopharyngeal angiofibromas in a female. Arch. Otolaryng. *82*:629–632, 1965.

Pang, L. Q.: Carcinoma of the nasopharynx. Arch. Otolaryng. *82*:622–628, 1965.

Papavasiliou, C. G.: Intrathoracic spread of nasopharyngeal carcinoma. Cancer *21*:940–944, 1968.

Parkhill, E. M.: Tumors of the palatine tonsil. AFIP Fascicle 10b, Section IV. Tumors of the oral cavity and pharynx. Nat. Acad. Sci., Washington, 1968, pp. 243–270.

Patterson, C. N.: Juvenile nasopharyngeal angiofibroma. Arch. Otolaryng. *81*:27–277, 1965.

Paymaster, J. C.: Some observations on oral and pharyngeal carcinoma in the state of Bombay. Cancer *15*:578–583, 1962.

Paymaster, J. C.: Cancer and its distribution in India. Cancer *17*:1026–1034, 1964.

Perez, C. A., Ackerman, L. V., Neill, W. B., Ogura, J. H., and Powers, W. E.: Cancer of the nasopharynx. Factors influencing prognosis. Cancer *24*:1–17, 1969.

Petersen, H.: A rare cyst of the pharynx. Acta Otolaryng. *54*:154–158, 1962.

Pierce, W. S., and Johnson, J.: Squamous cell carcinoma arising in a pharyngoesophageal diverticulum. Cancer *24*:1068, 1969.

Prior, J. T., and Stoner, L. R.: Sarcoma botryoides of the nasopharynx. Cancer *10*:957–963, 1957.

Raven, R. W.: Cancer of the hypopharynx and its surgical treatment. Brit. Med. J. *1*:951–953, 1952.

Rodriguez, H.: A new surgical approach to nasopharyngeal angiofibroma. Cancer *19*:458–460, 1966.

Rominger, C. J., and Santore, F. J.: Juvenile nasopharyngeal fibroma in female adults. Arch. Otolaryng. 88:177-179, 1968.

Rosenberg, M. M.: Dermoid cyst of tonsil. Arch. Otolaryng. 22:631-633, 1935.

Rubenfeld, S., Kaplan, G., and Holder, A. A.: Distant metastases from head and neck cancer. Amer. J. Roentgen. 87:441-448, 1962.

Sanford, D. M., and Becker, G. D.: Tuberculosis of the tonsil. Arch. Otolaryng. 84:343-345, 1966.

Sasaki, C. T.: Lung metastases by lymphatic spread from nasopharynx. Arch. Otolaryng. 87:396-399, 1968.

Scanlon, P. W., Gee, V. R., Erich, J. B., Wethaus, H. L., and Woolner, L. B.: Carcinoma of the palatine tonsil. Amer. J. Roentgen. 80:781-786, 1958.

Schermer, K. L., Pontius, E. E., Dziabis, M. D., and McQuiston, R. J.: Glomus jugulare and glomus tympanicum tumors. Cancer 19:1273-1286, 1966.

Schindel, J., and Markowicz, H.: Chordoma arising from ectopic notochord cells. Arch. Otolaryng. 84:441-443, 1966.

Seda, H. J., and Snow, J. B.: Carcinoma of the tonsil. Arch. Otolaryng. 89:756-761, 1969.

Seymour-Jones, A.: Hemangioma of pharynx. J. Laryng. 73:396-398, 1959.

Shahrokh, D. K., Devine, K. D., and Harrison, E. G.: Statistical evaluation of 115 cases of carcinoma of the epiglottis. Amer. J. Surg. 102:781-788, 1961.

Shapiro, J. J., and Mix, B. S.: Heterotopic brain tissue in palate. Arch. Otolaryng. 87:522-526, 1968.

Shaw, H. J., and Epstein, S. S.: Cancer of the epiglottis. Cancer 12:246-256, 1959.

Shedd, D., Van Essen, C. F., and Eisenberg, H.: Cancer of the nasopharynx in Connecticut. Cancer 20:508-511, 1967.

Slaughter, D. P., and de Peyster, F. A.: Pharyngeal neurilemmomas of cranial nerve origin. Arch. Surg. 59:386-397, 1949.

Smant, M. S., and French, A. J.: Prognosis of pseudoadenomatous basal cell carcinoma (cylindroma). Arch. Path. 72:107-112, 1961.

Snook, T.: The later development of the bursa pharyngea, homo. Anat. Rec. 58:303-319, 1934.

Sohn, D., and Feuerstein, S. S.: Fibromatous polyp of the hypopharynx presenting from the mouth. Arch. Otolaryng. 86:61-65, 1967.

Sollee, A. N.: Nasopharyngeal teratoma. Arch. Otolaryng. 82:49-52, 1965.

Sonn, M. L., and Peimer, R.: Postcricoid carcinoma as a sequel to radiotherapy for laryngeal carcinoma. Arch. Otolaryng. 62:428-431, 1955.

Soule, E. H.: Tumors of the oral cavity and pharynx. AFIP Fascicle 10b, Section IV, Washington, D. C., 1968.

Sternberg, S. S.: Pathology of juvenile nasopharyngeal angiofibroma — a lesion of adolescent males. Cancer 7:15-28, 1954.

Stobbe, G. D., and Dargeon, H. W.: Embryonal rhabdomyosarcoma of head and neck in children and adolescents. Cancer 3:826-836, 1950.

Stout, A. P., and Murray, M. R.: Hemangiopericytoma. Ann. Surg. 116:26-33, 1942.

Sturton, S. D., Wen, H. L., and Sturton, O. G.: Etiology of cancer of nasopharynx. Cancer 19:1666-1669, 1966.

Szanto, P. B., and Hollender, A. R.: Tuberculosis of the nasopharynx. Ann. Otol. 53:508-521, 1944.

Teloh, H. A.: Cancer of the tonsil. Arch. Surg. 65:693-701, 1952.

Teoh, T. B.: Epidermoid carcinoma of nasopharynx among Chinese: A study of 31 necropsies. J. Path. Bact. 73:451-465, 1957.

Timmis, P.: Chondroma of nasopharynx. J. Laryng. 73:383-387, 1959.

Tsukamoto, K., and Tazaki, E.: Four cases of hypopharyngeal carcinoma after cervical radiation. Gann 45:248-249, 1954.

Vaeth, J. M.: Nasopharyngeal malignant tumors: 82 consecutive patients treated in a period of 22 years. Radiology 74:364-472, 1960.

Vaheri, E., and Harma, R.: Simple fibromas of pharynx. Acta Otolaryng. 47:536-539, 1957.

Walker, E. A., Rigual, J. R., and Hough, J. V. D.: Teratomas of the pharynx. Amer. Surg. 29:219-226, 1963.

Wang, C. C., and James, A. E.: Chordoma with widespread metastases: Brief review of the literature and report of a case. Cancer 22:162-167, 1968.

Wang, C. C., Little, J. B., and Schulz, M. D.: Cancer of the nasopharynx. Cancer 15:921-926, 1962.

Webb, H. E., Harrison, E. G., Masson, J. K., and ReMine, W. H.: Solitary extramedullary myeloma (plasmacytoma) of upper part of respiratory tract and oropharynx. Cancer 15:1142-1155, 1962.

Weed, L. A., and Parkhill, E. M.: The diagnosis of histoplasmosis in ulcerative disease of the mouth and pharynx. Amer. J. Clin. Path. 18:130-140, 1948.

Wendling, D.: Acinic cell adenocarcinoma of the base of the tongue. Laryngoscope 78:64-67, 1968.

Wilkinson, H. F.: Pathologic changes in tonsils. A study of ten thousand pairs with special reference to presence of cartilage, bone, tuberculosis, and bodies suggestive of actinomycosis. Arch. Otolaryng. 10:127-151, 1929.

Withalm, A.: Zur Pathologie und Histologie des Epiglottiskarzinoms. Z. Laryng. Rhinol. Otol. 32:182-187, 1953.

Woolner, L. B.: Tumors of the epiglottis. AFIP Fascicle 10b, Section IV, Nat. Acad. Sci., Washington, D. C., 1968, pp. 271-286.

Wynder, E. L., Hultberg, S., Jacobson, F., and Bross, I. J.: Environmental factors in cancer of the upper alimentary tract (special reference to Plummer-Vinson syndrome) (Paterson-Kelly syndrome). Cancer 10:470-487, 1957.

Wynder, E. L., Dodo, H., Bloch, D. A., Gautt, R. C., and Moore, O. S.: Epidermiologic investigation of multiple primary cancer of upper alimentary and respiratory tracts. I. A retrospective study. Cancer 24:730-739, 1969.

Yarington, C. T., Smith, G. S., and Benzmiller, J. A.: Value of histologic examination of tonsils. Arch. Otolaryng. 85:680-681, 1967.

Yeh, S. H. U.: A histologic classification of carcinomas of the nasopharynx with a critical review as to the existence of lymphoepitheliomas. Cancer 15:895-920, 1962.

Larynx

Alexander, F. W., and Cassady, C. L.: 306 Laryngeal carcinomas: staging and end results. Arch. Otolaryng. 83:602-606, 1966.

Ash, J. E., and Raum, M.: Larynx (Chaps. 24 and 25) An Atlas of Otolaryngic Pathology. Amer. Acad. Ophthal. Otolaryng., Washington, D.C., A.F.I.P., 1956, pp. 306-355.

Ash, J. E., and Schwartz, L.: The laryngeal (vocal cord) node. Trans. Amer. Acad. Ophthal. 48:323-332, 1944.

Auerbach, O., Hammond, E. C., and Garfinkel, L.: Histologic changes in the larynx in relation to smoking habits. Cancer 25:92-104, 1970.

Baker, D. C., and Savetsky, L.: Congenital partial atresia of larynx. Laryngoscope 76:616-620, 1966.

Barton, R. J.: Observation on the pathogenesis of laryngeal granuloma due to endotracheal anesthesia. New Eng. J. Med. 248:1097-1099, 1953.

Battifora, H. A., Eistenstein, R., and Schild, J. A.: Rhabdomyoma of larynx. Cancer 23:183-190, 1969.

Baxter, J. D.: Glomus tumor (chemodectoma) of the larynx. Ann. Otol. 74:813–820, 1965.

Baxter, J. D.: Acute epiglottitis in children. Laryngoscope 77:1358–1367, 1967.

Bergstrom, J., Moberg, A., and Orell, S. R.: On the pathogenesis of laryngeal injuries following prolonged intubation. Acta Otolaryng. 55:342–346, 1962.

Bienenstock, H., Ehrlich, G. E., and Freyberg, R. H.: Rheumatoid arthritis of the cricoarytenoid joint. Arthritis Rheum. 6:48–63, 1963.

Bloom, W., and Fawcett, D. W.: A Textbook of Histology. 9th ed., Philadelphia, W. B. Saunders Company, 1968.

Brandenburg, J. H., Harris, D. D., and Bernett, M.: Chondrosarcoma of the larynx. Laryngoscope 77:752–762, 1967.

Butler, R. M., and Moser, F. H.: Padded dash syndrome: blunt trauma to larynx and trachea. Laryngoscope 78:1172–1182, 1968.

Capo, O. A.: Oxyphilic adenoma (oncocytoma) of larynx. Arch. Otolaryng. 82:42–44, 1956.

Castleman, B., and McNeely, B. V.: Tuberculosis of larynx and trachea. New Eng. J. Med. 279:423–430, 1968.

Chamberlain, D.: Metastatic malignant melanoma of larynx. Arch. Otolaryng. 83:231–232, 1966.

Cherry, J., and Margulies, S. I.: Contact ulcer of the larynx. Laryngoscope 78:1937–1940, 1968.

Cole, F.: Acute epiglottitis in the young. New Eng. J. Med. 276:1381–1382, 1967.

Cracovaner, A. J., and Opler, S. R.: Granular cell myoblastoma of larynx. Laryngoscope 77:1040–1046, 1967.

Delahunty, J. E., and Cherry, J.: Experimentally produced vocal cord granulomas. Laryngoscope 78:1941–1947, 1968.

Daly, J. F.: Relapsing polychrondritis of the larynx and trachea. Arch. Otolaryng. 84:570–573, 1966.

Dekelbaum, A. M.: Laryngeal papillomas. Arch. Otolaryng. 81:390–397, 1965.

Devine, K. D.: Sarcoidosis and sarcoidosis of the larynx. Larynx 75:533–569, 1965.

Donnelly, W. H.: Histopathology of endotracheal intubation. Arch. Path. 88:511–520, 1969.

Ellis, M. P., and Liderman, M.: Carcinoma of the larynx and pharynx. Trans. Med. Soc. London 76:48–63, 1960.

Ferguson, G. B.: Laryngocele. Laryngoscope 77:1368–1375, 1967.

Fields, J. A.: Renal carcinoma metastatic to larynx. Laryngoscope 76:99–101, 1966.

Glyn-Jones, D., and Gabriel, C. E.: The incidence of carcinoma of the larynx in persons under 20 years of age. Laryngoscope 79:251–255, 1969.

Goethals, P. L., Dahlin, D. C., and Devine, K. D.: Cartilaginous tumors of the larynx. Surg. Gynec. Obstet. 117:77–82, 1963.

Goethals, P. L., and Lillie, J. C.: Neurilemmoma of epiglottis. Arch. Otolaryng. 74:181–184, 1961.

Goldman, J. L., Bloom, B. S., Zak, F. G., Friedman, W. H., Gunsberg, M. J., and Silverstone, S. M.: Serial microscopic studies of radical neck dissections. Arch. Otolaryng. 89:620–628, 1969.

Goldman, J. L., Cheren, R. V., Zak, F. G., and Gunsberg, M. J.: Histopathology of larynges and radical neck specimens in a combined radiation and surgery program for advanced carcinomas of the larynx and laryngopharynx. Ann. Otol. 75:313–335, 1966.

Hedden, M., Ersoz, C. J., Donnelly, W. H., and Sofar, P.: Laryngotracheal damage after prolonged use of orotracheal tubes in adults. J.A.M.A. 207:703–708, 1969.

Heiner, E. R.: Primary amyloidosis of the larynx. Arch. Otolaryng. 87:413–415, 1968.

Himalstein, M. R., and Humphrey, T. R.: Pleomorphic carcinoma of the larynx. Arch. Otolaryng. 87:389–395, 1968.

Holinger, P. H.: Carcinoma in situ of the larynx. Editorial. Arch. Otolaryng. 83:303–304, 1966.

Holinger, P. H., and Cohen, L. L.: Neurofibromatosis with involvement of larynx. Laryngoscope 60:193–196, 1950.

Holinger, P. H., Schild, J. A., and Maurizi, D. G.: Laryngeal papilloma: review of etiology and therapy. Laryngoscope 78:1462–1474, 1968.

Hora, J. F., and Weller, W. A.: Chondroma of larynx. Arch. Otolaryng. 74:67–69, 1961.

Huizenga, C., and Balogh, K.: Cartilaginous tumors of the larynx. Cancer 26:201–210, 1970.

Iglauer, S.: Myoblastoma of the larynx. Ann Otol. 51:1089–1093, 1942.

Jackson, C.: Contact ulcer granuloma and other laryngeal complications. Anesthesiology 14:425–436, 1953.

Kaufman, R. S., and Balogh, K.: Verrucas and juvenile laryngeal papillomas. Arch. Otolaryng. 89:748–749, 1969.

Kean, H.: Cancer and trichinosis of larynx. Laryngoscope 76:1766–1768, 1966.

Kirchner, J. A.: Papilloma of the larynx with extensive lung involvement. Laryngoscope 61:1022–1029, 1951.

Kirchner, J. A., and Malkin, J. S.: Cancer of the larynx: 30 year survey. Arch. Otolaryng. 58:19–30, 1953.

Kroe, D. J., Pelcock, J. A., and Cocke, E. W.: Oncocytic papillary cystadenoma of the larynx. Arch. Path. 84:429–432, 1967.

Kuhn, A. J., Devine, K. D., and McDonald, J. R.: Cervical metastases from squamous cell carcinoma of larynx. Laryngoscope 67:169–190, 1957.

Lang, W. S.: Diphtheria at the present time. Laryngoscope 75:1092–1102, 1965.

Leonard, J. R., Chambers, R. G., and Trail, M. L.: Paralaryngeal cysts. Laryngoscope, 77:386–396, 1967.

Macfie, D. D.: Asymptomatic laryngoceles in wind-instrument bandsmen. Arch. Otolaryng. 83:270–275, 1966.

Majoros, W., Devine, K. D., and Parkhill, E. M.: Malignant transformation of benign laryngeal papillomas in children after radiation therapy. Surg. Clin. N. Amer. 43:1049–1061, 1963.

Martinson, F. D.: Chemodectoma of "glomus laryngicum inferior." Arch. Otolaryng. 86:70–73, 1968.

Mazzarella, L. A., Pina, L. H., and Wolff, D.: Asymptomatic metastasis to larynx. Laryngoscope 76:1547–1554, 1966.

McMillan, W. G., and Duvall, A. J.: Congenital subglottic stenosis. Arch. Otolaryng. 87:272–278, 1968.

McNelis, F. L.: Laryngeal carcinoma, classified by clinical staging. Arch. Otolaryng. 82:173–180, 1965.

Minckler, D. S., Meligro, C. H., and Norris, H. T.: Carcinosarcoma of the larynx. Case report with metastases of epidermoid and sarcomatous elements. Cancer 26:195–200, 1970.

Neffson, A. H.: Acute laryngotracheobronchitis: 25 year review. Amer. J. Med. Sci. 208:524–547, 1944.

New, G. B., and Erich, J. B.: Benign tumors of larynx (722 cases). Arch. Otolaryng. 28:841–910, 1938.

Ogura, J. H.: Surgical pathology of cancer of the larynx. Laryngoscope 65:867–926, 1955.

Pantazopoulos, P. E.: Primary malignant melanoma of the larynx. Laryngoscope 74:95–102, 1964.

Pappas, D. G., and Johnson, L. A.: Laryngeal myositis ossificans. Arch. Otolaryng. 81:227–231, 1965.

Pearson, C. M., Kline, H. M., and Newcomer, V. D.: Relapsing polychondritis. New Eng. J. Med. 263:51–58, 1960.

Perez, C. A., Holtz, S., Ogura, J. H., Dedo, H. H., and Powers, W. E.: Radiation therapy of early carcinoma of the true vocal cords. Cancer 21:764–771, 1968.

Polliack, A.: Benign mucous membrane pemphigoid with laryngeal stenosis in patient with thyroid carcinoma. Arch. Path. 86:48–51, 1968.

Pope, T. H.: Laryngeal myoblastoma. Arch. Otolaryng. 81:80–82, 1965.

Pratt, L. W., and Goodof, I. I.: Hemangioendotheliosarcoma of larynx. Arch. Otolaryng. 87:484–489, 1968.

Putney, F. J.: Laryngocele. Laryngoscope 78:749–755, 1968.

Putney, F. J., and Moran, J. J.: Cartilaginous tumors of larynx. Arch. Otolaryng. 81:422, 1965.

Ritter, F. N.: Hypothyroidism effect on larynx of rat: an explanation for hoarseness associated with hypothyroidism in the human. Arch. Otolaryng. 81:423–424, 1965.

Rogers, W. P., Jr., Reynolds, C., and Yatsuhashi, M.: Cancer of the larynx. New Eng. J. Med. 274:596–599, 1966.

Ross, J. A. T.: Special problems in acute laryngotracheobronchitis. Laryngoscope 79:1218–1226, 1969.

Sabri, J. A., and Hajjar, M. A.: Malignant mixed tumor of the vocal cord. Arch. Otolaryng. 85:332–334, 1967.

Scarpelli, D. G., McCoy, F. W., and Scott, J. K.: Acute lupus erythematosus with laryngeal involvement. New Eng. J. Med. 261:691–694, 1959.

Schneider, C., Gould, W. J., and Mirani, R.: Granular cell myoblastoma of larynx. Arch. Otolaryng. 89:873–877, 1969.

Sherwin, R. P., Strong, M. S., and Vaughn, C. W., Jr.: Polypoid and junctional squamous cell carcinoma of tongue and larynx with spindle cell carcinoma (pseudosarcoma). Cancer 16:51–60, 1963.

Shilling, B. B., Abell, M. R., and Work, W. P.: Leukemic involvement of larynx. Arch. Otolaryng. 85:658–665, 1967.

Smith, I. I., and Bain, A. D.: Congenital atresia of larynx. Ann. Otol. 74:338–349, 1965.

Smith, R. O., Hemenway, W. G., English, G. M., Black, F. O., and Swan, H.: Post intubation subglottic granulation tissue: Review of problems and evaluation of radiotherapy. Laryngoscope 79:1227–1251, 1969.

Sprinkle, P. M., Allen, M. S., and Brookshire, P. F.: Osteosarcoma of larynx. Laryngoscope 76:325–333, 1966.

Stein, A. A., Quebral, R., Boba, A., and Landwesser, C.: Post mortem evaluation of laryngotracheal alteration associated with intubation. Ann. Surg. 151:130–138, 1960.

Suehs, O. W., and Powell, D. B.: Congenital cyst of larynx in infants. Laryngoscope 77:654–662, 1967.

Tedeschi, L. G., and Cheren, R. V.: Laryngeal hyperkeratosis due to primary monilial infection. Arch. Otolaryng., 87:82–84, 1968.

Titche, L. L.: Carcinoma of the larynx following carcinoma of the lung. Arch. Otolaryng. 83:598–601, 1966.

Tonkin, J. P., and Harrison, G. A.: The effect on the larynx of prolonged endotracheal intubation. Med. J. Austral. 2:581–587, 1966.

Toomey, J. M.: Adenocarcinoma of the larynx. Laryngoscope 77:931–961, 1967.

Trible, W. M., and Kahauer, H.: Cancer of the larynx and pharynx. Arch. Otolaryng. 89:617–619, 1969.

VerMeulen, V. R.: Laryngeal carcinoma in the young. Laryngoscope 76:1724–1727, 1966.

Von Essen, C. F., Shedd, D. P., Connelly, R. R., and Eisenberg, H.: Cancer of the larynx in Connecticut 1935–1959. Cancer 22:1315–1322, 1968.

Ward, P. H., Engel, E., and Nance, W. E.: The larynx in the cri du chat (cat cry) syndrome. Laryngoscope 78:1716–1733, 1968.

Way, W. W., and Sooy, F. A.: Histologic changes produced by endotracheal intubation. Ann Otol. 74:799–812, 1965.

Esophagus

Allison, P. R.: Peptic ulcer of esophagus. Thorax 3:20–42, 1948.

Baker, L. A., Smith, C., and Lieberman, G.: The natural history of esophageal varices. Amer. J. Med. 26:228–237, 1959.

Barrett, N. R.: Chronic peptic ulcer of esophagus and esophagitis. Brit. J. Surg. 38:175–182, 1950.

Basque, G. J., Boline, J. E., and Holyoke, J. B.: Malignant melanoma of the esophagus: first reported case in a child. Amer. J. Clin. Path. 52:609–611, 1970.

Bigelow, N. H.: Carcinoma of esophagus developing at site of lye stricture. Cancer 6:1159–1164, 1953.

Bikhazi, H. B., Thompson, E. R., and Shumrick, D. A.: Caustic ingestion: current status. Arch. Otolaryng. 89:770–773, 1969.

Bishop, H. C., and Koop, C. E.: Surgical management of duplications of the alimentary tract. Amer. J. Surg. 107:434–442, 1964.

Block, G. E., and Lancaster, J. R.: Adenocarcinoma of the cardioesophageal junction. Arch. Surg. 88:852–859, 1964.

Bloom, W., and Fawcett, D. W.: A Textbook of Histology. 9th ed., Philadelphia, W. B. Saunders Co., 1968, pp. 544–546.

Blount, R. F., and Lachman, E.: *In* Schaeffer, J. P. (ed.): Morris' Human Anatomy, New York, McGraw-Hill Book Co., 1953, pp. 1337–1342.

Bluestone, C. D., Kerry, R., and Sieber, W. K.: Congenital esophageal stenosis. Laryngoscope 79:1095–1104, 1969.

Blumberg, J. B., Stevenson, J. K., LeMire, R. J., and Boyden, E. A.: Laryngotracheoesophageal cleft: the embryologic implications. Surgery 57:559–575, 1965.

Bosher, L. H., and Taylor, F. H.: Heterotopic gastric mucosa in the esophagus with ulceration and stricture formation. J. Thoracic Surg. 21:306–312, 1951.

Bosher, L. H., Burford, T. H., and Ackerman, L. V.: Pathology of experimentally produced lye burns and strictures of esophagus. J. Thorac. Cardiov. Surg. 21:483–489, 1951.

Boyd, D. P., Adams, H. D., and Salzman, F. A.: Carcinoma of the esophagus. New Eng. J. Med. 258:271–274, 1958.

Boyd, D. P., Meissner, W. A., Yelkoff, C. L., and Gladding, T. C.: Primary melanocarcinoma of esophagus (case report). Cancer 7:266–270, 1954.

Bremer, J. L.: Diverticula and duplications of the intestinal tract. Arch. Path. 38:132–140, 1944.

Burgess, H. M., Baggenstoss, A. H., Moersch, H. J., and Clagett, O. T.: Cancer of the esophagus: a clinicopathologic study. Surg. Clin. N. Amer. 31:965–976, 1951.

Cassella, R. R., Brown, A. L., Sayre, G. P., and Ellis, F. H.: Achalasia of esophagus: pathologic and etiologic considerations. Ann. Surg. 160:474–487, 1964.

Castell, D. O., and Harris, L. D.: Hormonal control of gastroesophageal sphincter strength. New Eng. J. Med. 282:886–889, 1970.

Conn, H. O., and Lindemuth, W. W.: Prophylactic porto-caval anastomosis in patients with esophageal varices. N. Eng. J. Med. *279*:725–732, 1968.

Desai, P. B., Borges, E. J., Vohra, V. G., and Paymaster, J. C.: Carcinoma of the esophagus in India. Cancer *23*:979–989, 1969.

Desforges, G., and Streider, J. W.: Esophageal cysts. New Eng. J. Med. *262*:60–64, 1960.

Dobbins, W. O.: Mallory-Weiss syndrome: a commonly overlooked cause of upper gastrointestinal bleeding. Gastroenterology *44*:689–695, 1963.

Facer, J. C.: Osteophytes of cervical spine causing dysphagia. Arch. Otolaryng. *86*:341–345, 1967.

Fraser, G. M., and Kinley, C. E.: Pseudosarcoma with carcinoma of esophagus. Arch. Path. *85*:325–330, 1968.

Freeark, R. J., Norcross, W. J., Baker, R. J., and Strohl, E. L.: The Mallory-Weiss syndrome: increasing surgical significance. Arch. Surg. *88*:882–887, 1964.

Gates, O., and Warren, S.: Radiation induced experimental cancer of the esophagus. Amer. J. Path. *53*:667–685, 1968.

Goldfarb, T. G.: Esophageal gland adenocarcinoma of the midesophagus. Amer. J. Clin. Path. *48*:281–285, 1967.

Goyal, R. K., Glancy, J. J., and Spiro, H. M.: Lower esophageal ring. New Eng. J. Med. *282*:1298–1305, 1355–1362, 1970.

Hagarty, G.: A classification of esophageal hiatus hernia with special reference to sliding hernia. Amer. J. Roentgen. *84*:1056–1060, 1960.

Haight, C.: Congenital atresia of esophagus with tracheo-esophageal fistula. Ann. Surg. *120*:623–655, 1944.

Heitzman, E. J., Heitzman, G. C., and Elliott, C. F.: Primary esophageal amyloidosis. Arch. Intern. Med. *109*:595–600, 1962.

Hurst, E. E.: Malignant tumors in Alaskan eskimos: Unique predominance of carcinoma of esophagus in Alaskan eskimo women. Cancer *17*:1187–1195, 1964.

Hurst, A. F., and Rake, G. W.: Achalasia of the cardia (so-called cardiospasm). Quart. J. Med. *23*:491–508, 1930.

Imbrie, J. D., and Doyle, P. J.: Laryngotracheoesophageal cleft, report of case and review of literature. Laryngoscope *79*:1252–1274, 1969.

Ingelfinger, F. J., and Kramer, P.: Dysphagia produced by contractile ring in the lower esophagus. Gastroenterology *23*:419–430, 1953.

Janes, R. M.: Diverticula of lower thoracic esophagus. Ann. Surg. *124*:637–652, 1946.

Kay, S.: A ten year appraisal of the treatment of squamous cell carcinoma of the esophagus. Surg. Gynec. Obstet. *117*:167–171, 1963.

Kay, S.: Mucoepidermoid carcinoma of the esophagus. Cancer *22*:1053–1059, 1968.

King, B. T.: New concepts of the etiology and treatment of diverticula of the esophagus. Surg. Gynec. Obstet. *85*:93–97, 1947.

Kiviranta, U. K.: Korrosion des Oesophagus und des Ventrikels. Acta Otolaryng. (Suppl.)*81*:1–128, 1949–50.

Lane, N.: Pseudosarcoma (polypoid sarcoma-like masses) associated with squamous cell carcinoma of the mouth, fauces and larynx. Cancer *10*:19–41, 1957.

Laubscher, F. A.: Esophagocardiac fistula, report of a case. New Eng. J. Med. *282*:794–795, 1970.

Lichtiger, B., Mackay, B., and Tessmer, C. F.: Spindle cell tumors of the head and neck: An ultrastructural study. Amer. J. Path. *59*:41A–42A, 1970.

Liebowitz, H. R.: Pathogenesis of esophageal varix rupture. J.A.M.A. *175*:874–879, 1961.

MacGregor, A. R.: Pathology of Infancy and Childhood. London, E. & S. Livingstone, 1960, pp. 184–186.

Mahour, G. H., and Harrison, E. G.: Osteochondroma of esophagus (tracheobronchial choristoma). Cancer *20*:1489–1493, 1967.

Mallory, G. K., and Weiss, S.: Hemorrhages from lacerations of the cardiac orifice due to vomiting. Amer. J. Med. Sci. *178*:506–515, 1929.

Marcial-Rojas, R. A., and Vallecillo, L. A.: Primary adenoid cystic carcinoma of esophagus. Arch. Otolaryng. *70*:197–201, 1959.

Martinez, I.: Cancer of esophagus in Puerto Rico. Cancer *17*:1279–1288, 1964.

Minielly, J. A., Harrison, E. G., Fontana, R. S., and Payne, W. S.: Verrucous squamous cell carcinoma of esophagus. Cancer *20*:2078–2087, 1967.

Moersch, H. J., and Harrington, S. W.: Benign tumor of the esophagus. Ann. Otol. *53*:800–817, 1944.

Moses, H. L., and Cheatham, W. J.: The frequency and significance of human herpetic esophagitis. Lab. Invest. *12*:663–669, 1963.

Mottet, N. K.: Physiologic metaplasia of esophageal epithelium (light and electron microscopic observations). Amer. J. Path. *52*:15a, 1968.

Perrone, J. A.: Dysphagia due to massive cervical exostoses. Arch. Otolaryng. *86*:346–347, 1967.

Plass, E. D.: Congenital atresia of esophagus with tracheo-esophageal fistula. Johns Hopkins Hosp. Rep. *18*:259–286, 1919.

Polk, H. C., Camp, F. A., and Walker, A. W.: Dysphagia and esophageal stenosis, manifestation of metastatic mammary cancer. Cancer *20*:2002–2007, 1967.

Prolla, J. C., Taebel, D. W., and Kirsner, J. B.: Current status of exfoliative cytology in diagnosis of malignant neoplasms of esophagus. Surg. Gynec. Obstet. *121*:743–752, 1965.

Rake, G. W.: On the pathology of achalasia of the cardia. Guy Hosp. Rep. *77*:141–150, 1927.

Rector, L. E., and Connerley, M. L.: Aberrant mucosa in the esophagus in infants and children. Arch. Path. *31*:285–294, 1941.

Robbins, S. L.: Pathology. Philadelphia, W. B. Saunders Co., 1967, pp. 818–826.

Rosenak, B. S., and VanVactor, H. D.: Extramucosal intramural enteric cyst of esophagus: a case report. Amer. J. Roentgen. *66*:81–86, 1951.

Rosenthal, A. H.: Congenital atresia of esophagus with tracheoesophageal fistula. Arch. Path. *12*:756–772, 1931.

Scarpa, F. J.: Polypoid squamous cell carcinoma of esophagus (carcinosarcoma). Cancer *19*:861–866, 1966.

Schatzki, R., and Gary, J. E.: Dysphagia due to diaphragm-like localized narrowing in lower esophagus ("lower esophageal ring"). Amer. J. Roentgen. *70*:911–922, 1953.

Schmidt, H. W., Clagett, O. T., and Harrison, E. G.: Benign tumors and cysts of the esophagus. J. Thorac. Sug. *41*:717–732, 1961.

Schridde, H.: Über Magenschleimhaut-Inseln im obersten Oesophagusabschnitt. Virchow's Arch. *175*:1–16, 1904.

Shamma, M. H., and Benedict, E. B.: Esophageal webs. A report of 58 cases and an attempt at classification. New Eng. J. Med. *259*:378–384, 1958.

Stembien, S. J., and Dogradi, A. E.: Dysphagia, odynophagia, and phagodynia. New Eng. J. Med. *276*:527, 1967.

Stout, A. P., Humphreys, G. H., II, and Rottenberg, L. A.: Carcinosarcoma of the esophagus. Amer. J. Roentgen. *61*:461–469, 1949.

Stout, A. P., and Lattes, R.: Tumors of the esophagus. Section V, Fascicle 20, Atlas of Tumor Pathology. Washington, D.C., Armed Forces Institute of Pathology, 1957.

Talerman, A., and WooMing, M. O.: The origin of squamous cell carcinoma of the gastric cardia. Cancer 22:1226–1232, 1968.

Tenta, L. T., and Ford, L. H.: Congenital H type T-E fistula in a young adult. Arch. Otolaryng. 85:675–679, 1967.

Toreson, W. E.: Secondary carcinoma of the esophagus as a cause of dysphagia. Arch. Path. 38:82–84, 1944.

Totten, R. S., Stout, A. P., Humphreys, G. H., II, and Moore, R. L.: Benign tumors and cysts of the esophagus. J. Thorac. Cardiovasc. Surg. 25:606–622, 1953.

Turnbull, A. D. M., and Goodner, J. T.: Primary adenocarcinoma of esophagus. Cancer 22:915–918, 1968.

Underwood, L. J., Montgomery, H., and Broders, A. C.: Squamous cell epithelioma that simulates sarcoma. A.M.A. Arch. Dermat. 64:149–158, 1951.

Ushigomi, S., Spjut, H. J., and Noon, G. P.: Extensive dysplasia and carcinoma in situ of esophageal epithelium. Cancer 20:1023–1029, 1967.

Weiss, S., and Mallory, G. K.: Lesions of cardiac orifice of stomach produced by vomiting. J.A.M.A. 98:1353–1355, 1932.

Weitzner, S.: Mucoepidermoid carcinoma of esophagus. Arch. Path. 90:271–273, 1970.

Wolf, S., and Almy, T. P.: Experimental observations on cardiospasm in man. Gastroenterology 13:401–421, 1949.

Wynder, E. L., and Bross, I. J.: A study of etiological factors in cancer of the esophagus. Cancer 14:389–413, 1961.

Yates, D. R., and Koss, L. G.: Paget's disease of esophageal epithelium. Arch. Path. 86:447, 1968.

The Trachea and Bronchi

Agnos, J. W., and Starkey, G. W. B.: Primary leiomyosarcoma and leiomyoma of the lung. New Eng. J. Med. 258:12–17, 1958.

Al-Saleem, T., Peale, A. R., and Norris, C. M.: Multiple papillomatosis of the lower respiratory tract. Cancer 22:1173–1184, 1968.

Anderson, A. E., and Foraker, A. G.: Eosinophilic granuloma of lung. Arch. Intern. Med. 103:966–973, 1959.

Anspach, W. E.: Atelectasis and bronchiectasis in children. Amer. J. Dis. Child 47:1011–1050, 1934.

Archer, R. L., Harrison, R. W., and Moulder, P. V.: Granular cell myoblastoma of trachea and carina. J. Thorac. Cardiov. Surg. 45:539–547, 1963.

Ashley, D. J. B., and Davies, H. D.: Histology and biologic behavior of carcinoma of lung. Cancer 20:165–174, 1967.

Auerbach, O., Hammond, E. C., Kirman, D., Garfinkel, L., and Stout, A. P.: Histologic changes in bronchial tubes of cigarette-smoking dogs. Cancer 20:2055–2066, 1967.

Auerbach, O., Stout, A. P., Hammond, E. C., and Garfinkel, L.: Changes in bronchial epithelium in relation to sex, age, residence, smoking and pneumonia. New Eng. J. Med. 267:111–125, 1962.

Auerbach, O., Stout, A. P., Hammond, E. C., and Garfinkel, L.: Multiple primary bronchial carcinomas. Cancer 20:699–705, 1967.

Bates, D. V.: Chronic bronchitis and emphysema. New Eng. J. Med. 278:546–551; 600–605, 1968.

Bauermeister, D. E., Jennings, E. R., Beland, A. H., and Judson, H. A.: Pulmonary blastoma, a form of carcinosarcoma. Amer. J. Clin. Path. 46:322–329, 1966.

Baum, G. L., Donnerberg, R. L., Stewart, D., Mulligan, W. J., and Putnam, L. R.: Pulmonary sporotrichosis. New Eng. J. Med. 280:410–413, 1969.

Beckers, J. N., Beuchner, H. A., and Ekman, P. J.: Pulmonary eosinophilic granuloma: its natural history and prognosis. Amer. Rev. Resp. Dis. 85:211–219, 1962.

Belanger, R., LaFleche, L. R., and Picard, J. L.: Congenital cystic adenomatoid malformation of the lung. Thorax 19:1–11, 1964.

Bennett, D. E., and Sasser, W. F.: Bronchiolar carcinoma: a valid clinicopathologic entity. Cancer 24:876–887, 1969.

Bennett, D. E., Sasser, W. F., and Ferguson, T. B.: Adenocarcinoma of the lung in men. Cancer 23:431–439, 1969.

Bensch, K. G., Corrin, B., Paniute, R., and Spencer, H.: Oat cell carcinoma of the lung; its origins and relationship to bronchial carcinoid. Cancer 22:1163–1172, 1968.

Bergmann, M., Ackerman, L. V., and Kemler, R. L.: Carcinosarcoma of lung. Cancer 4:919–929, 1951.

Berkheiser, S. W.: Carcinoma in situ of the lung of peripheral origin. Amer. J. Clin. Path. 46:315–321, 1966.

Black, H.: Fibrosarcoma of the bronchus. J. Thorac. Cardiovasc. Surg. 19:123–134, 1950.

Bloom, W., and Fawcett, D. W.: A Textbook of Histology. 9th ed., Philadelphia, W. B. Saunders Company, 1968.

Borrie, J., Lichter, I., and Rodda, R. A.: Intralobar pulmonary sequestration. Brit. J. Surg. 50:623–633, 1963.

Buffmire, D. K., Clagett, O. T., and McDonald, J. R.: Papillomas of larynx, trachea and bronchi. Mayo Clin. Proc. Staff meet. 25:595–600, 1950.

Butler, C., and Kleinerman, J.: Pulmonary hamartoma. Arch. Path. 88:584–592, 1969.

Cardell, B. S., and Pearson, R. S. B.: Death in asthmatics. Thorax. 14:341–352, 1959.

Cottrell, J. C., Becker, K. L., Matthews, M. J., and Moore, C.: The histology of gonadotropin secreting bronchiogenic carcinoma. Amer. J. Clin. Path. 52:720–725, 1969.

Daniels, A. C., Conner, G. H., and Straus, F. H.: Primary chondrosarcoma of tracheobronchial tree. Arch. Path. 84:615–624, 1967.

Decker, H. R.: Alveolar cell carcinoma of lung (pulmonary adenomatosis). J. Thorac. Cardiov. Surg. 30:230–247, 1955.

Drapanas, T., Siewers, R., and Feist, J. H.: Reversible poststenotic bronchiectasis. New Eng. J. Med. 275:917–921, 1966.

Duke, M.: Tumoral amyloidosis of lungs. Arch. Path. 67:110–117, 1959.

Dunnill, M. S.: The pathology of asthma with special reference to changes in the bronchial mucosa. J. Clin. Path. 13:27–33, 1960.

Ebert, R. V., and Pierce, J. A.: Pathogenesis of pulmonary emphysema. Arch. Intern. Med. 111:34–43, 1963.

Ellman, P., and Whittaker, H.: Primary carcinoma of trachea. Thorax 2:153–162, 1947.

Eraklis, A. J., Griscom, N. T., and McGovern, J. B.: Bronchiogenic cysts of the mediastinum in infancy. New Eng. J. Med. 281:1150–1155, 1969.

Evans, R. W.: Histological Appearances of Tumours. 2nd ed., Baltimore, The Williams & Wilkins Co., 1966, pp. 1089–1130.

Falor, W. H., Gordon, M., and Kaczala, O. A.: Chromosomes in bronchoscopic biopsies from patients with bronchial adenoma, bronchiogenic carcinoma and from heavy smokers. Cancer 24:198–209, 1969.

Fetterman, G. H., Sherman, F. E., Fabrizio, N. S., and Studvicki, B. S.: Generalized cytomegalic inclusion disease of the newborn. Arch. Path. 86:86–94, 1968.

Field, C. S.: Bronchiectasis in childhood. Pediatrics 4: I. Clinical Signs, 21–45; II. Etiology and Pathogenesis, 231–248; III. Prophylaxis, Treatment and Prognosis 355–372; 1949.

Fletcher, C. M.: Chronic bronchitis; its prevalence, nature and pathogenesis. Amer. Rev. Resp. Dis. 80:483, 1959.

Fontana, R. S., Carr, D. T., Woolner, L. B., and Miller, F. K.: An evaluation of methods of inducing sputum production in patients with suspected cancer of lung. Mayo Clin. Proc. 37:113–121, 1962.

Fox, T. F.: Argentaffinoma and bronchial adenoma. Lancet 2:355–356, 1960.

Frank, H. D., and Lieberthal, M. M.: Carcinoid syndrome originating in bronchial adenoma. Arch. Intern. Med. 111:791–798, 1963.

Galofre, M., Payne, W. S., Woolner, L. B., Clagett, O. T., and Gage, R. P.: Pathologic classification and surgical treatment of bronchogenic carcinoma. Surg. Gynec. Obstet. 119:51–61, 1964.

Garston, B.: The natural history, pathology and treatment of chronic bronchitis. Dis. Chest 40:530–538, 1961.

Gerle, R. D., Jaretzki, A., Ashley, C. A., and Berne, A. S.: Congenital bronchopulmonary foregut malformation. New Eng. J. Med. 278:1413–1419, 1968.

Goodner, J. T., Berg, J. W., and Watson, W. L.: The nonbenign nature of bronchial carcinoids and cylindromas. Cancer 14:539–546, 1961.

Gottlieb, P. M.: Changing mortality in bronchial asthma. J.A.M.A. 187:276–280, 1964.

Gowenlock, A. H., Platt, D. S., Campbell, A. C. P., and Wormsley, K. G.: Oat cell carcinoma secreting 5-hydroxytryptophan. Lancet 1:304–306, 1964.

Green, R. A., and Nichols, N. J.: Pulmonary involvement in leukemia. Amer. Rev. Resp. Dis. 80:833–844, 1959.

Gregorie, H. B., Othersen, H. B., and Moore, M. P.: The significance of sarcoid-like lesions in association with malignant neoplasm. Amer. J. Surg. 104:577–586, 1962.

Guillan, R. A., and Zelman, S.: Giant cell carcinoma of the lungs. Amer. J. Clin. Path. 46:427–432, 1966.

Guillan, R. A., Zelman, S., and Alonso, R. A.: Adenocarcinoma of the lungs. Amer. J. Clin. Path. 47:580–584, 1967.

Hajdu, S. I., Huvos, A. G., Goodner, J. T., Foote, F. W., Jr., and Beattie, E. J.: Carcinoma of the trachea. Cancer 25:1448–1456, 1970.

Haroutuman, L. M., Fisher, A. M., and Smith, E. W.: Tuberculosis and sarcoidosis. Bull. Johns Hopkins Hosp. 115:1–28, 1964.

Hausman, D. H., and Weimann, R. B.: Pulmonary tumorlet with hilar lymph node metastasis. Cancer 20:1515–1519, 1967.

Hentel, W., Longfield, A. W., Vincent, T. N., Filley, G. F., and Mitchell, R. S.: Fatal chronic bronchitis. Amer. Rev. Resp. Dis. 87:216–227, 1963.

Herman, D. L., Bullock, W. K., and Waken, J. K.: Giant cell adenocarcinoma of lung. Cancer 19:1337–1346, 1966.

Herout, V., Vortel, V., and Vondrackova, A.: Herpes simplex involvement of the lower respiratory tract. Amer. J. Clin. Path. 46:411–419, 1966.

Hodges, F. V.: Hamartoma of the lung. Dis. Chest 33:43–51, 1958.

Karnberg, S., Laitman, B. S., and Haltz, S.: Amyloidosis of the tracheobronchial tree. New Eng. J. Med. 266:587–591, 1962.

Karpas, C. M., and Blackman, N.: Adenocarcinoma arising in hamartoma of bronchus associated with multiple benign tumors. Amer. J. Clin. Path. 48:383–388, 1967.

Karrer, H. E.: The ultrastructure of mouse lung. J. Cell Biol. 2:241–252, 1956.

Kato, Y., Ferguson, T. B., Bennett, D. E., and Burford, T. H.: Oat cell carcinoma of lung. Cancer 23:517–524, 1969.

Kaufman, G., and Klopstock, R.: Papillomatosis of the respiratory tract. Amer. Rev. Resp. Dis. 88:839–846, 1963.

Kay, S., and Brooks, J. W.: Benign mixed tumor of the trachea with 7 year follow up. Cancer 25:1178–1182, 1970.

Kern, W. H., Jones, J. C., and Chapman, N. D.: Pathology of bronchogenic carcinoma in long term survivors. Cancer 21:772–780, 1968.

Kohn, D., Bensch, K., Liebow, A. A., and Castleman, B.: Multiple minute pulmonary tumors resembling chemodectomas. Amer. J. Path. 37:641–672, 1960.

Koss, L. G., Melamed, M. R., and Goodner, J. T.: Pulmonary cytology, a brief survey of diagnostic results from July 1, 1952, until December 31, 1960. Acta Cytol. 8:104–113, 1964.

Kramer, R.: Myoblastoma of bronchus. Ann. Otol. 48:1083–1086, 1939.

Kroe, D. J., and Pitcock, J. A.: Benign mucous gland adenoma of the bronchus. Arch. Path. 84:539–542, 1967.

Laubscher, F.: Solitary squamous cell papilloma of bronchial origin. Amer. J. Clin. Path. 52:599–603, 1969.

Levine, S.: Unusual bronchial foreign body. Arch. Otolaryng. 89:540–541, 1969.

Lieberman, J.: Heterozygous and homozygous alpha-1-antitrypsin deficiency in patients with pulmonary emphysema. New Eng. J. Med. 281:279–284, 1969.

Liebow, A. A., and Castleman, B.: Benign "clear cell tumors" of the lung. Amer. J. Path. 43:13a–14a, 1963.

Liebow, A. A., and Hubbell, D. S.: Sclerosing hemangioma (histiocytoma, xanthoma) of lung. Cancer 9:53–75, 1956.

Low, F. N.: The pulmonary alveolar epithelium of laboratory animals and man. Anat. Rec. 117:241–263, 1953.

Low, F. N., and Sampaio, M. M.: The pulmonary alveolar epithelium as an entodermal derivative. Anat. Rec. 127:51–63, 1957.

Lumpkin, S. M. M.: Bronchiogenic cysts. Arch. Otolaryng. 84:346–348, 1966.

MacMahon, H. E., Werch, J., and Sorger, K.: Tumorlet of bronchus. Arch. Path. 83:359–363, 1967.

Mallory, T. B.: The pathogenesis of bronchiectasis. New Eng. J. Med. 237:795–798, 1947.

Markel, S. F., and Abell, M. R.: Adenocystic basal cell carcinoma of the trachea. J. Thorac. Cardiov. Surg. 48:211–225, 1964.

Markel, S. F., Abell, M. R., Haight, C., and French, A. J.: Neoplasms of bronchus commonly designated as adenomas. Cancer 17:590–608, 1964.

McCarter, J. H., and Vazquez, J. J.: The bronchial basement membrane in asthma. Immunohistochemical and ultrastructural observations. Amer. J. Path. 48:37a, 1966.

McDonald, J. R., Harrington, S. W., and Claggett, O. T.: Hamartoma of lung. J. Thorac. Cardiov. Surg. 14:128–143, 1945.

McDonald, J. R., Moersch, H. J., and Tenney, W. S.:

Cylindroma of the bronchus. J. Thorac. Cardiov. Surg. *14*:445–453, 1945.

Melamed, M. R., Koss, L. G., and Cliffton, E. E.: Roentgenologically occult lung cancer diagnosed by cytology. Cancer *16*:1537–1551, 1963.

Miglets, A. W.: Primary tracheal carcinoma. Laryngoscope *75*:1853–1860, 1965.

Minken, S. L., Craver, W. L., and Adams, J. T.: Pulmonary blastoma. Arch. Path. *86*:442–446, 1968.

Moffat, A. D.: Congenital cystic disease of the lungs and its classification. J. Path. Bact. *79*:361–372, 1960.

Norris, R. F., and Tyson, R. M.: Pathogenesis of congenital polycystic lung and its correlation with polycystic diseases of other epithelial organs. Amer. J. Path. *23*:1075, 1947.

Novick, W. H.: Traumatic stenosis of the trachea in children. Laryngoscope *77*:1351–1357, 1967.

Ogilvie, A. G.: Natural history of bronchiectasis. Arch. Intern. Med. *68*:395–465, 1941.

Ozla, C., Christopherson, W. M., and Allen, J. D.: Mucoepidermoid tumors of the bronchus. J. Thorac. Cardiov. Surg. *42*:24–31, 1961.

Payne, W. S., Ellis, F. H., Woolner, L. B., and Moersch, H. J.: The surgical treatment of cylindroma (adenoid cystic carcinoma) and mucoepidermoid tumors of the bronchus. J. Thorac. Cardiov. Surg. *38*:709–726, 1959.

Pierce, J. A., Eisen, A. Z., and Dhingra, H. K.: Pathogenesis of emphysema in antitrypsin deficiency. Clin. Res. *17*:477, 1969.

Plachta, A., and Hershey, H.: Lipoma of the lung. Amer. Rev. Resp. Dis. *86*:912–916, 1962.

Reid, J. D., and Mehta, V. T.: Melanoma of lower respiratory tract. Cancer *19*:627–631, 1966.

Reid, L.: Chronic bronchitis and emphsema: A symposium; III. Pathological findings and radiological changes in chronic bronchitis and emphysema. Brit. J. Radiol. *32*:291–305, 1959.

Robbins, L. L.: The roentgenological appearance of parenchymal involvement of the lung by malignant lymphoma. Cancer *6*:80–88, 1953.

Robbins, S. L.: Pathology. 3rd ed. Philadelphia, W. B. Saunders Company, 1967.

Rojer, C. L.: Multicentric endobronchial myoblastoma. Arch. Otolaryng. *82*:652–655, 1965.

Romanoff, H., and Milwidsky, H.: Primary plasmacytoma of the lung. Brit. J. Dis. Chest. *56*:139–143, 1962.

Rosen, S. H., Castleman, B., and Liebow, A. A.: Pulmonary alveolar proteinosis. New Eng. J. Med. *258*:1123–1142, 1959.

Russell, W. O., and Chang, S. C.: A new technique for detecting malignant cells in sputum. Cancer *20*:681–686, 1967.

Russell, W. O., Neidhardt, H. W., Mountain, C. F., Griffith, K. M., and Chang, J. P.: Cytodiagnosis of lung cancer. Acta. Cytol. *7*:1–44, 1963.

Saltzstein, S. L.: Pulmonary malignant lymphomas and pseudolymphomas: classification, therapy and prognosis. Cancer *16*:928–955, 1963.

Sardana, D. S.: Congenital tracheal stenosis. Laryngoscope *76*:1615–1622, 1966.

Scadding, J. G.: Myocobacterium tuberculosis in the aetiology of sarcoidosis. Brit. Med. J. *2*:1618–1623, 1960.

Schmidt, H. W., Clagett, O. T., and McDonald, J. R.: Broncholithiasis. J. Thoracic Surg. *19*:226–245, 1950.

Smith, J. F., and Dexter, D.: Papillary neoplasms of bronchus of low grade malignancy. Thorax *18*:340–349, 1963.

Stoutter, L., Sniffen, R. C., and Robbins, L. L.: Clinical survey of adenomas of trachea and bronchus in a general hospital. J. Thoracic Surg. *28*:412–430, 1954.

Spain, D. M., Bradess, V. A., Tarter, R., and Matero, A.: Metaplasia of bronchial epithelium: effect of age, sex and smoking. J.A.M.A. *211*:1331–1334, 1970.

Spencer, H.: Pathology of the Lung. 2nd ed., New York, The Macmillan Co., 1968, pp. 778–869.

Spjut, H. J., Fier, D. J., and Ackerman, L. V.: Exfoliative cytology and pulmonary cancer. J. Thoracic Surg. *30*:90–107, 1955.

Sternberg, W. H., Sidrausky, H., and Ochsner, S.: Primary malignant lymphomas of lung. Cancer *12*:806–819, 1959.

Talamo, R. C., Blennerhassett, J. B., and Austin, K. F.: Familial emphysema and alpha anti-trypsin deficiency. New Eng. J. Med. *275*:1301–1304, 1966.

Talbott, J. H.: Alpha-1-antitrypsin deficiency emphysema. J.A.M.A. *210*:1094–1095, 1969.

Thurlbeck, W. M.: Pulmonary emphysema. Amer. J. Med. Sci. *246*:332–353, 1963.

Titus, J. L., Harrison, E. G., Clagett, O. T., Anderson, M. W., and Knaff, L. J.: Xanthomatous and inflammatory pseudotumors of the lung. Cancer *15*:522–538, 1962.

Toker, C.: Carcinoid adenoma of bronchus. Cancer *19*:1943–1948, 1966.

Turkington, R. W., Goldman, J. K., Ruffner, B. W., and Dobson, J. L.: Bronchiogenic carcinoma simulating hyperparathyroidism. Cancer *19*:406–414, 1966.

Ventura, J., and Domaradzki, M.: Pathogenesis of experimental bronchiectasis in laboratory rats. Arch. Path. *83*:80–85, 1967.

Vincent, T. N., Satterfield, J. V., and Ackerman, L. V.: Carcinoma of the lung in women. Cancer *18*:559–570, 1965.

Warner, R. R. P., Kirschner, P. A., and Warner, G. M.: Serotonin production by bronchial adenomas without carcinoid syndrome. J.A.M.A. *178*:1175–1179, 1961.

Watson, W. L., and Farpour, A.: Terminal bronchiolar or "alveolar cell" cancer of the lung. Cancer *19*:776–780, 1966.

Weiss, L., and Ingram, M.: Adenomatoid bronchial tumors. Cancer *14*:161–178, 1961.

Wenzel, F. J., Emanuel, D. A., and Zygowicz, P. M.: Simplified serologic test for farmers' lung. Amer. J. Clin. Path. *49*:183–185, 1968.

Whitwell, F.: Tumourlets of lung. J. Path. Bact. *70*:529–541, 1955.

Wigger, H. J., and Blanc, W. A.: Fatal hepatic and bronchial necrosis in adenovirus infection with thymic alymphoplasia. New Eng. J. Med. *275*:870–874, 1966.

Williams, E. D., and Azzopardi, J. G.: Tumors of lung and the carcinoid syndrome. Thorax *15*:30–36, 1960.

Winter, L. E.: Multiple primary carcinomas of the airways. Arch. Otolaryng. *83*:468–471, 1966.

Zarocostas, G.: An interesting case of tracheal stenosis. Laryngoscope *76*:555–560, 1966.

Zizmor, J., Naiberg, D., and Noyek, A. M.: Tracheobronchiomegaly: A case report. Arch. Otolaryng. *82*:294–295, 1965.

Zunker, H. O., Moore, R. L., Baker, D. C., and Lattes, R.: Adenoid cystic carcinoma of the trachea. Cancer *23*:699–707, 1969.

Section Seven

SURGICAL PRINCIPLES OF OTOLARYNGOLOGY

Chapter 21

FLUIDS AND ELECTROLYTES

by Donald G. McQuarrie, M.D., Ph.D.

Most otolaryngology patients pose no problem in maintenance of fluid and electrolyte balance. This is a mixed blessing. The rarity of a severe fluid problem simplifies the working day, but it tends to produce a complacency which will lead to unquestioning, stereotyped fluid management.

Fixed-formula fluid orders will result in an occasional iatrogenic misadventure which poises the unfortunate victim in an unnecessarily precarious position. If salvage is accomplished, it is time-consuming and expensive in terms of hospital costs but, most importantly, it can start a chain of complications which eventuate in death long after the patient is "in balance."

The "trick" is not to employ dazzling therapeutics in the salvage of a disaster. The ideal is to understand the underlying physiology, to recognize the patients who require more alert management, to balance the patient's fluids and electrolytes from the beginning of your care and, finally, to learn to deal with those established fluid and electrolyte problems which may be presented to you. These are the broad aims of this chapter. Space does not allow an encyclopedic discussion. The references at the end of the chapter were selected for pragmatic clinical usefulness and can fill in the many vacancies.

BODY FLUID COMPARTMENTS AND FACTORS INFLUENCING ELECTROLYTE DISTRIBUTION

Body Water

Body metabolism is carried out in an aqueous medium with a dynamic steady-state balance rigidly controlling the pH and the electrolyte distribution. The amount of water in each individual varies with the fat content of his body.

The soft lean tissues of the body have a water content of about 73 per cent. The rest of the body consists of bone and nonaqueous fat. In looking at patients one should develop the habit of estimating total body water at 45 to 50 per cent of body weight in the rotund fat female. Estimates should be adjusted upward in the lean young man to about 70 per cent of body weight as water. A loss of 4 L. of body water in a short, fat, 80-kg. person is proportionately more serious than the same loss in an 80-kg. lean, muscular individual.

The total body water is distributed into a number of compartments. The size of these compartments has been estimated by using various chemical substances with radioactive tags which are distributed in, and confined to, certain physiologic spaces. The approximate measurements are listed in Table 1. When the tracer is uniformly distributed to a particular space, the volume of distribution is determined by the general formula:

$$\text{Volume distribution} = \frac{(\text{Amount of tag given}) - (\text{quantity excreted})}{\text{Concentration}}$$

The values given in Table 1 may vary since authors differ in what is included in extracellular water. Some earlier tables include transcellular water, which embraces cerebrospinal fluid, intraocular, pleural, and peritoneal contents, the secretions of the salivary and digestive glands, and the fluid in the alimentary tract. Identification of this space is important since equilibration rates may be slow. In cer-

TABLE 1. *Distribution of Body Water*

COMPARTMENT	% OF TOTAL BODY WATER	AGENT USED FOR ESTIMATION
Total body water	100	DHO, THO, Antipyrine
Intracellular water	55	Difference between total body water and extracellular water
Extracellular water	35	Inulin, SO_4^-, Cl^-, Br^-
ECW = { Plasma volume	7.5	T1824, ^{131}I albumin
Interstitial fluid	27.5	Difference between extracellular water and plasma volume
Inaccessible bone water	7.5	Special techniques
Transcellular water	2.5	Special techniques

tain medical and surgical conditions there can be a massive enlargement of the transcellular space with an associated depletion of the active and circulating components of the extracellular volume.

Electrolyte Distribution

The simplest and most reasonable way to express electrolyte concentrations in body fluids and exogenously administered solutions is in terms of milliequivalents/liter. The relation between *milliequivalents* and *millimoles* is simple. A *mole* is the atomic weight of a substance in grams. An *equivalent* weight can be described as the atomic weight of a substance divided by its valence. A *milliequivalent* is simply 1/1000 of this amount. The conceptual convenience in relating the milliequivalent concentration of body fluid electrolytes is clear. If an ion is univalent, an equivalent is the same as a mole, or 1 milliequivalent equals a millimole. However, if an ion is bivalent, such as calcium, 1 mole equals 2 equivalents, and 1 millimole equals 2 milliequivalents.

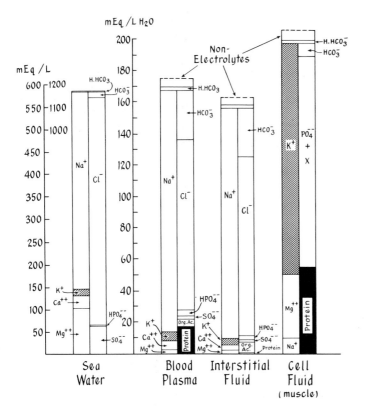

Figure 1. This diagram redrawn from Gamble shows the electrolyte composition of plasma, interstitial fluid and muscle. The assumption is made that the intracellular constituents exist in an aqueous phase.

The solute composition of the aqueous phases of the body has been estimated in various ways. For working clinical purposes, present-day estimates *are* quite good, and the composition is shown in Figure 1. In the purest sense, our present views require that certain assumptions be made in tracer substance distribution, and even larger assumptions must be made when disease states are considered. It is probably fair to assume that not all intracellular fluid is the same. Such a condition as potassium depletion does not affect the intracellular compartment of liver as much as it does skeletal muscle. Since muscle is over 87 per cent of the lean parenchymal cell mass and since it is affected more in nutritional and electrolyte imbalance, it is chosen as the representative of the cellular electrolyte composition. In examining Figure 1 the striking similarity of our internal aqueous environment to sea water becomes apparent. The hypertonicity (445 mEq. Na$^+$) as well as the magnesium and sulfate levels would prevent a tolerable equilibration of the human organism to sea water.

The plasma and interstitial fluid have Na$^+$ as their chief anion, while K$^+$ constitutes the principal anion of the intracellular environment. How body water and solutes are distributed between the interstitial space, plasma, and cells is dependent on a series of equilibria determined by osmotic pressure, hydrostatic events, molecular diffusion, Gibbs-Donnan equilibrium, active cellular transport, and renal exchange mechanisms.

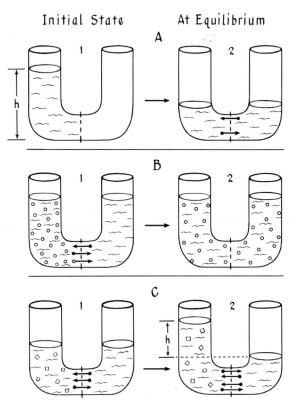

Figure 2. A diagrammatic simplification of osmotic equilibria across a semipermeable membrane. Diffusible solute is represented by open circles and nondiffusible solute is shown as open squares, See text for explanation.

OSMOLALITY AS A CONCEPT

If two compartments are separated by a membrane which is permeable only to water, and if one compartment is then filled with water, a state of equilibrium will soon be reached (Fig. 2 *A*). At equilibrium there will be equal motion of water molecules from side to side over any one period of time. If a freely permeable solute is added to one side (Fig. 2 *B*), it will distribute itself through both compartments in a short interval of time. As a result, the partial molal volume of water will have been decreased; hence, the activity of the water molecules will have been decreased, and fewer water molecules will move from one compartment to another in a unit of time. If a solute which cannot traverse the membrane is added to one side, as in Figure 2 *C*-1, the activity of the water molecules on the left side is reduced by an amount proportionate to the

molal concentration of the impermeable solute. As a result, more water molecules will move to the left than to the right. This will produce the situation seen in Figure 2 *C*-2. Water will enter the chamber on the left hand side of the membrane until a hydrostatic pressure is developed. The pressure increases the molecular activity of the water at the membrane level, which forces water in the reverse direction. The pressure developed in the column of our hydrostatic model at equilibrium is a measure of osmotic pressure (the pressure of the column marked h). The difference in osmotic pressure of two solutions may be defined as the pressure that must be imposed on one solution to bring the activity of the molecules of water to the same level as in the other solution.

Osmotic forces are important in the fluid equilibria in the body. In clinical circumstances membrane premeability varies, solute concentrations are disturbed by therapy, and active transport may be rate-limited in restoring the desired balance. A practical example might be seen in a patient who is overhydrated,

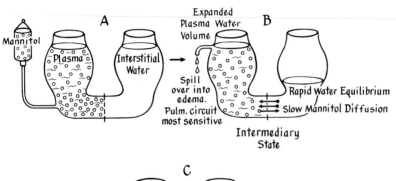

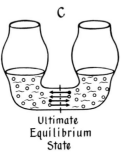

Figure 3. The effect of varying diffusion rate of water and mannitol across the capillary membrane. The chamber on the left represents the vascular space and the chamber on the right represents the interstitial space. See text for explanation.

with renal failure and compromised cardiac reserve. When a "well meaning" dose of mannitol is given as an osmotic diuretic, the mannitol penetrates many body compartments at a rate slower than water. In this instance we see first (Fig. 3 *A*) that the slowly diffusible solute is added to the circulating plasma volume, reducing the molecular activity of plasma water. As a result, more water is added to the plasma from the extravascular space than leaves. In the intermediary state (Fig. 3 *B*) plasma volume has expanded to a threatening degree before significant diffusion of the solute has taken place. The ultimate equilibrium (Fig. 3 *C*) will be reached many hours later if the patient survives the misadventure. In planning fluid therapy, consideration must be given to the types of fluids given and the forces which will distribute them in the body.

Volume Equilibrium

Osmotic activity is one of the factors participating in the distribution of water in the familiar concept outlined by Ernest Starling in 1896 to describe the forces which refill the vascular space after hemorrhage. This concept is outlined in Figure 4 as a refresher and should need no further review.

Ionic Equilibrium

The distribution of diffusible ions is maintained by active membrane transport of ions and **passively** and actively by the Gibbs-Donnan equilibrium. Gibbs-Donnan ratio stems from a simple thermodynamic rule enunciated by J. Willard Gibbs, the great American physicist and father of chemical thermodynamics, that the product of the concentration of any pair of diffusible cations and anions on one side of a membrane is equal to the product of the same pair of ions on the other side. For example:

$$Na^-_{(plasma)} \times Cl^-_{(plasma)} = Na^+_{(ISF)} \times Cl^-_{(ISF)}$$

This expression would be true if only these ions existed alone in an aqueous solution. However, we see in Figure 1 that plasma contains significant amounts of protein (P^-), which has negatively charged end groups. Hence, to

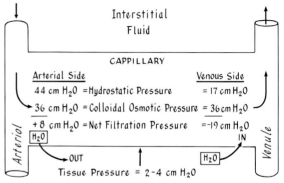

Figure 4. The concept outlined by Starling in 1896 to explain fluid movement across capillaries. The values are approximate estimates and may vary considerably in disease states.

ceptors, possibly
nary veins. Hemc
a powerful stimul
ing to the best
allows the distal
ing tubule to bec
allowing water
dients into the h
stitium. In the tot
ic urine in the r
made. Three hyp
ADH action: Fi
of hyaluronidase
bule membrane.
tor sites to open
acts with adeny
from ADP, proc
known mechanis
port all three the
In man a sec
one, significantly
ance. A small d
into an experim
antidiuresis afte
enhances sodi
increased potas
tion. The distal
regulatory influc
It has been th
ADH release a
lowing head and
but are very tra
thoracic or abd
evidence is sc
prolonged anti
retention.
For an exte
tion, see one
at the end of t

CLINICAL
PROBLEM

So far this
physiologic pc
some significa
would be to a
agement probl
an otolaryngo
cause problen
who impairs tl
discover "tut
natremic deh)
er extreme, a
with deglutiti
mor may be

maintain electrical neutrality, some of the sodium ions must be associated with the protein.

Hence the osmotic concentrations are shown at the bottom of this page. However, the product remains the same.

In the body the osmolar concentration is slightly greater in the protein-containing side, which increases the osmotic pressure (Fig. 1). The Gibbs-Donnan ratio is really not too great. It is 100 (plasma)/95 (ISF) for cations and 100 (plasma)/105 (ISF) for anions.

Active Transport

A more powerful force in distributing ions between body spaces is active membrane transport. Active transport of Cl^- and K^+ have been considered. Active transport of H^+ in the stomach and kidneys is well known. Nevertheless, it is the "sodium pump" which is the chief determinant of fluid space electrolyte composition. When you consider *how* ions are moved across a membrane against a concentration gradient, one is safe in saying "the manner whereby the cellular and extracellular fluids maintain their major compositional differences is poorly understood, and is currently under investigation." No matter whether you think of sodium being excluded from cells by "little red demons" or by ATP-powered lipoprotein reversing layers, it must be remembered that sodium is not completely excluded from cells, and the quantity of Na^+ in cells may increase with injury and disease, especially with marked nutritional wasting. Maintenance of a differential gradient requires metabolic energy.

The total exchangeable Na^+ in the body is 40 mEq./kg., or about 2800 mEq. in an adult. A large part of this is extracellular. With potassium, the total exchangeable K^+ is about 47 mEq./kg., or about 3200 mEq. About 98 per cent of this K^+ resides in the lean tissue mass, most of which is striated muscle. Since only 60 mEq. of the 3200 mEq. of K^+ is found in the extracellular fluid it is not surprising that serum K^+ determinations are a poor estimate of normalcy or depletion of total body K^+.

ACID-BASE REGULATION

The fundamentals of the acid-base regulation in the body fluids are clearly put forth in Davenport's classic small monograph, "The A.B.C. of Acid-Base Chemistry," and other texts. A few short paragraphs can only emphasize several clinically salient points. First, pH is a *logarithmic* expression of hydrogen ion concentration. A change of one pH unit actually represents a tenfold change in hydrogen ion concentration. Alteration of the pH by 0.3 units from the original pH doubles or halves the hydrogen ion concentration. Raising the pH from 7.10 to 7.40 requires that twice as many hydrogen ions be removed as when changing the pH from 7.40 to 7.70, although the pH interval is 0.3 in both instances. See Table 2.

In the management of the acid end products of metabolism, the body has only two routes of excretion, the kidneys and the lungs. Under normal conditions, carbonic acid and water are the usual end products of caloric production. In terms of quantity of excretion, the lungs of an average adult excrete over 800 mM. of carbon dioxide per day. Although renal mechanisms make minor but important quantitative adjustments so that the ratio HCO_3^-/H_2CO_3 which is normally 20:1 is minimally altered, HCO_3^- alone or pH alone is not adequate to determine the clinical status of a patient. Two of the three factors in the Henderson-Hasselbalch equation must be known to appraise a patient's acid-base status. This is commonly done by knowing the blood pH and the pCO_2 of arterial plasma.

An alternative common method is to derive the values from accurately determined pH of the patient's blood equilibrated with two differ-

TABLE 2. Hydrogen Ion Concentration

Difference = 40 mμ moles	7.10 7.20 7.30 7.40	= = = =	80 63 50 40	Nano equivalents/L.
Difference = 20 mμ moles	7.50 7.60 7.70	= = =	32 25 20	

$$\left.\begin{array}{l}[Na^+]_{(Plasma)} + [Cl^-]_{(Plasma)} \\ [Na^+]_{(Excess)} + [P^-]\end{array}\right\} = [Na^+]_{ISF} + [Cl^-]_{ISF}$$

ent gas mixtur
of CO_2 (Astru
There are tl
neys can adju
residue.

Conservatio
proximal tubι
from the tubι
leaving H^+ H
bule. Carbon
back into the
for reuse. "B
reconstitution
molecular HC

Phosphate
most of the ti
maximum pH
cells can excl
in the tubule.
hydrogen pho
(at a ratio of !
the mono to t
of 1:160 mor

Ammonia
formed from
in the distal t
tubule lumen
to produce
$(NH_3 + H^+ $
cess of ammc
ly available
takes several
subsides slov
not availabl
increase in a
a period of ε

RENAL

The classi
1935 showe
dium, becaι
almost exclι
regulator of
neys work
plasma whic
of body wa
largely dep(
operate in t
volume and
average day
may lose a:
routes. Wit
kidneys wil
170,000 ml
glomeruli. (

mon cause of a problem is the unthinking application of a "formula" to the "routine" fluid orders hastily written on morning rounds. A "routine" order for a postoperative patient with moderate mitral stenosis may be something like "2500 cc. D5W with 75 mEq. NaCl per liter and 20 ml. KCl per liter." This is topped off with a dash of some vitamin preparation containing ascorbic acid, and the fluid for the day is started without the physician's cerebral cortex having once been stirred by the process. Yet if you told the same physician that you were ordering a diet containing 12 Gm. of salt for this same patient with mitral heart disease, he would have fits of consternation. Having some secure "formula" or "routine order" to cling to seems to prevent any thinking about the patient's particular problems.

The most significant step which can be made in acquiring skills in fluid and electrolyte management is to recognize what peculiarities a patient may present which make *that* patient different from any other patient. One useful way of individualizing management is to use a fluid balance sheet. Much like music when you have practiced it long enough, the sheet itself is no longer necessary and a rational method of thinking is established. A format which I have found useful is shown in Figure 6. As seen in the figure, it can be constructed on any sheet of lined paper. Coupled with a few simple estimates of the electrolyte composition of the body fluids which may be lost, intelligent esti-

mates can be made of net change. For information, a brief table (Table 4) is added as adapted from Gamble's data. These daily estimates can be revised on the basis of laboratory determinations. In the patient with normal renal function and no complications, a number of assumptions can be made which simplify management. As we noted before, potassium excretion in the urine is relatively independent of volume and amounts to about 40 to 50 mEq. per day. Modest excesses of K^+ are well tolerated and excreted in the urine with no adverse effects. Unless the patient is secreting large amounts of acid gastric juice, you may estimate H^+ and Na^+ to be about equal in nasogastric (NG) suction. One must be alert for such ambiguities as may arise when an NG tube is threaded into the duodenum. The presence of bile in NG returns suggests that Na^+ content may be higher as a result of the presence of duodenal secretions in the aspirate.

For most practical purposes Na^+ and Cl^- content of the urine can be estimated at about 50-60 mEq./L. of each, recognizing that the Na^+ may be minimal during the time of aldosterone effect in the immediate postoperative period. On the other hand, it may be massive with salt loading.

Insensible water loss increases as body temperature increases. Osmotic work for the production of perspiration begins at about 100° F. It is hard to estimate the effect of the ambient ward environment, except by the physician's own response. A rule of thumb which is accu-

Fluid	DAY #1				DAY #2				DAY #3				DAY #4			
	VOLUME	Na	K	Cl	VOLUME	Na	K	Cl	VOLUME	Na	K	Cl	VOLUME	Na	K	Cl
INSENSIBLE	1000	-	-	-												
URINE	1500	90	40	90												
NASOGASTRIC	750	45	10	70												
T: Tube	500	75	5	50												
ILIOSTOMY	250	35	5	25												
TOTAL FLUID LOSS	4000	245	60	235												
TOTAL FLUID GIVEN	3000	225	60	285												
NET DIFFERENCE	-1000	-20	0	+50												
LAB VALUES	WT 165 Na 135 Cl 101 K 4.5 HCO₃ 25															

Figure 6. This crude figure is shown to emphasize that it is not necessary to have a fancy sheet in order to maintain a complex balance sheet for a patient. With only a minimum of effort, complex problems can be reduced to simpler management. For added precision in adults and children, it can be added up every 12 hours, instead of every 24 hours. If there is a question of sodium or potassium loss for any of the fluids, aliquots can be sent to the lab for accurate analysis of electrolyte content.

TABLE 4. Electrolyte Composition of Intestinal Secretions

		Na	K	Cl
Gastric	Average	59.0	9.3	89
(Fasting)	Range	6–157	0.5–65	13–167
	⅔ cases	31– 90	4.3–12	52–124
Small bowel	Average	105	5	100
(Miller Abbot)	Range	20–157	1–11	43–156
	⅔ cases	72–128	3.5–68	69–127
Ilium	Average	116	5	105
(Miller Abbot)	Range	82–147	2–8	60–137
	⅔ cases	91–140	3–7.5	82–125
Ileostomy	Average	129	16.2	110
(Recent)	Range	92–146	3.8–98	66–136
	⅔ cases	112–142	4.5–14.0	93–122
Bile	Average	145	5.2	100
	Range	122–164	3.2–9.7	77–127
	⅔ cases	134–156	3.9–6.3	83–110
Pancreas	Average	141	4.6	79
(3 patients)	Range	113–153	2.6–74	54–95

rate enough for most practical purposes is that an average healthy afebrile 70 kg. man will lose about 600 ml. of insensible water per day with no significant electrolyte content. A tracheostomy may reduce this slightly. Being on a respirator with full humidity will further reduce insensible water loss to under 200 ml./day. Insensible loss by sweating may be increased about 500 ml./24 hours for each degree of fever. (This presumes the temperature is constant over the 24 hours. A mental integration of the area under the temperature curve can be made to arrive at an estimate.) When active osmotic work is done by the sweat glands, the sodium and chloride content of sweat is in the range of 50 mEq./L. All these little generalities are nice for the uncomplicated adult patient. However, there are a number of problems which may occur on an ENT service which require more than average vigilance. I have tried to select several instances which seem to pose the most frequent problems in otolaryngology patients. Reviewing the physiology of these problems may serve as a stimulus to reduce the occurrence of such errors and to pursue a study of other problem areas.

THE NUTRITIONALLY DEPRIVED

It is not uncommon to have to operate upon a thin, wasted patient giving a history of 20 to 30 pound weight loss. Significant weight loss will follow impairment of deglutition in the oropharynx, esophageal obstruction, protracted sepsis, and numerous other disease entities. As the patient is first studied, a chronically low serum sodium level may be a prominent feature. Unlike acute dilutional hyponatremia, serum sodium levels in this chronic state are relatively well tolerated even when the serum sodium hovers around 125 mEq/L. The dangers of management come from a narrow-minded focus on the serum sodium alone. The inexperienced person will follow a reasoning cycle of: "low sodium $\rightarrow$ give concentrated saline or salt." This eventuates in edema and further complication of a debilitated state. The problem is more complex. The real question is, "Why is the extracellular sodium low?" In chronic starvation with weight loss, the energy sources must come from some fat and the lean body mass. The total body cell mass is depleted; both intracellular and extracellular protein are lost with depletion. Since intracellular protein contributes a significant portion of the *intracellular* osmotic activity, the total osmotic activity of the extracellular and intracellular environment is decreased. Figures for such a typical patient might reveal the following: Fat equal to less than 10% of body weight

Serum Na$^+$ = 130 to 135 mEq./L.
Increased extracellular water
Increased intracellular water

Total body water = 80% of the lean body mass when normally it should be about 70%

Osmolality of plasma = 259 mOsm/L, when normal is about 290 mOsm.

Total body potassium = 32 to 35 mEq./kg. (exchangeable K) when the normal is about 45 to 47 mEq./kg.

Hyponatremia, *by itself*, will impair the kidney's ability to secrete a water load. Exogenously administered Na^+ will distribute largely in the extracellular water. Since the body osmolality is determined in this instance by the osmolality of the cell, there will be an osmotic balance re-established by water leaving the cell. This will expand the extracellular fluid volume. If the amount of Na^+ is sizeable, edema will be produced and the serum sodium will still be low. Treatment of this chronic low-sodium state is to restore a positive nitrogen balance by establishing alimentation, by parenteral supplementation, or by controlling septic processes.

ACUTE WATER INTOXICATION

This is seen most commonly in the postoperative period either alone or in conjunction with some nutritional impairment. This problem requires the intervention of medical personnel for its production. In the postoperative period, vasopressin levels in the blood go from resting values of 2-5 μg./ml. to as high as 50-150 μg./ml. following a major operative procedure. ADH causes increased permeability of the distal tubule with the resultant transfer of water into the medullary interstitium. ADH levels usually stay elevated for 24 to 72 hours postoperatively following a major procedure such as a gastrectomy. There are no direct data of the ADH blood levels following oral and cervical surgical procedures. It has been the author's impression that hypertonicity of the urine usually fades by 48 hours after major ablative oropharyngeal and cervical surgery.

Clinical problems occur when a large water load is given to the debilitated patient while there is a significant ADH effect and the kidneys are unable to excrete the water load. Acute water intoxication is most commonly seen between 12 and 48 hours after surgery. When serum sodium is acutely lowered to 125-115 mEq./L., rapidly changing stupor, mental confusion, irrationality, and even generalized seizures may occur. One sure way of lowering the epileptic seizure threshold is to administer vasopressin and give water. In this circumstance body water is acutely diluted and osmolality is reduced.

Management is by one of two modes: First, give hypertonic sodium. This can be tolerated in a young, vigorous patient, but in an elderly patient with marginal cardiopulmonary reserve, an acute massive expansion of vascular fluid volume results. The second and more desirable method is water restriction. Water intoxication arises in the operating room and in the initial postoperative orders. Sensible fluid orders can prevent it.

Early Recognition of Acute Renal Failure

Therapeutic misadventures with excess water loads, excessive Na^+ administration, and acute pulmonary edema are frequently a result of a faulty recognition of renal failure. Given a postoperative patient with oliguria, there are usually no good preoperative data on renal function (such as creatinine clearance). The pattern of disaster is typical. The patient is brought into the hospital before surgery for workup and diagnostic tests over a period of several days and nights and given nothing by mouth. The night of surgery he is kept on nothing by mouth and given no supplementary hydration. He may receive variable amounts of fluid during surgery. Postoperative oliguria is noted. A misguided enthusiast gives 3 to 4 L. of fluids on the day of the patient's surgery with no results. This can be followed by a 500 ml. water "flush" and topped off by mannitol or, even worse, a mercurial diuretic. All these trial-and-error methods are followed in an attempt to distinguish between acute tubular damage, ADH effect, simple dehydration, inadequate circulating blood volume, and chronic marginal renal function. By the time a clear answer is obtained, the patient has a fluid overload of 4 to 6 L. What is a better approach? First, the clinical history: Try to pick out the patients with previous diseases suggesting renal involvement, i.e., pyelonephritis, diabetes, obstructive uropathy. Recognize those patients in whom there is a higher risk of renal damage as a result of blood loss, bacteremia, hypotensive episodes, and so forth. When oliguria is noted, the differentiation between dehydration or ADH effect and acute tubular necrosis is relatively simple. First of all, with simple dehydration there is maximal water conservation by functioning renal tubules. A serum osmolality will be normal or slightly elevated. A serum sodium will be normal to elevated. Urine osmolality will be high—usually 600-900 mOsm./L.—a clear separation between the concentrated urine and serum values. With acute tubular necrosis from any cause the tubules do no osmotic work on the small amount of urine which is formed. Hence, it has the same osmolar values as an ultrainfiltrate of plasma, i.e., about 300 mOsm./L. In the example of the water-loaded patient with oliguria, the serum sodium gives a clue. In a nondebilitated patient a dilution of the extracellular water resulting from failure of free water excretion is reflected in a lowered serum Na as well as a lowered osmolality.

Urine specific gravity is useful only when its many shortcomings are known. In acute tubular necrosis the specific gravity will be in the range of 1.010 *only* if no sugar is cleared, if there has been no evaporation of the specimen, if mannitol has not been given, if no dextran has been given, or if there is no proteinuria or hemoglobinuria. After administration of mannitol or dextran specific gravity can be 1.040+ in the face of acute tubular necrosis. If there is a question of acute tubular damage, check the osmolalities. Modern apparatus has made this a simple determination which is available in most larger hospitals.

What steps can be taken to prevent acute tubular necrosis? First, avoid dehydration. Many studies have shown that the hydrated secreting tubule is less susceptible to the damage of transient hypoxemia and reduced renal blood flow. The patient scheduled for a major procedure should arrive in the operating room with an established water diuresis. Second, recognize and treat bacteremic episodes promptly. Third, treat hypotension promptly. Finally, when oliguria occurs, arrive at a definitive diagnosis early and begin active management before a patient has been pushed to pulmonary edema. Many times a patient can be managed without dialysis through a period of tubular recovery *if* he has not had a fluid overload.

TUBE FEEDING PITFALLS

When a patient is unable to swallow and requires all feeding by gastrostomy or by a Levine tube, an unusual circumstance is established in which his internal environment is at the mercy of the intellect of his attending physician. He is unable to respond to thirst by drinking water. It should be unnecessary for every physician to discover iatrogenic hyper-osmolar, hypernatremic dehydration for himself.

The normal adult on a 2000 calorie diet excretes about 60 gm. of solid per day, which corresponds roughly to 1200 mOsm. of solute. The load can be sharply increased if the diet is high in sodium. Thirty grams of urea will contribute about 500 mOsm., in which 30 gm. of NaCl would contribute about 1200 mOsm. per L. A rough calculation of solid load which a patient is receiving can be made from the following:

$$\frac{\text{Last 2 figures of specific gravity at 25° C.}}{1000} \times (2.6) \times \frac{\text{24 hour urine vol.}}{}$$

$$= \text{Total solids in gm./day}$$

When specific gravity is 1.020 and urine volume is 1000 the solids amount to: (gm./24 hrs.) $= 20 \times 2.6 \times \frac{1000}{1000} = 52$ gm.

The figures in textbooks suggesting a maximum urine concentration to 1400 mOsm./L. with water deprivation were obtained on healthy adults. In children the maximum urinary concentration may approach only 800 mOsm./L. Similarly, older hospitalized patients rarely show an ability to concentrate above 800 mOsm./L.

When high calorie liquid feedings are given to an adult in the concentration of 1 calorie per ml., a 2000 calorie diet is contained in much less than 1800 ml. of water, even when the 300 ml. of water of combustion is added. Insensible water loss then uses 500 to 600 ml. of water. This leaves 1200 ml. of water to excrete the obligatory osmotic load. Assuming a maximum ADH effect, and no further aggravation of free water loss by hypotonic sweating, this would allow urine excretion at about 1000 mOsm. per L. This degree of concentration can be achieved only with excellent kidney function. The problem can be aggravated further with tube feedings having a higher solute load because of the use of partially hydrolyzed products, soluble carbohydrates, and more electrolytes. The usual 2000 calorie, high protein tube feeding produces about 1200 mOsm. of solute which must be excreted. Heavier calorie loads will push the osmotic load higher. It can be seen that if the osmotic load is high and the ability to concentrate urine is limited, there will be a deficit of water which must be made up from the total body water, both intracellular and extracellular. Clinically the patient usually loses weight, becomes comatose and somnolent. Muscle weakness supervenes. Oral and respiratory mucous membranes are desiccated. Cough and respiration are impaired. Even if the condition is recognized, the patient is already in severe jeopardy. The most usual complication is pneumonia. *Prevention of the problem is the key to therapy.* When the patient is unable to augment his water needs by oral intake, adequate water volume must be provided with the feedings. Two approaches are satisfactory: First, never give tube feedings over 1/2 calorie per ml., or, second, give enough plain water by gastrostomy or tube (or IV as 5 per cent dextrose in water) to produce a net water excess; usually this is a volume approximately equal to the concentrated 1 calorie/ml. feeding. When there is a question, keep urine under 500 mOsm./L. An understanding of this simple problem can prevent the frequently lethal complications which follow pushing a serum sodium to 165 mEq./L.

A second problem follows the use of concentrated tube feedings, and this is a simple osmotic diarrhea. When over 50 per cent of tube feeding calories are present as small carbohydrate molecules, they represent a large hyperosmolar load placed in the intestine. As the feeding is osmotically equilibrated by water transport into the gut, there is an intraluminal volume expansion. Thus, the carbohydrate, electrolyte, and other compounds act just as a saline cathartic, stimulating increased peristalsis and visceral emptying before balanced absorption is complete. The net effect is water, sodium, and bicarbonate loss as well as failure of nutritional absorption of the food introduced into the gastrointestinal tract. Again, the management consists of making these feedings nearer the osmolarity of body fluids, or making the feeding from more slowly hydrolyzed foodstuffs so that osmotic equilibration can occur slowly.

PATIENTS WHO RETAIN SALT AND WATER

The response of surgical patients to trauma by excretion of aldosterone is magnified in several conditions; two examples are cirrhosis of the liver and congestive heart failure. The more sensitive patients are those with rheumatic valvular disease of the left heart.

In the cirrhotic patient, particularly those with ascites, there is much empirical data and a confusion of opinion. The term "hepatorenal syndrome" has been used to place the patient in a category without explaining mechanisms. The cirrhotic patient's predilection to retain

salt and water can stem from lowered plasma colloidal osmotic pressure, increased antidiuretic activity, altered permeability of membranes, and altered tubular sodium resorption associated with increased aldosterone secretion. The fact is, sodium is retained. It produces an iso-osmolar expansion of extracellular volume. There is probably some "secondary" aldosteronism resulting from an inability of the damaged liver to inactivate circulating aldosterone.

The second large group of patients who require vigilance in management are those who have congestive heart failure, who have had it in the past, or who have such marginal cardiac reserve that they can be crowded easily to congestive failure by minimal blood volume expansion. Several factors may be operating to produce the salt and water retention. These factors are diagrammed in Figure 7.

In the patient with congestive heart failure there is a total body excess of sodium. This sodium may be within cells as well as in the extracellular fluid. There may also be a deficit of cell potassium. Which of the several mechanisms (Fig. 7) is dominant is uncertain. Nevertheless, the practical message is clear—more sodium is retained in a patient with congestive failure, and an excess sodium load is not excreted so well.

As stated earlier, the purpose of this chapter is to produce an awareness not only of areas of

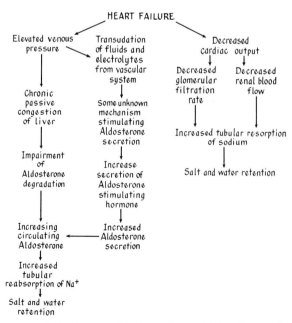

Figure 7. A theoretic scheme for explaining decreased capacity to excrete sodium by people with heart failure. Any or all of these mechanisms may be operating.

clinical problems, but also the physiologic mechanisms that may underlie empiric fluid and electrolyte management. Discussions have been presented only to illustrate the necessity of tailoring management to each patient's needs. Even so brief a chapter can point to some of the more interesting concepts and problems and suggest additional source materials.

REFERENCES

Davenport, H. W.: The A.B.C. of Acid-Base Chemistry. 4th ed. Chicago, University of Chicago Press, 1958.

Drucker, W. R., and Wright, H. K.: Physiology and pathophysiology of gastrointestinal fluids. Curr. Probl. Surg., May, 1964.

Gamble, J. L.: Chemical Anatomy, Physiology, and Pathology of Extracellular Fluid. Cambridge, Harvard University Press, 1964.

Hill, F. S.: Practical Fluid Therapy in Pediatrics. Philadelphia, W. B. Saunders Company, 1954.

Moore, F. D.: Metabolic Care of the Surgical Patient. Philadelphia, W. B. Saunders Company, 1959.

Muntwyler, E.: Water and Electrolyte Metabolism and Acid-Base Balance. St. Louis, The C. V. Mosby Co., 1968.

Pitts, R. F.: The Physiologic Basis of Diuretic Therapy. Springfield, Charles C Thomas, 1959.

Zimmerman, B.: Postoperative management of fluid volumes and electrolytes. Curr. Probl. Surg., Dec., 1965.

Chapter 22

WOUND HEALING

by Thomas K. Hunt, M.D.

Repair and regeneration are processes fundamental to life. Without them surgery could not be done. Contributions to the understanding of repair during the past two centuries, such as the discovery of antisepsis, have made modern surgery possible. A century ago surgeons had no choice but to accept open, infected wounds; however, since Lister's application of antisepsis, knowledge of the mechanism of healing has grown. Although the surgeon is not yet able to control healing, he now can at least modify it. The surgeon who has detailed knowledge of the reparative process will be able to influence healing to the benefit of his patient.

THE NATURE OF THE WOUND

"Wound" is a difficult word to define since many physiological events not ordinarily considered as part of "wounding" have properties similar to the classic incised injury. "Wound" might well be defined as any event which is followed by healing. Tissue changes consistent with healing are found in numerous conditions. Atheromata, for instance, are composed of fibrous tissue, and early in their evolution are indistinguishable from granulation tissue. The venous thrombus heals as it "organizes." "Healing" occurs around the scirrhous cancer of the breast, accounting for its hardness. The common denominators of all these processes are necrosis of cells, disturbance of tissue nutrition, and disruption of normal tissue architecture. These events are almost always followed by an increased permeability of local microvasculature, inflammation, collection of fibroblasts, fibroplasia, and regeneration of a local microcirculation.

What triggers inflammation and proliferation of fibroblasts is unknown. Menkin (1950) and several others have theorized that "wound hormones" exist, with specific actions of attracting white cells and causing vasodilatation, but the evidence is not conclusive. It seems possible that environmental conditions which exist after the disruption of tissue nutrition stimulate proliferation of fibroblasts. On the other hand, it is possible that the proteolysis which follows wounding releases low molecular weight peptides which may signal the need for a regenerative process. For example, bradykinin, a low molecular weight peptide which causes relaxation of smooth muscles and local vasodilatation, has been found in large quantities in burned tissue (Goodwin et al., 1963).

FORMS OF HEALING

It is customary to divide the types of healing into first, second, and third intentions. First intention healing is defined as normal healing following clean incision and reapproximation of tissue. Second intention healing occurs when an open wound is allowed to heal without approximation or suture of the edges but rather through the formation of granulation tissue* and eventual coverage (if the wound is on a surface) by migration of epidermal cells. Healing by third intention, a rarely used term, occurs when a wound is left to accomplish the

---

*Granulation tissue is the red, rather granular-appearing tissue which appears during healing of open wounds. Microscopically it is a mixture of new collagen, blood vessels, fibroblasts and macrophages.

first three to five days of healing while open and is then closed to finish healing as if by primary intent. This mechanism can be used clinically to avoid suppurative infection in contaminated wounds and is often the treatment of choice under these conditions. Closure of a wound by skin graft is also an example of third intention healing.

THE PHASES OF HEALING

It is customary to divide normal primary healing into three phases: the substrate phase, the proliferative phase, and the resorptive phase. These phases overlap and cannot be defined precisely. As our knowledge increases, the description of healing by "phases" becomes less satisfactory. Nevertheless, it is still the best division available.

Substrate Phase. The substrate phase occurs during the first three to five days after wounding, when the wounded tissue is prepared for subsequent healing. Damaged vascular structures thrombose, and plasma and lymph exude into the damaged area. Inflammation begins and dying tissue is lysed and removed. Mucopolysaccharides appear in a pattern typical of the wound. Collagen lysis, particularly the removal of pre-existing collagen, is apparently of great importance during these first few days.

Proliferative Phase. The proliferative phase begins as the first fibroblasts appear, which can be as soon as two days after wounding. Collagen synthesis can be detected shortly thereafter. By the fifth or sixth day many fibroblasts have appeared and collagen synthesis accelerates, hence the name proliferative phase. This rapid synthesis occurs until the end of the second or third week. During the first few days of the proliferative phase, which overlap the last days of the substrate phase, wound healing becomes something of a struggle between the lysis and the synthesis of collagen. It is at this time that any exaggeration of lysis of old collagen or delay or diminution of synthesis of new collagen can lead to dehiscence of the wound or leakage of an anastomosis (Fig. 1). If all goes well, however, tensile strength increases rapidly after five or six days and approaches the holding strength of the sutures by the end of the first week. Wounds in the gastrointestinal tract may, at this stage, be even stronger than normal tissue. However, wounds in skin fascia and tendons have gained only about 20 per cent of their ultimate strength. In the prolif-

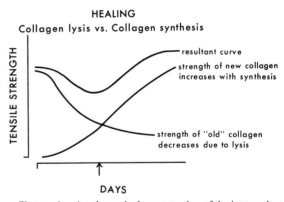

HEALING
Collagen lysis vs. Collagen synthesis

resultant curve
strength of new collagen increases with synthesis

strength of "old" collagen decreases due to lysis

TENSILE STRENGTH

DAYS

Figure 1. A schematic demonstration of the interaction of collagen synthesis and lysis. Pathological healing is likely to result if the synthesis curve is delayed (moved to the right) or if lysis is exaggerated and its curve is moved downward.

erative phase, the "healing ridge"* appears (Pareira and Serkes, 1962). Its absence may be the first sign of inadequate healing and impending wound disruption. The normal wound becomes slightly red and warm in about one week.

Resorptive Phase. In the final or resorptive phase the hyperplastic wound tissue, with its large numbers of fibroblasts, capillaries, and young collagen, starts to resorb, and the wound begins to resemble normal tissue more closely. The point which separates the proliferative and the differentiation phases might be defined as the point at which net accumulation of collagen ceases and net loss of collagen begins. The amorphous young collagen fibers gradually coalesce, become larger and longer, and intertwine with the original collagen fibers at the edges of the wound. The wound appears less active, but even though there is a net resorption of connective tissue, synthesis of collagen still occurs more rapidly than in normal tissue for approximately six months. Tensile strength increases despite the net resorption of connective tissue (Forrester et al., 1969). Wounds of the intestinal tract may be stronger than normal tissue at this time. However, in highly organized connective tissues in which strength is a fundamental property, the wound rarely reaches normal strength. Skin and fascia, for instance, regenerate to approximately 80 per cent of normal strength (Fig. 2). Mechanical properties, including elasticity, probably never return to normal (Forrester et al., 1969).

*The "healing ridge" is an indurated ridge along the wound deep to the skin and extending about 1 cm. on each side of the wound. Dehiscences tend to occur in wounds which have not developed this ridge along their entire length.

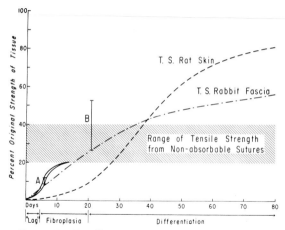

Figure 2. Tensile strength curve of a healing wound. The major portion of strength is regained after the first several weeks.

COMPONENTS OF REPAIR

The important components of healing are: (1) epithelization, (2) connective tissue regeneration and repair, and (3) wound contraction. All repair includes one or more of these processes. Connective tissue repair includes not only collagen and mucopolysaccharide synthesis but also vascular and lymphatic regeneration. Regeneration or hyperplasia of the existing cells of an organ may also occur to accommodate for the loss of cellular function in the damaged area. Liver and kidney are the prime examples of these processes in the human.

Epithelization. Epithelial cells at the edge of a wound proliferate and migrate. In primary healing, mitoses appear in the basal layer of the squamous cell epithelium a few days after the wounding, and the epithelial cells advance across the wound surface and into a favorable plane between dead and living tissue at the edge of the wound. The new epithelium is often thinner and less pigmented than normal.

Connective Tissue Regeneration. Connective tissue repairs and regenerates itself largely through the activity of the fibroblast. This is a large, plump cell liberally endowed with protein-synthesizing endoplasmic reticulum. Fibroblasts synthesize collagen and probably mucopolysaccharides as well (Dunphy, 1963). According to current theory, the fibroblast synthesizes the basic molecule of the collagen polymer, a long thin molecule 2890 by 14 Å. This molecule, or possibly its components (the single chains which eventually form the triple helix), are secreted into the extracellular fluid where they slowly polymerize to form large, strong, insoluble fibers (Fig. 3).

During the early stage of collagen synthesis, proline is incorporated into the growing polypeptide chain. After this chain is completed and separated from the ribosome, a fixed number of the proline molecules are converted to hydroxyproline by protocollagen hydroxylase. This vital step is essential to the synthesis of collagen (Udenfriend, 1966). Lysine is incorporated and hydroxylated in a similar manner. The reaction has certain obligatory requirements, including iron, ascorbic acid, alpha-keto-glutarate, and molecular (dissolved) oxygen. The hydroxylated molecules apparently are important in subsequent intramolecular bonding.

This suggests that severe iron deficiency, ascorbic acid deficiency, and states of local tissue hypoxia will interfere with healing. The literature confirms these predictions. Simple iron deficiency anemia in the adult, however, does not impair healing. Ascorbic acid and oxygen deficiencies are well known for their

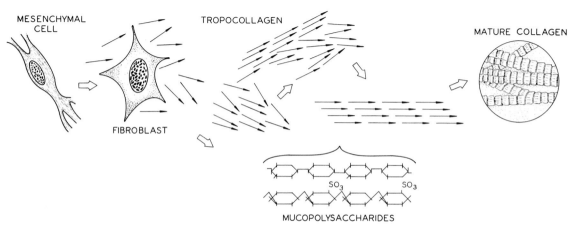

Figure 3. Diagrammatic representation of collagen synthesis and polymerization.

deleterious effects on healing (Dunphy, 1956; Hunt and Zederfeldt, 1969).

When the collagen molecule is finally assembled into its triple helix it is called "protocollagen." These molecules then polymerize to form the familiar collagen fiber. Adjacent molecules overlap approximately 25 per cent, thus aligning certain amino acid groups and accounting for the characteristic cross-banding seen on electron microscopy.

The process of bridging a wound with collagen fibers can be visualized as similar to the outward growth of a bridge from a river bank, gaining strength and span as each steel beam goes into place. Intermolecular and intramolecular cross-linking, the ultimate source of tensile strength, probably occurs gradually. For example, the natural rubber polymer "cures" for a time before its elastic properties develop. During the differentiation phase of healing this constant "tightening" of collagen fibers apparently occurs, accounting for the fact that tensile strength increases even though the total collagen content of the wound decreases. The "remodeling," as one would expect, is influenced by the mechanical stresses which may act upon healing tissue. Such stresses partially determine the amount, form, and architecture of the final product (Krippaehne et al., 1962).

Polymerization and remodeling must occur in an environment favorable for alignment and approximation of the molecules. It is presumed that the ground substance, composed of sulfated and nonsulfated mucopolysaccharides of very high molecular weight, provides this environment. Mucopolysaccharides account for the metachromatic staining in healing tissue. The synthesis of these substances is probably also a function of the fibroblast (Dunphy, 1963).

Nutritional substances necessary for collagen formation must be delivered to the healing site. However, as noted previously, the circulation to wounded tissue has been disrupted. Pre-existing (and functioning) capillaries at the edge of the wound send capillary buds toward the wound edge, and these buds advance with (but slightly behind) the edge of healing tissue. The capillary buds meet other buds to form arches of new circulation. Circulation is eventually established across the wound. The regenerating capillaries are fragile and easily injured. They must stay within the support of newly synthesized collagen so that they will not burst from the effects of transmitted blood pressure and at the same time they must stay near the advancing front of the healing tissue in order to supply its needs. This tenuous circulation provides a clue to other possible determinants of healing, namely, blood volume and arterial oxygen tension (Hunt and Zederfeldt, 1969).

Wound Contraction. Contraction is a rather mysterious process by which open wounds on certain portions of the body spontaneously shrink and close. The process involves the full thickness of the wound and is perhaps better called "intussusceptive healing." Contraction differs from contracture, which is loss of joint motion from shrinking scar tissue. Contraction involves the entire thickness of a wound and in the human is best seen in the back of the neck and in the region of the trunk and face. Wounds of the extremities contract less well and depend more on connective tissue formation and epithelization for eventual healing. The contractile force has been measured and is compatible with forces exerted by other cellular systems (Higton and James, 1964). It is, however, independent of collagen formation and other measurable biochemical components of the wound (Abercrombie et al., 1961). The wise clinician remains patient and relies on contraction to close wounds in favorable areas so that large defects may heal with small scars. If skin grafts are prematurely placed on a rapidly contracting wound, contraction will be inhibited or even abolished, and a large skin graft scar will result where previously the wound was destined to become covered by normal skin.

HEALING OF SPECIAL TISSUES

The pattern of connective tissue healing is similar in all areas of the body, differing only in rate and extent. More specialized tissues heal in different ways.

Nerves. The distal portions of wounded peripheral nerves degenerate, whereas neural sheaths reanastomose. The axon then regenerates through the healed sheaths, advancing as much as several centimeters per week. This explains the delayed but often remarkable reappearance of function in the end-organ. Unfortunately the individual nerve sheath is unable to seek out and rejoin its original distal end. Therefore, regenerating motor fibers, for example, may find themselves filling sensorineural sheaths and grow in vain into sensory end-organs. The best regeneration, therefore, is found in the "purer" peripheral nerves.

Intestines. Intestinal healing has not been well studied. The rate of healing apparently varies from one portion of the intestine to the other. Clinical experience has shown that wounds in the colon and in the esophagus are the most dangerous of all. Usually the intestinal anastomosis regains strength rapidly; by a week to ten days it is even stronger than normal intestine (Hermann et al., 1964). The colon and esophagus contain little collagen. Since the normal reaction to injury includes collagen lysis, there is a critical period, usually from the fourth to seventh day after healing, when anastomoses are likely to leak. The balance between collagen synthesis and lysis is shown in Figure 2. Any event which delays synthesis or exaggerates lysis is likely to increase the risk of bursting. Meticulous surgical technique can assure better healing by reducing tissue injury. Furthermore, trauma, even distant from the wound, tends to excite a collagen lysis reaction in the nearby intestine (Hawley, unpublished data). Because of this loss of tissue, perforation is as likely to occur near an anastomosis as in the anastomosis itself. Local infection, which often occurs near esophageal or colon anastomoses, will increase the lysis of local collagen and increase the likelihood of perforation.

Bone. The healing of bone depends largely upon the synthesis of collagen. However, bone healing includes a unique process, the condensation of hydroxyapatite crystals on specific points in the collagen fiber. A long time is required for full calcification and attainment of final strength. The time lapse, however, is really in the same range as that experimentally noted for full development of fibrous tissue strength in soft tissue wounds. The clinical importance of calcification is so vital that the impression is gained that bone healing is protracted. Many textbooks give detailed descriptions of bone healing, and it will not be discussed in further detail here. The most recent comprehensive reviews of wound healing were written by Peacock in 1967 and Schilling in 1968.

Skin Grafts. The skin graft is a rather special tissue. The circulation to the graft is totally interrupted. The original vascular supply in the dermis, where the skin is separated, is composed mainly of arterioles or capillaries. The critical three or four days which follow the placement of the graft see a remarkable inosculation of the small vessels of the host to those of the graft. When enough vessels have joined, circulation to the skin graft is re-established, and the graft lives. After re-establishment of circulation, the immune mechanisms can now attack a homograft. In the accelerated form, this usually occurs in four to seven days, indicating that circulation is relatively complete at that time. The autograft eventually is remodeled, and a competent circulation is permanently attained.

SUTURE MATERIALS AND PROSTHESES

The properties of the ideal suture material are difficult to determine. Wire is one of the most inert suture materials and maintains its tensile strength for a long time. However, wire sutures are painful and sometimes difficult to tie. Plastic sutures, particularly nylon, are inert and may retain their tensile strength even longer than wire. However, plastic sutures often come untied, and some plastic fibers are so inert that they are not fixed in tissue. Silk is an animal protein and is nearly inert in human tissue. It loses its tensile strength over a long period, making it unsatisfactory for suturing arteries or cardiac valves. Silk sutures, because of their multifiber construction, are a haven for bacteria, although even contaminated wounds sutured with silk will usually heal without infection. On occasion silk sutures will form a nidus for small abscesses, which migrate to the surface and are discharged. Many plastic fibers will do the same, despite belief to the contrary.

Catgut, which is made from the submucosa of sheep intestine, will eventually resorb, but the resorption time is variable. Catgut provokes considerable inflammatory reaction. A new technique in absorbable suture manufacture involves the reconstitution of bovine collagen. These "collagen sutures" appear to cause less inflammation and are somewhat more constant in their absorptive properties.

The more reactive a suture is, the more likely it is to be the site of inflammation and infection. Postlethwait and his associates (1959) have performed a number of studies on the properties of sutures.

New prosthetic materials are constantly being tested. Among the metals, vitallium and titanium alloys have been the most successful. Solid implants of these metals, such as new joint components, have worked well. Metal mesh prostheses to restore form or to repair hernias allow good healing, but the mesh eventually fractures from fatigue and disintegrates.

Plastic fibers are longer lasting. Teflon and nylon are almost inert. Teflon, however, has an unwettable surface and in finer mesh prevents the growth of connective tissue into the interstices. Solid prostheses of nylon, silicone, or Teflon have the same property and, consequently, may migrate. Dacron has a more wettable surface and allows penetration by connective tissue.

Migration has been one of the worst problems with plastic inserts. When migration is limited by the proximity of bone or when a formed prosthesis can actually be sutured into place at a fixed point, success has been more uniform. Even the best of plastics is still a foreign body, and infection around plastic prostheses remains a major problem. Autologous tissue, when its use is technically feasible, is preferred for grafting in an infected or potentially infected area.

FACTORS AFFECTING HEALING

A number of investigators have studied the relationship of nutrition to wound healing. Healing has a high priority in the body economy, and mild to moderate nutritional deficiencies do not affect it. However, major nutritional depletion retards healing.

The most critical and best known nutritional deficiency affecting healing is scurvy. Ascorbic acid depletion arrests healing in early fibroplasia. As noted previously, ascorbic acid is necessary for the hydroxylation of proline. Scurvy arrests healing in the early phase of fibroplasia (Dunphy et al., 1956).

Protein depletion (as opposed to protein starvation) also retards healing if weight loss exceeds 20 per cent of original body weight. Classic experiments by Localio et al. (1948) show that the simple administration of methionine largely returns healing to normal. Wound dehiscence and infection tend to occur more often in patients who have lost significant amounts of weight and who have low serum albumin concentrations.

Recently zinc deficiency has been related to retarded wound healing. An indolent wound with a yellow-gray exudate suggests zinc deficiency. The administration of zinc sulfate, 220 mg. three times daily, appears to be safe and effective in returning wound healing to normal. The mechanism of the effect of zinc is not known (Pories et al., 1967).

Diabetes retards healing. The actual mechanism is not clear. Diabetic vascular disease leads to oxygen deficiency which can retard healing. Poor circulation may also lower the temperature of the wound and impede healing. Carbohydrate metabolism is prominent in healing tissue and probably fulfills its energy requirements. If carbohydrate metabolism is interfered with, possibly through poor insulin supply, healing would be expected to slow.

Tests of healing in poikilothermic animals have shown that the rate of healing is dependent on temperature (Reddan and Rothstein, 1965). Presumably for this reason, cutaneous wounds on the extremities heal less rapidly than those on the warm trunk.

Wounds in ischemic tissue heal poorly or not at all. Obviously many factors are involved in ischemia. Recent research has shown that hypoxia is a constant feature of wounded tissue (Hunt et al., 1967a) and suggests that oxygen supply may govern the rate of healing under certain conditions. As noted before, molecular oxygen is necessary for the hydroxylation of proline upon which all subsequent processes in collagen formation depend. If wounds are closed under tension, or if shock or hypotension occurs, healing may not proceed.

Cortisone is well known for its depressive effect on healing. Patients who are taking cortisone at the time of operation run a great risk of wound infection. Recent information shows that administration of vitamin A can counteract the effects of cortisone on wound healing (Ehrlich and Hunt, 1968). The effect is seen with both systemic and topical administration of vitamin A. However, systemic use of vitamin A in patients who are receiving cortisone for control of inflammatory disease must be undertaken with caution since, if vitamin A can counteract the effects of cortisone on the wound, it also can presumably counteract the anti-inflammatory effects of cortisone.

INFECTION AND RESISTANCE

The wound presents an ideal site for bacterial growth inasmuch as the carbon dioxide tension is high, the oxygen tension is low, and the environment is moist and dark. Yet wounds obviously have some resistance to infection, since virtually all wounds are contaminated while they are open, yet relatively few wounds become infected. Numerous studies have shown that there are three prerequisites for wound infection: (1) a receptive host, (2) contamination by microorganisms, and (3) a culture medium in the wound. In the prevention of infection the patient's resistance and the state of the wound must be considered as much as the degree of bacterial contamination. "Trauma to the wound is as important a cause of postoperative infection as is the introduction of bacteria" (Dykes and Anderson, 1961).

The more organisms there are contaminating the wound, the more likely is an infection (Hunt et al., 1967b). However, many other factors are involved. For instance, clostridial infections will occur unless dead tissue is present in the wound. Antibiotics obviously influence the type of bacteria which may cause infection. Cortisone and diabetes diminish resistance to infection. Sutures also increase susceptibility. Recent studies on nonsuture closure of skin show that the number of infections was decreased when skin sutures were avoided (Connolly et al., 1969).

CARE OF THE WOUND

Postoperative local care of the closed wound involves simple cleanliness and protection from trauma. Wounds can be infected by external application of bacteria, particularly in the first three or four days. Most wounds can be exposed to the atmosphere safely at any time after operation. However, if a wound is likely to be contaminated or traumatized, it should be protected by some sort of dressing for at least the first four days. Protection from contamination may require repeated cleansing as well as dressings.

Care of the wound starts in the preoperative period and ends only months later. One must be clean, gentle and skillful in surgical technique, and attentive to postoperative protection of the wound. The wound is susceptible to major systemic physiological disorders such as hypovolemia, anoxia, shock, hypotension, starvation, and drug administration. "Although wound healing is in many ways a local phenomenon, the ideal care of the wound is essentially the ideal care of the patient." (Hunt and Dunphy, 1967).

REFERENCES

Abercrombie, M., Jones, D. W., and Newcombe, J. F.: The role of contraction in the repair of excised wounds of the skin. In Slome, D.: Wound Healing. Proceedings of a Symposium held on November 12-13, 1959, at the Royal College of Surgeons of England. New York, Pergamon Press, Symposium Publications Division, 1961.

Connolly, W. B., Hunt, T. K., Zederfeldt, B., Cafferata, H. T., and Dunphy, J. E.: Clinical comparison of surgical wounds closed by suture and adhesive tapes. Amer. J. Surg. *117*:318, 1969.

Dunphy, J. E.: The fibroblast—An ubiquitous ally for the surgeon. New Eng. J. Med. *268*:1367, 1963.

Dunphy, J. E., Udupa, K. N., and Edwards, L. C.: Wound healing: A new perspective with particular reference to ascorbic acid deficiency. Ann. Surg. *144*:304, 1956.

Dykes, E. R., and Anderson, R.: Atraumatic technic—The sine qua non of operative wound infection prophylaxis. Cleveland Clin. Quart. *28*:157, 1961.

Ehrlich, H. P., and Hunt, T. K.: Effects of cortisone and vitamin A on wound healing. Ann. Surg. *167*:324, 1968.

Forrester, J. C., Zederfeldt, B. H., Hayes, T. L., and Hunt, T. K.: Mechanical, biochemical and architectural features of repair. *In* Dunphy, J. E., et al. (ed.): Repair and Regeneration. New York, McGraw-Hill Book Co., Inc., 1969.

Goodwin, L. G., Jones, C. R., Richards, W. H. G., and Kohn, J.: Pharmacologically active substances in the urine of burned patients. Brit. J. Exper. Path. *44*:551, 1963.

Hawley, P.: Unpublished data.

Herrmann, J. B., Woodward, S. C., and Pulaski, E. J.: Healing of colonic anastomoses in the rat. Surg. Gynec. Obstet. *119*:269, 1964.

Higton, D. I. R., and James, D. W.: The force of contraction of full thickness wounds of rabbit skin. Brit. J. Surg. *51*:462, 1964.

Hunt, T. K., and Dunphy, J. E.: Wound healing. *In* Wells, C., and Kyle, J.: Scientific Foundation of Surgery. London, Heinemann, Ltd., 1967.

Hunt, T. K., and Hawley, P.: Surgical judgment and colon anastomosis. Dis. Colon Rectum *12*:167, 1969.

Hunt, T. K., Jawetz, E., Hutchinson, J. G. P., and Dunphy, J. E.: A new model for the study of wound infection. J. Trauma *7*:298, 1967a.

Hunt, T. K., Twomey, P., Zederfeldt, B., and Dunphy, J. E.: Respiratory gas tensions and pH in healing wounds. Amer. J. Surg. *114*:302, 1967b.

Hunt, T. K., Zederfeldt, B., and Goldstick, T. K.: Oxygen and healing. Amer. J. Surg. *118*:521, 1969.

Krippaehne, W. W., Hunt, T. K., Jackson, D. S., and Dunphy, J. E.: Studies on the effect of stress on transplants of autologous and homologous connective tissue. Amer. J. Surg. *104*:267, 1962.

Localio, S. A., Morgan, M. E., and Hinton, J. W.: The biological chemistry of wound healing. I. The effect of dl-methionine on the healing of wounds in protein-depleted animals. Surg. Gynec. Obstet. *86*:582, 1948.

Menkin, V.: Newer Concepts of Inflammation. Springfield, Ill., Charles C Thomas, 1950.

Pareira, M. D., and Serkes, K. D.: Prediction of wound disruption by use of the healing edge. Surg. Gynec. Obstet. *115*:72, 1962.

Peacock, E. E., Jr.: Dynamic aspects of collagen biology. I. Synthesis and assembly. J. Surg. Res. *7*:433, 1967.

Pories, W. J., Henzel, J. H., Rob, C. G., and Strain, W. H.: Acceleration of healing with zinc sulfate. Ann. Surg. *165*:434, 1967.

Postlethwait, R. W., Schauble, J. F., Dillon, M. L., and Morgan, J.: Wound healing: II. An evaluation of surgical suture material. Surg. Gynec. Obstet. *108*:555, 1959.

Reddan, J. R., and Rothstein, H.: Influence of temperature on wound healing in a poikilotherm. Exper. Cell. Res. *40*:442, 1965.

Schilling, J. A.: Wound healing. Physiol. Rev. *48*:374, 1968.

Udenfriend, S.: Formation of hydroxyproline in collagen. Science *152*:1335, 1966.

Chapter 23

THE PHYSIOLOGY AND TREATMENT OF SHOCK DUE TO VOLUME LOSS (TRAUMA), SEPSIS, OR MYOCARDIAL DAMAGE*

by Richard C. Lillehei, M.D., Ph.D.,
Ronald H. Dietzman, M.D., George J. Motsay, M.D., and
Leonard S. Schultz, M.D.

After a generation of use of synthetic vaso-pressors, we still find ourselves with the same mortality rate (70 to 90 per cent) from shock due to bacterial sepsis (particularly gram-negative infections) or to acute or chronic cardiac failure (Lillehei et al., 1964, 1967; Dietzman and Lillehei, 1968). In contrast, there has been a dramatic reduction in the mortality rate from traumatic shock; (shock due to volume loss) this is not due to the use of pharmacological agents, but to the liberal use of blood, plasma, plasma substitutes, and saline solutions. Thus, we must still deal with the unsolved problems of treating patients in septic and cardiogenic shock, and also with the dilemma of treating patients suffering from traumatic shock who do not respond to volume replacement. Moreover, with the increasing age of the population and with the increasing complexity of surgical procedures on the aged, we frequently see combinations of traumatic, septic, and cardiogenic shock in the same patient. The problem of treatment is further complicated because most physicians feel each of these types of shock is distinct and requires a separate and different protocol for treatment even though patients in shock show a characteristic alteration in the microcirculation, which is often independent of the cause of the shock.

Initially there is vasoconstriction in arterioles and venules, causing ischemic anoxia, which is followed after a variable period of time by loss of tone in arterioles and obstruction to outflow in venules owing to a combination of persisting venular constriction, aggregation of blood cells within the stagnant microcirculation, and probable microthrombosis as a late or terminal phase of shock (Figs. 1 and 2) (Dietzman and Lillehei, 1968a).

Whether stagnant anoxia occurs or persists depends on the severity of the original insult, which may be blood or fluid loss, sepsis or cardiac damage, the perpetuation of the insult, and the general condition of the patient. It is important to emphasize that this vasoconstrictive response in the microcirculation does not occur in all organs; that is, it is not an all-or-none phenomenon but is restricted initially to the viscera and skin, more specifically, the microcirculation of the skin, liver, lung, gut, and kidney—all organs which are adrenergically innervated and responsive to catecholamines. Epinephrine and norepinephrine are the naturally occurring catecholamine substances that are involved in

*Supported by U.S.P.H.S. grant HE02941-14 and U.S. Army grant Da-49-193-MD-2539.

623

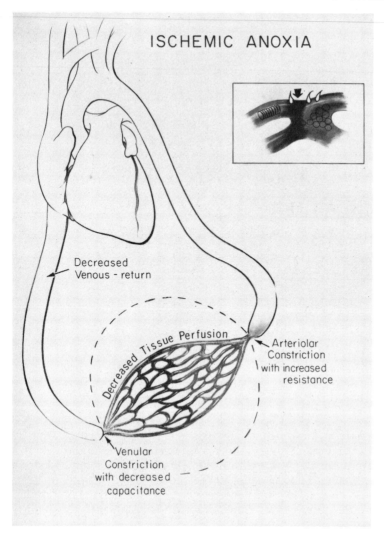

ISCHEMIC ANOXIA

Decreased
Venous - return

Decreased Tissue Perfusion

Arteriolar
Constriction
with increased
resistance

Venular
Constriction
with decreased
capacitance

Figure 1. Schema for the response of the microcirculation to the stress of trauma, myocardial damage, or gram-negative bacterial sepsis. In the initial response to stress there is constriction of arterioles and venules throughout the microcirculation of the viscera (including the lung) and skin. In this phase there is a decrease in intravascular hydrostatic pressure, whereas colloid osmotic pressure tends to remain unchanged. Thus, there is a net influx of fluid into the vascular system as a result of this response. This mechanism for autotransfusion can take care of volume deficits up to 1 L. in the average adult, if the loss has not been too rapid.

most cases, but any related compounds, natural or synthetic, may also initiate or intensify this response.

How is it that seemingly diverse stimuli such as bleeding and infection and cardiac damage lead to this common microcirculatory response? The response is initiated by the baroreceptors of the aorta and great vessels and probably also by baroreceptors which are now known to be present throughout the vascular system (Figs. 3 and 4).

When blood volume is depleted from any cause, venous return to the heart decreases and the cardiac output falls, followed by a fall in the blood pressure. Baroreceptors respond to decreased arterial pressure by decreased tone, which activates the sympathetic nerve centers in the brain stem. Increased sympathetic activity causes an outpouring of epinephrine

from the adrenal medulla and norepinephrine from the postganglionic sympathetic nerve endings. The microcirculations of the skin and viscera are supplied with alpha receptors that respond to epinephrine and norepinephrine, causing vasoconstriction in arterioles and venules. The microcirculation of the brain, heart, and voluntary muscles have few, if any, such alpha receptors and do not constrict; therefore, these organs receive a greater percentage of the reduced cardiac output. The heart and voluntary muscles do have beta receptors, however, which are also stimulated by the epinephrine and norepinephrine, and this results in an increased rate and force of contraction of the heart (inotropic and chronotropic effect) and dilatation of arterioles and venules in the voluntary muscles. The cerebral circulation has neither alpha nor beta receptors, but during shock

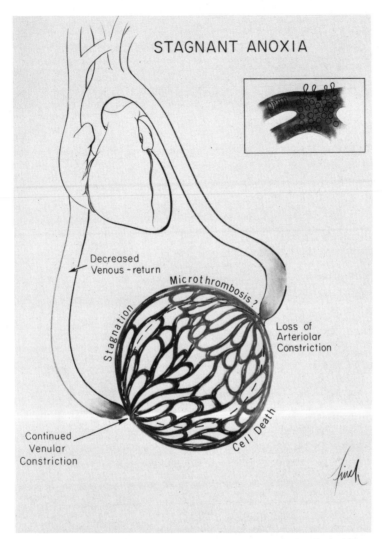

Figure 2. If the initial stress or insult is severe, or the recipient unusually susceptible, or if there are combinations of insults of trauma, myocardial damage or sepsis, then ischemic anoxia gives way to stagnant anoxia. The period of time for this transition to occur is variable; it may occur in minutes following overwhelming sepsis or may even extend over a period of years, as in congestive heart failure.

The appearance of the microcirculation now is different from that Figure 1. While there is a continued venular constriction, arteriolar constriction is less prominent and in some instances may even be absent. This allows blood to get into the microcirculation but it cannot get out. As a result there is stagnation and pooling and an increase in hydrostatic pressure which tends to force fluid out of the vascular system. Edema, particularly in the lungs, characterizes this stage of the response to shock. Moreover, as the anoxia and acidosis increase, the membranes of the vasculature of the microcirculation begin to lose their integrity and allow blood cells to leave the vascular system, which results in the typical hemorrhagic lesions of late shock seen in the abdominal viscera and in the lungs.

No exact explanation has been given for the loss of tone of arterioles before the venules, but perhaps the fact that the venular side of the circulation is normally exposed to lower oxygen tensions and a more acid pH would account for their ability to maintain their tone longer than arterioles in this stage of stagnant anoxia. This stage of stagnant anoxia has sometimes been called "irreversible shock," but this is a misnomer since it is possible, experimentally and clinically, to salvage the organism from this state of cardiovascular deterioration.

Another prominent finding in stagnant anoxia is aggregation of the cellular components of the blood with the possibility that disseminated intravascular coagulation may occur with the using up of clotting elements of the blood. This is signaled by bleeding from mucous membranes and wounds and is more often a late complication of septic shock than of traumatic or cardiogenic shock.

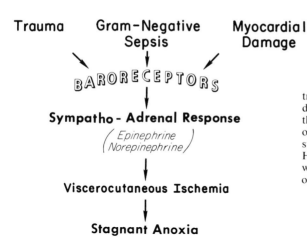

Figure 3. The common diverse insults causing shock, trauma, gram-negative bacterial endotoxins and myocardial damage elicit a common response in the microcirculation of the viscera and skin because they affect the baroreceptors of the great vessels. Thus, the nature of the response to stress does not distinguish between these various insults. However, the intensity of the response will certainly vary with the intensity of the insult as well as with the condition of the responding organism.

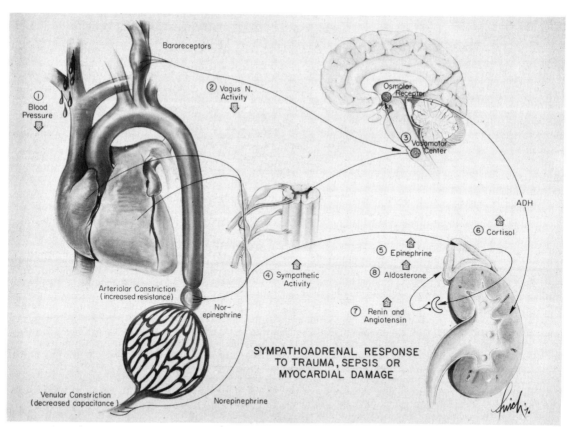

Figure 4. The sympathoadrenal response results when blood pressure is lowered, which decreases the number of impulses in the nerve fibers connecting the baroreceptors of the great vessels and the sympathetic centers in the brain stem. These nerve fibers are carried within the vagus nerve. The result is a sympathoadrenal stimulation, with outpouring of epinephrine from the adrenal medulla and norepinephrine from the postganglionic sympathetic nerve endings. The adrenal cortex also takes part in the sympathoadrenal response, and there is an increase in cortisol production by the cortex.

it benefits from the effects of these receptors elsewhere by receiving a greater proportion of the reduced cardiac output, since no vasoconstriction occurs within the cerebral circulation. These vascular responses are apparently evolutionary in nature and designed for preservation of life.

This response to stress was labeled the "fight or flight reaction" by Cannon, almost half a century ago; (Cannon, 1923) an equally descriptive term for the phenomenon might be "nature's first aid." The term "nature's first aid" will serve to remind the physician that he need not and should not persist in continued first aid measures that involve the use of synthetic agents such as levarterenol, metaraminol, or related substances which cause further vasoconstriction. Such a course of action accelerates the progression from ischemic to stagnant shock. This progression will also occur if the conditions which caused the shock are not corrected, if the insult is extremely severe, or if the recipient of the insult is weakened for any reason (for example, a very young or very old patient). More specifically, stagnant shock seems to occur when arterioles are no longer able to maintain their constriction because of anoxia and acidosis. In contrast, venules appear to retain tone for longer periods, perhaps because of their exposure to lower oxygen tension and a lower pH in the normal state. This persistence in venular tone, abetted by increased platelet adhesiveness and blood cell aggregation which has taken place because of slow flow, blocks the outflow from the microcirculation of the viscera and skin. Microthrombosis is believed by some investigators to further aggravate the problem by causing further outflow obstruction and by using up clotting factors so that bleeding from mucous membranes, stomach, gut, or wounds may occur in the late stage of shock (McKay and Hardaway, 1963; Hardaway, 1968).

The advent of stagnation within the microcirculation further reduces the effective circulating blood volume. Moreover, rising hydrostatic pressures within the stagnant pools of blood forces plasma into the interstitial spaces. The end result of this process, if it is not corrected, is a loss of integrity of the cells with bleeding into the tissues. The skin, lung, liver, gut, and kidney of patients dying from severe and/or prolonged shock may show varying manifestations of this process. It should be noted also that the organ which is most severely damaged may vary among various mammalian species. Thus, in man the lung appears to be the most sensitive organ in shock, followed by the kidney. In contrast, the canine gut is more sensitive than the kidney, but the lung of the dog is also easily damaged in shock whether the cause is blood loss, endotoxins, or cardiac damage. The rabbit lung is similar to the canine lung in its sensitivity. The gut of the rat is also damaged in shock. Among primates, the lung, kidney, and perhaps the liver seem to be the most sensitive organs in shock.

The series of events described earlier is well documented in the experimental laboratory with a variety of animals, and most physicians now agree that this sequence of events is correct for hemorrhagic shock in experimental animals and man. Few, however, appreciate the fact that a similar picture also occurs in septic and cardiogenic shock.

SEPTIC SHOCK

What happens in septic and cardiogenic shock? Do the conditions in the laboratory simulate those which occur in man? Presently, most patients suffering shock from sepsis have a gram-negative infection. All gram-negative bacteria—*Escherichia coli*, *Klebsiella-Aerobacter*, *Pseudomonas*, *Proteus*, coliform species, and so on, are the most common—contain a complex lipopolysaccharide called endotoxin in their cell walls. The endotoxin is released upon death of the bacteria. It then combines with some element in the blood, probably complement or leukocytes or both, to become a potent sympathomimetic substance which causes intense vasospasm in the viscerocutaneous microcirculation.

Because of the great potency of the endotoxin there is a rapid progression from an ischemic to a stagnant microcirculation; and the deterioration of the microcirculation, which takes hours to occur in hemorrhagic shock, can occur in seconds or minutes following exposure to endotoxin. The loss of effective circulating blood volume in the stagnant microcirculation reduces the venous return, cardiac output, and blood pressure. Once again, the baroreceptor response is brought into play, and the increased sympathetic activity mediated through the sympathetic centers further increases stagnation in the viscerocutaneous microcirculation. There is also some evidence that the endotoxin-blood combination acts on the central nervous system directly to cause disorientation or coma, or both, tachypnea, and tachycardia (Motsay et al., 1969). The picture now is not significantly different from that already described in detail for hemorrhagic shock, but it is more severe, the principal difference being in the accelerated deterioration of the microcirculation following exposure to endotoxin. The organs principally damaged in the dog are the lung and gut and in primates the lung, liver, and kidney. The description given here is one derived from experiments in the laboratory with a variety of experimental animals and endotoxins from various gram-negative bacteria.

The picture in man is similar, but there is one important difference which has troubled most investigators: the normal or high cardiac output and normal or low total peripheral resistance usually seen in patients suffering septic shock. Only very late in septic shock does the cardiac output fall if the heart has previously been normal. Despite these hemodynamic findings, which differ from those seen in hemorrhagic or cardiogenic shock, the clinical signs of septic shock in man following gram-negative bacterial sepsis are similar to those found in the other types of shock: hypotension, cold, pale or cyanotic skin of the extremities, and oliguria or anuria.

The disparity between measured values and clinical observations has caused many physicians to believe that the experimental animal reacts differently to endotoxins than does man. Furthermore, some of these same investigators have used this finding to discount the value of all observations on shock in experimental animals.

Recently we and others have gathered information which apparently explains this diversion between experimental and clinical observations (Motsay et al., 1969; Lillehei et al., in press). The first piece of evidence in unraveling this puzzle was provided by Weil, who noted the high cardiac output and low total peripheral resistance in cirrhotic patients in septic shock. Arteriovenous shunting in the liver of cirrhotics is an anatomical phenomenon, and this apparently accounted for the high output and low resistance in this group of patients (Weil et al., 1964). Yet, it does not explain why this same hemodynamic picture also occurs in patients who do not have cirrhosis. Observations on arteriovenous oxygen differences and oxygen uptakes which we have made on patients in septic shock suggest that shunting does occur in patients without cirrhosis and that the lung is often the site of this admixture. But the conditions which cause pulmonary admixture or arteriovenous shunting probably operate elsewhere in the body as well.

Why does arteriovenous shunting occur in septic shock in man but not in experimental animals? Is it because endotoxin acts differently in man than in other mammals? Or is it because in the experimental laboratory endotoxin derived from killed gram-negative bacteria is used rather than living bacteria so that the inflammatory process induced by the living bacteria is absent?

In man the source of gram-negative sepsis is usually inflammation in the lungs, abdominal viscera, peritoneum, soft tissues, or within the genitourinary tract. The inflammatory aspect of infection and its relation to arteriovenous shunting in the microcirculation of the affected areas was noted by Metchnikoff many years ago (Metchnikoff, 1893). He thought this a result of local hormone production, but that the increasing resistance to flow in the stagnant normal pathways must also be a factor. This resistance to flow through normal channels may then exceed the critical opening pressure of arteriovenous shunts, which open and stay open until obstruction to normal pathways is relieved. This attractive explanation has received confirmation in studies on experimental animals in which a focus of inflammation has been produced along with injection of living bacteria. When this is done, there is a fall in resistance and increased cardiac output indicative of shunting (Hermreck and Thal, 1969). It is interesting that the injection of living bacteria, similar to the injection of endotoxin, will not produce the high output–low resistance picture in experimental animals if inflammation is absent (Motsay, unpublished).

More recently, the kinens have been indicted as initiators of this local arteriovenous admixture. These substances are activated by the interaction of plasma globulins and factors released from damaged tissue.

More work is required before the complete explanation of this process is clear; yet, the effect on tissue anoxia from such a shunting in septic shock is readily apparent. Stagnant anoxia produces a profound drop in nutritional blood flow to the tissues, and arteriovenous shunting compounds this insult by diverting nutritional blood flow away from or around these stagnant beds. Perhaps this twofold basis for anoxia in septic shock is responsible for the suddenness with which shock occurs in sepsis and the profound deterioration of hepatic, renal, and pulmonary function which so often results in death (Fig. 5).

Figure 5. Arteriovenous admixture or shunting is particularly prominent in gram-negative infections. It is, apparently, not related specifically to the endotoxin of the gram-negative bacteria since experimental animals injected with endotoxin from killed gram-negative bacteria do not show such admixture. When inflammation is provoked in the experimental animal with living gram-negative bacteria, however, then admixture or shunting does occur. The exact mechanism for the appearance of admixture is not clear but appears to involve the interaction of living bacteria and tissue. Bradykinins have been implicated as the agents released by tissue which may cause local arteriovenous admixture. The effect on the cell of such arteriovenous admixture is further oxygen deprivation in addition to that already resulting from the stagnant anoxia induced by endotoxin.

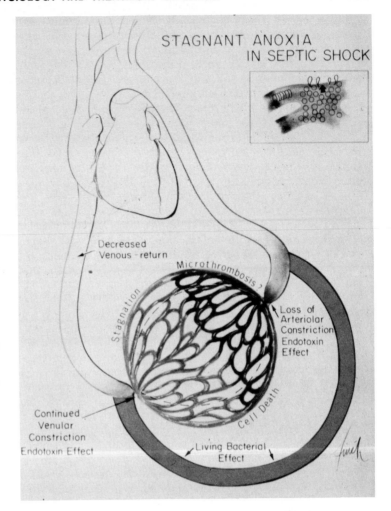

CARDIOGENIC SHOCK

We will now discuss the last of the three most common causes of shock—cardiac damage. Why should a central insult such as cardiac damage, whether it be acute or chronic, result in a peripheral response similar to that caused by volume loss or by endotoxins of gram-negative bacteria? Again, baroreceptors are involved. With cardiac damage, cardiac output falls, leading to a fall in blood pressure, and baroreceptors pass this information onto the sympathetic centers within the brain stem. The sympathoadrenal response initiated by these sympathetic centers is identical in every way with that which occurs following a decrease in venous return due to volume loss or sepsis. Moreover, when cardiac damage occurs over a prolonged period of time, then the same peripheral changes which occur are called "congestive failure." But the changes in congestive heart failure are identical with those of stagnant anoxia. There is increased total peripheral resistance and a decreased cardiac output. Moreover, as the term congestion implies, there is a stagnation within the microcirculation and the viscerocutaneous areas are again involved. Pulmonary edema, hepatic congestion, low cardiac output, cold, poorly perfused extremities, and oliguria are characteristic of both acute cardiogenic shock and chronic congestive failure. The only significant difference is in time; stagnant anoxia occurs in minutes or hours, whereas congestive heart failure may take years to occur.

In summary, the viscerocutaneous response to the stress of trauma (volume loss), sepsis, or cardiac damage is mediated through the sympathoadrenal system, which results in a clinical picture of cold extremities, oliguria, and, in a variable period of time, hypotension.

What use can be made of this information in

the treatment of shock in man, if indeed the common forms of shock are related by a common response of the microcirculation of the viscera and skin? First, it is apparent that there is a twofold deficit in stagnant shock whatever its cause—a decrease in the effective circulating blood volume and a disturbance in the microcirculation itself. In most instances, this means that additional volume must be given. The nature of the fluid used—blood, plasma, plasma substitutes, dextrans, or crystalloid solutions—will depend on the nature of the deficit. In most cases of traumatic shock, substantial quantities of blood will be required, supplemented with one of the crystalloid solutions. In septic shock it is more likely that plasma, dextrans, and salt solutions will be required if the hematocrit is over 35 per cent (hemoglobin, 11 gm.).

In cardiogenic shock one must be far more cautious in the administration of fluids. Yet here again, the judicious use of volume may be lifesaving, as has now been shown in several clinical studies, particularly that of Langsjoin (Langsjoin and Inmon, 1968).

Correction of stagnant anoxia can be done in a variety of ways. We have had most of our experience working with the alpha adrenergic blocking agent phenoxybenzamine and with massive doses of glucocorticosteroids, which also cause vasodilatation but by means other than alpha blockade.

Phenoxybenzamine is one of the most potent alpha adrenergic blocking agents known. When given intravenously, its effect occurs within minutes and lasts for 24 or more hours. There are two problems presently associated with its use. The first is that its effect is so rapid that it will magnify any pre-existing hypovolemia; hence, it is imperative that right atrial or central venous pressure observations be continuously made when phenoxybenzamine is used, and added volume is usually given to the extent that the central venous pressure will allow. A more important practical problem associated with the use of phenoxybenzamine is that this drug is still an investigational one and, therefore, not available to the great majority of physicians.

The corticosteriods are far more subtle than phenoxybenzamine in causing vasodilatation, the vasodilatation being mediated through different pathways. From our own studies we know at least three ways in which the circulation is affected by massive doses of corticosteriods. In studies in the dog we found that a massive dose of a synthetic glucocorticosteroid such as methylprednisolone (30 mg. per kg.) slows nerve impulse transmission in postgang-

lionic sympathetic nerves (Dietzman, unpublished). Similarly, isolated Pappenheimer paw preparations or studies on bowel sgements show that the corticosteriods in massive doses also preserve the integrity of small vessels so that there is less leakage from the microcirculation (Motsay et al., 1970). Finally, there is also evidence that pharmacological doses of corticosteriods decrease platelet adhesiveness and preserve their integrity, important factors in preventing or correcting the stagnant anoxia in the microcirculation.

It is important to emphasize that the glucocorticosteriods are used in shock not for physiological replacement, but for their pharmacological effects, three of which are listed just previously; but there are undoubtedly other effects that are as yet unknown. There is no evidence in shock, with rare exceptions, that the adrenal cortex does not respond with increased cortisol output for physiological needs just as the adrenal medulla increases its epinephrine output. We have found that the doses of corticosteriods which cause vasodilatation must be massive; physiological doses have no effect. This is an area of misunderstanding which deserves much emphasis.

Figure 6 illustrates a comparison of vasodilators and vasoconstrictors, while Figure 7 shows a protocol for the use of such agents alone or in combination with other vasoactive drugs.

Figure 8 presents the essence of our approach to the treatment of shock. Pressure is a product of flow times resistance. The problem of shock is a deficiency in nutritional blood flow such that cells and organs cannot function normally. It is Pyrrhic victory at best to raise pressure merely by further increasing resistance because nutritional blood flow is further decreased and the degree of stagnation is increased. Flow is increased by adding volume, by mobilizing stagnant volume, or both, a process which is enhanced by using vasodilators such as methylprednisolone in massive doses (30 mg. per kg. I.V.). Experimental studies, which have involved hemorrhagic, endotoxic, and cardiogenic shock, have shown conclusively that survival can be increased by such an approach (Lillehei et al., 1964, 1967; Dietzman and Lillehei, 1968,1968a; Lillehei et al., 1967; Motsay et al., 1969, 1970). In contrast, the promiscuous use of vasopressor drugs does not increase survival of the experimental animal in shock whatever the cause. These dismal results in the laboratory using vasopressors alone mirror the results in humans, in whom there has been no significant increase in sur-

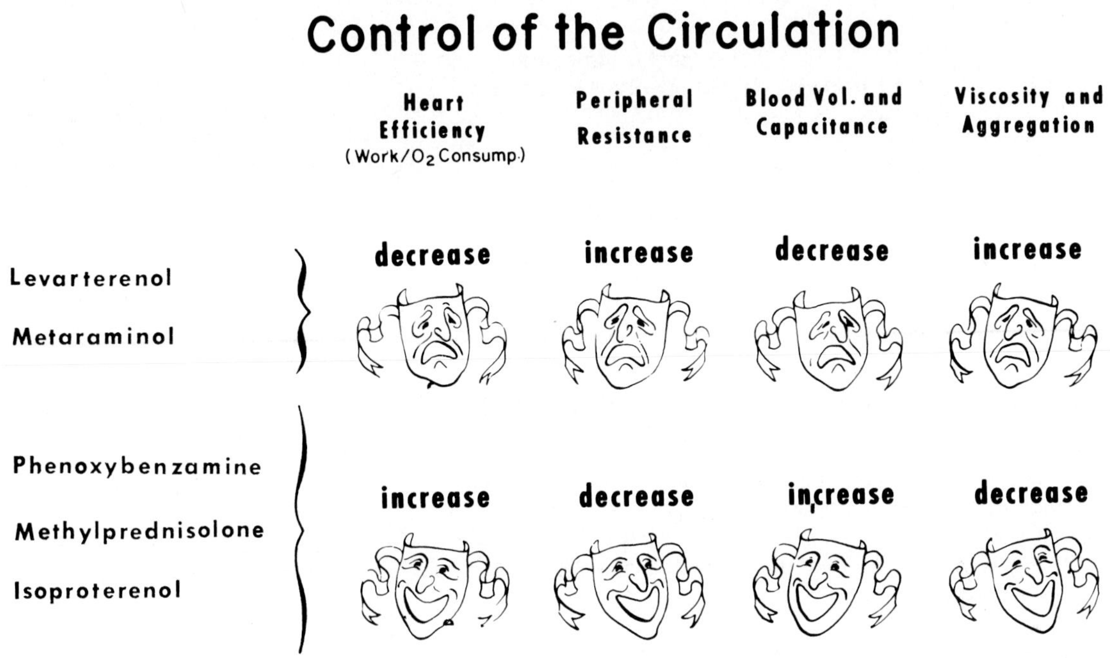

Control of the Circulation

	Heart Efficiency (Work/O$_2$ Consump.)	Peripheral Resistance	Blood Vol. and Capacitance	Viscosity and Aggregation

Levarterenol

Metaraminol

> decrease   increase   decrease   increase

Phenoxybenzamine

Methylprednisolone

Isoproterenol

> increase   decrease   increase   decrease

Figure 6. In discussing the effects of various drugs on the circulation it is important to emphasize their effects both on the heart and the peripheral circulation. For the most part the "vasoconstrictors" have an adverse effect on the peripheral circulation, and while they increase the force and/or rate of myocardial contraction, the efficiency of the heart is decreased because of the increased arteriolar and venular resistance.

The "vasodilators" generally have a salutary effect on the peripheral circulation by decreasing arteriolar and venular constriction, which improves myocardial function. Massive doses of methylprednisolone or phenoxybenzamine also exert a modest inotropic effect on the myocardium. Isoproterenol causes its vasodilatation principally in the microcirculation of the voluntary muscles through its effect on beta receptors. Thus, while overall total peripheral resistance decreases with isoproterenol, the decrease does not always occur in those areas such as viscera and skin where it is most needed. Perhaps this is the reason that isoproterenol has not been as useful as hoped in the treatment of shock.

Protocol for Use of Vasodilators

A. Methylprednisolone 30 mg/kg I.V. bolus

B. Repeat in 2–4 hours if no or waning response

C. If no response or continued vasodilation required, switch to phenoxybenzamine 1mg/kg I.V. drip in one hour (in 100 ml D$_5$W)

D. Aggressive volume replacement with either methylprednisolone or phenoxybenzamine

E. If cardiac index remains below 2 L/m^2 then add to 100 ml D$_5$W microdrip:

     1. Glucagon   5.0 mg
     2. Isoproterenol   0.4 mg
     3. Levarterenol   4.0 ml
            or
     4. Metaraminol   10.0 mg

Figure 7. A protocol for the use of the various vasoactive agents in combination with volume replacement in the treatment of shock.

Systolic B.P. kept under 110 mmHg

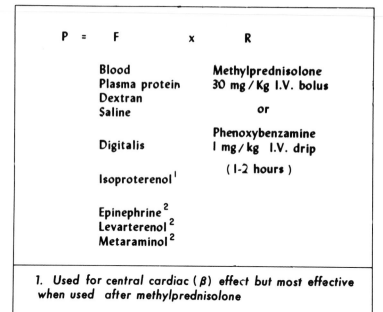

$$P = F \times R$$

Blood Plasma protein Dextran Saline	Methylprednisolone 30 mg / Kg I.V. bolus
	or
Digitalis	Phenoxybenzamine 1 mg / kg I.V. drip
	(1-2 hours)
Isoproterenol[1]	
Epinephrine[2] Levarterenol[2] Metaraminol[2]	

1. Used for central cardiac (β) effect but most effective when used after methylprednisolone

2. Used also for central cardiac (β) effect after blockade of peripheral (α) effect with methylprednisolone

Figure 8. The essence of our approach to the treatment of shock is to raise flow rather than resistance in order to raise pressure. This is best done with a combination of volume replacement and a massive dose of methylprednisolone for its beneficial effect on arterioles and venules of the microcirculation of the viscera and skin. Inotropic agents are used in small doses solely for their central cardiac effect. By using these agents in combination with massive doses of steroids, we find that we can use much smaller doses of the inotropic agent and avoid the deleterious side effects of these agents.

vival in either septic or cardiogenic shock when vasopressors have formed the keystone of treatment.

DIAGNOSIS OF SHOCK

There are many criteria for diagnosing shock but the three most reliable are a systolic blood pressure below 90 mm. Hg in a previously normotensive patient or 30 mm. Hg below the usual preoperative systolic pressure in hypertensive patients. This is usually accompanied by cold, pale, or cyanotic skin of the lower extremities, a drop in urine output, and a cooling of the extremities many hours prior to the fall in blood pressure. This should alert the physician to forestall hypotension by prompt use of intravenous volume. In contrast, one occasionally sees a systolic blood pressure below 90 mm. Hg in a patient who has a normal urine output and warm skin. Often an intra-arterial pressure in such a patient is within the normal range, and the problem lies in the blood pressure cuff or in the fact that the patient has an unusually fat arm.

Recently we have added another criteria for diagnosing shock, or perhaps more properly "impending shock," due to trauma or cardiac damage. If the cardiac index is below 2 L. per min./m^2 and remains so for an hour or more, even in the face of a normal blood pressure, then the patient will usually suffer a fall of blood pressure in a few hours. By beginning treatment when the cardiac index is at or below 2 L. per min./m.^{2}, our survival results from traumatic and cardiogenic shock are far better than when we have waited for hypotension to occur.

THE PLAN OF TREATMENT

In treating shock in man we follow the format shown in Figures 7 and 8. Most patients suffering from postoperative shock do not have an adequate effective circulating blood volume; hence, adding volume is usually the single most important measure to raise flow and pressure. This has been emphasized in the treatment of traumatic or burn shock; but it is equally important in the treatment of septic shock, and even in cardiogenic shock carefully added fluids are usually of value and may be all that is needed to resuscitate the patient. The choice of fluids will depend upon the type of fluid believed to have been lost.

But what can be done when fluid alone does not solve the problem, as is occasionally the case in traumatic shock and often the case in septic or cardiogenic shock? Here the use of vasodilators to reduce resistance is of great value in our experience. We have now made hemodynamic and metabolic observations on over 200 patients suffering shock from varying problems in which vasodilators of one form or another have been used.

The physiological basis for the use of vasodilators was presented earlier, and specific examples of such use of vasodilators in combination with fluids and other measures will best illustrate our treatment.

Traumatic Shock

A 62 year old man suffered shock following surgery for removal of an abdominal aortic aneurysm (Fig. 9). Blood pressure, central venous pressure, cardiac index, and urine output were low. The skin of the peripheral extremities was cool and pale and the total peripheral resistance was high.

Blood was given, and the cardiac index rose and total peripheral resistance fell. Blood pressure increased, indicating that the pressure increased owing to increased flow rather than to increased resistance. The urine output increased and the skin warmed. Metabolically the blood lactate initially rose slightly because of a washout of accumulated lactate in the vis-

cerocutaneous circulation and then fell as additional oxygen was available for metabolism of the accumulated lactate. After this prompt resuscitation the patient was returned to the operating room and found to be bleeding from the back wall of the aneurysm, which had been left in place.

In the situation presented in Figure 9 volume alone restored pressure, but in the situation shown in Figure 10 we see that volume alone was not enough. This man suffered shock from a bleeding peptic ulcer. Venous pressure rose in the face of blood transfusion, but blood pressure and cardiac index remained low. The patient remained oliguric and his skin was cool. Digitalization was begun but with little effect. A bolus of methylprednisolone (30 mg. per kg.) was given intravenously over a five-minute period. Over the next two hours the venous pressure gradually fell, and it was possible to instill additional blood, which restored blood pressure, cardiac index, urine output, and skin temperature toward normal. In this patient the microvascular changes in the viscerocutaneous circulation had apparently reached the early stages of stagnation, which cannot always be reversed by volume alone and requires some agent to correct the disturbance in arterioles and venules. Corticosteroids in massive doses

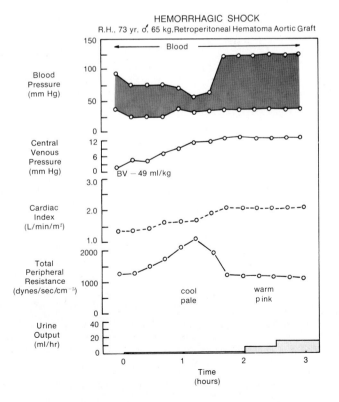

HEMORRHAGIC SHOCK
R.H., 73 yr, ♂, 65 kg, Retroperitoneal Hematoma Aortic Graft

Figure 9. Typical traumatic shock resulting from postoperative blood loss from the bleeding posterior wall of an abdominal aortic aneurysm. Almost all patients suffering hypovolemic shock will respond to volume alone if treatment is prompt, the source of blood loss is eliminated, and other complications such as infection or cardiac failure do not occur. With any of these complications, however, it is advisable to use vasodilator drugs to correct this disturbance in the microcirculation which has resulted in the stagnation. (See Figure 10.)

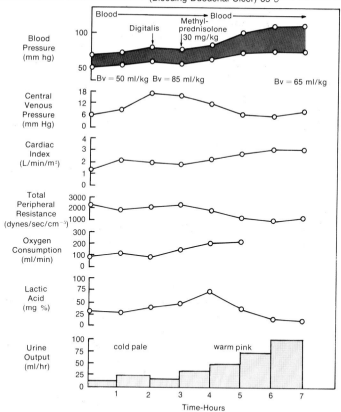

Figure 10. This 65 year old man was suffering from blood loss from a bleeding peptic ulcer. Despite adequate transfusion of blood, blood pressure and cardiac index remained low with poor peripheral perfusion as manifested by oliguria and cool skin. Moreover, the problem was complicated by a rise in central venous pressure, indicating congestive failure. Digitalis was used but with only minimal response. To correct this patient's problem, arterial resistance was lowered and venous capacitance increased with a bolus of methylprednisolone, 30 mg. per kg. This enabled us to give more blood and to restore the normal viscerocutaneous perfusion, resulting in a rise in urine output, warming skin and a rise in blood pressure as a result of an increased cardiac index or output.

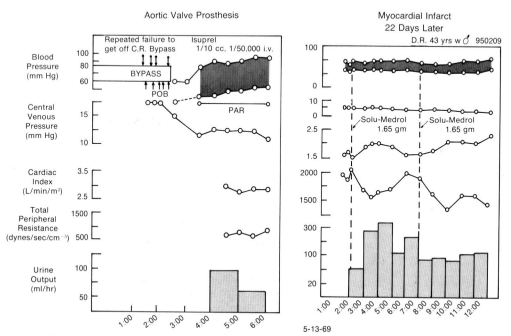

Figure 11. This patient suffered a myocardial infarction three weeks following replacement of an aortic valve for rheumatic aortic stenosis. The infarction was complicated by hypotension and congestive heart failure. Added digitalis was given without effect and isoproterenol was also tried. A bolus of 30 mg. per kg. of methylprednisolone was then given intravenously, which led to a gradual improvement in all hemodynamic and metabolic indicies. This patient recovered and left the hospital. We have not seen any significant differences in response to massive doses of corticosteroids between patients suffering shock or low output as a result of myocardial infarction and those suffering shock or low output syndrome following cardiac surgery. (See Figure 12.)

634

are the most readily available, safe drugs to use in correcting the microcirculatory stagnation of shock.

Cardiogenic Shock

A patient suffered a myocardial infarction and shock some three weeks following replacement of an aortic valve for rheumatic aortic stenosis (Fig. 11). The patient was suffering congestive failure along with shock; he had a high central venous pressure, low cardiac index, and low arterial pressure. Added digitalis was without effect, as was isoproterenol. The patient was given 30 mg. per kg. of methylprednisolone intravenously as a bolus, and over the next two hours the cardiac index gradually rose above 2 L. per min. per m.² and the central ve-

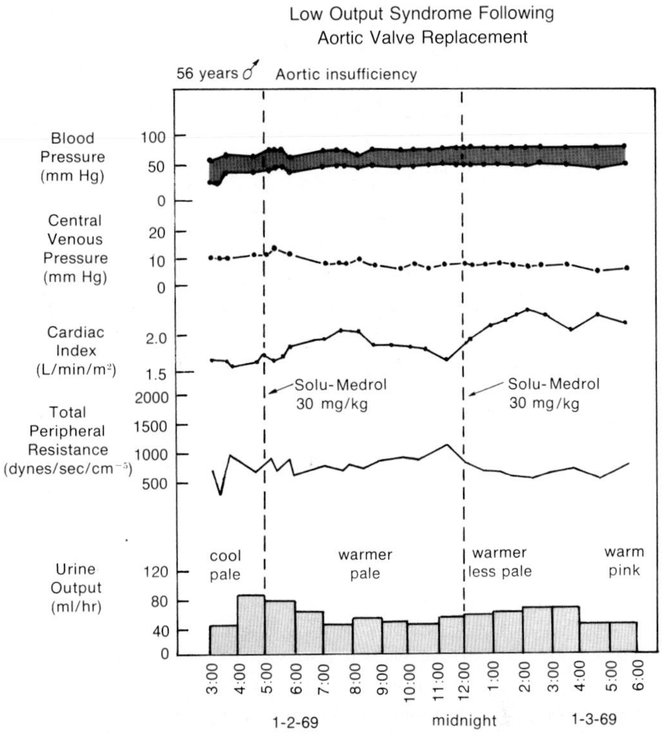

Figure 12. *A*, This patient was in low output syndrome or shock following aortic valve replacement. Two doses of 30 mg. per kg. of methylprednisolone intravenously, as shown, resulted in a gradual return toward normal of all the hemodynamic and metabolic indices measured and the patient recovered.
B, A comparison of the hemodynamic and metabolic responses of patients suffering shock from myocardial infarction or shock following cardiac surgery for acquired or congenital heart disease.

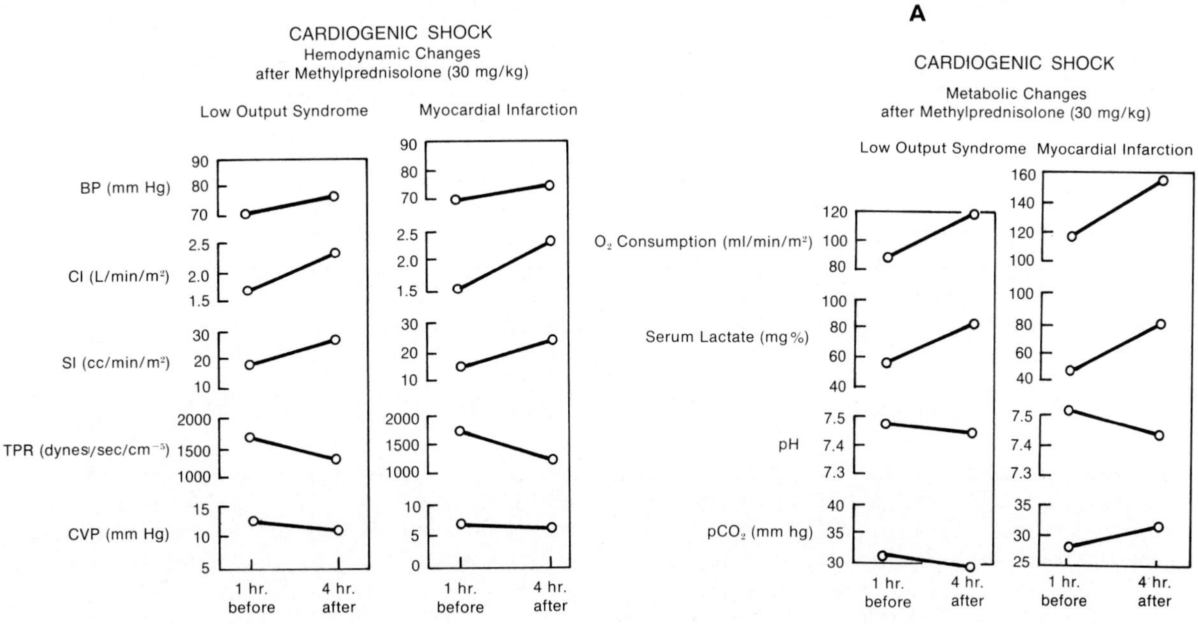

nous pressure decreased. Arterial pressure then rose, urine output increased, and the skin warmed. Metabolically, oxygen consumption increased markedly as cardiac index increased. This led to a washout of accumulated blood lactate in the stagnant microcirculation. The patient went on to make a complete recovery.

Still another type of cardiogenic shock seen more frequently in recent years is that following various procedures for correction of congenital and acquired cardiac defects, including coronary artery obstructions. In these patients, as in those suffering shock from myocardial infarction, the problem is usually one of low cardiac index and high central venous pressure indicative of congestive failure. Patients suffering the "low output syndrome" following cardiac surgery have suffered the same high mortality as patients suffering the low output syndrome, or shock, following myocardial infarction—70 or 90 per cent—when conventional means of therapy employing vasopressors are used.

Our results have been far better when we have used agents to reduce the characteristically high resistance found in the low output syndrome. In the patient pictured in Figure 12, who suffered low output syndrome following valve replacement, resistance was lowered with a dose of methylprednisolone (30 mg. per kg.) given intravenously. This resulted in a slow rise in cardiac index and a fall in central venous pressure and total peripheral resistance. A second dose of methylprednisolone was given some six hours later when the cardiac index again began to decrease. Usually one or two doses of the methylprednisolone is all that is necessary to help the patient suffering cardiogenic shock unless he has a massive infarction of the ventricle or a mechanical problem such as obstruction of the outflow tract by a prosthetic valve.

We have seen no adverse effects from administration of large doses of corticosteroids on wound healing, susceptibility to infection, gastrointestinal bleeding, or adrenocorticol suppression. Only corticosteriods given for prolonged periods of time induce these toxic effects.

Septic Shock

In septic shock we are dealing with a more complex condition than either traumatic or cardiogenic shock. This is because of the inflammatory effect of the living bacteria on tissue and the probable production of local hormones which lead to arteriovenous admixture or "physiological shunting." Thus, we have the paradox of patients suffering profound shock with oliguria, acidosis, and hypotension in the face of normal or high cardiac indices and low total peripheral resistances. It is important to emphasize that this increased cardiac index is not nutritional because the blood is not reaching the cells. This phenomenon is best illustrated in the lung, where it is often impossible to increase oxygen tensions to normal levels in the arterial blood despite the use of a respirator and 100 per cent oxygen. Blood may bypass over one half the alveoli in septic patients because of physiological shunting around the alveoli. The lung is a site for this shunting in many septic patients, but shunting may also occur in any areas of inflammation, and anatomical shunts may already exist in cirrhotic patients. Perhaps this is the reason that cirrhotic patients suffering septic shock have nearly a 100 per cent mortality. Indeed, it was in cirrhotic patients that high cardiac indices and low resistance were first noted to occur in septic shock, as was discussed earlier.

In septic shock a third factor is introduced in the treatment of shock after regulation of volume and use of vasodilators: the control of infection and elimination of the source of continued bacterial contamination of the blood. It is equally important in septic shock to restore the effective circulating blood volume and to correct the microcirculatory stagnation which characterizes septic shock and which is due to the endotoxins of the gram-negative bacteria.

An example of septic shock due to *Escherichia coli* is shown in Figure 13. This patient had multiple fistulas and peritonitis following surgery for regional enteritis. His blood pressure was low, he was oliguric, and his peripheral skin was cool. In the face of this, he had a low normal cardiac index and a very low peripheral resistance. His central venous pressure was in the normal range. We were unable to raise the oxygen tension of his arterial blood above 65 mm. Hg despite the use of a respirator and 100 per cent oxygen. As expected, his oxygen consumption under these conditions was low. Plasma fractions and balanced salt solutions were used to restore the effective circulation volume to normal. At the same time a massive dose of methylprednisolone (30 mg. per kg.) was given intravenously to aid in the correction of the stagnation in the viscerocutaneous circulation and to mobilize pooled blood trapped in these areas. Kanamycin was given in-

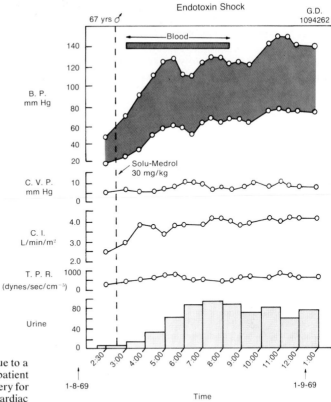

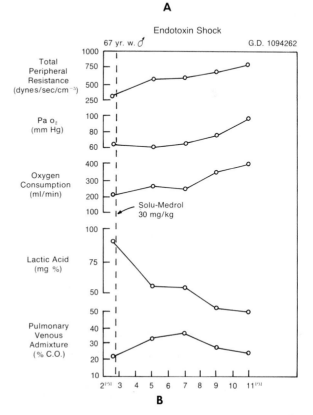

Figure 13. Typical example of septic shock due to a gram-negative bacteria, *Escherichia coli*. This patient had multiple fistulas and peritonitis following surgery for regional enteritis. He showed the typical high cardiac output, low total peripheral resistance of septic shock occurring in the face of severe hypoxia as manifested by low oxygen consumption, lactic acidosis, and a disturbed sensorium, along with the usual signs of shock: hypotension, oliguria, and cool skin of the extremities.

Treatment included kanamycin to take care of the living bacterial factor, a massive dose of methylprednisolone to correct the stagnation in the microcirculation caused by the bacterial endotoxin, and elimination of the source of contamination by bypassing the fistulas and placing the patient on his abdomen for dependent drainage.

Note the low oxygen tension of the arterial blood in the face of assisted respiration and 100 per cent oxygen. Admixture within the lungs as calculated by Berggren's formula reached almost 50 per cent. As the disturbances caused by the living bacteria and their endotoxins were corrected by these therapeutic measures, the resulting hemodynamic and metabolic effects of the disturbances also were corrected. Note also that the arteriovenous admixture in the lungs fell toward normal levels of under 15 per cent and it was now possible to raise the oxygen tension of the arterial blood to normal levels.

travenously in a 500 mg. dosage after blood and urine cultures were taken. Finally, abscesses were drained and the patient placed on his abdomen to prevent accumulation of intestinal contents in the peritoneal cavity. The proper institution of these measures resulted in a rapid resuscitation and eventual recovery of this patient. The effects of the therapy can be seen in the rise in blood pressure, increasing urine output, and warming of the skin. The cardiac index fell slightly and resistance rose, probably a result of decreasing arteriovenous admixture in lungs and peritoneum as the inflammatory process was eliminated. Coincident with this we were now able to bring the oxygen tension of his arterial blood to normal levels, and oxygen consumption rose. Accumulated lactate within the previously stagnant visceral cutaneous circulation was washed out and metabolized.

One final word. A large part of a decreased effective circulating blood volume in septic shock is due to the stagnation within the circulation. Hence, as this volume is mobilized, venous return increases, in addition to that provided by the infusion of fluids. Congestive failure may then occur in such patients after their resuscitation if the patient is not carefully watched. Usually the kidney will take care of excess volume in the 48 hours after resuscitation, but if renal damage has occurred, then reduction of intravenous infusions to avoid congestive failure and use of diuretics will be necessary.

The Use of Other Drugs

We have not completely abandoned the use of synthetic sympathomimetic agents such as levarterenol, metaraminol, or isoproterenol, which is a synthetic derivative of the catecholamines. Rather, these agents are used as needed for their central inotropic affect. Levarterenol and metaraminol have both an alpha and beta effect. The alpha (or peripheral viscerocutaneous constricting) effect can be blocked by the massive dose of methylprednisolone. This leaves the beta central effect on the heart relatively unaffected. In cardiogenic shock we employ small doses of levarterenol or metaraminol occasionally for an additional boost of cardiac index. In this manner, lower concentrations are used and toxic side effects are less common.

A better drug for the inotropic effect is probably isoproterenol, which is a pure beta stimulator. Nonetheless, we have found that its effect is potentiated by prior use of a vasodilator such

as methylprednisolone. Then isoproterenol can be given in smaller doses with fewer toxic side effects, such as tachycardias or arrhythmias, and with less evidence of the development of tachyphylaxis.

Inotropic agents are rarely necessary in septic shock unless there are complicating cardiac factors because of the already high outputs found in this condition.

Digitalis is often indicated in these patients even in the absence of previous history of heart disease. Often we begin digitalization along with the measures listed previously. The digitalization is then completed or discontinued, depending on the subsequent course of the patient. In the absence of significant arrhythmias and a normal serum potassium, there is little risk to the use of digitalis in this way. Digitalis is the only drug which causes an inotropic effect on the myocardium without increasing myocardial oxygen demand.

Other Vasodilating Drugs

There are many other drugs, in addition to the corticosteroids, which can be used for vasodilatation, yet most of them have one or more problems which lessen their usefulness. Phenoxybenzamine is the most potent alpha blocking agent that we have available. Its effect is almost immediate and may last for 24 or more hours. Unfortunately it is not available to most practicing physicians. But, even if it were available, the rapid onset of its effect has some drawbacks since it will accentuate the effects of a pre-existing hypovolemia by rapid expansion of the venous capacitance. Yet it is a valuable drug in certain situations such as acute congestive failure. Another alpha blocking agent is phentolamine, but this substance, in contrast to phenoxybenzamine, has a very short period of action and must be given as a continuous drip for the entire period that vasodilatation is desired.

Chlorpromazine has an alpha blocking effect and can be used for vasodilatation, but its depressing effect on the central nervous system has made it less useful than the corticosteroids. In the laboratory, doses of chlorpromazine, which will achieve vasodilatation equal to that of the corticosteroids or phenoxybenzamine, are in the area of 25 mg. per kg. or more. In man this dose will cause serious central nervous system depression and coma. Still, other investigators have reported that small doses of chlorpromazine, 5 or 10 mg. total dose, given intravenously at frequent intervals, will cause vasodilatation. Unfortunately no hemodynamic or metabolic measurements have been made by these investigators to support the use of chlorpromazine in this dosage (Laborit, 1955). Finally, there are other newer drugs, dopamine and glucagon, for example, which appear to be primarily inotropic agents. These show some promise in the laboratory as agents to treat shock, but experience with their use in man is still limited.

Diuretics

More recently potent diuretics such as ethacrynic acid and furosemide have become available. These agents often result in a diuresis even in the face of a low renal blood flow. Thus, we now see the paradox of a dying patient who is still secreting urine. This finding should not obscure the fact that the primary focus in shock is to increase the nutritional blood flow in the manner detailed earlier. Nonetheless, these diuretics can play a valuable adjuvant role when combined with administration of volume and use of vasodilators. We usually give, initially, 100 mg. of furosemide intravenously in an oliguric patient and follow this with additional doses as needed. Furosemide seems to have fewer side effects on the eighth cranial nerve than ethacrynic acid and is our choice for this reason.

Results of Therapy

Figure 14 shows the results of treating patients with the protocol of restoration of volume, vasodilators and, occasionally, inotropic agents. Overall survival is over 70 per cent. In previous experience with similar patients, we, and others, have had a *mortality* rate of 70 per cent using vasoconstrictors; thus, a complete turnabout has resulted from use of this program of volume regulation and vasodilators. It is important to note that the number of patients in hemorrhagic or traumatic shock is small since we have included in this group only patients in traumatic shock who did not respond to control of bleeding and administration of blood and other fluids. This emphasizes that most patients in traumatic shock can be resuscitated by volume control alone.

With this plan of treatment the majority of patients can be resuscitated from their shock, whatever its cause, with restoration of good nutritional blood flow as evidenced by hemodynamic and metabolic measurements and clinical

Shock in Man

Survival Following
Vasodilator[1.] – Volume
(positive inotropic[2] therapy when necessary)

	TRAUMATIC[3.]	SEPTIC[4.]	CARDIOGENIC
No. Patients	15	52	115
Survival[5.]	11 (73%)	36 (70%)	78 (68%)

1. Methyl prednisolone 30 mg/kg I.V. or phenoxybenzyamine 1 mg/kg I.V.
2. Levarterenol, Metaraminol, Isoproterenol or Glucagon
3. Unresponsive to volume alone
4. All with positive blood culture
5. Left hospital

Figure 14.

observations of skin temperature and urine output. If, in addition, the offending agent or source of the problem can also be eliminated, such as bleeding, infection, or continued cardiac damage, then the patients will recover completely.

What About Patients Who Do Not Respond to This Program?

We have found that patients who do not respond to a program of fluids, vasodilators, and inotropic agents when necessary are usually suffering from either a massive myocardial infarction, involving most of the left ventricle, or have some unrecognized abdominal catastrophe such as splenic, hepatic, or pancreatic rupture or gangrenous, perforated bowel, or both. When a patient does not respond within four hours to this protocol, we immediately suspect one of these problems and take measures to rule them out by use of a peritoneal tap and lavage or laparotomy.

SUMMARY

The usual causes of shock occurring during and following operative surgery are associated with a decrease in effective circulating blood volume, which may be due to external blood loss or pooling within the circulation, or both, as commonly occurs in gram-negative septic shock or congestive failure with cardiac damage. All these conditions elicit a viscerocutaneous vasoconstrictive response mediated through baroreceptors. The later stages of this response are characterized by stagnation in the microcirculation of the viscera and skin with loss of tone in arterioles, and venous outflow obstruction due to venular constriction or aggregation or both, or microthrombi within the stagnant circulation. The problems resulting from such a process include a decrease in the effective circulating blood volume, which may represent an actual loss of blood volume or pooling of large volumes within the circulation, and a disturbance in the microcirculation. Effective treatment must include restoration of effective circulating blood volume, which usually means the administration of additional fluids and the correction of the microcirculatory disturbance by use of a vasodilator. The most effective, safe vasodilators presently available are glucocorticosteroids, given in massive doses. The usual dosage has been 30 mg. per kg. of methylprednisolone, given as an intravenous bolus. Inotropic agents, such as levarterenol, metaraminol, and isoproterenol, are occasionally used for their inotropic or chronotropic effects, but only after peripheral vasodilatation with methylprednisolone. In this situation we have found that these inotropic agents become more effective in smaller doses and have less toxicity. A protocol utilizing this plan of treatment has resulted in an overall survival of more than 70 per cent of patients suffering traumatic, septic, or cardiogenic shock or combinations of these problems.

REFERENCES

Cannon, W. B.: Traumatic Shock. New York, D. Appleton Company, 1923.

Dietzman, R. H.: Unpublished Data.

Dietzman, R. H., and Lillehei, R. C.: The treatment of cardiogenic shock. IV. The use of phenoxybenzamine and chlorpromazine. Amer. Heart J. *75*:136 (January), 1968.

Dietzman, R. H., and Lillehei, R. C.: The treatment of cardiogenic shock. V. The use of steroids. Amer. Heart J. *75*:274 (February), 1968*a*.

Hardaway, R. M.: Clinical Management of Shock. Springfield, Ill., Charles C Thomas, 1968. Chapt. 17, Blood Coagulation Aspects of Shock.

Hermreck, A. S., and Thal, A. T.: Mechanisms for the high circulatory requirements in sepsis and septic shock. Ann. Surg. *170*:677, 1969.

Laborit, H.: Le choc traumatique. Sem. Hôp. Paris *31*:1, 1955.

Langsjoen, P. H., and Inmon, T. W.: Hermorrhalogic observations in acute myocardial infarction. Angiology *19*:247, 1968.

Lillehei, R. C., Dietzman, R. H., and Movsas, S.: Visceral circulation in shock. Gastroenterology *52*:468–471, 1967.

Lillehei, R. C., Dietzman, R. H., Movsas, S., and Bloch, J. H.: Treatment of septic shock. Modern Treatment *4*:321–326, 1967.

Lillehei, R. C., Longerbeam, J. K., Bloch, J. H., and Manax, W. G.: Nature of irreversible shock: Experimental and clinical observations. Ann. Surg. *160*:682, 1964.

Lillehei, R. C. (ed.): Shock in high and low flow states. Excerpta Medica, in press.

McKay, D. G., and Hardaway, R. M.: Thrombosis of Arterials, Capillaries and Venules: Experimental Considerations. Monograph 4, p. 259. "The Peripheral Blood Vessels." International Academy of Pathology. Baltimore, The Williams & Wilkins Company, 1963.

Metchnikoff, E.: Lectures on the Compared Pathology of Inflammation. Translated from the French by F. A. Starling and E. H. Starling. London, Kegan, Paul, Trensch Truber and Co., 1893.

Motsay, G. J.: Unpublished observations.

Motsay, G. J., Alho, A., Jaeger, T., Dietzman, R. H., and Lillehei, R. C.: Effects of corticosteroids on the circulation in shock: Experimental and clinical results. Fed. Proc. *29*:1861, 1970.

Motsay, G. J., Dietzman, R. H., and Lillehei, R. C.: Treatment of endotoxin shock. Rev. Surgery. *26* (6): 381–399, 1969.

Weil, M. H., Shubin, H., and Bittle, M.: Shock caused by gram negative microorganisms: Analysis of 169 Cases. Ann. Intern. Med. *60*:384, 1964.

Chapter 24

NUTRITIONAL CONSIDERATIONS IN HEAD AND NECK SURGERY

by Henry Buchwald, M.D., Ph.D., and Richard L. Varco, M.D., Ph.D.

At times the patient who has had head and neck surgery is limited in his ability to eat and drink as a result either of his primary disease process or, secondarily, from necessary surgical intervention. Thus, the otolaryngologist may be presented with a patient suffering from chronic starvation and/or protein depletion; e.g., a person with a carcinoma of the tongue may be unable to masticate adequately and to eat solid foods. Such an individual should be restored to a state of proper nutrition and nitrogen balance before extensive therapy is undertaken. At other times the surgeon will be faced with a patient temporarily or permanently denied oral alimentation; e.g., one with an incurable upper esophageal carcinoma. This necessitates use of another route for nutriment intake for days or even months. Thus, knowledge of caloric values, food constituent requirements, tube and parenteral feeding preparations, as well as those operative techniques and technical factors involved in their use, should be part of the armamentarium of any physician who desires to provide appropriate care to this group of patients.

The purpose of this chapter is to review certain general aspects of nutrition with particular reference to specific means of providing for head and neck patients those proteins, carbohydrates, fats, vitamins, fluids, and electrolytes required for optimum preoperative dietary preparation, postoperative recovery and healing, and, when indicated, acceptable long-term sustenance.

GENERAL ASPECTS OF PATIENT NUTRITION

Energy Values of Foods

Specific measurements of those calories available to man from intermediate metabolism of food have been calculated to be 4.1 calories per gram for carbohydrates, 9.45 calories per gram for fats, and 4.35 calories per gram for protein. The common Atwater convention of 1903 rounds these values off to 4 calories per gram for carbohydrates and proteins and 9 calories per gram for fats. It is, therefore, possible to calculate rapidly the energy potential of a food substance or of a meal from tables on food constituents. The daily basal caloric requirement for an adult man is about 1500 calories per 24 hours. This energy is needed for muscle tone and to maintain the basal circulatory, respiratory, digestive, glandular, and cellular activity. For the amount of work required to move, sit up, cough, and so forth, with a person otherwise on complete bed rest, approximately 2000 calories total per day are needed, and for one restricted to ambulation in his room the requirement is roughly 2250 calories per day. Additional precise information in this area of energy consumption, tables, and body surface formulas can be found in most textbooks of nutrition and calorimetry.

Proteins

In 1838 Mulder isolated a nitrogenous substance which he described as the basic constituent of living tissue; he gave this material the name "protein," taking its derivation from the Greek verb "to take the first place." These high molecular weight compounds are built from 22 known amino acids. Of these the 10 considered to be essential are so designated because they cannot be synthesized by man in amounts adequate to promote new tissue growth. Proteins have been classified as complete, partially complete, or incomplete, as a relative function of their content of these essential amino acids (arginine, histidine, isoleucine, leucine, lysine, methionine, phenylalanine, threonine, tryptophan, and valine). Examples of complete proteins are casein and lactalbumin from milk, egg ovalbumin and ovelvitellin, glycinin from soybeans, and certain proteins derived from the cereal grains.

Protein absorption from the gastrointestinal tract generally occurs as amino acids, following its enzymatic hydrolysis through successive stages (proteins → proteans → metaproteins → proteoses → peptones → peptides → amino acids). The smaller the protein molecule or protein derivative presented to the intestine, the more rapid will be its absorption. That is to say, the farther along the hydrolysis sequence from proteins to amino acids, the less time will be required for ultimate enzymatic digestion and the greater will be the quantitative proportion of amino acids available for absorption relatively high in the intestinal tract. If intestinal absorptive capacity is reduced by reason of bowel shortening or malabsorption, the amount of fat in the intestinal tract assumes an important role in protein absorption. When the amount of fat presented to the intestinal absorptive surface per unit area increases, the absorptive capacity of that area for amino acids proportionally decreases. Thus, when the total absorptive functional intestinal surface area is substantially decreased, then the presence of larger amounts of fat seriously interferes with amino acid absorption.

The recommended minimum protein requirement for an adult man is approximately one gram per kilogram of body weight per day. Two- or threefold this amount is suggested for the growing child, the cancer victim, or a post-operative patient. In addition to demonstrated increased protein requirements of healing tissues, the surgeon should recall that exudative sites can lose large amounts of proteins as serum, white blood cells, or whole blood.

Carbohydrates

Carbohydrates provide the greatest total weight or calories of available energy in the diets of most people. They constitute the most abundant and the most economical foods in the world. Fortunately they are the easiest food substance for the body to digest and absorb. Intravenous infusions of carbohydrate products are also well utilized.

Again, on considering assimilation from the intestinal tract, the simpler the organic form of the carbohydrate presented to the intestinal wall, the more rapidly will a given amount be absorbed. Carbohydrate digestion also consists of a series of enzymatic hydrolyses, proceeding from the more complex and larger molecular weight carbohydrates of the starches to the dextrins and, finally, after several intermediate stages to the monosaccharides, the six carbon sugars that are the end-products of carbohydrate digestion. Thus, since the enzymatic hydrolysis time to the monosaccharide level for complicated carbohydrates exceeds that of dextrins, absorption per unit surface area will be a function of the state of hydrolysis of the carbohydrate. Knowledge of the form of carbohydrate present in a food (e.g., a candy bar) will, therefore, permit estimation of the rapidity with which the sugar is available for energy.

Finally, the monosaccharides (glucose, fructose, mannose, galactose) are absorbed at individual rates by active and specific mucosal transport mechanisms. As early as 1900 Reid, and more recently Fisher (1953), demonstrated the duodenum as the most active site of glucose absorption per unit mucosal area.

Fats

Fats yield the most energy per unit weight and are thus an important calorie source to a patient. However, adequate fat absorption requires no less than 75 per cent of a normal small intestine. Enzymatic fat hydrolysis to fatty acids and glycerol as end-products to be absorbed is intrinsically slow. Also, whereas amino acids and simple sugars (monosaccharides) are rapidly absorbed, this is not true for the fatty acids and glycerol. These substances have a slow rate of transfer into the mucosal cell. Additional delay occurs since they must then be reconstituted (re-esterified) within the cell to triglycerides (the combination of three fatty acids and glycerol) before they are free to pass via the lacteals and into the circulation. Furthermore, the capacity of the intestinal mucosa to absorb fat products decreases per unit area from jejunum to ileum. Attempts at increasing the fat load excessively to up the amount absorbed are self-defeating. This will result in steatorrhea, plus a greater loss of water, electrolytes, proteins, fat soluble vitamins, and calcium.

A change in intestinal flora also seriously interferes with the digestion of fats. Intestinal antibiotics of the broad-spectrum variety have been used to reverse this form of steatorrhea.

In the early 1930's a syndrome of scaly dermatitis, ecchymosis, alopecia, growth inhibition, and impaired reproduction and lactation was demonstrated in rats on a diet devoid of the unsaturated fatty acids linoleic or linolenic and arachidonic by Burr and co-workers (1932) and Evans and associates (1934). Similar effects caused by a dietary or absorptive deficit of these essential fatty acids (that is, fatty acids that cannot be synthesized from the body acetate pool) have not been well documented in man.

Though excellent amino acid protein hydrolysates have been manufactured in the United States for intravenous infusion, a clinically sound pyrogen-free lipid emulsion for intravenous use is not yet available in this country.

Fluid and Electrolytes

Consideration of fluid and electrolyte balance is presented elsewhere in this volume and will not be discussed in this chapter. However, in association with the discussion of fat absorption and the fat dietary load, the paradox should be pointed out that since the formation of calcium fatty acid soaps serves as the vehicle for normal absorption of the insoluble calcium ion, in the patient with fat malabsorption the very formation of this soap complex interferes with calcium assimilation and results in the loss of large amounts of calcium in the feces. Note of warning: the sodium content of whole milk is 550 mg./L. When large amounts of milk are consumed the danger exists, especially in the care of the patient with cardiac disease, of an excessive sodium load.

Vitamins and Minerals

Any chronically malnourished patient may have either subclinical or manifest avitaminosis. If the clinical picture or laboratory tests establish that diagnosis, specific vitamin therapy is indicated. In the absence of a specific deficiency requiring therapy, three vitamin supplements should be routinely considered in the overall surgical care: thiamine (vitamin B_1), C, and K.

Thiamine. Thiamine (vitamin B_1) participates in those enzyme systems which are essential to carbohydrate metabolism and also maintains normal gastrointestinal activity. Therefore, in any nutritional preparation requiring an intake of large quantities of carbohydrate, 10 to 20 mg. daily of thiamine is advised.

Vitamin C. The contribution of vitamin C to wound healing has been clearly established. A low tissue concentration of vitamin C is positively correlated with poor wound healing and increased wound disruption (Pollack, 1952). In certain head and neck patients vitamin C intake can be low. This situation is worsened by augmented vitamin C losses from raw wound surfaces of sizable dimension. The calculated normal basic daily requirement of vitamin C is 75 mg.; however, in the surgical patient 500 mg. daily may be a reasonable dose.

Vitamin K. Vitamin K is largely produced by the normal intestinal flora. It is also contained in certain green leaves, egg yolk, and soybeans. This fat soluble vitamin requires, therefore, adequate fat absorption or parenteral vitamin K supplementation to insure the amount required by the liver to form prothrombin. Otherwise, hypoprothrombinemia, interference with blood clotting at the thrombin conversion stage, and excessive bleeding can develop. The most readily available laboratory test to evaluate these circumstances is the direct prothrombin time measurement. Numerous oral and parenteral preparations of vitamin K are available for supplementation purposes.

Iron. The recommended daily iron allowance for adult men is 10 mg. and for adult premenopausal women, 12 to 15 mg. Any patient who has to rely on liquid oral nutrition can exhibit a negative iron balance. There are less than 5 gm. of iron in a healthy adult, and since much of this is in stores poorly mobilized, iron depots can readily be exhausted. Thereafter the patient can develop an iron deficiency anemia without blood loss. A source of iron in its most usable form is, of course, blood transfusion, and it may be well to plan preoperative transfusion to achieve a hemoglobin concentration of at least 12 gm. per 100 ml. prior to elective major operations. For long-term maintenance the physician must think more in terms of iron supplementation rather than the continued use of blood transfusions. There are a great variety of parenteral and oral preparations available to the physician, and reference to them may be found in the annual PDR publication.

Trace Minerals. The trace minerals, manganese, cobalt, copper, magnesium, and so forth, are generally present in adequate amounts in the diets of people on normal oral alimentation and without excessive stool losses. However, these substances may be diminished or absent from the diet of patients on parenteral feeding or modified liquid diets. For these patients provision for mineral supplementation should be made. Syndromes have been described in association with low blood levels of specific trace minerals. These events may arise because these substances serve as catalysts for various enzymatic processes. The most striking is the syndrome of hypomagnesemia. This deficiency state is characterized by fatigue, generalized muscle weakness, tingling of the lips, nose, and extremities, pre-tetany with a positive Chvostek sign and, finally, frank tetany with carpal-pedal spasms despite a normal serum calcium concentration.

SPECIFIC MEANS OF AIDING NUTRITION IN THE HEAD AND NECK PATIENT

Total Parenteral Nutrition

Parenteral nutrition, adequate to meet daily caloric needs, is customarily used for only brief periods of time, since the glucose solutions produce local venous thromboses. Alternatively, long-term use of a central venous catheter can be followed by intravascular sepsis. Yet it is appreciated that in the head and neck patient, oral alimentation may be particularly difficult or, at times, indeed impossible.

Francis D. Moore, in *Metabolic Care of the Surgical Patient* (1959), takes a rather pessimistic view of long-term total parenteral nutrition for adults as evaluated by true body weight gain and an anabolic state. Scattered reports by Beal and associates (1957) and Holden and co-workers (1957) had shown, however, that positive nitrogen balance could be achieved during short periods of total intravenous feedings. More recently, Dudrick and associates (1968) have documented that apparently normal growth, development, and certainly a positive nitrogen balance can be achieved in beagles receiving only intravenous nutrition (1968). Indeed, the puppies fed totally by the venous route seemed to outgrow their orally fed littermates. Subsequent application of their method has been nutritionally successful in certain patients with intra-abdominal problems (e.g., multiple intestinal fistulas). They have reported parenteral nutritional management associated with weight gain, normal development, and wound healing in infants with gastrointestinal anomalies treated for 10 to 210 days. They credit their ability to maintain safe long-term venous infusions to very careful catheter maintenance care techniques. The skin surrounding the catheter is cleansed with ether or acetone, scrubbed with tincture of iodine solution, and a broad-spectrum antibiotic ointment reapplied to the catheter exit site; the occlusive dressing is changed (aseptically) every few days.

The Dudrick formula, assembled in a hospital pharmacy, is 165 gm. of anhydrous glucose in 860 ml. of 5 per cent glucose with 5 per cent fibrin hydrolysate solution (Aminosol, Abbott). This yields 1 L. containing 1000 calories and 6 gm. of amino acid-peptide nitrogen. Preparation requirements include sterile mixing facilities in a laminar airflow room. This is unlikely to be available in many hospitals. A modified preparation plan consists of aseptically mixing commercially available bottled solutions on the nursing stations just prior to patient delivery. This can be achieved by adding 750 ml. of a 5 per cent casein hydrolysate (Amigen, Baxter) to 250 ml. of a 50 per cent glucose solution. This combination yields 800 calories and 5.23 gm. of amino acid–peptide nitrogen per liter. Sodium, potassium, chloride, calcium, magnesium, and phosphorus can be added to the daily fluids as indicated by the needs of the individual patient. For its desired anabolic effect and for the building of new cells with high concentrates of intracellular potassium, it is necessary to provide 40 to 60 mEq. of potassium chloride per liter of parenteral solution. The commercial casein hydrolysate solution contains 35 mEq. of sodium, 18 mEq. of potassium, 5 mEq. of calcium, 2 mEq. of magnesium, 30 mEq. of phosphate, and 22 mEq. of chloride per liter. All these electrolyte values must be considered in calculating the total daily requirements. Addition of a vitamin mixture to each 1000 ml. unit of parenteral solution is recommended; this can readily be achieved by adding 1 ml. of a commercially available water soluble vitamin preparation. Also, iron, vitamin B_{12}, vitamin K, folic acid, and the trace elements such as zinc, copper, manganese, cobalt, and iodine can be either added to the intravenous solution or given as intramuscular injections when indicated. Though the precise requirements for essential fatty acids has not been determined, addition of a unit of plasma weekly is suggested as the best means for supplying these substances.

We have employed up to 7000 ml. of the amino acid–glucose mixture daily, utilizing this preparation both as daily maintenance fluid and for fluid replacement of fistula losses, gastric aspiration loss, and so forth. We have, therefore, used this mixture for the total fluid requirement for patients over many weeks. The use of this preparation at such high volumes, or as only a portion of the daily intravenous fluids, requires careful attention to certain precautions: It is possible to achieve an osmotic diuresis and dehydration secondary to the high glucose content of the solution. The amount of daily urine should be carefully charted, as well as the qualitative presence of sugar in the urine; serum and urine quantitative glucose determination should be obtained at least every third day. If the daily urine volume exceeds one half the venous infusion volume or the glucose content of the urine is in excess of 50 gm. daily, the intravenous glucose concentration should be reduced. The long-term effect of this high glucose delivery on the pancreas and pancreatic function has not as yet been determined. The patient with normal kidneys will be able to handle the amino acid load without any difficulties. However, persistent use of this mixture, especially in patients with impaired renal function, might result in azotemia. It is well, therefore, to monitor renal function by obtaining a BUN and/or a serum creatinine every other day and at an early stage of this therapy to obtain a more precise measure of quantitative renal function, e.g., a creatinine clearance. Periodic serum electrolyte determinations must certainly be carried out, and the dangers of an intolerable sodium or potassium load, especially in the patient with borderline cardiac reserve, should be kept in mind. Complications can be minimized by daily recalculation of the electrolyte content of the intravenous solution and the patient's daily losses.

As a rule, intravenous nutrition is best supplied through an indwelling superior vena cava or subclavian catheter by straight drip. However, under certain situations in the adult, and more commonly in the pediatric age group, a constant volume infusion pump in the delivery circuit is indicated. By using a pump a more careful control of minute to minute, hour to hour infusion is obtained; in babies it is often essential to utilize the pump flow pressure to offset the venous circulatory back-pressure that babies generate on crying. The pump is also needed to force the solution through the very fine openings in a bacterial millipore filter inserted into the system for additional control of bacterial contamination during long-term intravenous feeding regimens.

In addition to amino acid–glucose solutions, our currently available intravenous nutrition preparations include ethyl alcohol and probably will soon include pyrogen-free solutions of fatty acids. Satisfactory fatty acid solutions are currently available in Europe and may eventually be cleared for use in the United States. Those intravenous lipid-containing compounds previously marketed in the United States often were associated with impurities, variability in lipid concentrations, and febrile side effects. The sedative effect of intravenous ethyl alcohol, 5 per cent solution, may be desirable in the management of certain patients.

A word concerning clyses and intraperitoneal fluid infusions; a brief word indeed: do not use them. Their usefulness is short-lived, their delivery is uncomfortable, and for nutritional purposes they are inadequate.

Principles of Alimentary Feedings

Four routes of administration have been used in the management of patients with impairment of the normal mechanical and physiological mechanisms of food ingestion, digestion and emulsification, and propulsion: (1) liquid and semiliquid oral feeding; (2) standard diet ingestion and mastication, swallowing, and bag collection from an esophagostomy, with reinjection distally into the gastrointestinal tract; (3) gastrointestinal tract tube feedings; and (4) enema feedings. Since factors of retention and expulsion tend to make caloric uptake by rectal feeding unpredictable and difficult to control, and since the colon is poorly suited for the absorption of proteins in contrast to the small bowel, we find no real application for nutriment enemas. We have, however, utilized the other three methods successfully preoperatively, immediately following operation, and during a prolonged postoperative period, while attempting to select the mode of alimentation best suited to the problem and to the personality of the individual.

The entire daily caloric, electrolyte, mineral, vitamin, and fluid requirements of the patient can be delivered to the intestinal tract or, when diarrhea poses a problem, supplemental intravenous infusion can be utilized to minimize the intestinal water load. For example, certain patients with head and neck disorders combined with a shortened or malfunctioning small intestine can absorb adequate amounts of calories through their gastrointestinal tract if the volume is low. However, if such a patient is also given large amounts of fluids via the gastrointestinal route, massive diarrhea and malabsorption could result.

In patients with nonbacterial diarrhea we have successfully used for both bowel control and for hyperalimentation a diet high in protein, low in carbohydrate, low in fat, and low in fiber content. This consists of a curd-forming mixture of peanut butter, cheddar cheese, dry cottage cheese, and boiled skim milk, diluted for delivery with varying proportions of water. It can be adapted for tube feeding. Minimization of the carbohydrate content in this mixture to less than 20 per cent by weight reduces the osmotic shift of fluid into the bowel lumen (secondary to the enzymatic hydrolysis of the carbohydrates to the simple sugars). The low fat content of this diet is important since fat interferes with the availability of the mucosal surface interface for absorption of other food substances, in particular amino acids. Too, rapid transit of the meal is to be avoided since that allows the fat to reach the colon partially hydrolyzed and with cathartic properties due to the high content of partially hydrolyzed triglycerides or free fatty acids. The high calcium concentration of the diet seeks to minimize the diarrheagenic action of fat by binding these lipids as soaps. Elimination of a high fiber content results in decreasing the bulk of the intestinal bolus, allowing relatively greater mucosal surface contact time for absorption of nutrients and slower intestinal transit time.

Commercial purées and blended diets, of a wide variety and high palatability, are available for the patient with a normally functioning gastrointestinal tract and the ability to swallow liquids and semiliquids but with inability to chew. Or, as an alternative, a balanced, high caloric, high protein diet can be prepared in the kitchen of hospital or home and treated in a blender until it can be taken either from a cup or through a straw. Recently the elemental diet developed by NASA has been adapted for clinical use by Stephens and Randall (1969). This is a concentrated mixture of l-amino acids, simple sugars, electrolytes, vitamins, and minerals. It is absorbed without further digestive breakdown and is free of bulk-forming fiber content.

A special variation of oral feeding may be considered in the patient able to handle foodstuffs orally, with normal mastication and deglutition, but unable to provide esophageal transit, e.g., the patient with a mid or low esophageal carcinoma with either temporary or permanent disruption of intestinal continuity. If the ability to eat and the enjoyment of food is important to this patient, he can eat, collect the swallowed food in a bag connected to a cervical esophagostomy stoma, and reinject the contents into a gastrostomy tube. This compromise with reality may seem unimportant to the physician, yet to the patient such a technique might facilitate his own adjustment to a harsh reality.

Feedings can be introduced into the alimentary tract by a nasogastric tube or through a catheter inserted into a distal cervical esophagostomy, a gastrostomy, or an enterostomy. The nutrient material can be delivered by intermittent or continuous drip, by a constant volume pump, or by intermittent injections of "feedings." For the ambulatory patient with normal gastrointestinal function, the intermittent delivery of fairly large amounts of formula proves to be the least burdensome and incapacitating. If hyperalimentation for body building and wound healing is desired, then continuous around-the-clock delivery can yield better results.

In preparing tube feeding formulas the dietitian has the advantage of not having to consider palatability or taste variability. Formulas for high caloric, high protein mixtures using common foods homogenized in a blender can be made readily available. There are also acceptable commercial preparations (e.g., Meritine, Coyle; Sustagen, Mead Johnson, etc.). In patients free of diarrhea, the addition of short and medium chain triglycerides (Portagen, Mead Johnson) for augmentation of the caloric load should be considered. The shorter the hydrolyzed fatty acid chain, the more rapid is the rate of absorption. It is to be stressed that all tube feedings require the cooperation and dedication of the nursing personnel, the patient, the patient's family, and the attending physician. Successful tube feeding programs should not be ordered but rather be instituted, explained, and carefully managed.

Specific Surgical Procedures to Aid in Nutrition

Cervical Esophagostomy. In the patient with an intact alimentary system from the cervical esophagus on down, feeding via a cervical esophagostomy is feasible. Since a cervical esophagostomy usually involves a stoma at the skin level, a permanent indwelling catheter for tube feedings is not necessary and the patient can insert the catheter at the time of feeding for administration of the diet either by drip or direct low pressure injection. This procedure at times is preferable to a feeding gastrostomy. A distal cervical esophagostomy involves stomatization also of the proximal esophagus and, thereby, creates the problem of salivary drainage, a situation often annoying socially to the patient. In select patients this problem can be circumvented or minimized by construction of a side-on stoma with a flaplike cutaneous outlet, allowing the salivary secretions to pass down the esophagus. A cervical esophagostomy can be performed on either the right or the left side; this decision is often based on the location of the patient's primary disease. The procedure is facilitated by having a nasogastric tube in place. General intubation anesthesia is preferable since it avoids laryngospasm secondary to manipulation of the larynx or the trachea. If, however, general anesthesia is contraindicated, the operation can be performed under local infiltration anesthesia.

A linear incision parallel to the anterior border of the sternocleidomastoid muscle is made, and the incision is deepened through the platysma and the anterior layer of the deep cervical fascia. The anterior border of the sternocleidomastoid muscle is then mobilized and the belly of the muscle is retracted medially. This retraction will bring into view the lateral and posterior surface of the thyroid gland. The dissection must remain inferior to the gland. Anterior exposure of the gland signifies an approach through an incorrect tissue plane. The middle deep cervical fascia is then incised (essentially the carotid sheath in this area), exposing the internal jugular vein, the vagus nerve, and the common carotid artery. At this stage of the procedure, in order to facilitate exposure, it is often necessary to doubly ligate and divide the inferior thyroid artery. The contents of the carotid sheath are retracted posteriorly, thereby exposing the esophagus. Care must be taken not to injure the recurrent laryngeal nerve, which will lie in a groove between the lower esophagus and the overlying trachea. It is now possible to elevate the esophagus from its bed by a combination of sharp and blunt dissection. Palpation of the nasogastric tube within the lumen of the esophagus aids the surgeon in passing a full curved clamp beneath the esophagus and encircling the esophagus with a rubber catheter. The esophagus should be freed superiorly and inferiorly for a distance adequate to allow it to be brought to skin level through the dissection plane used for its exposure.

If it is elected to bring out separate proximal and distal stomas, the esophagus is divided and the cut mucosal margins are tacked directly to the skin. If, on the other hand, it is elected to make a side window in the esophagus, this is constructed with longitudinal division of the esophageal fibers, placing anchoring sutures at either end of the incision to prevent tearing; again, the cut mucosal margin is anchored to the skin surface. Hemostasis must be well controlled prior to closure. If the wound is thoroughly irrigated, bleeding points can become more apparent. It should not be necessary to insert a drain; closure of the deep layers is not indicated. The platysma and subcutaneous closure is carried out with inverted 4-0 chromic catgut sutures, and fine skin approximation is accomplished with interrupted sutures of a nonabsorbable 5-0 material. If two stomas are constructed it is desirable to leave a small skin bridge between them. The esophageal stoma or stomas are best secured flush to the skin with interrupted 4-0 or 5-0 nonabsorbable sutures to be removed in five to seven days.

Feeding Gastrostomy. The feeding gastrostomy is probably the simplest technical procedure for tube feedings. The cutaneous orifice is not visible in the dressed patient. The feeding catheter can be kept clean and inconspicuously taped to the left upper quadrant of the abdomen.

Several basic gastrostomy procedures and modifications are described in atlases of operative technique. We have preferred the Witzel gastrostomy. Correct performance of this type of operation virtually insures against the leakage that leads to the serious sequelae of wound infection, local abscess, and peritonitis. The operation can be performed under local or general anesthesia. Access to the stomach is obtained through a midline, paramedian, or transverse rectus dividing incision. We are guided in this choice by the individual patient's anatomy, e.g., angle of rib flare, other abdominal scars, etc. We prefer to bring the gastrostomy tube out separately rather than through the incision.

When the abdominal cavity is entered the anterior surface of the mid or upper stomach is clasped with Babcock clamps and brought into the operative field. In order to construct a generous tunnel approximately 6 to 7 cm. long, it is necessary to visualize well about 10 cm. of the anterior gastric wall. About midway between the lesser and greater curvatures one is less likely to encounter large vessels. With the placement of each suture a conscious effort should be made to avoid puncturing a vessel and thereby producing a hematoma of the gastric wall. A purse string suture is placed through the seromuscular layers of the exposed gastric wall using 4-0 nonabsorbable suture. If feasible, a second purse string suture is placed around the perimeter of the first. An incision is then made through the muscularis, and the mucosa is picked up with forceps and incised. Care is taken not to dissect the mucosa from the gastric wall upon insertion of the feeding catheter. The purse string sutures are tied, and an attempt made to funnel the gastric wall inward around the catheter. The catheter tunnel is then constructed by folding the anterior gastric wall around the catheter for a distance of at least 6 cm. proximal to the site of entry, using Lembert sutures and employing generous rolls of gastric wall above and below the catheter. In addition, it is essential to place one or two stitches distal to the site of entry to insure a tight seal.

Further security of the line of closure and prevention of leakage can be obtained by suturing the gastric wall at the proximal end of the tunnel to the peritoneum of the anterior abdominal wall. To insure that the catheter is not inadvertently removed or does not fall out prior to establishment of a tract, we have anchored the catheter by a direct stitch of nonabsorbable suture through the gastric wall and then tied around the catheter at the point of exit from the seromuscular tunnel. It is essential to anchor the tube to the skin with a nonabsorbable suture. The cutaneous exit for the tube should be a stab wound just large enough to permit passage of the catheter. The abdominal wound is closed separately, utilizing non-absorbable sutures.

We have employed various catheters in construction of feeding gastrostomies: a straight nasogastric tube with multiple openings within the gastric lumen, a Foley catheter with inflation of the balloon to insure anchorage, a Malecot or a mushroom catheter, and, finally, a large T-tube with extra fenestrations cut in both limbs. In most circumstances we prefer a large diameter (No. 18 French) nasogastric tube in adults. For prolonged gastrostomy feedings it will be necessary from time to time to change the catheter because of deterioration of the rubber. Nevertheless, rubber catheters are generally preferable to plastic tubes since they remain flexible longer. Feeding of the patient may begin within 24 to 48 hours, but should usually be delayed until signs of effective bowel activity are present. Until then the gastrostomy tube is attached to low pressure suction. It is best to initiate feeding with a sterile solution of 5 per cent dextrose in water and then to progress to skim milk and finally to a tube diet.

Feeding Jejunostomy. In certain circumstances it may be impossible to construct a feeding gastrostomy, and it then becomes necessary to achieve alimentation via a more distal site – a feeding jejunostomy. This should be constructed as far proximal as permitted by the disease process. If feasible, the first loop of jejunum beyond the ligament of Trietz is best utilized. Either upper quadrant is a reasonable operative site and, again, we suggest bringing the tube out through a separate opening. The jejunostomy is constructed along the antimesenteric border and here, too, we prefer the use of the Witzel principle. Care should be taken not to obstruct the smaller diameter of the jejunum by the amount of bowel infolded.

Drug Aids in Furthering Nutrition

Antiemetics. Head and neck cancers, the presence of necrotic or purulent tissue, and the effects of radiation therapy, singly or in combination, will be responsible for nausea and emesis in certain patients. For acute parenteral management of this problem we have utilized prochlorperazine (Compazine, Smith, Kline & French), chlorpromazine (Thorazine, Smith, Kline & French), promazine hydrochloride (Sparine, Wyeth), and hydroxyzine (Vistaril, Pfizer). These compounds also provide tranquilizing effects. Selection of which drug to employ is usually based on the individual patient's tolerance and response to that agent and the previous conditioning experience of the physician using that particular compound. These drugs can reveal such adverse reactions associated with their use as central nervous system depression, potentiation of the actions of narcotics and barbiturates, and facilitation of hypotension. They should be used cautiously in patients with pre-existing cerebral depression or orthostatic hypotension, and in those receiving antihypertensive medication.

For prolonged ambulatory care oral preparations of these drugs are available. We have also satisfactorily employed less potent agents such as meclizine hydrochloride (Bonine, Pfizer) and trimethobenzamide hydrochloride (Tigan, Roche). These two compounds are generally well tolerated and have few, if any, side effects other than drowsiness. Trimethobenzamide is available in an intramuscular preparation; meclizine hydrochloride is not. Trimethobenzamide may have to be taken as 250 mg. three or four times daily to achieve the desired effect, whereas meclizine hydrochloride in doses of 25 to 100 mg. may need to be given only once or twice every 24 hour period.

Anorexia. Unfortunately to date there is no preparation which will directly stimulate the hunger center of the hypothalamus. This is unfortunate since many cancer patients, in particular those undergoing x-ray therapy, have little or no appetite. The antiemetics may be helpful in removing the nauseous sensations which so often accompany anorexia. The ingestion of alcoholic beverages has often been recommended for appetite induction, though solid scientific evidence for this mode of treatment is lacking.

Other Problems. For particular patients antacids, antispasmodics, and anticonstipation agents might be indicated. One side effect of tube feeding and/or radiation therapy can be diarrhea. Any medicinal approach to treating this problem should be based on full consideration of the potentially initiating circumstances. For the patient with increased bowel motility, a combination of diphenoxylate hydrochloride with atropine sulfate (Lomotil, Searle) has been shown to be of value. This product is supplied in both tablet and liquid form, with each tablet and each teaspoon of liquid containing 2.5 mg. of diphenoxylate hydrochloride. Though this compound is potentially addictive, we have not found patient addiction with use for as long as two years. The recommended dose is up to 8 tablets daily; however, we have employed this drug with satisfactory results for short periods at a dosage of 4 tablets four times a day. For acute episodes of severe diarrhea codeine, paregoric, or tincture of opium is recommended. However, none should be used on a prolonged basis in patients with curable lesions since each is habit forming and truly addictive. If the bowel problem is primarily one of watery evacuations, a nonabsorbable bulk hydrophilic material such as psyllium hydrophilic mucilloid (Metamucil, Searle) can be used to advantage. When it is believed that the rapid transit of bile acids (the natural cathartic) or excessive quantities of partially hydrolyzed fatty acids in the colon are primarily responsible for the diarrhea, additional calcium as the gluconate, chloride, or carbonate will form heavy ion soaps with less activity as mucosal irritants.

CONCLUSIONS

The patient undergoing head and neck surgery, and in particular the patient with a cancer of the head and neck region, often presents the responsible physician with challenging problems related to adequate nutrition and sound wound healing. Indeed, the efforts of the most skilled surgeon can be nullified by patient malnutrition. The principles of adequate nutrition and the means and methods to deliver nutrients must be intrinsic to the knowledge and skills of the practicing surgeon and will often provide the margin of difference between success and failure, comfort and distress.

REFERENCES

Atwater, W. O., and Benedict, F. G.: A Respiration Calorimeter with Appliances for the Direct Determination of Oxygen. Carnegie Institution of Washington, D. C., 1905.

Beal, J. M., Payne, M. A., Gilder, H., Johnson, G., and Craver, W. L.: Experience with administration of an intravenous fat emulsion to surgical patients. Metabolism 6:673, 1957.

Burr, G. O., Burr, M. M., and Miller, E. S.: On the fatty acids essential in nutrition. J. Biol. Chem. 97:1, 1932.

Dudrick, S. J., Wilmore, D. W., Vars, H. M., and Rhoads, J. E.: Long-term total parenteral nutrition with growth, development, and positive nitrogen balance. Surgery 64:134, 1968.

Evans, H. M., Lepkovsky, S., and Murphy, E. A.: Vital need of the body for certain unsaturated fatty acids: Reproduction and lactation upon fat-free diets. J. Biol. Chem. 106:431, 1934.

Fisher, R. B., and Parsons, D. S.: Galactose absorption from the surviving small intestine of the rat. J. Physiol. 119:224, 1953.

Holden, W. D., Krieger, H., Levey, S., and Abbott, W. E.: The effects of nutrition on nitrogen metabolism in the surgical patient. Ann. Surg. 146:563, 1957.

Moore, F. D.: Metabolic Care of the Surgical Patient. Philadelphia, W. B. Saunders Company, 1959.

Mulder, G. J.: Action de l'acide hydrochlorique sur la proteine. Bull. Sci. Phys. Nat. (Leyde), 153, 1838.

Pollack, H., and Halpern, S. L.: Therapeutic Nutrition. Washington, D. C., National Academy of Sciences National Research Council, No. 234, 1952, p. 37.

Reid, E. W.: On intestinal absorption, especially on the absorption of serum, peptone, and glucose. Phil. Trans. Roy. Soc., *192*:211, 1900.

Stephens, R. V., and Randall, H. T.: Use of a concentrated, balanced, liquid elemental diet for nutritional management of catabolic states. Ann. Surg. *170*:642, 1969.

Wilmore, D. W., Graff, D. B., Bishop, H. C., and Dudrick, S. J.: Total parenteral nutrition in infants with catastrophic gastrointestinal anomalies. J. Pediat. Surg. *4*:181, 1969.

Chapter 25

BASIC PRINCIPLES OF PLASTIC SURGERY IN THE HEAD AND NECK

by Byron J. Bailey, M.D.

The basic tenet of the philosophy of regional surgery is that concentration upon the special anatomic features and physiologic complexities of a given body region are necessary in order for an individual to acquire therapeutic expertise in the management of disorders in that region. In regard to surgical therapy, this understanding of basic structure and function must be coupled with sound knowledge of surgical concepts and principles.

This chapter's purpose is to provide a review of basic principles of head and neck plastic surgery as they relate to elective procedures and the management of trauma and cancer. The subsequent information is presented with the emphasis on breadth of subject rather than depth in the hope that it will serve to stimulate further study in many of these areas.

We shall present information gathered from many sources as we attempt to correlate basic knowledge with useful surgical principles.

ANATOMY OF THE SKIN

It would be fair to say that many surgeons show a lack of comprehension and respect for the integumentary system and view it as a barely alive obstruction in the path to the primary surgical target. Rather than being a nuisance which must be divided, laboriously re-

tracted, and casually sutured, it is a complex, dynamic organ which must be understood and pampered.

The skin varies in thickness, elasticity, texture, and mobility in different parts of the body. It is thinner in the female than in the male, and in infancy and old age than in the middle years of life. Average skin thickness measurements in the head and neck are in the range of 0.080 to 0.090 inch over the nape of the neck, approximately 0.065 inch over the brow, 0.030 to 0.040 inch over most of the face, to approximately 0.013 inch over the upper eyelid.

The facial-cervical skin is patterned into lines of expression and wrinkles which are of great importance when it is desirable to hide scars. The facial lines of expression develop perpendicularly to the direction of facial muscle fibers and differ from the "lines of Langer," which were determined from cadaver studies and are related to the orientation of elastic fibers in the skin. In the areas where these lines do not coincide, a more favorable cosmetic result will follow when incisions are made in the lines of expression (also called the lines of election) (Fig. 1).

The integumentary system has many functions including the following: It serves as a barrier against bacteria and is a waterproof covering, permitting our fluid bodies to exist in a dry atmosphere (keratin). It protects the body against excessive ultraviolet radiation (melanin) and participates in the regulation of body temperature and excretion (sweating). It produces vitamin D during exposure to ultraviolet light.

The skin consists of three basic layers, the *epidermis,* the *dermis,* and the *subcutaneous fatty layer* (panniculus adiposus). In most mammals there is a fourth layer which is a discontinuous sheet of striated muscle, the panniculus carnosus, just deep to the subcantaneous fatty layer. It is of interest that this fourth layer is vestigial in man, with the exception of the neck, where the platysma muscle is the only human representation of the panniculus carnosus.

The *epidermis* is comprised of five distinct layers, which may be listed and characterized as follows (from superficial to deep): The *stratum corneum* is made up of flattened, dry,

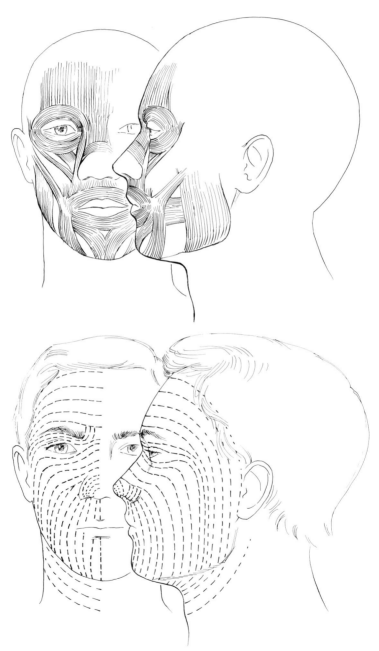

Figure 1. The "favorable lines" (lines of election) of the face and neck. Generally, these lines are at right angles to the direction of the fibers of the underlying facial muscles (note the exceptions above and below each eye). Incisions placed in these lines or in facial-cervical creases will heal with minimal scarring.

scalelike dead cells, whereas the *stratum lucidum* is a thin, eosinophilic, densely cellular layer. The *stratum granulosum* is usually two to four cell layers thick. The cells are oval in shape with basophilic intracellular granules. The *stratum spinosum* (malpighian layer, prickle cell layer) consists of polyhedral-shaped cells with oval nuclei which lie parallel to the skin surface. The cells grow larger as they become more superficial. The *stratum germinativum* (basal layer) is one or two cells thick with much mitotic activity.

The *dermis* (corium) is the next layer deep to the epidermis. It contains primarily collagen fibers, elastic fibers, and ground substance. It is divided into the superficial *papillary layer* (looser connective tissue populated with vascular tufts adjacent to the rete pegs) and the deeper *reticular layer* (thicker, more dense, and traversed by the larger vessels traveling superficially).

The blood supply to the skin is arranged into two flat arterial networks. The deeper of the two (rete cutaneum) lies in the subcutaneous layer just beneath the dermis. This plexus sends arterial branches up through the dense reticular layer of the dermis where they branch out to form the more superficial vascular network (rete subpapillare). More superficial extensions of these perforating vessels branch out like candelabras to provide 10 to 12 vascular tufts adjacent to nearby rete pegs (Fig. 2).

The changes of aging are seen dramatically in the skin. The rate at which these changes become noticeable varies considerably on an individual basis, but in general they are accelerated rapidly by exposure to the actinic rays of the sun. The histologic alterations have been described as follows: (1) loss of subcutaneous fat, (2) atrophy of skin glands, (3) atrophy and fragmentation of collagen fibers, (4) decreased elastic fibers, (5) homogenization of the ground substance, and (6) decreased tissue hydration.

These changes result in a loss of elasticity and subsequent inability of the facial skin to return to a relaxation state after muscular contraction. The consequence of this loss is the formation of wrinkles, squint lines and frown lines. Further, the facial muscles as well as the skin exhibit a loss of tone which allows gravity to reshape many areas into "sags, bags, and wattles."[4] In many patients these changes become either the basis for elective surgical intervention in the form of the face-lift operation or an important consideration in the planning and execution of the successful closure of traumatic wounds or surgical incisions.

Specific principles related to skin anatomy include the following: Whenever possible, incisions should be placed in the lines of expres-

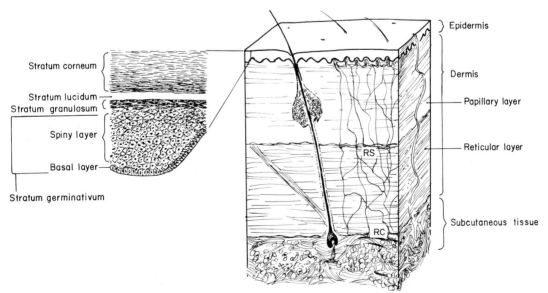

Figure 2. The skin is comprised of the epidermis and the dermis. Note that the dermis is divided into a superficial *papillary layer* and a deep *reticular layer*. The tough connective tissue of the dermis provides the holding strength for the skin sutures. The blood vessels are arranged into a deep subdermal plexus, the *rete cutaneum,* and a superficial plexus, the *rete subpapillare.*

sion or natural skin creases of the head and neck. Undermining and flap elevation are accomplished with greater safety beneath the dermis deep in the subdermal layer, with care being taken to limit injury to the rete cutaneum. The deep (reticular) layer of the dermis is tough and is the proper level for placement of subcuticular sutures. The subcutaneous layer is looser and is susceptible to strangulation by sutures.

It is advisable to bevel a vertical incision through the brow in the direction of the slant of the hair follicles in order to avoid noticeable permanent loss of adjacent hair. You may shave the hair of the scalp if necessary, but *do not* shave the brows.

Meticulous hemostasis must be stressed when dealing with aged skin which has lost much of its elasticity. Even minimal bleeding may result in an extensive hematoma in the elderly patient.

WOUND HEALING

This subject has been covered extensively in Chapter 22, but several key points will be reviewed and emphasized.

The healing of a wound is a body response to tissue injury and parallels the classic "inflammatory reaction." It begins with a *lag phase* (first to fifth day) during which time the following events take place: The wound fills with a coagulum of lymph and plasma. Some fibrin may appear in the depth of the wound. There is then increased blood flow in the adjacent tissues, increased capillary permeability, and a shift downward in pH to about 6.4. The wound becomes "a metabolic pool," with increased amounts of intracellular and extracellular fluids (edema) (Moore, 1959). Leukocytes, histiocytes, and macrophages travel into the wound and remove cellular debris and bacteria by phagocytic and enzymatic digestion. Adjacent

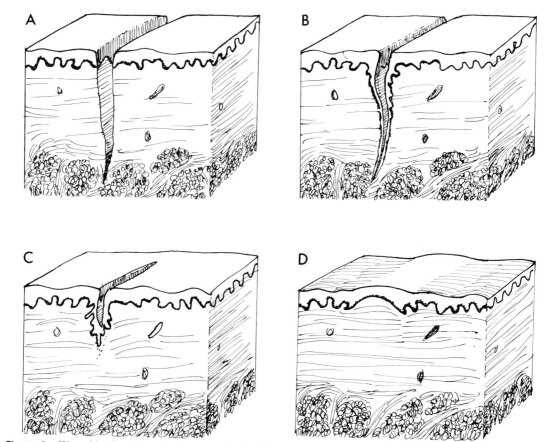

Figure 3. Wound healing shown in diagrammatic drawings of the sequential events after a surgical incision and suture closure. *A,* Shows the histologic appearance a few hours after repair; *B,* about one week later; *C,* two weeks later; and *D,* at one month. We see that the epithelium migrates into the depths of the wound and is pushed out as the healing takes place (primarily from the subdermal layer). (Lindsay, W. K., and Birch, J. R.: Card. J. Surg. 7:297, 1964.)

epithelium migrates deep into the cleft of the wound, and there is minimal proliferation of endothelial capillary buds in the subcutaneous layer (Ham, 1969). This first response may be initiated by the release of leukotaxine from the injured cells.

The second stage is that of *fibroplasia* (fifth to fourteenth day), which is characterized by the following events: There is further proliferation of capillaries from the subcutaneous layer, resulting in superficial extension of the reparative process. Fibroblasts migrate up into the dermis, secreting collagen and reticulum as they go. Other collagen may form from tropocollagen in the ground substance, and mucopolysaccharide ground substance becomes more abundant. The tensile strength of the wound is provided at first primarily by the collagen and increases rapidly as the fibroblasts align themselves along the lines of stress of the wound.

The third stage is that of *scar contracture*, and may last up to a year. During this period the cicatrix contracts in all its dimensions and increases in tensile strength. As the contraction progresses, it compresses the capillary vessels within the scar and there is a gradual blanching in appearance. Histologic patterns of the stages of wound healing are shown diagrammatically in Figure 3.

Many factors may lead to abnormal or delayed wound healing. These include: (1) protein deficiency and vitamin deficiency (especially vitamin C); (2) impaired wound oxygenation (edema, vessel injury, anemia, or radiation effect); (3) infection or foreign material in the wound (hematoma, suture); (4) systemic diseases (diabetes, cirrhosis, uremia); (5) old age; and (6) excessive steroids (apparently they produce a defect in the sulfation of mucopolysaccharides).

Two specific forms of abnormal healing are hypertrophic scars and keloids. They may be considered to be benign tumors of dense scar which has undergone hyalinization. Another concept views these two processes as abnormal prolongations of the fibroplastic second phase of normal wound healing. The hypertrophic scar is seen clinically as a widened cicatricial area which blanches more slowly than usual and has a very thin epithelial cover, but usually is level with the skin surface or only slightly elevated. The keloid is seen as a more florid example of fibroplasia, with the production of a more vascular, bulging tumor which involves adjacent areas of uninjured skin in some instances. Keloids develop more frequently in Negroes and dark-skinned Caucasians and are more common in the region of the face and neck. They arise most often during the second decade of life.

Effective management of keloids has been described with use of radiotherapy, surgical excision, topical and systemic steroids, and intralesional injection of steroids. Several studies have suggested that triamcinolone is the most potent agent available for the prevention of keloid formation and that it produces regression in the size of most mature keloids. (Grabb and Smith, 1968).

General principles in regard to normal and abnormal wound healing include the following: Preoperative evaluation of the patient's nutritional status and the detection of any systemic disorders are essential steps in the total management of the candidate for major surgery. Delayed wound healing is to be anticipated in elderly patients and in those who have been receiving high doses of steroids. Excessive tension on skin sutures may result in a hypertrophic scar, such scars being more common in children (especially when lacerations or incisions run across the lines of expression) and are prone to widen as the child grows. A dense scar over the nose or mandible may require revision in order to prevent interference with bone growth. A careful history and physical examination will identify most "keloid formers." Steroid injection with or without radiation therapy appears to be very effective in preventing keloids when employed early in the course of wound healing.

BASIC PRINCIPLES OF WOUND CLOSURE

The purpose of wound closure is to approximate the soft tissue accurately and gently so that it may heal per primum (by first intention) with minimal scarring. The task is accomplished by the use of the proper instruments, the proper suture material, and the proper surgical techniques.

When closing wounds in the head and neck, the surgeon should select a short (four- to six-inch), lightweight needle holder. Those designed by Webster or Castroviejo are excellent for this purpose. When tissue forceps are required, less trauma will be produced if the surgeon uses those designed with numerous fine, sharp teeth such as the Brown-Adson forceps. Most of the tissue manipulation can be accomplished using delicate skin hooks. These

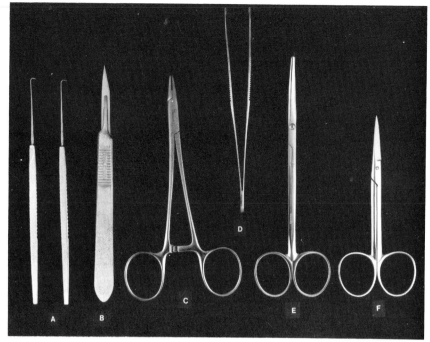

Figure 4. Basic instruments which are useful for careful, gentle soft tissue work include: (A) Cottle skin hooks, (B) Bard-Parker knife handle with a #11 blade which is ideal for careful skin incisions, (C) a lightweight, 5-inch Hegar-Baumgartner diamond jaw needle holder, (D) toothed Brown-Adson forceps, (E) curved 5½ inch Metzenbaum scissors, and (F) straight, sharp-pointed Knapp iris scissors.

are very useful for retraction and stabilization of the wound edges. In relatively long, linear wounds, a skin hook can be placed in each end and pulled away from the wound to aid in accurate approximation of the apposing sides. Examples of these instruments are shown in Figure 4.

Decisions in regard to the selection of suture material are based on the properties of size, strength, knot-holding characteristics, and the reaction produced in the local tissue. The least reactive materials are stainless steel, monofilament synthetic strands, and braided synthetic sutures. Slightly more reaction is produced by silicone-coated silk, regular silk, and cotton. Plain catgut and chromic catgut produce the greatest tissue reaction. Chromic catgut produces less reaction initially, but ultimately initiates a greater tissue response. Silk is usually preferred for closing accessible mucous membrane wounds (tongue, oral cavity) because of ease of handling and excellent knot-holding ability.

Wound closure technique begins with accurate approximation of the apposing edges, taking special care to align key landmarks. Areas

requiring meticulous care include the eyebrow, eyelid margins, nasal alar margins, and vermilion border of the lip.

The purpose of the subcutaneous tissue closure is to take the tension off the skin sutures during the period of healing. In the neck, simple interrupted sutures of 3-0 catgut are placed about 1 cm. apart, taking care to bury the knot. Facial wounds are closed with a minimum number of 4-0 plain catgut sutures which are placed in the subcutaneous tissue and just catch the deeper portion of the dermis. The first suture is placed in the middle of the incision, and subsequent sutures bisect the remaining distances to be closed in order to avoid the creation of a "dog-ear" at the end of the wound. The knots are tied with sufficient tension to approximate the edges, but not tightly enough to produce tissue strangulation.

Skin sutures of the smallest appropriate size are placed close together and close to the wound margin. Simple sutures are placed by engaging the skin surface at a 90 degree angle with the needle and then passing the needle into the wound by rotating the wrist in the arc of the needle. The needle is then regrasped in the

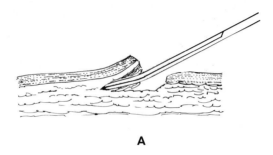

A

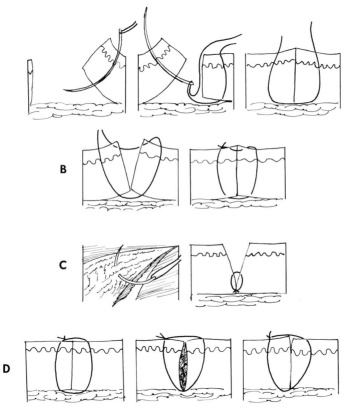

B

C

D

Figure 5.   Eversion is accomplished by (*A*) undermining the wound edges slightly, then (*B*) placing the suture slightly closer to the wound margin superficially than it is in the deeper layers. Alternating vertical mattress sutures with simple sutures facilitates eversion. (*C*) represents the technique of "burying the knot" and (*D*) shows common errors in suturing technique.

wound and passed through the tissue of the opposite side, taking care to include exactly the same amount of soft tissue on both sides. Slight eversion of the wound is desirable in order to produce a scar that will be level with the adjacent skin after contraction is complete (McGregor and Illingworth, 1968). Eversion is accomplished by undermining the wound edges slightly (Fig. 5); taking slightly more of the deep soft tissue in the simple sutures; and interspersing vertical mattress sutures with simple sutures.

General principles in wound closure include the following: Speed in wound closure is much less important than accuracy, careful planning, and the gentle handling of tissue. Use of "crosshatch" marks in long surgical incisions insures accurate reapproximation. Many small sutures placed close together and close to the wound margin minimize the scarring. In tying surgical knots, the rule is "approximate; don't strangulate." The headlight is most useful during the repair of intranasal and intra-oral wounds, and the operating microscope may be very helpful in the repair of *key* areas.

PRINCIPLES FOR MINIMIZING TISSUE INJURY

The surgeon must be aware constantly that minimal tissue injury is a key factor in the final cosmetic result. On a microscopic level, tissue injury often produces small islands of tissue necrosis which lead to the formation of microabscesses and local fibrosis. The end result of this sequence is excessive scarring.

In order to minimize tissue injury, it is essential that meticulous attention be given to many details. Skin hooks should be used for retraction and stabilization of tissue, and when tissue forceps must be used, only those with multiple fine teeth should be employed. Wound edges should be grasped at the level of the subcutaneous tissue, rather than on the skin surface. Only sharp knife blades and scissors should be used for incisions and debridement. Suture material with a swaged-on needle is preferable to separate needle and suture.

In achieving hemostasis, one should avoid taking excessively large bites of tissue in the hemostat and also overuse of electrocautery

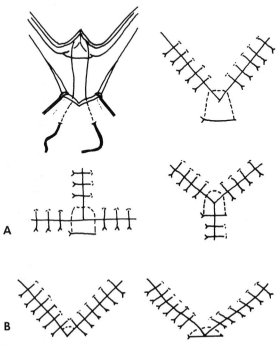

Figure 6. *A,* The half-buried horizontal mattress stitch (Gillies) produces minimal injury and vascular compromise in areas with tenuous blood supply. *B,* Illustrates two common errors in placing corner sutures which may cause necrosis of a small tongue of tissue.

and ligatures. Pressure and time are sufficient to control most small bleeding vessels. Excessive size, numbers, and tension in placing and tying sutures should be avoided. A half-buried mattress stitch (Gillies' corner stitch) should be used to close an angle of a wound (Fig. 6).

In summary, it is essential that the surgeon cultivate a microscopic concept of the tissue trauma which he creates in handling soft tissue and strive to minimize this injury.

PRINCIPLES OF OPTIMAL WOUND CARE

In order to achieve an optimal final result, we must consider several details of total wound management.

The first phase of total care begins with the preoperative preparation of the wound. Meticulous cleansing is essential, not only for the prevention of infection, but also to avoid tatooing by foreign material. Usually most of the particles will be removed by scrubbing, but on occasion it will be necessary to use a sharp scalpel blade to lift out tiny bits of debris. When one is dealing with traumatic lacerations and abrasions, it is not uncommon for the time required to prepare the wound to exceed the time necessary for closure.

During the wound closure, aseptic technique is mandatory.

During the operative period, there are several key rules of technique which should be observed. Both patient and surgeon must be comfortable during the repair. In this regard, there must be adequate regional anesthesia (e.g., 1 per cent lidocaine with 1:100,000 epinephrine). The surgeon should be seated, with his arms braced against the table if possible. Meticulous hemostasis is a cardinal feature of successful wound management.

Accurate and complete approximation of wound edges is the key to avoiding "dead space" in a wound. In turn, this is essential in order to prevent seromas and hematomas, which predispose to major wound infections. Proper wound drainage is equally important in preventing hematomas and seromas. Large neck wounds may be drained effectively by using small perforated tubing and negative pressure (such as the Hemovac unit*). Smaller wounds in the face and neck may be drained with ¼-inch Penrose drains, a sterile rubber

band, No. 90 polyethylene tubing, or a size 0 sterile silk suture. Pressure dressings serve an important function in preventing the accumulation of blood and serum under extensive skin flaps. The cotton bolus pressure dressing is effective in immobilizing skin grafts and thereby enhancing the probability of "take." In rhinoplasty the common tape and metal splint pressure dressing serves to stabilize bone and cartilage during the early phase of healing.

Several other less important practices have been followed as part of our routine of wound care. During the first few days after the dressing is removed, ointment is applied to the wound daily. This appears to limit crust formation and itching and to improve the appearance of the local area. There seems to be no significant difference between the use of a combination steroid-antibiotic ointment and A & D ointment. Skin sutures are removed four to five days postoperatively. This time interval is increased to eight to 12 days if there is evidence of delayed healing. At discharge the patient is advised to begin massaging the wound once or twice daily with a lanolin cream or cocoa butter. This appears to soften the scar and may prevent adhesions between the superficial wound and deeper tissue layers.

MINIMIZING THE VISUAL IMPACT OF SCARRING

We have all observed that the visible end result in terms of scarring after similar injuries or surgical procedures in the head and neck may vary dramatically from one patient to another. Putting aside the individual patient's differences in healing and the varying degrees of surgical skill or care in handling tissue wounds, we are left with two major activities which contribute to this observation: the first is the matter of planning surgical incisions; the second is the use of techniques of scar revision and camouflage.

In the planning of incisions about the face and neck, the surgeon has at least four options which will minimize the visual impact of the resultant scar. He may hide the incision where it will not be seen (e.g., inside the hairline, in the brow). The incision may be placed in a wrinkle or skin crease (line of expression) in the face or neck. The incision may be placed where it can be seen, but won't be noticed, such as the junction of two anatomic regions (e.g., the parotidectomy incision at the junction of the face and the ear). The incision may be placed in a

*Hemovac is manufactured by the Zimmer Company,

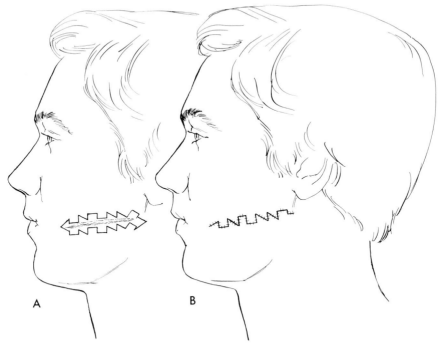

Figure 7. Zigzagplasty is designed to break up the long straight scar into many short segments. The visual improvement is significant in most scars longer than 2 cm.

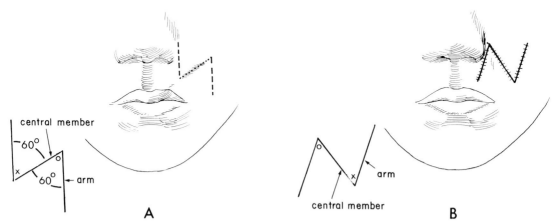

Figure 8. A scar is shown at right angles to the nasolabial fold. A 60-degree angle Z-plasty is outlined which has been designed (*A*) to replace the line of tension in the nasolabial fold (*B*) in order to decrease the deformity of the upper lip and improve the cosmetic appearance.

region where the resulting scar will not cast a shadow on the face or neck when the light is from directly overhead (e.g., below such prominences as the brow and the jaw). Surgical revision and camouflage techniques should be considered for any disfiguring or detracting scars on the face or neck.

Wide scars are usually amenable to correction by excision and undermining with careful closure in layers. The subcutaneous sutures must be placed in a manner which will avoid excessive tension on the skin sutures. In some instances it will be advisable to perform a Z-plasty in order to reposition the line of the scar within or parallel to the lines of expression. This is a versatile technique which has many uses in the head and neck (Bernstein, 1969).

The visual impact of a long linear scar is reduced by breaking the straight line into short, irregular segments which are less noticeable. This is accomplished by the technique of zigzagplasty (Fig. 7).

Checkrein scars can be managed by excision of the elevated cicatrix and performance of a Z-plasty repair to prevent re-formation of the checkrein across a depression. Figure 8 shows the use of the 60 degree angle Z-plasty in altering the deforming effect of scar contracture around the mouth.

The Z-plasty technique is also useful in improving the appearance of the "trap-door" type of deformity. When the trap-door flap is hinged superiorly, the Z-plasty is done in the center of the inferior portion of the curved scar. It serves to break up the long curved line visually.

Dermabrasion is quite useful in the management of depressed scars. The effect of this procedure is to lessen the sharp slope of the edges of the depression and to produce a visual blending of the scar with the adjacent normal skin.

COMPREHENSIVE EVALUATION OF THE INJURED PATIENT

The increase in the incidence of serious head and neck trauma in our country during the past two decades has drawn otolaryngologists into this area of activity. Successful management of the trauma victim begins with a complete and accurate evaluation of all the obvious and possibly obscure injuries.

Several general principles have been suggested for the period of evaluation and in-clude the following (A.C.S., 1961): A careful history should be taken and a thorough physical examination performed. "Always look for the second injury" and determine the priority of care when there are multiple injuries. The patient must be handled carefully to avoid further injury and to avoid further contamination of any open wound. The injured part or parts should be placed at rest. Open wounds should receive prompt treatment.

Further specific principles of the evaluation of head and neck injuries have been defined. There are six steps which must be taken in the Emergency Room in every patient with severe maxillofacial trauma: (1) be certain that the airway is unobstructed; (2) identify the source and control all bleeding; (3) check the vital signs and insert a large bore intravenous needle if there is evidence of impending shock; (4) rule out possible intrathoracic and abdominal injury; (5) rule out possible fractures of the extremities and the spine; and (6) evaluate the status of the central nervous system. Periorbital ecchymosis, hematoma over the mastoid tip (Battle's sign), and hemotympanum suggest a basal skull fracture. Clear fluid from the nose or ear indicates a cerebrospinal fluid leak.

When this phase of the evaluation has been completed, one may turn his attention to a further defintion of the maxillofacial trauma. Palpation for areas of tenderness, crepitation, and false motion will provide important clues regarding possible fractures of the facial bones, larynx, and trachea (Dingman and Natrig, 1964). Roentgenographic studies are then undertaken to clarify the exact location and nature of any fractures.

Laryngotracheal trauma is frequently overlooked when it occurs in combination with more obvious injuries. Because of the vital importance of early repair and stenting, special care must be taken to inspect the larynx and trachea in any patient with hoarseness, hemoptysis or respiratory difficulty (Shumrick, 1967).

Another problem occurs in regard to the evaluation of possible vascular injury in the neck in cases of blunt trauma. Serial measurements of neck circumference and arteriography may be required in order to determine the necessity of exploration.

There are *specific principles* governing management of traumatic wounds. Debridement of the skin, cartilage, and bone is minimized in the head and neck because of the excellent blood supply. If soft tissue injuries occur in conjunction with skeletal fractures, whenever practical the soft tissue repair is delayed until the definitive management of the bony injury has been completed. Proper tetanus prophylaxis should be an integral part of the total management of the trauma patient. Postreduction roentgenograms should be obtained soon after the surgical repair of facial fractures. Photographic documentation of injuries and surgical results is extremely valuable. The psychological impact of serious maxillofacial trauma should always be taken into account. Thorough explanation of injuries and surgical procedures and counseling of the patient and his family should be routine.

AWARENESS OF DANGER AREAS AND SPECIAL PROBLEMS

Lacerations and surgical incisions in certain regions may be associated with serious complications. These sites are designated as danger areas and are worthy of more detailed consideration.

If lines are drawn posteriorly and inferiorly from the lateral canthus of the eye, any laceration in this region of the face requires close inspection for possible injury to the parotid salivary duct or major branches of the facial nerve. When there is evidence of laceration of the parotid duct, it should be cannulated with No. 90 to No. 120 polyethylene tubing and repaired with 8-0 arterial silk, using the operating microscope. A pressure dressing is useful in stabilizing the wound and in helping to prevent a salivary gland-cutaneous fistula.

When there appears to be an injury to a major branch of the facial nerve, it is advisable to identify the main trunk of the nerve at the stylomastoid foramen and trace it out to the cut end. The distal end is then found by using the facial nerve stimulator, and the sheath of the nerve is sutured with 8-0 arterial silk. The operating microscope and fine otosurgical alligator forceps facilitate this difficult repair.

Other danger areas are the infraorbital region because of the possibility of developing an ectropion, and the medial canthus area because of the risk of associated injury to the lacrimal drainage system. Any facial (periorbital, paranasal) or cervical concavity may develop checkrein scar contractures during the late phase of wound healing. Stenosis may develop in the nasal vestibule and valve areas and the external auditory canal with resultant impairment of function. Stenting is often advisable in these locations.

Special problems are encountered oc-

casionally and require extraordinary management. These problems include through-and-through lacerations of the cheek or lip which require a three- or four-layer closure. The mucosal surface is repaired first, using 4-0 silk; then the muscle and subcutaneous layers are approximated with plain 4-0 catgut and the skin is sutured. Through-and-through defects of the lip or cheek are handled by suturing skin to mucosa and allowing the wound to heal. Delayed repair of the defect is accomplished using a skin flap, which must take into consideration the lining tissue, the supporting tissue, and the external covering. Partial or total avulsion injuries of the face and neck are managed by reattaching the soft tissue if it has not been injured too severely.

Trap-door lacerations are sutured initially. Those which are based superiorly will usually become quite edematous, and a Z-plasty will probably be required at a later date. Lacerations of the auricle must be cleaned meticulously to avoid perichondritis. We prefer to backcut the cartilage 1 to 2 mm. and use only perichondrial and skin sutures. An immobilizing otoplasty-type dressing is used.

Human bites are prone to cause infection. For this reason, one should use a minimal number of subcutaneous sutures in closing such wounds and place the patient on broad spectrum antibiotics.

Untreated wounds in the head and neck which are not grossly contaminated may be closed up to 24 hours after injury because of the excellent blood supply. Subcutaneous sutures are minimized; nylon monofilament sutures are used in the skin.

RECONSTRUCTIVE PRINCIPLES FOR SKIN AND DERMAL GRAFTS

Considerations of skin grafts and their use must begin with several definitions.

A *full-thickness skin graft* (Wolfe's graft) consists of the epidermis plus all the dermis.

Split-thickness skin grafts are epidermis plus a portion of the dermis. These may be subclassified as follows: thin—0.010 inch in thickness, translucent, also known as Thiersch's graft; intermediate—0.017 inch thick; and thick—0.025 inch thick, opaque.

A *dermal graft* is comprised primarily of dermis. It can be obtained by elevating the superficial skin (approximately 0.012 inch thick) and then taking the underlying layer (approximately 0.015 inch thick).

TABLE 1. Characteristics of Skin Grafts and Dermal Grafts

	NUTRITIONAL	CONTRACTION	APPEARANCE	DURABILITY	DONOR SITE	BEST USES
Thin skin grafts 0.010–0.012 inch	Require less nourishment; better "take" in recipient site with compromised blood supply	More contraction	Poor color and texture match; atrophic, glistening	Less protection and resistance to subsequent trauma	Usually heals readily	1. Line maxillectomy defect 2. After heavy irradiation 3. On a fatty bed 4. Over periosteum or perichondrium 5. To cover burns
Intermediate grafts 0.015–0.017 inch						1. Line flaps 2. Eyelid defects
Thick skin grafts 0.025 inch	Greater requirements; poorer "take"	Less contraction	Better color and texture match; may grow hair if quite thick	More durable	Donor site occasionally heals slowly and may require subsequent grafting	1. To fill in defects in the face where color and texture match are needed 2. To line oral cavity defects when scar contracture must be minimized 3. When greater durability is required
Dermal grafts 0.012–0.018 inch	Apparently similar to thin skin graft; early vascularization	Probably similar to intermediate skin graft	Becomes dry if exposed to air; remains moist in mucous membrane areas	Intermediate	Usually heals readily	1. Carotid artery protection 2. Cover large mucosal surface defects 3. Reinforce oropharyngeal suture lines. 4. May be buried to fill defects

A *composite graft* usually consists of a layer of cartilage sandwiched between two layers of skin covering. This is often obtained by taking a full-thickness wedge from the posterior margin of the auricle. There are numerous other examples of composite grafts, including dermis-fat grafts and skin-cartilage-perichondrial grafts.

Skin grafts of different thicknesses vary considerably in their characteristics. Thin grafts have the advantages of requiring less nourishment and, hence, they "take" better when there is a compromised blood supply in the recipient site. Thin grafts have the disadvantages of greater contraction and less resistance to injury. Thick grafts have the advantages of better color and texture match; they contract less, and they resist subsequent trauma better. They have the disadvantages of poorer "take"; they occasionally grow hair (if the donor site was a hair-bearing region); and the donor site may require subsequent grafting.

Skin grafts have several general disadvantages. They usually will not survive on bare cortical bone or cartilage, and they may not "take" on infected granulation tissue, fat, or a recipient site that has been irradiated. Skin grafts are a very poor cover for an exposed carotid artery and are prone to crusting when they are used to cover a mucous membrane defect.

There are many situations, however, in which skin grafts are extremely useful (Farrior, 1966). Thin grafts are used to cover burns and to line extensive defects after major cancer surgery. Intermediate grafts are used to line flaps and the beds from which they have been raised. They are also ideal for grafting the upper lid since they are thin enough to permit folding when the lid is elevated. Thick split-thickness grafts may be used on the face when full thickness grafts of sufficient size are not practical and a good color and texture match is needed. They are also useful in relining the oral cavity when minimizing graft contraction is a key factor. Full-thickness grafts are ideal for small defects on the face because of the excellent color and texture match when they are obtained from the postauricular region, upper lid, or supraclavicular area.

Dermal grafts have been used in many situations. They may be rolled up and implanted beneath the skin to fill small defects. These grafts have proved to be of value in providing protection of the carotid artery when it becomes exposed by breakdown of the overlying skin cover (Reed, 1965). This event may be anticipated when a full course of radiation therapy has been

delivered to the region preoperatively. Dermal grafts have also been suggested as being applicable for covering large raw oropharyngeal surfaces, and may be useful in the repair of nasal septal perforations and oral-antral fistulas (Reed, 1968). Table 1 summarizes the characteristics of skin grafts and dermal grafts.

Composite grafts are used in the head and neck in several specific situations. They are usually taken from the ear and are used to repair defects of the nasal alar margin. Extreme care must be taken to handle the graft and recipient tissue gently. The graft should not be larger than 2 cm. in its greatest dimension. Successful repair of a through-and-through laryngocutaneous defect using an auricular composite graft has been reported. Full-thickness defects of the upper lid may be repaired by using a composite graft (one half the width of the defect) taken from the opposite upper lid.

RECONSTRUCTIVE PRINCIPLES FOR LOCAL AND REGIONAL FLAPS

A skin flap is a regional sheet of skin and subcutaneous tissue which is moved to another location while a portion remains attached to its vascular supply in one area. Skin flaps are used when wounds are too extensive for primary closure or when skin grafts cannot be employed for some reason such as: (1) inadequate vascularity in the bed of the wound, (2) the requirement for a thicker tissue covering, (3) the need to repair a full-thickness defect, or (4) the likelihood that further surgical procedures will be necessary beneath the area to be covered. Again, several definitions are required for the subsequent discussion.

Advancement Flap. This is usually a square or rectangular flap adjacent to the defect which is undermined and moved forward into the defect by virtue of the skin's elastic properties or by employing Burow's triangles alongside the lateral incisions. Modifications of the simple advancement flap are the V-Y advancement flap and the bipedicle advancement flap.

Rotation Flap. A curved flap is undermined immediately adjacent to the defect and then pivoted along its arc to cover the defect. A Burow's triangle is usually necessary to prevent a "dog ear" in the tissue adjacent to the flap at its proximal end.

Transposition Flap. This is usually a rectangular flap which is raised adjacent to a defect and pivoted into the defect. As a rule, this leaves a secondary raw surface which must be covered with a skin graft. The standard Z-plasty and the bilobed flap are modifications of the transposition flap.

Interpolation Flap. This is similar to the transposition flap except that it is rotated into a nearby defect, but not one which is immediately adjacent to the flap. The pedicle is divided in two to three weeks. The *arterial island flap* is a specialized type of interpolation flap in which an island of skin and subcutaneous tissue is raised along a major artery and vein. A portion of this flap is denuded of its skin in order that the flap can be passed through a tunnel and the skin at the distal end can be used to fill a nearby defect. The *tubed pedicle flap* is another modification of the interpolation flap in which the proximal end of the flap is "tubed" by suturing the lateral margins of the flap together to prevent drainage, infection, and contraction. It is used when the surgeon needs to use only the distal end of the flap to cover a defect.

Specific details regarding the anatomy, use, and limitations of the flaps used commonly in head and neck surgery may be found in excellent articles by Bakamjian (1965), Shumrick (1969), Ogura (1969), and Sisson and Goldstein (1970).

When local and regional flaps are used, the major flaps must be planned carefully, raised accurately, and handled very gently if the transfer is to be successful. In planning the flap, it must be remembered that the "pivot" point of the flap is its site of attachment most distant from the recipient site. It is important to avoid kinking the attachment of the flap.

The greatest single factor in flap necrosis is excessive tension. Adequate venous drainage is more important to flap survival than arterial inflow. For this reason, it is wiser to select flaps which are based inferiorly rather than superiorly whenever possible. Key factors in flap survival are the patient's nutritional state and hematocrit. If a long tenuous transfer is planned, it may be prudent to transfuse the patient up to a hematocrit of 40 per cent.

Tubed pedicle flaps require judgment in terms of the amount of subcutaneous fat enclosed in the tube. If too much fat is included, it may compromise the venous return; if too much is removed, there may be excessive injury to the vital arterial vessels in the subcutaneous layer. The maximum length to width ratios for pedicle flaps vary rather widely. A general rule may be stated that single pedicle flaps without a named vascular supply should not exceed a length to width ratio of 2:1; bipedicle flaps should not exceed 3:1; single pedicle flaps based on a named vascular supply should not exceed 4:1. The vascular supply to a flap can be increased by outlining incisions, partial undermining, complete elevation and resuturing in place, and staging with a two- to three-week delay. Pedicle flaps should be tested for adequate blood supply ("challenged") before the attachment is divided. The vascular supply to a flap is decreased by previous irradiation, infection, or the development of a hematoma beneath the flap. Rotation flaps are stronger (have a better vascular supply) than other types of flaps because of their relatively larger base and their lower length to width ratio. The surgeon should plan to make pedicle flaps approximately 15 per cent longer than appears necessary in order to lessen the tension and avoid kinking of the flap. When a staged, tubed pedicle flap is being planned, 20 to 25 per cent should be added to the length for each move which is planned ("waltzing" the tube).

Careful selection of the simplest and strongest flap in a given reconstructive situation is the key to a favorable outcome.

CONCLUSION

This chapter represents our effort to organize and review many of the principles of regional plastic surgery of the head and neck.

Basic science information has been summarized and correlated with appropriate clinical problems in order to illustrate both the surgical principle and its foundation whenever possible.

We have emphasized the general precept of gentleness in the handling of tissue and the priority that accuracy has over speed.

In otologic surgery we have grown accustomed to seeing the diseases, surgical results, and complications displayed in the form of microscopic slides. This has led us to an understanding of these problems and processes on a cellular level. Further, we have accepted the use of the operating microscope as a common and essential aid in the surgical procedure. Now we must extend our ability to think and work on a cellular level to the field of facial plastic surgery. We need to develop our awareness of the "micro" scars which develop from "micro" trauma and take the steps to avoid them.

Finally, we would stress that the purpose of

this chapter is to provide an overview of the subject and a stimulus for deeper and more detailed study by otolaryngologists working in this area.

REFERENCES

American College of Surgeons: Early Care of Acute Soft Tissue Injuries. 2nd ed. W. B. Saunders Company, Philadelphia, 1961.

Bakamjian, V. Y.: A two-stage method for pharyngoesophageal reconstruction with primary pectoral skin flap. Plast. Reconst. Surg. *36*:173, 1965.

Bernstein, L.: Z-plasty in head and neck surgery. Arch. Otolaryng. *89*:574, 1969.

Conley, J.: Face-lift Operation. Springfield, Ill., Charles C Thomas, 1968.

Dingman, R. O., and Natvig, P.: Surgery of Facial Fractures. Philadelphia, W. B. Saunders Company, 1964.

Farrior, R. T.: Rehabilitation by skin grafting. Arch. Otolaryng. *83*:120, 1966.

Grabb, W. C., and Smith, J. W.: Plastic Surgery: A Concise Guide to Clinical Practice. Boston, Little, Brown and Company, 1968.

Ham, A. W.: Histology. 6th ed. Philadelphia, J. B. Lippincott Co., 1969, Chapter 23.

McGregor, I. A., and Illingworth, Sir C.: Fundamental Techniques of Plastic Surgery and Their Surgical Applications. 4th ed. Baltimore, The Williams & Wilkins Co., 1968.

Moore, F. D.: Metabolic Care of the Surgical Patient. Philadelphia, W. B. Saunders Company, 1959.

Ogura, J. H. (ed.): Symposium on cancer of the head and neck. Otolaryng. Clin. N. Amer. *2* (No. 3), 1969.

Reed, G. F.: Use of dermal grafts in otolaryngology. Ann. Otol. *74*:769, 1965.

Reed, G. F., et al.: Self-epithelization of dermal grafts. Arch. Otolaryng. *87*:518, 1968.

Shumrick, D. A.: Trauma of the larynx. Arch. Otolaryng. *86*:691, 1967.

Shumrick, D. A.: Reconstructive flaps in head and neck surgery. Otolaryng. Clin. N. Amer. *2* (No. 3):685, 1969.

Sisson, G. A., and Goldstein, J. C.: Flaps and grafts in head and neck surgery. Arch. Otolaryng. *92*:599, 1970.

Chapter 26

PRE- AND POSTOPERATIVE CARE

by W. B. Hofmann, M.D.

PREOPERATIVE CARE

General Considerations

Initial Workup and Planning

The preoperative care and evaluation of a patient actually begins with the initial office contact. A history with good detail should be solicited from the patient, or the parent if the patient is a child. It should include questions that probe for clues to disease in all otolaryngologic areas, not just the one involved in the chief complaint. Ideally a general medical history should also be obtained so that the practitioner has a clear mental picture of the patient's past and present health problems. The history should be followed by a careful physical examination. In the case of the otolaryngologist, this is limited to the head and neck area; however, provision should be made for general medical examination by the patient's family physician and the ENT specialist should always be ready to examine those areas which might show findings that could be coupled to head and neck disorders. After the examination is completed and a reasonable diagnosis has been made, a course of action is formulated, with a definitive plan that will resolve the problem as quickly and as completely as possible.

Patient Understanding

A meaningful relationship between the physician and his patient will reinforce the patient's confidence. The patient should be given a clear understanding, in terms he is able to understand, of what the doctor feels the problem is and what will be necessary in the way of workup and treatment to resolve it. Too often this vital portion of medical care is not carried out as thoroughly as it might be. A patient should not only understand what can be done for his problem; he should also know what *can't* be done. He should know the possible consequences and side effects of surgery other than the intended result. Lack of understanding is probably the commonest cause of lawsuits, and in today's world this is no small problem.

The Otologic Patient

Clinical Examination

The ear should be carefully evaluated on the first office visit. Ideally this should include examination under the microscope. Any discharge should be sent for culture and sensitivity studies, and an attempt should be made to control drainage by the use of various antibiotic eardrops or powders. Several visits, with cleaning of the ear on each occasion, may be necessary to determine whether it is possible to "dry up" the ear. The microscope gives a much better idea as to type and limits of the various ear disorders. It gives the examiner a better opportunity to evaluate the status of the middle ear mucosa, to decide whether there is squamous epithelium in the middle ear, to test the mobility of the ossicles as well as possible ossicular damage, and to determine the presence or absence of tympanosclerosis. Tuning fork tests and the fistula test should always be done in suspected cases of ear disease, especially in a patient with a chronic draining ear.

Audiometric Evaluation

At the first opportunity, and after being certain that the external auditory canal is clean, an audiogram should be carried out. It should include air and bone testing as well as speech reception thresholds and speech discrimination scores. It should always be completed before any contemplated surgery.

Eustachian Tube Function

Eustachian tube function is difficult to evaluate preoperatively in the chronically infected ear since the tissues are inflamed. One can get some idea as to past function from the type of ear disease that is present. Chronic adhesive otitis with cholesteatoma, for instance, suggests a poor record for that eustachian tube. Nasal diseases, particularly nasal allergy, should be adequately investigated prior to ear surgery, and an attempt should be made to clear up sinus problems as conservatively as possible.

Radiologic Evaluation

Sinus films are helpful in ruling out sinus disorders that may have a bearing on eustachian function and, secondarily, the middle ear. Routine mastoid films should probably be obtained prior to ear surgery, although they are unlikely to influence the decision on whether to operate. Polytomography is an expensive but valuable tool in some cases.

The Maxillofacial Patient

Facial Fractures

Clincal Examination. For the otolaryngologist, the clinical examination of a patient with a facial injury usually begins in the emergency room or in some other nonplanned emergent situation. He usually will be asked to see the patient in consultation after an initial evaluation has been made by a traumatologist or general surgeon. Occasionally he will be the first physician to see the patient and, in this instance, should assume the primary role of patient care until other needed specialty services can be provided.

The clinical examination of the facial bony structure may reveal any or all of the following findings in cases of suspected fracture:

1. Edema and ecchymosis anywhere about the head and neck, but especially around the eyes and in the upper or lower buccal sulcus on either side.

2. Anesthesia or paresthesia over the chin or anterior facial areas, suggesting injury to the mental or inferior alveolar nerves in the case of mandibular fractures, and to the infraorbital nerve with orbital rim or blowout fractures.

3. Epistaxis, which may be unilateral or bilateral.

4. Diplopia, usually present in upward gaze, suggesting orbital floor injury.

5. Flattened appearance to malar eminence, suggesting fracture of the zygoma.

6. Mobility of the palate with ill fitting dentures or teeth that do not "feel right," suggesting midfacial injury.

7. Crepitation over fracture sites.

8. "Step-off," which is noted when there is orbital rim fracture and these areas are palpated.

9. Subcutaneous emphysema.

10. Obvious deformities of the mandible to palpation or inspection as well as mandibular malocclusion.

11. The pupils may be on different levels in suspected cases of fractured zygoma.

12. Difficulty in closing the mandible completely may suggest impingement of the coronoid process on a fractured zygomatic arch.

It goes without saying that any injured patient deserves the best available general physical examination. Other injuries of a neurosurgical, surgical, ophthalmologic and orthopedic nature take precedence over facial fracture repair. The otolaryngologist should be certain that the injured patient's airway is adequate. To minimize edema and if other injuries allow, the patient is kept in a high semi-Fowler's position until surgery.

Radiologic Examination. This has been explained in detail in the chapter on facial fractures. The one most important view to be obtained, in cases of suspected facial injury, is the plain or stereo waters film.

Photography. Adequate initial photography is often useful, at a later date, to illustrate the extent of the original injury. "One picture is worth a thousand words" was never a truer statement than it is in the case of facial injury. These pictures frequently have a bearing on various types of litigation and are sometimes helpful in planning reconstructive procedures.

Dental Considerations. One of the prime considerations in the repair of facial fractures is to restore the teeth or dentures to their normal, occlusive state. Accordingly all attempts should be made to preserve as many of the patient's own teeth as possible and to repair damaged dentures. If the patient is completely or partially edentulous and has no dentures, a prosthodonist is invaluable in the construction of a Gunning splint or other device that will maintain normal or near normal intermaxillary relationships until healing can occur.

The Head and Neck Surgery Patient

Clinical Evaluation

The patient with a head and neck cancer problem should be carefully evaluated in the office on the first visit. Usually the clinician can obtain a pretty good idea as to the extent and location of the cancerous area by inspection and indirect examination of the pharynx and larynx. Since one out of ten patients may have a "double" primary, a thorough search of the remainder of the respiratory tract should be instituted. A complete general evaluation by an internist is in order. This should be followed by direct laryngoscopy and biopsy of the suspected area. Direct nasopharyngoscopy, esophagoscopy and bronchoscopy are done as indicated. At endoscopy, the lesion should be carefully mapped and described so that everyone who has a part in treatment understands the extent of the tumor. The radiotherapist should be consulted and informed if preoperative radiotherapy is planned.

Radiologic Evaluation

Certainly any x-rays deemed necessary in the general workup of a patient with head and neck cancer, such as gall bladder, gastrointestinal and other films, should be obtained as needed. One would hate to miss an adenocarcinoma of the bowel while treating a head and neck tumor. Head and neck films that should more or less be routinely obtained are sinus survey, skull series, and films of the cervical spine. Frequently laminograms may be helpful in delineating what is involved and what is not. This is especially true in maxillary or other sinus cancers as well as in nasopharyngeal lesions. Special x-ray studies, such as a sialogram or laryngogram, are also frequently of value. The laryngogram should be obtained in suspected cases of laryngeal cancer *before* the biopsy, since edema and infection surrounding the biopsy site tend to obscure the true findings of a laryngogram. The sialogram may help to differentiate between tumor and infection and probably should be employed whenever possible to help in the diagnosis of salivary gland problems.

Anticipation of Problems

The prime objective of head and neck surgery is to extirpate the lesion and to reconstruct the patient physiologically and cosmetically. Healing by primary intention is the goal; frequently it cannot be achieved for many reasons. Take the not infrequent example of the patient who has been irradiated, unsuccessfully, as the primary form of treatment for a lesion of the tongue or tonsil. Is the old adage, "we can always operate," true? Perhaps it is, but we certainly cannot operate without expecting a significant number of problems with the healing of irradiated tissue. These problems should be anticipated prior to surgery and steps taken to counteract or perhaps to help to prevent wound breakdown. In large lesions one might consider a planned pharyngotomy initially, followed by staged reconstruction. Perhaps a forehead flap or Bakamjian flap, at the time of the original surgery, will promote healing by bringing fresh tissue to an irradiated bed. In any event, no surgical planning is complete without taking reconstruction into consideration prior to the operation.

Problems with the patient and his family can also be significant. Both should have a thorough understanding of the possible difficulties prior to surgery.

Dental Considerations

The teeth should be carefully evaluated prior to irradiation therapy. Those which are in a poor state should be removed and the bony alveolar ridge rendered smooth prior to the initiation of therapy. A period of several days should be allowed for healing before therapy is started. The remaining teeth should be cleaned and filled when indicated. Supervoltage therapy allows less absorption and scattering in bone and is somewhat better tolerated by connective tissues and skin. This being the case, dental complications such as caries alveolar bone resorption and necrosis are seen much less often than with older forms of treatment. Routine removal of all teeth prior to start of therapy is to be condemned.

POSTOPERATIVE CARE

General Considerations

Immediate Postoperative Care

Until the patient is safely recovered from anesthesia, postoperative care is the domain of the anesthesiologist unless a local anesthesic has been used by the otolaryngologic surgeon. Vital signs should be monitored at frequent intervals for the first few hours. The patient is usually kept in a semi-Fowler's position with bedside rails in the up position. The various tubes, such as nasogastric, urinary catheter and particularly the drainage tubes placed in any operative wound, should be quickly attended to after transfer to the recovery room. Stasis in a Hemovac drain frequently results in clotting that may necessitate changing the tube; therefore, continuous suction should be maintained during transfer to recovery. The n-g tube, if one is present, should be either clamped or hooked to gomco suction. These activities should be supervised by the physician, since a multitude of various tubes is sometimes confusing to the nursing staff.

Fluids and Feeding

Perhaps the greatest nutritional problem the ENT specialist faces is in a patient with advanced head and neck cancer who has undergone weight loss and is anorexic as well. In a patient with a poor general nutritional status, wound healing is certainly jeopardized. One might consider the use of intravenous hyperalimentation prior to surgery to help reverse this trend.

Aside from this, nutritional problems are not common in most ENT patients. Electrolyte imbalance is a rare problem for the otolaryngologist, except perhaps in a patient with a chylous fistula. Nasogastric suction is seldom employed except in the head and neck surgery patient when one wishes to prevent vomiting for 12 to 24 hours after surgery. It is discontinued after the danger of nausea and vomiting are past, and soon thereafter tube feedings can be started.

Tube feedings can maintain the nutrition of the average head and neck patient quite well. Most standard hospital tube feedings contain somewhat less than one calorie per ml. of fluid and, when given in adequate amounts, are suf-ficient to maintain the caloric requirements of a recovering patient. Adequate water should be given along with the tube feeding. Dehydration can result in the tube feeding syndrome of hypernatremia, hyperchloremia and azotemia.

Intravenous fluids are seldom needed beyond 24 to 48 hours following surgery in the ENT patient except perhaps as a vehicle for the intravenous administration of antibiotics.

Soft diets, easy to chew and swallow, are frequently indicated for those patients for whom IV and tube feedings are not needed. Swallowing can be difficult following nasal surgery with packing of the nose, and in this instance a soft diet can be of some value. Patients who have had procedures in and around the pharynx, such as tonsillectomy, pharyngeal flap procedure, etc., also do better when given a soft diet.

Ambulation

Otolaryngologic patients should be ambulated as quickly as possible following surgery. Getting a patient up and walking is probably easier to accomplish following ENT procedures than in any other specialty since all surgery is above the clavicles. Patients with a history of phlebitis should be protected with ace bandages or elastic stockings during and after surgical procedures.

Pain Control

Alleviation of postoperative pain is usually not a prominent problem in the ENT patient. Frequently, pain may be less than it was in the preoperative state, as for instance following drainage of a peritonsillar abscess or after removal of a large fungating tongue cancer. Radical neck dissection eliminates much of medication needed to control pain. Minor degrees of discomfort can usually be controlled with codeine or Darvon, with or without APC type additives. Dilaudid is excellent for relief of severe pain and is administered in doses of 2 mg. IM or subcutaneously. It produces less nausea, vomiting, and sedation than either morphine or Demerol.

The Care of the Tracheostomy

Tracheostomy care should begin in the recovery room with adequate suctioning. It should be remembered that an endotracheal tube is an irritant and, as such, causes an increased amount of tracheobronchial secretion, much of which may be rather thick and glairy. In addition, bypassing the upper airway with a tracheostomy renders the patient's natural protective function, the cough, rather inefficient and ineffective. It becomes the job of paramedical personnel to keep the tracheobronchial tree clean, and this is accomplished by adequate tracheobronchial suctioning. The answer to the frequent question, "How often shall I suction the patient?" is, "As often as necessary." This may be every 15 minutes in some patients, in some circumstances. Suctioning should be preceded by slow instillation of sterile saline, perhaps 3 to 5 ml., in the trachea. This is followed by suctioning. The catheter should be introduced as far as possible into the tracheobronchial tree gently, and without suction. Suction is then applied as the catheter is slowly withdrawn. This may have to be done three or four times. Adequate time should be allowed between each withdrawal to permit the patient to catch his breath. Remember that the catheter is competing with the patient for his oxygen. Following suctioning, a small amount of saline should be reintroduced to lessen the viscosity of the sputum.

Antibiotics

There are instances in which antibiotics are obviously indicated postoperatively, as after drainage of a peritonsillar abscess. In other situations, however, there seems to be a difference of opinion as to whether antibiotics should be administered. It is the author's feeling that they should be used after head and neck surgery in which the oral cavity has been violated, after ear surgery, and after the repair of extensive facial fractures.

The Otologic Patient

Dressings

A standard mastoid type dressing should be routinely employed for those patients who have had a postaricular incision; it is also helpful in children even if a postaricular incision has not been employed. Children seem to have a knack for undoing what the surgeon has carefully done, and nothing is more discouraging than to find external auditory canal packing pulled loose and hanging down the child's neck. Mastoid dressings should be firmly attached and taped in place so that they cannot rotate. Care should be taken not to have a narrow band of dressing going across the upper forehead, since necrosis has resulted from too tight a dressing.

Dizziness

Dizziness may follow some ear surgery, notably stapedectomy, for several days. It is best treated with Dramamine, Bonine or perhaps Inovar as well as bed rest.

Wound Care and Suture Removal

Ordinarily it is better to change a mastoid dressing on the second postoperative day. If the wound is clean and uninfected, it need not be redressed until the skin sutures are removed, in about seven days. The time to remove packing from the external auditory canal seems to vary with each ear surgeon. Outer canal packing may be removed in about two weeks from an ear that has been grafted and when there is a posterior canal flap to hold in place. Rosette packings directly against a temporalis fascia or other type of graft may be removed in three weeks. Some Cortisporin Otic Drops or other suitable eardrops may be used a few days before removal of a rosette to help to loosen it from the underlying graft.

Follow-up Care

Initially the ear patient should be seen as often as deemed necessary by the otologist. The operated ear may need to be cleaned at fairly frequent intervals. After healing takes place it is well to check hearing from time to time in the reconstructed ear. Ordinarily in a successful reconstruction the graft will "thin" over a period of months with a concomitant slight increase in the hearing acuity. A successfully operated ear should be watched intermittently for the rest of the patient's life. These visits may, in the final analysis, be necessary only every six to 12 months.

The Maxillofacial Patient

Dressings

Dressings are seldom if ever used on the patient with a facial fracture, nor are they required after plastic procedures, as a general rule, except after otoplasty, rhinoplasty, and as a means of immobilizing a skin graft. An otoplasty dressing is essentially a bilateral mastoid dressing. Care should be taken to keep the reformed helix far enough lateral to the mastoid area of the skull. Generally about four to five gauze or Telfa pads properly cut out to the contour of the ear and placed between the helix and the skull are sufficient to maintain the ear in good position. Twenty-four hours after surgery the dressing should be split in the midforehead area and swung laterally on each side to allow inspection of the ears. The dressing is again closed and taped in the midforehead area where it was originally split. Usually the dressing is worn for approximately seven to 10 days and may be changed if this is deemed necessary. The rhinoplasty may be thought of as a controlled fracture and, like any fracture, immobilization is necessary until healing has occurred. This is usually accomplished by placing dental base plate wax stents (or other suitable material such as Supramyd) against the nasal septum on either side to hold it in position. The nasal cavities are then carefully packed, usually with petrolatum gauze, in such a manner that the bony and cartilaginous portions of the nasal pyramid are held snugly in position from the inside. The nose is suitably taped around the nares, and an external cast or stent is placed around the nasal pyramid and taped into place. There are many types of preformed nasal stents, and some surgeons simply use plaster. The total effect of the dressing is to hold the pyramid in place between the packing inside and the "cast" outside. There are as many variations of the rhinoplasty dressing as there are people doing the procedure.

Wound Care and Suture Removal

Surgical wounds incurred during maxillofacial surgery need constant gentle care. It is well to clean the wound three or four times a day with hydrogen peroxide. Any accumulations of crust should be removed from the sutures and the line of incision. This may be followed by the application of a thin layer of an antibiotic-steroid ointment such as Cortisporin. These measures help to achieve good healing with minimal scar tissue. Sutures may be removed in stages. Frequently every other suture can be removed on the third day and the remaining sutures over the next one to two days.

Photography

Daily or twice daily pictures of a healing maxillofacial patient are the best form of documentation as to his progress. They are an excellent complement to the preoperative photography.

Follow-up Care

These patients should be followed as often as deemed necessary by the attending otolaryngologist. Nasal packing following rhinoplasty can usually be removed on the fifth or sixth day. It is well to have the patient wear his "cast" for perhaps two to three weeks following the surgery. It offers some means of protection and also lets others know that the patient has had a nasal problem. It is also well to have the patient keep glasses elevated from the healing bridge of his nose. This may be conveniently done by placing a piece of Scotch tape about the bridge of the glasses and taping it to the forehead. Contact lenses are ideal in this situation. For the otoplasty patient, one should consider the use of fine chromic sutures to close the skin incision. This is especially helpful in children, since the chromic need not be removed and the ears can be quite painful until healing occurs. The patient may wear a stocking cap over the ears at night to help to maintain good position. The upper part of a lady's discarded stocking will serve well for this purpose.

The Head and Neck Surgery Patient

Dressings

There are those who believe in bulky pressure type dressings following the head and neck cancer surgery, and those who do not. The author feels that, generally, dressings should not be employed, at least initially, following surgery. As far as the head and neck wound is concerned, the primary aim for the first 48 to 72 hours is to keep it decompressed and not to allow blood or serum to accumulate under the flaps. Raw surface needs to be apposed to raw surface, and if this condition can be met for three days, the unirradiated wound will probably heal. Needless to say, the development of a hematoma during this time can be disastrous. Without a dressing, the wound can be more adequately inspected and any stasis of the drains with hematoma formation can be quickly diagnosed.

Perhaps the best drainage system is the popular Hemovac. To help to prevent stasis or clotting, suction should be applied to the tubes as soon as they are introduced into the wound. Prior to placing the last subcutaneous suture in the wound, it is well to gently suction the corners of the wound with a nontraumatic suction tip such as a tonsil suction. As soon as transfer to the recovery room is completed, the Hemovac system should be attached to the wall suction. It is well to "break" the wall suction every two hours, attach the tube to an intermittent Gomco, and gently massage or roll the wound. This is conveniently done by rolling a cling dressing from the superior and posterior aspects of the wound toward the supraclavicular area. This may break up small clots and keep the system functioning normally. None of these things can be done well when a dressing has been applied.

If after three or four days it becomes obvious that a wound is not going to heal, and that flaps are not seating (as perhaps in a patient who has had irradiation), then a pressure dressing is indicated to try to get as much as possible of the wound to heal.

Wound Care and Suture Removal with Primary Healing

Head and neck wounds may be kept clean with the intermittent daily use of hydrogen peroxide followed by an antibiotic-steroid ointment. Sutures are usually removed within seven days.

Wound Care After Wound Breakdown

Wound breakdown in head and neck surgery is not uncommon, especially in those patients who have had irradiation prior to being operated on. It is less common when the irradiation has been done in a planned fashion. Breakdown is bad for these basic reasons:

1. It can lead to, or be accompanied by fistula formation.

2. It can lead to carotid artery rupture with its attendant problems of death and stroke.

3. It greatly prolongs morbidity and frequently necessitates extensive reconstructive surgery requiring months of hospitalization.

As soon as nonhealing becomes evident, the surgeon should try to salvage what he can. Any "tented" areas of the flap should be released and packed down to the underlying tissue with a pressure dressing. Any necrotic tissue should be carefully debrided. A small indirect fistula may heal with good, constant, normal debridement followed by pressure dressings. Large fistulas, which are direct, always require secondary reconstruction. Rupture of the carotid artery requires immediate care. Local pressure will usually suffice to stop the bleeding until the patient can be typed, cross matched, and taken to the operating room for ligation of the artery. The incidence of carotid rupture is greatly lessened when the artery is protected, at the time of surgery, with a dermal graft or levator scapulae muscle pedicle.

Follow-up Care

Head and neck cancer patients should be followed every month for 12 to 18 months. If there are no signs of recurrence, they may be seen every six to eight weeks for the next 12 to 18 months, at which time they are seen every three months for the next one to two years. At the end of five years they are seen every six months for life.

Chapter 27

BIOPSY OF HEAD AND NECK LESIONS

by Donald A. Shumrick, M.D.

An amazing awareness of physical disability is revealed in many ancient drawings. As these drawings attest, the occurrence of lesions of the head, and especially the neck, was recognized by Chinese healers as early as the 13th century. Such masses undoubtedly presented more problems to those early healers than they do to modern physicians. Perhaps the doctor of today, knowing of the many benign and malignant diseases that occur in the head and neck region, is more apprehensive about the management of these problems than were his predecessors (Fig. 1).

Early recognition and categorization of disease is mandatory if an increase in the number of cures is to be achieved (Moore, 1968). Both benign and malignant lesions of the head and neck are usually seen first by the family physician. If he has a high index of suspicion and a desire for accurate diagnosis, he will frequently perform a biopsy in the case of skin and oral mucosal lesions, even though he may be sure of the clinical diagnosis. The basic aim of the biopsy is to provide the pathologist with tissue for cellular study, tissue culture, or possibly both. This is the first and most direct step in the management of a patient with a lesion of the head or neck. The ideal biopsy material is a section of the suspect area plus a cuff of surrounding tissue if its origin is from skin or mucosa.

Biopsies may be performed in the physician's office as an outpatient procedure for lesions involving the skin or structures in the oral cavity. If an endoscopic procedure is required to obtain a pharyngeal, laryngeal, bron-

chial or esophageal biopsy, the safest and most convenient method is to admit the patient to the hospital in the afternoon and, with appropriate preoperative medications, to perform the endoscopic procedure and biopsy the following morning under a combination of topical and light general anesthesia. Frequently an Emergency Room or clinic area may be utilized for

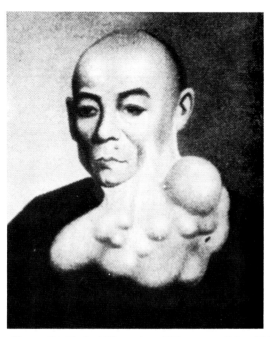

Figure 1. Early 13th century Chinese scroll in which an unknown artist depicts a massive cervical neck lesion.

small biopsies performed under local or topical anesthesia, thus allowing better utilization of inpatient facilities.

NECK MASSES

In the main, the neck masses of most patients who consult their family physician are the result of inflammatory processes. This is especially true in children. This fact, however, should never deter the physician from searching for early or silent primary malignant disease in the head and neck structures. The incidence of primary malignancies of the head and neck that metastasize to the cervical area has been estimated to range from 79 to 93 per cent (Slaughter, 1949).

In certain malignant diseases a cervical mass appears as the first symptom. This is especially true of lesions of the nasopharynx, half of which are detected because of the cervical mass. The neck mass is the first sign in 28 per cent of tonsil malignancies, 30 per cent of tongue cancers and 10 per cent of floor of the mouth lesions. In these cases the primary malignancy may be completely overlooked by the patient; his only complaint is the mass in the neck (Martin et al., 1952).

The age of the patient and the position of the neck mass must be considered in the evaluation of each case. A frequent mistake by those not well versed in this field is the removal of a lymph node from the cervical neck without an adequate investigation for a primary lesion, which may be readily available.

To categorize the possible causes of neck masses (excluding those of thyroid origin) and to estimate the probable results of treatment, a division of patients into age groups is useful. These lesions lend themselves well to such categorization. Classification of patients in this way is often helpful in the differential diagnosis.

The diagnostic probabilities should be considered in three main age groups: children (infancy to 20 years), young to middle-aged adults (21 to 40 years), and middle-aged to aged adults (41 or more years).

Cervical Masses in Children

The overwhelming majority of neck masses in this age group are the result of inflammatory processes. Cervical neck masses found in children often enlarge to an alarming size and, of course, the greater the size, the more one suspects malignancy. Complete examination of such a patient reveals that the cervical masses are usually multiple, occasionally tender, bilateral and shotty, or singular; on the other hand, they may be lobulated or matted together. Frequently the tonsils and pharyngeal lymphoid tissues are hyperplastic and usually indicate an upper respiratory infection of bacterial origin. If other systemic signs are present, such as axillary and inguinal lymphadenopathy with leukopenia, a viral etiology is most likely. Infectious mononucleosis is most common among teen-agers and college students. This is easily ruled out by serologic tests.

Congenital cysts such as thyroglossal duct cysts, brachiogenic cysts and cystic hygromas account for the remainder of the cystic neck masses in this age group. Most solid malignant tumors of children that occur in the head and neck area are rhabdomyosarcomas involving the eye, middle ear, antrum and soft palate; the benign tumors include lipomas, schwannomas and, rarely today, tuberculous lymph nodes. Aside from abdominal tumors, children tend to have nonsolid malignancies such as leukemia.

Cervical Masses in Young to Middle-aged Adults

This group may continue to exhibit congenital lesions, but by this age most will have been corrected. In the main, unilateral masses occurring in the 21 to 40 year old age group are malignant. The commonest is the lymphoma. These cervical masses may represent a local manifestation of a systemic disease. The mass is lobulated or appears to be a series of nodes matted together. A complete physical examination plus systemic evaluation is mandatory prior to investigation of an enlarged lymph node.

Cervical Masses in Middle-aged to Aged Adults

Metastatic malignant diseases account for the majority of neck masses in the over 40 age group (Martin et al., 1952). In 80 per cent of these patients the primary malignancy occurs above the clavicle. A symmetrical enlargement of a cervical lymph node indicates a localized process. These masses may well be the external manifestation of a small silent lesion of the oral cavity or hypopharynx (Fig. 2).

All too frequently a biopsy of an enlarged cervical lymph node is taken under local anes-

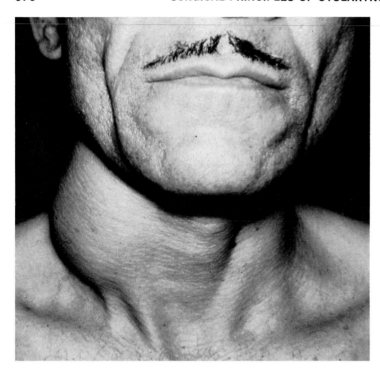

Figure 2. A cervical metastasis from an occult malignancy of the hypopharynx.

thesia as an outpatient procedure or in the office. If the procedure is performed under general anesthesia, it is possible that the anesthesiologist might call to the surgeon's attention a mass in the floor of the mouth, an ulceration of the tongue, or a fungating lesion of the larynx that the patient has failed to mention.

BIOPSY

In all instances the biopsy of a suspicious lesion of the mucosa or skin should precede any surgical investigation of a cervical mass. Removal of an enlarged node should be undertaken as the last step in diagnosis, not the first (Shumrick, 1965). A thorough examination of the head and neck should include: skin, scalp, ears, nose, oral cavity, nasopharynx, hypopharynx and larynx; when indicated esophagoscopy and bronchoscopy should be carried out. Biopsy should be made of cervical masses only after each of these areas has been thoroughly investigated at least twice to rule out the existence of primary tumor. In lesions of the scalp, skin and oral cavity, excisional biopsy is advisable if the area is small.

FROZEN SECTIONS

The use of cryostat frozen sections makes it possible to obtain accurate and immediate biopsy results. This technique may be employed in patients in whom multiple biopsies are required, so that it will not be necessary for the patient to return to the operating room for further biopsies, as in the case of a report of "nondiagnostic tissue" or "acute and chronic inflammation" which is received several days after regular sections are obtained. In addition, safe surgical margins may be ascertained by frozen sections during excision of a head or neck tumor.

ANESTHESIA

Biopsy of lesions of the skin, the mucosa of the oral cavity and the anterior nasal cavity may be made with the use of topical anesthesia. Mucosa overlying a lesion may be anesthetized with topical 10 per cent cocaine applied with a cotton pack. This anesthetic agent remains the most effective and the safest if properly applied. A drying agent such as 0.6 mg. of atropine along with a quick-acting barbiturate should be administered intramuscularly an hour before the biopsy. (Cocaine, as well as any other topical agent, is ineffective if a sea of saliva covers the underlying tissues.) The biopsy may be taken after five minutes since cocaine will not only induce anesthesia but, because of its vasoconstricting qualities, will

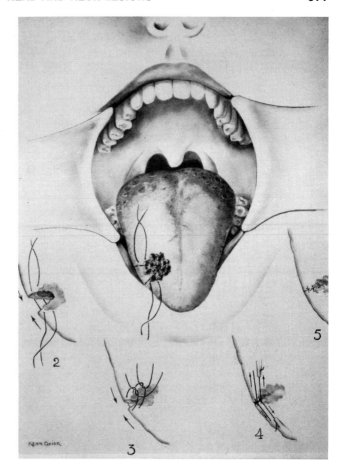

Figure 3. Hemostasis may be achieved by drawing the opposing edges together with chromic suture.

reduce bleeding. Local anesthesia, using 1 per cent lidocaine (Xylocaine) with or without epinephrine, may be employed for an incisional biopsy that is deep and requires adequate noninvolved mucosa in the biopsy specimen. The mucosa is ballooned around the desirable site for the biopsy, and a wedge may be removed, including adjacent normal tissue. Bleeding is frequently minimized by local anesthetics and is most often controlled with a pressure or hemostatic pack. If it continues, 3-0 chromic sutures may be used to appose the edges of the biopsy site. The sutures should be placed superficially, with care being taken that the surrounding tissues are not seeded with tumor cells. If the suspected lesion is in the tongue, the sutures may be placed through adjacent normal tissue before the biopsies are taken. When the section has been removed, the sutures are drawn together for hemostatsis much as in a liver biopsy (Fig. 3).

BIOPSY TECHNIQUES

Excisional Biopsy

Small lesions that do not appear by palpation to infiltrate deeper structures and are under 0.5 cm. in greatest diameter may be removed in toto as a biopsy. This can usually be accomplished with topical, local or regional anesthetic blocks. The specimen should include 0.25 to 0.5 cm. of apparently normal mucosa or skin. The resulting defect may be closed primarily and further treatment, if needed, determined after the pathologist's report. Excisional biopsies are particularly applicable for ulcers in the oral cavity and for small skin lesions of the face and neck that do not involve either the vermilion borders of the lips or the lids of the eye. Incisions for skin lesions can frequently be placed in normal skin lines, thus minimizing unsightly scars. In most lesions of the head and neck, this biopsy technique and that utilizing incisional specimens offer the most accurate and the quickest source of information for the clinician.

Incisional Biopsies

A common biopsy performed in the head and neck area is one in which a specimen that includes part of the suspect tissue plus a normal cuff of adjacent tissue is removed. Frequently this is accomplished by infiltrating the surrounding tissue with local anesthetic and using a scalpel such as a No. 11 or 15 Bard-Parker blade, to remove a pie-shaped specimen, with the apex of the "pie" being wide enough to include a representative and diagnostic sample of the tumor. This tissue should give not only a positive diagnosis but, in the case of epidermoid carcinoma, a fair chance of defining the degree of differentiation. Most lesions of the oral cavity are associated with a break in the mucous membrane and thus are inflamed and infected, making diagnosis difficult because of the associated edema and inflammatory cell changes. As in the case of excisional biopsies, the incision should, when feasible, be placed in such a manner that the

resultant scar could be included with a definitive primary surgical procedure or with a neck dissection if the biopsy report should be "lymph node with metastatic malignancy" (Fig. 4). Large tumors of the oral cavity, such as epidermoid carcinomas of the tonsil, tongue and palate, frequently outgrow their blood supply and become necrotic. A superficial biopsy may return a pathological diagnosis of acute and chronic inflammation with tissue necrosis. If the clinical signs indicate a suspected lesion may be malignant, a clinician should never accept such a report as being final. Repeated biopsies should be performed until a positive report is returned or the physician is satisfied that no malignant disease is present. On occasion, a near tonsillectomy may be performed by the physician whose responsibility it will be to administer definitive surgical treatment. An injudiciously placed biopsy scar may require the removal of large amounts of skin or mucosa which would present a real burden in the surgical closure at the time of definitive care.

Another problem area is in the diagnosis and management of hyperkeratosis of the oral mucosa. Frequently these lesions may be widespread and actually cover the entire buccal surface of the cheek. To attempt excisional biopsy

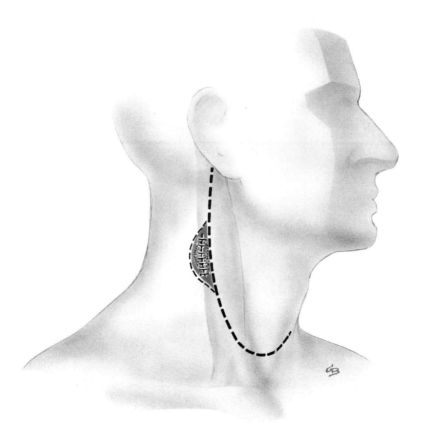

Figure 4. Biopsy incision of a neck mass should be planned so that the scar can be excised at the time of definitive neck dissection.

would be difficult because of the problem of resurfacing such a large area. This lesion, however, cannot be ignored, and the possibility of an invasive carcinoma lurking in the depths of these horny, plaque-like growths must be ruled out. This is best accomplished by multiple, deep, incisional biopsies of any and all areas that are thought to be atypical hyperkeratosis or to have changed to a more fleshy appearance since last observed. The possibility of such a patient's being subjected to many biopsy procedures over a long period of time is so high that the entire problem should be discussed with the patient prior to the first biopsy (Guenta et al., 1969).

Cutaneous Biopsy

This is a version of the incisional biopsy and may be used in an outpatient situation. Most practitioners of this type of biopsy use a skin punch (Peterson et al., 1969). This instrument is similar to a miniature cookie cutter, the two being employed in a similar manner. In a biopsy of a potential malignancy this technique is of limited value, and in some instances may necessitate repeated cutaneous biopsies or even an incisional biopsy. If deeper biopsies are indicated, a scalpel and skin sutures may be required. As with most punch or aspiration techniques, the tissue may be compressed or distorted to such a degree that a histological diagnosis is impossible. The added disadvantage in malignant lesions of the head and neck is that a corridor of tissue, the width of the punch, is now potentially seeded with tumor cells and must be removed when definitive treatment is administered. In addition, an occasional lesion of the head and neck may be an unpigmented melanoma, which should be removed by an excisional biopsy, with further treatment planned after the pathological report.

In general, the value of cutaneous punch biopsies is certainly questionable in light of other available techniques.

Cellular and Smear Biopsies

This method of definitive diagnosis has been disappointing. The number of false negative specimens obtained definitely limits its value. The technique involves the use of fluids that have been subjected to centrifuge and, after proper fixation, imbedding, sectioning and staining; a diagnosis is based upon individual cellular abnormalities. An adjunct of this method is the smearing of a suspected lesion or the cut edge of a biopsy specimen on a clean glass slide. The slide is subjected to immediate fixation before drying.

Most clinicians prefer to await the results of a permanent histological diagnosis made from the cut edge of the smear biopsy specimen before initiating definitive treatment of a suspected head or neck lesion.

Aspiration Biopsy

This technique is defined as a procedure in which negative pressure is created in a syringe and, as a result of the pressure differences, cellular material is drawn from the tissues through the needle into the syringe. Much recent literature has dealt with this subject. It would seem that the positive advantages over incisional or excisional biopsy are meager, if they exist at all (Engzell et al., 1970). In needle or aspiration biopsies the penetrating instrument often passes through the deep cervical fascia of the neck into cervical masses, thus violating the facial compartment that contains the lymph nodes draining the head and neck area and thereby contaminating a region not accessible to treatment (Fig. 5). Even in the best of hands, the needle biopsy often yields insufficient amounts of tissue and a second or a third attempt is necessary. Hematoma resulting from needle biopsy frequently presents problems. In addition, it must be assumed that a corridor of tissue from the skin down to the biopsy area is contaminated with tumor cells. If the specimen proves positive, this corridor must be removed with the specimen, and frequently the puncture made with the biopsy needle has become indistinguishable from the surrounding tissue, which is an advantage in a benign lesion but may be disastrous in a malignant one.

Endoscopic Biopsies

Endoscopic biopsies utilize special types of anesthesia and special instruments. These should be done as inpatient procedures in the operating room. The ideal anesthesia for laryngoscopies and bronchoscopies is a good topical block of the oral and pharyngeal mucosa with cocaine or Dyclone. The superior laryngeal nerves should also be blocked, plus the laryngeal surface of the epiglottis and the true vocal cords. If a general anesthetic is desired, the apneustic technique is one of the most useful

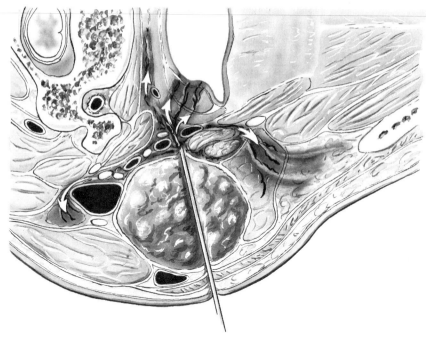

Figure 5. Needle biopsy, even when skillfully performed, may pass through the tumor and contaminate the deeper fascial planes.

for endoscopic procedures contemplated to last no longer than three to five minutes in patients free of cardiopulmonary disease. Prior to the induction, the patient is denitrogenated by breathing high flows of oxygen for five to ten minutes. During this time a baseline blood pressure and pulse rate are obtained, a precordial stethoscope is applied, and an intravenous infusion is begun. A hypnotic dose of thiopental is then injected intravenously, followed by 60 to 80 mg. of succinylcholine. After one minute of hyperventilation with oxygen, the endoscopic procedure begins. For the technique to be satisfactory, a high partial pressure of oxygen must be maintained in the airway to prevent dilution of alveolar oxygen tension by air. This can be accomplished by running six to eight liters per minute of oxygen through the side arm of the bronchoscope or nasal catheter placed in the oropharynx during laryngoscopy. The use of excessive suction draws air into the endoscope, thereby diluting the oxygen tension in the airway. The patient with advanced pulmonary disease who already has a high carbon dioxide tension plus ventilation-perfusion imbalance is a poor candidate for this technique. Should the endoscopy take longer than the contemplated time or should there be a change in rate or rhythm of the pulse, the laryngoscope should be removed and the patient ventilated for one minute. If a bronchoscope is

being used, it should be withdrawn to the carina (unless it is a ventilating bronchoscope) and positive pressure breathing administered by intermittent occlusion of the viewing end of the bronchoscope, with the oxygen flush valve of the anesthesia machine fully open. After the patient is ventilated to lower the alveolar carbon dioxide tension, the endoscopist may continue for another three to five-minute period while additional hypnotic doses of thiopental and succinylcholine are given as needed to maintain apnea. The endoscopist must be willing at any time, when so directed by the anesthetist, to cease his operative efforts and to allow the patient to be ventilated.

If a bronchoscopy is to be performed, instillation of 5 cc. of 5 per cent cocaine or 0.5 per cent Dyclone into the trachea and main stem bronchi will achieve adequate anesthesia. It must be recalled the right main stem bronchus is embryologically a continuation of the trachea and that the two form a gentle 120 degree angle. The left main stem bronchus is almost at right angles to the trachea. Instillation of an anesthetic agent is much more difficult on the left side, since it does not drop in naturally, and this is accomplished by positioning the patient to the right or left during instillation. Occasionally the surgeon may be approached by an anesthesiologist who is knowledgeable in regional anesthesia and who suggests use of transtracheal and superior laryngeal blocks. The use of these procedures in patients with suspected malignant disease in the head and neck region is definitely contraindicated. The possibility of direct involvement of a primary pharyngeal or laryngeal tumor or an undetected metastatic node which may be encountered with the injection needle is too great a risk when other satisfactory techniques are available. The addition of a light general anesthetic or the use of such agents as Inovar is advisable and applicable since the topical anesthetic blocks abolish manipulative stimulation and deep anesthesia is not required. Prior to any instrumentation, a routine chest film and bronchogram should be obtained. The edema created by bronchoscopy alone prevents any adequate study with contrast dye.

Laryngoscopy

The basic instruments used with this examination include a plastic (universal) mouth gag for special protection of the maxillary incisor teeth. This may be obtained from a prosthodontist; if used frequently it should be replaced every four to six months. The gag resembles a plastic upper dental plate or prosthesis. The Hollinger anterior commissure laryngoscope is the best all-purpose instrument for hypopharyngeal and laryngeal examinations. The protruding superior lip of this instrument allows the operator to use the laryngoscope much as a long finger and to move folds of mucosa in examining the pyriform sinus and postcricoid area and to efface false and true vocal cords in the search for hidden malignant nodules. The recent addition of fiber optic illumination with its incredible natural light has made laryngoscopy the most important tool in the otolaryngologist's hands. The examination and biopsy of all other lesions of the head and neck may be satisfactorily performed by members of other medical disciplines, but only the otolaryngologist has really mastered the use of this most important instrument and technique. The anterior commissure laryngoscope is applicable not only to examination, but also to biopsy as well as treatment. Nodules and lesions of the true vocal cords, similar types of disease of the epiglottis, pyriform sinus, aryepiglottic folds and postcricoid area may all be examined and biopsies taken using this most versatile instrument. This is also the instrument of choice for examination and biopsy of the pharynx. The suspension laryngoscope as devised by Lynch and later revised by Roberts has added a dimension to laryngoscopy not hitherto available. For the first time the operator has both hands free and excellent endoscopic exposure. Because of the extremely complicated equipment required for Lynch suspension laryngoscopy, plus the need for a general anesthesia, the technique has not gained widespread use. During World War II, with its shortage of medical assistants, the Sam Roberts Chest Suspension laryngoscope became very popular. A single operator can use the equipment; biopsy or treatment can be carried out under local anesthesia. The laryngoscope has a bilateral light carrier with a wide aperture. When natural light fiber optic illumination was added, it made this type of instrument ideal for laryngeal endoscopy. It must be understood that this instrument is for treatment and diagnosis not for exploration, since, once in place, it is completely immobile. For examination of the trachea and bronchi, the Broyles' bronchoscope is most suitable. The esophagus may be examined with the Jesberg esophagoscope. The instruments used for the actual biopsies are either straight-biting or up-biting cup forceps. They range in size from 2 to 6 mm. in diameter.

SUMMARY

In general, biopsies of facial, intra-oral, pharyngeal, laryngeal, bronchial and esophageal lesions should be carried out in the early part of the diagnostic investigation. Biopsies of neck masses should definitely be performed only after an exhaustive search for a primary lesion has been concluded. This may even include upper and lower gastrointestinal studies, IVP's, skull films, and so forth.

REFERENCES

Engzell, U., et al.: Aspiration biopsy of tumors of the neck. Acta Cytol. *14*(No. 2):51–57, 1970.

Giunta, J., et al.: The accuracy of the oral biopsy in the diagnosis of cancer. Os. Om. Op. *28*(No. 4):552–556, 1969.

Martin, H., et al.: The diagnostic significance of a "lump in the neck." Postgrad. Med. *2*:491–500, 1952.

Moore, S. E.: When do you pull the plug? J.A.M.A. *205*: 29, 1968.

Peterson, W. C., et al.: Dermatology—Self-induced eruptions. Minn. Med. *52*:103–104, 1969.

Shumrick, D. A.: Lump in the neck. G. P. *31*:110–117, 1965.

Slaughter, D. P.: Excision of the mandible for neoplastic disease. Surgery *26*:507–522, 1949.

Section Eight

MEDICAL PRINCIPLES OF OTOLARYNGOLOGY

Chapter 28

HEMATOLOGY

by John J. Will, M.D.

ANEMIA

Anemia is an abnormal state in which the oxygen-carrying capacity of the blood per unit volume is below normal for age and sex. To the physician anemia exists if there is a reduction in the circulation of either hemoglobin or erythrocytes. Anemia is always a manifestation of a more fundamental disorder, which may be genetic, inflammatory, nutritional, endocrinologic, immunologic, neoplastic, vascular, or toxic in type. The recognition and identification of the underlying cause of anemia are essential for the best management of the patient. The failure to do so before initiating therapy often results in ineffective treatment, in the need for a more complex diagnostic investigation and, occasionally in irreparable injury to the patient.

Diagnosis of Anemia

Diagnosis is facilitated by an understanding of the mechanisms causing anemia. The erythrocyte has a finite life span of about 120 days (Berlin et al., 1959). Metabolic alterations associated with erythrocyte aging lead to a reduction in adenosine triphosphate and available cellular energy, to diminished cation transport, to alterations of membrane lipid and, ultimately, to cellular death (Jandl, 1966). In health the daily destruction of senescent erythrocytes is balanced precisely by the release of an equal number of red blood cells from the bone marrow. Anemia will occur if the erythropoietic capacity of the bone marrow is less than normal or if blood loss or blood destruction is in excess of its functional capacity. The normal bone marrow can compensate for moderate increases in blood destruction by increasing erythrocyte production as much as sixfold (Crosby, 1955).

Morphologic alterations in erythrocytes occur with anemia, and a characterization of the anemia based upon the size and hemoglobin content of the red cell is very helpful in diagnosis (Table 1). The erythrocyte volume and hemoglobin concentration are readily calculated from formulas devised by Wintrobe in 1932. A skillful examination of a properly prepared stained blood film will allow confirmation of the Wintrobe indices and identification of abnormal erythrocyte forms which may give important clues to the etiology of an anemia (Fig. 1).

A systematic approach to the problem of anemia is required for proper diagnosis. First, the existence of anemia must be recognized. Mild anemia and slowly developing anemia of greater severity are often asymptomatic and recognizable only if blood counts are obtained. If anemia is symptomatic the patient may complain of weakness, fatigue, dyspnea with exertion, or of postural faintness. A history of blood loss is of obvious importance. Jaundice, fever, and abdominal and skeletal pain suggest a hemolytic anemia. Dietary inadequacy of vitamins, minerals, and protein call attention to the possibility of a nutritional anemia, whereas a family history of anemia may indicate a genetic cause. Pallor or icterus of mucous membranes and of skin, atrophy of the papillae of the tongue, cardiac enlargement, tachycardia, systolic murmurs over the pulmonic and apical areas, increased pulse pressure, hepatosplenomegaly, neuritis and posterolateral column disease are important physical alterations in anemia.

TABLE 1. Classification of Anemia

CLASS AND TYPE	RETICULOCYTE RESPONSE TO ANEMIA
I. **Normocytic and normochromic anemias**	
MCV 80–94 cμ MCHC > 30%	
A. Acute blood loss	Increased
B. Increased blood destruction	Increased
1. Intracorpuscular abnormalities	
2. Extracorpuscular abnormalities	
C. Impaired blood production	Decreased
1. Anemia of chronic disorders	
2. Anemia of bone marrow failure	
a. Marrow hypoplasia or aplasia	
b. Marrow hyperplasia	
3. Myelophthisic anemia	
II. **Hypochromic and microcytic anemias**	
MCV < 80 cμ MCHC < 30%	
A. Iron deficiency anemia	Normal to decreased
B. Thalassemia	Normal to increased
C. Pyridoxine-responsive anemia	Normal to decreased
III. **Macrocytic and normochromic anemia**	
MCV > 94 cμ MCHC > 30%	
A. Megaloblastic anemias	Decreased
1. Vitamin B_{12} deficiency	
2. Folic acid deficiency	
B. Normoblastic anemias	
1. Macrocytic anemia of chronic liver disease	Normal to increased
2. Hypothyroidism	Decreased
3. Increased blood destruction with brisk reticulocytosis	Increased

Second, the morphology of the red cells and the mechanism causing the anemia must be established. A complete blood count and a reticulocyte count are essential; from these data the Wintrobe indices are calculated. Most anemias can then be classified into one of three morphologic groups, either normocytic and normochromic, microcytic and hypochromic, or macrocytic and normochromic. The reticulocyte count is a helpful indicator of mechanisms which cause anemia. Reticulocytosis in the presence of anemia indicates a bone marrow response to the anemia and, by inference, suggests either blood loss or increased blood destruction as causal. On the other hand, reticulocytopenia indicates impaired erythropoietic function. These classifications have limitations because the morphologic features and physiologic mechanisms do not always fit completely into single groupings. Despite these limitations they are important and useful in diagnosis.

Third, to complete the diagnosis of anemia, the underlying disorder must be found. In most instances an etiologic diagnosis can be synthesized from the historical facts, the physical abnormalities, and the laboratory data.

Normocytic Normochromic Anemias

Normocytic and normochromic anemia is the morphologic type encountered most frequently. Acute blood loss, increased blood destruction, and impaired blood production must be considered in its etiology.

Acute Blood Loss

The signs and symptoms of acute blood loss depend upon the rate and quantity of bleeding. They are determined chiefly by a series of physiologic events that follow hypovolemia and not by the reduced oxygen-carrying capacity of the blood. The erythrocytes are normocytic and normochromic, thrombocytosis and leukocytosis occur within hours after hemorrhage, and reticulocytosis commences 24 to 48 hours later.

Increased Blood Destruction

Disorders characterized by increased destruction and shortened survival of erythrocytes are referred to as hemolytic states. Either intracorpuscular abnormalities or extracorpuscular factors may cause the shortened erythrocyte survival. Hemolytic states in which bone marrow hyperplasia maintains a normal erythrocyte mass are compensated, and those with inadequate bone marrow hyperplasia to maintain normality are uncompensated. Hemolytic anemias are the least common of the normocytic and normochromic anemias. The symptoms and signs vary with the cause, rate, and severity of the hemolysis. In mild or compensated hemolytic states there may be no symptoms; whereas in acute, severe hemolysis, life-threat-

ening manifestations occur. A history of chills, fever, jaundice, abdominal or skeletal pain, or red-brown colored urine in an anemic patient indicates the likelihood of hemolysis. Drug or chemical exposure in the patient or a family history of anemia, jaundice, or splenomegaly may indicate a cause for hemolysis. Pallor associated with icterus, skeletal anomalies, splenomegaly, or chronic leg ulcers are important physical findings in hemolytic anemias.

Laboratory examination is critical in the diagnosis of hemolytic anemia. A brisk reticulocytosis with a normocytic and normochromic anemia in the absence of acute bleeding or recent hematinic therapy suggests hemolysis. The presence of polychromasia, spherocytes, sickle cells, target cells, helmet cells, erythro-

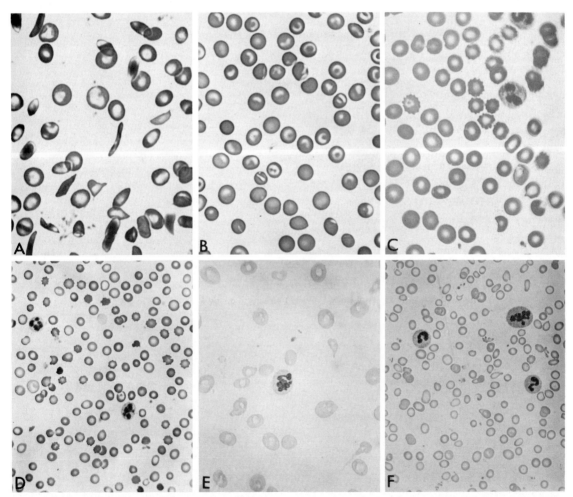

Figure 1. Morphologic abnormalities in peripheral blood films. *A*, Sickled erythrocytes in sickle cell anemia; *B*, target cells in sickle cell–hemoglobin C disease; *C*, burr cells in chronic renal disease; *D*, contracted, distorted and fragmented erythrocytes in cardiac hemolytic anemia; *E*, macrocytosis of erythrocytes and a hypersegmented neutrophil in pernicious anemia; and *F*, dimorphic appearance of erythrocytes and hypersegmented neutrophil in megaloblastic anemia of pregnancy.

cyte fragments, or normoblasts in the blood film signals the probability of hemolysis and gives a clue to its cause. Bone marrow examination reveals erythroid hyperplasia. With severe intravascular hemolysis, plasma hemoglobin is increased, methemalbumin is formed, and serum haptoglobin is absent. The plasma is red to brown in color, and hemoglobinuria and hemosiderinuria follow. In chronic extravascular hemolysis the serum bilirubin is increased chiefly in the form of unconjugated bilirubin bound to albumin. The serum haptoglobin content is decreased, and the fecal excretion of urobilinogen is increased. Once the existence of hemolysis has been established by the demonstration of increased hemoglobin catabolism and bone marrow erythroid hyperplasia, the exact etiology must be found. More sophisticated laboratory procedures are often necessary. These include hemoglobin electrophore-

sis, osmotic fragility, Coombs test and other antibody identification procedures, tests for cellular enzyme deficiencies and ^{51}Cr tagging of erythrocytes for survival and splenic sequestration studies.

Intracorpuscular Abnormalities

Anemias resulting from intracorpuscular defects of erythrocytes most frequently are of genetic origin. Only the most important of these anemias will be discussed, although a complete classification is given in Table 2.

Hereditary Spherocytosis. Hereditary spherocytosis is inherited as a mendelian dominant characteristic. The erythrocytes have a spherical shape, are readily trapped, and are eventually destroyed in the spleen. The nature of the cellular defect remains elusive, but there is an abnormal permeability of the cell membrane

---

TABLE 2. Classification of Hemolytic Disease

I. Due to intracorpuscular defects
  A. Hereditary
    1. Spherocytosis
    2. Elliptocytosis
    3. Stomatocytosis
    4. Hemoglobinopathies
    5. Thalassemia
    6. Disorders due to erythrocyte enzyme deficiencies:
      glucose-6-phosphate, glutathione synthetase, glutathione reductase, pyruvate kinase, triosephosphate isomerase, and others
    7. Unstable hemoglobin hemolytic disease
  B. Acquired
    1. Paroxysmal nocturnal hemoglobinuria
    2. Hemolytic anemia associated with myeloid metaplasia
    3. Deficiency of vitamin B_{12}, folic acid, or iron

II Due to extracorpuscular defects
  A. Infectious agents
    Malaria, virus infections, bacterial septicemia
  B. Chemical and drug agents
    Lead, alpha-methyldopa, penicillin, cephalothin, quinidine, stibophen, phenacetin, sulfonamides, and others
  C. Physical agents
    1. Cardiac hemolytic anemia
    2. Microangiopathic hemolytic anemia
    3. March hemoglobinuria
    4. Burns
  D. Antibody-induced hemolytic anemia
    1. Isoantibodies
      a. Transfusion reactions
      b. Hemolytic disease of the newborn
    2. Autoantibodies
      a. Idiopathic
      b. Associated with systemic lupus erythematosus, chronic lymphocytic leukemia, malignant lymphoma, and other diseases
  E. Nonimmune hemolytic anemia associated with other diseases
    1. Associated with splenomegaly—congestive, infiltrative, or inflammatory
    2. Chronic liver disease
    3. Neoplasia
    4. Thrombotic thrombocytopenic purpura

---

to sodium resulting in osmotic swelling and ultimately in hemolysis (Jacob, 1965).

Anemia is most often mild or even compensated, although on occasion it is severe. It may be discovered in the evaluation of asymptomatic jaundice, splenomegaly, or cholelithiasis. With infection, anemia may increase because of transient bone marrow aplasia. Mild icterus, slight pallor, and splenomegaly are the usual physical findings.

Spherocytes, although sometimes infrequent, can be identified on the blood film. Reticulocytosis is variable; unconjugated bilirubin is increased in the serum. The osmotic fragility of the erythrocytes is increased but may not be demonstrable until the cells are stressed by a 24 hour incubation at 37° C. (Young, 1955).

Hemoglobinopathies. Hemoglobinopathies result from inherited alterations of the structure of human hemoglobin (Heller, 1966). In adult life there are three hemoglobin components: a major component, hemoglobin A; and two minor components, hemoglobin A_2 and hemoglobin F. Hemoglobin A_2 comprises about 2.5 per cent of the total hemoglobin, and hemoglobin F occurs in trace amounts. These hemoglobins have a similar gross structure of their globin moiety consisting of two structurally distinct pairs of peptide chains. One of these pairs, the alpha chain, is identical in hemoglobin A, A_2 and F, while the non-alpha chains differ in each of these hemoglobins. Alpha chains are combined with beta chains in hemoglobin A, with delta chains in hemoglobin A_2, and with gamma chains in hemoglobin F (Weatherall et al., 1969). Hemoglobin variants arise from the substitution in these chains of one amino acid for another. Over 30 genetic variants due to alpha chain substitutions have been reported; almost twice as many beta chain mutants have been studied (Jones, 1968).

Clinically important hemoglobinopathies in the United States are the beta chain variants, hemoglobins S and C. In hemoglobin S, valyl replaces the glutamyl residue in position 6 of the beta chain. In hemoglobin C, lysyl is substituted for the glutamyl residue in the same position. Hemoglobin S and hemoglobin C occur in about 8.5 and 2 per cent, respectively, of American Negroes and are inherited as mendelian recessive characteristics. In general, the heterozygous carrier of either of these hemoglobins has slightly less than half his hemoglobin as the variant type and is asymptomatic.

The individual who is homozygous for S hemoglobin develops a severe disorder, sickle cell anemia. From 75 to nearly 100 per cent of his hemoglobin is of the S variant, hemoglobin A_2 is normal in amount, and the remaining hemoglobin is hemoglobin F. Anemia develops early in life. Intravascular sickling causes increased blood viscosity, plugging of capillary beds and repeated episodes of chest, abdominal, and skeletal pain. Jaundice, cardiomegaly, systolic heart murmurs, hepatomegaly, and skeletal deformities are the rule. Splenomegaly may be present in the first decade of life, but repeated infarction results in "autosplenectomy." The disease is ultimately fatal.

The hemolytic anemia is associated with leukocytosis and often with thrombocytosis. Sickled erythrocytes are seen on the stained blood film. Jaundice is due chiefly to unconjugated bilirubin, but liver dysfunction and intrahepatic obstructive disease may develop. Then conjugated bilirubin is also increased in the serum. Hemoglobins S and F can be identified and quantitated by electrophoresis.

Homozygous hemoglobin C disease occurs in about one in 6000 American Negroes (Terry, 1954). The hemolytic state is usually mild or fully compensated; splenomegaly is present. The most prominent feature of the stained blood film is the presence of numerous target cells. In wet preparations of blood, especially after splenectomy, intraerythrocytic crystals of hemoglobin can be seen (Wheby et al., 1956). Hemoglobin C is easily identified by electrophoresis.

Sickle cell-hemoglobin C disease occurs in individuals who are heterozygous for both these beta chain variants, and is the most frequent of the double heterozygous combinations in American Negroes. The severity of the hemolytic anemia is intermediate between sickle cell anemia and hemoglobin C disease. Splenomegaly occurs in two thirds of the patients. Target cells are prominent in the stained blood film. Diagnosis is established by the electrophoretic demonstration of S and C hemoglobins.

Thalassemia. The thalassemias are a group of hereditary anemias all having in common a retardation in the rate of production of normal globin chains. The primary defect appears to be in the mechanism controlling the rate of globin synthesis. Depending on which peptide chain is affected, the anemias are designated as alpha, beta, gamma, or delta thalassemia (Fessas, 1968). The thalassemic syndromes occur most frequently in people of Mediterranean origin, particularly those from Italy, Sicily, and Greece, but they occur worldwide and are found in people from the Near East and the

Far East, and in the American Negro. Because hemolysis is a feature of thalassemia, it is discussed in this section even though the erythrocytes are characteristically microcytic and hypochromic. Several recent reviews of thalassemia have been published, and only the most frequently occurring syndromes are discussed here (Weatherall, 1965; Nathan, 1966).

Homozygosity for beta-thalassemia major results in classic Cooley's anemia, a serious disorder beginning in infancy. Pallor, icterus, mongoloid facies, growth retardation, and hepatosplenomegaly are features of this disease. The anemia is severe, and the red cells show marked microcytosis and hypochromia, aniso-poikilocytosis, polychromasia, basophilic stippling, and some targeting. Normoblasts are numerous in the peripheral blood. The hemoglobin pattern is characterized by a decreased to absent hemoglobin A, by a marked increase in hemoglobin F, and by low, normal, or increased hemoglobin A_2. The anemia is a result of ineffective erythropoiesis and shortened erythrocyte survival (Sturgeon and Finch, 1957).

Heterozygosity for beta-thalassemia (beta-thalassemia minor) produces a wide spectrum of disease. At one extreme are cases with severe chronic anemia and splenomegaly clinically indistinguishable from beta-thalassemia major, in the middle are cases with mild anemia and leg ulcers, and at the other extreme, the asymptomatic carriers. In the latter, anemia may develop during pregnancy or with the stress of injury or infection. The characteristic red cell is microcytic and slightly hypochromic, but on the stained blood film, cells can vary from a nearly normal to a very abnormal appearance resembling thalassemia major. Erythrocyte osmotic fragility is decreased. In most cases hemoglobin A_2 is increased to levels of 4 to 6 per cent; in one half the patients hemoglobin F may be slightly increased, with values under 5 per cent. Erythrocyte survival is normal or slightly reduced, and anemia, if present, is largely a result of ineffective erythropoiesis.

There is overlap in the populations in which structural hemoglobin variants and thalassemia are found. In the American Negro hemoglobin S or hemoglobin C may be found in combination with beta-thalassemia. In the doubly heterozygous individual the production of normal beta chains is markedly curtailed, and little or no hemoglobin A is produced. Accordingly, the hemoglobin pattern consists chiefly of the hemoglobin variant associated with slight increases in hemoglobins A_2 and F. Diagnosis rests with careful hematologic evaluation of the patient and his family. Quantitative hemoglobin electrophoretic analysis is essential.

Alpha-thalassemia is difficult to identify. The homozygous state results in fetal death; the heterozygous state causes little abnormality. At birth inclusions may be found in erythrocytes and several unstable hemoglobins can be identified by electrophoresis. These abnormalities disappear after birth as adult hemoglobin synthesis takes over (Yet et al., 1967).

Hereditary Hemolytic Disease Due to Enzyme Deficiency. Hereditary deficiencies of erythrocyte enzymes occur rarely but are important causes of drug-induced hemolysis and chronic hemolytic anemia. Normal red cells are deficient in stored energy. They depend on glycolysis via the anaerobic Embden-Myerhof and the oxidative phosphogluconate pathways to provide compounds of high potential energy and reductive capacity which keep the red cells functioning and alive. A deficiency of an essential enzyme for glycolysis causes a susceptibility of the red cell to hemolysis. Glucose-6-phosphate dehydrogenase and pyruvate kinase deficiencies occur most frequently, but at least 11 other enzyme deficiencies have been reported in cases of hemolytic disease (Beutler, 1969).

Glucose-6-phosphate dehydrogenase deficiency is inherited as a sex-linked recessive characteristic in Negroes and in people from the Mediterranean basin area. The clinical expression of this abnormality is variable and relates to quantitative and qualitative differences of the enzyme. In the Negro male hemolytic episodes occur only in association with drug ingestion, infection, or acidosis (Table 3). In most heterozygous females the susceptibility to hemolysis is slight. In the Mediterranean type of deficiency, hemolytic disease of the newborn may occur and persist as a chronic hemolytic anemia (Salvidio et al., 1967).

TABLE 3. **Compounds Associated with Hemolysis of G6PD-Deficient Red Cells***

Antimalarials: primaquine, pamaquine, quinacrine, quinine†
Sulfonamides: sulfanilamide, sulfisoxazole, sulfamethoxypyridazine, salicylazosulfapyridine, and others
Sulfones: sulfoxone, diaphenylsulfone, and others
Analgesics: acetanilid, acetylsalicylic acid, acetophenetidin
Nonsulfonamid antibacterials: nitrofurazone, nitrofurantoin, chloramphenicol†
Other: naphthalene, menadione, quinidine,† fava beans†

_____

*For a complete compilation, see Beutler, 1969.
†Hemolysis only in Caucasians.

Pyruvate kinase deficiency is inherited as an autosomal recessive characteristic. Only the homozygote manifests anemia, which may be mild, moderate, or severe. Splenomegaly occurs. On the blood film some red cells show dense, irregularly contracted, and crenated forms.

Hereditary red cell enzyme deficiency should be considered in all patients with a nonspherocytic hemolytic anemia, especially if there is a history of drug ingestion. Screening tests are available for the identification of the specific enzyme deficiency (Beutler, 1966).

Paroxysmal Nocturnal Hemoglobinuria. This acquired form of hemolytic anemia is extremely rare but is interesting because of the unusual mechanism of hemolysis. The classic patient has a chronic hemolytic anemia, with hemoglobinuria more marked at night and clearing during the day. Despite the hemolytic process, leukopenia and thrombocytopenia are common. Rarely, pancytopenia and marrow hypoplasia may precede the onset of hemolytic anemia (Letman, 1952). The basic mechanism of hemolysis in PNH remains an enigma (Hartman and Jenkins, 1965). Erythrocyte acetylcholine esterase is regularly decreased, but its role in hemolysis is unknown. Presumably the red cell membrane is at fault and the late acting hemolytic components of complement can attach directly to it and induce hemolysis (Rosse et al., 1965). The diagnosis of PNH is substantiated by demonstrating hemolysis of the PNH red cells in acidified serum or in low ionic strength sucrose solutions (Hartman and Jenkins, 1966).

Extracorpuscular Abnormalities

Hemolytic states occur because of extracorpuscular factors inducing a random destruction of normal erythrocytes. Disorders of this type are acquired, and the causes are diverse. They include immunologic illness, infections, drugs, chemicals, physical agents, mechanical trauma, and hyperfunction of an enlarged spleen.

Isoimmune and Immune Blood Group Antibodies and Hemolysis. Naturally occurring 19-S, IgM isoantibodies of the ABO blood systems are capable of inducing severe intravascular hemolysis in transfusion reactions caused by incompatibility. Immune antibodies which develop from stimulation by blood group antigens (ABO, Rh, MNS, P, etc.) may be either IgM, IgG, or IgA immunoglobulins. The IgG immune blood group antibodies are 7S globulins, have a molecular weight of 150,000, and can pass the placental barrier. Hemolytic disease of the newborn in either ABO or Rh incompatibility is a result of this type of immune antibody.

Autoimmune Hemolytic Anemia. Erythrocyte autoantibodies distinguish the autoimmune hemolytic anemias (AIHA). These antibodies for the most part are IgG immunoglobulin. They have maximum agglutinating activity at 37° C. in the presence of human antiglobulin serum and often have a specificity for antigens of the Rh system. Warm IgM antibodies are not infrequent, but IgA antibodies are rare (Engelfreit et al., 1968). In some instances red cell sensitization is due to coating with components of serum complement which can be identified by an anticomplement antiserum.

The fundamental cause of autoimmune disease remains unknown. However, several observations are of importance. The graft versus host reaction is an experimental model of an immunologic disorder frequently accompanied by AIHA. In this model a graft of immunologically competent cells fails to recognize the antigens of the host and mounts an immunologic attack against various tissues of the host, including red cells (Porter, 1960). It has been proposed that in spontaneous autoimmune disease a "forbidden clone" (Burnet, 1959) arises from a deletion of a genetic locus for a single histocompatibility antigen. The mutant clone then reacts to all normal cells as antigenic. The occurrence of AIHA and other immunological disorders in a strain of New Zealand Black mice (Bielschowsky et al., 1959) and the recognition in man of the existence of AIHA and other autoimmune disease in multiple family members indicate the possibility of a genetic predisposition. The development of red cell autoantibodies in patients receiving long-term treatment of hypertension with alpha-methyldopa points to environmental factors also contributing to the appearance of immunologic disease (Carstairs et al., 1966).

Autoimmune hemolytic anemia in man may be either idiopathic or a manifestation of another disease. The frequency of idiopathic and secondary AIHA is about equal. In some instances AIHA is the first symptom of a disease which may not be identified until later. These include chronic lymphocytic leukemia, Hodgkin's disease and other malignant lymphoma, acute disseminated lupus erythematosus and other connective tissue diseases, as well as a group of miscellaneous disorders. Autoimmune hemolytic anemia may be acute or chronic, fulminating or mild. The symptoms are often a reflection of the severity of the anemia. Fever and jaundice are common, and slight splenomegaly is present in at least one half the patients. In secondary AIHA many of the symptoms and physical signs are a result of the underlying disease. Laboratory abnormalities are those common to all hemolytic anemia, but the hallmark of AIHA is the presence of a positive antiglobulin test (Coombs test). In secondary AIHA lymph node biopsy, serum immunoelectrophoresis, antinuclear antibody identification, and lupus cell preparations assist in the identification of the primary disorder.

Hemolytic anemia caused by cold agglutinins is rare. The high titer cold autoantibodies which give rise to the cold hemagglutinin syndromes are IgM immunoglobulin. Most often they are monoclonal proteins, fix complement, and have anti I specificity. Cold hemagglutinin disease may be either idiopathic or associated with mycoplasma pneumonia infection, virus infection, or lymphoreticular malignancies. Pallor, acrocyanosis, Raynaud's phenomena and, often, hemoglobinuria occur after exposure to cold. Diagnosis rests on the demonstration in vitro of a high titer of cold agglutinins and often of cold hemolysins at a pH of 6.5 to 7.0 (Schubothe, 1966).

Another distinct type of cold autoantibody is the Donath-Landsteiner antibody found in cases of paroxysmal cold hemoglobinuria. This antibody is an IgG immunoglobulin, fixes complement, and can be identified by the classic Donath-Landsteiner test.

Certain drugs cause immunologic hemolysis of normal erythrocytes (Beutler, 1969). Stibophen was the first drug reported to do this. It forms a drug-protein complex which attaches to red cells, fixes serum complement, and results in hemolysis. Erythrocytes coated in this fashion usually gave a positive Coombs test of the nongamma type. Penicillin, in very large doses, is capable of inducing hemolytic anemia in some persons. The erythrocyte is an innocent bystander. Normal red cells bind penicillin, and in those penicillin-treated patients producing antipenicillin antibodies of the IgG type, hemolytic anemia may occur. These patients will have a positive anti-IgG antiglobulin test. The antihypertensive drug alpha-methyldopa produces a hemolytic anemia indistinguishable from idiopathic AIHA. About 20 to 30 per cent of the patients receiving alpha-methyldopa develop antibodies, but the number developing hemolytic anemia is less than 1 per cent.

The antibodies are of the IgG type, combine with the erythrocyte in the absence of the drug, usually have specificity for the Rh blood system, and give a positive anti-IgG antiglobulin test. Other drugs reported to produce an immune hemolytic anemia are quinidine, para-aminosalicylic acid, phenacetin, and the sulfonamides. When drug-induced immune hemolytic anemia is suspected, a Coombs test should be made with a broad-spectrum human antiglobulin serum.

Cardiac Hemolytic Anemia. The advent of cardiac surgery led to the recognition of hemolytic anemia associated with cardiac disease (Marsh et al., 1969). In severe aortic stenosis and occasionally in mitral stenosis, mechanical hemolytic anemia occurs. It also occurs with Teflon patches and aortic and mitral valve prostheses. The anemia may become severe with prosthetic valve malfunction. The anemia is normocytic and normochromic, becoming hypochromic in longstanding hemolysis because of iron loss from hemosiderinuria. Burr cells, helmet cells, microspherocytes, and other red cell fragments are present in stained blood films.

Impaired Blood Production

Normocytic and normochromic anemia results from impaired erythropoiesis. The red cell has a normal or only slightly shortened survival time, but the functional capacity of the bone marrow is inadequate to maintain a normal red cell mass. The erythropoietic defect may be primary to the bone marrow or may be exogenous.

Anemia of Chronic Disorders. A mild nonprogressive anemia often accompanies chronic infection, cancer, chronic liver disease, and rheumatoid arthritis (Cartwright, 1966). It is called "secondary" or "simple chronic" anemia and is one of the most commonly encountered forms of anemia. The pathogenesis is complex. A slight shortening of the red cell life span occurs, but inadequate bone marrow erythropoiesis is the major cause of the anemia. Erythropoietin does not increase in response to the anemia. Iron absorption is decreased, and the reticuloendothelial system develops an increased avidity for iron. As a consequence, hypoferremia follows and, if the anemia is longstanding, hypochromia and microcytosis ensue.

The anemia is characteristically asymptomatic. The hemoglobin is most often greater than 9 gm. per 100 ml. The red cells are normocytic and normochromic, but slight microcytosis and hypochromia can develop. The serum iron and transferrin values are low, while bone marrow hemosiderin is normal to increased. Diagnosis is readily made from the clinical situation and the alterations in iron metabolism.

The anemia of renal disease is similar in many respects to the anemia of other chronic disorders. In acute nephritis with azotemia, expansion of the plasma volume may cause an apparent anemia without any reduction of the red cell mass. Mild anemia may develop from blood loss. In chronic renal disease with azotemia, anemia may become severe (Loge et al., 1958). The major defect is a failure of erythropoiesis, although bleeding and hemolysis are sometimes contributing causes. Both intracorpuscular and extracorpuscular defects are factors in the hemolysis (Mann et al., 1965). Erythropoietin levels are low in uremia, and the diseased kidney is either unable to produce or to activate this erythropoietic-stimulating hormone. This deficiency as well as other undetermined factors contribute to the bone marrow impairment (Gordon, 1968). The anemia of uremia is normocytic and normochromic, and a slight to moderate relative reticulocytosis occurs. Burr cells and polychromasia are commonly seen on the blood films of these patients.

Anemias of Bone Marrow Failure. Anemias of bone marrow failure constitute a heterogenous group of severe anemias which may be congenital in origin or acquired. The cardinal feature of these anemias is impaired erythropoiesis, which in some instances is associated with impaired granulocytopoiesis and thrombocytopoiesis. Pancytopenia may then be present. The bone marrow may be aplastic, hypoplastic, or hyperplastic, but regardless of its cellularity its functional capacity is impaired.

Congenital hypoplastic anemia. Most often this anemia has its onset in the first year of life, after the third or fourth month. Rarely, the onset is delayed until adolescence or even adulthood. The symptoms and physical abnormalities are those of a chronic anemia. Cardiomegaly and congestive heart failure are frequent complications. Splenomegaly and hepatomegaly are late complications of hemosiderosis, and in some instances hemochromatosis occurs. The anemia is normocytic and normochromic, and reticulocytes are decreased or absent. Leukopenia and thrombocytopenia occur only with the development of hypersplenism. The bone marrow has a striking absence of nucleated precursors of the erythrocytes but retains a normal granulocytic and megakaryocytic activity. During the course of the illness the number of erythroid precursors may increase somewhat or even become hyperplastic, although erythropoiesis remains ineffective. Spontaneous remissions of the anemia have occurred after periods ranging from six months to 13 years (Diamond et al., 1961). The etiology is unknown. In childhood the anemia has occurred in association with other developmental defects including cystic kidneys, skeletal abnormalities, and aberrations of tryptophan metabolism (Altman et al., 1961). In adults "pure" red cell anemia may be associated with thymoma (Jahsman et al., 1962).

Congenital pancytopenia. This rare form of anemia, first reported by Fanconi in 1927, is characterized by pancytopenia, bone marrow hypoplasia, and a number of congenital anomalies, including brown pigmentation of the skin, dwarfism, hypogenitalism, renal defects, strabismus, ear anomalies and deafness, mental retardation, and multiple neurological abnormalities. The hematological abnormalities usually appear between the ages of four and 12 years. Congenital pancytopenia is transmitted as an autosomal recessive characteristic with incomplete penetrance. A number of chromosomal aberrations, including a specific type of polyploidy, have been reported (Bloom et al., 1966). Siblings of the patients with anemia often possess other congenital anomalies without blood changes. A high incidence of leukemia is found in the families of these patients (Garriga and Crosby, 1959). Familial hypoplastic anemia without associated anomalies has also been reported (Estren and Dameshek, 1947).

Acquired aplastic anemia. Aplastic anemia refers to a group of refractory anemias characterized by severe pancytopenia and by hypoplasia or aplasia of the bone marrow. Aplastic anemia is caused by drugs, chemicals, and ionizing radiation in about 50 per cent of the patients (Table 4). In the remaining cases no

TABLE 4. **Drugs Frequently Associated with Aplastic Anemia***

Chloramphenicol
Phenylbutazone
Mephenytoin
Gold compounds
Tolbutamide
Sulfamethoxypyridazine
Quinacrine
Chlorpropamide
Chlorpromazine

*For a complete compilation see Bithell and Wintrobe, 1967.

cause can be found and they are classified as idiopathic.

The onset may be abrupt or insidious. In addition to the symptoms of anemia, purpura, epistaxis, retinal hemorrhage, gingival bleeding, melena, and hematuria are manifestations of thrombocytopenia. Neutropenia is associated with ulcerative stomatitis and pharyngitis, and fever resulting from infection is frequent. The spleen, liver, and lymph nodes are not usually enlarged. Diagnosis rests on finding hypoplasia or aplasia of the bone marrow in association with pancytopenia. A careful search must be made for exposure to toxic agents in the patient's work and in his home. Particular attention should be directed to medications taken by the patient.

Refractory anemia with hyperplastic bone marrow. Refractory anemia with hyperplastic bone marrow describes a group of diseases characterized by severe anemia and, at times, by pancytopenia (Vilter et al., 1963). The etiology is unknown. The problem is primary to the bone marrow since no systemic disease has been found that can be held accountable. In most instances the bone marrow is hypercellular, but erythropoiesis is ineffective. In some instances erythroid hypoplasia is the only abnormality, and in other instances the bone marrow is hypoplastic in some areas and hyperplastic in others. Other features of the bone marrow include mast cell hyperplasia, hemosiderosis, ringed sideroblasts, and megaloblastoid erythropoiesis. Refractory anemia with these features has been called refractory sideroblastic anemia (Heilmeier et al., 1958). Another type of refractory anemia is characterized by pancytopenia, extreme megaloblastoid erythropoiesis, and maturation defects in granulocytopoiesis. Ringed sideroblasts are uncommon, but normoblasts contain a polysaccharide stained by the periodic acid-Schiff stain. This disease usually terminates quickly as myelomonoblastic leukemia, panmyelosis with myelofibrosis, erythroleukemia, or aplastic anemia. The diagnosis of refractory anemia with hyperplastic bone marrow requires the exclusion of diseases causing anemia and the demonstration by biopsy of the cytologic abnormalities of the bone marrow.

Myelophthisic anemia. This type of anemia is associated with space-occupying disorders of the bone marrow and is encountered with metastatic carcinoma, multiple myeloma, granulomatous disease, Hodgkin's disease, and other malignant lymphomas. The anemia is variable in severity. The most significant abnor-

mality is the presence of normoblasts in the blood out of proportion to the severity of the anemia. Immature granulocytic cells and bizarre platelet forms may be present. A bone marrow examination is helpful in diagnosis.

Hypochromic Microcytic Anemias

Hypochromic microcytic anemia is caused most frequently by chronic iron deficiency, but morphologically similar anemias occur in thalassemia and pyridoxine responsive anemia.

Iron Deficiency Anemia. Iron is essential to human life. It plays critical roles in oxygen transport via hemoglobin and myoglobin and in oxidative metabolism via the heme enzymes, cytochromes, catalases, and peroxidases (Polycove, 1966). A normal adult has a total body content of 3 to 5 gm. of elemental iron. The iron is distributed as follows: 70 per cent in red cells; 25 per cent in storage iron as hemosiderin and ferritin; less than 1 per cent in enzymes, plasma, and extracellular fluid; and the remainder unaccounted for. Iron balance is maintained by controlled iron absorption rather than by excretion. Iron is absorbed in the duodenum, where the epithelial cells of the mucosa play an important role in control (Bothwell and Carlton, 1968). Iron transport across mucosal cells is an active metabolic process. A proportion of the iron in the gut is transported quickly across the mucosa to the plasma where it is bound to the iron-binding protein, transferrin. Much of the remaining iron is deposited in the mucosal cells as the iron protein complex, ferritin. If unneeded, this iron is lost into the gut by cellular exfoliation. Mucosal transport of iron is enhanced by a deficiency of iron in the body and by increased erythropoiesis, but the exact mechanisms regulating the mucosal transport have not been identified.

Iron excretion from the body is limited to the quantities lost by cellular desquamation from the gastrointestinal tract, by secretion in bile, urine, and sweat, and by menstruation. This amounts to 0.5 to 1.0 mg. per day in men and 0.8 to 2.0 mg. per day in women during reproductive years. An average American diet is estimated to contain 12 to 18 mg. of iron, of which 5 to 10 per cent is absorbed by an adult. The nutritional intake of iron in a man is adequate to maintain balance, but in an adolescent girl and a menstruating female iron balance may be precarious.

Iron deficiency anemia is the most common anemia (Brown, 1966). It occurs in infancy and adolescence when growth outstrips the supplies of dietary iron. Pregnant women are another high risk group in whom iron requirements may exceed dietary supplies. In the American adult, however, chronic blood loss is the most important factor in the development of iron deficiency. Menorrhagia is the single most frequent cause of iron deficiency, but blood loss from epistaxis, peptic ulcer, hiatus hernia, gastritis, diverticulosis, polyps, neoplasm and hemorrhoids are commonplace.

The symptoms of iron deficiency anemia are diverse, and its recognition may be by chance examination. When symptoms occur, they are usually insidious in onset and are those common to all anemias. Pallor of the mucous membranes and skin is the outstanding physical finding. Mild glossitis may occur. Longitudinal ridging, brittleness, and spooning of the nails occur infrequently in iron deficiency as seen in the United States. Splenomegaly is seen only in cases of long standing.

Iron deficiency, regardless of its cause, results in mobilization of iron from stores in the reticuloendothelial cells to provide metal for hemoglobin synthesis and essential heme enzymes. Depletion of iron stores is associated with a fall in serum iron content, a rise in serum transferrin level, and an increased absorption of iron. When the supply of iron becomes inadequate for heme synthesis, anemia soon appears. The red cells are at first hypochromic, but as erythropoiesis is further restricted microcytosis appears, reflecting excessive cell division before bone marrow release (Leventhal and Stohlman, 1966). Reticulocytes are normal or reduced in number unless recent hemorrhage has occurred. Platelets may be increased in number. Bone marrow samples stained for hemosiderin by the Prussian blue technique show decreased or absent stainable iron granules.

Pyridoxine-Responsive Anemia. A group of microcytic and hypochromic anemias occur which have in common impaired erythropoiesis, iron overload, ringed sideroblasts in the bone marrow, and a variable response to vitamin B_6 therapy. In spite of these similarities many differences exist in individual cases.

In its rare and "typical" form, a severe microcytic and hypochromic anemia with striking poikilocytosis of the red cells afflicts young adults or middle-aged males (Horrigan and Harris, 1968). Abnormalities in tryptophan metabolism occur in about one half the patients. Anemia or tryptophan metabolic abnormalities often are found in male relatives of the patient. Serum iron values are high, transferrin levels are reduced, and the saturation of the iron-binding protein markedly increased. Response to vitamin B_6 therapy is partial. The abnormalities in red cell shape persist even though the anemia improves. Some of these patients respond to an indolic compound found in crude liver extracts.

"Atypical" cases of pyridoxine-responsive anemia are found more frequently. These occur beyond middle age and are often associated with malnutrition, with primary disease of the bone marrow or liver or, occasionally, with the administration of isoniazid, cycloserine, or pyrazenoic acid (McCurdy et al., 1966). About 10 per cent of the atypical patients have megaloblastic erythropoiesis. The response to vitamin B_6 or combined vitamin B_6 and folic acid therapy may be partial or complete.

The etiology and pathogenesis of these anemias are not fully understood. The "typical" cases, in part, may be a hereditary sex-linked inborn error of metabolism. The "atypical" cases are considered to be acquired, the metabolic error being precipitated by the development of some primary disease or by drug ingestion.

Macrocytic and Normochromic Anemia

Macrocytic anemias fall into two main groups. The most striking macrocytosis is accompanied by megaloblastic erythropoiesis and is a result of folic acid or vitamin B_{12} deficiency. Macrocytosis associated with normoblastic erythropoiesis is found in chronic liver disease, hypothyroidism, and in other anemias with intense erythropoiesis and reticulocytosis.

Macrocytic Megaloblastic Anemias. Megaloblastic anemias occur because of a deficiency of vitamin B_{12} or of folic acid. The macrocytic red blood cell is thought to appear because of skipped cell divisions of its bone marrow progenitors, the megaloblasts. A megaloblast is larger than its normal marrow counterpart, and the maturation of its nucleus lags behind the maturation of its cytoplasm. Its nuclear chromatin is fine and widely separated, and nucleoli are well defined in the earlier stages of maturation. Similar chromatin changes and bizarre nuclear shapes occur in band cells, metamyelocytes, and even in megakaryocytes.

Erythropoiesis is ineffective (Finch, 1959) and the primary defect is in the synthesis of precursors of DNA which are required for rapid doubling of cellular DNA prior to mitosis. Mitosis occurs less frequently than normal, and the cell grows large and full of RNA during a prolonged resting stage (Glazer et al., 1959). Studies with bacteria, animals, and human beings indicate important roles for folic acid and vitamin B_{12} in nucleic acid metabolism. Folic acid, in its tetrahydrofolate coenzyme forms, is capable of accepting or donating one-carbon units in chemical reactions involved in the biosynthesis of purines and in the reduction of deoxyuridylate to thymidylate (Bertino and Johns, 1968). Vitamin B_{12} is indirectly related to nucleic acid metabolism, as it seems to be a factor without which tetrahydrofolate coenzyme forms cannot be formed or function effectively (Vilter et al., 1963).

A number of clinical syndromes ascribed to a deficiency of these hematopoietic vitamins have been described and must be considered in the diagnosis of megaloblastic anemia. Pernicious anemia is the most frequent megaloblastic anemia resulting from vitamin B_{12} deficiency. This deficiency also occurs after total gastrectomy, in fish tapeworm anemia, in intestinal blind pouch anemia, and in vegans. Folic acid deficiency is a more common deficiency and is seen in megaloblastic anemia of pregnancy and of infancy, in drug-induced megaloblastic anemia, in nutritional macrocytic anemia, in sprue and in other malabsorption syndromes.

LEUKEMIA AND LYMPHOMA

Neoplastic diseases of the hematopoietic and lymphopoietic tissues remain a major challenge to the investigator. There has been no lack of research or of speculation about their cause, but the etiology of human leukemia and lymphoma is still unknown.

The role of genetic factors in the etiology of these diseases has been under intensive study and several recent reviews are available (Mac-Mahon, 1966; Zuelzer and Cox, 1969; Fraumeni, 1969). Familial aggregation of single types of leukemia among adults is suggestive of an important genetic influence in leukemogenesis. This occurs most frequently in chronic lymphocytic leukemia, but the number of these family clusters is unimpressive when compared with the overall frequency of this disease. The importance of genetic factors is more clearly indicated in studies of concordance of leukemia in twins and in nontwin sibs of leukemic children. A concordance rate of about 20 per cent was reported in identical twins (MacMahon and Levy, 1964), and concordance among nontwin sibs was shown to exceed the normal expectation (Miller, 1964). However, Miller in 1968 did not confirm this excess risk in nontwin sibs, but this discrepancy may be explained by the brief period of observation in the later study.

Familial Hodgkin's disease has been recognized and concordance in three sets of twins reported, but the data are not convincing evidence for a genetic role in its cause (Mac-Mahon, 1966). Rigby et al. in 1968 reported 39 multiple family cases of leukemia or lymphoma, with 91 involved close relatives. Concordance was noted in cases of Hodgkin's disease, malignant lymphoma, chronic lymphocytic leukemia, acute leukemia, and multiple myeloma.

Ethnic differences are recognized in the occurrence of leukemia. Chronic lymphocytic leukemia is rare in Japanese and other non-Caucasians. In the United States the incidence of all types of leukemia is high in Jews. On the other hand, a comparative study of mortality in childhood leukemia and lymphoma among the immigrants and native born in Israel demonstrated a higher rate of leukemia in the foreign born and little difference in the rates of lymphoma in both groups (Royston and Modan, 1968). These conflicting observations would suggest that other factors than race are involved. An appraisal of all genetic data seems to indicate that familial predisposition to these neoplastic diseases occurs in a few instances but is not of major importance in all.

Disorders associated with chromosomal abnormalities increase the risk of leukemia. The association of leukemia and Down's syndrome is well recognized. Here the chromosomal defect is trisomy 21, resulting from meiotic nondisjunction. This association suggests that extra chromosomes play a role in leukemogenesis. Sporadic cases of leukemia have also been reported in association with Klinefelter's syndrome, in the D-trisomy syndrome, and in other congenital disorders associated with aneuploidy. Susceptibility to acute leukemia occurs in Bloom's syndrome, Fanconi's anemia, and ataxia telangiectasia. These diseases are inherited as autosomal recessive characteristics and are all associated with chromosomal breakage and rearrangement. The manner in which chromosomal instability predisposes to leukemia, however, remains a matter for speculation.

Chromosomal abnormalities in leukemic cells occur frequently. A deletion of chromosomal material involving one of the smallest acrocentric chromosomes, the G-21 Philadelphia chromosome (Ph'), is a diagnostic feature of most cases of chronic myelogenous leukemia (Whang-Peng et al., 1968). Despite the unique specificity of this defect, it has not been established whether this chromosome alteration is a cause or an effect of the disease. In acute leukemia in relapse, aneuploidy, pseudodiploidy, and marker chromosomes occur frequently, but there is no consistency of defects among cases of a specific type of leukemia. The role of these chromosomal aberrations in leukemogenesis remains uncertain.

Malignant lymphoma occurs excessively in congenital and acquired disorders characterized by immunologic deficiency. Lymphoreticular neoplasms are reported in association with ataxia telangiectasia, Wiskott-Aldrich syndrome, sex-linked and Swiss types of agammaglobulinemia, immunosuppressive therapy following renal transplant, and in other acquired immunoglobulin deficiency states. The common denominator in these diseases is immunoglobulin deficiency, and it has been proposed that these patients have an inadequate defense for oncogenic viruses.

Although numerous studies have established clearly that fowl leukoses, murine leukemia and lymphoma, cat leukemia, cattle leukemia, and other animal neoplasms are of viral origin, a similar relationship in human leukemia and lymphoma has not been established (Rauscher et al., 1966). Virus particles have been demonstrated by electron microscopy in lymph nodes, bone marrow, and plasma of patients with lymphoma and leukemia. Established tissue culture lines of neoplastic cells from leukemia and lymphoma patients contain viruses which resemble the herpes virus. Burkitt lymphoma, first reported in Ugandan children, is of particular interest in this regard. This occurs in endemic proportions in Central Africa where malaria, yellow fever, and dengue are also endemic. It has been proposed that this tumor might be caused by an infectious agent transmitted by an arthropod vector. The Epstein-Barr virus (E.B.V.) has been demonstrated in cell cultures from African Burkitt lymphoma, in American Burkitt lymphoma cell lines, and in other cell lines of hematologic neoplasms (Epstein et al., 1964). High titers of E.B.V. antibodies can be demonstrated in the sera of patients with Burkitt lymphoma, but antibodies to this virus also occur in subjects without neoplastic disease. Recently high titers of E.B.V. antibodies have been recognized in infectious mononucleosis (Henle et al., 1968). All these observations in man and animal make attractive the proposal that viruses are etiologically important in human leukemia and lymphoma, but at this time the evidence is only circumstantial.

Other environmental factors are known to cause leukemia. Chronic myelogenous and acute leukemia can follow radiation exposure. The evidence for this has been obtained from epidemiologic studies of patients receiving partial body radiation for treatment of ankylosing spondylitis (Court Brown and Doll, 1965) and from survivors of the atomic blasts in Hiroshima and Nagasaki (Bizzozero et al., 1966). Many case reports and occupational surveys incriminate benzene exposure as a cause of acute leukemia (Vigliani and Saita, 1964). Chloramphenicol may also have leukemic properties. These chemicals as well as radiation exposure injure bone marrow and cause chromosomal damage. Cellular mutation may follow and a new cell line develop which has a selective advantage over normal hematopoietic tissue.

These facts appear to indicate a heterogeneity in the etiology of hematopoietic and lymphoreticular neoplasms. A series of complex interactions between host and environmental factors may culminate in a malignant mutation of a somatic cell. The survival of this mutation and its development into a significant neoplasm may be determined also by the interaction of additional host and environmental forces. A simple cause and effect hypothesis of oncogenesis is untenable.

Acute Leukemia

Acute leukemia is a fatal neoplastic disorder characterized by an infiltration of the bone marrow and other tissues by immature leukocytes, chiefly blast cells. Abnormal cell release and disordered hematopoiesis result in the appearance of immature leukocytes in the blood and in the development of anemia, granulocytopenia, and thrombocytopenia.

The kinetics of leukemic cell proliferation in all stages of the disease are unknown (Cronkite, 1967). It is estimated that at least 10^{11} leukemic cells must be present in the bone marrow before the diagnosis can be made. Therefore, studies of kinetics made after the diagnosis of leukemia is established reflect characteristics of advanced disease and do not necessarily indicate the early events in leukemogenesis. Clearly leukemic cell proliferation is a diversion from the normal steady state of leukopoiesis in which death and production of new cells are equal. The traditional concept of acute leukemia as a rapidly proliferating autonomous population of cells does not appear to be correct. Leukemic cells have been shown to have generation times equal to, or more prolonged than, normal bone marrow cells. Tritiated thymidine labeling of bone marrow cells indicates that the population of actively dividing cells within the leukemic marrow is lower than normal. Mauer and his associates in 1968 showed that only large leukemic blast cells are labeled early after administration of thymidine. The larger population of small blast cells becomes labeled only as the intensity of the label in the larger cells diminishes, indicating the production of small blast cells from division of large blast cells. These small cells presumably could constitute a population of resting cells capable of being transformed into dividing cells if given the proper stimulus. They would have the capacity for self-renewal and, in a sense, serve as stem cells for the leukemic process. The emergence of labeled cells from the marrow into the blood is more rapid in leukemic than in normal persons, but the turnover of leukocytes in blood is lower than normal. These comparisons of leukemic and normal leukocyte kinetics suggest that leukemia may be an accumulative disorder rather than a proliferative one (Bierman, 1967). In acute leukemia, defective maturation and marrow release of leukocytes exist, but the factors controlling these processes are unknown.

Leukemia is the commonest neoplasm of childhood and is predominantly acute lymphoblastic in type (Table 5). It has a peak incidence in the third and fourth years of life and then rapidly declines in frequency. Acute myeloblastic leukemia and its variants occur at all ages and exceed acute lymphoblastic leukemia in incidence after age 20. In children and adults the onset of acute leukemia can be sudden, often following an upper respiratory infection. The onset also can be insidious, and in some instances anemia, leukopenia, or pancytopenia can be present for months before the true nature of the illness is apparent. The latter state has been called the "preleukemic" stage of leukemia and occurs more often in adults than in children. Malaise, fever, purpura, epistaxis, bone pain, and pallor are common symptoms. Mild to moderate enlargement of lymph nodes, spleen, and liver can occur in acute lymphoblastic leukemia, but these changes are less conspicuous in acute myeloblastic leukemia. Lesions of the mouth, nose, and throat are among the commonest manifestations of acute leukemia. Bleeding gums, gingival hypertrophy and necrosis, petechial and ulcerative lesions of the buccal membranes and tongue, tonsilar enlargement and ulceration, herpetic lesions of the nares and lips, as well as bacterial and fungal infections of the mouth, nose, and throat occur (Love, 1936).

The rising incidence of infections by subvirulent or nonvirulent organisms in acute leukemia has coincided with the more extensive use of antileukemic agents, corticosteroids, and broad-spectrum antibiotics. The untoward effects of this therapy can be attributed to interference with antibody production, to poor localization of infection, to granulocytopenia, and to the overgrowth and dominance of viruses, bacteria, and fungi insensitive to antibiotics. Moniliasis, herpes simplex, or pseudomonas infection of the nose, oral pharynx, or mouth may portend a more serious invasion and dissemination of infection. Systemic infection with cytomegalovirus, herpes zoster virus, staphylococcus, *Clostridium perfringens*, *Escherichia coli*, *Klebsiella pneumoniae*, aspergillus, phycomycetes (mucormycosis), *Cryptococcus neoformans*, *Pneumocystis carinii*, or other organisms often develops as a complication of acute leukemia. Hemorrhage into the middle or inner ear, or leukemic infiltration of the auditory nerve can cause deafness or labyrinthine disturbances (Shanbrom and Finch, 1958). Hemorrhages in the conjunctivae, sclera, and retina of the eyes are commonplace. Leukemic infiltration can involve salivary glands, thyroid, thymus, kidney, liver, testicle, central nervous system, and other organs.

Blood findings typically include normocytic and normochromic anemia, thrombocytopenia, and the presence of leukocyte blast cells. The total leukocyte count can be low, normal, or high. Diagnosis of acute leukemia is facilitated by aspiration of a bone marrow specimen. Most often the bone marrow is diffusely hypercellular as a result of a marked increase in blasts and other immature leukocyte forms. Normoblasts and megakaryocytes are decreased in number. Rarely, the marrow specimen can appear hypoplastic and indistinguishable from aplastic anemia. A needle or surgical biopsy should be performed in such cases. Special histochemical stains are useful in establishing a morphologic diagnosis (Hayhoe et al., 1964).

Will, 1969). Leuke[r]
structures in the r
ment on the osti
results in tinnitus,
ing. Leukemic inf
and its intracranial
turbances in audit
of the eighth crani

Any part of th
involved as a re
thrombosis, demy[
leukemic cells. T[
include cranial ner
nal cord and nerve
thesias, hyporefl
multifocal leukoe
changes, visual lo
kemic involvemer
types of leukemia
ic lymphocytic l
may be localized
tion of the larynx
dium, stomach, s
bladder, and oth[
relentless extensi
leukemia. With
weight loss, rec[
anemia, and thr[
rhage complicate
of patients with c
develop autoimn
hemolytic anemia
mune thrombocyt

Serum protein
chronic lymphoc[
emia may be pre
"monoclonal" in
roglobulins occur
as the disease pr[
els fall below n[
synthesis. The f
antigenic stimula
(von Furth, 196[
In most cases
mia, leukocytosi[
ic granulocytic
are under 100,00
thirds of patient[
et al., 1966). Th
population of sn
prise 80 to 99 pe
When anemia d
normochromic.
sis, reticulocyt[
polychromatoph[
red blood cells
The Coombs tes

TABLE 5. *Classification of Neoplastic Disorders of Hematopoietic Tissues*

CLASS AND TYPE	VARIANTS	ALTERNATIVE TERMINOLOGY
Acute leukemia		
Myeloblastic	Promyelocytic	
	Myelomonocytic	
	Erythroleukemia	Acute erythremic myelosis (di Guglielmo)
Lymphoblastic	Acute leukemia of childhood (stem cell)	
Monoblastic		
Chronic leukemia		
Myelocytic		
Lymphocytic		
Monocytic		
Malignant lymphoma*		
Lymphocytic, differentiated	Follicular variants occur in all classes of malignant lymphoma	Lymphosarcoma, differentiated
Lymphocytic, undifferentiated		Lymphosarcoma, undifferentiated
Mixed type		Lymphocytic and reticulum cell sarcoma
Reticulum cell sarcoma differentiated		Stem cell lymphoma
Reticulum cell sarcoma, undifferentiated		Histiocytic lymphoma
Hodgkin's disease		
	Lymphocyte predominence	Hodgkin's paragranuloma
	Nodular sclerosis	Hodgkin's granuloma
	Mixed cellularity	Hodgkin's granuloma
	Lymphocyte depletion (reticular, diffuse fibrosis)	Hodgkin's sarcoma
Gammopathies		
Multiple myeloma		Plasma cell myeloma
Macroglobulinemia of Waldenström		
Heavy chain disease		Franklin's disease
Other		
Polycythemia vera		Erythremia, Osler's disease
Myelofibrosis with extra-medullary hematopoiesis		Agnogenic myeloid metaplasia
"Primary" thrombocytosis		Hemorrhagic thrombocythemia

*Braunstein and Gall, 1962; Rappaport, 1966; Lukes et al., 1966.

The periodic acid-Schiff stain is positive in blast cells in lymphoblastic and erythroleukemia but is negative or weak in myeloblastic leukemia. Peroxidase positivity is present in myeloblastic leukemia and erythroleukemia but is negative in lymphoblastic leukemia. In some cases of myeloblastic and erythroleukemia Auer bodies, rod-shaped cellular inclusions, can be seen in Romanowsky stained preparations of blood and bone marrow. They do not occur in lymphoblastic leukemia.

Chronic Leukemia

Chronic forms of leukemia usually have a longer course than occurs in acute leukemia, and the leukemic leukocytes are more mature. Chronic myelocytic and chronic lymphocytic leukemia comprise the bulk of the cases of chronic leukemia and are found in about equal incidence in the United States. Rarely, chronic leukemia is of a monocytic type.

Chronic myelocytic leukemia occurs primarily between the ages of 20 and 45 years but is recognized in all ages. Studies of granulocytic kinetics indicate a breakdown in the equilibrium between leukocyte production and destruction. The bone marrow mitotic pool is greatly expanded in size, but cell division occurs no more frequently than in normal bone marrow. The generation times of mitotic cells in the pool are normal or even slightly prolonged. The expanded mitotic pool could result from a greater than normal input of undifferentiated stem cells into the myeloid compartment, but there is no conclusive evidence for this. Studies with tritiated thymidine and ^{32}P indicate that immature granulocytes in the bone marrow have a ready access to the blood and a prolonged intravascular circulation time (Boggs, 1967). On the other hand, the bone

marrow capa
granulocytes
demonstrated
1967). None
normalities c
for the profou
it is evident t
is not a pro
mitotic activit
of granulocyti

Chronic my
ious in its o
cede any othe
the earliest sy
early satiety i
may occur, ca
a friction rub
of the spleen
frequent, but
common. Le
bone, periost
number of pa
ment is rare.
kemic infiltrat
Shilling et al.
cytic leukemi
nosis is reaso
can be achiev
survival time
three years. A
in about one

Leukocytos
per cu. mm. v
phonuclear n
myelocytes is
al blood. Eo
frequently. M
terminal blast
the predomin
disease progr
mal or increas
and thromboc
manifestation.
hypercellular,
roid ratio. A
are present, a
the number of
karyocytic hy
ulocytic hyper
some can be
marrow or bl
alkaline phos
kocytes is ve
which is hel
from a leuke
phosphatase
vated.

elderly, males again have a greater incidence (2:1). Age-corrected survival rates are much better for young adults than for persons over 50. In the former group, nodular sclerosis and lymphocyte predominance are the most frequent histologic patterns, and in the latter group a reticular pattern with lymphocyte depletion is the lesion found commonly.

Hodgkin's disease has long been considered a disease of multicentric origin, but a more recent viewpoint holds that it is unicentric in origin, with an orderly progression from single node areas, to multiple node areas, to widespread disease (Rosenberg and Kaplan, 1966). This viewpoint, if correct, indicates the importance of early diagnosis and the need for assessing the extent of the neoplasm. It also offers the hope of a cure of Hodgkin's disease by early, aggressive, and extensive radiation treatment (Kaplan, 1966). In addition to cytologic classification of Hodgkin's disease, clinical staging of the disease is important in determining the size and location of radiation ports and in evaluating the results of therapy. The recommendations for staging proposed at a symposium in New York (Wilder, 1966) are now used frequently and are as follows:

Stage　　I: Limited to one anatomic region, or two contiguous anatomic regions, but all on the same side of the diaphragm.

Stage　II: Disease present in more than two anatomic regions but all on the same side of the diaphragm.

Stage III: Disease present on both sides of the diaphragm but not extending beyond involvement of lymph nodes, spleen, or Waldeyer's ring.

Stage IV: Involvement of bone marrow, lung or pleura, liver, bones, kidneys, gastrointestinal tract, or other organs in addition to lymph nodes, spleen, or Waldeyer's ring.

All stages are further classified into subgroups A or B to indicate the absence or presence of systemic symptoms.

Characteristically the patient with Hodgkin's disease has excellent health until the onset of disease (Ultman et al., 1966). Usually painless enlargement of one or more lymph nodes occurs without any systemic symptoms. The lymphadenopathy, at the outset, is localized in at least 25 per cent of patients and occurs most frequently in the cervical lymph nodes. Less commonly it is localized in the mediastinal,

axillary, or inguinal lymph nodes. Retroperitoneal periaortic node involvement occurs frequently but is not usually an early or an isolated finding. Primary splenic Hodgkin's disease is rare, but the spleen is involved initially in up to 30 per cent of patients and, eventually, in 80 per cent. As the disease progresses more node areas become involved, and the lungs, liver, bones, or central nervous system may be invaded. Systemic symptoms of lassitude, fever, anorexia, pruritus, weakness, and weight loss accompany disseminated disease.

Almost any organ may be involved initially or in advanced Hodgkin's disease, including skin, thyroid, breast, ovary, cervix, vulva, and bladder and other portions of the urinary tract. Involvement of the tonsil or Waldeyer's ring may occur initially (Jackson et al., 1936; Neiger, 1964); less commonly and usually as a late manifestation, nasal or laryngeal involvement may cause obstruction of respiratory pathways, epistaxis, deafness, or hoarseness (Cahn, 1948; Lautz, 1958; Shilling et al., 1967).

"Simple chronic" anemia occurs commonly as the disease progresses; less often anemia is due to either secondary hypersplenism or to autoimmune disease. The changes in the leukocytes are neither constant nor diagnostic. Neutrophilic leukocytosis occurs in over 50 per cent of the patients. Monocytosis and lymphocytopenia develop as the disease advances. Eosinophilia, occasionally marked, may be seen. Platelets are normal or increased in number early in the disease. Granulocytic hyperplasia of the bone marrow occurs, and when marrow involvement with Hodgkin's disease is present, Reed-Sternberg cells can be identified in marrow films and sections.

Immunologic abnormalities occur in Hodgkin's disease. Hyperglobulinemia occurs in over 70 per cent of patients early in the illness, but over 50 per cent with advanced disease have hypogammaglobulinemia. Relative anergy to several common allergens (tuberculin, mumps virus, oidiomycin, trichophytin) occurs in about 50 per cent of patients (Chase, 1966). The level of anergy can fluctuate and, in part, relates to the activity and extent of Hodgkin's involvement. These immunologic deficits contribute to the increased susceptibility of the Hodgkin's patient to infection, including bacterial septicemia, tuberculosis, fungal infections, and both localized and systemic viral infections. Infectious complications are the cause of death in about one fifth of patients.

The diagnosis of Hodgkin's disease rests

upon biopsy of either involved lymph nodes or other organs. When possible, the surgeon should obtain several nodes for pathological examination and should use care in clamping specimens to prevent crushing artifacts. Once the diagnosis has been established, careful clinical staging must be done. To do this, chest x-ray including tomography, lymphangiography to demonstrate retroperitoneal lymphadenopathy, bone marrow biopsy, and liver function studies (BSP excretion, serum alkaline phosphatase determination, serum protein electrophoresis) plus, if abnormal, liver biopsy are essential.

Lymphocytic and Reticulum Cell Types of Malignant Lymphoma

The incidence of lymphosarcoma and of reticulum cell sarcoma is very low in the first two decades of life but then increases linearly throughout life to age 75. These neoplasms are slightly more frequent in males than in females, with the sex difference more striking in younger age groups.

The commonest presenting symptom is painless lymphadenopathy but, in contrast to Hodgkin's disease, cervical node enlargement is associated early with node enlargement in axillary, inguinal, or other areas. Involvement of extranodal sites is not uncommon in bringing these diseases to the attention of the physician (Rosenberg et al., 1961). The tonsil and other structures of the oronasopharynx are the second most common site for the appearance of lymphosarcoma. These sites include the lingual tonsils, the pharyngeal lymphoid tissues, and the gingiva. Involvement of the nasal sinuses or of the parotid and lesser salivary glands rarely may be initial locations of the neoplasm. The skin, gastrointestinal tract, and bone are other important sites of involvement which may be either primary or part of widespread disease. Symptoms of malaise, fever, sweating, pruritus, or weight loss occur at the outset in about 20 per cent of patients with lymphosarcoma and reticulum cell sarcoma.

Burkitt's tumor requires special mention. This form of lymphosarcoma is predominantly extranodal and has a predilection for the jaw and facial bones of children under 14 years of age. The disease is usually multifocal, with involvement of one or more of the following sites: abdominal or pelvic viscera, retroperitoneal soft tissues, thyroid gland, salivary glands, and central nervous system (Carbone et al., 1969). Leukemic manifestations in the peripheral blood are rare. The neoplasm consists predominantly of undifferentiated lymphoblasts, among which histiocytic cells are interspersed, producing the characteristic "starry-sky" pattern. Burkitt's tumor constitutes 50 per cent of all malignant tumors of children in central equatorial Africa but it also occurs in the United States and elsewhere throughout the world (Dorfman, 1965; O'Conner et al., 1965; Sachs, 1966).

Clinical staging of lymphosarcoma and reticulum cell sarcoma is less useful than it is in Hodgkin's disease because of the tendency for early dissemination. If lymphangiography is performed in patients who clinically have only peripheral node enlargement apparent, 80 to 90 per cent will be shown to have intra-abdominal disease.

Of the nonspecific changes in the blood, anemia is the most important. It is present in one third to one half of the patients with lymphosarcoma but is much less common in patients with reticulum cell sarcoma. Autoimmune hemolytic anemia occurs as a complication of lymphosarcoma and is rarely the presenting manifestation of the disease. Peripheral blood changes of leukemia occur in about one third of patients with lymphosarcoma and much less frequently in reticulum cell sarcoma. Platelets may be normal or decreased in number. The bone marrow may be normal, focally involved, or diffusely infiltrated with neoplastic cells.

Hypogammaglobulinemia is very common, and poor antibody response is an important factor in the susceptibility of these patients to bacterial, viral, and fungal infections. Impaired "cellular" immunity is less frequent than in Hodgkin's disease.

As in Hodgkin's disease, the diagnosis must be made by biopsy of either an involved lymph node or other organ. The extent of the disease usually can be determined from the physical examination supplemented by a chest x-ray, an upper and lower gastrointestinal x-ray, and intravenous pyelogram, and a bone marrow aspiration. Lymphangiography is often unnecessary if these diagnostic examinations are performed.

GAMMOPATHIES

The gammopathies constitute a group of diseases characterized by hyperplasia of plasma cells or of similar related cells and by the synthesis of large amounts of monoclonal immunoglobulins (paraproteins).

The abnormal protein which can be found in the serum of a patient with a gammopathy shows a sharp peak on electrophoresis, resulting from the large amount of the single, homogeneous, abnormal protein and the frequently reduced amounts of normal immunoglobulins (Alper et al., 1966). The peak or spike is often referred to as the M component, a term stressing the most common occurrence of these proteins in myeloma and macroglobulinemia. All M components are structurally unique for the patients in whom they occur. Immunoelectrophoresis of the M components has shown that they may belong to any one of the major immunoglobulin classes, IgG, IgA, IgM, or IgD. M components may consist also of immunoglobulin fragments, i.e., Bence Jones protein or Fc fragments (Franklin et al., 1964). In contrast to normal immunoglobulins which have two antigenically distinct types of light chains designated as kappa or lambda chains, M components have a single type of light chain, of either the kappa or lambda variety.

The increased use of electrophoresis and immunoelectrophoresis for the analysis of serum proteins has fostered the identification of an increasing number of disorders associated with monoclonal immunoglobulin components. In a large series of sera containing M components, 50 per cent were found to be associated with multiple myeloma, 15 per cent with Waldenström's macroglobulinemia, 2 per cent with leukemia or lymphoma, 4 per cent with carcinomas, and 6 per cent occurred in persons without apparent disease (Waldenström, 1961).

Rarely, M components have been reported in association with rheumatoid arthritis, disseminated lupus erythematosus, periarteritis, Sjögren's disease, Felty's syndrome, scleroderma, autoimmune hemolytic anemia, dermatitis ulcerosis, tuberculosis, nocardiosis, sarcoidosis, infectious mononucleosis, cytomegalovirus disease, cirrhosis, Gaucher's disease, Paget's bone disease, and in allergic reactions to drugs (Michaux and Heremans, 1969).

In all these heterogeneous disorders it is postulated that the monoclonal immunoglobulin production represents the activity of "escaped" clones of immunoglobulin-secreting cells. These clones may result from neoplastic proliferation, from prolonged and intense stimulation of the immunoglobulin forming tissues, or from genetic variations.

HEMOSTASIS

Blood is normally fluid and circulates under pressure in the vascular system. A complex and orderly system of physiologic and biochemical reactions prevents spontaneous hemorrhage and helps to control traumatic hemorrhage. Normal hemostasis involves vascular factors, platelets, and plasma coagulation factors. The prevention of clotting and the resolution and removal of the products of coagulation are equally important to the normal state. The vascular endothelium, the circulation of plasma coagulation factors in an inactive form, and the presence of inhibitors contribute to keeping blood fluid and to limiting clotting to sites of vascular injury. A number of recent reviews present in detail the biochemical and physiologic concepts of hemostasis (Spaet, 1966; Williams, 1968; Davey and Lüscher, 1968).

Blood Vessels

Unfortunately there are large gaps in our knowledge of the function of blood vessels in hemostasis during health and in disease. The location, size, and supporting tissues of blood vessels influence the pattern of hemostasis after injury. When arteries, in which blood pressure is high, or large veins are injured, blood flow cannot be controlled without the use of pressure or surgical intervention. In smaller vessels, venules, and capillaries, hemostasis is accomplished by adhesion of endothelial surfaces, retraction and constriction of vessels, and formation of platelet plugs. These early events occur rapidly and are followed later by much slower phases of hemostasis.

Blood Platelets

The platelets serve a variety of functions. They help to maintain normal vascular integrity, plug holes in small vessels, release factors influencing vascular contractility and permeability, and are necessary for the activation of the intrinsic clotting pathway. Little is known about the activity of platelets in normal vascular integrity, but the thrombocytopenia and thrombocytopathy clearly are associated with increased capillary fragility and abnormal bleeding.

More is known about their role in hemostasis after vascular injury. Platelets quickly adhere to collagen, which has been exposed in the damaged vessel (Hugues, 1960). Platelets continue to accumulate upon this original aggregate as a result of the release of adenosine diposphate (ADP) by the platelets themselves (Gaarder et al., 1961). A plasma cofactor, probably fibrinogen, is necessary for the aggregation of platelets by ADP.

At this stage of platelet clumping their membranes remain intact and the aggregate is easily broken up. With continuing aggregation, clot-promoting activity evolves, leading ultimately to the formation of thrombin. As a result of thrombin activity the platelets fuse in a process of viscous metamorphosis. This irreversible aggregation is associated with a massive release of intracellular granules along with vaso-active amines, adenine nucleotides, proteins, and phospholipids. The phospholipids of the platelet granules, and perhaps of the platelet membrane as well, assist in the generation of enzymatic activity leading to formation of more thrombin (O'Brien, 1969). Platelet Factor III is a phospholipid complex which is the essential procoagulant derived from platelets. It plays a role in the generation of thromboplastin activity via the intrinsic pathway. Other substances with clotting activity released from platelets are largely plasma coagulation factors adsorbed onto the platelet.

Once thrombin has been generated, the platelet aggregate contracts through a mechanism dependent upon a contractile protein of platelets called thrombasthenin. Thrombasthenin functions enzymatically as a magnesium-dependent adenosine triphosphatase, thereby releasing more ADP, which furthers the process of platelet aggregation.

Platelet aggregates also adhere to fibrin threads within the fibrin meshwork formed during the last stage of clotting. Platelets are necessary for clot retraction to take place, but the exact mechanism for this reaction is unknown.

Plasma Coagulation System

The most complex part of the hemostatic mechanism is the plasma coagulation system. Plasma factors circulate as procoagulants and are converted to active enzymes during the process of clotting (Table 6). It is clear that blood coagulation consists of a series of auto-catalytic events in which a small quantity of active enzyme converts a larger inactive substrate into an active enzyme (Fig. 2). A series of such reactions results in an increasingly rapid production of a relatively large amount of enzyme which ultimately converts fibrinogen to fibrin. This concept has been called the enzyme cascade or waterfall sequence of blood clotting (Macfarlane, 1964; Davie and Ratnoff, 1964).

In the first stage of clotting, thromboplastin activity is generated. Two pathways exist for the formation of this prothrombin converting principle. The intrinsic pathway begins with the activation of Factor XII. Foreign surfaces including glass, silica, collagen fibers, and others, activate this factor in vitro but the in vivo mechanism of activation is unknown. Factor XIIa, in turn, activates factor XI, and a chain of reactions begins from which thromboplastin activity slowly evolves. The extrinsic pathway bypasses the early steps of coagulation and thromboplastin activity is elaborated rapidly. Tissue factors in the presence of Factor VII and calcium activate Factor X. From this point coagulation proceeds in a common pathway. In the second stage of clotting, prothrombin is converted to thrombin in the presence of calcium. In the third stage thrombin then converts fibrinogen to fibrin, which is stabilized by Factor XIIIa (Duckert and Beck, 1968).

TABLE 6. *International Nomenclature for Clotting Factors*

NUMERAL IDENTIFICATION		NAME
Procoagulant	*Active Form*	
Factor I	Ia	Fibrinogen
Factor II	IIa (thrombin)	Prothrombin
Factor III		Thromboplastin (tissue)
Factor IV		Calcium
Factor V	Va	Proaccelerin, labile factor
Factor VI	This term is obsolete	
Factor VII		Proconvertin, stable factor
Factor VIII	VIIIa	Antihemophilic factor
Factor IX	IXa	Plasma thromboplastin component
Factor X	Xa	Stuart-Prower factor
Factor XI	XIa	Plasma thromboplastin antecedent
Factor XII	XIIa	Hageman factor, contact factor
Factor XIII	XIIIa	Fibrin-stabilizing factor

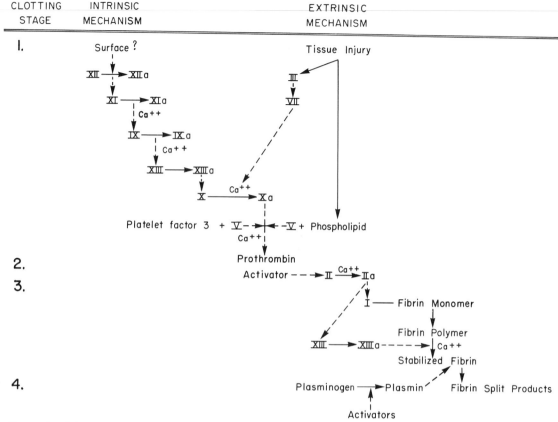

Figure 2. Schematic model of blood coagulation. Broken arrow indicates an enzymatic activity; solid arrow indicates a transformation of a coagulation factor.

In the fourth stage of clotting fibrin deposits are destroyed by a proteolytic enzyme system termed the "plasminogen-plasmin" system. Plasminogen can be activated to plasmin by a number of activators found in tissues and plasma and in eosinophils. Plasmin hydrolyzes fibrin and fibrinogen to soluble digestion products having anticoagulant activity. As part of the normal repair process, fibrinolysis is restricted to the site of fibrin deposition. In the general circulation antiplasmins rapidly complex plasmin and neutralize its activity. The fibrinolytic system has been the subject of several reviews (Ambrus, 1966; Niewiarowski, 1968).

Disorders of Hemostasis

Bleeding syndromes occur because of inherited or acquired defects involving blood vessels, platelets, or plasma coagulation factors (Tables 7 and 8). The defects may either be quantitative or qualitative, although the former occur more frequently. The hemostatic mechanism is so effective that often it must be compromised at several sites before bleeding occurs. However, spontaneous hemorrhage does occur with single, severe defects of the type found in hemophilia and in other inherited deficiencies of coagulation factors.

TRANSFUSION THERAPY

Transfusion therapy has burgeoned since World War II. Surgeons discovered the usefulness of blood and plasma transfusions to support their patients during prolonged and difficult surgery. Increased knowledge of the numerous blood groups, improved techniques in cross-matching the donor and recipient, the availability of the antiglobulin sensitization test (Coombs test) for detection of incomplete antibodies, the development of plastic containers, and the improvement of preservatives for storing blood have all combined to make progress in blood transfusion one of the outstanding accomplishments of modern medicine. The advent of specialized and automated equipment

TABLE 7. *Hereditary Defects of Hemostasis*

NAME	CHARACTERISTICS	TESTS USEFUL IN DIAGNOSIS*
Blood Vessels		
Hereditary hemorrhagic telangiectasis (Osler-Rendu-Weber disease)	Multiple elevated, dilated capillaries and venules, pinpoint to several millimeters in size. Distributed over skin and mucous membranes and may occur in parenchyma of liver, lung and other organs. Epistaxis, hematemesis, melena, and hematuria are frequent. Autosomal dominant.	None
von Willebrand's disease, Types 1, 2, & 3	Capillary abnormality in skin and mucous membranes. Abnormal capillary contractility in nail beds. Factor VIII and platelet adhesiveness decreased. Spontaneous bleeding, mild to severe; may be severe with surgery. Autosomal dominant.	Bleeding time and partial thromboplastin time prolonged. Thromboplastin generation test normal to long. Platelet adhesiveness normal to decreased. Factor VIII assay decreased. Great variability in laboratory abnormalities in individual cases.
Platelets		
Congenital hypoplastic thrombocytopenia	Spontaneous bleeding associated with congenital anomalies. Variant of Fanconi syndrome. Autosomal recessive.	Bleeding time prolonged. Platelet count decreased. Bone marrow megakaryocytes decreased to absent.
Aldrich's syndrome	Thrombocytopenia eczema, and recurrent infections in first years of life. Sex-linked recessive.	Bleeding time prolonged. Platelet count decreased. Bone marrow megakaryocytes normal in number.
Plasma factors		
Factor I	Rare disorder. Spontaneous bleeding and hemorrhage with minor trauma. Hemarthrosis. Autosomal recessive.	Clotting time, prothrombin time, and thrombin time are prolonged. Fibrinogen assay, trace or absent.
Factors II, V, VII, X	Rare disorders. Occur as single deficiencies which must be identified by laboratory examination. Spontaneous bleeding and hemorrhage with minor trauma. Menorrhagia. Probably autosomal recessive.	Prothrombin time prolonged in II, V, VII, X deficiencies. Thromboplastin generation test abnormal in V and X deficiencies. TAMe assay of prothrombin abnormal in II deficiency. Specific assays for Factors V, VII, X will identify defect.
Factors VIII, IX	Most common hereditary defects. Severe spontaneous bleeding and hemorrhage with minor trauma. Hemarthrosis crippling. Sex-linked recessive.	Clotting time normal to prolonged. Partial thromboplastin time prolonged. Thromboplastin generation test abnormal. Specific deficiencies identified by Factor VIII and IX assays.
Factor XI	Rare disorder. Bleeding after trauma or surgery. Nearly all patients Jewish. Autosomal recessive.	Clotting time normal to slightly long. Partial thromboplastin time prolonged. Thromboplastin generation test abnormal.
Factor XII	Rare disorder. Remarkable absence of clinical bleeding. Autosomal recessive.	Clotting time, partial thromboplastin time prolonged. Thromboplastin generation test abnormal and corrected by celite adsorbed serum.
Factor XIII	Rare disorder. Bleeding after trauma.	Thromboelastography.

*Sirridge, 1967.

TABLE 8. Acquired Defects of Hemostasis

NAME	CHARACTERISTICS	TESTS USEFUL IN DIAGNOSIS
Blood vessels		
Trauma	Petechiae, ecchymoses, hemorrhage. Form determined by type of trauma and size of vessel.	None.
Vitamin C deficiency	Follicular hyperplasia, perifollicular hemorrhage, confluent ecchymoses, periarticular hemorrhages, gingival hemorrhage.	Ivy bleeding time prolonged. Capillary fragility increased.
Senile purpura, corticosteroid purpura, purpura of uremia, diabetes, infection, drugs, etc.	Bleeding limited to skin or mucous membranes. Mechanism unknown. May be associated with platelet and plasma factor abnormalities in uremia.	Inconsistent abnormalities in Ivy bleeding time and capillary fragility.
Allergic purpura (Henoch-Schönlein)	Purpura, urticaria, erythema, arthralgia, periarticular swelling, abdominal pain, and renal hemorrhage.	Capillary fragility normal to increased. Bleeding time, clotting time, platelet function, normal.
Platelets		
Thrombocytopenia— idiopathic, secondary, thrombotic	Petechiae and ecchymoses on skin and mucous membranes, gingival bleeding, epistaxis, hemoptysis, hematemesis, melena, hematuria. Bleeding usually from multiple sites, but may be localized, as epistaxis, hematuria, etc.	Stained blood film—platelets decreased or absent. Platelet count decreased, clot retraction poor, prothrombin consumption decreased.
Thrombocytopathia in polycythemia vera, essential thrombocytosis, leukemia, uremia disseminated lupus erythematosus, etc.	Bleeding manifestations similar to thrombocytopenic states.	Stained blood film—platelets normal in number, but vary in size and shape. Bleeding time prolonged, clot retraction normal to abnormal, platelet adhesiveness and aggregation abnormal.

Plasma factors				
Factor I			*D.I.C.*	*Fibrinolysis*
Deficient in abruptio placentae; amniotic embolization; fetal death; abdominal, thoracic and open heart surgery; carcinoma of pancreas, prostate, etc.; sepsis; shock; phlebitis; cirrhosis*	Abrupt onset of severe bleeding from mucous membranes into skin, and from kidneys. Part of disseminated intravascular coagulation (D.I.C.) or of activation of fibrinolytic system or both. Occasionally process is chronic. Multiple deficiencies predominate in D.I.C. while pure fibrinolysis results in lysis of fibrin, Factor I, and to a lesser extent, of Factors V and VIII.	Clotting time	Prolonged	Prolonged
		Prothrombin time	Prolonged	Prolonged
		Partial thromboplastin time	Prolonged	Prolonged
		Fibrinogen	Low	Low
		Thrombin time of test/normal plasma mixtures	Normal	Prolonged
		Ethanol gelation	Positive	Negative
		Platelet count	Decreased	Normal
		Fibrinolysin	Absent or present	Present

*Breen and Tullis, 1968.

to separate platelets, leukocytes, erythrocytes, and plasma has made it practical to prepare blood components tailored to fit the patient's needs. The number of useful plasma protein fractions has also increased, making possible specific replacement therapy for coagulation factor deficiencies. Greenwalt and Perry in 1969 declared that whole blood transfusion should be relegated to the limbo of the "shotgun" prescription. The ideal in transfusion practice is to separate each unit of blood into several therapeutically useful components. A single donor would then serve multiple recipients.

Indications for Transfusion Therapy

The clinician cannot be expected to be fully cognizant of all aspects of immunohematology and of blood preservation since these are areas of increasing technical complexity. However, he prescribes the transfusion therapy, carries the responsibility for the results and should have a clear concept of the objectives of transfusion as well as of the harmful effects (Hoxworth, 1960).

The purpose of transfusion therapy is to replace some portion or function of blood which is lacking or inadequate. The following situations are indications for transfusion therapy.

Massive Bleeding. Acute severe blood loss results in hypovolemia, a decreased oxygen-carrying capacity, shock, and metabolic acidosis. Whole blood is the best therapeutic product, since the erythrocytes combat hypoxia and plasma supports the circulation. Plasma expanders, including serum albumin, clinical dextran, and 5 per cent protein solutions, are extremely valuable in the emergency treatment of acute blood loss and shock.

Anemia. Anemia is not an indication for

TABLE 8. *Acquired Defects of Hemostasis (Continued)*

NAME	CHARACTERISTICS	TESTS USEFUL IN DIAGNOSIS
Factors II, VII, IX, X Deficient in the newborn, in vitamin K deficiency, liver disease, obstructive jaundice, sprue and other diarrheal states, broad-spectrum antibiotic therapy, coumarin and salicylate therapy	Mild to moderate deficiencies are asymptomatic or associated with occult bleeding. Severe deficiencies cause hemorrhage from nose, gastrointestinal tract, genitourinary tract, or retroperitoneally. A deficiency of these factors in apparently healthy medical personnel should indicate the possibility of coumadin ingestion.	Prothrombin time prolonged. See Table 7 for tests to identify individual factors. An isolated Factor IX deficiency does not prolong the one stage prothrombin time.
Factor V Deficient in liver disease, fibrinolysis, and disseminated intravascular clotting.	Factor V deficiency is usually associated with multiple deficiencies of Factors II, V, IX, X.	Prothrombin time prolonged. Factor V assay identifies the deficiency.
Inhibitors of stage 1 of clotting Factor VIII inhibitors occur most frequently in hemophiliacs, rarely in postpartum period, and in older patients without apparent cause	Inhibitors of Factor VIII are the most common. Inhibitors of Factors IX and XI are rare. Bleeding severe, resembling that of hemophilia.	Blood clotting time prolonged. Partial thromboplastin time prolonged. Thromboplastin generation test abnormal. Test/normal plasma mixtures are abnormal in above tests.
Inhibitors of stage 2 of clotting Occur in disseminated lupus erythematosus, penicillin reactions, and other hypersensitivity states.	Rare. Bleeding may not occur or may be moderate. Most often they inhibit thromboplastin activity, rarely Factors V or VII.	One stage prothrombin time prolonged. Partial thromboplastin time prolonged. Test/normal plasma mixtures are abnormal in above tests.
Inhibitors of stage 3 of clotting Heparinlike inhibitors occur in urticaria pigmentosa, neoplastic disease and disseminated lupus erythematosus; fibrin formation abnormal in multiple myeloma macroglobulinemia, etc.	Heparinlike inhibitors are rare and are active in all stages of clotting. Paraproteins inhibit normal fibrin formation and contribute to the multifactorial causes of hemorrhage in plasma cell dyscrasias.	Blood clotting time prolonged. Thrombin time prolonged. One stage prothrombin time, partial thromboplastin time and thromboplastin generation test are abnormal with heparinlike inhibitors.

transfusion, and the goal of maintaining the hemoglobin at an arbitrary minimum value is not justified. Transfusion is indicated when the oxygen-carrying capacity of the blood is reduced to a level which produces severe symptoms of cerebral, cardiac, or pulmonary embarrassment. The limits of physiological tolerance are fairly broad and the patient with slowly developing anemia seldom needs transfusion, especially if placed at rest. If immediate treatment is required, the component of choice is packed erythrocytes. Severely anemic patients may be in impending heart failure and infusion of whole blood could result in overt decompensation.

Thrombocytopenia. Serious hemorrhage, including melena, hematemesis, hematuria, and intracranial bleeding, may occur when the platelet count falls below 50,000 per cu. mm. Platelet transfusions are now used prophylactically in patients with thrombocytopenia undergoing surgery; in patients with leukemia, aplas-

tic anemia, and septicemia complicated by thrombocytopenia; and, rarely, in idiopathic thrombocytopenic purpura (Stefanini and Dameshek, 1953). Repeated platelet transfusions have limited effectiveness because isoimmunization occurs in recipients who are not receiving immunosuppressive drugs. Platelets may be given as platelet-rich plasma, but platelet concentrates are more effective and conveniently used.

Neutropenia. Replacement therapy with granulocytes is desirable since neutropenia is frequently associated with fulminating sepsis. Unfortunately the procurement of granulocytes in adequate numbers from normal donors is technically difficult. Furthermore, the brief intravascular time of normal granulocytes necessitates daily transfusion of these cells. The use of donors with chronic myelogenous leukemia and the development of the NCI-IBM blood cell separator circumvent some of these difficulties (Freireich et al., 1965). However, granulocyte transfusion remains in a developmental stage at this time.

Plasma protein deficiency. A deficiency of plasma proteins occurs in acute blood loss, severe burns, protein-losing enteropathies, nephrosis, cirrhosis, malnutrition, and other conditions. The use of liquid or lyophilized pooled plasma as a source of plasma proteins is no longer acceptable because of the high risk of viral hepatitis. In the controlled study of Redeker and associates in 1968, hepatitis occurred in 12 of 120 recipients of plasma which had been commercially bulk pooled, stored at 30 to 32° C., and ultraviolet irradiated. Purified or partially purified proteins are available which can withstand heating at 60° C. for 10 hours in order to eliminate the hazard of hepatitis. These include 5 per cent albumin solutions, salt poor 25 per cent concentrations of albumin, and partially purified solutions of human albumin and alpha and beta globulins.

Plasma Coagulation Factors. Replacement therapy in bleeding disorders requires the provision of a useful amount of a deficient clotting factor. Fresh or fresh frozen plasma contains in low concentrations all known clotting factors except platelets. The effectiveness of plasma infusions is limited by the extremely large volumes needed to raise the deficient factor to a hemostatic level. Today more concentrated forms of some of the blood coagulation factors are available. Purified fibrinogen, cryoprecipitated and amino acid-precipitated concentrates of human Factor VIII, and a concentrate of the prothrombin complex (Factors II, VII, IX, and X) are available and make possible the effective treatment of acquired and congenital coagulation factor deficiencies (Wagner et al., 1964; Pool and Shannon, 1965; Tullis et al., 1965).

Complications of Transfusion Therapy

Transfusion therapy always constitutes a risk which must be weighed against the benefits which may be achieved from its use. The dangers include reactions resulting from incompatibility, transmission of disease, circulatory overload, reactions from leukoagglutinins, and allergic reactions.

Hemolytic reactions resulting from incompatibility within the ABO, the Rh, the Kell, and the other antigenic systems may result from technical or clerical errors within the laboratory, from erroneous identification of recipients' samples brought to the laboratory, or from confusion of units of blood at the time of transfusion.

Manifestations of a severe hemolytic transfusion reaction include chills and fever, pain in the back and chest, respiratory distress, rapid pulse and shock, hemoglobinemia and hemoglobinuria, oliguria, and anuria. A severe reaction may occur from the transfusion of as little as 50 ml. of incompatible blood. For this reason close observation of the patient in the first 15 minutes of transfusion should never be neglected. If symptoms occur, the immediate termination of the blood transfusion may be lifesaving. In anesthetized patients incompatibility reactions are difficult to detect and may be manifest only by the development of unusual bleeding or shock.

If a hemolytic reaction occurs, the suspected unit of blood along with a sample of the recipient's blood should be returned to the laboratory for comparison with the pretransfusion samples, compatibility studies, and antibody detection. The patient's blood is observed for serum bilirubin content, and cultures and smears for bacteria are made on the used unit.

The commonest diseases transmitted by transfusion are viral hepatitis, malaria, and bacterial infection. Hepatitis is the most important hazard of transfusion therapy. It can be transmitted by whole blood, cellular components, plasma, and concentrates of coagulation factors. The incidence of icteric hepatitis in patients transfused with blood alone has been estimated in the United States to vary from 0.16 to 3.0 per cent (Young, 1955). The only method of prevention is the careful screening of prospective donors for recent jaundice or exposure to hepatitis. Unfortunately the incidence of anicteric hepatitis is high and goes unrecognized in the blood donor population.

The transmission of malaria by blood transfusion may become an increasingly important problem because of increased world travel and deployment of military personnel in areas where malaria is endemic (Chojnacki et al., 1968). Here too, careful history taking from the prospective donor concerning his residence in endemic malarial areas and the occurrence of chills and fever is the only preventive measure.

Bacterial contamination of blood is, fortunately, rare. Especially dangerous are gram-negative bacilli capable of growing at refrigerator or room temperatures and containing endotoxins (Brande et al., 1955). Transfusion of bacterially contaminated blood will produce chills, fever, and rapid circulatory collapse that may prove fatal even when recognized early and treated vigorously. In addition to the cleansing precautions taken at the time of blood collection, blood should be kept refrigerated until shortly before use. Blood that appears grossly hemolyzed or unusually cloudy should not be used.

Chills and fever occurring during or after transfusion of blood components may also be caused by bacterial contamination of the product. Multiple entrances into the blood container, which are necessary in the preparation of some components, increase the chance for contamination.

Circulatory overload is a frequent and dangerous consequence of transfusion. It is produced easily in the normovolemic, anemic patient by the too rapid transfusion of too large a volume of whole blood. It may go unrecognized in the anesthetized patient until pulmonary edema and circulatory collapse occur. The manifestations of circulatory overload are restlessness, distended veins, feelings of fullness in head and chest, dyspnea, pulmonary edema, cough productive of frothy secretions, cyanosis, and hypotension. Circulatory overload can be avoided best by careful monitoring of the patient with a central venous pressure line and by use of selected component therapy in place of whole blood.

Severe febrile reactions may occur in some patients who have had repeated blood transfusions (Brittingham and Chaplin, 1957). These reactions are a result of isosensitization and the development of leukocyte agglutinins or, less commonly, platelet agglutinins. This type of reaction may be avoided either by the use of blood from which the buffy coat has been removed or by the use of washed packed erythrocytes.

Allergic reactions occur in about 1 per cent of blood transfusions and can follow the use of any blood components. Fortunately these reactions are mild and usually consist of itching, urticaria, and fever. The allergic reaction may result from antibodies carried in the donor plasma or from antigens in the hypersensitive recipient. Prospective donors with a history of allergy or recent immunologic therapy should be rejected.

Special problems occur with massive blood transfusion and with the use of blood to prime devices of extracorporeal circulation. These include citrate and heparin toxicity, potassium toxicity, excessive body cooling, and thrombocytopenia (Bayon and Howland, 1963; Young, 1964; Burton, 1968).

REFERENCES

Alper, C. A., Rosen, F. S., and Janeway, C. A.: Medical progress. The gamma globulins II. Hypergammaglobulinemia. New Eng. J. Med. 275:591, 1966.

Altman, K. I., and Miller, G.: A disturbance of tryptophan metabolism in congenital hypoplastic anemia. Amer. J. Dis. Child. 102:416, 1961.

Ambrus, J. L.: Pharmacology Society symposium. The fibrinolysin system. Fed. Proc. 25:28, 1966.

Amromin, G. D.: Pathology of Leukemia. New York, Hoeber Division, Harper & Row, 1968.

Bayon, C. P., and Howland, W. S.: Cardiac arrest and temperature of bank blood. J.A.M.A. 183:58, 1963.

Berlin, N. I., Waldman, T. A., and Weisman, S. M.: Life span of red blood cell. Physiol. Rev. 39:577, 1959.

Bertino, J. R., and Johns, D. G.: Folate metabolism in man. Plenary Session Papers, XII Congress, International Society of Hematology, New York, 1968, p. 133.

Beutler, E.: A series of new screening procedures for pyruvate kinase deficiency, glucose-6-phosphate dehydrogenase deficiency, and glutathione reductase deficiency. Blood 28:553, 1966.

Beutler, E.: Drug induced hemolytic anemia. Pharmacol. Rev. 21:73, 1969.

Bielschowsky, M., Hyler, J., and Howie, J. B.: Spontaneous hemolytic anemia in mice of the NZB/Bl strain. Proc. Univ. Otago Med. School 37:9, 1959.

Bierman, H.: The leukemias—proliferative or accumulative. Blood 30:238, 1967.

Bithell, T. C., and Wintrobe, M. W.: Drug induced aplastic anemia. Seminars Hemat. 4:194, 1967.

Bizzozero, O. J., Jr., Johnson, K. G., and Ciocco, A.: Radiation-related leukemia in Hiroshima and Nagasaki, 1946-1964. I. Distribution, incidence and appearance time. New Eng. J. Med. 274:1095, 1966.

Bloom, G. E., Warner, S., Gerald, P. S., and Diamond, L. K.: Chromosome abnormalities in constitutional aplastic anemia. New Eng. J. Med. 274:8, 1966.

Boggs, D. R.: The kinetics of neutrophilic leukocytes in health and disease. Seminars Hemat. 4:359, 1967.

Boggs, D. R., Sofferman, S. A., Wintrobe, M. M., and Cartwright, G. E.: Factors influencing the duration of survival of patients with chronic lymphocytic leukemia. Amer. J. Med. 40:243, 1966.

Bothwell, T. H., and Carlton, W. R.: Current concepts concerning iron balance. Plenary Session Papers, XII Congress, International Society of Hematology, New York, 1968, p. 144.

Brande, A. I., Carey, F. J., and Siemienski, J.: Studies of bacterial transfusion reactions from refrigerated blood: The properties of cold growing bacteria. J. Clin. Invest. 34:311, 1955.

Braunstein, H., and Gall, E. A.: The cytologic and histochemical features of malignant lymphoma. In Tocantins, L. M. (ed.): Progress in Hematology. Vol. III New York, Grune & Stratton, 1962, p. 136.

Breen, F. A., Jr. and Tullis, J. L.: Ethanol gelation: A rapid screening test for intravascular coagulation. Ann. Intern. Med. 69:1197, 1968.

Brittingham, T. E., and Chaplin, H., Jr.: Febrile transfusion reactions caused by sensitivity to donor leukocytes and platelets. J.A.M.A. 165:899, 1957.

Brown, E. B.: Clinical aspects of iron metabolism. Seminars Hemat. 3:314, 1966.

Buckton, K. E., Court Brown, W. M., and Smith, P. G.: Lymphocyte survival in men treated with X-rays for ankylosing spondylitis. Nature (London) *214*:470, 1967.

Burnet, M.: Autoimmune disease. I. Modern immunological concepts. Brit. Med. J. *2*:645, 1959.

Burton, G. W.: Some problems of massive blood transfusion. Proc. Roy. Soc. Med. *61*:687, 1968.

Cahn, H. L.: Hodgkin's disease involving the nose. New York. J. Med. *48*:2622, 1948.

Carbone, P. P., Berard, C. W., Bennett, J. M., Ziegler, J. L., Cohen, W. H., and Gerber, P.: Burkitt's tumor. Ann. Intern. Med. *70*:817, 1969.

Carson, P. E., and Frischer, H.: Glucose-6-phosphate dehydrogenase deficiency and related disorders of the pentose phosphate pathway. Amer. J. Med. *41*:744, 1966.

Carstairs, K. C., Breckenridge, A., Dollery, C. T., and Worlledge, S. M.: Incidence of a positive direct Coombs test in patients on alpha-methyldopa. Lancet *2*:133, 1966.

Cartwright, G. E.: Anemia of chronic disorders. Seminars Hemat. *3*:351, 1966.

Chase, M. W.: Delayed-type hypersensitivity and the immunology of Hodgkin's disease with a parallel examination of sarcoidosis. Cancer Res. *26*:1097, 1966.

Chaudhry, A. P., Sabes, W. R., and Gorlin, R. J.: Unusual oral manifestations of chronic lymphatic leukemia. Oral Surg. *15*:446, 1962.

Chojnacki, R. E., Brazinsky, J. H., and O'Neill, B., Jr.: Transfusion-introduced falciparum malaria. New Eng. J. Med. *279*:984, 1968.

Court Brown, W. M, and Doll, R.: Mortality from cancer and other causes after radiation for ankylosing spondylitis. Brit. Med. J. *2*:1327, 1965.

Craddock, C. G.: Kinetics of lymphoreticular tissue with particular emphasis on the lymphatic system. Seminars Hemat. *4*:387, 1967.

Cronkite, E. P.: Kinetics of leukemic cell proliferation. Seminars Hemat. *4*:415, 1967.

Crosby, W. H.: The metabolism of hemoglobin and bile pigment in hemolytic disease. Amer. J. Med. *18*:112, 1955.

Dacie, J. V., and Worlledge, S. M.: Autoimmune haemolytic anemias. *In* Brown, E. B., and Moore, C. V. (ed.): Progress in Hematology. Vol. VI. New York, Grune & Stratton, 1969, p. 82.

Dameshek, W.: Chronic lymphocytic leukemia—an accumulative disease of immunologically incompetent lymphocytes. Blood *29*:566, 1967.

Davey, M. G., and Luscher, E. F.: Biochemical aspects of platelet function and hemostasis. Seminars Hemat. *5*:5, 1968.

Davie, E. W., and Ratnoff, O. D.: Waterfall sequence for intrinsic blood clotting. Nature (London) *145*:1310, 1964.

Diamond, L. K., Allen, D. M., and Magill, F. B.: Congenital (erythroid) hypoplastic anemia; a 25 year study. Amer. J. Dis. Child. *102*:403, 1961.

Dorfman, R. F.: Childhood lymphosarcoma in St. Louis, Missouri, clinically and histologically resembling Burkitt's tumor. Cancer *18*:418, 1965.

Duckert, F., and Beck, E. A.: Clinical disorders due to deficiency of factor XIII (fibrin stabilizing factor, fibrinase). Seminars Hemat. *5*:83, 1968.

Engelfreit, C. P., van der Borne, A. E. G., Jr., van der Giessen, M., Becker, D., and van Loghem, J. J.: Autoimmune haemolytic anaemias. I. Serological studies with pure anti immunoglobulin reagents. Clin. Exp. Immun. *3*:605, 1968.

Epstein, E., and MacEachern, K.: Dermatologic manifestations of the lymphoblastoma-leukemia group. Arch. Intern. Med. *60*:867, 1937.

Epstein, M. A., Achong, B. G., and Barr, Y. M.: Virus particles in cultured lymphoblasts from Burkitt's lymphoma. Lancet *1*:702, 1964.

Estren, S., and Dameshek, W.: Familial hypoplastic anemia of childhood. Amer. J. Dis. Child. *73*:671, 1947.

Fanconi, G.: Familiare infantile pernizo-saartige anamie (pernizoises Blutbild und Konstitution). Jahrle Kindern. *117*:257, 1927.

Fessas, P.: The heterogeneity of thalassemia. Plenary Session Papers, XII Congress, International Society of Hematology, New York, 1968, p. 52.

Finch, C. A.: Some quantitative aspects of erythropoiesis. Ann. N.Y. Acad. Sci. *77*:410, 1959.

Ford, W. L., and Gowans, J. L.: The traffic of lymphocytes. Seminars Hemat. *6*:67, 1969.

Franklin, E. C., Lowenstein, J., Bigelow, B., and Meltzer, M.: Heavy chain disease. A new disorder of serum and gamma globulins. Amer. J. Med. *37*:332, 1964.

Fraumeni, J. F.: Clinical epidemiology of leukemia. Seminars Hemat. *6*:250, 1969.

Freireich, E. J., Judson, G., and Levin, R. H.: Separation and collection of leukocytes. Cancer Res. *25*:1516, 1965.

Gaarder, A., Jonsen, J., Laland, S., Hellem, A., and Owren, P. A.: Adenosine diphosphate in red cells as a factor in the adhesiveness of blood platelets. Nature (London) *192*:531, 1961.

Garriga, S., and Crosby, W. H.: The incidence of leukemia in families of patients with hypoplasia of the marrow. Blood *14*:1008, 1959.

Glazer, H. S., Mueller, J. F., Jarrold, T., Sakurai, K., Will, J. J., and Vilter, R. W.: The effect of vitamin B_{12} and folic acid on nucleic acid composition of the bone marrow of patients with megaloblastic anemia. J. Lab. Clin. Med. *43*:905, 1959.

Gordon, A. S.: Hormonal relations to erythropoiesis. Plenary Session Papers, XII Congress, International Society of Hematology, New York, 1968, p. 288.

Greenwalt, T. J., and Perry, S.: Preservation and utilization of the components of human blood. *In*, Brown, E. B., and Moore, C. V. (ed.): Progress in Hematology. Vol. VI. New York, Grune & Stratton, 1969, p. 148.

Hartman, R. C., and Jenkins, D. E., Jr.: Paroxysmal nocturnal hemoglobinuria: Current concepts of certain pathophysiologic features. Blood *28*:850, 1965.

Hartman, R. C., and Jenkins, D. E., Jr.,: The "sugar-water" test for paroxysmal nocturnal hemoglobinuria. New Eng. J. Med. *275*:155, 1966.

Hayhoe, F. G. J., Quaglino, D., and Doll, R.: The cytology and cytochemistry of acute leukaemias. Medical Res. Council Special Report Series, No. 304. London, Her Majesty's Stationery Office, 1964.

Heilmeier, L., Keiderling, W., Bilger, R., and Bernauer, H.: Über chronische refraktäre Anamien mit sideroblastischem Knochenmark (Anaemia refractoria sideroblastica). Folio Haemat. *2*:49, 1958.

Heller, P.: Hemoglobinopathic dysfunction of the red cell. Amer. J. Med. *41*:799, 1966.

Henle, G., Henle, W., and Diehl, V.: Relation of Burkitt's tumor-associated herpes type virus to infectious mononucleosis. Proc. Nat. Acad. Sci. *59*:94, 1968.

Hines, D. D., Halsted, C. H., Griggs, R. C., and Harris, J. W.: Megaloblastic anemia secondary to folate deficiency associated with hypothyroidism. Ann. Intern. Med. *68*:792, 1968.

Horrigan, D. L., and Harris, J. W.: Pyridoxine responsive anemias in man. *In* Harris, R. S., Wool, I. G., and

Loraine, J. A. (ed.): International Symposium on Vitamin Related Anemias. New York, Academic Press, 26:549, 1968.

Hoxworth, P. I.: Physician's responsibility in blood transfusion. Surg. Gynec. Obstet. 110:237, 1960.

Hugues, J.: Accolement des plaquettes au collagéne. C. R. Soc. Biol. 154:866, 1960.

Jackson, H., Jr., and Parker, A. B., Jr.,: Hodgkin's Disease and Allied Disorders. New York, Oxford University Press, 1947.

Jackson, H., Parker, F., and Brues, A. M.: Malignant lymphoma of the tonsil. Amer. J. Med. Sci. 191:1, 1936.

Jacob, H. S.: Hereditary spherocytosis: A disease of the red cell membrane. Seminars Hemat. 2:139, 1965.

Jahsman, D. P., Monto, R. W., and Rebuck, J. W.: Erythroid hypoplastic anemia (erythroblastopenia) associated with benign thymoma. Amer. J. Clin. Path. 38:152, 1962.

Jandl, J. H.: Pathophysiology of hemolytic anemia. Amer. J. Med. 41:657, 1968.

Jarrold, T., and Vilter, R. W.: Hematologic observations in patients with chronic hepatic insufficiency, sternal bone marrow morphology and bone marrow plasmacytosis. J. Clin. Invest. 28:286, 1949.

Jones, R. T.: Mechanisms underlying polymorphisms in hemoglobins and other proteins. Plenary Session Papers, XII Congress, International Society of Hematology, 1968, p. 64.

Kann, H. E., Jr., Mengel, C. E., Meriwether, W. D., and Ebbert, L.: Production of in vitro characteristics of paroxysmal nocturnal hemoglobinuria erythrocytes in normal erythrocytes. Blood 32:49, 1968.

Kaplan, H. S.: Evidence for a tumoricidal dose level in the radiotherapy of Hodgkin's disease. Cancer Res. 26:1221, 1966.

Katz, R., Velasco, M., Guzman, C., and Allessandri, H.: Red cell survival estimated by radioactive chromium in hepatobiliary disease. Gastroenterology 46:399, 1964.

Keitt, A. S.: Pyruvate kinase deficiency and related disorders of red cell glycolysis. Amer. J. Med. 41:762, 1966.

Kowalski, E.: Fibrinogen derivatives and their biologic activities. Seminars Hemat. 5:45, 1968.

Lautz, H. A.: Nasal and laryngeal involvement in abdominal Hodgkin's disease. Arch. Otolaryng. 67:78, 1958.

Lester, R., and Schmid, R.: Bilirubin metabolism. New Eng. J. Med. 270:729, 1964.

Letman, H.: Possible paroxysmal nocturnal hemoglobinuria with development of aplastic anemia. Blood 7:842, 1952.

Leventhal, B., and Stohlman, F., Jr.: Regulation of erythropoiesis XVII. Determinants of red cell size in iron deficiency states. Pediatrics 37:62, 1966.

Loge, J. P., Lange, R. D., and Moore, C. V.: Characterization of the anemia associated with chronic renal insufficiency. Amer. J. Med. 24:4, 1958.

Love, A. A.: Manifestations of leukemia encountered in otolaryngologic and stomatologic practice. Arch. Otolaryng. 23:173, 1936.

Lukes, R. J., Craver, L. F., Hall, T. E., Rappaport, H., and Ruben, P.: Obstacles to the control of Hodgkin's disease. Report of the Nomenclature Committee. Cancer Res. 26:1311, 1966.

Macfarlane, R. G.: An enzyme cascade in the blood clotting mechanism, and its function as a biochemical amplifier. Nature (London) 202:498, 1964.

MacMahon, B.: Epidemiology of Hodgkin's disease. Cancer Res. 26:1189, 1966.

MacMahon, B., and Levy, M. A.: Prenatal origin of childhood leukemia. Evidence from twins. New Eng. J. Med. 270:1082, 1964.

Mann, D. L., Donati, R. M., and Gallagher, N. I.: Erythropoietin assay and ferrokinetic measurements in anemic uremic patients. J.A.M.A. 194:1321, 1965.

Marsh, G. W., and Lewis, S. M.: Cardiac haemolytic anaemia. Seminars Hemat. 6:133, 1969.

Marshall, R. A., and Jandl, J. H.: Responses to "physiologic" doses of folic acid in the megaloblastic anemia. Arch. Intern. Med. 105:352, 1960.

Mauer, A. M., Saunders, E. F., and Lampkin, B. C.: The nature and causes of variability of proliferative activity in marrow cell population in human acute leukemia. In The Proliferation and Spread of Neoplastic Cells. Baltimore, The Williams & Wilkins Company, 1968, p.358.

McCurdy, P. R., Donohoe, R. F., and Magovern, M.: Reversible sideroblastic anemia caused by pyrazinoic acid (pyrazinamide). Ann. Intern. Med. 64:1280, 1966.

Michaux, J., and Heremans, J. F.: Thirty cases of monoclonal immunoglobulin disorders other than myeloma or macroglobulinemia. Amer. J. Med. 46:562, 1969.

Miller, R. W.: Radiation, chromosomes and viruses in the etiology of leukemia. New Eng. J. Med. 271:30, 1964.

Miller, R. W.: Deaths from childhood cancer in sibs. New Eng. J. Med. 279:122, 1968.

Mollison, P. L.: Blood Transfusion in Clinical Medicine. 4th ed. Philadelphia, F. A. Davis Company, 1967.

Nathan, D. G., and Gunn, R. B.: Thalassemia: The consequences of unbalanced hemoglobin synthesis. Amer. J. Med. 41:815, 1966.

Neiger, M., von: Hodgkin's disease of Waldeyer's tonsilar ring. Pract. Otorhinolaryng. 26:375, 1964.

Nelson, M. A., Jr., and Stiff, R. H.: An unusual manifestation of lymphoma. Oral Surg. 23:351, 1967.

Niewiarowski, S.: Physiologic implications of fibrinolysis. Plenary Session Papers, XII Congress, International Society of Hematology, New York, 1968, p. 330.

O'Brien, J. R.: The properties of the platelet membrane in dynamics of thrombus formation and dissolution. In Johnson, S. A., and Guest, M. M. (ed.): Dynamics of Thrombus Formation and Dissolution. Philadelphia, J. B. Lippincott, 1969.

O'Conner, G. T., Rappaport, H., and Smith, E. B.: Childhood lymphoma resembling "Burkitt tumor" in the United States. Cancer 18:411, 1965.

Polycove, M.: Iron metabolism and kinetics. Seminars Hemat. 3:235, 1966.

Pool, J. G., and Shannon, A. E.: Production of high-potency concentrates of antihemophiliac globulin in a closed-bag system: Assay in vitro and in vivo. New Eng. J. Med. 273:1443, 1965.

Porter, K. A.: Immune hemolysis: A feature of secondary disease and runt disease in the rabbit. Ann. N.Y. Acad. Sci. 87:391, 1960.

Rappaport, H.: Tumors of the hematopoietic system. Washington, D.C., A.F.I.P., Sec. 3, Fasc. 8, 1966.

Rauscher, F. J., Carrese, L. M., and Baker, C. G.: Survey of viral oncology with particular reference to lymphomas. Cancer Res. 26:1176, 1966.

Redeker, A. G., Hopkins, C. E., Jackson, B., and Peck, P.: A controlled study of the safety of pooled plasma stored in the liquid state at 30-32° C for six months. Transfusion 8:60, 1968.

Rigby, P. G., Pratt, P. T., Rosenlof, R., and Lemon, H. M.: Genetic relationship in familial leukemia and lymphoma. Arch. Intern. Med. 121:67, 1968.

Rosenberg, S. A., Diamond, H. D., Jaslowitz, B., and

Craver, L. F.: Lymphosarcoma: A review of 1269 cases. Medicine *40*:31, 1961.

Rosenberg, S. A., and Kaplan, H. S.: Evidence for an orderly progression in the spread of Hodgkin's disease. Cancer Res. *26*:1225, 1966.

Rosse, W. F., and Dacie, J. V.: Complement and paroxysmal nocturnal haemoglobinuria red cell. *In* Wolstenholme, G. E. W., and Night, J. (ed.): Ciba Foundation Symposium on Complement. Boston, Little, Brown and Company, 1965, p. 343.

Royston, I., and Modan, B.: Comparative mortality of childhood leukemia and lymphoma among the immigrants and native born in Israel. Cancer *22*:385, 1968.

Sachs, R. L.: Burkitt's tumor (African lymphoma syndrome) in California. Oral Surg. *22*:621, 1966.

Salvidio, E., Pannacciulli, I., Tizianello, A., and Azinar, F.: Nature of hemolytic crises and fate of G-6-PD deficient, drug damaged, erythrocytes in Sardinians. New Eng. J. Med. *276*:1339, 1967.

Schubothe, H.: The cold hemagglutinin disease. Seminars Hemat. *3*:27, 1966.

Shanbrom, E., and Finch, S. C.: The auditory manifestations of leukemia. Yale J. Biol. Med. *31*:144, 1958.

Shilling, B. B., Abel, M. R., and Work, W. P.: Leukemic involvement of larynx. Arch. Otolaryng. *85*:658, 1967.

Silberstein, E. B.: The Schilling test. J.A.M.A. *208*:2325, 1969.

Sirridge, M. S.: Laboratory Evaluation of Hemostasis. Philadelphia, Lea & Febiger, 1967.

Spaet, T. H.: Hemostatic homeostasis. Blood *28*:112, 1966.

Stefanini, M., and Dameshek, W.: Collection, preservation, and transfusion of platelets. New Eng. J. Med. *248*:797, 1953.

Steg, R. F., Dahlin, D., and Gores, R. J.: Malignant lymphoma of the mandible and maxillary region. Oral Surg. *12*:128, 1959.

Sturgeon, P., and Finch, C. A.: Erythrokinetics in Cooley's anemia. Blood *12*:64, 1957.

Terry, D. W., Motulsky, A., and Rath, C. E.: Homozygous hemoglobin C.: New hereditary hemolytic disease. New Eng. J. Med. *251*:365, 1954.

Tullis, J. L., Melin, M., and Jurigian, P.: Clinical use of human prothrombin complexes. New Eng. J. Med. *273*:667, 1965.

Ultman, J. E., Cunningham, J. K., and Gellhorn, A.: The clinical picture of Hodgkin's disease. Cancer Res. *26*:1047, 1966.

Valentine, W. N., Hsin-soon, H., Paglia, D. E., Anderson, H. M., Baughan, M. A., Jaffe, E. R., and Garson, M. O.: Hereditary hemolytic anemia associated with phosphoglycerate kinase deficiency in erythrocytes and leukocytes. New Eng. J. Med. *280*:528, 1969.

von Furth, R.: The formation of immunoglobulins by circulating lymphocytes. Seminars Hemat. *6*:84, 1969.

Vigliani, E. C., and Saita, G.: Benzene and leukemia. New Eng. J. Med. *271*:872, 1964.

Vilter, R. W., Will, J. J., Wright, T. L., and Rullman, D.: Interrelationships of vitamin B_{12}, folic acid, and ascorbic acid in the megaloblastic anemias. Amer. J. Clin. Nutr. *12*:130, 1963.

Wagner, R. H., McLester, W. D., Smith, M., and Brinkhouse, K. M.: Purification of antihemophiliac factor (Factor VIII) by amino acid precipitation. Thromb. Diath. Haemorrh. *11*:64, 1964.

Waldenström, J.: Studies on "abnormal" serum globulins (M components) in myeloma, macroglobulinemia and related diseases: Clinical diagnosis and biochemical findings in material of 296 sera with M-type marrow gamma globulins. Acta Med. Scand. *170*:110, 1961.

Weatherall, D. J.: The Thalassemia Syndromes. Oxford, Blackwell Scientific Publications, Ltd., 1965.

Weatherall, D. J., and Clegg, J. B.: The control of human hemoglobin synthesis and function in health and disease. *In* Brown, C. B., and Moore, C. V. (ed.): Progress in Hematology. Vol. VI. New York, Grune & Stratton, 1969, p. 261.

Whang-Peng, J., Canellos, G. P., Carbonne, P. P., and Tijio, J. H.: Clinical implications of cytogenetic variants in chronic myelocytic leukemia (CML). Blood *32*:755, 1968.

Wheby, M. S., Thorup, O. A., and Leavell, B. S.: Homozygous hemoglobin C disease in siblings: Further comment on intraerythrocytic crystals. Blood *11*:266, 1956.

Wilder, J. W.: Obstacles to the control of Hodgkin's disease. Cancer Res. *26*:1046, 1966.

Will, J. J.: Personal observation, 1969.

Williams, W. J.: Recent concepts of the clotting mechanism. Seminars Hemat. *5*:32, 1968.

Wintrobe, M. M.: The size and hemoglobin content of the erythrocyte. J. Lab. Clin. Med. *17*:899, 1932.

Yet, W. K., Allen, A., and Lowenstein, L.: Hydrops fetalis with alpha-thalassemia. New Eng. J. Med. *276*:18, 1967.

Young, L. E.: Hereditary spherocytosis. Amer. J. Med. *18*:486, 1955.

Young, L. E.: Complications of blood transfusion. Ann. Intern. Med. *61*:136, 1964.

Zuelzer, W. W., and Cox, D. E.: Genetic aspects of leukemia. Seminars Hemat. *6*:228, 1969.

Chapter 29

BASIC PRINCIPLES OF
IMMUNOLOGY

by Richard Hong, M.D.

Competent immunity represents the end result of appropriate cellular processing of foreign substances (antigen) introduced into the body by infection, injection, or ingestion and causing the production of antibody proteins (immunoglobulins) and/or the proliferation of a specific cell population, both end-products having the capacity to combine with the specific inducing substances. This combination generates another series of events which generally leads to the elimination of the inducer by mechanisms such as phagocytosis or lysis. Two types of immunity can be differentiated, that which is mediated and can be transferred by immunoglobulins (humoral) and that which is mediated and can be transferred by cells (cellular immunity). Viewed in this way the dogma of immunity can be pictured schematically as in Figure 1.

Afferent Limb

The afferent limb is charged via the macrophage with the responsibility of categorizing ingested materials as antigenic or not (recognition), and after making this initial decision, it must appropriately interact with the invader in a "processing" step. This step is all-important since the unprocessed material cannot directly cause the effector cells of the efferent limb to exert their immunological prowess and, in part, results in an antigen-RNA complex yielding what has been termed by some, "super-antigen" (Fishman and Adler, 1963; Askonas, 1965). "Super-antigen" loses its potency upon exposure to RNAse. Although it was at first tempting to postulate that an appropriate message was being carried to an as yet incomplete antibody template, characterization of the

Figure 1. Afferent and efferent limbs of immunity.

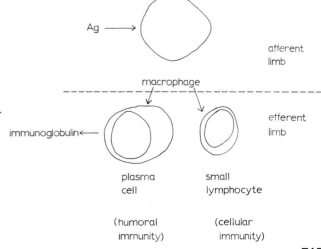

715

RNA involved (i.e., size and base sequence) excludes an informational role for the ribonucleoprotein (RNP). A distinctive RNP found only in macrophages combines with the antigen, however. So it seems most likely that the RNA expresses the specific adjuvant effect of the macrophage (Gottlieb, 1969). In fact, most antigen is probably "processed" without an intermediate RNA step.

It follows from reference to Figure 1 that disordered immunity can result from deficiency in two main areas—viz., afferent or efferent. To date, few clinical examples of inability to appropriately recognize and process antigen (afferent abnormality) have been uncovered. The notable exception is the Aldrich syndrome (see later) in which response to carbohydrate antigens is impaired and, as a result, the patients uniformly lack isohemagglutinins (Cooper et al., 1968). Most immunological deficiency involves the efferent side. It is, therefore, appropriate to consider this in greater detail.

Efferent Limb

The cells of importance in the final delivery of immune processes result from maturation and differentiation under the influence of organ(s) known as "central" lymphoid tissues. We envision a cell of dual capability trafficking to a site of differentiation where it receives appropriate instruction to determine its final fate. In chickens, two organs are involved; the thymus controls those cells responsible for cellular immunity (thymic dependent), and the bursa of Fabricius, an outpouching of the gut, controls those cells concerned with immunoglobulin production (thymic independent system). To date, a perfect analog of the bursa of Fabricius has not been found in mammals, but the independence of cellular and humoral immunity suggests that a similar dual control system also exists. Laboratory studies and analogy with the chicken model suggest that the controller of humoral immunity in mammalian species is also gut-associated. The primitive stem cell originates in the bone marrow. These relations are shown in Figure 2 (Peterson et al., 1965; Micklem et al., 1966; Good et al., 1969).

IMMUNITY ACTIVATING MECHANISMS

Both immune systems follow a similar scheme in attaining full expression. Surprising-

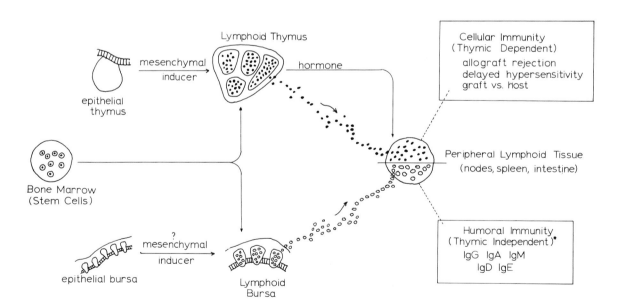

Figure 2. Pathways of differentiation leading to immunity. Bone marrow cells come under the influence of inductive organs (central lymphoid tissues) which direct their ultimate fate and residence in the peripheral lymphoid tissues. The major protective roles provided by each type of immunity are shown.

*Recent data show an interrelationship between the thymus and previously considered "thymic independent" antibody production (Claman et al., 1966).

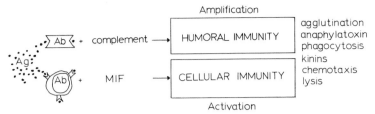

Figure 3. Amplification of the initial antigen-antibody interaction. Activation of complement components or generation of MIF (see text) increases the number and magnitude of biologic effects (far right-hand column).

ly, the initial antigen-antibody reaction is relatively impotent biologically and by itself does little to produce the lethal environment necessary for both lysis or destruction of the invading organism. Thus, both systems require an "activator." This substance essentially initiates the sequence of events we know as inflammation, i.e., diapedesis, chemotaxis, generation of kinins, etc. The activating mechanisms also involve amplification so that one antigen-antibody interaction generates hundreds of activator molecules or activator cells. The essential steps in efferent immunity, then, are accomplished by mediators and activators (Fig. 3).

Humoral Immunity

The mediators of the humoral system are a group of globulins known collectively as immunoglobulins (Ig's). Older appellations designating immunoglobulins by electrophoretic characteristics are of little clinical value and, hence, terms such as gamma or beta globulins should not be widely used. Three major classes comprise nearly 100 per cent of the total serum immunoglobulins: IgG, 85 per cent; IgA, 10 per cent; and IgM, 5 per cent. Trace

amounts of two others, IgD and IgE, are also present. Because of differing efficiency in various biological functions (agglutination, lysis, complement fixation, etc.) and different anatomical localization, the various major classes seem to be structurally and functionally modified for different roles in humoral antibody protection (Table 1). Present information suggests that IgM is most concerned with rapid response to infectious agents and may serve as a first line of defense. IgG is best suited to provide long-term protection and passive protection from mother to fetus (Uhr, 1964). The IgA system is of unknown significance in serum reactions, but much understanding has come from the work of Tomasi (1968) and South (1966). Its predominant localization to secretions of luminal surfaces which receive nonhematogenous antigenic stimulation and its independence of response from serum IgA levels suggest that its primary role is somehow involved in surface protection phenomena. Whereas 85 per cent of the serum immunoglobulins are of the IgG class, at least 85 per cent (and in some cases nearly all) the immunoglobulins of saliva, tears, nasal, intestinal, bladder, and biliary secretions are of the IgA class.

Immunization by usual systemic methods

TABLE 1.   Comparison of Ig's*

	IgG	IgM	IgA	IgE	IgD
Agglutination	1[†]	750[a]	?	?	
Phagocytosis	1	2000[b]	?	?	
Complement fixation	1	2[c]	0	?	
Placental passage	1	0	0	0	
Half-life	13–25 days	4–7 days	3–7 days		2–5 days
% I.V. distribution	48–62	65–100	40		63–86
$S_{20,W}$	6.5–7.0	18–20	7,10,13,15,17	8.0	6.2–6.8
		30			
MW	140,000	850,000	370,000 (11S)	200,000	~180,000

*See also Cohen and Milstein, 1967.

†Numbers = relative efficiency, assigning to IgG a relative value of 1; thus, IgM is 750 times as efficient in agglutination as IgG.

?unknown.

[a]Greenbury et al., 1963.

[b]Rowley and Turner, 1966.

[c]Borsos and Rapp, 1965.

produces appropriate serum antibody levels which are of importance in prevention of systemic infection; such immunization, however, produces little or no local protection, and challenge by means of a nonhematological route (nasal instillation or orally) results in infection. Local immunization, on the other hand, produces appropriate protective responses, and the antibody responsible has been shown to be IgA. Nevertheless, a few isolated reports of normal individuals with selective IgA deficiency have thrown doubt upon the indispensable nature of IgA in these areas. These controversies are partly resolved by observations demonstrating compensatory IgM secretion in some of the above mentioned and by consideration of other compensatory mechanisms (e.g., cellular defenses) (reviewed by Tomasi, 1968). Recent studies implicate a possible role of IgE in protection from sinopulmonary disease (Cain et al., 1969); the modulating role of other, perhaps as yet undescribed, immunoglobulins must also be considered in evaluating the whole problem of local immunity. Ishizaka and Ishizaka, (1968) and Stanworth et al. (1967) have shown that reaginic antibody capable of initiating allergic reactions is primarily of the IgE class. No beneficial IgD role has as yet been described.

Antibodies exert their protective effects via various mechanisms such as neutralization of exotoxins, lysis, and rendering of organisms more susceptible to phagocytosis. The synergistic and complementary effects of other se-rum factors, as well as cellular immunity, play roles of varying importance, depending on the organism involved. Another role of antibodies as protective coverings is suggested by recent studies. In hypogammaglobulinemic patients who receive gamma globulin intravenously there is a high incidence of anaphylactic reactions. Following the injection, however, gamma globulin can be readministered intravenously without any symptoms. The theory is that the initial injection covers receptor sites capable of initiating anaphylactic reactions, so that subsequent injections are without effect. Similarly, aggregated gamma globulin in untreated guinea pigs produces anaphylaxis, but this can be prevented by prior injection of rheumatoid factor. This nonantibody role of immunoglobulins may be of great importance in modifying host response to hypersensitive reactions (see later) (Barandun et al., 1962; Gough and Davis, 1966).

Immunoglobulin Structure

All immunoglobulins in man and other species studied to date show the same basic molecular structure. The primary unit is composed of two identical pairs of polypeptide chains. One of each pair (light chain) is smaller, with a molecular weight of approximately 22,000, and is identical for all the major immunoglobulin classes in man and shows striking homologies with other species. The other chain (heavy chain) is about twice as large and ac-

TABLE 2. Chemical Formulation of Immunoglobulins

Ig	FORMULA		
	Heavy Chain	Light Chain	Whole Molecule
IgG	γ	κ	$\gamma_2 \kappa_2$
	γ	λ	$\gamma_2 \lambda_2$
Serum IgA	α	κ	$\alpha_2 \kappa_2$ or $(\alpha_2 \kappa_2)_2$
	α	λ	$\alpha_2 \lambda_2$ $(\alpha_2 \lambda_2)_2$
IgM	μ	κ	$(\mu_2 \kappa_2)_5$
	μ	λ	$(\mu_2 \lambda_2)_5$
IgD	δ	κ	$\delta_2 \kappa_2$
	δ	λ	$\delta_2 \lambda_2$
IgE	ϵ	κ	$\epsilon_2 \kappa_2$
	ϵ	λ	$\epsilon_2 \lambda_2$
Secretory IgA	α	κ	+ "T" = $(\alpha_2 \kappa_2)_2 \cdot$ T*
(11S)	α	λ	+ "T" = $(\alpha_2 \lambda_2)_2 \cdot$ T

*T = "piece"; see text.

counts for the biological and chemical differences between each major Ig class. Its size varies, with molecular weight about 50,000 for IgG, 65,000 for IgA, and 70,000 for IgM and IgE (Table 2). Major differences in biological activity such as complement fixation, placental passage, and half-life (also see later) are conferred upon the molecule by the heavy chain. Both chains appear to participate in the combining site. The immunoglobulins are synthesized in plasma cells and lymphocytes, and one cell apparently synthesizes only one immunoglobulin.

The major classes also vary in their tendency to polymerize the four-chain unit. IgM exists normally in a pentameric state, the five units arranged in a ring shape with combining sites pointing outward. The molecular weight thus approximates 850,000, and the protein settles very rapidly in an ultracentrifugal field, giving rise to the older designation, 19S gamma. The large size seems to enhance agglutination and phagocytic capabilities of the molecule. In certain pathologic states (e.g., lupus erythematosus), the monomeric form of IgM, 7S IgM, is found in the serum. Intravascular IgA is nearly all monomeric, but small amounts of polymerized dimer and trimer forms are present. The IgA present in secretions is unique, existing primarily as 11 and 17S polymers (dimer or trimer) with only minor amounts of 7S components. Another feature of the secretory IgA is that it is not antigenically identical with the serum counterpart. Extra antigenic determinants are found in the secretory protein and have been ascribed to a small protein which is thought to be added to the 11S dimer during or after its synthesis in the plasma cells of the lamina propria of the gut or other secretory tissue. This unusual biological event is thought to represent a structural modification to enhance the biological vigor of IgA, which must function in a relatively unphysiologic environment such as the milieu of the intestinal stream. This small addition is known as "secretory piece," "transport piece," or "T-chain," among other things. The variable nomenclature indicates the degree of uncertainty relative to its true biological role (Tomasi, 1968). It has been suggested that the "piece" is involved in secretion into lumina and protection from proteolysis (South, 1966; Tomasi, 1968).

Much understanding of the structure-function relationships of the immunoglobulin molecules has been obtained by studying subunit portions of the proteins. The subunits are obtained by enzyme cleavage or reduction of the disulfide bonds which help to bind the component chains together. Various structure-function relationships are shown in Figure 4 and have recently been reviewed by Cohen and Milstein (1967).

Since the immunoglobulin molecules are composed of two sets of polypeptide chains, it can be expected that improper assembly can yield aberrant molecules (see discussion of hemoglobinopathies). The heavy and light chains are synthesized on separate polyribosomes under independent genetic control. In malignant states, such as certain forms of myeloma, suppression of light chain synthesis leads to production of only heavy chain molecules (H-chain disease); involvement of the heavy chain ribosomes produces the converse situation, light chain disease. In both these disorders, increased amounts of the abnormal product (paraprotein) appear in the serum and usually are excreted in the urine. The excess production of the abnormal immunoglobulin subunit is usually associated with diminished synthesis of normal functionally competent immunoglobulins, accounting for the antibody deficiency and predisposition to infection often encountered in these and other myelomatous states. It is not to be inferred from this that myeloma proteins lack specific antibody function; indeed, myeloma proteins with antibody activity have been described (Eisen et al., 1967; Metzger, 1967). However, almost invariably, for whatever reason, the marked proliferation of myeloma cells precludes the synthesis of immunoglobulins derived from cell lines not involved in the neoplastic process, so that other immunoglobulins (antibodies) are inadequately generated.

Subgroups of the major classes also exist, differing antigenically one from the other; the antigenic specificity is carried by both heavy and light chains. Thus, kappa and lambda types of light chains exist, as well as four types of IgG heavy chains (γG1-4), two types of IgA heavy chains, and two types of IgM heavy chains. Small differences in biological capability are found among the IgG subgroups; e.g., γG4 cannot bind complement, and γG2 cannot fix to skin. It seems that the detectable differences between the various subtypes of the immunoglobulins (known as "isotypes") serve to indicate minor structural changes between immunoglobulin molecules which have undergone some specialization of function during evolution. Despite the numerous possible mixtures of polypeptide chains, a given immu-

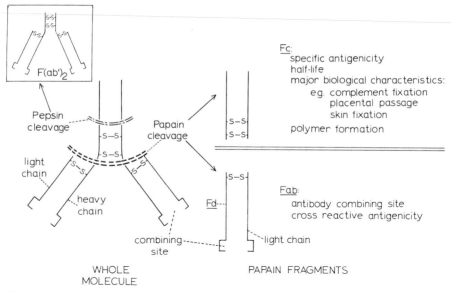

Figure 4. Enzymatic subunits of IgG produced by papain or pepsin. Papain cleaves "below" the inter-heavy chain disulfide bonds, yielding one Fc and two Fab fragments. The biologic activities localized to the fragments are shown. The half of the heavy chain which remains attached to the lights chains to form "Fab" is called "Fd." The inset shows the main product obtained by pepsin cleavage. Since the heavy chains remain connected, the portion of the molecule remaining after digestion is divalent like the original. The divalent F (ab')₂ can form a precipitate, whereas the Fab cannot; however, Fab is a "blocking" antibody, having complete ability to combine with antigen.

noglobulin seems to be restricted to having only one antigenic type of heavy chain and one antigenic type of light chain per molecule (Table 2) (Natvig et al., 1967; Franklin and Frangione, 1969).

Ontogeny of Immunity

Contrary to earlier beliefs, vigorous synthesis of immunoglobulin is possible early in life, even in utero. However, nearly all the antibody synthesized during intrauterine life and in the immediate postnatal period is of the IgM class. Thus, elevation of serum IgM, the levels of which are normally very low to absent at birth, serves to signal an intrauterine or perinatal infection. Occasionally similar antigen exposure will also result in detectable levels of IgA in the serum. The tendency for IgM to respond fully so early in life is reflected in the normal ontogenetic pattern of serum immunoglobulin levels. Serum IgM attains adult levels by the first year of life, while IgG does so at approximately four years of age, and IgA not until adolescence (West et al., 1962; Stiehm and associates 1966, a and b).

IgM and IgG, but not IgA, have the capacity to fix complement. When IgM and IgG molecules combine with their inducing antigens they undergo certain structural changes which give them the capacity to also combine with the first of the nine components of the complement system. After this combination, the remaining eight components are activated in this order: $C\bar{1}$, $\bar{4}$, $\bar{2}$, $\bar{3}$, $\bar{5}$, $\bar{6}$, $\bar{7}$, $\bar{8}$, $\bar{9}$.* $C\bar{3}$ is not added directly to the antigen-antibody $\bar{1}$, $\bar{4}$, $\bar{2}$ complex. Rather, this aggregation activates hundreds of $C\bar{3}$ molecules so that they can finish generating the remainder of the sequence. Thus, for a few molecules of antigen and antibody, many complete activated complement sequences are generated, providing the amplification alluded to previously. Biologically active peptides such as chemotactic factor, kinins, and anaphylotoxin form as a direct result of activation of the various components. When the ninth and final complement factor is added, lysis can occur (Müller-Eberhard, 1967).

Humoral immunity is most concerned with protection from extracellular pyogenic pathogens (staphylococcus, streptococcus, pneumococcus, etc.), and deficiency of this system results primarily in septic episodes due to those invaders.

---

*A bar over the numerical designation of the complement component is used to indicate that the component is in the activated state (Austen, 1968).

Cellular Immunity

Cellular immunity is mediated by small lymphocytes ($< 7\ \mu$ diameter) which are also morphologically different from medium and large lymphocytes, having a denser nuclear chromatin structure and a higher nuclear-cytoplasmic ratio. All cellular immune reactions require cellular integrity and are most appropriately transferred with preparations of intact cells. However, substances (transfer factor) can be extracted from the small lymphocyte which have the capacity to interact with normal unsensitized lymphoid cells to convert them to an immune state (Lawrence, 1955). Complement may play some role in reactions of cellular immunity, but it does not assume the same degree of importance as in humoral immune reactions (Perlmann et al., 1969). The activation of cellular immunity is probably accomplished by a substance known as migration inhibition factor (MIF). This protein of approximate molecular weight of 65,000 exerts chemotactic action and causes localization of macrophages and their subsequent activation to a state at which they have the capacity to destroy normal as well as infected tissue and also the cells directly engaged in the immune reaction. One sensitized lymphocyte can activate and attract over 100 macrophages (David et al., 1964; Bennett and Bloom, 1968). Cellular immunity provides the major protective mechanism for tuberculosis, fungi, and certain viruses (vaccinia, varicella, measles). Cellular immunity also is mostly involved in homograft rejection (Lawrence, 1957). The major role of cellular immune mechanisms in the rejection of solid grafts leads to consideration of this system as of prime importance in tumor rejection. Neoantigens may form on malignant cells as a result of the malignant process, and failure to eliminate these cells as a result of inadequate cellular immunity may allow tumor engraftment as suggested by the high incidence of malignancy in immunological deficiency states (Good and Finstad, 1968; Benacerraf and Green, 1969).

Tolerance and Autoimmunity

It is appropriate to consider here the phenomenon of tolerance. Tolerance may be defined operationally as the failure to respond with an immune reaction following adequate antigenic stimulation in an individual whose component parts of the immunological apparatus are intact. Thus, tolerance is usually restricted to a single class or small groups of antigens, and the response to other antigens is entirely appropriate and complete. Few examples of human disease states can be definitely ascribed to tolerance. In the Aldrich syndrome, tolerance of carbohydrate antigens is present (see later). It has been suggested that in malignant states the tumor is tolerated, representing a failure of the normal surveillance mechanism to eliminate the neoplastic tissue. Another interesting hypothesis, recently proposed by Burnet (1968), is that tolerance to measles virus leads to subacute sclerosing panencephalitis. Increasing awareness of tolerance as a pathogenetic mechanism will undoubtedly shed light on many as yet undefined disease entities.

The fact that our own competent immunological system seems to avoid responding to all the antigens contained within our bodies represents a form of tolerance. A loss of the tolerant stage is associated with the various autoimmune disorders. The true mechanism of achieving tolerance is poorly understood, but the brilliant observations of Burnet and Fenner (1949), and Billingham, Brent and Medawar (1953) suggested strongly that, in some way, the exposure of the immunocompetent system to an antigen at an early stage of development (i.e., in utero) inhibits its ability to respond. This tolerant stage, however, can be abrogated by minor alteration of the self-antigen or in association with the production of antibodies to an antigen (usually obtained from a different species) which bears partial immunologic identity to the self-product. Thus, Weigle (1967) showed that chemical modification of an animal's own thyroglobulin could lead to antithyroglobulin antibodies and thyroiditis. Subsequently he demonstrated that injection of rabbits with unaltered thyroglobulin obtained from cows led to antibodies directed against the heterologous thyroglobulin, the animals' own thyroglobulin, and thyroiditis.

In human situations, antigenic modification can come about as a result of viral modification of red cell membranes (e.g., leading to cold agglutinin disease) or ultraviolet modification of DNA (lupus erythematosus) (Tan, 1968). Antibodies formed in response to streptococci have been purported to be involved in the development of rheumatic heart lesions and poststreptococcal glomerulonephritis because the streptococci share antigens with normal heart and kidney tissues (Markowitz et al., 1960; Kaplan, 1963). Although the formation of antibodies reacting with tissue components clearly represents a loss of the tolerant state, the actual mechanism by which the antibodies lead to the tissue destruction (if, in fact, they do) is in general still a matter of conjecture (Zabriskie, 1967). The fact that passive transfer of autoantibodies of the types described previously does not lead to disease places strong doubt upon their direct role in autoimmune disorders. In systemic lupus erythematosus, for example, the passive transfer of serum from an affected mother to her child as well as from a patient to a normal volunteer does not lead to the disease. It seems clear that the presence of autoantibodies signals the loss of tolerance and serves to indicate that the host is susceptible to or actually undergoing an autoaggressive attack, but the antibodies may not necessarily be directly involved in the pathogenetic mechanism.

The kidney, however, seems susceptible to a special form of attack when antibodies are combined with their antigen in certain proportions (slight antigen excess). In these cases the antigen-antibody system may or may not bear antigenic relationship to the kidney. It is thought that the special flow characteristics of the glomerulus which are necessary for filtration favor the entrapment of the complexes in the glomerular tuft. The physicochemical nature of the complexes as well as the state of activity of the reticuloendothelial system and the liberation of vasoactive amines may also play a role. Subsequent attraction of complement leads to inflammation and destruction of renal mass (Unanue and Dixon, 1967). It is assumed, but less rigidly shown, that antigen-antibody complexes can play a role in other hypersensitivity diseases, localizing in joints, vessel walls, etc.

Thus, although most immunologic reactions serve to protect the individual from harm, when uncontrolled and not self-limited, the magnitude and chronicity of the destructive reaction can be such as to lead to damage to the host out of proportion to that expected, considering the nature of the invading agents. Reactions of this sort account for the bulk of diseases known collectively as autoimmune or collagen diseases. As described previously, certain organs (e.g., kidney, blood vessels) bear the brunt of these attacks, however, and no well-defined diseases of the otorhinolaryngologic system can be assigned to this mechanism. (See discussion of Wegener's granulomatosis.)

ALLERGY – IMMEDIATE HYPERSENSITIVITY

Another means by which an unfortunate antibody reaction results in troublesome symptomatology for the host involves the allergic diathesis. The major steps involved in the generation of allergic phenomena include attachment of the antibody (reagin) to specific target-cell receptor sites, combination with the inciting antigen (allergen), with subsequent release from the target cell of agents which are either pharmacologically active or able to activate precursors. Again, as alluded to in previous discussions, the initiating antigen-antibody reaction gains amplification and activation through the components generated by the combination. At present, four cellular products are recognized: histamine, slow-reacting substance (SRS-A), plasma kinins, and serotonin. Histamine is derived primarily from mast cells, platelets, leukocytes, and the parietal cell region of the stomach. SRS-A is released primarily from polymorphonuclear leukocytes. In addition to its platelet source, serotonin can be obtained from the mucosal layer of the gastrointestinal tract and from cerebral tissue. Specific tissue receptor sites seem to be involved on the target cell (Austen and Humphrey, 1963; Becker and Austen, 1968). These sites can be pre-empted by prior absorption of the tissue with normal gamma globulins, preventing the specific antibody from attachment upon the cell. Despite the therapeutic approach which this finding suggests, double blind studies have shown no benefits derived from gamma globulin injections in allergic states (Abernathy et al., 1958; Biozzi et al., 1959). Recent work has shown that in humans a class of antibodies known as IgE (see previous discussion) is primarily involved. Although present in only nanogram quantities in normal serum, elevated levels are detected in allergic patients and in patients with parasitic infestation by malaria or Ascaris (Johansson et al., 1968). IgE has a marked affinity for cell surfaces (homocytotropic antibody). When located on mast cells and combined with its inducing antigen (e.g., ragweed), IgE has the capacity to release histamine. In mice IgG_a causes release of SRS-A from polymorphonuclear leukocytes (Austen and Humphrey, 1963). Desensitization is thought to induce the formation of "blocking" antibodies. Evidence indicates that the blocking antibodies are of the IgG class in serum and IgA class in secretions and operate by having a greater binding affinity for the allergen, thus preventing the combination of allergen with IgE and the subsequent release of histamine (Osler et al., 1968). Some clinical improvement attends increased blocking antibody formation (Lichtenstein et al., 1968; Sadan et al., 1969). Of interest in this regard also, is the fact that cases of severe intractable asthma in association with selective IgA deficiency have been recorded (West et al., 1962).

OTHER DEFENSE MECHANISMS

Although beyond the scope of this discussion, it should be remembered that in addition to host defense mechanisms based on immunologic mechanisms, supportive and perhaps alternative pathways exist for elimination of invading agents, e.g., phagocytosis. In addition, the inflammatory reactions designed to contain hostile invaders represent the sum total of a complex set of pharmacological reactions, improper integration of which may permit entry of such magnitude that immunological mechanisms are overwhelmed (reviewed in Forscher, 1968). The ability of engulfing cells to kill the ingested agents is also of importance in limiting the invasion. A recently defined disease of white cells, chronic granulomatous disease, seems to represent this fault (Holmes et al., 1966).

IMMUNOLOGICAL DEFICIENCY STATES

It is reasonable for an immunological deficiency state to be suspected in a patient with a history of recurrent infections. In actual practice, however, most children with such a history will be found to have no detectable immunologic disorder, but will have an allergic diathesis. Less common but more diagnostic manifestations of altered immunity include severe intractable atopic eczema, persistent oral moniliasis despite adequate therapy, and any blood disorder, e.g., neutropenia, lymphocytopenia, thrombocytopenia, anemia, and so forth. Although a time-honored method for making the diagnosis, paper electrophoretic techniques are of little value and tend to lead to too many false-positive diagnoses. At the low levels of gamma globulins, where accuracy is needed, electrophoretic techniques even on newer supporting media (e.g., cellulose acetate) are grossly inadequate.

Readily available in nearly all cities are the facilities for immunologic quantitation of the immunoglobulins. Complete kits requiring minimal laboratory skill are obtainable commercially. However, a note of caution should be sounded here. Depending upon the nature of the standards and the antiserums employed, widely differing values are obtained in different laboratories across the country. It is recommended that corroboration of one's standards (usually a pool of normal sera) be obtained from a reference center.* For routine clinical use, however, when the clinician is primarily interested in low values, this may not be necessary. The clinician should avoid overinterpretation of borderline values since normal ranges vary widely. Usually if a patient has a serious immune deficiency, the IgG levels are 1-200 mg./100 ml.; IgM and IgA, 0-10 mg./100 ml. During the first year of life, IgA and IgM levels are normally quite low (Stiehm and Fudenberg, 1966). In some immune deficiency syndromes, IgM is elevated rather than decreased, but in these cases the IgA and IgG values remain markedly diminished.

Levels of immunoglobulins just slightly below published values require correlation with other tests of immunologic competence before being judged of clinical significance. Since gamma globulin is antigenic and anaphylactic reactions have been observed, its empirical use cannot be condoned. One of the simplest means of assessing the true significance of immunoglobulin levels is to perform a functional assay. Tests for antibodies to which reasonable exposure can be expected (e.g., isohemagglutinins, polio) or a Schick test can be accomplished easily and, if positive for antibody presence, the actual Ig levels can be ignored for all practical purposes.

Cellular immunity can be assessed by enumerating small lymphocytes (< 7 μ) and using skin tests for delayed hypersensitivity. This assessment is fraught with some danger. In some children with cellular deficiency, adequate numbers of lymphocytes are present ($>$ 1500/cu. mm.). However, on careful examination, it can be seen that they do not possess the condensed nuclear chromatin and high nuclear cytoplasmic ratio seen with the true small lymphocyte (Fig. 5). Skin tests have no meaning if sufficient exposure to the infectious agent has not occurred. The most reliable assay for small lymphocyte competence is the response to

---

*NCI Reference Center, 6715 Electronic Drive, Springfield, Virginia 22151.

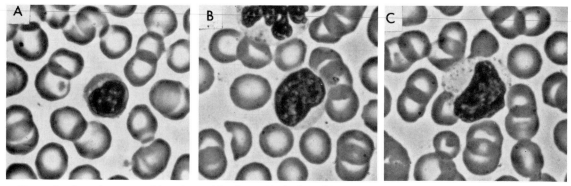

Figure 5. Lymphocytes and lymphocytoid cells. *A*, Typical small lymphocyte. The dense nuclear chromatin and high nuclear-cytoplasm ratio is evident. *B*, Large lymphocyte as evident by comparison with erythrocyte diameter. The nuclear chromatin is fine. Virtually all lymphocytes in cellular immune deficiencies, if present at all, are of this variety and phytohemagglutinin stimulation is usually negative. *C*, Cell commonly designated as lymphocytoid monocyte or monocytoid lymphocyte, having features of both lymphocytes and monocytes. It partially accounts for the monocytosis seen in cellular immune deficiency and is frequently present in large numbers. Phase contrast microscopy. ($\times$ 1000.)

phytohemagglutinin stimulation. A normal response (i.e., 60 to 90 per cent blast transformation) virtually rules out cellular immune deficiency. Other tests of cellular competence are more difficult to perform and do not generally fall within the province of the routine lab.

Immunologic disorders of special interest to otorhinolaryngologists are now considered.

An intriguing combination of eczema, thrombocytopenia, and recurrent ear infection occurring in families and following an X-linked pattern of inheritance is known as the Wiskott-Aldrich syndrome (Aldrich et al., 1954). Patients with this syndrome have severe frequent recurrent otitis media leading to draining ears. The outcome is usually fatal, death occurring from bleeding, *Pneumocystis carinii* pneumonia, generalized herpes infection, or lymphoma. The patients have been shown to lack the ability to respond to carbohydrate antigens, leading to a characteristic absence of isohemagglutinin titers despite elevated IgG levels. Usually immunoglobulin levels assume a distinctive pattern: normal to elevated IgG, markedly elevated IgA, and diminished IgM. This pattern may not develop until late in the course of the disease (Cooper et al., 1968; Blaese et al., 1968).

Ataxia telangiectasia is a familial autosomal recessive disorder characterized by progressive cerebellar ataxia, often beginning in infancy, and associated with varying degrees of chronic sinopulmonary infection leading to severe respiratory insufficiency. The presence of telangiectasia of the exposed bulbar conjunctiva is a major diagnostic feature, and a halting irregular conjugate gaze (oculomotor apraxia) is found. Over 60 per cent of the patients have a combined IgA and IgE deficiency; occasional cases of marked IgA elevation or deficiency of all immunoglobulins are seen. Deficiencies of cellular immunity are usually present also. An impressive list of abnormalities involving many systems can be compiled for this disease. In addition to vascular, cerebellar, and lymphoid abnormalities, aminoaciduria and lesions of the cerebral ventricles, pituitary gland and ovaries have been described. Death from lymphoma, a common terminal event of immunological deficiency states, may occur. The pathogenesis of this varied symptom complex remains unknown (Boder and Sedgwick, 1957; Peterson et al., 1963).

Wegener's granulomatosis is a polyangiitic process which usually begins with midline lesions which may be mistaken for nasal polyps. Relentless progression with rapid death resulting from renal involvement and failure is the usual outcome, but limited forms with confinement to the upper respiratory tract are seen. Cases have been observed in renal transplant patients receiving immunosuppressive therapy, suggesting an infectious etiology (Carrington and Liebow, 1966).

The widespread epidemic of rubella in 1964 led to the birth of many infants who had been infected in utero. It soon became apparent that the classic triad of heart disease, deafness, and cataracts formed only a small part of the total symptom complex. Involvement of nearly every system has been described; in addition, immunologic deficiency states occur, ostensibly due to impaired differentiation of the lymphoid stem cells. The usual abnormality has been humoral deficiency with elevation of IgM and diminution of IgA and IgG levels; however, combined cellular as well as humoral defects are known (Soothill et al., 1966; Cooper, 1968).

It should be appreciated that some patients with total hypogammaglobulinemia can be amazingly symptom-free, except for upper respiratory infections, and may present themselves to a physician for treatment of recurrent or chronic sinusitis. A lack of a history of life-threatening infections should not lull the clinician into discarding the diagnosis of immunological deficiency. Such patients may well have hypogammaglobulinemia or isolated IgA deficiency.

Reasonable indications for tonsillectomy and adenoidectomy include eustachian tube or upper airway obstruction from pharyngeal lymphoid tissues. The recent appreciation of gut-associated lymphoid tissues as playing important roles in controlling differentiation and final expression of the immunoglobulin-producing cell lines has led to speculation that the tonsils might function as central lymphoid tissue (Peterson et al., 1965). No clear evidence exists that an immune deficiency results from tonsillectomy, however. The central controller of the immunoglobulin system in man would seem to be more widespread in distribution, being not restricted to a single organ, and it is unlikely that removal of tonsils (or appendices or intestinal resections for that matter) can measurably affect the immunoglobulin production apparatus. Furthermore, peripheralization of the competent cells allows postnatal removal or ablation of central tissues with minimal effects in most cases.

REFERENCES

Abernathy, R. S., Strem, E. L., and Good, R. A.: Chronic asthma in childhood. Double blind controlled study of treatment with gamma globulin. Pediatrics 21:980–993, 1958.

Aldrich, R. A., Steinberg, A. C., and Campbell, D. C.: Pedigree demonstrating a sex-linked recessive condition characterized by draining ears, eczematoid dermatitis and bloody diarrhea. Pediatrics 13:133–139, 1954.

Askonas, B. A., and Rhodes, J. M: Immunogenicity of antigen-containing ribonucleic acid preparations from macrophages. Nature (London) 205:470–474, 1965.

Austen, K. F.: Nomenclature of complement. Bull. WHO 39:935–938, 1968.

Austen, K. F., and Humphrey, J. H.: In vitro studies of the mechanism of anaphylaxis. Advances Immun. 3:1–96, 1963.

Barandun, S., Kistler, P., Jeunet, F., and Isliker, H.: Intravenous administration of human gamma globulin. Vox Sang. 7:157–174, 1962.

Becker, E. L., and Austen, K. F.: Anaphylaxis. In: Miescher, P. A., and Müller-Eberhard, H. J. (ed.): Textbook of Immunopathology. New York, Grune & Stratton, 1968, pp. 76–93.

Benacerraf, B., and Green, I.: Cellular hypersensitivity. Ann. Rev. Med. 20:141–154, 1969.

Bennett, B., and Bloom, B. R.: Reactions in vivo and in vitro produced by a soluble substance associated with delayed-type hypersensitivity. Proc. Nat. Acad. Sci. USA 59:756–762, 1968.

Billingham, R. E., Brent, L., and Medawar, P. B.: "Actively acquired tolerance" of foreign cells. Nature (London) 172:603–606, 1953.

Biozzi, G., Halpern, B. N, and Binaghi, R.: The competitive effect of normal serum proteins from various animal species on antibody fixation in passive cutaneous anaphylaxis in the guinea pig. J. Immunol. 82:215–218, 1959.

Blaese, R. M, Strober, W., Brown, R. S., and Waldman, T. A.: The Wiskott-Aldrich syndrome: A disorder with a possible defect in antigen processing or recognition. Lancet 1:1056–1060, 1968.

Boder, E., and Sedgwick, R. P.: Ataxia-telangiectasia. Familial syndrome of progressive cerebellar ataxia oculocutaneous telangiectasia and frequent pulmonary infection. Pediatrics 21:526–554, 1957.

Borsos, T., and Rapp, H. J.: Complement fixation on cell surfaces by 19S and 7S antibodies. Science 150:505–506, 1965.

Burnet, F. M.: Measles as an index of immunological function. Lancet 2:610–613, 1968.

Burnet, F. M., and Fenner, F.: Production of Antibodies. 2nd ed. London, The Macmillan Company, 1949.

Cain, W. A., Ammann, A. J., Hong, R., Ishizaka, K., and Good, R. A.: IgE deficiency associated with chronic sinopulmonary infection. J. Clin. Invest. 48:12a, 1969.

Carrington, C. B., and Liebow, A. A.: Limited forms of angiitis and granulomatosis of Wegener's type. Amer. J. Med. 41:497–527, 1966.

Claman, H. N., Chaperon, E. A., and Triplett, R. F.: Thymus-marrow cell combinations; synergism in antibody production. Proc. Soc. Exp. Biol. Med. 122:1167–1169, 1966.

Cohen, S., and Milstein, C.: Structure and biological properties of immunoglobulins. Advances Immun. 7:1–91, 1967.

Cooper, L. Z.: Rubella: A preventable cause of birth defects in intrauterine infections. In: Good, R. A., and Bergsma, D. (ed.): Immunological Deficiency Diseases in Man. Birth Defects Original Article Series, Vol. IV, No. 1. New York, The National Foundation Press, 1968, pp. 23–25.

Cooper, M. D., Chase, H. P., Lowman, J. T., Krivit, W., and Good, R. A.: Wiskott-Aldrich syndrome: An immunologic deficiency disease involving the afferent limb of immunity. Amer. J. Med. 44:499–513, 1968.

David, J. R., Lawrence, H. S., and Thomas, L.: Delayed hypersensitivity in vitro. II. Effect of sensitive cells on normal cells in the presence of antigen. J. Immun. 93:274–278, 1964.

Eisen, H. N, Little, R. R., Osterland, C. K., and Simms, E. S.: A myeloma protein with antibody activity. Cold Spring Harbor Symp. Quant. Biol. 32:75–81, 1967.

Fishman, M., and Adler, F. L.: Antibody formation initiated in vitro. II. Antibody synthesis in X-irradiated recipients of diffusion chambers containing nucleic acid derived from macrophages incubated with antigen. J. Exp. Med. 117:595–602, 1963.

Forscher, B. K. (ed.): Chemical biology of inflammation. Biochem. Pharm. (Suppl.), March, 1968.

Franklin, E., and Frangione, B.: Immunoglobulins. Ann. Rev. Med. 20:155-174, 1969.

Good, R. A., and Finstad, J.: The association of lymphoid malignancy and immunologic functions. In: Zarafonetis, C. J. D. (ed.): Proceedings of the International Conference on Leukemia-Lymphoma, Philadelphia, 1968, pp. 175-197.

Good, R. A., Finstad, J., Cain, W. A., Fish, A., Perey, D. Y. E., and Gatti, R. A.: Models of immunologic diseases and disorders. Fed. Proc. 28:191-205, 1969.

Gottlieb, A. A.: Studies on the binding of soluble antigens to a unique ribonucleoprotein fraction of macrophage cells. Biochemistry 8:2111-2116, 1969.

Gough, W. W., and Davis, J. S., IV: Effects of rheumatoid factor on complement levels in vivo. Arthritis Rheum. 9:555-565, 1966.

Greenbury, C. L., Moore, D. H., and Nunn, L. A. C.: Reaction of 7S and 19S components of immune rabbit antisera with human group A and AB red cells. Immunology 6:421-433, 1963.

Holmes, B., Quie, P. G., Windhorst, D. B., and Good, R. A.: Fatal granulomatous disease of childhood: An inborn abnormality of phagocytic function. Lancet 1:1225-1228, 1966.

Ishizaka, K., and Ishizaka, T.: Human reaginic antibodies and immunoglobulin E. J. Allerg. 42:330-363, 1968.

Johansson, S. G. O., Mellein, T., and Vahlquist, B.: Immunoglobulin levels in Ethiopian preschool children with special reference to high concentration of immunoglobulin E (IgND). Lancet 1:1118-1121, 1968.

Kaplan, M. H.: Immunologic relation of streptococcal and tissue antigens. J. Immun. 90:595-606, 1963.

Lawrence, H. S.: The transfer in humans of delayed skin sensitivity to streptococcal M substance and to tuberculin with disrupted leucocytes. J. Clin. Invest. 34:219-230, 1955.

Lawrence, H. S.: Similarities between homograft rejections and tuberculin-type allergy: A review of recent experimental findings. Ann. N. Y. Acad. Sci. 64:826-835, 1957.

Lichtenstein, L. M., Norman, P. S., and Winkenwerder, W. L.: Clinical and in vitro studies on role of immunotherapy in ragweed hay fever. Amer. J. Med. 44:514-524, 1968.

Markowitz, A. S., Armstrong, J. S., and Kushner, D. S.: Immunological relationships between the rat glomerulus and nephritogenic streptococci. Nature (London) 187:1095-1097, 1960.

Metzger, H.: Characterization of a human macroglobulin, V. A. Waldenström macroglobulin with antibody activity. Proc. Nat. Acad. Sci. 57:1490-1497, 1967.

Micklem, H. S., Ford, C. E., Evans, E. P., and Gray, J.: Interrelationships of myeloid and lymphoid cells: Studies with chromosome-marked cells transfused into lethally irradiated mice. Proc. Roy. Soc. 165:78-102, 1966.

Müller-Eberhard, H. J.: Chemistry and reaction mechanisms of complement. Advances Immun. 8:2-72, 1968.

Natvig, J. B., Kunkel, H. G., and Litwin, S. P.: Genetic markers of the heavy chain sub-groups of human gamma G globulin. Cold Spring Harbor Symp. Quant. Biol. XXXII Antibodies. New York, 1967, pp. 173-180.

Osler, A. G., Lichtenstein, L. M., and Levy, D. M.: In vitro studies of human reaginic allergy. Advances Immun. 8:183-228, 1968.

Perlmann, P., Perlmann, H., Müller-Eberhard, H. J., and Manni, J. A.: Cytotoxic effects of leucocytes triggered by complement bound to target cells. Science 163:937-939, 1969.

Peterson, R. D. A., Blaw, M., and Good, R. A.: Ataxia-telangiectasia: A possible clinical counterpart of the animals rendered immunologically incompetent by thymectomy. J. Pediat. 63:701, 1963.

Peterson, R. D. A., Cooper, M. D., and Good, R. A.: The pathogenesis of immunologic deficiency diseases. Amer. J. Med. 38:579-604, 1965.

Rowley, D., and Turner, K. J.: Number of molecules of antibody required to promote phagocytosis of one bacterium. Nature (London) 210:496-498, 1966.

Sadan, N., Rhyne, M. B., Mellits, E. D., Goldstein, E. O., Levy, D. A., and Lichtenstein, L. M.: Immunotherapy of pollinosis in children: Immunologic basis of improvement. New Eng. J. Med. 280:623-627, 1969.

Soothill, J. F., Hayes, K., and Dudgeon, J. A.: The immunoglobulins in congenital rubella. Lancet 1:1385-1388, 1966.

South, M. A., Cooper, M. D., Wollheim, F. A., Hong, R., and Good, R. A.: The IgA system. I. Studies of the transport and immunochemistry of IgA in the saliva. J. Exp. Med. 123:615-627, 1966.

Stanworth, D. R., Humphrey, J. H., Bennich, H., and Johansson, S. G. O.: Specific inhibition of the Prausnitz-Küstner reaction by an atypical myeloma protein. Lancet 2:330-332, 1967.

Stiehm, E. R., Ammann, A. J., and Cherry, J. O.: Elevated cord macroglobulins in the diagnosis of intrauterine infections. New Eng. J. Med. 275:971-977, 1966.

Stiehm, E. R., and Fudenberg, H. H.: Serum levels of immune globulins in health and disease: A survey. Pediatrics 37:715-727, 1966.

Tan, E. M: Antibodies to deoxyribonucleic acid irradiated with ultraviolet light: Detection by precipitins and immunofluorescence. Science 161:1353-1354, 1968.

Tomasi, T., and Bienenstock, J.: Secretory immunoglobulins. Advances Immun. 9:1-96, 1968.

Uhr, J. W.: The heterogeneity of the immune response. Science 145:457-464, 1964.

Unanue, E. R., and Dixon, F. J.: Experimental glomerulonephritis. Advances Immun. 6:1-79, 1967.

Weigle, W. O.: Natural and Acquired Immunologic Unresponsiveness. Cleveland, The World Publishing Co., 1967.

West, C. D., Hong, R., and Holland, N. H.: Immunoglobulin levels from the newborn period to adulthood and in immunoglobulin deficiency states. J. Clin. Invest. 41:2054-2064, 1962.

Zabriskie, J. B.: Mimetic relationships between group A streptococci and mammalian tissues. Advances Immun. 7:147-187, 1967.

Chapter 30

ENDOCRINOLOGY

by Frank N. Ritter, M.D.

A classic concept of human physiology is that all cellular activities of the body are controlled and integrated by the endocrine glands and the central nervous system. The endocrine system accomplishes its effects by the liberation of hormones into the blood stream. Hormones are proteins or polypeptides that act as catalysts to control the metabolic processes of various specific tissues, termed target tissues. The result is usually an increased activity of these tissues, which might be located in either an anatomical organ or region. In some instances the target is another endocrine gland, so that instead of increased metabolism the liberation of a second hormone is the effect of the primary stimulating hormone. The degree of tissue response depends upon the rate and amount of the stimulating hormone, but overactivity does not normally occur because excessive metabolism in the target cells checks the additional release of the stimulating hormone. This finely controlled reciprocal reaction that exists in the axis between target tissue and hormone is termed negative feedback.

THE PITUITARY GLAND

The pituitary gland is an illustration of the joint control of body tissues by the endocrine and central nervous systems. This gland, the hypophysis, has a dual embryonic origin. The anterior part is derived from a pharyngeal evagination termed Rathke's pouch, whereas the posterior portion develops from the hypothalamus of the central nervous system. The pars anterior is composed of three types of epithe-

lioid cells: The acidophils, the basophils and the chromophobe cells. These cells secrete hormones: the acidophilic cells, growth and luteotropic hormones; and the basophilic cells, luteinizing and follicle-stimulating hormones, corticotropin and thyrotropin. Recent research definitely indicates that a secretion also occurs from the chromophobe cells, but the exact hormone is not as yet identified (Rovner, 1970). These anterior pituitary hormones are released upon liberation of neurosecretory substances from the hypothalamus. Their target tissues are other endocrine glands.

The posterior pituitary secretes two hormones: oxytocin and the antidiuretic hormone. These pituitary hormones are released when the pituitary is stimulated by the hypothalamus over neural connections between these structures.

Thus, growth and renal, adrenal, ovarian, and thyroid function are only a few bodywide expressions of this neural and endocrine relationship (Best and Taylor, 1966; Guyton, 1968).

Pituitary Surgery

Pathological lesions of the pituitary produce abnormalities usually manifested in other organ systems of the body. Yet because the gland is anatomically adjacent to the sphenoid air sinus, the rhinologist may be summoned to perform a hypophysectomy. This sphenoid approach is not the only surgical route to the pituitary, but it results in less postoperative morbidity than the intracranial approach. Specific technical points of the surgery are covered elsewhere, but some points should be covered here because of the endocrinological changes that occur pre-or post-operation.

The often quoted indications for hypophysectomy are: (1) increased secretion of any pituitary cell groups or pituitary tumors with abnormal secretions, acidophilic and basophilic adenomas; (2) pituitary tumors which cause symptoms by expansion, chromophobe adenoma; (3) to lessen pituitary hormonal stimulation of a sex endocrine gland which, in turn, secretes sex hormones that promote the growth of a malignant neoplasm; and (4) in diabetic retinopathy.

Symptomatically, pituitary tumors cause headaches and visual disturbances. The headaches are dull in type and located deeply within the head, atop the vertex or at the occiput. The visual disturbance is the field defect of a progressive bitemporal hemianopsia. This results when the lesion expands superiorly against the optic chiasm.

Increased secretion from the acidophilic cells or a tumor composed of these cells causes either giantism or acromegaly. Prior to adolescence, giantism occurs. After puberty, when the long bones have fused, only the membranous ones can enlarge, and acromegaly results. To the otorhinolaryngologist this means that the nasal bones, mandible, maxilla, and laryngeal cartilages may enlarge. Usually this growth does not disturb the physiology in any of these anatomical areas except the larynx. At this location growth of the thyroid alae causes the vocal cords to elongate, and the pitch of the voice deepens. Cordal motion is not impaired.

Endocrine Changes Following Pituitary Ablation

Some endocrine changes result immediately after hypophysectomy. The first and most serious is severe weakness and endocrine-induced shock. These symptoms result from interference in the pituitary-adrenal axis, specifically from lack of production of corticotropin by the anterior pituitary. This hormone stimulates the adrenal cortex, which, in turn, liberates mineralocorticoids and glucocorticoids. Of these the more important is the decrease in the glucocorticoids, the loss of which does not permit adrenaline to maintain normotension of the peripheral vascular system. For this physiological reason, supplemental exogenous cortisone is administered prior to and after hypophysectomy, and the patient is maintained on this hormone indefinitely. The night preceding surgery 100 mg. of cortisone acetate is administered intramuscularly. Immediately prior to surgery 100 mg. of the steroid is parenterally administered, and during surgery or immediately thereafter 100 to 200 mg. is given in a slow intravenous drip. Postoperatively the dosage is diminished and titrated until a proper level of blood pressure, general activity, and strength can be maintained. Usually 200 mg. is given in divided doses the first postoperative day. The amount is decreased each day thereafter, giving 150 mg., then 100 mg., and so on, until a physiological normotensive end point is maintained. Since steroids are diabetogenic, the serum blood sugar level should be determined periodically in the postoperative period. Cortisone may also break down scar formation and retard healing, so reactivation of a duodenal ulcer or a healed pulmonary tubercular lesion may occur. (See The Adrenal Gland later in this chapter for more details.)

A second early symptom following pituitary surgery is a severe diuresis. This symptom is due to loss of the antidiuretic hormone of the posterior pituitary. Normally the hormone promotes water resorption by the distal renal tubule. Without it, the quantity of diuresis is several liters daily and the specific gravity of the urine is very low. The diuresis is controlled by injections of vasopressin (Pitressin tannate) in oil, 5 units every other day. Depending upon the degree of diuresis and following healing of the operative site, Pitressin is administered in a nasal spray or as a snuff (Rovner, 1970).

Thyroid replacement may be needed after pituitary ablation. Several weeks after surgery the patient may become languid and dull, showing signs of weakness and inactivity. Anticipatory treatment should not be instituted, but a diagnosis of the degree of the hypothyroid state should be made by determining the basal metabolic rate and the serum protein bound iodine and cholesterol levels. The treatment is the administration of exogenous thyroid extract or chemically purified thyroglobulin. The patient's response should be gauged by a clinical appraisal of activity and the previously cited laboratory tests until they are within a range accepted as normal.

Sex hormones are liberated by the gonads in response to stimulus by the pituitary. Unless the surgical hypophysectomy was performed to halt the advance of a sex hormone-dependent malignancy, feminizing or masculinizing hormones are administered to maintain secondary sex characteristics and libido.

THE THYROID GLAND

The thyroid gland, a shield-shaped structure in the lower anterior neck, produces thyroxine, a hormone which profoundly influences both the growth and metabolic activity of all body tissues. The hormone is assimilated in the thyroid gland from elemental iodine and four tyrosine amino acid molecules. Several chemical conjugations are necessary to yield tetraiodothyronine which, combined with a globulin, is stored in the follicles as colloid. The release of thyroxine is by stimulus of thyrotropin from the anterior pituitary. A reciprocal feedback in the pituitary-thyroid axis exists, for overproduction of thyroxine checks any further release of thyrotropin.

The adequacy of thyroid function is determined by measuring the patient's growth, the metabolic rate, and the serum level of circulating thyroxine. Growth comparisons provide some estimate of adequate thyroid function, but the basal metabolic rate and the blood serum level of the circulating iodine bound to protein (protein bound iodine) are more accurate. A relatively new test is the T3 red cell uptake, which permits an exact measurement of circulating triiodothyronine, the most active portion of thyroxine.

Hypothyroidism

Hypothyroidism may be congenital or acquired. Congenital athyreosis, resulting from absence of thyroid tissue or lack of elemental iodine in the diet, is termed cretinism. These patients are dwarfs with reduced mental function. The syndrome is rare, but the defect is suspected when a child fails to grow. Diagnosis is confirmed by obtaining low values on the thyroid function tests. Supplemental iodine, thyroid extract, or a synthetic hormone will reverse the physical changes, but the mental retardation usually persists.

Ear, Nose, and Throat Findings in Cretinism
The ear. One author who describes these patients states that the auditory canals and tympanic membranes are not abnormal, but a severe hearing loss often exists. Another reports that the ossicles and/or inner ear are undeveloped (Benda, 1949). Very old temporal bone reports on this illness shed little light upon the aural findings, and no recent temporal bone report exists (Alexander, 1909). Animal research on the defect favors an inner ear lesion as a cause for the deafness. In the developing chick embryo the sensory cells of the acoustic organ are deformed and their supporting cells are watery or edematous in appearance (Ritter and Lawrence, 1960); supposedly this watery material is hyaluronic acid.

The larynx. Clinically these dwarfs are supposed to have high pitched voices, but the disorder of the voice has not been described (Alexander, 1909). Research also fails to provide an answer. The tongue of the cretin infant is large, and this aggravates any existing voice problem.

Myxedema. When hypothyroidism is an acquired illness following thyroiditis, thyroidectomy, or irradiation with ^{131}I, it most often occurs after growth has been attained. Thus, changes are confined to decreased cellular metabolism, and growth is unaffected. As a result, in chronic hypothyroidism all the body's tissues accumulate excess acid mucopolysaccharides and are puffy. This generalized state of increased tissue fluid is called myxedema. Laboratory tests reveal a decreased basal metabolic rate (BMR), and a lowered protein bound iodine determination.

The ears, nose, and throat share this generalized myxedematous accumulation, and manifest changes and symptoms dependent upon its severity.

The larynx. The best documented of the otorhinolaryngological changes in myxedema are found in the larynx. Fluid occurs just under the mucosa and causes the vocal cord to appear puffy (Hilger, 1956). These clinical changes have been documented experimentally in laboratory animals (Figs. 1 and 2) (Ritter, 1964). Therapy consists in reversing the hypothyroid state with thyroid extract or one of the synthetic substitutes and stripping the vocal cord of the myxedematous tissue.

The nose. The nasal tissues accumulate acid mucopolysaccharides in the submucosa similar to that which occurs in the larynx. This finding has been demonstrated in both man and laboratory animals (Proud and Lange, 1957; Weisskopf, 1960). Patients complain of chronic excess nasal discharge and nasal stuffiness. The chronicity of symptoms without concomitant infection, allergy, neoplasm, or sensitivity to chemicals should alert one to the possibility of hypothyroidism as a cause of these nasal complaints. Diagnosis can be made both by noting decreased laboratory values of thyroid function and by biopsy of the nasal tissues, usually a portion of the inferior turbinate; staining the tissue with a colloidal iron technique will show increased accumulation of acid mucopolysaccharides (Weisskopf, 1960). These

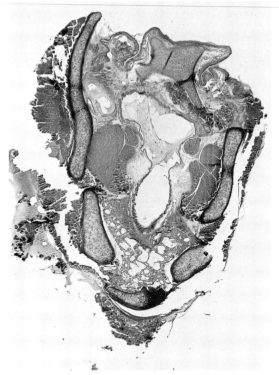

Figure 1. A coronal section of a rat larynx. This control animal was 160 days of age at sacrifice. The supraglottic laryngeal lumen is partially filled with debris.

deposits in the mucosa and submucosa are located around blood vessels and glandular elements, which explains the altered nasal discharge and nasal stuffiness. Therapy is systemic, utilizing thyroid extract or a purified synthetic derivative.

Because postnasal drip is a feature of the nasal changes in hypothyroidism and responds to medication, thyroid extract has been empirically used to decrease the nonpathogenic postnasal drip that afflicts many people; for this purpose, however, the use of thyroid extract has been unrewarding.

The ear. In the ear the site of the myxedematous change determines the type of hearing loss encountered. Should the eustachian tube or middle ear mucosa become invaded with heavy deposits of acid mucopolysaccharides, a serous yellow effusion develops in the middle ear cleft (McMahon, 1947). The hearing loss is conductive in type. Sometimes the acid mucopolysaccharide deposit does not develop in these areas, but instead a sensorineural loss occurs. The loss is usually moderate, but audiologically it is difficult to determine if it is cochlear or retrocochlear (DeVos, 1963). Human temporal bone studies are not available to

clarify this point. Animal studies suggest a lesion either in the spiral ganglion cells or in the Claudius or Boettcher cells of the external sulcus (Figs. 3 and 4) (DeVos, 1963; Ritter, 1967b). In each study all these cells seemed to contain vacuolated or watery areas. Possibly these are areas of increased deposition of acid mucopolysaccharides. Both kinds of hearing loss in myxedema, conductive and sensorineural, are reversible upon proper systemic treatment of the hypothyroid state.

Hyperthyroidism and diseases of the parathyroid glands do not sufficiently alter the structures of the ear, nose, and throat to cause symptoms. Thus, the pathological behavior of these endocrine glands is discussed with their surgery in another chapter.

THE ADRENAL GLAND

The adrenal gland lying atop the superior pole of each kidney has an outer cortex and a central medulla. The cortex develops from me-

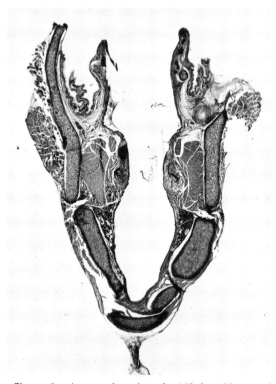

Figure 2. A coronal section of a 160 day old rat made hypothyroid with radioiodine.[9] The submucosal tissue of the true vocal cord stains dark with colloidal iron, demonstrating the deposition of increased amounts of acid mucopolysaccharide.

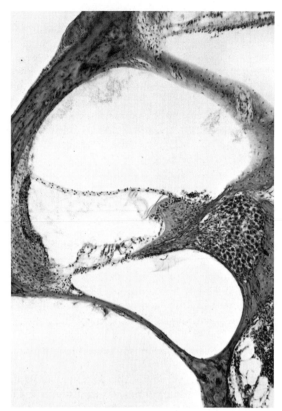

Figure 3. The organ of Corti in a control rate of 200 days' age.

soderm, and the medulla is neuroectodermal in origin. Anatomically the gland is divided, and physiologically the medulla and cortex secrete various hormones, over 30 in number. The principal ones (Rovner, 1970):

Medulla (catecholamines)
    Dopamine
    Norepinephrine
    Epinephrine
Cortex (corticosteroids)
Mineralocorticoids (mineral and water metabolism)
    Aldosterone
Glucocorticoids (carbohydrate, fat, and protein metabolism; anti-inflammatory effect)
    Cortisol, hydrocortisone (compound F)
    Corticosterone (compound B)
    Cortisone (compound E)
Androgenic corticoids

Prednisone, prednisolone, methylprednisolone (Medrol), triamcinolone (Aristocort) and others are synthetic derivatives of cortisone or hydrocortisone and have more potent glucocorticoid and anti-inflammatory qualities, but few mineralocorticoid traits, thus minimizing salt and water retention by the patient.

The release of the adrenal hormones is dependent upon the environmental stress surrounding the individual. The stress is monitored via the hypothalamus and central nervous system. Medullary hormones are liberated upon stimulus of the sympathetic nervous system, and cortical hormones are liberated from the basophilic cells of the anterior pituitary by stimulation by corticotropin.

The Adrenal Medulla

Adrenaline is the most effective of the hormones of the adrenal medulla. In general, but not always, it causes vasoconstriction. For example, it constricts the arterioles of skin and kidneys, but in smaller doses dilates vessels of skeletal muscles, liver, and the coronary artery system. Systolic blood pressure is elevated because of its effect of increasing cardiac output. It acts on the smooth muscles of the bronchi as a bronchodilator. This pharmacological effect of vasoconstriction makes it a helpful adjunct in clinical medicine and leads to its use in local

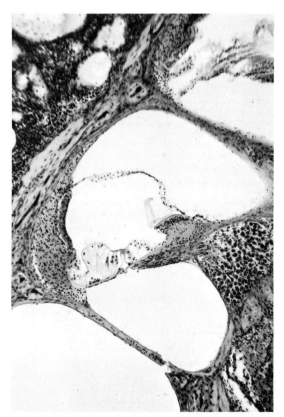

Figure 4. The organ of Corti in a 220 day old rat rendered hypothyroid with radioiodine.[14] The cells of the external sulcus are larger than the control animal and this may in some way cause a hearing loss.

anesthetics to decrease blood loss. In rare instances, should too much adrenaline be administered, and headache, palpitation, and cardiac output be increased beyond tolerance, phentolamine (Regitine) is given as an antidote, 5 mg. slowly intravenously.

Clinically adrenaline is also useful in anaphylaxis. Sensitivity to allergens and various medications may cause nasal, laryngeal, and tracheobronchial symptoms. Histamine release occurs in the antigen-antibody reaction of anaphylaxis and this, in turn, causes edema in these sites. Choking, airway obstruction, and shock can develop quickly. To overcome these effects, oxygen is of prime importance, but adrenaline is administered rapidly to negate the effect of histamine upon the tissues, lessening edema and overcoming the airway problem by producing bronchodilatation. Usually 1 mg. (1 ml. of 1:1000 adrenaline) is administered intramuscularly. If necessary the drug is given intravenously diluted in 10 ml. of normal saline. In addition, cortisone 100 to 250 mg. I.M. or I.V., aqueous diphenhydramine 5 to 20 mg. I.V., and aminophylline 500 mg. I.V. is given. The medication is titrated to overcome the symptoms and effects of anaphylaxis; it may be necessary that these drugs be given in gradually decreasing amounts until the symptoms have completely subsided (Chatton et al., 1968).

The Adrenal Cortex

The Mineralocorticoids. As a group these hormones are concerned primarily with salt and water balance. The most active and potent mineralocorticoid is aldosterone. This hormone controls salt and water excretion via the kidney in two ways: by increasing the renal tubular resorption of sodium, and by increasing the renal excretion of potassium. When the hormone fails to act, as after adrenal atrophy or surgery or after pituitary gland surgery, sodium is lost from the body in large amounts but potassium is retained. The loss of sodium will slowly result in weakness, diminished peripheral vascular resistance, and lowered blood pressure. If potassium is not excreted, its elevated serum level will result in cardiac irregularities, and shock and death may result.

The Glucocorticoids. This hormonal group is responsible for proper function of carbohydrate, fat, and protein metabolic cycles. Two additional important functions are an anti-inflammatory effect and a "permissive" effect upon the vascular tone of blood vessels which is required to permit the catecholamines (chiefly noradrenaline) to act upon them to exert normotension. The usual daily excretion of glucocorticoids does not significantly affect inflammation and healing, but larger amounts will block all stages of the process. The effects range from prevention of tissue fluid loss at the time of the acute inflammation or injury, to the inhibition of collagen being laid down in the fibroblast during healing.

This anti-inflammatory effect is the main reason steroid therapy has gained such a wide use in clinical practice. Hormones have been synthesized that now have potent anti-inflammatory qualities but few mineralocorticoid effects. The otorhinolaryngologist has shared in the benefits of the steroids. To name a few: nasal allergy improves and nasal polyposis is lessened (Baker and Strauss, 1962). The laryngeal edema resulting from trauma and infection may be diminished (Durcan, 1963; Ritter, 1967a). The strictures of corrosive burns in the air and food passages have been lessened (Cardova and Daly, 1964). In the ear they are effective in lessening pain, edema, and the granulation tissue response from infection. The dosage and route of steroid therapy depend upon the clinical need. There are few contraindications to their immediate use, and large amounts can be tolerated safely.

The use of exogenous steroids for a period of time locally or by the systemic routes may result in suppression of the patient's normally functioning adrenal gland. When the exogenous steroid is discontinued it is tapered slowly over days, or weeks, depending upon the length of time the steroid has been administered. This permits the patient's adrenal glands to assume their production of cortisone. Sometimes it is necessary to wilfully impose stress (a surgical operation) on patients who have been taking maintenance levels of steroids. Because of the patient's inability to quickly synthesize sufficient adrenal hormones, the exogenous hormones are administered in an increased amount. This rapid administration is called a "steroid prep" or "steroid burst." The tabulated form on the following page outlines the essentials.

All doses are in milligrams. The duration of therapy is for 10 days postoperative. It may be tapered more quickly to five days without risk unless the patient has been on steroids for a prolonged period of time.

When a doubt exists as to whether to prepare a patient before surgery by giving exoge-

| | | CORTISONE ACETATE | | | | | HYDRO-CORTISONE I.V. |
| | I.M. | | Oral | | | | |
	7 A.M.	7 P.M.	8 A.M.	12	4 P.M.	8 P.M.	
Day before surgery		100					
Day of surgery	100	50					200
Postop. day 1	50	50					100–150
2	50	50					50–100
3	50	50	25		25		
4	50		25	25	25		
5			25	25	25	25	
6			25	25	25		
7			25	12.5	25		
8			25	12.5	12.5		
9			25		12.5		
10			25		12.5		

nous cortisone, it is always safer to prepare preoperatively than chance the onset of shock during or after surgery. The few contraindications to cortisone therapy are active tuberculosis, psychosis, and active peptic ulcer. Relative contraindications may be severe diabetes, acute viral or bacterial infection, congestive heart failure, and uremia. Yet if these medical conditions are known and treated vigorously at the time steroids are given, the degree of contraindication is lessened.

THE OVARY

The ovarian sex hormones, estrogen and progesterone, sometimes exert otorhinolaryngologic effects in female patients. These are variable in degree and inconsistent in occurrence. Vicarious menstruation in the form of epistaxis may occur in some pubertal females around the menses. The epistaxis is caused by vascular congestion secondary to the circulating estrogen serum level. The bleeding is almost always located in Little's area and is easily controlled with chemical or electrical cautery.

The stuffy nose of pregnancy is a more common illness and is due to high progesterone levels. Rhinoscopy reveals congestion of the nasal tissues, and the best therapy is the topical use of 0.25 per cent phenylephrine nose drops. Several weeks post partum the nasal obstruction will diminish spontaneously as the progesterone level decreases.

The synthetic female hormones, used as oral contraceptives, are responsible for a feeling of plugged ears, nasal congestion, and vertigo in some patients. These symptoms are probably due to fluid retention in the structure involved. The use of a different "pill" often relieves this complaint (Schiff, 1968).

REFERENCES

Alexander, G.: Das Dehorogan der Kretinen. Arch. Ohrenheilk. *78*:59–128, 1909.

Baker, D. C., and Strauss, R. B. Intranasal injection of long acting corticosteroids. Trans. Amer. Laryng. Ass. *83*:166–173, 1962.

Benda, C. E.: Mongolism and Cretinism. New York, Grune & Stratton, 1949.

Best, C. H., and Taylor, N. B. (ed.): The Physiological Basis of Medical Practice. 8th ed. Baltimore, The Williams & Wilkins Co., 1966.

Cardova, J. C., and Daly, J. F. Management of corrosive esophagitis. Analysis of treatment, methodology and results. New York J. Med. *64*:2307–2313, 1964.

Chatton, M. J., Margen., and Brainerd H. (ed): Handbook of Medical Treatment. Los Altos, California, Lange Medical Publications, 1968.

DeVos, J. A.: Deafness in hypothyroidism. J. Laryng. *77*:390–414, 1963.

Durcan, D. J : Tracheal stricture successfully treated by dilatation and steroids. J. Laryng. *77*:351–352, April 1963.

Guyton, A. C.: Textbook of Medical Physiology. 3rd ed. Philadelphia, W. B. Saunders Company, 1968.

Hilger, J. A.: Otolaryngologic aspects of hypometabolism. Ann. Otol. *65*:395–413, 1956.

McMahon, B. J.: Influence of constitutional factors in otological conditions. Ann. Otol. *56*:298–304, 1947.

Proud, G. O., and Lange, R. D.: The effect of thyroidectomy on the nasal mucosa of experimental animals. Laryngoscope *67*:201–207, 1957.

Ritter, F. N.: The effect of hypothyroidism on the larynx of the rat. Ann. Otol. *73*:404–416, 1964.

Ritter, F. N.: Subglottic stenosis following cricothyrotomy. Trans. Amer. Acad. Ophthal. Otolaryng. *71*:792–801, 1967a.

Ritter, F. N.: The effects of hypothyroidism upon the ear, nose and throat. Laryngoscope *78*:1427–1479, 1967b.

Ritter, F. N., and Lawrence, M.: Reversible hearing loss

in human hypothyroidism and correlated changes in the chick inner ear. Laryngoscope *60*:393–407, 1960.

Rovner, D.: Personal communication, 1970.

Schiff, M: The "pill" in otolaryngology. Trans. Amer. Acad. Ophthal. Otolaryng. *72*:76–84, 1968.

Scott-Brown, W. G., Ballantyne, J., and Grooves, J. (ed.): Diseases of the Ear, Nose and Throat. 2nd ed. Chapter 15, Volume I. New York, Appleton-Century, Crofts, Inc., 1965.

Weisskopf, A.: Connective tissue: A synthesis of modern thought and its impact on understanding of nasal diseases. Laryngoscope *60*:1029–1059, 1960.

Chapter 31

GENERAL PRINCIPLES OF GENETICS, INCLUDING COUNSELING

by Lee E. Schacht, Ph.D.

It has long been apparent to man that when he closely compares individuals within a population they are unlike in their physical and mental characteristics. Man has attempted for centuries to find an explanation for these differences and has finally concluded that they result from two forces—heredity (nature) and environment (nurture). Until quite recently there was great controversy as to which of the two forces was paramount in determining individual uniqueness. It is now obvious that the either/or concept of nature versus nurture is indefensible and that a more reasonable question is, "How much of the variability in a given trait is due to heredity, how much to environment, and how much to an interaction between the two?"

When we attempt to determine the etiology of a trait or a characteristic common to a group of individuals, it is the variation in expression of that trait and not the trait itself that is studied. Sometimes there are two or three very specific classifications into which these variations fall. At other times one observes a large number of small variations that are distributed in a continuous series, e.g., weight, height, intelligence. From the study of variations in phenotypic expression of a trait within a population we are able to make ascertainments as to the extent and interaction of the genetic and environmental forces.

Many clinical entities that appear as isolated events are also often part of a syndromal picture. For example, in Alport's syndrome there are two major clinical characteristics, hearing loss and kidney disease. In otolarnygology, many of the patients seen have multiple anomalies that fit into specific syndromes. The etiology of some diseases may be clearly environmental (e.g., rubella syndrome), or clearly genetic and due to a chromosomal abnormality (Down's syndrome) or a single defective gene (mandibulofacial dysostosis). Other diseases or anomalies may be the result of a genetic potential expressing itself within a specific environmental situation (cleft lip with or without cleft palate; schizophrenia). This chapter will attempt to provide some basic information on the genetic component in the causation of disease.

CHROMOSOMES AND GENES

Chromosomes

The cytological study of experimental animals has provided us with basic knowledge of the structure and arrangement of genetic information. The area of human cytogenetics, that is, the morphological study of the chromosomes in the cells of man, has taken great strides in the past decade. It is now known that specific chromosome abnormalities cause certain diseases; with time, the number of these associations will increase. Although human cytogenetics is not yet comparable to the sophisticated cytogenetics of Drosophila and maize, it is still a useful tool in confirming genetic principles and diagnosing syndromes, and serves as a stepping stone in the development of finer techniques that will produce more specific information.

The number and morphology of the normal chromosome complement of man is well known. Figure 1 shows the metaphase chromosomes from a single human cell. Figure 2 is a diagrammatic representation of these chromosomes, showing them arranged in the standardized pattern for analysis and evaluation. The 46 chromosomes are compared to each other and then placed in one of seven groups (lettered A, B, C, D, E, F and G). This grouping is done on the basis of (1) overall chromosome length, (2) position of the centromere or constriction, and (3) length of the two arms in relationship to each other (Fig. 3).

Figure 4 shows the actual karyotype of Figure 1, and one can see that it is not always possible to clearly identify each chromosome. Group A chromosomes are the longest and have centrally placed constrictions (metacentric). Within Group A, pairs 1, 2 and 3 can be clearly distinguished from one another. Group B chromosomes, pairs 4 and 5, are not mor-

phologically distinguishable from each other. Group C chromosomes, which include the X-chromosome and pairs 6 through 12, are essentially indistinguishable from one another (Fig. 2). Chromosomes 13, 14 and 15 are acrocentric (i.e., the centromere or constriction is very near the end of the chromosome) and are placed in Group D. These three pairs of chromosomes are not easily distinguishable from one another on most slides. Group E includes chromosomes 16, 17 and 18, and in good preparations each of these pairs can be distinguished. Group F includes chromosomes 19 and 20 (metacentric), and these are not distinguishable as specific pairs. Group G is composed of the shortest chromosomes and, like the D Group, they have the centromere near the very end of the chromosome; this group includes 21, 22 and the Y-chromosome. Chromosome pairs 21 and 22 are not morphologically distinguishable from each other; however, the Y-chromosome can usually be identified. Females have two X-chromosomes and thus show a karyotype pattern with 16 chromosomes in the C group and 4 chromosomes in Group G. Males have an X- and a Y-chromosome and show a karyotype pattern of 15 in Group C and 5 in Group G.

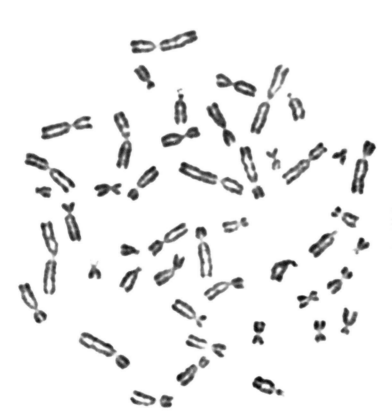

Figure 1. Metaphase chromosome spread from leukocyte culture of human male. (Courtesy of Human Genetics Unit, Minnesota Department of Health.)

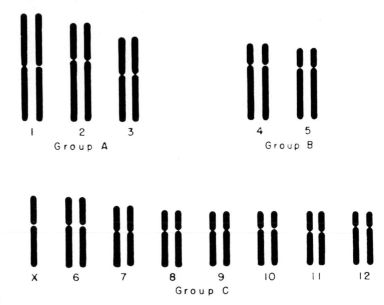

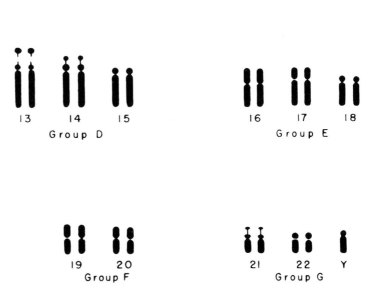

Figure 2. Idiogram of human chromosomes.

As indicated, there are 23 pairs of chromosomes, of which 22 pairs are termed autosomes and one pair sex chromosomes. One of each pair of chromosomes is inherited from the mother and the other from the father, but it is impossible to determine which chromosome of each pair is maternal in origin and which is paternal. An exception is the sex chromosomes, because the X in the male must be maternal in origin since the only source for the Y is the father. As with the autosomes, the two X-chromosomes in the female cannot be differentiated as to origin. The two chromosomes that form a pair are called *homologous chromosomes*.

Genes

Arranged in a linear order along the length of each chromosome, but not visible to the eye, are a series of hereditary "units" called *genes*. These units are the basic modules of hereditary transmission and may be defined as a unit of function or structure. Each chromosome carries the same genes for specific traits in exactly the same linear order as its homologous chromosome. The position of the gene on the chromosome is called a *gene locus* (Fig. 3); thus, there are two genes present at a locus on a pair of homologous chromosomes.

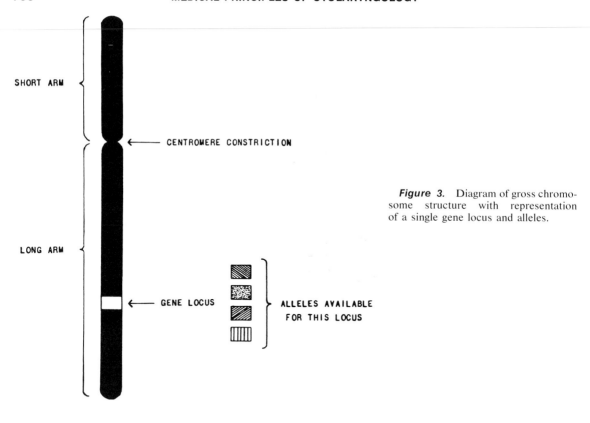

SHORT ARM

← CENTROMERE CONSTRICTION

Figure 3. Diagram of gross chromosome structure with representation of a single gene locus and alleles.

LONG ARM

← GENE LOCUS

ALLELES AVAILABLE
FOR THIS LOCUS

Alleles

Within a population it is possible for several different "forms" of a gene to be present. These various gene "forms" that produce different effects upon the same trait and occupy the same locus are called *alleles*. It is these alleles with their different effects on the trait that provide the hereditary variability within a population. Although there may be two, three or more alleles present in a population, an individual carries only two of these at any one time. They may be identical to each other, or they may be different, in their effect on that specific trait. As an example we might use the ABO blood group system in which there are three possible alleles, designated I^A, I^B and I^O. An individual who has two I^A alleles or one I^A and one I^O is typed as A. The I^O allele does not express itself in the presence of I^A or I^B in routine blood grouping procedures. An individual with two I^B alleles or one I^B and one I^O is typed B. The individual who has two I^O alleles is typed O; the one who has both an I^A and I^B allele is typed AB. When both alleles at a gene locus are identical, the individual is said to be *homozygous* for that locus. When the two alleles at the gene locus are different in their effect upon the trait, the individual is said to be *heterozygous* for that locus.

Mutation

In discussing the alleles of a specific gene locus the question naturally arises as to the source of new alleles. The primary source of new alleles is a phenomenon called mutation. Mutation is a permanent, heritable change in the basic molecular (nucleotide) sequence of a gene. These changes can either occur spontaneously or be induced by such mutagens as chemicals or radiation. Most, though not necessarily all, mutations are detrimental. Through the course of time some mutations have occurred that are advantageous to the individual within the environment in which he is living. In the process of evolution, the alleles that are best adapted for survival within the present environment have increased in frequency through natural selection. Mutations, then, continue to provide new material for natural selection in an ever-changing environment. If a mutation occurs that results in a detrimental dominant gene, this gene is usually eliminated within one or two generations, be-

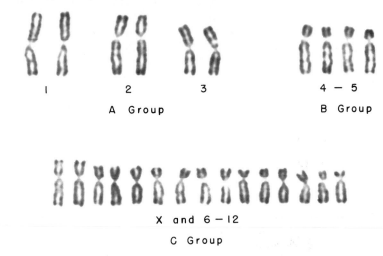

I   **2**   **3**   **4 — 5**

A Group   B Group

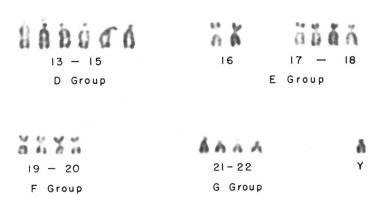

X and 6 — 12

C Group

Figure 4. Karyotype of Figure 1.

13 — 15   **16**   **17 — 18**

D Group   E Group

19 — 20   **21 - 22**   **Y**

F Group   G Group

cause the individual carrying this gene is in most instances nonreproducing. Recessive alleles may be maintained in a population because they produce little or no reduction in the viability of the individual carrying this allele in the heterozygous state. Thus, detrimental alleles may be maintained in a population at a specific frequency that is determined by an equilibrium between the forces of selection and mutation.

PATTERNS OF INHERITANCE

Autosomal Dominant

Let us now consider how these two alleles affecting the same trait interact with each other to produce the hereditary component of the trait. When one of the two alleles present at a locus expresses itself with a clinically detectable characteristic, that allele is said to be dominant to the other allele. An example of an autosomal dominant pattern of inheritance is mandibulofacial dysostosis. The gametes of an affected individual are equally likely to carry the deleterious or the normal allele to the next generation. Therefore, one can expect that 50 per cent of the offspring of such an affected individual will show the same trait. A family history shows that transmission is from an affected parent to affected offspring, generation by generation, without regard to sex of the affected individuals. Unaffected sibs of the patient rarely, if ever, have affected children.

Autosomal Recessive

If the allele for a detrimental effect does not express itself when present in a single dose, it is said to be recessive to the allele for normal development. An individual must then have two alleles for the detrimental effect at that locus before a clinical picture is seen. This type of inheritance is termed autosomal recessive. Many of the hereditary types of hearing loss as well as most of the inborn errors of metabolism are inherited as autosomal recessives; that is, the individual is homozygous for the detrimental allele and this allele is recessive to the normal allele. A family history of these diseases usually shows neither parent with the clinical disease, although in fact each one does carry one gene for the trait and is classified as a *carrier*. Parents are usually unaware that they each carry a recessive gene for the same trait until a child is born with the disease. After such an event there is a 25 per cent risk of recurrence of the disease with each subsequent pregnancy without regard to the sex of the offspring. When one reviews the medical history of the family for several generations there is usually no indication of the presence of this gene on either side. Because the frequencies of such detrimental genes in the population are usually quite low, the chance that a carrier will marry another carrier is small. When the partners of a marriage are related to each other, i.e., a consanguineous mating, the chance of having detrimental genes in common is greater.

SEX-LINKED RECESSIVE. A third common inheritance pattern is termed sex-linked recessive. In this case the recessive gene is located on the X-chromosome. As far as we are able to determine the Y-chromosome carries no homologous genes. If a detrimental recessive gene is present on an X-chromosome in a female, it is usually clinically masked by the "normal" allele on the homologous X. However, in a *hemizygous* male with no homologous X-chromosome, the presence of the one sex-linked recessive gene will produce a clinical picture. In this type of inheritance pattern, one usually finds only males affected, with transmission through a carrier female. On the average, one half of the sons of a carrier female will be affected. Hemophilia is a classic example of a disease that is transmitted by a sex-linked recessive gene.

With the rapid development of new laboratory and diagnostic techniques, especially in the areas of biochemical genetics and cytogenetics, the classic definition of some common genetic terms used to describe various phenomena may need to be refined. There are now a number of recessive diseases in which the carrier individuals, usually showing no demonstrable clinical features of the disease, can be identified. These individuals may show some abnormal response to a stress situation. With this ability to identify the recessive heterozygous genotype it may be necessary to revise the definitions of dominant and recessive. At this time these terms are used with respect to how the genotype is clinically expressed in a normal environmental situation.

Forms of Genetic Action

Other terms which are often used to describe observed genetic action are as follows:

Penetrance. It has been observed, especially in diseases that have a dominant inheritance pattern, that an individual who must carry the gene does not develop a clinical phenotype. These unaffected individuals usually have an affected parent and affected sibs, as well as affected children, so that the gene has been transmitted through an individual who did not show the disease. This phenomenon is referred to as lack of penetrance. In some cases the degree of penetrance, expressed as a percentage, has been calculated. Penetrance then refers to an all-or-nothing situation with regard to the clinical expression of a genotype.

Expressivity. There are a number of diseases or syndromes that show several often unrelated clinical symptoms. It has been noted that two individuals with the same clinical diagnosis do not show exactly the same expression of the clinical features. This situation has been observed in single families in which the various affected members may show a rather wide variation in expression of the clinical features of the disease. For example, in the disease osteogenesis imperfecta, four major clinical symptoms may appear: fragile bones, blue sclerae, deafness and loose ligaments. Although this disease is due to a single dominant gene, the expression of these four symptoms in any affected individual may vary with regard to which are present, as well as the degree of severity for each symptom. Thus, expressivity denotes variation in the expression of the symptoms of a disease within an affected individual.

Age of Onset. Although the genotype of an individual is established at the time of fertilization, the genes may express themselves at different times during the life of the individual. Many genetic diseases are clearly diagnosable at the time of birth, but there are also a large number that show no clinical manifestation until much later. Huntington's chorea is a good example of this situation. Although in some cases the onset of this autosomal dominant disease has been in early childhood or in the seventies, these extremes are rare exceptions.

The usual age of onset and clinical diagnosis is 40 ± 10 years of age. In attempting to determine whether a patient has a genetic disease, the usual age of onset of that disease must be borne in mind.

Genetic Heterogeneity. There are a number of genetic diseases that appear to be the result of mutations at different gene loci, but nevertheless produce the same general clinical picture. Retinitis pigmentosa is an example of such genetic heterogeneity. The medical and genetic literature clearly demonstrates that this genetic disease may be inherited as an autosomal recessive, autosomal dominant or sex-linked recessive. In this situation it is important that an accurate family history be obtained so that the pattern of inheritance can be established. The family history is most important in determining the prognosis for other family members.

Sex Ratio. In some diseases the ratio of affected males to females is consistently divergent from unity. Although an aberrant sex ratio might indicate that the gene in question is located on the X-chromosome, other explanations may be possible. The sexual constitution of the individual has broad influence on the development and function of many tissues and organs; thus, an unusual sex ratio may occur. For example, an abnormal sex ratio occurs in the congenital malformation cleft lip with or without cleft palate, in which approximately twice as many males are affected as females. Possible explanations for this phenomenon may be that one sex is more susceptible than the other or that one affected sex is more likely to survive to term than the other.

In attempting to evaluate the genetic factors involved in any disease or anomaly all factors must be considered before ruling out a genetic etiology. When a patient is an isolated case of a known or possible new disease or syndrome, the physician should consider not only the possibility of a recessive inheritance pattern but also the possibility that the patient may represent a new mutation.

Quantitative Traits

Thus far we have been dealing with clear-cut hereditary patterns in which the individuals fall into one, two or three clinical categories with little or no diagnostic problem. Unfortunately many of the most interesting and complex traits do not fit the simple patterns of inheritance. Traits which show a continuous series of variations, e.g., intelligence, height, weight, are called quantitative traits. In dealing with these quantitative traits it is difficult to determine the degree to which the genetic and environmental forces contribute to the phenotype, at least with the methods of measurement now available. From the genetic point of view, the primary difficulty appears to be that these traits are not caused by a single gene, but may involve several pairs of alleles at different loci and on different chromosomes. It is usually assumed that the genetic factor in the etiology is composed of many genes having small, similar and cumulative effects. The environmental factors acting on this genotype produce more of the phenotypic variation observed in the population than is the case with single gene traits. This pattern of inheritance has been variously termed *multifactorial, polygenic* or *quantitative*.

GENETIC COUNSELING

Genetic counseling is an attempt to provide a patient or his family with an understanding of the hereditary factors involved in a particular disease. Such counseling should be available to all patients and their families who are concerned about the transmission of an anomaly from generation to generation. Whether the physician involved with this patient does the genetic counseling or whether he refers the patient to a genetic counseling service depends on several factors.

Good genetic counseling requires:

1. As accurate a diagnosis of the patient as it is possible to obtain, including all special diagnostic procedures available, such as biochemical or cytogenetic evaluation.

2. A complete medical history of the family encompassing not only the patient but his sibs, parents, nieces, nephews, aunts, uncles, first cousins and grandparents. The history should include specific medical information on other affected or suspected family members, and this information should be confirmed by medical or other records.

3. An evaluation of the acquired information in view of what has been reported in the literature.

4. A basic knowledge of genetics and specific knowledge of the genetic factors involved in the disease or trait in question.

5. The time, the ability, and the interest to discuss with the family the genetic factors involved in the causation of the disease under discussion in a manner which will make this

information comprehensible. Counseling without understanding on the part of the patient is pointless.

6. Information concerning community sources, such as family planning clinics, mental health center, educational resources, and so forth, which are available to the family.

Because each case differs as to the time and effort necessary to provide genetic counseling, it may not always be possible for one person to fulfill all the requirements listed. Consequently, genetic counseling is often the result of a team approach, utilizing multiple services available within the community and working under the overall direction of the physician. In this instance, the question of who does the final genetic counseling with the family should depend on which member of the team has established the best rapport. This may be the referring physician or may very well be the geneticist, the nurse or the social worker.

Because a great many anomalies are environmentally caused or do not appear to have a genetic etiology, many couples or patients can be reassured that subsequent children will not be affected. However, when the risk of recurrence is 25 to 50 per cent, a patient is entitled to knowledge of this risk. It is the purpose of genetic counseling to provide patients and their families with accurate, understandable information concerning reproductive outcome and to help them to reach responsible decisions with regard to reproduction.

CONCLUSION

Because a large number of patients seen by the otolaryngologist have multiple abnormalities involving other tissues or organs, it is important that the physician view the total clinical picture when attempting to evaluate the genetic etiology of the disease or syndrome. In many instances a family history going back several generations can be most helpful. Although the field of medical genetics is relatively young, advances are being made in technology and in the understanding of the biochemical basis of gene action. Few practicing physicians, however, have received more than a cursory view of genetics during their academic years and most, because of the pressure of practice, have had little opportunity to keep abreast of new developments. Therefore, when the genetic aspects of the disease under study are being considered either to aid in the establishment of diagnosis or to provide genetic counseling to the patient and his family, reference should be made to published material or to a genetic counseling and evaluation center.

REFERENCES

Brown, K. S.: The genetics of childhood deafness. *In* McConnell, F., and Ward, P. H. (ed.): Deafness in Childhood. Nashville, Tenn., Vanderbilt University Press, 1967.

Gorlin, R. J., and Pindborg, J. J.: Syndromes of the Head and Neck. New York, McGraw-Hill Book Company, 1964.

Konigsmark, B. W.: Hereditary deafness in man. New Eng. J. Med. *281*(13):713–720, 1969.

Lynch, H. T., and Bergsma, D. (ed.): International Directory of Genetic Services. 2nd. ed. New York, The National Foundation, Inc., 1969.

McKusick, V. A.: Mendelian Inheritance in Man. 2nd. ed. Balt more, Johns Hopkins Press, 1968.

McKusick, V. A.: Human Genetics. 2nd. ed. Englewood Cliffs, New Jersey, Prentice-Hall, Inc., 1969.

Sorsby, A.: Clinical Genetics. 2nd. ed. London, Butterworth & Co., Ltd., 1971.

Thompson, J. S., and Thompson, M. W.: Genetics in Medicine. Philadelphia, W. B. Saunders Company, 1966.

Chapter 32

HEAD AND NECK SYNDROMES

by Robert J. Gorlin, D.D.S.

In a text such as this only a few of the more common syndromes of the head and neck may be considered, since their number is legion. Syndromes of deafness are reviewed elsewhere. The reader who desires amplification of material presented here or information on syndromes not considered in these pages is referred to texts devoted exclusively toward that end, such as those of Leiber and Olbrich (1966), Gorlin and Pindborg (1964), McKusick (1968), Becker (1964-1968), Gellis and Finegold (1968), Smith (1970) and Goodman and Gorlin (1970). The Birth Defects Original Article Series (1969-1972) is an incomparable source of information concerning new and unusual disorders.

ACROCEPHALOSYNDACTYLY

(Apert's Syndrome)

Acrocephalosyndactyly is a rare variant among the craniostenoses, characterized by (1) oxycephaly (acrocephaly) and (2) syndactyly of hands and feet. The syndrome was mentioned as early as 1942 by Baumgartner, though eponymic credit is given to Apert for his presentation of the syndrome in 1906. In 1938 Valentin thoroughly reviewed 93 cases from the literature, and in 1960 Blank established distinct criteria for the syndrome and estimated the incidence to be 1 in 160,000 live births, with an equal distribution between sexes. Because of the high infant mortality, he found the frequency decreased to about 1 in 2,000,000 in the general population. Over 150 cases have been reported.

The majority of cases of acrocephalosyndac-

tyly are sporadic. The syndrome may be transmitted by an autosomal dominant gene. Chromosomal studies have revealed a normal complement without evidence of gross chromosomal abnormality. An advanced paternal age effect has been demonstrated.

The middle third of the face appears flat and underdeveloped, producing a relative prognathism. The nose is sometimes small and somewhat parrot-shaped. Hypertelorism and strabismus are often noted. The orbits are flattened, and the eyes tend to be proptosed. A horizontal groove extends across the forehead just above the supraorbital ridges in some cases.

The cranium has a characteristic oxycephalic appearance. It is ovoid and brachycephalic, with a high, prominent, steep forehead. The frontal and temporal areas bulge. The apex of the cranium is located near or anterior to the bregma, the occipital region being flat and in the same vertical place as the neck. A number of patients possess an open anterior fontanel which, at times, continues to an open frontal suture. There is irregular early obliteration of cranial sutures. Roentgenographically the fusion of the coronal suture is most often found, alone or together with fusion of the sagittal suture. Marked accentuation of digital markings is usually observed. The majority of affected patients have an intelligence distinctly below normal.

The symmetrical syndactyly varies in the degree from partial fusion of the skin to a true progressive osseous syndactyly of metacarpals, metatarsals, and phalanges. When the three middle fingers are completely fused, there is often a common nail that gives the hand the appearance of a mitten (middigital hand mass).

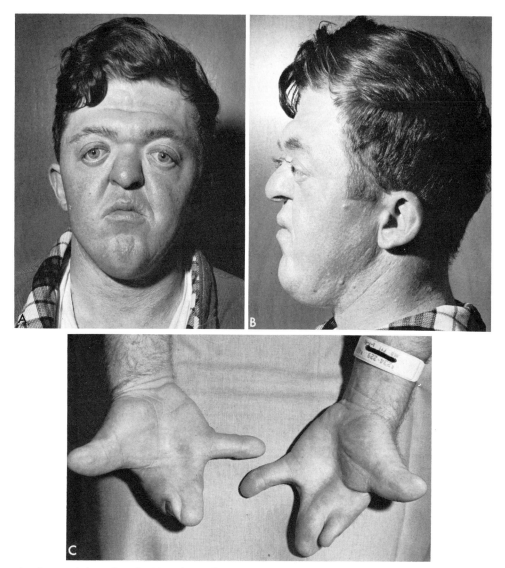

Figure 1. Acrocephalosyndactyly (Apert's syndrome). *A*, Twenty-eight-year-old male with ocular hypertelorism, antimongoloid obliquity of palpebral fissures. *B*, Note pronounced supraorbital ridges, exophthalmos, midfacial hypoplasia, beaked nose and low-set ears. *C*, Middigital hand mass due to fusion of second, third and fourth digits.

Illustration continued on opposite page.

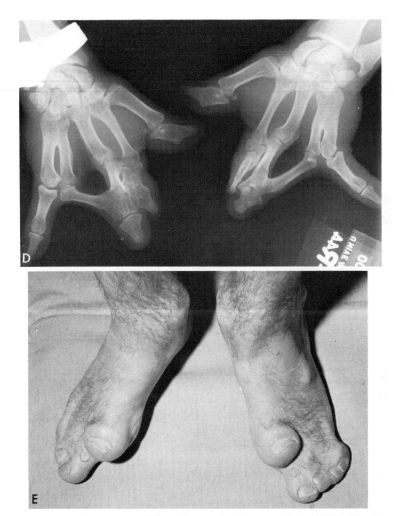

Figure 1. *Continued. D*, Roentgenogram exhibiting fusion of phalanges within middigital hand mass, proximal fusion of fourth and fifth metacarpals, absence of proximal phalanx of thumb and middle phalanx of fifth fingers. *E*, Hypoplasia of halluces, syndactyly of second through fifth toes. (Courtesy of John Opitz, Madison, Wisconsin.)

Other skeletal abnormalities have been noted: aplasia or ankylosis of several joints, especially elbow, shoulder and hip, ankylosis of vertebrae, and spina bifida.

Frequently observed is a high-arched palate with a marked median furrow. Posterior cleft palate or bifid uvula is found in at least 25 per cent of these patients. Associated with hypoplastic maxilla is relative mandibular prognathism and compression of the upper arcade, which becomes V-shaped, leading to an irregular positioning of the teeth. Crowding of the teeth may lead to a marked thickening of the alveolar process. The pointed arcade may cause protrusion of the middle portion of the upper lip.

CRANIOFACIAL DYSOSTOSIS

(Crouzon's Syndrome)

Crouzon's syndrome is characterized by: (1) cranial synostotic malformations, (2) bilateral exophthalmus with external strabismus, (3) parrot-beaked nose, and (4) relative mandibular prognathism with drooping lower lip.

The syndrome is inherited as an autosomal dominant trait without complete penetrance. Not uncommonly sporadic cases have been reported, i.e., with a negative genetic history, thus representing new mutations.

The facies is easily recognized; it is characterized by marked exophthalmus, ocular hypertelorism, and hypoplastic maxilla. This last feature produces a marked relative mandibular prognathism and short upper lip. The cranium is brachycephalic, with frontal bossing and ridging of the sagittal suture. Roentgenographically the coronal, sagittal, and lambdoidal sutures are prematurely synostosed. Increased digital markings are almost always present.

Exophthalmus is a constant feature, probably being due to shallow orbits. At times there is spontaneous luxation of the globes. Eighty per cent of affected individuals have optic nerve damage. Nystagmus and mental retardation are seen occasionally.

Oral manifestations include hypoplastic maxilla, a V-shaped palatal arch in contrast to the normal U-shaped form, dental malocclusion and, rarely, clefting of the palate.

CLEIDOCRANIAL DYSOSTOSIS

The syndrome was probably first described by the poet Homer. Accurate descriptions were made by Scheuthauer in 1871 and by Marie and Sainton in 1897. Cleidocranial dysostosis is transmitted as an autosomal dominant trait, although in less than one half the patients it arises spontaneously, perhaps as a result of mutation or of a gene with poor penetrance.

Individuals with the syndrome are short in stature and have long necks and narrow shoulders. The face appears small, the nasal bridge is depressed, and the nose is broad at the base.

The skull is brachycephalic, with marked frontal, parietal, and occipital bossing. Fontanels and sutures remain open, often for life. Wormian bones are formed through secondary centers of ossification in the suture lines.

The clavicles may be unilaterally or bilaterally aplastic or hypoplastic, generally at their acromial end. Because of this bony defect patients with the condition are able to approximate their shoulders in front of the chest.

Other observed bony anomalies include congenital dislocation of the hip, underdevelopment of the pelvis, coxa vara or coxa valga, genu valgum, scoliosis, kyphosis, and cervical ribs.

Several oral manifestations are present in the syndrome, such as supernumerary teeth and hypoplastic maxilla. The so-called pseudonanodontia is the result of delayed eruption and impaction of deciduous, permanent, and supernumerary teeth. Probably the most prominent oral manifestation is the number of supernumerary teeth present, which at times simulates a third dentition.

The paranasal sinuses are often underdeveloped or absent. The mastoids are usually not pneumatized because of altered function of the sternocleidomastoid muscles.

MANDIBULOFACIAL DYSOSTOSIS

(Treacher Collins Syndrome, Franceschetti-Zwahlen-Klein Syndrome)

Treacher Collins (name often erroneously hyphenated) described the essential components of the syndrome. Franceschetti and coworkers during the 1940's published extensive reviews of this syndrome, employing the name mandibulofacial dysostosis.

It is inherited as an autosomal dominant with incomplete penetrance and variable expressivity. About 300 cases have been described to date.

The facial appearance is quite characteristic. The sloping palpebral fissures, sunken cheek

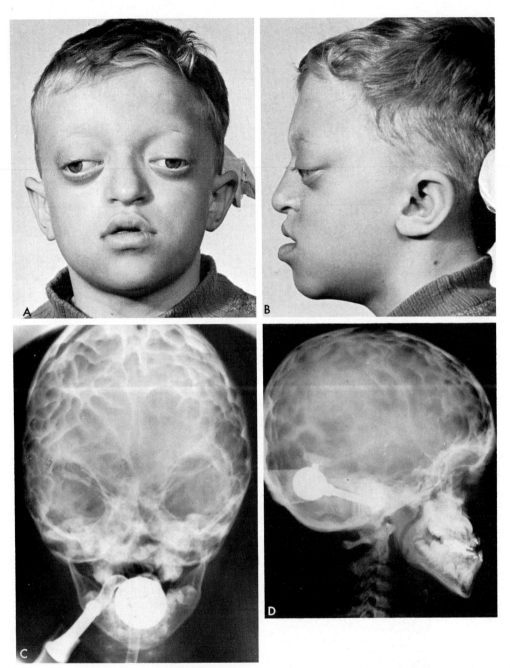

Figure 2. Craniofacial dysostosis (Crouzon's disease). *A*, Ocular hypertelorism, exophthalmos, strabismus evident. *B*, Midfacial hypoplasia. *C* and *D*, Note shortening of anteroposterior diameter of skull and marked digital impressions.

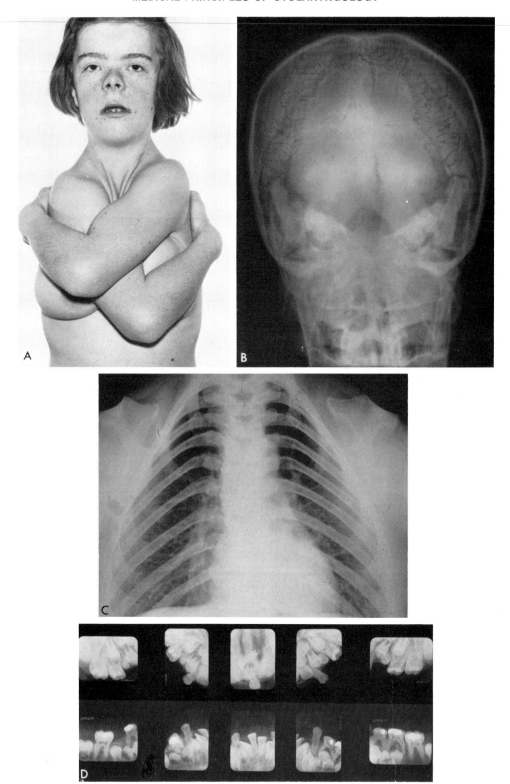

Figure 3. Cleidocranial dysostosis. *A*, Ocular hypertelorism. Note patient's attempt to approximate the shoulders. *B*, Numerous Wormian bones found in lambdoidal sutures. *C*, Note complete bilateral aplasia of clavicles. *D*, Roentgenogram of jaws exhibits numerous supernumerary teeth. Often, many teeth fail to erupt. (*A* from M. Fons, Acta Otolaryngologica *67*:483, 1969. *B* to *D*, from R. J. Gorlin and J. J. Pindborg, Syndromes of the Head and Neck, McGraw-Hill, 1964, New York.)

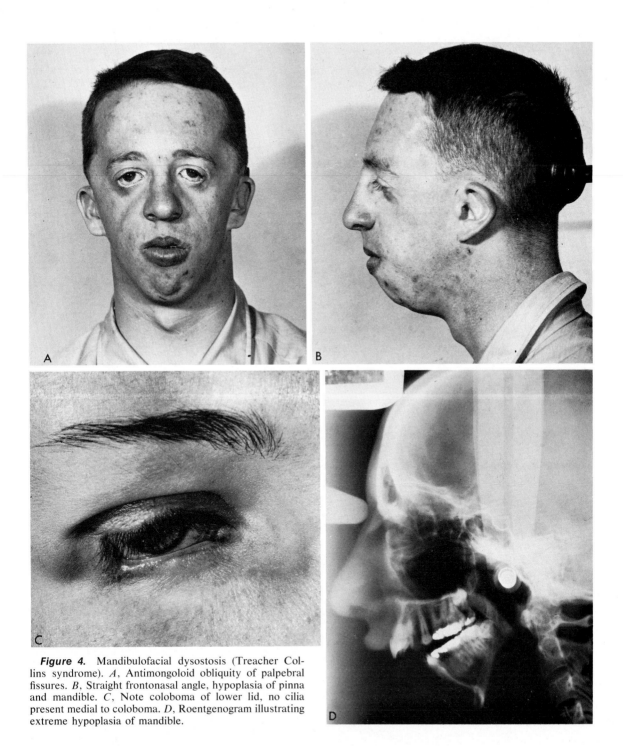

Figure 4. Mandibulofacial dysostosis (Treacher Collins syndrome). *A*, Antimongoloid obliquity of palpebral fissures. *B*, Straight frontonasal angle, hypoplasia of pinna and mandible. *C*, Note coloboma of lower lid, no cilia present medial to coloboma. *D*, Roentgenogram illustrating extreme hypoplasia of mandible.

bones, deformed pinna, receding chin, and large fishlike mouth present a clinical picture that once seen is unforgettable.

The supra-orbital ridges are poorly developed, and often there are increased digital markings. The body of the malar bones may be totally absent, but more often they are grossly and symmetrically underdeveloped, with non-fusion of the zygomatic arches. The mastoids are not pneumatized and are frequently sclerotic. The paranasal sinuses are often small and may be completely absent. The lower margin of the orbit is noted to be defective.

The palpebral fissures slope laterally downward (antimongoloid obliquity) and often (about 75 per cent) there is a coloboma in the outer third of the lower lid. About one half of the patients have a deficiency of cilia medial to the coloboma.

The pinna is often deformed, crumpled forward, or misplaced. Over one third have absence of the external auditory canal or an ossicle defect accompanied by deafness. Roentgenographic studies have shown sclerosis of the middle and inner ears with poor delineation of their structure. Extra ear tags and blind fistulas may occur anywhere between the tragus and the angle of the mouth.

The nasal-frontal angle is usually obliterated and the bridge of the nose raised. The nose appears large because of the lack of malar development. The nares are often narrow and the alar cartilages hypoplastic.

The mandible is almost always hypoplastic. Roentgenographic studies have shown that the angle is more obtuse than normal and that the ramus may be deficient. The undersurface of the body of the mandible is often pronouncedly concave. The coronoid and condyloid processes are flat or even aplastic. The palate is noted to be cleft in about 30 per cent of the cases we have reviewed.

OCULOMANDIBULODYSCEPHALY WITH HYPOTRICHOSIS

(Hallermann-Streiff Syndrome)

The syndrome consists of (1) dyscephaly, (2) parrot nose, (3) mandibular hypoplasia, (4) proportionate nanism, (5) hypotrichosis, and (6) bilateral congenital cataracts.

There appears to be no genetic basis for this syndrome.

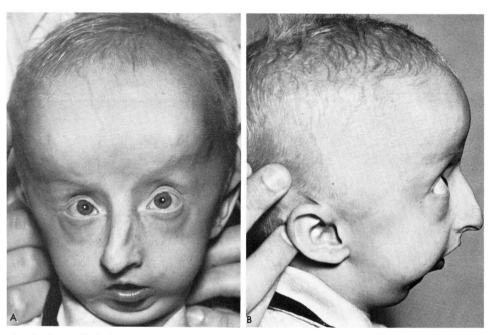

Figure 5. Oculomandibulodyscephaly (Hallermann-Streiff syndrome). *A*, Exophthalmos, strabismus, infantile cataracts. *B*, Low-set ears, severe micrognathia. Mandibular condyle is separated from ear canal by block of bone. (*A*, Courtesy of D. Hoefnagel, Hanover, N. H. *B*, from Hoefnagel, D., and Benirschke, K.: Arch. Dis. Child. *40*:57–61, 1965.)

The face is small, with a characteristic parrot-nose, receding chin, and brachycephaly (rarely scaphocephaly or microcephaly). Open fontanels and gaping of the longitudinal and lambdoidal sutures are frequent findings.

Ocular anomalies include microphthalmia, blue sclerae, and b lateral congenital cataracts that often rupture spontaneously and resorb. The majority of patients have been noted to manifest nystagmus or strabismus.

The nose is thin, pointed, and curved and, combined with the mandibular hypoplasia, gives the individual a parrotlike appearance. Hypotrichosis, especially of the scalp, brows, and cilia, is a constant feature. Axillary and pubic hair are also scant. Alopecia is most prominent in the frontal and occipital areas.

Other associated findings include osteoporosis, cutaneous atrophy, lordosis or scoliosis, and spina bifida.

The most common oral finding is hypop asia of the mandible, generally accompanied by a "double" cutaneous chin with a central cleft or dimple. Roentgenograms of the temporomandibular joint area show the joint to be displaced approximately 2 cm. forward. The palate is high and narrow, and the mouth is usually stated to be small. Dental anomalies, such as malocclusion, malformation of teeth, and natal teeth commonly occur.

OSTEOGENESIS IMPERFECTA AND DENTINOGENESIS IMPERFECTA, CLEAR (BLUE) SCLERAE, OTOSCLEROSIS, AND LOOSE LIGAMENTS

The syndrome consists of: (1) fragile bones, (2) clear or blue sclerae, (3) deafness, (4) loose ligaments, and (5) a dentinogenesis imperfecta-like alteration.

The syndrome is inherited as an autosomal dominant trait. However, only about one third of affected patients present a familial history of the condition. The remaining two thirds comprise largely sporadic cases and, rarely, patients with family pedigrees that possibly suggest autosomal recessive inheritance. Those having a family history are inclined to have the disease in a milder form and to manifest it later in life. Only about one in three patients presents the complete syndrome.

The degree of expressivity is variable. Of patients having blue sclerae, about 60 per cent have the bone disease and possibly only about 30 per cent have otosclerosis.

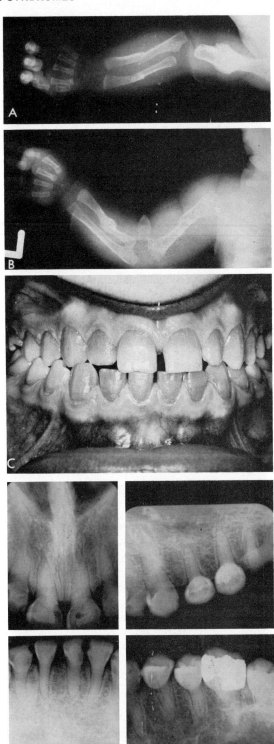

Figure 6. Osteogenesis imperfecta. *A*, Note micromelia. Child had multiple intrauterine fractures, blue sclerae. *B*, Multiple fractures and calluses of long bones. *C*, Opalescent teeth. *D*, Note reduced size of roots, obliteration of root canals. (*A*, *B* and *D* from Gorlin, R. J., and Pindborg, J. J., Syndromes of the Head and Neck. New York, McGraw-Hill Book Co., Inc., 1964.)

In the congenital type of osteogenesis imperfecta, intrauterine fractures may be so numerous that the child may be born dead or may survive for only a short time. Micromelia is often quite striking.

The skull is large, especially in the anteroposterior direction. The forehead is broad and bossed, with a temporal bulge and an overhanging occiput giving the skull a "mushroom" appearance. Roentgenographic examination reveals remarkably thin calvaria and the presence of numerous wormian bones in the occipital area.

The long bones, especially those of the legs, are bowed. Subperiosteal fractures of the shaft and multiple microfractures at the epiphyses are often seen, as well as kyphoscoliosis and pectus carinatum and excavatum. Laxity of ligaments, resulting in habitual dislocations of joints and flatfoot, is not uncommon, being seen in at least 25 per cent of affected individuals.

Clear (blue) sclerae are the most constant feature of the syndrome. The intensity of blueness varies from family to family and from patient to patient. The blue color is apparently due, in part, to thinning of the sclerae, which allows the choroid color to be transmitted, and also to increased translucency related to a thinner fibrous coat, a deficiency in collagen fibers, or an increase in mucopolysaccharide content.

Deafness is one of the more frequent findings, usually beginning in the third decade and increasing progressively with time; it is otosclerotic in nature. Fewer than one half the patients with the heritable form of osteogenesis imperfecta are deaf, while only 20 per cent of those without a familial history are so affected. Rarely is complete deafness observed, but hearing appears to be more severely impaired in patients with serious bone involvement. In some patients the tympanic membrane has been found to be thinned and bluish in color.

The deciduous teeth are affected in about 80 per cent of the patients, the permanent teeth in only about 35 per cent. There does not appear to be any relationship of dentin impairment to the degree of bone involvement. The crown of the tooth is usually vertically smaller than normal. Upon eruption the teeth are noted to be translucent or opalescent. The color darkens with age, becoming gray, pink, amber, or bluish. The enamel, while clinically normal, usually cracks off. Roentgenographically the roots are thin, fine, and disproportionately shortened. The pulp chamber and canal are greatly diminished in size or even totally absent.

CRANIOMETAPHYSEAL DYSPLASIA AND CRANIODIAPHYSEAL DYSPLASIA

Buried under various designations such as leontiasis ossea and osteopetrosis, craniometaphyseal dysplasia consists of (1) alterations in the metaphyses of long bones somewhat similar to those seen in metaphyseal dysplasia (Pyle's disease), i.e., increased diaphyseal density and widened metaphyses with reduced density; and (2) bony overgrowth of the face and jaws, especially evident in the paranasal areas.

The condition may be transmitted as an autosomal recessive trait, but is more often inherited as a dominant trait. Comprehensive reviews are those of Jackson et al. (1954), Spranger et al. (1965), Graf (1965), Millard (1967) and Gorlin et al. (1969).

A head which appears rather large, with an extremely broad and flat nasal bridge, ocular hypertelorism, and open mouth, gives the patient a vacuous expression. The mouth is kept open because of nasal blockage. Blindness resulting from optic atrophy in early infancy is not uncommon in the recessive form. Ocular hypertelorism has been a relatively constant finding.

Generalized late motor development has been usual in this syndrome. Several patients have shown marked mental retardation, headache, vomiting, and irritability. Facial nerve paralysis and deafness have also been common features, presumably the result of overgrowth of the foramina.

Soon after birth the skull exhibits marked thickening and increased density of the vault, with elimination of the diploë, especially in the frontal and occipital areas. The paranasal sinuses are similarly obliterated. The bones of the skull base, the maxilla, and the mandible also become enlarged, thickened, and increased in density.

The long bones, especially the femurs, assume an "Erlenmeyer flask" shape in the metaphyseal area, with decreased density. The diaphyseal area is increased in density, the medullary bone being porotic and lacking the usual trabecular pattern. Similar changes are seen in the metacarpals and phalanges.

The blood count and serum calcium, phosphorus, and alkaline phosphatase are normal and may be used to exclude several entities.

What appears to be a different disease, yet having several facets in common with craniometaphyseal dysplasia, is what we should like to call craniodiaphyseal dysplasia. Examples of

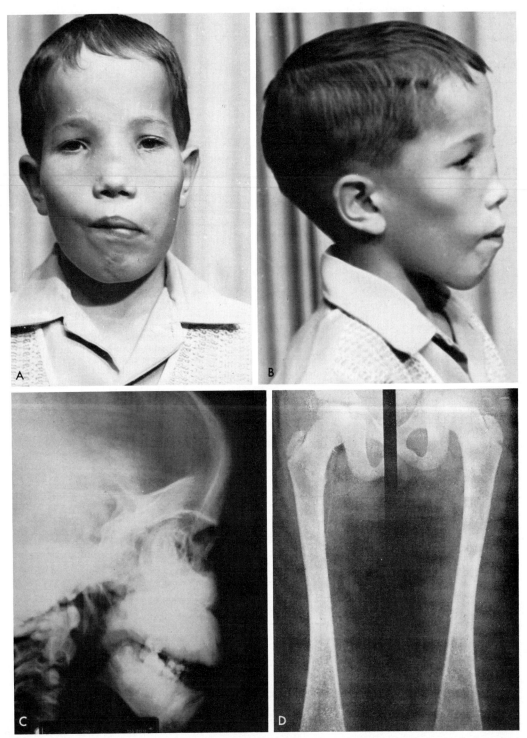

Figure 7. Craniometaphyseal dysplasia. *A* and *B*, Characteristic facies exhibiting ocular hypertelorism, elimination of frontonasal angle, marked broadening of nasal bridge and left lower facial paralysis. *C*, Note block of bone in nasal area. *D*, Roentgenograms illustrating flaring of metaphyseal region of femora.

this condition are illustrated in the cases of Halliday (1949-1950), Joseph et al. (1958) and Stransky (1962). It is much more severe, producing marked facial distortion and severe mental retardation. The disorder is inherited as an autosomal recessive trait. The parents of the child described by Halliday were first cousins. Nasal obstruction and facial alteration are noticeable within the first few years. Vision fails by the seventh or eighth year.

There is marked sclerosis of the calvaria and facial bones, and the paranasal sinuses are overgrown. The ribs are widened and extremely dense, the clavicles being most severely involved and thickened in the midportions. The vertebrae, for the most part, are not involved. The long bones are straight, with a thin cortex and a remarkably uniform thickness of the shaft. In the metacarpals and metatarsals similar changes are seen. There is some degree of ballooning of the midportion of the shaft. The cortex is thinner than normal except for the first metacarpal, which shows some osteosclerosis.

PYCNODYSOSTOSIS

Pycnodysostosis has been defined as a syndrome consisting of (1) dwarfism, (2) osteopetrosis, (3) partial agenesis of the terminal digits of the hands and feet, (4) cranial anomalies, such as persistence of fontanels and failure of closure of cranial sutures, (5) frontal and occipital bossing, and (6) hypoplasia of the angle of the mandible.

In a recent survey of the literature Sedano and Gorlin (1968) found a total of 75 cases in 53 families. It is inherited as an autosomal recessive trait. The consanguinity rate among the parents of the affected patients was 36 per cent. There is good evidence to suggest that Toulouse-Lautrec had this disease.

The adult height is reduced, being 53 to 60 inches in most cases. The terminal digits of the fingers and toes may present a drumstick appearance.

Increased bone density is responsible for multiple fractures in these patients, but this peculiarity tends to disappear after puberty.

The head is rather large because of frontal and occipital bulging, and the chin recedes. Parrotlike nose is a constant finding, as is agenesis of the angle of the mandible. Facial bones are usually underdeveloped, with pseudoprognathism.

The skull is dolichocephalic, with frontal and occipital bossing. Most cranial sutures and fontanels are open, especially the parieto-occipital. Wormian bones are commonly observed.

The frontal sinuses are consistently absent and the other paranasal sinuses are hypoplastic or missing. The mastoid air cells are often not pneumatized.

There is increased radiopacity of all bones, but especially of the long bones, spine, and skull base. The terminal digits of the fingers and toes are markedly hypoplastic, exhibiting fragmentation of the heads with preservation of the bases, underdevelopment of the unguiculate processes, or narrowing of the ends of otherwise normal terminal phalanges.

THE ORAL-FACIAL-DIGITAL (OFD-I) SYNDROME

The syndrome of (1) multiple hyperplastic frenula, (2) cleft tongue, (3) dystopia canthorum, (4) hypoplasia of nasal alar cartilages, (5) median cleft of the upper lip, (6) asymmetric cleft palate, (7) various digital malformations, and (8) mild mental retardation was first defined by Papillon-Leage and Psaume in 1954. Similar cases had been reported earlier under various names.

The OFD-I syndrome is inherited as an X-linked dominant trait limited to females and lethal in males (Gorlin and Psaume, 1962; Fuhrmann et al., 1966; Gorlin, 1968).

The facies is characteristic, presenting lateral displacement of the inner canthi, hypoplasia of the alar cartilages and broad nasal root. The upper lip is short, presenting a pseudocleft in the midline.

Evanescent milia of the face and ears are common, but they disappear before three years of age. Dryness and/or alopecia of the scalp is present in about 65 per cent of affected individuals.

Several digital malformations are associated with the syndrome, such as clinodactyly, syndactyly, and brachydactyly in decreasing order of frequency. Toe malformations are less common and include unilateral hallucal polysyndactyly, variable syndactyly, and brachydactyly. Roentgenograms of hands and feet show the short tubular bones to be shorter and thicker than normal, with some degree of osteoporosis. The cranial base angle (nasion-sella-basion) is increased, being about 140 degrees (normal value, 131 degrees).

One third to one half of the patients are mentally mildly retarded (IQ, 70 to 90). Rarely mental retardation is severe and there may be hydrocephalus or porencephaly.

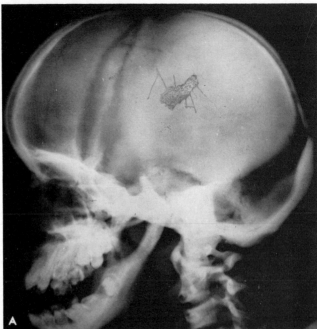

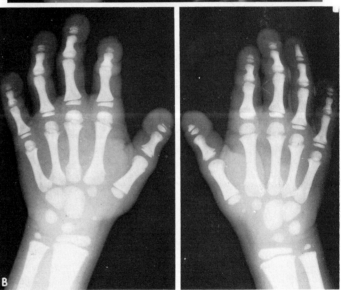

Figure 8. Pycnodysostosis. *A*, Open sutures, especially lambdoidal, absence of mandibular angle. *B*, Increased density of bone, dysplasia of terminal phalanges.

Oral manifestations include a thick hyperplastic upper central frenum which, in part, eradicates the mucobuccal fold in the area. The frenum also extends through the upper lip beyond the vermilion border, producing a small midline "cleft." Lateral clefts of the palate are produced by bilateral grooves arising from the maxillary buccal frenula. The palate is then divided into an anterior segment (behind the canines) and two posterior processes. The soft palate often presents a complete asymmetric cleft.

The lower mucobuccal fold is traversed by thick fibrous bands, especially in the region of the lower lateral incisors, which produce clefting of the alveolar process and, by extension, bi-, tri-, or tetrafurcation of the tongue.

About 50 per cent of patients present a small, whitish hamartoma between the lobes of the divided tongue. This mass is formed by fibrous connective tissue, salivary gland tissue, a few striated muscle fibers and, rarely, cartilage. One third of the patients may present ankyloglossia.

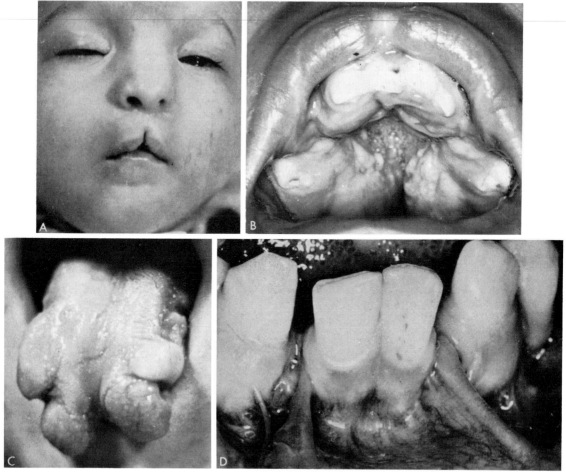

Figure 9. Oral-facial-digital syndrome I. *A*, Pseudocleft in middle of upper lip, one nostril smaller. *B*, Note lateral clefts in premolar area. Patient had asymmetric cleft of soft palate. *C*, Tetrafurcation of tongue. *D*, Hyperplastic frenula traverse mucobuccal fold in region of missing lower lateral incisors. (Gorlin, R. J., and Psaume, J.: J. Pediat. *61*:520–530, 1962.)

A somewhat similar syndrome (OFD-II, Mohr syndrome) is inherited as an autosomal recessive trait. These people have bilateral polysyndactyly of the halluces and manual hexadactyly (Rimoin and Edgerton, 1967).

CLEFT PALATE, SMALL DYSPLASTIC MANDIBLE, AND GLOSSOPTOSIS

(Robin's Syndrome)

The syndrome of cleft palate, small dysplastic mandible, and glossoptosis was recognized as early as 1822 by St. Hilaire. Although the syndrome is named after Robin (1923, 1934), and the corrective procedure is named for Douglas (1946, 1956), the condition and its treatment were both thoroughly described by Shukowsky in 1911.

There is no evidence of single gene inheritance for the syndrome. It probably represents arrested intrauterine development and is probably multifactorial. During the tenth to twelfth weeks in utero, the maxilla grows rapidly and, by the fourth to fifth month, the disparity between the upper and lower jaws is quite apparent. The syndrome has been produced experimentally in laboratory animals.

Congenital murmurs and/or heart disease have been observed in 15 to 20 per cent of these patients, and about an equal number have been found to have major mental retardation (Smith and Stowe, 1961).

The "Andy Gump" facies is quite distinctive. Dyspnea and periodic cyanotic attacks associated with retraction of the sternum and ribs are evident during the inspiratory phase of respiration, especially when the infant is in the supine position. The difficulty is usually noted

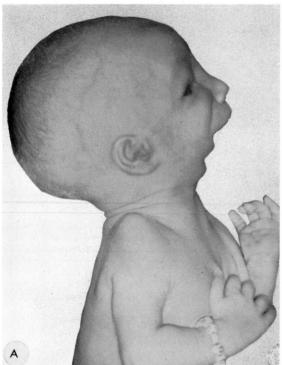

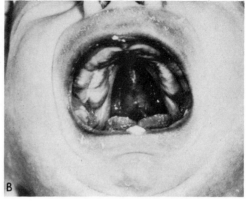

Figure 10. Robin's syndrome. *A*, Severe micrognathia leading to glossoptosis and respiratory embarrassment. *B*, Cleft of hard and soft palates.

at birth. Pruzansky and Richmond (1954) and Kiskadden and Dietrich (1953) demonstrated that if the infant survives the initial period, his subsequent mandibular growth catches up so that a normal profile is achieved by four to six years of age.

Pruzansky (1969) described the mandible as having a foreshortened body with a characteristic ratio of ramus to mandibular body length. Presumably the primary defect lies in the dysplastic growth of the mandible. This prevents the normal descent of the tongue from between the palatal shelves.

The exact physiologic mechanism by which the asphyctic episodes are produced is not known, but most investigators have suggested that the symmetrical lack of lower jaw growth prevents adequate support of lingual musculature, allowing the tongue to fall downward and backward (glossoptosis). This obstructs the epiglottis, permitting egress of air but preventing inhalation, much as a ball valve.

CLEFT LIP-PALATE AND CONGENITAL LIP FISTULAS

The syndrome of cleft lip-palate and congenital lip fistulas has been recognized for over 100 years. An extensive recent survey has been carried out by Červenka et al. (1967).

The syndrome is transmitted as an autosomal dominant trait (Van der Woude, 1954) with 80 per cent penetrance, but there is a possibility that the type of cleft present is influenced by modifying genes. The syndrome is seen with a frequency of about 1:75,000 to 1:100,000 live births and affects both sexes equally. Figures calculated on the basis of 38 pedigrees (Červenka et al., 1967) showed that affected individuals have a 22 to 40 per cent chance of having an affected child with a cleft with or without lip pits.

Usually bilateral, symmetrically located depressions are observed on the vermilion portion of the lower lip. The fistulas may be as large as 3 or more mm. in diameter or so small as to barely permit the introduction of a hair probe. The dimple may be circular or may present as a transverse slit. Rarely, they may be located at the apex of nipplelike elevations. The depressions represent blind sinuses which descend through the orbicularis oris muscles to a depth of 0.5 to 2.5 cm. and communicate with underlying minor salivary glands through their excretory ducts. These fistulas often transport a viscid saliva to the surface, either spontaneously or upon pressure (Koberg, 1966).

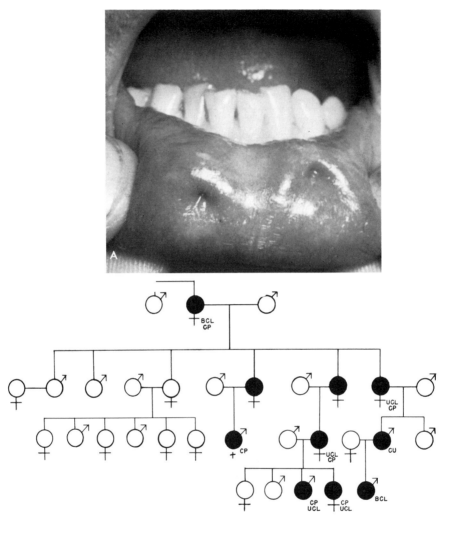

● = LIP FISTULAS
C P = CLEFT PALATE
UCL = UNILATERAL CLEFT LIP
BCL = BILATERAL CLEFT LIP
CU = CLEFT UVULA

Figure 11.   Cleft lip-palate and congenital lip fistulas. *A*, Bilateral paramedian pits of lower lip. *B*, Autosomal dominant transmission. (Gorlin, R. J., and Pindborg, J. J.: Syndromes of the Head and Neck. New York, McGraw-Hill Book Co., Inc., 1964.)

The pits may be an isolated finding (about 33 per cent) or associated with cleft lip-palate (approximately 67 per cent). When associated with lip-palate clefts, the clefts are bilateral in over 80 per cent of the patients.

A few cases have been reported in which there has been but a single pit. Adhesions between maxilla and mandible and filiform ankyloblepharon have also been noted (Gorlin and Pindborg, 1964; Červenka et al., 1967).

Warbrick et al. (1952) suggested that the congenital lip pits arose from persistence of embryonal sulci normally present in the mandibular arch of the 5 to 6 mm. embryo but disappearing by the 10 to 16 mm. stage.

Associated anomalies of the extremities have included talipes equinovarus, syndactly and popliteal pterygia. Congenital lip pits have also been seen in association with the oral-facial-digital syndrome (Gorlin and Pindborg, 1964).

MULTIPLE MUCOSAL NEUROMAS, PHEOCHROMOCYTOMA, AND MEDULLARY CARCINOMA OF THE THYROID

Pheochromocytoma may occur in combination with neurofibromatosis or with various brain tumors (cerebellar hemangioblastoma, ependymoma, astrocytoma, meningioma, spongioblastoma). A considerable number of reports have been published on the association of pheochromocytoma and multiple endocrine adenomas. Still another is the syndrome of *multiple mucosal neuromas, medullary carcinoma of the thyroid, and pheochromocytoma* (Williams and Pollack, 1966; Gorlin et al., 1968).

Pheochromocytoma, either alone or in combination with other tumors, may be inherited as an autosomal dominant trait.

The mucosal neuromas principally involve the lips and anterior tongue, although buccal, gingival, nasal, conjunctival, and laryngeal lesions have been described. Labial involvement produces a "blubbery" appearance. The oral and labial component appears first and often is evident during the first few years of life. Microscopically the mucosal nodules are plexiform neuromas.

Numerous white medullated nerve fibers traverse the cornea to anastomose in the pupillary area. They can be seen with ease under slit-lamp examination. The upper eyelid is often thickened and everted (Schimke et al., 1968).

The pheochromocytoma may produce weakness, choking and flushing, pounding headache, hypertension, palpitation, profuse sweating, and intractable diarrhea. The attacks may last from minutes to hours and may terminate in shock or death. The tumors are often (approximately 60 per cent) bilateral. They may be evident as early as puberty but, in most cases, occur before the fourth decade.

Medullary carcinoma of the thyroid, a tumor derived from cells from the ultimobranchial body, elaborates both amyloid, histaminase, and calcitonin. These cells probably originally migrated into the ultimobranchial body from the neural crest. The tumor may appear as early as the 14th year but, in most cases, will become manifest before the 35th year. In several patients it has metastasized, causing death.

Some patients have had megacolon, and others have had neurofibromatous lesions of Auerbach's and Meissner's plexuses. Most of the patients have had an asthenic build.

MULTIPLE OSTEOMAS, FIBROUS AND FATTY TUMORS OF THE SKIN AND MESENTERY, EPIDERMOID INCLUSION CYSTS OF THE SKIN, AND MULTIPLE POLYPOSIS

(Gardner's Syndrome)

This syndrome was first extensively described by Gardner and co-workers in 1953 and 1954. It is inherited as an autosomal dominant trait with rather marked penetrance and variable expressivity.

Epidermoid inclusion cysts of the skin are one of the most frequent manifestations of the syndrome. They may be present on the face, trunk, and extremities, usually appearing after puberty. Fibromas and desmoid tumors of the skin and/or mesentery also may be present, as well as lipomas and lipofibromas.

The characteristic feature of the syndrome is the presence of multiple polyposes of the colon and rectum, with a marked tendency to malignant degeneration. The polyps may be present before puberty.

Multiple osteomas may be found in the calvaria and facial skeleton. The osteomas generally precede the appearance of intestinal polyposis. Frontal bone, maxilla, and mandible are most frequently involved. Histologically the bone shows a mature appearance and well developed haversian systems. Long bones also may be the site of osteomas, but these are

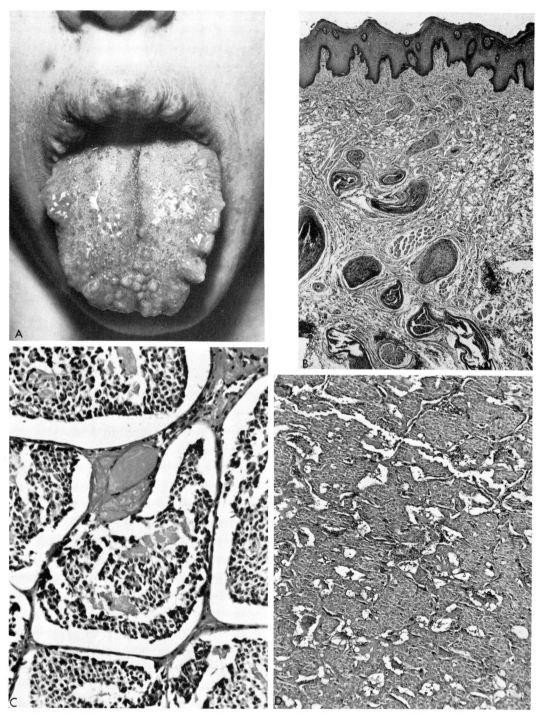

Figure 12.   Multiple mucosal neuromas, pheochromocytoma and medullary carcinoma of the thyroid. *A*, Macrocheilia; note numerous nodules on anterior tongue. *B*, Mucosal neuromas. *C*, Medullary carcinoma of thyroid, note amyloid deposits. *D*, Pheochromocytoma. (Gorlin, R. J., et al.: Cancer *22*:293–299, 1968.)

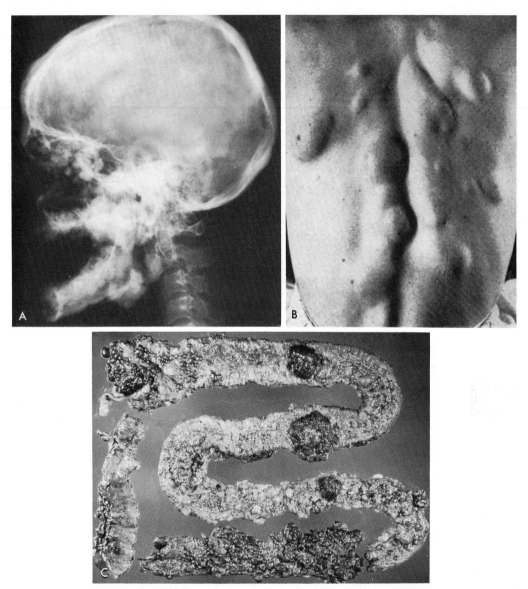

Figure 13. Gardner's syndrome. *A*, Note osteomas of mandible and paranasal sinuses. *B*, Numerous epidermoid inclusion cysts of back. *C*, Multiple polyposis of large bowel. (Gorlin, R. J., and Pindborg, J. J.: Syndromes of the Head and Neck. New York, McGraw-Hill Book Co., Inc., 1964.)

small and may mimic osteomyelitis (Gorlin and Chaudhry, 1960; Thomas et al., 1968).

Roentgenologically, besides the polyposis of the large bowel, the most striking feature is that of osteomas of the head. Radiopaque, diffuse areas can be seen throughout the calvaria, especially in the frontal and temporoparietal region. The maxilla and the mandible are involved as well. The osteomas expand and may obliterate the paranasal sinuses. They are especially common in the sphenoid and ethmoid sinuses. (It would indeed be interesting to follow up a large compendium of published case reports of "osteomas of the paranasal sinus" to see how many of them had this syndrome!)

NEVOID BASAL CELL CARCINOMA SYNDROME

The major components of the syndrome are (1) multiple nevoid basal cell carcinomas, (2) cysts of the jaws, (3) vertebra and rib anomalies, chiefly bifid rib, (4) calcification of the falx cerebri, and (5) medulloblastoma (Gorlin et al., 1965; Berlin et al., 1966).

The nevoid basal cell carcinomas generally appear in childhood or at puberty and involve the nose, eyelids, cheeks, trunk, arms, and neck. They are flesh-colored to pale brown. Microscopically they cover the wide spectrum of basal cell and adnexal carcinomas: superficial, multicentric, pigmented, adenoid, and solid. Milia are often intermixed with the skin carcinomas.

Bifurcation and/or splaying may involve more than one rib and be bilateral. Shortened fourth metacarpal, bridging of sella, calcification of the falx cerebri, spina bifida occulta in the cervicothoracic area, and kyphoscoliosis are also frequent findings.

Various associated eye anomalies have been reported: congenital cataract, glaucoma, and coloboma of the choroid and optic nerve.

The jaws show numerous cysts varying in size from microscopic to several centimeters which are lined by a uniform layer of keratinized or parakeratinized stratified squamous epithelium. They have a marked tendency to recur after surgical removal.

Medulloblastoma has been reported in several instances and, in some families, a sibling of an affected individual had died in early childhood of medulloblastoma.

The syndrome is inherited as an autosomal dominant trait, with high penetrance and variable expressivity.

MUCOCUTANEOUS MELANOTIC PIGMENTATION AND GASTROINTESTINAL POLYPOSIS

(Peutz-Jeghers Syndrome)

The most important component of the syndrome is the polyposis of the gastrointestinal tract. The polyps are hamartomatous in origin. The following sites, in order of frequency, are involved: jejunum, ileum, large bowel, rectum, stomach, duodenum, and appendix (Klostermann, 1966).

Polyps may produce intussusception and occasionally lead to severe intestinal obstruction and death. The age of onset cannot be precisely determined, but generally there is a history of gastrointestinal problems before the third decade of life.

There is no evidence that the polyps are premalignant. Some patients have had polyps of the bladder, nose, cervix, and bronchi, but this is unusual.

Fifty per cent of affected individuals exhibit discrete, brown to bluish black macules of the skin, chiefly around the oral, nasal, and orbital orifices. The number of pigmented spots varies in different patients. Pigmentation of the extremities can also be found.

The lips, especially the lower, and the buccal mucosa are involved with pigmented macules in about 98 per cent of the patients, less frequently the gingiva and palate. The melanotic spots are larger than those on the skin. The cutaneous pigmented macules tend to fade after puberty, but the intraoral pigmentation is more stable.

Granulosa-theca cell tumors have been noted in several females with the syndrome.

HYPOHIDROTIC ECTODERMAL DYSPLASIA

The major components of the syndrome are (1) hypodontia, (2) hypotrichosis, and (3) hypohidrosis. Principally affected are structures of ectodermal origin.

The syndrome is usually transmitted as an X-linked recessive trait. However, at least 30 females have manifested the complete syndrome. The increased parental consanguinity in these cases suggests autosomal recessive inheritance and illustrates the genetic heterogeneity of this syndrome (Gorlin et al., 1970). Dominant hidrotic forms of ectodermal dys-

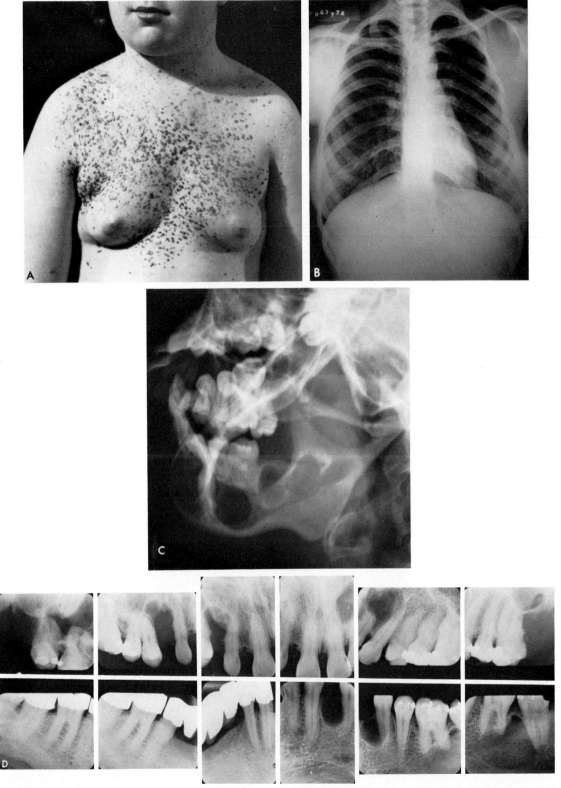

Figure 14. Nevoid basal cell carcinoma syndrome. *A*, Numerous basal cell carcinomas over chest of pubescent girl. (Courtesy of J. B. Howell and M. R. Caro, A. M. A. Arch. Dermat., *79*:67, 1959.) *B*, Note several bifid ribs. *C*, Extensive cystic alteration of mandible. *D*, Another patient with several cysts adjacent to the teeth. (Gorlin, R. J., and Goltz, R.: New England J. Med., *262*:908, 1960.) (Gorlin, R. J., and Pindborg, J. J.: Syndromes of the Head and Neck. New York, McGraw-Hill Book Co., Inc., 1964.)

763

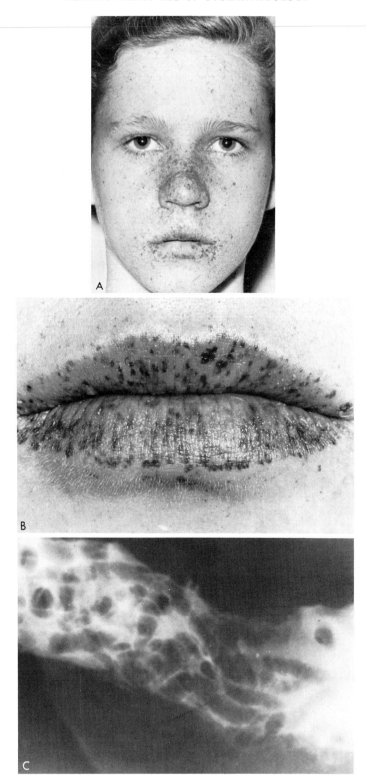

Figure 15. Peutz-Jeghers syndrome. *A,* Note periorificial spotty pigmentation. *B,* Mucosal involvement is usually quite marked. *C,* Numerous polyps of small bowel. (*A* from G. Klostermann, Stuttgart, Germany. *B* from M. Zingsheim, Hautarzt *17:*85–86, 1966.)

plasia are different syndromes from the one considered here.

The facies is quite characteristic, different affected individuals looking enough alike to be considered brothers. The skull resembles an inverted triangle. Marked frontal bossing, depressed nasal bridge (simulating the saddle nose of congenital syphilis), protuberant lips, and obliquely inserted ears are the most prominent facial feature.

The syndrome may not be manifested until the second year of life and, because the physical features are not so apparent, the child may present with a "fever of unknown origin." The inability to sweat, because of marked aplasia of the eccrine sweat glands, results in intolerance to heat, with severe hyperpyrexia. The skin is soft and thin, presenting severe dryness because of the absence of sebaceous glands. Eczema and asthma are common. Linear wrinkles are seen about the eyes and mouth. Small hyperkeratotic plaques are frequently noted on the palms and soles. At birth the body is devoid of lanugo hair; after puberty the beard is generally normal, but axillary and pubic hair are scant. The scalp hair is generally blond, fine, stiff, and short. The eyelashes and especially the eyebrows are often entirely missing. The finger- and toenails are usually normal or slightly spoon-shaped.

The most striking oral finding is hypodontia or, in several cases, anodontia. The few teeth that may be present are often retarded in eruption and have a conical crown form.

ERYTHEMA MULTIFORME EXUDATIVUM

(Stevens-Johnson Syndrome)

The syndrome is seen mainly in young adults, predominantly males. It is a self-limited, frequently recurrent disease with an acute onset and may last from one to several weeks. The initial manifestation is usually an upper respiratory infection (tonsillitis, rhinitis, pharyngitis, bronchitis) associated with headache, nausea, malaise and/or arthralgia. Fever may be present in the early stage.

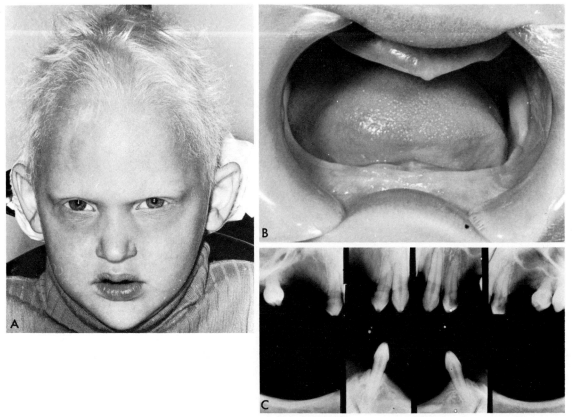

Figure 16. Hypohidrotic ectodermal dysplasia. *A,* Note sparse fine hair, fine wrinkles about eyes. *B,* Complete anodontia. *C,* Another patient with severe oligodontia; few remaining teeth have conical crown form.

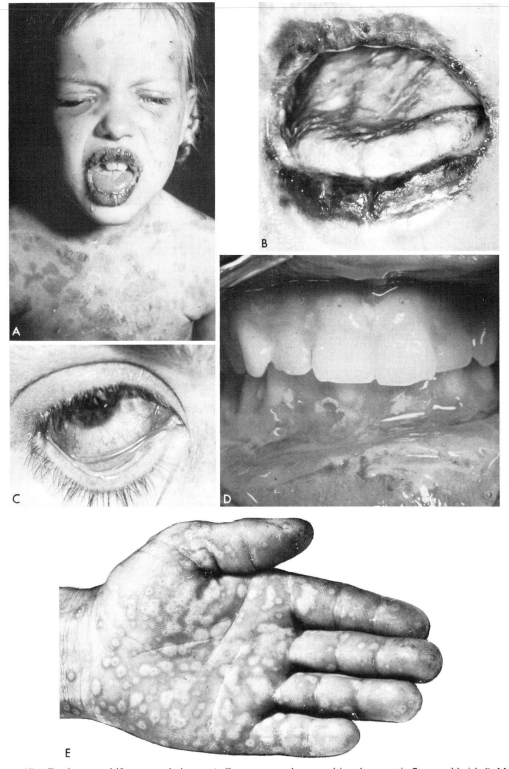

Figure 17. Erythema multiforme exudativum. *A*, Cutaneous and mucosal involvement in 7-year-old girl. *B*, Mucosal involvement of palpebral conjunctiva. *C*, Extensive labial and lingual lesions. *D*, Note friability of oral mucosa. *E*, Iris-like appearance to palmar lesions. (*B* and *C* from Gorlin, R. J., and Pindborg, J. J.: Syndromes of the Head and Neck. New York, McGraw-Hill Book Co., Inc., 1964).

Skin lesions may occur anywhere, but appear predominantly on the dorsum of hands and feet. The basic skin lesions show an annular pattern that may vary in size and form from maculopapular to vesiculobullous; they are usually symmetrically distributed.

The conjunctiva shows a fibrinomembranous type of involvement. Other mucous membranes may also be involved, those of the mouth (see below), penis and vulva being most frequently affected. Bronchitis, bronchopneumonia, and ulceration of the gastrointestinal tract occur.

Oral lesions usually appear after the skin involvement. However, in some patients, this sequence is reversed. Oral lesions occur on the lips, buccal and gingival mucosa, tongue, and hard and soft palate. The ruptured oral vesicles become confluent, forming shallow erosions covered by a necrotic pseudomembrane. The lesions are secondarily infected, thus complicating the clinical picture. Extensive crust formation occurs on the lips. Occasionally one can see oral involvement without cutaneous manifestations.

The etiology of the disease is obscure; in some cases there may be a history of allergy or drug idiosyncrasy. The majority of cases, however, are idiopathic.

REFERENCES

General

Becker, P. E.: Humangenetik– Ein kurzes Handbuch in fünf Bänden, Stuttgart, George Thieme Verlag, 1964–1968.
Gellis, S. S., and Finegold, M.: Atlas of Mental Retardation Syndromes. Washington, D.C., U.S. Department of Health, Education, and Welfare, 1968.
Goodman, R., and Gorlin, R. T.: The Face in Genetic Disorders. St. Louis, The C. V. Mosby Co., 1970.
Gorlin, R. J., and Pindborg, J. J.: Syndromes of the Head and Neck. New York, McGraw-Hill Book Co., 1964.
Leiber, B., and Olbrich, G.: Wörterbuch der klinischen Syndrome. 4th ed., Berlin, Urban and Schwarzenburg, 1966.
McKusick, V. A.: Mendelian Inheritance in Man. 2nd ed., Baltimore, The Johns Hopkins Press, 1968.
Smith, D. W.: Recognizable Patterns of Human Malformation. Philadelphia, W. B. Saunders Company, 1970.

Acrocephalosyndactyly

Blank, C. E.: Apert's syndrome (a type of acrocephalosyndactyly). Observations on a British series of thirty-nine cases. Ann. Human Genet. *24*:151–164, 1960.
Lewin, M. L.: Facial and hand deformities in acrocephalosyndactyly. Plast. Reconstr. Surg. *12*:138–147, 1953.
Woolf, R. M., et al.: Acrocephalosyndactyly — Apert's syndrome. Plast. Reconstr. Surg. *24*:201–208, 1959.

Craniofacial Dysostosis

Dodge, H. W., et al.: Craniofacial dysostosis: Crouzon's disease. Pediatrics *23*:98–106, 1959.
Krause, A. C., and Buchanan, D. N.: Dysostosis craniofacialis (Crouzon). Amer. J. Ophthal. *22*:140–144, 1959.
Schiller, J. G.: Craniofacial dysostosis of Crouzon. A case report and pedigree with emphasis on heredity. Pediatrics *23*:107–112, 1959.

Cleidocranial Dysostosis

Fitchet, S. M.: Cleidocranial dysostosis. Hereditary and familial. J. Bone Joint Surg. (Amer.) *11*:838–866, 1929.
Kunrad, R., and Ache, D.: Zur Frage der Dysostosis cleidocranialis. Arch. Kinderheilk. *167*:82–91, 1962.
Soule, A. B.: Mutational dysostosis. J. Bone Joint Surg. (Amer.) *28*:81–102, 1946.
Zellweger, H., et al.: Über die Dysostosis cleidocranialis. Helvet. Paediat. Acta *5*:264–278, 1950.

Mandibulofacial Dysostosis

Franceschetti, A., and Klein, D.: Mandibulo-facial dysostosis. New hereditary syndrome. Acta Ophthal. *27*:143–224, 1949.
Harrison, S. H.: Treacher Collins syndrome. Brit. J. Plast. Surg. *3*:282–290, 1951.
Hunt, P. A., and Smith, D. I.: Mandibulo-facial dysostosis. Pediatrics *15*:190–197, 1955.
McKenzie, J., and Craig, J.: Mandibulo-facial dysostosis (Treacher Collins syndrome). Arch. Dis. Child. *30*:391–395, 1955.
Pavsek, E. J.: Mandibulofacial dysostosis (Treacher Collins syndrome). Radiology *79*:598–602, 1958.
Stovin, J. J., et al.: Mandibulofacial dysostosis. Radiology *74*:225–231, 1960.
Thier, C. J.: Symptomenkomplexe in Rahmen der mandibulofacialer Dysplasien. Klin. Monatsbl. Augenheilk. *13*:378–388, 1959.
Wildervanck, L. S.: Dysostosis mandibulo-facialis (Francheschetti-Zwahlen) in four generations. Acta Genet. Med. (Roma) *9*:447–451, 1960.

Oculomandibulodyscephaly With Hypotrichosis

Casperson, I., and Warburg, M.: Hallermann-Streiff syndrome. Acta Ophthal. *46*:385–390, 1968.
Hoefnagel, D., and Benirschke, K.: Dyscephalia mandibulo-oculo-facialis. (Hallermann-Streiff syndrome). Arch. Dis. Child. *40*:57–61, 1965.
Lamy, M., et al.: La dyscephalie (syndrome de Hallermann-Streiff-François) Arch. Franc. Pediat. *22*:929–938, 1965.
Srivastava, S. P., et al.: Mandibulo-oculo-facial-dyscephaly. Brit. J. Ophthal. *50*:543–549, 1966.

Osteogenesis Imperfecta

Evans, H. D.: Severe osteogenesis imperfecta with pregnancy. Obstet. Gynec. *28*:394–396, 1966.
Gorlin, R. J., and Pindborg, J. J.: Syndromes of the Head and Neck. New York, McGraw-Hill Book Co., 1964.
Walter, J. R., and MacVicar, J. E.: Blue sclerae, brittle bone and retinal detachment. J. Pediat. Ophthal. *4*:13–16, 1967.

Craniometaphyseal and Craniodiaphyseal Dysplasia

Gorlin, R. J., et al.: Genetic craniotubular bone dysplasias and hyperostoses: A critical review. Birth Defects, Original Article Series *5*(4):79–95, 1969.

Graf, K.: Die Bedeutung des Pyle-Syndroms (Leontiasis ossea) für die Oto-Rhino-Laryngologie. Laryng. Rhinol. Otol. *44*:438–445, 1965.

Halliday, J.: A rare case of bone dysplasia. Brit. J. Surg. *37*:52–63, 1949-1950.

Joseph, R., et al.: Dysplasie cranio-diaphysaire progressive. Ses relations avec la dysplasie diaphysaire progressive de Camurati-Engelmann. Ann. Radiol. *1*:477–490, 1958.

Millard, D. R., et al.: Craniofacial surgery in craniometaphyseal dysplasia. Amer. J. Surg. *113*:615–621, 1967.

Mori, R. A., and Holt, J. F.: Cranial manifestation of familial metaphyseal dysplasia. Radiology *66*:335–343, 1956.

Spranger, J., et al.: Die kraniometaphysäre Dysplasie (Pyle). Kinderheilk. *93*:64–79, 1965.

Stransky, E., et al.: On Paget's disease with leontiasis ossea and hypothyreosis starting in early childhood. Ann. Paediat. *199*:393–408, 1962.

Pycnodysostosis

Giedion, A., and Zachmann, M.: Pyknodysostose. Helv. Paediat. Acta *21*:612–621, 1966.

Maroteaux, P., and Lamy, M.: La pycnodysostose. Presse Méd. *70*:999–1002, 1962.

Schuler, S. E.: Pycnodysostosis. Arch. Dis. Child. *38*:620–625, 1963.

Sedano, H., and Gorlin, R. J.: Pycnodysostosis. Amer. J. Dis. Child. *116*:70–76, 1968.

Oral-Facial-Digital Syndrome I

Doege, T. C., et al.: Studies of a family with the oral-facial-digital syndrome. New Eng. J. Med. *271*:1073–1080, 1964.

Fuhrmann, W., Stahl, A., and Schroeder, T. M.: Das oro-facio-digitale Syndrom. Humangenetik. *2*:133–164, 1966.

Gorlin, R. J.: The oral—facial—digital (OFD) syndrome. Cutis *4*:1345–1352, 1968.

Gorlin, R. J., and Psaume, J.: Orodigitofacial dysostosis: A new syndrome. A study of 22 cases. J. Pediat. *61*:520–530, 1962.

Rimoin, D. L., and Edgerton, M. T.: Genetic and clinical heterogeneity in the oral-facial-digital syndrome. J. Pediat. *71*:94–102, 1967.

Cleft Palate, Small Dysplastic Mandible, and Glossoptosis

Dennison, W. M.: The Pierre Robin syndrome. Pediatrics *36*:336–341, 1965.

Kiskadden, W. S., and Dietrich, S. R.: Review of the treatment of micrognathia. Plast. Reconstr. Surg. *12*:364–376, 1953.

Pruzansky, S.: Not all dwarfed mandibles are alike. Birth Defects, Original Article Series 5(2):120–129, 1969.

Pruzansky, S., and Richmond, J. B.: Growth of the mandible in infants with micrognathia. Amer. J. Dis. Child. *88*:29–42, 1954.

Randall, P., et al.: Pierre Robin and the syndrome that bears his name. Cleft Palate J. *2*:237–246, 1965.

Smith, J. L., and Stowe, F. R.: The Pierre Robin syndrome. A review of 39 cases with emphasis on associated ocular lesion. Pediatrics *27*:128–133, 1961.

Cleft Lip-Palate and Congenital Lip Fistulas

Červenka, J., et al.: The syndrome of pits of the lower lip and cleft lip and/or palate. Genetic considerations. Amer. J. Human Genet. *19*:416–432, 1967.

Gorlin, R. J., and Pindborg, J. J.: *Syndromes of the Head and Neck*. New York, McGraw-Hill Book Co., 1964.

Koberg, W.: Zur Kenntnis der kongenitalen Unterlippen-fisteln. Oest. Z. Stomat. *63*:60–74, 1966.

Van der Woude, A.: Fistula labii inferioris congenita and its association with cleft lip and palate. Amer. J. Human Genet. *6*:244–256, 1954.

Warbrick, J. G., et al.: Remarks on the etiology of congenital bilateral fistulas of lower lip. Brit. J. Plast. Surg. *4*:254–262, 1952.

Multiple Mucosal Neuroma Syndrome

Gorlin, R. J., et al.: Multiple mucosal neuromas, pheochromocytoma and medullary carcinoma of the thyroid—A new syndrome. Cancer *22*:293–299, 1968.

Schimke, R. N., et al.: Pheochromocytoma, medullary thyroid carcinoma and multiple neuromas. New Eng. J. Med. *279*:1–7, 1968.

Williams, E. D., and Pollack, D. J.: Multiple mucosal neuromas with endocrine tumors. A syndrome allied to von Recklinghausen's disease. J. Path. Bact. *91*:71–80, 1966.

Gardner's Syndrome

Gardner, E. J., and Richards, R. C.: Multiple cutaneous and subcutaneous lesions occurring simultaneously with hereditary polyposes and osteomatosis. Amer. J. Human Genet. *5*:139–147, 1953.

Gorlin, R. J., and Chaudhry, A. P.: Multiple osteomas, fibromas, lipomas and fibrosarcomas of the skin and mesentery, epidermoid inclusion cysts of the skin, leiomyomas and multiple intestinal polyposis. New Eng. J. Med. *263*:1151–1158, 1960.

Plenk, H. P., and Gardner, E. J.: Osteomatosis (leontiasis ossea). Hereditary disease of membraneous bone formation associated in one family with polyposis of colon. Radiology *62*:830–840, 1954.

Thomas, K. E., et al.: Natura history of Gardner's syndrome. Amer. J. Surg. *115*:218–226, 1968.

Multiple Nevoid Basal Cell Carcinoma Syndrome

Berlin, N. I., et al.: Basal cell nevus syndrome. Ann. Intern. Med. *64*:403–421, 1966.

Gorlin, R. J., et al.: The multiple basal cell nevi syndrome. Cancer *18*:89–104, 1965.

Mills, J., and Foulkes, J.: Gorlin's syndrome. A radiological and cytogenetic study of nine cases. Brit. J. Radiol. *40*:366–371, 1967.

Zackheim, H. S., et al.: Basal cell carcinoma syndrome. Arch. Derm. *93*:317–323, 1966.

Peutz-Jeghers Syndrome

Bartholomew, L. G., et al.: Intestinal polyposis associated with mucocutaneous melanin pigmentation; Peutz-Jeghers syndrome. Review of literature and report of six cases with special reference to pathologic findings. Gastroenterology *32*:434–451, 1957.

Klostermann, G. F.: Peutz-Jeghers syndrome. Arch. Klin. Exp. Derm. *226*:182–198,1966.

Laumonier, R., et al.: Pathologie du syndrome de Peutz-Jeghers. Ann. Anat. Path. *10*:75–98, 1965.

Zegarelli, E. V., et al.: Atlas of oral lesions observed in the syndrome of oral melanosis with associated intestinal polyposis (Peutz-Jeghers syndrome). Amer. J. Dig. Dis. *4*:479–489, 1959.

Hypohidrotic Ectodermal Dysplasia

Glicklich, L. G., and Rosenthal, I. M.: Anhidrotic ectodermal dysplasia. J. Pediat. *54*:19–26, 1959.

Gorlin, R. J., and Pindborg, J. J.: *Syndromes of the Head and Neck*. New York, McGraw-Hill Book Co., 1964.

Gorlin, R. J., et al.: Hypohidrotic ectodermal dysplasia in

females. A critical analysis and argument for genetic heterogeneity. Z. Kinderheilk. *108*:1–11, 1970.

Sarnat, B. G., et al.: Fourteen year report of facial growth in case of complete anodontia with ectodermal dysplasia. Amer. J. Dis. Child. *86*:162–169, 1953.

Erythema Multiforme

Bradtzaeg, P.: Erythema multiforme exudativum. A review of the literature with special reference of oral manifestations. Odont. T. *72*:362–390, 1964.

Shklar, G.: Oral lesions of erythema multiforme. Arch. Derm. *92*:495–500, 1965.

Soll, S. N.: Eruptive fever with involvement of the respiratory tract, conjunctivitis, stomatitis and balanitis: An acute clinical entity, probably of infectious origin: Report of twenty cases and review of the literature. Arch. Intern. Med. *79*:475–500, 1947.

Stevens, A. M., and Johnson, C. F.: A new eruptive fever associated with stomatitis and ophthalmia. Amer. J Dis. Child. *24*:526–533, 1922.

Section Nine

OTOLARYNGOLOGY AND CLOSELY RELATED DISCIPLINES

Chapter 33

ANESTHESIA

ANESTHESIA FOR OTOLARYNGOLOGIC PROCEDURES

by

John Adriani, M.D.

LOCAL VERSUS GENERAL ANESTHESIA

Various techniques of anesthesia embodying combinations of drugs have been introduced for performing otolaryngeal procedures. The fact that new techniques and drugs are tried, have periods of enthusiastic use, and then are forgotten indicates that no wholly satisfactory method of anesthesia is available for a given procedure or group of procedures and that an ideal does not exist. Many otolaryngologic procedures in adults may be performed without difficulty with regional methods of anesthesia—infiltration, nerve block, or topical anesthesia—provided the operator is capable, gentle, and skillful. The operator who uses regional methods must instill a high degree of confidence in a patient if the method is to be successful. Nonetheless, some patients are not psychically suited to have any surgical procedure performed with regional anesthesia. They are unable to offer the necessary cooperation, irrespective of the skill and psychologic approach of the operator. Patients who are apprehensive, delirious, psychoneurotic, or psychotic must, therefore, be given general anesthesia. Infants and children are, almost without exception, apprehensive and uncooperative when otolaryngologic procedures are performed using local anesthesia. Under these circumstances general anesthetics or other drugs which produce immobilization are indicated.

Patients undergoing operations for otolaryn-gologic procedures must be evaluated and studied in the same manner and care as patients for any major surgical procedure. A complete history and physical examination are essential features of the preoperative work-up. The presence of systemic diseases is of equal significance in the management of the otolaryngologic patient as any other. In addition, certain points in the history and physical examination are peculiar to the otolaryngologic patient, such as allergy with excess secretions, asthma, lymphoid tissue, postnasal drip, polyps, and benign and malignant neoplasia which cause bleeding, aspiration, or obstruction.

One overlooked factor of extreme importance, particularly when laryngoscopic and bronchoscopic procedures are performed, is that pulmonary function and ventilatory reserve may be low. The mere introduction of a bronchoscope into the bronchus of a diseased lung may reduce ventilation to an intolerable level and the patient, if conscious, struggles to survive.

AVAILABLE TECHNIQUES AND DRUGS

As one reviews the history of the various drug combinations and techniques that have been introduced for anesthesia for otolaryngologic procedures over the past several decades, it is obvious that the majority consist of a combination of a local anesthetic as the primary agent and some form of basal narcosis as the secondary agent, or a general anesthetic as the primary agent and a local anesthetic as a secondary agent. The term basal narcotic refers to the use of nonvolatile drugs which, when given intravenously, rectally, or intramuscularly, induce a deep state of hypnosis with amnesia but do not abolish reflex activity completely. Which is the primary agent and which is the secondary depends upon the potency of the primary general anesthetic agent.

Morphine-Scopolamine

One of the earliest techniques used for endoscopic and other otolaryngologic procedures consisted of morphine combined with scopolamine and a barbiturate as the basal analgesic-amnesic secondary agent, with the topical application of cocaine, tetracaine, or other surface-acting local anesthetic as the primary agent, or nerve block or infiltration of the appropriate area. Complete amnesia and adequate relief of pain were obtained. In appropriate cases, although satisfactory, this procedure had a number of drawbacks, the most notable being that some disorientation occurred in the postoperative period. It has been revived and is still used by some. Instead of morphine, the scopolamine is combined with meperidine (Demerol) by many workers. Others use dihydromorphinone (Dilaudid), oxymorphone (Numorphan), or other narcotics. The end result is the same. Patients undergoing bronchoscopy or laryngoscopy have, as a rule, some degree of respiratory distress or airway obstruction. Morphine, other narcotics, and central nervous system depressants diminish ventilation and interfere with gaseous exchange. The scopolamine acts as an amnesic as well as a drying agent. It is, therefore, highly efficacious when combined with a narcotic as an adjunct for local anesthesia and for regional anesthesia also.

INHALATION ANESTHESIA

Ether

For many years the most common inhalation technique, but far from ideal, was the open drop technique. Anesthesia was induced by using open cone ethyl chloride or vinyl ether followed by drop ether, followed by insuf-flation of ether and air or nitrous oxide combined with ether. This technique and its modifications is still used in some areas of the country for performing otolaryngologic procedures in infants and children. In most hospitals it has gradually been relegated into obsolescence, where it rightfully belongs. The hazard of fire is ever present. Still more important is the danger from asphyxia from respiratory obstruction or aspiration, resulting from lack of control of airway or inhaled concentrations or overdosage.

When ether is properly administered, the disagreeable aspect has disappeared. However, it should be used with a nasotracheal or orotracheal catheter in all types of head and neck surgery to avert the danger of asphyxia. In spite of its pungency, ether is not "irritating" to the lungs and injurious to the mucosa of the upper airway or the alveoli. Nitrous oxide combined with ether, administered by mask, and induction followed by insufflation of ether and nitrous oxide and oxygen during maintenance, was also popular but is now seldom used except in isolated areas because other techniques have supplanted it.

Rectal Anesthesia

In the mid-1920's tribromoethanol (Avertin) was introduced as a basal narcotic. Tribromoethanol produces unconsciousness and amnesia but does not obtund the pharyngeal and tracheobronchial reflexes. It was, therefore, inadequate as a primary agent and unsuitable as a sole agent. It was objectionable for a number of reasons: (1) Tribromoethanol depresses the medullary, respiratory, and vasomotor centers. Respiratory depression and hypotension occur frequently. (2) Patients remain narcotized, with depressed reflex activity, for some time after the procedure is completed because the drug has to be metabolized. The respiratory depression is undesirable because most patients undergoing otolaryngologic surgery have airway problems and respiratory insufficiency. (3) The technique of rectal administration is cumbersome and time-consuming. The agent was used with a certain degree of success in performing bronchograms. An endotracheal tube was introduced after the pharynx and larynx were anesthetized topically with a local anesthetic. Nitrous oxide was used as a supplement, since nonflammable agents must be used in x-ray units. Apnea was produced by hyperinflation of the lung after instillation of the contrast media area at the time of exposure of the film.

Avertin likewise has also been combined with ether, nitrous oxide, and cyclopropane without a local anesthetic. However, many operators found that less Avertin and ether were necessary if topical anesthesia was used as an adjunct. Even though tribromoethanol is seldom used, its history is reviewed at this point to emphasize the inadequacies of "rectal anesthesia."Other drugs have been used in the same manner as tribromoethanol. Among these have been chloral hydrate, paraldehyde, and hexobarbital (Evipal). These are not recommended. Hexobarbital was supplanted by thiopental (Pentothal) and more recently by methohexital (Brevital). The barbiturates used rectally have the same drawbacks and disadvantages as the older basal narcotics, with the additional objection that they are laryngospasmogenic. Severe and often fatal laryngo- and bronchospasm may be precipitated from secretions and instrumentation in the upper airway. They are not completely anesthetic and the patient may move about when instrumentation is attempted.

Cyclopropane

Cyclopropane was introduced in the early 1930's. It likewise was used and is still used for general anesthesia for otolaryngologic procedures. Its chief drawback is its flammability, and many procedures require use of the microscope, cauteries, stimulators, and other devices which may cause sparks or flames, thus precluding its use. A nonflammable agent must be selected under these circumstances. Cyclopropane is best administered intratracheally. For endoscopy, anesthesia is induced in the usual manner with a mask; the larynx is exposed to introduce the bronchoscope, after which cyclopropane and oxygen are insufflated in the side arm of the bronchoscope. Objections are raised by the operator that the visibility is poor because the index of refraction of the stream of cyclopropane and oxygen differs from that of air and the image is distorted. Explosions have occurred when cyclopropane, ether, and other flammable anesthetics have been used, from static electricity or breakage as a result of some defect of the bulb or the light carrier during endoscopic procedures.

Cyclopropane is often combined with ether. The mixture has many advantages. A pharmacologic attribute of cyclopropane is its tendency to depress respiration which, in turn, causes respiratory acidosis. In addition, it causes the release of norepinephrine, which in the presence of excess carbon dioxide sensitizes the pacemaker cells of the heart. Ectopic foci become active and arrhythmias result. Ether possesses a stimulating action on respiration because of the local effects on the alveolar receptors which overcome this acidosis and arrhythmogenic effect. Epinephrine, norepinephrine, and isoproterenol (Isuprel) have a stimulating effect on the pacemaker cells. When these catecholamines are used simultaneously with cyclopropane, serious ventricular arrhythmias develop, such as ventricular tachycardia. In the highly irritable heart ventricular fibrillation may result. Halogenated anesthetics behave in a similar manner, but this arrhythmogenic activity is most pronounced with cyclopropane. In the order of decreasing activity, next to cyclopropane are chloroform, trichloroethylene, ethyl chloride, halothane, and methoxyflurane. Fluroxene, vinyl ether, and ethyl ether may be used simultaneously with these catecholamines.

Halothane

Halothane (Fluothane) is presently one of the most widely used inhalation anesthetics for all types of surgical procedures. It is a chlorinated, brominated, and fluorinated hydrocarbon. Halogenation of hydrocarbons reduces or completely abolishes flammability. In addition, halogenation causes varying degrees of cardiotoxicity and hepatotoxicity. Shortly after induction of halothane anesthesia, hypotension develops. This has been ascribed to a number of factors, the most important of which are: (1) its myocardial depressant effect, (2) its failure to release norepinephrine (unlike cyclopropane), (3) vasodilation as a result of central depression of the vasomotor center, and (4) some degree of ganglionic blockade. Halothane is one of the most potent of the inhalation anesthetics. In fact, it surpasses chloroform in potency. It is nonpungent and not laryngo-or bronchospasmogenic and is, therefore, highly desirable when laryngospasm and bronchospasm are a possibility. Induction time is rapid. Recovery likewise is rapid—five to ten minutes, depending upon the duration of the period of administration. Unlike chloroform or ether, relaxation is in most cases not adequate unless unsafe concentrations are used; therefore, muscle relaxants should be used as adjuncts. It is useful for virtually any type of otolaryngologic procedure. Intubation is not only strongly recommended but almost mandatory. Little oozing or bleeding occurs because of the hypotension. When blood pressure is normal, bleeding differs in no way from other anesthetics.

It is advisable not to use halothane in combination with epinephrine because it may cause ventricular fibrillation if excessive quantities of the vasoconstrictor are used. The limits of dosage of epinephrine are difficult to establish. Much debate exists at the present time concerning the hepatotoxic potential of halothane. The drug is not considered to be directly hepatotoxic like chloroform; the lesions in the liver are not reproducible in animals, as they are with chloroform. In man hepatitis has occurred from time to time. The present concept is that some degree of sensitization occurs, and the reaction in the liver is of an allergic nature. The evidence and absolute proof for this are lacking, however. Hepatitis may occur more often after repeated administrations rather than after single usage. The drug should not be used in patients with known liver or renal dysfunction. Halothane has been used by the mask technique followed by insufflation into the arm of the bronchoscope or with the Sanders ventilating bronchoscope. It is a satisfactory agent for this purpose because it is not spasmogenic. Halothane is a bronchial dilator and is not flammable. Relaxation for intubation and insertion of the bronchoscope is obtained by using succinylcholine or some other neuromuscular blocking agent.

Methoxyflurane

Methoxyflurane (Penthrane), the most recent addition to the list of inhalation anesthetics, has an advantage over some of the other volatile agents for certain otolaryngologic procedures. It is a fluorinated and chlorinated ether. It resembles ethyl ether in many respects and halothane in others, and one could rightfully categorize it as being a cross between the two. It is not flammable. It is pleasant to inhale. Induction time, like that of ether, is lengthy and recovery likewise is slow. The slow recovery may be of advantage because anesthesia may be terminated when the surgical levels are reached, and endoscopic and other examinations may proceed without further use of the agent. Muscle relaxation using the agent alone is adequate for the introduction of the laryngoscope and bronchoscope; neuromuscular blocking agents are not necessary adjuncts. If topical anesthesia precedes the general, lighter levels of anesthesia are required. The analgesia is longer lasting and allows the operator sufficient time to leisurely complete the procedure. The drug is alleged to have a nephrotoxic potential as well as a hepatotoxic one. Arrhythmias are less apt to occur than with halothane when methoxyflurane is combined with epinephrine, but they have been reported when the quantity of epinephrine was not strictly curtailed. If other agents are available, the combination is best not used. Like halothane, methoxyflurane causes myocardial depression and hypotension.

Trichloroethylene

Trichloroethylene is an old drug introduced as an analgesic several decades ago primarily to relieve pain due to trigeminal neuralgia. Its value for this purpose was doubtful and it fell into disuse. Its use was revived in the early 1940's when it was introduced as an inhalation anesthetic. Its chief virtue was lack of flammability. It is a halogenated hydrocarbon and possesses the same attributes as do other drugs in this category, namely, cardiotoxicity and hepatoxicity. It vaporizes slowly because of a relatively high boiling point, and for this reason induction is slow and accompanied by excitement. It undergoes some degree of biodegradation in the body and is not stable in the presence of soda lime, which is commonly used in anesthesia apparatus. It is used to some extent to fortify nitrous oxide, allowing the use of greater quantities of oxygen and avoiding asphyxia, and as an analgesic combined with air. Various types of hand inhalers are available for self-administration of the vapors by obstetrical patients. These may also be used for analgesia during removal of dressings following mastoidectomy and similar procedures of short duration not requiring full surgical anesthesia. Like cyclopropane, it may not be combined with epinephrine.

Fluroxene

Fluroxene (Fluoromar) is a fluorinated ether chemically allied to vinyl ether but manifesting decreased flammability because of the presence of the fluorine atoms on its molecule. Since it is conceded to be flammable, it has not received widespread acceptance. It lacks the ability to produce profound muscle relaxation.

Its chief virtue is that it does not sensitize the heart to epinephrine and norepinephrine; for this reason is used when these agents are required for hemostasis.

INTRAVENOUS ANESTHESIA

Intravenous Ether

Ether dissolved in saline has been used intravenously in combination with heavy sedation and topical anesthesia for endoscopy. Large volumes of the solution of ether are necessary for effective anesthesia. The solution is cooled in order that more ether will dissolve in a given volume of saline; as much as 6 per cent will dissolve by cooling. Hemolysis resulted from the use of the mixture and it has been abandoned. Its use is revived from time to time but it is not recommended.

Thiopental, Thiamylal, and Methohexital

Intravenous thiopental and other ultrashort-acting barbiturates (thiamylal, methohexital) are seldom used alone for surgical anesthesia of any type. Generally they are combined with nitrous oxide and a muscle relaxant or are used as a basal or preliminary agent for other anesthetics. Their use as a sole agent for endoscopy has been tried but was quickly abandoned because they proved to be extremely hazardous. The tracheobronchial reflexes are not only not obtunded by the ultrashort-acting barbiturates, but they are even exaggerated by these drugs. The combination of thiopental and topical anesthesia was and still is used by some endoscopists. Even though the topical anesthesia is effective, the tracheobronchial reflexes continue to be active, and even though the local stimulus is gone, severe bronchospasm is still a possibility. The presence of secretions in the lower respiratory tract, particularly in cases of suppurative diseases, may initiate the response.

Intravenous Alcohol

Intravenous alcohol was used as an anesthesia in the early 1940's. It was not effective, and understandably so, because alcohol is a poor analgesic agent. Even when combined with local anesthesia, it was not satisfactory because the patient's reflex activity was not abolished and the sensorium was clouded. Both of these factors made the patient uncooperative.

Intravenous Local Anesthetics

Procaine, lidocaine, and other local anesthetics have been used intravenously for endoscopy with a limited degree of success. Procaine was first used, but the quantities required to abolish tracheobronchial reflexes were so great that serious systemic reactions occurred. Intravenous lidocaine is still used by some anesthetists. It appears to provide a greater degree of analgesia and obtunds the tracheobronchial reflexes to a greater degree than procaine. Even though it is better, it still does not provide adequate anesthesia for most otolaryngologic procedures. The same objections apply to tetracaine (Pontocaine), mepivacaine (Carbocaine), dibucaine (Nupercaine), and other local anesthetics.

Neuromuscular Blocking Agents

Muscle relaxants have been used as adjuncts to anesthesia for several decades. Not all muscle relaxants are suitable, however. Muscle relaxants fall into several categories: those which act centrally in the cortex and other subcortical areas, such as the psychosedatives (tranquilizers) and those which act at polysynaptic neurones in the brain and spinal cord (mephanesin, meprobamate, etc.); those which act at the myoneural junction (neuromuscular blocking agents); and those which act directly on striated muscle to depress its activity (quinine). Of these only the neuromuscular blocking agents satisfactorily relax striated muscle for surgical purposes and are capable of producing paresis and complete paralysis. Two pharmacologic types are recognized: the nondepolarizers, which include tubocurarine, the active principle in curare, and gallamine (Flaxedil); and the depolarizers, which include succinylcholine (Anectine, Sucostrin). It must be stressed that the neuromuscular blocking agents are merely adjuncts to anesthesia. They are not analgesic or anesthetic and in no way block sensory impulses from peripheral receptors. They must be used in combination with analgesic and amnesic agents. The combination of thiopental or one of its pharmacologic relatives (Surital, methohexital) and nitrous oxide is widely used. The safety of inhalation anesthesia is increased since the deeper levels required to obtain muscle relaxation can be avoided. They have certain drawbacks, however. Neuromuscular blocking agents do not penetrate lipid capsules of the liver microsomes and therefore are not easily detoxified by the liver. With the exception of succinylcholine, which is quickly hydrolyzed by the pseudocholinesterases in plasma of normal individuals, all these drugs are excreted by the kidney. Succinylcholine is given by the drip technique. Some persons have an atypical enzyme which does not readily hydrolyze the drug. Cases of prolonged apnea have resulted and have lasted many hours when succinylcholine drip has been used in these patients.

The muscle relaxants combined with thiopental (Pentothal) or other ultrashort-acting barbiturates and topical anesthesia have been used and are still used by some anesthetists for endoscopic procedures. This technique is satisfactory only if adequate ventilation can be assured at all times. Unfortunately the relaxant paralyzes the intercostal muscles and the diaphragm, and apnea or hypoventilation results. Chest respirators of various sorts, cuirasses, "raincoat" modifications of the tank respirator, and various ventilating bronchoscopes have been introduced to artificially ventilate the patient during this period of inadequate ventilation. Chest ventilators have proved to be far from satisfactory. Chest movements occur but they are no index of the adequacy of ventilation. Vigorous inspiratory and expiratory movements may be mechanically produced, yet the upper airway may be partially or incompletely obstructed, particularly when laryngeal surgery is being performed, and asphyxia results. The anesthetist must stand at the patient's side rather than at the head of the table and is therefore not able to determine whether the airway is completely patent. It is possible for complete obstruction to be present and one not be aware of it.

The ventilating bronchoscope recently introduced by Sanders, however, obviates many of the aforementioned difficulties, particularly that of providing an adequate airway. The desired anesthetic agent is insufflated into the bronchoscope by a device operated manually which releases gas from a pressure gauge. Gallamine, tubocurarine, or succinylcholine is used in conjunction with thiopental in performing the bronchoscopy with this instrument. This combination is the secondary or basal agent, and topical anesthesia the primary agent. The use of topical anesthesia is almost mandatory because it obtunds the tracheal and bronchial reflexes. These are accentuated by thiopental, and without topical anesthesia severe bronchospasm could result. The neuromuscular blocking agents have no effect on smooth muscle and do not alleviate the spasm. In fact, tubocurarine releases histamine, which augments the bronchospasm. The combination may also be used for esophagoscopy. A cuffed endotracheal catheter of the noncollapsible type should be used when performing esophagoscopy. The catheter may be attached to a closed anesthetic circuit with the carbon dioxide absorption system and ventilation maintained by manual or mechanical compression of the breathing bag.

As a general rule, indications for the continued use of a neuromuscular blocking agent throughout most otolaryngologic procedures are seldom present. The relaxant is administered to facilitate introduction of endotracheal tubes. Few procedures in otolaryngology require muscle relaxation except intubation. The relaxants are abused by some anesthetists and are used more for convenience than necessity. Some anesthetists paralyze the patient to avoid movements if anesthesia inadvertently becomes too light or because they prefer to use mechanical ventilators, thereby avoiding the use of assisted respiration, which requires greater attention and effort on their part. All this may decrease safety as far as the patient is concerned.

MISCELLANEOUS AGENTS

Hydroxydione

The steroid, Viadril, introduced in the mid-1950's, appeared to be adequate as a secondary agent for basal narcosis when combined with nitrous oxide and other anesthetics or with topical anesthesia as a primary agent for endoscopic procedures. Nitrous oxide was insufflated into the side arm of the bronchoscope in some cases. The agent, popular at first, is now little used and is gradually being relegated into obsolescence. Venous thrombosis and phlebitis have occurred frequently. Besides, dosage was difficult to determine.

Lytic Cocktail

Combinations of psychosedatives such as promethazine (Phenergan), secobarbital (Seconal), chlorpromazine (Thorazine), and meperidine (Demerol) have been used in combination with local and topical anesthesia. This mixture, once referred to as "the lytic cocktail," is still used but has the disadvantages of morphine and scopolamine. Hypotension resulting from use of the narcotic and the phenothiazine, and respiratory depression due to the narcotic are the most objectionable features. The phenothiazines as a class block adrenergic receptors, and the receptors are therefore not responsive to epinephrine, norepinephrine, and other vasopressors. It is sometimes used for diagnostic procedures, endoscopy, changes of dressings, etc. It may be supplemented with nitrous oxide insufflated into the side arm of the bronchoscope or by mask for other procedures.

Innovar

The newest anesthetic is a fixed-ratio combination known by the proprietary name of Innovar. This mixture consists of a psychosedative, droperidol (Inapsine), pharmacologically similar to but not chemically allied to the phenothiazines; and a recently introduced narcotic, fentanyl (Sublimaze), in a ratio of 50 parts of the psychosedative to one part of narcotic. It has found acceptance among some clinicians as an anesthetic for otolaryngologic procedures, but not all who use it are fully aware of its drawbacks. The combination is satisfactory as a basal narcotic because it decreases reflex activity, and movement and struggling are avoided. The mixture cannot be used as a sole agent, however. The primary agent, as is the case with other combinations, is actually nitrous oxide, a local anesthetic, administered by nerve block or topically. Innovar induces a state referred to as neuroleptanalgesia. The patient responds to auditory, tactile, and visual stimuli, but the mixture causes amnesia and the patient has little recollection of events occurring during the procedure. Severe muscle rigidity, hypotension, and respiratory failure may occur.

The drawbacks of the combination are gradually being recognized as its use becomes more widespread. It is illogical to assume that two drugs, each having dissimilar action, can be used in a fixed ratio for all patients; tolerance for each varies from one patient to the next. The combination is suited primarily as a basal and is not a true anesthetic. Both agents are now available individually, and it is not only more logical but wiser to use each individually and to adjust dosage to suit individual patients. Respiration is usually depressed. Muscle rigidity caused by the fentanyl interferes with ventilatory movements and must be overcome with a muscle relaxant. This means adding another drug with a hazardous potential and causing further depression or respiration or even apnea. At the conclusion of anesthesia an antinarcotic is usually required to overcome respiratory depression and muscle rigidity. The action of droperidol often outlasts the effects of fentanyl by several hours; supplements, therefore, should be made by adding fentanyl without droperidol to avoid cumulative effects.

Ketamine (Ketalar)

Ketamine (Ketalar) is a recently introduced drug which has not been thoroughly evaluated. This drug has both a cataleptic and an analgesic effect. Onset of action is rapid and duration is brief. It is devoid of sedative and hypnotic properties. Presumably it causes dissociation within the cerebrum, and pain impulses are not transmitted over the usual pathways.

Chemically the compound is unlike other analgesics, being a chlorophenyl methylamino cyclohexanone. The drug is rapidly metabolized. An intravenous dose of 1 mg. per pound of body weight induces surgical anesthesia within one minute so is suitable for brief surgical procedures. Small increments are added for longer procedures. The drug, as is the case with other psychosedatives, has some antiarrhythmic properties whose value remains to be established. Concomitant use of barbiturates and other hypnotics and narcotics prolongs recovery time. The pharyngeal reflex, as is the case with many of the basal narcotics, is not abolished. Thus, the patient is able to maintain his airway, swallow secretions, and perform other reflex acts which are protective. Overdosage causes respiratory depression and apnea. Hallucination and confusional states occur postoperatively, particularly in middle-aged adults, and for this reason the drug is of limited usefulness in adults. It is used primarily for children. Elevation in blood pressure and increases in pulse rate occur, particularly on emergence from the anesthesia. Convulsions have been reported. It is used primarily for diagnostic and minor surgical procedures such as biopsies. Time will be required to properly evaluate its worth.

Apneic Oxygenation

A technique known as "apneic oxygenation," utilizing diffusion respiration, has been suggested as being useful for laryngoscopic and bronchoscopic procedures. Apnea is induced with a muscle relaxant, and oxygen is permitted to diffuse into the lung through the bronchoscope. Topical anesthesia and a basal dosage of thiopental are required for pain relief and patient comfort. The carbon dioxide does not diffuse so readily as oxygen and tends to be retained. To obviate this it is absorbed by a buffer called THAM, given intravenously, which is excreted in the urine. A severe alkalosis may result from the use of THAM, which is also characterized by other serious side effects.

Hypotensive Anesthesia

The term hypotensive anesthesia is actually a misnomer. More properly it should be called deliberately induced hypotension. This procedure is used as an adjunct in surgical procedures involving severe blood loss as a result of oozing not controllable by usual methods employed for hemostasis. The technique is based upon the fact that if vasodilatation is produced by sympathetic blockade, the capillary blood pressure will be maintained within normal limits even though the systemic blood pressure is reduced and thereby adequate perfusion will be maintained. The lowered systemic pressure reduces the amount of bleeding. The technique is used when surgery is performed in highly vascular areas, as for example when the maxilla is excised, or when a dry field is essential for success, as in the case of the fenestration operation. The peripheral resistance is reduced either by inducing a total spinal block by injecting a dilute solution of a local anesthetic or by using a ganglionic blocking agent or by using an alpha adrenergic blocking agent such as a phenothiazine or dibenzylene. Sodium nitroprusside relaxes vascular smooth muscle and it, too, is used by some workers. The commonest method is to use trimethephan (Arfonad) by intravenous drip. Primarily this causes a ganglionic blockade, although some peripheral action also occurs. The patient is anesthetized in the customary manner, and at the time of the anticipated bleeding, systolic pressure is reduced to a level of approximately 80 mm. Hg but no less than 60. The procedure has its dangers. Circulation time is prolonged and perfusion may not be adequate. Thrombosis of the coronary and cerebral vessels has been reported, as have anuria, cerebral ischemia, blindness, and reactionary hemmorhage. The technique is not justified in benign conditions.

LOCAL ANESTHESIA

The clinically useful topical local anesthetics fall into two categories: (1) the nitrogen-containing derivatives, which are largely amines, and (2) the hydroxy compounds or alcohols. The amino compounds are alkaline in nature because they are either secondary or tertiary amines. Their names, in most cases, end with the suffix "caine" or "ane." Hydroxy compounds are aliphatic (straight chained), cyclic, or aromatic (benzene ring) alcohols. The most important compounds in the alcohol group are benzyl alcohol, monobromosalicyl alcohol, menthol, chlorbutanol, phenol, and octyl alcohol. None of the alcohols is so effective as the nitrogen-containing derivatives with respect to duration of topical action or effectiveness. In addition, they are not suitable for injection because they are cytotoxic and cause local injury in therapeutic concentrations. The alcohols are not convulsants and do not, as a rule, cause systemic reactions characteristic of the amino type compounds. They are not ionized and their activity is not influenced by alkalinization.

The chemical configuration of the effective nitrogen-containing local anesthetics consists of a hydrocarbon nucleus (A), usually of the aromatic type, and an amino nitrogen (C), separated by an intervening two or three carbon chain (B).

The chain is usually referred to as the pivot. The hydrocarbon nucleus is attached to the pivot at X by an ester, amide, or ether linkage. Compounds that adhere closely to this configuration appear to be the most effective clinically, the least toxic locally, and the most toxic systemically. Departure from this configuration causes a diminution of both anesthetic potency and a systemic toxicity, and an increase in local toxicity. Dibucaine, cocaine, tetracaine, and lidocaine conform to this conventional configuration. These drugs are potent, relatively speaking, and are not cytotoxic in the recommended effective clinical concentrations. On the other hand, phenacaine, pramoxine, tripellennamine (Pyribenzamine), and dyclonine (Dyclone) depart from the conventional configuration. They are, relatively speaking, less potent topically. More concentrated solutions are required for effective anesthesia when this type is used. Slough, edema, and other local reactions may follow injection. Pyribenzamine has two nitrogen atoms in its structure, since it is a derivative of ethylenediamine. This configuration is a distinct departure from the so-called conventional configuration which has been described previously. A concentration of 4 or 5 per cent is required for topical anesthesia. Although it was enthusiastically hailed as a suitable topical anesthetic, clinical experience with the drug has been disappointing. It is nowhere near as effective as cocaine, dibucaine, tetracaine, lidocaine, or dyclonine as a topical anesthetic. Also, injection perineurally has caused irritation and even slough. The antihistamines, as is the case with local anesthetics, cause local sensitivity; therefore, repeated use may cause cutaneous or systemic allergy.

Absorption of Topical Anesthetics

The topical application of local anesthetics is a widespread practice. Many physicians in all specialty groups resort to their use in this manner. The application of local anesthetics to mucous membranes may be a hazardous procedure unless extreme caution is exercised. These drugs have a lethal potential which commands respect. The foremost, and a life-threatening, hazard of local anesthetics stems from the adverse systemic effects resulting from rapid absorption. Rapid absorption occurs in highly vascular areas more than in the nonvascular areas. In essence, systemic reactions result from overdosage. The majority of adverse reactions from local anesthetics occur when an excessive quantity of a drug gains access to the systemic circulation. It has been well established that the rise in blood levels after topical application to the mucosa of the pharynx, trachea, and bronchi is rapid, because these drugs readily penetrate the epithelial surfaces of the mucous membranes. Blood levels simulate, to a certain extent, those resulting from intravenous injection. However, the peak levels attained are intermediate between those resulting from intravenous injection and local infiltration. Absorption through the unbroken skin is

insignificant, and any relief afforded is most likely the result of a placebo effect. It is questionable that otic preparations used in the external ear are effective.

The ease of absorption of local anesthetics varies with the type of mucous membrane to which the drug is applied, the area of the surface exposed to the drug, and the concentration of the drug. Peak levels are attained most quickly after application of local anesthetics to the mucous membranes of the tracheobronchial tree; next, to the mucosa of the pharynx. They are poorly absorbed after esophageal or intragastric instillation. Blood levels may rise quickly after instillation of a drug into the posterior urethra, particularly if the surface has been traumatized by the passage of sounds, catheters, or other types of instrumentation. Some absorption may occur from the bladder but this is not significant. Absorption from the lower esophagus, stomach, and bladder is poor because the contents are acid. The drug exists in the form of its salt, and the salt is ionized and does not penetrate epithelial barriers. The urine is acid and any unmetabolized drug which is excreted exists in the ionized state and likewise is not absorbed. In addition to poor absorption because of ionization, the low blood level after gastric instillation is also the result of the greater likelihood of the drugs' being metabolized more rapidly than normally because they are transported via the portal system through the liver where they are either temporarily stored or undergo rapid metabolic degradation.

Absorption is extremely rapid from serous surfaces, such as the pleural spaces or peritoneal cavity. Blood levels rise almost as quickly from these sites and to the same level as if the drug were administered rapidly intravenously. Absorption from the alveoli likewise is rapid. Nebulized particles of local anesthetic solutions less than 3 μ in diameter reach and coat the alveolar surface. The hydrostatic pressures in the capillaries of the lung are of such values that any fluid in the alveoli is quickly drawn into the blood. Thus, a dry alveolar surface is always assured, and collection of fluid in the lung is averted. Particles less than 100 μ in diameter are baffled in the pharynx and mouth or on the tongue and do not pass into the trachea or bronchi.

Evaluation of Topical Anesthetics

The effectiveness of topical anesthetics in man has not been easy to assess. No wholly satisfactory method of comparing one drug with another under identical conditions has been available. The wide variations in response and tolerance between individuals, and the rate and degree of absorption in one part of the body as compared to another have made comparison difficult. Many drugs have been evaluated for their anesthetic effects on the cornea of rabbits, guinea pigs, and man. The data obtained from these studies have not been reliable indices of their effectiveness clinically for endoscopy in the trachea, pharynx, larynx, bronchi, and esophagus. The ability to suppress the cough reflex in the trachea has also been used as a means to assess topical activity, particularly in man. This method has certain obvious drawbacks. First, the activity of this reflex varies from one person to another. Second, it becomes exhausted and decreases progressively after a stimulus is repeatedly applied to a given area. The activity of the reflex is diminished in the aged; therefore, age is a variable factor.

The author and his co-workers devised a method for comparing the potency and effectiveness of topical anesthetics in man. They utilized a pulsatile electric current of low voltage and amperage delivered by a nerve stimulator. The current causes a tingling sensation when the electrode is applied to a mucous surface. The amperage and voltage necessary to elicit the response on the mucous membranes are far less than are required to elicit the same response on the skin. The tip of the tongue was found to be the most sensitive area in the body responding to an electrical current since it is heavily endowed with sensory receptors.

The author and his co-workers studied a series of 50 drugs. They found that cocaine, tetracaine, and dibucaine were the most potent and longest lasting agents in the entire series. The mean difference of the duration of action of the three drugs expressed in minutes was so small that it was not considered significant. It is difficult, therefore, to state categorically which of the three drugs is the longest lasting in the concentrations used. It appears that 0.5 per cent dibucaine is the most potent.

The duration of action of a given topical anesthetic varies from one mucous surface to another. For example, the duration of action in the conjunctival sac of the eye is twice that at the tip of the tongue. The duration of action of a topically applied drug is increased progressively as the concentration is increased until a maximal concentration is attained, after which no further increase in duration results. Exceed-

ing the concentration merely increases the possibility of overdosage and a systemic reaction. In fact, the duration of anesthesia is shortened when the maximum effective concentration is exceeded. The buffering mechanisms within the mucous membranes are less effective than those of other tissues. The acid released from the salt is adequately handled by the mucous membranes up to a given point, beyond which it no longer operates. When an excess is used, decreased activity results. This is due to lowering of the tissue pH by the excess acid released from the salt.

Correlation of the effective dose of a local anesthetic with the toxic dose is virtually impossible in man. Twenty per cent cocaine is equally as effective as 1 per cent tetracaine as far as duration of action is concerned. However, one would not recommend 20 per cent cocaine for routine use; therefore, distinctions must be made between the maximum effective concentration and the optimal concentration that is clinically safe. Reactions occur most frequently when the quantities used are excessive and exceed a tolerable maximum of a particular drug in a patient. The effectiveness of concentrations used in the studies at the tip of the tongue, however, are not necessarily a reflection of the concentration one would use clinically because such factors as dilution with saliva, loss due to baffling, and the total concentration of drug delivered to a given area introduce uncontrollable variations.

Clinicians frequently request specific figures from pharmacologists that indicate safe limits of dosage. Although tables indicating maximal tolerable quantities of local anesthetic drugs for clinical use are available, such values are, at best, approximations and serve only as general guides. Variable factors such as tolerance and technique of use, site of application, vascularity of the tissue, body temperature, etc., modify the dosage of drug applied. One cannot, therefore, place complete reliance upon tables of dosages recommended as limits. Reactions do not necessarily occur when recommended limits are exceeded; yet they may occur when less than the limit is used, because of variations in tolerance. Untoward responses may occur when less than the recommended maximum dose is used in patients who have diminished tolerance.

Effect of Tissue Buffers

Since local anesthetics are amines, they are basic and combine with acids to form salts.

Ordinarily the salt is the form dispensed for clinical use. This is so because salts are stable, water soluble, and easily sterilized. Tissue fluids have considerable buffering capacity, and the pH solution of a local anesthetic, whether it be acid or alkaline, becomes adjusted to that of the tissues.

Alkalinization of solutions of local anesthetics has been proposed to increase their effectiveness. This procedure is of no value for the injection techniques because the buffering potential of the tissues offsets the effect of alkalinization. The buffering capacity of the mucous membranes, however, is limited, and alkalinization may be of benefit. The free base is less soluble than that of the salt. The duration of action of the base topically applied, however, is less than that of the salt. Alkalinization of procaine hydrochloride, which is ineffective even in 20 per cent concentrations, causes some increase in effectiveness. Even though alkalinized, its duration averages not more than nine to ten minutes. Neither the duration of action nor the effectiveness of the procaine base is comparable to that of cocaine hydrochloride. Alkalinization appears to be a procedure of doubtful clinical importance. Injections of suspensions of the base are locally cytotoxic and cause neurolysis.

Period of Latency

A period of latency precedes the establishment of anesthesia irrespective of the site of application of the local anesthetic drug. The period of latency varies with the chemical nature of the drug. It is, as a rule, longer for longer lasting drugs. It is also directly related to the concentration used. The duration becomes progressively shorter as the maximum effective concentration is reached. The period of latency when 4 per cent cocaine is used at the tip of the tongue is four minutes; the overall duration is ten minutes. As the concentration approaches 20 per cent the period of latency is shortened to one minute and the duration is increased to 50 minutes. Some clinicians who consider 4 per cent cocaine unsatisfactory and prefer the 10 per cent solution have the erroneous impression that the greater efficacy is the result of retardation of absorption because of the vasoconstrictor action of cocaine. This, however, is not the case. The improvement in anesthesia and a shortening of the period of latency are the result of the increase in concentration and not of local vasoconstriction.

Use of Vasoconstrictors

For more than 70 years vasoconstrictors have been used extensively to retard absorption and to prolong the action of local anesthetics. Dozens of vasoconstrictors are available, but of the many which have been tried for regional anesthesia, epinephrine is the most effective. Vasoconstrictors are helpful when added to solutions for injection perineurally, peridurally, or intrathecally. For some reason not clearly understood, they are ineffective topically. The author and his co-workers found that topical norepinephrine was, like epinephrine, ineffective. Ephedrine and phenylephrine, which are slowly metabolized, likewise do not prolong the action. Therefore, failure to act is not due to breakdown of these substances. The polypeptide type vasoconstrictors, such as angiotensin, vasopressin, and octapressin, which act directly on the arteriolar smooth muscle or the capillaries themselves and not on the adrenergic receptors, as does epinephrine, are also ineffective. Angiotensin (Hypertensin) is ineffective when injected perineurally because it is metabolized by tissue enzymes. Vasopressin is not quickly detoxified locally. It possesses a vasoconstrictor activity which nearly equals that of epinephrine. Octapressin is a synthetic polypeptide that contains the same eight amino acids found in vasopressin but arranged in a different order. It is equally as effective as epinephrine intrathecally, subcutaneously, and perineurally, but it is not effective topically.

Effect of Nonanesthetic Substances

Supplementary nonanesthetic substances are often added to local anesthetic solutions in an attempt to intensify and prolong their effect. Substances recommended are various cations, vasodilators, enzymes such as hyaluronidase, demulcents, detergents, and agents that increase viscosity. The addition of cations to solutions of local anesthetics modifies the block and potentiates the action if such solutions are injected perineurally. Topically, however, they cause no change in duration. Calcium, potassium, sodium, magnesium, and ammonium ions in concentrations ranging from 2 to 5 per cent neither prolong nor increase the intensity of anesthesia when added to 1 per cent tetracaine or 10 or 15 per cent cocaine.

A mixture known as Forrestiere's solution, used by some otolaryngologists for endoscopic procedures in the nose, pharynx, and trachea, is alleged to be superior to 4 per cent cocaine. This solution is composed of phenol 0.25 per cent, epinephrine 1:100,000, cocaine 4 per cent and potassium chloride 2 per cent. Presumably the phenol acts additively with the cocaine. Apparently the epinephrine prolongs the action of the cocaine by inducing vasoconstriction and retarding absorption, and the potassium supposedly potentiates the effects of cocaine and phenol. Experimental data in man indicate that the duration of action of this mixture is essentially the same as that of 4 per cent cocaine alone.

Detergents, other surface-acting substances, and mucolytic agents have been added to solutions of topical anesthetics to lower surface tension and to facilitate penetration of the anesthetic into the tissues. Hexylresorcinol, tyloxapol, and hexachlorophene added to 4 per cent or 1 per cent tetracaine produced no significant effect. The duration of anesthesia is shortened but not significantly, clinically speaking. Hyaluronidase acts as a spreading factor when injected perineurally; however, it has no significant influence on duration or intensity of anesthesia.

Demulcents or colloidal substances are often added to prolong contact of the drug with the mucous surface. Gelatin, methylcellulose, polyethylene glycol, mucilloid, and similar agents added to aqueous solutions cause no significant prolongation of the action of tetracaine, cocaine, lidocaine, or benzocaine.

Vasodilators added to local anesthetics have little or no significant effect on duration of action. Histamine, nicotinic acid, and theobromine shortened the latent period and the overall duration of anesthesia less than 10 per cent of that of the control. One would expect the drug to be removed from the area much faster than usual if vasodilators produced any significant effect. Whether these are inactive topically and exert no influence upon duration of action has not been established.

Effects of Mixing Drugs

Mixing of two drugs at the maximum effective concentration causes no reinforcement of the activity of either the combination or of each individual drug. The intensity, latent period, and duration of anesthesia using a mixture of two drugs at the tip of the tongue or in the conjunctival sac is the same as the longer lasting of the two drugs. In fact, in some cases the duration of anesthesia with the combina-

tion is shorter than the duration of the longer lasting drug. For example, the overall duration and period of latency of 4 per cent lidocaine combined with 1 per cent tetracaine is the same as that following the use of 1 per cent tetracaine alone. Nothing is gained by combining two anesthetic drugs. The reason given for mixing two drugs is that a shorter acting one has a short latent period while the longer lasting ones have a long latent period. Mixing shortens the time of onset of anesthesia. The possibility of systemic reactions is enhanced when two drugs are combined. Laboratory studies indicate that the systemic effects of two local anesthetics are additive. In fact, some data available concerning work done in rats state that potentiation may even occur.

Reactions to Local Anesthetics

The perineural concentration of a local anesthetic necessary to interrupt conduction in a nerve fiber is many times greater than that tolerated if the drug is circulating in the plasma. The inadvertent intravascular injection of local anesthetics or the rapid uptake from highly vascular areas such as the scalp, mucous membranes, or gums produces a train of symptoms that clinicians refer to as a "reaction." The cardiovascular and central nervous system are the most vulnerable and those in which immediate effects are noted.

Overlapping action is noted between local anesthetics and certain antihistaminic, anticholinergic, narcotic, and adrenergic compounds. Examination of the structural configuration of these compounds reveals the chemical grouping that forms part of the molecule and is assumed to be responsible for local anesthetic activity, namely, an amino group and a hydrocarbon nucleus separated by an intervening chain of two or three carbon atoms.

Types of Reactions

Local

The adverse effects of local anesthetics may be local or systemic. Local effects are due to cytotoxicity; neurolysis, slough, and edema are the usual manifestations. Drugs proved to be locally toxic have been discarded.

Not all adverse effects can be ascribed to the drug itself, however. Sometimes adjuvants, potentiating agents, or preservatives may be responsible for unanticipated responses. Epinephrine, which is often added to an anesthetic preparation to retard absorption, may cause vasospasm, particularly in appendages such as the fingers, toes, ears, and penis. The addition of potassium ion to the molecule to potentiate the effects of the drug may cause edema and soreness. Hydrochloric acid, which is loosely bound with the base of certain drugs (for example, lidocaine), may act upon the metal plungers of syringes specially designed for regional anesthesia and may cause local irritation. Sodium sulfite, which is used to preserve epinephrine, phenol, benzyl alcohol, and similar agents incorporated to prolong the block, may be cytotoxic.

Drugs that are inherently cytotoxic, such as Eucupin and quinine, are obsolete and should not be used. Many local anesthetics are innocuous at low concentrations but are cytotoxic and cause slough at high concentrations. Therefore, it is advisable not to exceed the concentrations recommended for a particular drug.

Systemic

Systemic adverse reactions are most often due to overconcentration, resulting in high plasma levels, intolerance or diminished tolerance, allergic response, and idiosyncrasy. Most reactions are due to high plasma levels resulting from the rapid absorption of the drug or from exceeding the recommended dosage limit. Often these reactions are due to thoughtlessness or lack of appreciation of the hazards of these drugs.

Central Nervous System Effects

The initial effect usually observed from circulating high plasma levels is central excitation. Yawning, excitement (often termed hysteria), nausea, and vomiting may be the prodromata of developing excitation. Twitching of the small muscles merging into generalized tonic or clonic convulsions may follow. Convulsions are of short duration, as a rule. Their duration and severity will be influenced to a large extent by the total quantity of drug absorbed, the blood level, and the rapidity of clearance from the blood stream. Drugs such as procaine or chloroprocaine are rapidly hydrolyzed by the plasma esterases, and thus the excitation caused by these substances is short lived. Drugs such as lidocaine or mepivacaine are amides and therefore are not hydrolyzed in the plasma but, instead, are metabolized in the liver. They may not be cleared from the plasma so quickly as those hydrolyzed by esterase, and the ensuing convulsions may thus persist for longer periods of time.

The generalization that drugs that stimulate the nervous system will, if given in excess, cause depression of that system appears to hold true in the case of local anesthetics. The convulsions may be fleeting in some cases, and a comatose state, accompanied by respiratory failure and areflexia, develops. Electroencephalographic examination reveals that excitation is cortical in origin. It has been assumed that the stimulation occurs from above and proceeds downward. However, studies in animals using deep electrode implantation indicate that this is not necessarily so, because depression of one area of the brain may be occurring while stimulation may be taking place in another area. Whether this occurs in man and is the same for all drugs is not known.

The occurrence of convulsions has been well emphasized by pharmacologists and clinical teachers; because of this, therefore, most physicians are aware of their possible occurrence and the techniques of handling. The convulsions are, however, the more innocuous manifestations of systemic toxicity. Some drugs produce drowsiness, sleepiness, and amnesia without any other manifestation; lidocaine has been incriminated in this respect.

Cardiovascular Effects

The more serious and less emphasized manifestation of intoxication from local anesthetics is depression of the central nervous system and the cardiovascular system. It is generally assumed that the cardiovascular effects of local anesthetics are delayed and appear after the convulsions. However, cardiovascular depression may occur simultaneously with convulsions. This is often overlooked because the convulsions are more dramatic and frightening and thereby draw the attention of the physician to this aspect of the symptoms of systemic intoxication.

Some drugs affect the heart before they produce central excitation; in these instances, the first manifestation of intoxication may be syncope due to myocardial depression, or asystole, which may occur without the slightest suggestion of central excitation. Tetracaine behaves in this manner. Those reactions from tetracaine that are heralded by convulsions are inclined to be benign and amenable to treatment. Usually the less severe reactions are characterized by hypotension, bradycardia, and various types of arrhythmias. However, those cases in which the first manifestation is syncope generally are fatal. In these situations, even though resuscitative measures are instituted promptly, death invariably ensues. Data from animal studies strongly suggest that for each drug a dose exists which, if exceeded, will cause death irrespective of measures instituted to overcome its effect.

Allergic Effects

Adverse reactions are often blamed on allergy to local anesthetics, but actually allergy is an infrequent cause of reactions. However, a local anesthetic can act as a haptene and combine with body proteins to produce an antigen-antibody response on subsequent exposure to the drug. Allergic responses seldom occur after the initial use of a drug; usually there is a history of repeated exposure.

Convulsions and hypotension are not the usual manifestations of an allergic response, instead, dermatitis, edema, bronchoconstriction, and eczema are observed. Usually the response is delayed, relatively speaking, and occurs several hours after the use of the drug. The reaction commonly referred to as anaphylactoid is manifested by the sudden development of syncope, and death may result.

Allegedly the injection of an insignificant amount of drug could produce an allergic response. As little as one drop instilled into the conjunctival sac has been known to cause death. Such reactions are extremely rare; this is fortunate, since so little is known about their etiology and mechanism of action.

As already stated, allergy to local anesthetics occurs most often in patients repeatedly exposed to a drug; nurses, dentists, and physicians are affected most frequently. To support the fact that allergic responses are infrequent, it is worthy to note that when procaine penicillin G was used extensively, many patients who became sensitized to penicillin did not develop such a response to procaine.

The use of skin tests to determine whether one will react adversely to a local anesthetic is of doubtful value. A person who is allergic to the test drug may show a negative response when the drug is administered because the drug, acting as a haptene, combines with the proteins in the skin, which may differ from those elsewhere in the body. Also, the haptene may be a metabolite and not the drug itself. Time may be required for the necessary union to occur. Most difficulties arising from the use of local anesthetics are the result of overconcentration and not of allergy.

Idiosyncrasy

Too often the word idiosyncrasy has been used to describe reaction due to overconcentration. Idiosyncrasy to local anesthetics is an uncommon adverse response. Convulsions and cardiovascular depression are not characteristic of a reaction due to idiosyncrasy. The occurrence of tachycardia and hypertension following the use of small amounts of a local anesthetic, suggesting epinephrine release, has been the usual manifestation of this type of reaction.

Miscellaneous

Bone marrow depression may be placed under the miscellaneous category. Agranulocytosis has been reported after the continued use of procainamide. The possibility that related compounds may do likewise should not be disregarded, but this type of response is unlikely to occur since thses drugs are seldom used for long-term therapy. Methemoglobin may follow the use of local anesthetics. Benzocaine and its allies and prilocaine hydrochloride (Citanest) have also caused this type of response.

Tolerance to Local Anesthetics

Little attention has been given to the status of the patient and his systemic response to local anesthetics. A considerable amount of the data available on toxicity has been obtained from healthy animals, human volunteers, and patients whose physical status can be considered good; for example, patients undergoing hernioplasty or similar operations. Studies in animals and careful analysis of cases of intoxication in man strongly suggest that such factors as myocardial disease, electrolyte imbalance, acidosis, and anemia may be responsible for diminished tolerance to these drugs and that doses ordinarily considered reasonable and within the limits of safety may cause symptoms of overdosage when administered to susceptible patients. This is of utmost importance in surgery and should be strongly emphasized, because a local anesthetic is often selected for "poor risk" patients because it is considered innocuous, when actually it is not.

Treatment and Prophylaxis

The treatment of adverse reactions depends upon their type and cause. Central excitation is preferably combated by the judicious and cautious use of ultrashort-acting barbiturates such as thiopental sodium, sodium methohexital, and thiamylal sodium.

The use of oxygen as an antidote has been suggested, but the evidence that this in any way alleviates the severity of the reaction in the absence of anoxia is not convincing. In animals the duration of excitation and the severity of the cardiovascular response were in no way altered when oxygen was inhaled instead of air. Likewise, the toxic dose was not altered.

The use of neuromuscular blocking agents instead of barbiturates also has been advocated to control convulsions. The neuromuscular response is overcome by the paralysis, but electroencephalographic examination reveals that the excitation persists. Whether this produces irreversible changes in the neurons in the brain is a debatable point that needs clarification. The excitation disappears then thiopental is given.

The recommendation that a muscle relaxant be used is an ill advised one in some respects. Nearly all physicians at one time or another use local anesthetics, and more often than not they use them in situations in which resuscitative equipment and drugs are not immediately available. Furthermore, these reactions occur more frequently when used by inexperienced individuals, many of whom have had no experience in either the treatment of an adverse reaction to a local anesthetic or in the use of muscle relaxants. The muscle relaxants themselves are dangerous drugs since they cause apnea, which requires expert management.

The use of a barbiturate fractionated in small quantities and given slowly is safer. It is true that barbiturates may enhance myocardial depression, but this occurs when an excess is used and administered rapidly. The cardiovascular depressant effects of local anesthetics respond to the intravenous administration of vasopressors, particularly those that stimulate the heart muscle, such as ephedrine.

REFERENCES

Adriani, J.: Clinical pharmacology of local anesthetics. Clin. Pharmacol. Ther. *1*:645–673, 1960.

Adriani, J: Premedication: An old idea and new drugs. J.A.M.A. *171*:108, 1959.

Adriani, J., and Campbell, D.: Fatalities following topical application of local anesthetics to mucous membranes. J.A.M.A. *162*:1527–1530, 1956.

Adriani, J., Webb, C., and Steiner, L.: Preanesthetic medication: 1958 concepts. Southern Med. J. *52*:137, 1959.

Adriani, J., and Zepernick, R.: Comparative potency and duration of action of topical anesthetic drugs in man. Anesthesiology *24*:120–121, 1963.

Adriani, J., and Zepernick, R.: Clinical effectiveness of drugs used for topical anesthesia. J.A.M.A. *188*:711, 1964.

Adriani, J., and Zepernick, R.: Comparative potency and effectiveness of topical anesthetics in man. Clin. Pharmacol. Ther. *5*:49, 1964.

Adriani, J., Zepernick, R., and Hyde, E.: The influence of the status of the patient on the systemic effects of local anesthetic agents. Anesth. Analg. *45*:87, 1966.

Authement, E., and Adriani, J.: Untoward effects of surface and local anesthetics. J. Louisiana Med. Soc. *114*:334–339, 1962.

Kolodny, A. L., and McLoughlin, P. T.: Comprehensive Approach to the Therapy of Pain. Springfield, Ill., Charles C Thomas, 1966.

McNeil Laboratories package insert on Innovar.

Moore, D.: Regional Block: Handbook for Use in Clinical Practice of Medicine and Surgery. 3rd ed. Springfield, Ill., Charles C Thomas, 1964, p. 17.

New Drugs: Local anesthetics. Chicago, A.M.A. Press, 1967.

Pizzolato, P., and Mannheimer, W.: Histopathologic Effects of Local Anesthetic Drugs and Related Substances. Springfield, Ill., Charles C Thomas, 1961.

Steinhaus, J. E.: Comparative study of experimental toxicity of local anesthetic agents. Anesthesiology *13*:577–586, 1952.

GENERAL ANESTHESIA FOR EAR, NOSE, AND THROAT SURGERY

by

Roderick A. Malone, M.D.

A surgeon should clearly understand the scope and limitations of anesthesiology as it relates to his particular field. Advances in this branch of medicine over the past few years have made possible a striking reduction in the morbidity and mortality of surgical patients. Without close cooperation between surgeon and anesthesiologist, however, such improvement could not have been brought about and cannot be maintained. It must be emphasized that the responsibility of the anesthesiologist for the patient is not confined to the operative period, but begins when the decision is made to perform surgery and extends until the day of the patient's discharge from the hospital.

PREANESTHETIC EVALUATION

A complete physical examination, consideration of the patient's history, and knowledge of relevant laboratory data are essential prerequisites for adequate preanesthetic assessment, since impaired function of any major system may have an adverse effect on his course during and after anesthesia. It is in the patient's best interest to identify any significant pathological condition which either may necessitate postponement of surgery until it resolves spontaneously or is treated, or may modify the choice of anesthetic agents to be used. Abnormalities in this context may be termed deficits, and as such are readily classified.

Pulmonary Deficits

Infections

Recent upper respiratory tract infections are associated with accentuated respiratory reflexes, increased secretions and, occasionally, with occult myocarditis. Since encephalitis and ascending paralysis can be associated with viral infections, spinal and epidural anesthesia are inadvisable. Longstanding pulmonary infection, particularly if untreated, predisposes toward increased bronchial secretions and airway obstruction.

Hypoxia

1. Arterial pO_2 is decreased by atelectasis, abnormalities of the ventilation-perfusion ratio, and extrapulmonary shunts because of venous-arterial admixture.

2. Oxygen diffusion is impaired in left ventricular failure, pulmonary edema, and the adult respiratory distress syndrome.

3. Oxygen-carrying capacity is reduced by anemia.

Inadequate Ventilation

1. Airway resistance changes in the presence of tumor, excess secretions, chronic aspiration, bronchospasm, edema, or the airway collapse of emphysema. Expiratory airflow is reduced and cough is ineffectual.

2. Decrease in compliance may exist either because of pulmonary disease such as fibrosis or edema, or because of conditions which reduce thoracic wall mobility. Examples are ankylosis, skeletal deformity, or muscle splinting associated with pain.

Anatomical Aberrations

Features such as a short mandible; prominent upper incisors; short, thick neck; small mouth; and inability to extend the head or open the mouth are usually associated with difficulty in intubation and airway management and must be recognized preoperatively.

Cardiovascular Deficits

Myocardial Dysfunction

In the presence of arteriosclerotic heart disease and coronary insufficiency, anesthesia is associated with a greater likelihood of arrhythmia, decreased cardiac output, and postoperative myocardial infarction. Among patients with a history of recent infarction, the incidence of recurrence rises in inverse proportion to the elapsed time. If this is under six months, there is a 55 per cent chance of another episode; such early recurrences have a mortality rate of about 70 per cent. In all patients who are at risk in this category, the extent of myocardial reserve should be carefully estimated by evaluation of their exercise tolerance.

Hypertension

Some untreated hypertensive patients are hypovolemic. Blood pressure may fall precipitously, especially during induction of anesthesia. Hypertensive crises may also occur during surgery or in the immediate postoperative period. Electrolyte depletion and altered autonomic function may result from rigorous antihypertensive therapy.

Hypovolemia

Blood volume may be contracted because of chronic blood loss, poor nutrition, limited activity, prolonged bedrest, diuretics, and extensive or repeated bowel preparation.

Renal Deficits

General anesthesia for elective surgery is contraindicated in the presence of acute renal disease. Chronic disease is important when associated with any reduction of function, which will always become more marked during anesthesia. Significantly impaired function retards excretion of water, electrolytes, and many of the drugs commonly used in anesthesia such as muscle relaxants, barbiturates, and cardiac glycosides.

Hepatic Deficits

Any history of hepatitis, excessive use of alcohol or narcotics, poor nutrition, or the presence of hepatomegaly requires full laboratory documentation of liver function status. Protein and coagulation factor synthesis may be decreased and drug metabolism altered or impaired. These as well as maintenance of adequate hepatic blood flow during anesthesia are important considerations in the choice of agents to be used. The syndrome of halothane-associated hepatitis is described in the next section.

Metabolic Deficits

1. Endocrine disorders should be treated and stable control established. Uncontrolled diabetes mellitus is associated with cardiovascular and acid-base disturbances. Inadequately treated hyperthyroidism and myxedema also give rise to cardiovascular problems during anesthesia.

2. Patients who have had systemic corticosteroid therapy within the previous year require physiologic amounts, beginning the evening before surgery. In many instances the steroid can be discontinued soon after the procedure is completed.

3. Febrile patients should be treated aggressively to reduce body temperature toward normal.

Neuromuscular Deficits

Muscle relaxant drugs often bring about exacerbation of myopathies and of myasthenia gravis. Succinylcholine administration causes potassium flux from denervated muscle and elevates serum potassium, sometimes to dangerously high levels. Motor deficit following poliomyelitis is temporarily accentuated after the administration of a muscle relaxant, causing the patient great anxiety. If there has been bulbar involvement with respiratory insufficiency, such muscle weakness could be lethal if not recognized.

Drug Interaction

The greater the number of drugs prescribed for a patient, the greater is the likelihood of altered pharmacodynamics. One drug may affect the activity of another. Induction of hepatic microsomal enzymes occurs with chronic usage of alcohol, narcotics, barbiturates, and anticoagulants. Antihypertensive and psychotropic drugs change the patient's response to anesthesia and surgical stress by interfering with the function of the sympathetic nervous system. Myocardial depressants and peripheral vasodilators may also affect his response. Only through accurate documentation of the patient's medications can these problems be foreseen.

A preoperative checklist is not useful, since it soon becomes outdated. Anesthesia complications can often be avoided by timely preoperative consultation. It is far better to discuss any anticipated difficulty well beforehand rather than to wait until the night before surgery after preanesthetic rounds.

PHARMACOLOGY OF ANESTHESIA-RELATED DRUGS

Surgical anesthesia is ideally the minimal degree of cerebral depression required to block afferent impulses from surgical stimuli. The amount of anesthetic administered to maintain this state will change from time to time, depending upon what is being done in the surgical field. Since there is some delay before any such adjustment becomes effective in the brain, good communication between surgeon and anesthesiologist with regard to imminent alterations in levels of stimulation will facilitate optimal timing in this respect.

A summary of the pharmacologic action of drugs used in anesthesia will now be presented in order to emphasize the importance of understanding pathophysiologic mechanisms in the selection of appropriate techniques.

Inhalation Agents

Halothane

The most frequently used primary anesthetic is halothane. This drug provides smooth, rapid induction of and emergence from anesthesia. Anesthesia planes are not difficult to recognize and can be changed relatively easily. It is nonflammable. Halothane is a potent respiratory depressant, but not an irritant. Since it gives rise to little or no bronchospasm or laryngospasm, it is excellent for the patient with chronic obstructive pulmonary disease or asthma. It is a potent myocardial depressant, but compensatory sympathetic reflexes are usually not disrupted if light planes of anesthesia are maintained. Halothane, in common with all the other hydrocarbon anesthetics, is associated with a high incidence of cardiac arrhythmia. The concomitant use of epinephrine for local vasoconstriction increases this risk which, for arrhythmic potential in both categories, is dose-dependent. With epinephrine, the probability of arrhythmia is high when its concentration is greater than 1:100,000, or when the total dose exceeds 0.1 mg. in ten minutes or 0.3 mg. in one hour. The maximum safe dose during hydrocarbon anesthesia is probably no more than 20 ml. of a 1:200,000 solution.

High concentrations of halothane are sympatholytic, leading to peripheral vasodilation and expansion of the vascular space. This will be detrimental to the patient if hypovolemia is present, but otherwise results in improved tissue perfusion during anesthesia, and can be used as a diagnostic test of adequate volume replacement. All anesthetic agents reduce renal blood flow, and halothane is no exception. Although not itself a muscle relaxant, it poten-

tiates the action of drugs specific for this purpose. There is little postoperative nausea.

Recently the problem of hepatic microsomal sensitivity to halothane has been elucidated. Certain patients to whom it is administered for the first time become sensitized. If given halothane anesthesia again, they will develop hepatic damage which varies in severity from mild to the most severe and lethal form. It has been well documented that the process is a sensitization and not a dose-dependent direct hepatotoxic effect. The problem has been reviewed extensively in the report of the National Halothane Study Group. Allergic manifestations during the postoperative period such as arthralgia, rash, marked eosinophilia, unexplained fever, malaise, symptoms suggestive of influenza, or signs of hepatic dysfunction are all indications that a patient may have become sensitized, and halothane should not be used subsequently. The incidence of halothane-associated hepatitis is only one in 36,500 according to the National Halothane Study, and lower or even nonexistent in other retrospective studies. The syndrome has not been reported in children. Halothane continues to be a most useful drug in patients who do not give a history of previous sensitization.

Methoxyflurane

Methoxyflurane is a halogenated ether. It differs from halothane in that it is a better analgesic, obtunds airway reflexes more consistently at a given level of anesthesia, and can be administered safely in high temperature environments. In anesthetic doses there is some degree of muscle relaxation, and the dose of muscle relaxant may be reduced. Because methoxyflurane is highly soluble in blood and fat, induction and emergence may be prolonged, and residual effects may be present for as long as two or three days. Recently it has been used more as an analgesic supplement to nitrous oxide than as a primary anesthetic. It is a potent respiratory and myocardial depressant, sensitizing the myocardium to the actions of epinephrine. It is also sympatholytic. Since there is probably cross-sensitivity with halothane, methoxyflurane should not be given to a patient in whom halothane-induced hepatic sensitivity is suspected to have occurred.

There have been numerous reports of high output renal failure following administration of methoxyflurane. This is not related to the decrease in renal blood flow which occurs during anesthesia, but results from toxic action of fluorine, a metabolic breakdown product, on renal tubular epithelial cells. It is dose-dependent, is more common in obese patients, and has been associated with concurrent use of tetracyclines.

Fluoroxene

Fluoroxene is a halogenated ether. The greatest advantages are a sympathomimetic effect and relative absence of respiratory depression, features which are especially of benefit in the elderly or debilitated. The compound is flammable in concentrations greater than four volumes per cent but these are reached only during induction. Unfortunately postoperative nausea is relatively common.

Ether

The use of ether has declined progressively through the years because of its flammability, slow induction and emergence, and high incidence of postoperative nausea and vomiting. However, its advantages are that in surgical planes of anesthesia respiration is usually stimulated, and negative inotropism is offset by sympathetic stimulation.

Cyclopropane

Induction of anesthesia with cyclopropane is rapid. Cyclopropane is sympathomimetic, and blood pressure is maintained despite direct myocardial depression unless morphine is used as a premedicant. Many anesthesiologists prefer to use cyclopropane in a hypotensive patient because blood pressure is raised to normal or greater than normal by peripheral vasoconstriction; however, there are arguments against this concept of blood pressure maintenance at the expense of tissue perfusion. Cyclopropane is explosive. Cardiac arrhythmias occur, and the incidence is increased by simultaneous use of epinephrine. It is a potent respiratory depressant. Renal and hepatic blood flow are markedly reduced. For these reasons, cyclopropane is often reserved only for rapid induction in children.

Nitrous Oxide

Nitrous oxide is probably one of the most frequently used inhalation anesthetics. Some mildly depressive effects on the myocardium,

peripheral vasculature, kidney, and liver are rarely of clinical importance. It is slightly sympathomimetic. Although not a potent anesthetic, it provides sufficient analgesia to be useful as a carrier for more effective drugs.

Nitrous oxide is more soluble than nitrogen in blood. A gas-filled space (e.g., lung cyst, closed loop of bowel, air-filled ventricles, pneumothorax, or air embolism) will increase in volume when nitrous oxide is breathed. This occurs because nitrous oxide diffuses into it rapidly in order to reach equilibrium, whereas nitrogen diffuses out slowly. When the inspired concentration of nitrous oxide is 80 per cent, the amount of gas in the space will increase fivefold. A vein graft for tympanoplasty may be displaced when nitrous oxide diffuses into the closed middle ear space.

Intravenous Agents

Intravenous anesthetic agents are popular for induction because the stage of excitement is passed through rapidly or does not occur at all. If the patient's condition should deteriorate during administration of an inhalation agent, anesthesia can be rapidly lightened by elimination of the drug through the lung. With intravenous anesthesia, on the other hand, this safety feature does not exist. The action of most intravenous agents used for induction is rapid and usually of short duration, because immediate high brain-blood levels are quickly reduced by redistribution. However, as tissue stores become progressively saturated, duration of action is prolonged.

Thiobarbiturates

In the United States anesthesia is most frequently induced by a thiobarbiturate, because induction is rapid and pleasant. These drugs cause marked depression of respiration and myocardial function and may produce profound hypotension if the patient is hypovolemic or in poor general condition. Barbiturates are not ideal for maintenance of anesthesia because of the degree of cerebral depression required to block response to surgical stimulation.

Narcotics

Recently narcotics have been used in large doses as primary anesthetics because they cause little myocardial depression. When given in this manner, these drugs produce first a profound analgesia and eventually anesthesia. Peripheral resistance is decreased, so severe hypotension may occur in the hypovolemic patient. There is marked respiratory depression, and controlled ventilation is mandatory during anesthesia. However, in the postoperative period respiratory depression is advantageous if it is felt necessary to assist ventilation to assure adequate oxygenation in a patient with pulmonary complications.

Rapid administration of large doses of narcotics may cause generalized muscle rigidity which can be relieved by muscle relaxants. A new narcotic antagonist naloxone hydrochloride (Narcan) is now available for clinical use. Unlike other drugs in this category, it is a pure antagonist. In the absence of narcotics it exhibits essentially no pharmacological activity. It effectively antagonizes all the effects of narcotics, but excitement may occasionally follow its use.

Shorter acting narcotics allow more flexibility during anesthesia. Fentanyl, an analgesic 50 to 100 times more potent than morphine, has been introduced recently for clinical use in the United States. The analgesic effect of this drug lasts 30 to 40 minutes, which makes it particularly useful during anesthesia since the duration of narcotic action can be planned to terminate at the end of surgery so that postoperative respiratory depression does not occur.

Innovar

Neurolepsis is a tranquil state in which a person lies with eyes closed, has no interest in his environment, and is slow to respond to external stimuli. However, he is easily roused and is in full command of his intellectual functions.

Droperidol, which is a butyrophenone derivative, is a neuroleptic agent. It is also a potent antiemetic and has been found useful in the treatment of Meniere's syndrome and postoperative nausea. In large doses it may produce extrapyramidal symptoms; these can be controlled by benztropine (Cogentin).

Neuroleptanalgesia is produced by the administration of a neuroleptic drug together with a narcotic. A convenient combination is Innovar, which consists of droperidol and fentanyl in a 50:1 ratio. This is an excellent supplement to local anesthesia for certain procedures which require patient cooperation, such as endoscopy. If nitrous oxide is given during neuroleptanalgesia, general anesthesia results. Innovar is often associated with mild

hypotension. Respiratory depression, sometimes severe, is a side effect of its narcotic component. Marked muscle rigidity, which can be blocked by muscle relaxants, may develop if fentanyl is given rapidly. Innovar is contraindicated in myasthenia gravis, Parkinson's disease, and asthma.

Ketamine

Ketamine was introduced into clinical practice in 1970. It produces dissociative anesthesia, a condition in which afferent impulses from the surgical site reach the brain but are not perceived as pain. Visceral pain is less effectively blocked than that of somatic origin. After intravenous injection, anesthesia occurs in one circulation time and the patient awakens four to five minutes later, provided no other depressant drugs have been given. There does not seem to be a cumulative effect.

Ketamine is sympathomimetic. Cardiac output increases, peripheral resistance remains the same or decreases, and blood pressure rises. This may limit its use in hypertensive individuals. The airway is usually well maintained unless it is stimulated; then laryngospasm, bronchospasm, or coughing will often occur. This likelihood is increased in the presence of upper respiratory infection and in the heavy smoker. The drug is a poor choice for procedures in the mouth or airway. Muscle hypertonus and random movements are side effects. Patients must be undisturbed during emergence or they may go through a period of dissociation and hallucination. This does not appear to be a common problem in children, and use has been primarily in the younger age group for repetitive superficial procedures such as burn dressing changes. Ketamine should be used only by trained individuals, and complete anesthesia facilities should be at hand.

Muscle Relaxants

The introduction of muscle relaxant drugs drastically changed anesthesia practice; complete relaxation of the abdomen for surgery could be safely provided, ventilation easily controlled, and the concentration of primary anesthetic reduced.

There are two types of muscle relaxants: those which depolarize the neuromuscular end-plate (succinylcholine) and those which do not (d-tubocurarine, gallamine). With the former, neuromuscular block is maintained until the end-plate repolarizes; the latter act by competitively blocking the action of acetylcholine on the end-plate, thus causing paresis. Depolarizing muscle relaxants are usually short-acting. With higher doses a second phase of activity called desensitization, "dual" or Phase II block may occur in which the postjunctional membrane of the neuromuscular junction becomes progressively desensitized to acetylcholine and a block similar to that of the nondepolarizing drugs occurs. There is no antagonist for a depolarizing drug. Nondepolarizing drugs have a longer duration of action and can usually be antagonized by prostigmine. Persistence of curarization may occur with an overdose of relaxant. Each time a muscle relaxant is used, there is a chance that muscle tone may not return quickly to its preoperative state, and the possibility of inadequate respiratory effort must be borne in mind.

ANESTHESIA CONSIDERATIONS RELATED TO OPERATIVE PROCEDURES

Ear

Surgery of the inner ear is frequently performed under local anesthesia after prior sedation. Overzealous premedication to ensure patient cooperation can cause a degree of depression which is unsafe in the absence of an anesthesiologist. If local anesthesia is inadequate, it may be necessary to provide general anesthesia. Under these circumstances, an appropriate depth is difficult to maintain because dissection and manipulation move in and out of areas locally anesthetized, and the level of stimulus can change abruptly. If high concentrations or large amounts of epinephrine have been injected at the operative site, arrhythmia is likely to occur with inhalation anesthetics.

Procedures in the vicinity of the facial nerve should be done without muscle relaxants if muscle response to a nerve stimulus is required. High concentrations of nitrous oxide should not be used during tympanoplasty.

During microsurgery no spontaneous movement of the patient can be allowed. Alteration of the position of the head during light anesthesia or manipulation of the endotracheal tube must therefore be avoided.

Nose

Anesthesia for procedures in the nose offers no difficulties other than those described previously, i.e., patchy or inadequate local anesthetic infiltration, and the hazards of inordinate doses of epinephrine.

Pharynx

Every patient requiring pharyngeal surgery, including tonsillectomy and adenoidectomy, should be intubated routinely. This eliminates the possibility of airway obstruction or aspiration, even when surgery is in close proximity to the glottis. It is usually feasible, even in complicated surgical procedures such as pharyngeal reconstruction, to work around an endotracheal tube which has been passed through the nose or retracted by a mouth gag.

Endoscopy

Anesthesia for endoscopy presents a number of problems. Local anesthesia may be used. The same care and consideration must be taken as if the patient were to receive a general anesthetic. General anesthesia may be required because the patient is unable or unwilling to cooperate.

Of greatest concern to the anesthesiologist is the fact that the airway can be so easily compromised, so a technique must be chosen which will ensure adequate oxygenation at all times. Inhalation or intravenous anesthetics may be used with controlled ventilation, spontaneous breathing, or apnea. It is important, however, to develop a specific protocol acceptable to both the otolaryngologist and the anesthesiologist. The role that each will play during the procedure must be clearly understood.

Inhalation Techniques

Inhalation anesthesia for laryngoscopy can be provided with or without intubation. Insufflation of ether, methoxyflurane, or halothane has been advocated. Manipulation of the airway activates primitive reflexes that can be obtunded only by deep anesthesia. At this depth of anesthesia, ventilation is severely depressed when methoxyflurane or halothane is used; if ether is chosen, spontaneous ventilation may still be adequate. The presence of electrical connections and light sources around the mouth constitutes an explosion hazard during ether anesthesia. It is difficult to maintain a stable level of anesthesia with insufflation techniques, and on emergence there is often irritation of the airway, and some degree of laryngospasm may occur. For these reasons, this technique has been unacceptable in our department.

Many problems can be obviated if the trachea is intubated and ventilation is controlled. A small endotracheal tube must be used, which may make ventilation difficult. Even a small tube hampers proper examination of the larynx; furthermore, the tube is easily kinked and may be pulled out accidentally.

Inhalation techniques may be used during bronchoscopy if a Sanders ventilating bronchoscope is used. Esophagoscopy presents no problems when the patient is intubated, provided the esophagoscope does not compress the soft endotracheal tube. This can be avoided by the use of armored tubes.

Intravenous Techniques

Various groups have found neuroleptanalgesia together with topical anesthesia to be ideal for endoscopy. In the experience of the author, this technique has not always provided the total relaxation necessary for a thorough examination.

Apneic Oxygenation

Adequate oxygenation can be maintained by a nonventilating technique (apneic oxygenation). The patient's lungs are denitrogenated by having him breathe high flow oxygen for at least ten minutes. He is then anesthetized with an intravenous barbiturate and paralyzed with a short-acting muscle relaxant, and oxygen is insufflated into the pharynx, usually via a nasal catheter. Under these circumstances, arterial oxygen tension is maintained at a safe level for 20 to 30 minutes; of course, the carbon dioxide tension will rise, since carbon dioxide is not eliminated through the lungs. Adequate oxygenation can be maintained even though the airway may be completely occluded during this time. In chronic lung disease, especially if there is maldistribution of ventilation, the period of denitrogenation must be extended. Topical anesthesia with 4 per cent lidocaine will help to suppress hypertension and cardiac arrhythmias, which tend to occur during manipulation of the airway. The procedure should not exceed ten minutes and should be terminated at once if there is any evidence of hypoxia or if cardiac arrhythmias occur. Further attempts at the procedure must await adequate ventilation with oxygen.

The advantages of this method are good relaxation, unobstructed view of the larynx and pharynx, adequate oxygenation throughout the procedure, and lack of problems related to sharing the airway. The technique has been lifesaving in patients who manage to breathe adequately when they are awake but who, during anesthesia, become completely obstructed from tumor or surgical manipulation. Preoxygenation allows sufficient time for recovery from anesthesia and paralysis so that spontaneous breathing may resume, or for the airway to be obtained by other means.

Tracheostomy

The indications for tracheostomy are: (1) airway obstruction present or imminent, (2) inability to clear airway secretions, (3) protection of the airway from chronic aspiration, or (4) facilitation of therapy for respiratory insufficiency.

In acute airway obstruction the first necessity is to relieve asphyxia by ventilation with a mask and oxygen. Surgical manipulation or intubation in the hypoxic patient and the acute respiratory alkalosis which may accompany sudden relief of airway obstruction greatly increase the likelihood of fatal cardiac arrhythmias. Following oxygenation, emergency management of the airway may be facilitated by intubation. If tracheostomy is still indicated, ventilation of the intubated patient can be assured during the operative procedure. If the need for ventilatory assistance or management of secretions is expected to be of short duration, intubation alone may suffice. Tracheostomy is usually indicated if the patient has been intubated for 48 to 72 hours unless extubation is imminent. Prolonged intubation is better tolerated if the tube is passed by the nasotracheal route.

There are circumstances under which the patient should not be intubated first. If, because of edema, trauma, or tumor, the patient is barely able to maintain an airway, the anatomy may be so distorted that the glottis cannot be visualized. Repeated unsuccessful attempts at intubation may cause complete obstruction. In these instances, immediate tracheostomy while ventilation is assisted with mask and oxygen will be preferable.

Complications of endotracheal intubation in children such as glottic web, granulomatous reaction, or subglottic stenosis have been reported. The advantages and risks of intubation have to be weighed against those of tracheostomy in this age group. Neither intubation nor tracheostomy is indicated if the situation can be managed by other means.

Extubation

The safest time to extubate the patient is early in the day when the greatest number of personnel are available to help if there should be any difficulty. The individual who extubates the patient must be fully prepared to reintubate if necessary. Means of oxygenation and equipment for intubation must be available. Those responsible for the initial intubation should be informed before the tube is removed.

Tracheostomy Care

Good nursing care is of utmost importance to the patient with a tracheostomy. Aseptic technique is mandatory; a strict protocol must be set up and followed closely. A sterile glove should be worn on the hand holding the catheter and care should be taken to avoid contamination. If the catheter becomes blocked, it should be replaced; it should always be discarded after use. If the patient has severe pulmonary disease, ventilation with a bag and oxygen is necessary before and after each attempt to pass the catheter. A catheter of appropriate size should be chosen so that it will not completely block the lumen of the tube.

When the nose is bypassed, it is important to humidify the inspired gases artificially; otherwise the cilia of the tracheobronchial mucosa will lose their mucus covering and become inactive. Secretions will accumulate and become inspissated, and infection is prone to occur. The tracheal "collar" does not increase humidity adequately, especially when the inspiratory flow rate is large. This can be improved by the use of a "T-piece" reservoir with a volume equal to the patient's tidal volume. Optimal humidification of the tracheobronchial tree cannot be achieved if the patient is dehydrated.

There is currently much concern about tracheal stenosis following tracheostomy. This is related to infection and to ischemia of the tracheal wall caused by the cuff on the tube. Newer cuffs have a lower pressure which is distributed over a larger area of tracheal mucosa and will probably lead to a decrease in the incidence of this complication.

Oxygen

Oxygen is a toxic drug. High concentrations produce severe and often irreversible pulmonary damage. This probably occurs when the concentration is in excess of 60 per cent, but duration of exposure and the oxygen tension of arterial blood are also of importance. Inspired concentration should be no higher than that necessary to maintain arterial oxygen tensions between 80 and 100 mm. Hg. However, if these levels cannot be reached with less than 60 per cent oxygen, more must be used. Fortunately arterial tension can often be improved by other means, such as changing the patient's position, improving cardiac output, instituting chest physiotherapy, inducing diuresis to relieve pulmonary interstitial edema, giving positive pressure ventilation, or increasing functional residual capacity with positive end expiratory pressure.

Ventilation

The circumstances under which ventilation must be supported are as follows:

1. Inability to maintain ventilation as evidenced by rising arterial CO_2 tension. In acute respiratory insufficiency a pCO_2 of 60 mm. Hg or greater is used as a critical level to determine need for assisted ventilation.

2. Hypoxia which has not been relieved by less aggressive measures.

3. Prohibitive work of breathing secondary to factors such as increased physiologic dead space, change in pulmonary compliance (pulmonary edema), or thoracic compliance (severe abdominal distention). Whatever the cause of increased respiratory work, it is better to institute ventilation early rather than to wait until fatigue and obvious respiratory failure are present.

4. Loss of ventilation secondary to neurological (paralysis) or mechanical (flail chest) failure of the ventilatory apparatus.

Successful management of patients requiring assisted ventilation will depend upon adequate monitoring of respiratory parameters, attention to changes in cardiac as well as pulmonary status, good nursing care, and the frequent attendance of a physician. The patient is therefore best cared for in a specialized facility within the hospital such as an Intensive Care Unit or Respiratory Care Unit.

Major Head and Neck Surgery

Airway

Head and neck resections and reconstructive surgery generally do not present airway problems when carried out electively. Whether the patient will require tracheostomy or endotracheal intubation during the procedure will be determined by the area of dissection. In either case, the endotracheal tube should be sutured into place so that it cannot be displaced inadvertently.

Air Embolus

If the operative field is above the level of the heart, the possibility of air embolism exists. Negative pressure during inspiration is transmitted to veins in the operative field. If a vein is transected during this time, and especially if held open by tissue traction or adherence to surrounding structures, large volumes of air will be aspirated. Air embolism is always a possibility when the patient who is breathing spontaneously is placed in the semi-Fowler's position for surgery, and the risk increases during an inspiratory sigh. Significant aspiration of air is manifested by characteristic "machinerylike" or "gurgling" heart sounds and by hypotension secondary to decreased cardiac output. The following treatment must be instituted immediately:

1. Ligation or compression of the vein through which air has access to the circulation.
2. Aspiration through a central venous catheter, if one exists, in order to recover as much air as possible.
3. Cessation of nitrous oxide anesthesia to minimize expansion of the air which has been introduced.
4. If adequate amounts of air cannot be aspirated through a central venous catheter, the patient should be turned onto his left side and external cardiac massage applied. The purpose of cardiac massage in this position is to allow blood to bypass the serum froth which is obstructing right ventricular outflow, and by this means to restore cardiac output. Small amounts of air remaining in the right ventricle will eventually be forced into the pulmonary circulation and will be eliminated by the alveoli. Occasionally a significant bolus of air will gain access to systemic circulation through right to left cardiac or intrapulmonary shunts, and cerebral air embolism may occur. If brain stem embolization occurs, the patient frequently cannot be resuscitated.

Blood Replacement

Replacement of massive blood loss during surgery is fraught with several hazards. Mismatched transfusion and hepatitis are complications whose incidence will depend upon the quality of the blood bank service. Acid-citrate-dextrose preservative and duration of storage at low temperature are the cause of most of the other problems associated with transfusion. Platelets and labile coagulation Factors V and VIII are lost soon after the blood is drawn. The pH of stored blood, initially 6.9 to 7.0 as a result of acidification, may fall to 6.4 over a three-week period as lactic acid and carbon dioxide accumulate. Potassium levels rise, fibrin debris increases, and the oxyhemoglobin dissociation curve shifts to the left, with the result that smaller amounts of oxygen will be released to the tissues if the patient's arterial oxygen tension is lower than normal. The altered oxyhemoglobin curve has been related to loss of red cell 2,3-diphosphoglycerate. This material appears to increase in red cells of patients having chronic tissue hypoxia (e.g., anemia, chronic pulmonary disease, cardiac failure) as a compensatory measure. Multiple transfusions lowering 2,3-DPG may impair tissue oxygenation in these patients.

When blood is lost during surgery, blood volume may be restored with fluids. Hemodilution results, but provided cardiac output is adequate and the circulating volume maintained, the lowered hematocrit can be tolerated until hemostasis is achieved. At this time whole blood can be transfused to raise the red cell concentration.

Although in most instances there will be adequate reserves of platelets and labile clotting factors, blood replacement greater than the blood volume may deplete these elements. If the platelet count falls below 100,000 per cu. mm., or labile factors become sufficiently diluted, coagulation deficits occur. These can be corrected by the administration of fresh blood, fresh frozen plasma, or platelet concentrate.

Since citrate is added to the preservative to bind calcium, routine administration of calcium has been advocated during transfusion. However, citrate is readily metabolized except in the moribund patient, and most individuals have enough calcium stores available to maintain coagulability. Therefore, calcium should be given only during massive, rapid transfusion or when there is electrocardiographic evidence of calcium deficiency. Calcium chloride is completely ionized and will be effective immediately.

Coagulopathies occurring during surgery are not common but are potentially fatal. Primary fibrinolysis and disseminated intravascular coagulation have been known to be precipitated by decreased tissue perfusion, shock, intense adrenergic stimulation, the release of thromboplastin from traumatized tissues, hemolysis, and the infusion of particulate matter or debris. During surgery the coagulopathy usually presents as severe oozing with or without hypotension. Clot formation is delayed secondary to depletion of platelets, fibrinogen, and other clotting factors; clot lysis will occur in the presence of increased circulating fibrinolysins. The treatment of disseminated intravascular coagulation is replacement of depleted coagulation factors, together with general supportive measures. Heparinization to halt the consumption phenomenon has been advocated. Primary fibrinolysis without consumption phenomenon can be treated with epsilon-amino-caproic acid.

Metabolic acidosis may be present in patients who require major blood transfusion, since lactic acid accumulates in poorly perfused tissue. Restoration of adequate circulation will correct this. Because of the low pH of bank blood, routine administration of sodium bicarbonate has been advocated. However, a large part of the acidity of bank blood is the result of accumulated carbon dioxide, which is readily removed after transfusion by ventilation. Other factors are the citrate preservative and the accumulated lactic acid from red cell metabolism, both of which are metabolized to form bicarbonate. With routine administration of alkali, the patient may eventually develop metabolic alkalosis, which can be detrimental as the oxyhemoglobin dissociation curve is shifted to the left, which does not facilitate tissue oxygenation. It would seem wiser to give sodium bicarbonate only if significant base deficit has been determined by arterial blood gas measurements.

During storage of bank blood some of the cells hemolyze, releasing potassium. Also, red blood cells are less able to hold potassium at low temperature and low pH. As a result, serum potassium levels can be very high in blood which has been stored for three weeks. After the blood is administered, potassium tends to re-enter the cells as the blood warms and the pH rises. There may be some instances, however, when the hyperkalemia will result in characteristic EKG changes. If this should occur, it should be aggressively treated with sodium bicarbonate, hyperventilation, and the administration of ionized calcium and possibly intravenous glucose and insulin, all of which promote movement of potassium into the cell.

Blood Warmers

Blood or blood products should be warmed to body temperature before administration. Cold infusions result in lowered body temperature, especially in air-conditioned operating rooms. Lowered body temperature causes a shift to the left of the oxyhemoglobin dissociation curve, vasoconstriction, metabolic acidosis, and shivering, which results in increased oxygen consumption. Cold solutions infused rapidly, particularly through central venous catheters, produce a temperature gradient across the heart which may lead to fatal arrhythmias.

Induced Hypotension

Blood loss may be reduced and operative conditions improved by deliberate hypotension. Intravascular pressure can be lowered in the surgical field by:

1. Decreasing peripheral resistance with a ganglionic blocking agent.
2. Delaying full replacement of blood loss.
3. Raising the operative field above the level of the heart in order to reduce venous pressure.
4. Decreasing cardiac output with a ganglionic blocking agent, a myocardial depressant such as halothane, or by decreasing venous return to the heart with continuous positive airway pressure. The latter must be applied carefully to avoid distension of veins in the operative field.

Induced hypotension is particularly useful when surgery is performed in a highly vascular area or when hemostasis is otherwise difficult to achieve. An appropriate pressure is one at which capillary ooze is no longer evident.

Although the pressure head in the vascular tree is reduced, organ blood flow is usually maintained at about normal levels because of vasodilatation. Cerebral blood flow is kept normal by autoregulation unless the patient has severe cerebrovascular occlusive disease which renders blood flow to the affected areas pressure-dependent. Since cardiac work and oxygen consumption will be diminished, coronary perfusion is adequate. There is an increase in physiological dead space because pulmonary blood flow is reduced. Inspired oxygen concentration and tidal volume must be raised to compensate for this. When the mean blood pressure is 65 mm. Hg or above, renal blood flow will be adequate. Below this level, glomerular filtration almost stops and urinary output will fall noticeably. However, since blood flow to renal parenchyma is sustained, urinary output will recover as soon as adequate arterial pressure is re-established.

Great care must be taken when placing the patient in position on the operating table, because prolonged compression of soft tissues may result in complete ischemia. This is particularly true of the head. An assistant leaning on it for support may cause pressure necrosis of the scalp where it is in contact with the table; compression of the eye may result in blindness.

Although induced hypotension is often beneficial, certain risks must be kept in mind. Patients with significant cerebrovascular, cardiac, pulmonary, or renal disease are not candidates for this technique. It should be used only in those for whom a life-threatening situation exists and for whom the benefits of hypotension are expected to outweigh the possible hazards.

When surgery is carried out under induced hypotension, it is important before the wound is closed to return blood pressure toward the level which is normal for that patient in order to be assured of continuing satisfactory hemostasis.

Tracheal Resection and Reconstruction

Although tracheal resection may be performed for removal of tumors, it is usually carried out as part of a reconstruction procedure in patients who have developed stenosis at the site of a tracheostomy stoma or at the point of contact of an inflated tracheostomy cuff. Such patients may develop symptoms of airway obstruction insidiously or present with acute respiratory obstruction as a result of edema or inflammation related to an upper respiratory infection or bronchoscopy.

Before surgery the site and extent of stenosis must be accurately assessed. The following approach to anesthetic management is recommended: First, the lungs are denitrogenated with 100 per cent oxygen to provide maximum reserve in case the airway should subsequently become completely obstructed. An indwelling arterial catheter facilitates monitoring of blood pressure and sampling for blood gas analysis. Electrocardiographic monitoring is also advisable. Anesthesia is induced and the trachea intubated. When the trachea distal to the stenotic lesion has been opened, a sterile endotracheal tube is passed and connected to the anesthesia system with a sterile extension tube. The patient is allowed to breathe spontaneously throughout the procedure when possible, so that ventilation can be maintained if accidental extubation should occur. After resection of the lesion, the lower tube is removed, and the one which had been introduced through the larynx is then guided through the area of anastomosis. Following completion of the anastomosis, the tube can be withdrawn to a point proximal to the suture line. The patient's chin is frequently sutured to his chest to keep the neck flexed so

that tension on the anastomosis will be reduced. As this may compromise the airway, it is best to delay extubation until the patient is awake. If pulmonary complications should occur in the postoperative period, every effort should be made to avoid reintubation because of the risk of damage to the anastomosis. Careful attention should be paid to hydration of the patient to prevent the development of edema at the suture line.

The foregoing points cannot, by any means, encompass all the factors that might influence the patient undergoing otorhinolaryngological surgery. Careful preoperative evaluation, communication, attention to detail during the procedure, and rational postoperative support will minimize problems and improve patient care.

REFERENCES

Arkins, R. A., et al.: Mortality and morbidity in surgical patients with coronary artery disease. J.A.M.A. *190*:485, 1964.

Bunker, J. P.: Metabolic effects of blood transfusion. Anesthesiology 27:446, 1966.

Draper, W. B., et al.: Studies on diffusion respiration; alveolar gases and venous blood pH of dogs during diffusion respiration. Anesthesiology 8:524, 1947.

Eger, E., and Severinghaus, J.: Rate of rise of $PaCO_2$ in apneic unanesthetized patients. Anesthesiology 22:419–425, 1961.

Frumin, M. J., et al.: Apneic oxygenation in man. Anesthesiology 20:789, 1959.

Giffin, B., et al.: Anesthetic management of tracheal resection and reconstruction. Anesth. Analg. 48:884, 1969.

Goodman, L. S., and Gilman, A.: The Pharmacological Basis of Therapeutics. 3rd ed. New York, The Macmillan Co., 1965, Sections II and IV.

Heller, M. L., et al.: Apneic oxygenation in man: Polarographic arterial oxygen tension study. Anesthesiology 25:25–30, 1964.

Holmdahl, M. H.: Pulmonary uptake of oxygen, acid-base metabolism and circulation during prolonged apnea. Acta Chir. Scand. (suppl.) 212:1, 1956.

Katz, R., and Epstein, R. A.: The interaction of anesthetic agents and adrenergic drugs to produce cardiac arrhythmias. Anesthesiology 29:763, 1968.

Larson, A. G.: Deliberate hypotension. Anesthesiology 25:682, 1964.

McKay, D. G.: Trauma and disseminated intravascular coagulation. J. Trauma 9:646, 1969.

Miller, R. D., et al.: Coagulation defects associated with massive transfusions. Ann. Surg., Nov. 1971.

Miller, R. D., et al.: Effects of massive transfusion of blood on acid-base balance. J.A.M.A. 216:1762, 1971.

National Academy Sciences–National Research Council: Summary of national halothane study. J.A.M.A. 197:775, 1966.

Pontopiddon, H., et al.: Acute respiratory failure in the surgical patient. *In* Advances in Surgery Vol. 4. Chicago, Year Book Medical Publishers, Inc., 1970.

Scurr, C., and Fellman, S.: Scientific Foundations of Anaesthesia. Philadelphia, F. A. Davis Co., 1970, Section II, p. 121.

Topkins, M. J., et al.: Myocardial infarction and surgery. Anesth. Analg. 43:716, 1964.

REGIONAL BLOCK ANESTHESIA IN SURGERY OF THE HEAD AND NECK

by

Paul B. Borgesen, D.D.S., M.D., and Robert L. Maresca, M.D.

PREMEDICATION AND CONTINUOUS SEDATION IN CONJUNCTION WITH REGIONAL BLOCK ANESTHESIA*

In the late 1890's Ceci, of Genoa, Italy, suggested and used morphine and scopolamine as premedications for operations performed under local anesthesia. The advantages were obvious to the practicing surgeons at that time, and to date there has been no evidence to show that premedication is anything other than helpful to both the surgeon and the patient for such procedures. In addition to allaying apprehension, lowering the metabolic rate, and reducing reflex excitability, proper premedication diminishes the intensity of response to the actual painful stimuli attendant upon the injection of the local anesthetic drug and further diminishes the responses to stimuli, other than pain, either directly or indirectly connected with the operative procedure.

There is no standard "ideal" battery of premedicating drugs suitable for all patients. As a base line for kind of drug, amount, and time of administration, the following has proved successful for the authors for years. One of the barbiturates, sodium phenobarbital, is used by itself, and one of the true narcotics is combined with a parasympatholytic drug (in the authors' hands, meperidine and atropine) and, in the past 10 years, one of the tranquilizing drugs of the hydroxyzine variety is also used.

The time of administration of premedication is as follows: for the sodium phenobarbital, two hours prior to the anticipated time of incision; for the narcotic, parasympatholytic and tranquilizer, one hour prior to the time of incision. As to amount, a base line can be used, with modification to fit the individual situation. For most males between the ages of 25 and 50 and in otherwise good health except for the condition for which surgery is contemplated, 200 mg. of sodium phenobarbital, 100 mg. of Demerol and

0.4 mg. of atropine, with 100 mg. of hydroxyzine, is administered. Such modifications in dosage as are needed should be made. In planning such modifications, cardiovascular and pulmonary status, hepatic function, psychic status, and any existing concomitant disease upon which any of the drugs might be reasonably expected to have an adverse effect must be considered. In our opinion the use of scopolamine in a patient who is to remain awake is contraindicated because of the unpredictability of its effects on the excitability of the cerebral cortex from any form of psychic stimulation.

There is no question in the minds of the authors as to the desirability of the maintenance of an "ideal" state of sedation during the *entire* operative procedure. Therefore in the past five years over 2600 surgical procedures in the field of otolaryngology have been performed under local anesthesia with proper premedication supplemented by the intravenous administration of a solution consisting of 500 ml. of 5 per cent glucose and water containing 100 mg. of Demerol and 100 mg. of Benadryl and administered as a constant drip at varying rates of speed throughout the procedure, such rates being determined by the existing state of sedation of the patient. (It should be emphasized that sedation *only* is the goal, and to this end a 20-gauge needle, or smaller, is used to help to avoid inadvertently rapid administration.) This has proved very satisfactory, and indeed many major procedures have been performed with its use. These have included prolonged operations such as radical neck dissection with en bloc resection of oral and/or oropharyngeal structures. Surgery involving bony structures such as mandibular split or resection and mastoid surgery have not been a problem since well sedated patients tolerate the sound and vibration of the drill quite well. The use of continuing sedation in minor but long procedures, such as face lift, has produced more pleasant postoperative patient comment.

The individual surgeon should, of course, be alert to advances in the field of sedation and should be particularly alert in modern times to the fact that a certain percentage of his patients will already be taking some form of psychic sedation daily and may indeed be consuming

---

*This section deals with useful regional block procedures and will not include topical or infiltrative local anesthesic techniques, such as those employed for tonsillectomy and middle ear procedures since they are readily learned and frequently employed by all surgeons doing operations upon the head and neck.

quantities of alcohol which are indeterminate, two facts which will further modify the use of any of these drugs.

A list of questions is included, the answers to which should provide information to guide the surgeon in his choice of kind and amount of premedicating and maintenance sedative drug:

1. Do you have any diseases of the heart, lungs, kidney, or liver?

2. Do you have any diseases of the thyroid or adrenal glands?

3. Are you taking any medicine at this time for any condition?

4. Have you taken cortisone drugs during the past six months?

5. Do you have glaucoma?

6. Would you describe yourself as the kind of person who has an unusually violent response to pain or to exciting events?

SUPRAORBITAL AND SUPRATROCHLEAR NERVE BLOCK

These nerves, end branches of the first or ophthalmic division of the trigeminal, give sensory innervation to the forehead and upper eyelid. Block anesthesia of these nerves is useful in excision of lesions, the repair of lacerations, diagnostic procedures in facial pain, and in the delay or transfer of pedicle flaps.

Technique of Injection

A short, 17-gauge needle is used. In many patients a supraorbital notch is palpable, and in-

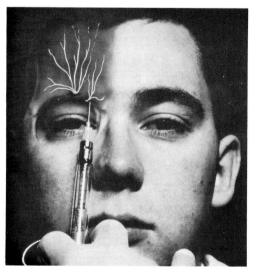

Figure 1. Supraorbital and supratrochlear block.

jection is made on the supraorbital rim at the notch. If a notch is not palpable, the foramen is located at the rim, 3 to 5 mm. medial to the pupil when the eye is in cardinal gaze position. One milliliter of solution usually suffices.

The supratrochlear nerve is injected at the supraorbital rim, halfway between the supraorbital nerve and the nasofrontal angle (lateral margin of the root of the nose) (Fig. 1).

INFRATROCHLEAR NERVE BLOCK

Block anesthesia of this small nerve is occasionally useful. It supplies the medial canthal area and the tissues over the lateral aspect of the bony dorsum of the nose.

Technique of Injection

A short, 27-gauge needle is used to deposit 1 to 2 ml. of anesthetic solution midway between the inner canthus and the dorsum of the nose. The point of injection is on a plane which is a horizontal continuation of the medial canthus.

BLOCK OF THE ANTERIOR AND POSTERIOR ETHMOIDAL NERVES

The anterior ethmoidal nerve is ordinarily "blocked" by a topically applied anesthetic on the lateral nasal wall, high in the dome and superior to the anterior end of the middle turbinate. True block anesthesia, though not often required, can be accomplished within the orbit at the anterior ethmoidal foramen.

Technique of Injection

A 1½-inch needle is introduced through a wheal 1 cm. above the medial canthal ligament. The needle closely follows the junction of the superior and medial orbital walls to a point 1.5 cm. deep to the superior orbital rim, where 1.5 to 2.0 ml. of solution is slowly deposited subperiosteally.

The *external nasal nerve* is merely the terminal external branch of the anterior ethmoidal nerve (Fig. 2). If anesthesia of the nasal tip and ala is all that is required, this branch may be blocked subcutaneously at the junction of the nasal bone and upper lateral cartilage, midway between the nasal dorsum and the base of the nose.

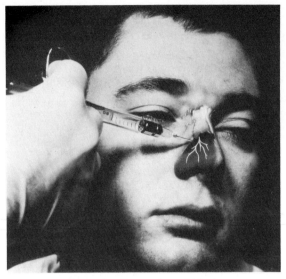

Figure 2. External nasal block.

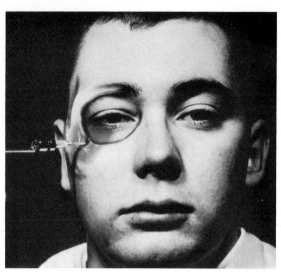

Figure 3. Zygomaticofacial block.

The posterior ethmoidal nerve may be blocked externally by an extension of the above procedure, by advancing the needle an additional 1.0 to 1.5 cm. posteriorly and making the injection at this point. Since the optic nerve lies at an average 4-cm. depth from the superior orbital rim, the needle depth at no point should exceed 3 cm.

Intranasal anesthesia of the posterior ethmoidal branches is ordinarily obtained by cotton strips or cotton applicators applied to the mucosa of the posterior portions of the middle and superior meatuses. Intranasal block is ordinarily not possible, since this nerve presents to the nasal cavity as several branches rather than as a single trunk.

The most neglected area of the internal nose as regards obtaining complete anesthesia is the posterior portion of the middle and inferior meatuses and posterior tip of the inferior turbinate. These areas are heavily innervated by the posterior nasal branches of the maxillary nerve. Special attention to infiltration or topical anesthetization of these areas is therefore occasionally required.

ZYGOMATIC (ZYGOMATICOFACIAL) NERVE BLOCK

Block anesthesia of this nerve is not often required but may be useful in maxillary surgery or repair of lacerations.

Technique of Injection

It is blocked at its foramen of exit from the orbit, which is at the junction of a vertical line along the lateral orbital rim and a horizontal line along the infraorbital rim (Fig. 3).

Intraorbital block of this branch may be useful during orbital exenteration. Here, an attempt at subperiosteal injection at the junction of floor and lateral wall of the orbit should be made 2 cm. deep to the orbital rim.

MAXILLARY NERVE BLOCK

The maxillary nerve, the second division of the trigeminal, innervates the skin and mucosa of the midface, including the maxilla, palate, and teeth. It is accessible to nerve block as it traverses the pterygopalatine fossa. Although extra-oral routes of injection are described, these are rather difficult to perform adequately, are usually painful, and generally are not necessary. The intra-oral route is rather painless and relatively simple to perform if one can visualize the anatomical structures involved. Indications for use of this nerve block are: extensive midfacial procedures such as partial maxillectomy, extensive antral surgery including vidian neurectomy and cryosurgical approach to the internal maxillary artery, palatal surgery, repair of midface fractures, and extensive dento-alveolar surgery.

The authors employ an intra-oral route which consists in anesthetization of the labiobuccal sulcus as it begins to curve postero-inferiorly just above and posterior to the third molar tooth. A small wheal is raised in the posterior-most point of the superior labiobuccal sulcus. A 25-gauge spinal needle is bent to an angle of 60 degrees at a point 4 cm. from the needle tip. The needle, attached to the syringe, is inserted into the wheal and passed superomedially, with slight inclination posteriorly, along the posterior margin of the maxillary tuberosity and advanced into the sphenomaxillary fissure and into the pterygopalatine fossa. Practice on a skull will serve to fix the spatial relationships in the operator's mind. If the needle meets bony obstruction prior to its complete entrance of 3 cm., it has usually abutted the base of the lateral pterygoid plate and should be partially removed and advanced in a more vertical path. Aspiration prior to injection is necessary, since intravascular injection (pterygoid venous plexus or internal maxillary artery) is a possibility. Two or 3 ml. of anesthetic solution is deposited slowly.

On rare occasions a temporary (hours) diplopia results owing to diffusion of the anesthetic solution into the superior orbital fissure. The patient is told of this possibility and that it is of no concern.

The authors have also employed this route in the diagnosis and temporary alleviation of vascular face pain of midfacial and retro-orbital distribution. The point of injection is just short of the pterygopalatine fossa. The solution used is a mixture of local anesthetic and corticosteroid. The rationale for this procedure is the perivascular diffusion of material, an end which is not difficult to obtain. This is a commonly successful technique, but vascular face pain is not in the scope of this chapter.

INFRAORBITAL NERVE BLOCK

The infraorbital nerve, which constitutes the direct continuation of the maxillary nerve, supplies the tissue of the lower eyelid, anterior cheek, and nasolabial fold area and mucosa above the nasal vestibule and is readily accessible to nerve block for use in surgical procedures and for diagnostic procedures in neuralgias with trigger zones in this area.

The nerve is usually anesthetized at its point of exit at the infraorbital foramen since entrance of the needle into the infraorbital canal itself is rarely indicated and may result in injury of the nerve with fibrosis and painful paresthesias. The foramen is located just medial to the midpoint of the infraorbital ridge, directly below, or directly below and a millimeter or two medial to, the pupil of the eye when the eye is in cardinal gaze position.

From an extraoral route (Fig. 4) a small wheal is raised in the skin approximately one finger breadth below the bony margin of the infraorbital rim and the needle advanced directly toward the bone and in a position angled slightly upward. The point of injection will be 0.5 cm. below the orbital ridge. Two milliliters of anesthetic solution usually suffice. It is not necessary to enter the canal itself.

When using the intra-oral route, the needle is inserted into the labiobuccal sulcus with the same landmarks being kept in mind, but necessarily with the needle angled in a more superior direction. If the needle point is not palpable, deposition of a small amount of the solution will enable the operator to feel the swelling beneath his fingertip for more accurate localization of the neurovascular bundle. Two milliliters of anesthetic solution is slowly deposited at the foramen after aspiration.

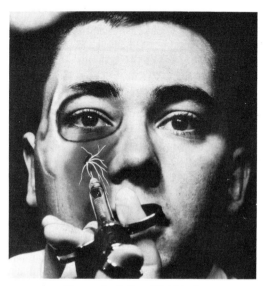

Figure 4.   Infraorbital block.

GREATER PALATINE AND NASOPALATINE NERVE BLOCKS

The greater palatine nerve leaves the maxillary nerve in the pterygopalatine fossa and descends in the pterygopalatine canal to emerge through the greater palatine foramen to give sensory innervation to all but the premaxillary segment of the palate. Lesser or posterior palatine nerves are also described as being separate branches; however, the point is didactic since anesthetization of the greater palatine nerve adequately blocks the lesser branches as well.

The nasopalatine nerve, one of the posterior nasal branches of the maxillary nerve, traverses the nasal septum to enter the palate through the incisive foramen, supplying the premaxilla portion of the palate.

Technique of Injection

The entire palate can be anesthetized by a bilateral greater palatine nerve block and a nasopalatine block.

The greater palatine foramen is located 1 cm. medial to the interspace between the second and third maxillary molars. Less than 0.5 ml. of solution is required, and entrance *into* the pterygopalatine canal is not necessary. Though passage through the pterygopalatine canal is a route to the main trunk of the maxillary nerve, its use is not highly recommended since the anesthesia obtained is usually not profound and the probability of postinjection paresthesias in the greater palatine distribution is fairly high.

The incisive canal and nasopalatine nerve are located deep to the nasopalatine papilla, in the midline just posterior to the central incisors. A few tenths of a milliliter of solution is all that is required to obtain profound anesthesia of the premaxillary segment of the palate.

MANDIBULAR AND LINGUAL NERVE BLOCKS

Regional block anesthesia of the mandibular or third division of the trigeminal nerve is an extremely useful and commonly employed procedure. To obtain complete anesthesia of the mandibular nerve requires considerations of its three major branches, namely, the inferior alveolar nerve, the lingual nerve, and the long buccal nerve. Generally speaking, the auriculotemporal branch is not anesthetized for procedures for which third division anesthesia is required.

Injection of the inferior alveolar nerve will obtain anesthesia of that half of the mandibular bone, the teeth as far as the midline, and the mental nerve which supplies the tissues of the corresponding half of the lower lip and anterior chin. Anesthesia of the lingual nerve will be limited to the anterior two thirds of the tongue on the corresponding side, the mucosa on the floor of the mouth and the gingival mucosa lingual to the teeth (Fig. 5). The long buccal nerve supplies general sensation to the buccal gingiva and the buccal mucosa itself as far superiorly as the orifice of Stenson's duct.

Technique of Injection

The needle employed is 1⅝ inch, preferably 25-gauge, although needles somewhat longer may be used. Since the end target of the injection will be the mandibular foramen just posterior to the lingula on the medial aspect of the ramus of the mandible, and considering that the mandibular foramen is in the approximate geometric center of the ramus, palpation with the fingers on both the anterior and posterior borders of the mandible will enable the operator

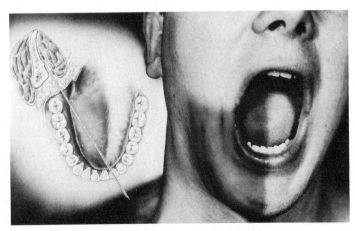

Figure 5. Anatomy of the third division (mandibular nerve) block.

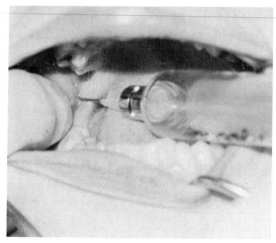

Figure 6.   Right mandibular block.

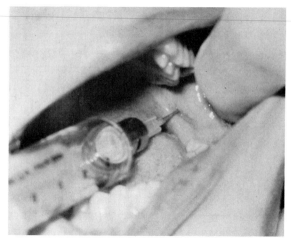

Figure 7.   Left mandibular block.

to stereognostically visualize this point. For a *right* mandibular block (Fig. 6), the thumb palpates the anterior border of the ramus immediately above the occlusal plane of the teeth, and the index, middle, and ring fingers palpate the posterior border of the mandible, with the small finger being placed along the inferior border of the mandible just anterior to the angle. The needle is introduced into the triangular space formed laterally by the anterior border of the ramus and medially by the pterygomandibular raphe. The point of entrance is in the center of this triangle, approximately 7 to 10 mm. above the occlusal surface of the teeth, which in most cases would be at the midsection of the operator's thumb. The barrel of the syringe lies in a horizontal plane and, with the needle just entering the mucosa, the posterior portion of the barrel lies across the bicuspid region on the opposite side of the mouth. Entrance is made to a depth of approximately 1 cm. where 0.5 to 1.0 ml. of the anesthetic solution is deposited to anesthetize the *lingual branch*. Advancement is then made to contact the bone in the geometric center of the ramus where 1 to 2 ml. of the solution is deposited. Because of the intense vascularity of the pterygoid area, aspiration is performed prior to injection and the injection is performed slowly. The needle is withdrawn and injection is made into the retromolar triangle (that space on the anterior surface of ramus formed by the external oblique line laterally and the internal oblique line medially) at the same level as the inferior alveolar and lingual injection, and 0.5 to 1.0 ml. of solution is injected to obtain anesthesia of the *long buccal branch*. (It crosses the anterior border of

the ramus into the buccal region at approximately this level.)

Injections on each side of the mandible are, of course, made identically; however, it should be noted that with the right-handed operator, a *left* mandibular injection (Fig. 7) can best be made with the operator's left arm curving over the patient's forehead and left side of the face, so that his thumb is again on the anterior border of the ramus but the index finger lies along the inferior border of the mandible just anterior to the angle, and the long, ring, and small fingers lie along the posterior border of the mandible. In this manner, the patient's head is entirely surrounded by the operator's arm, a technique long and successfully employed by dentists.

Additional Techniques

A technique of varying the position of the needle within the tissues of the pterygomandibular space is sometimes taught. This is technically unnecessary and on rare occasions results in a broken needle.

External block anesthesia of the mandibular nerve can be obtained through both a lateral entrance into the sigmoid notch and an inferior entrance from below the angle of the mandible. These are rarely necessary, are inaccurate, and will not in most cases obtain complete conduction anesthesia.

Bilateral mandibular nerve blocks are frequently of use to the otolaryngologist, primarily for biopsy purposes and for extensive intra-oral resections. The authors have utilized this type of anesthesia in conjunction with cervical plexus block to perform mandibular section with resection of a portion of tongue, floor of mouth, mandible, and radical neck en bloc.

MENTAL NERVE BLOCK

Anesthesia of the mental nerve can be obtained unilaterally or bilaterally for purposes of performing biopsies of the lower lip, wedge resections, and vermilion advancement techniques. Passage of the needle into the mental foramen itself will block the incisive nerves as well as the mental nerve should procedures including the anterior teeth be required.

Technique of Injection

The mental foramen is situated between the roots of the first and second bicuspid teeth approximately a centimeter from the lower border of the mandible. This point can be easily visualized by the operator and as such can be injected either from the intra-oral or extra-oral approach (Fig. 8). If anesthesia of the mucosa of the lower lip and the skin of the lower lip and jaw is all that is required, entrance of the needle into the canal is unnecessary and 1 to 2 ml. of anesthetic solution deposited against the bone in this area will result in profound anesthesia of these structures; however, if anesthesia of the contents of the mandibular canal anterior to this point is required, as for operations including the structures of the bone and teeth, entrance into the canal is desired and must be made from a posterior direction with the needle angled anteroinferiorly so as to actually enter the foramen. Only tiny amounts of anesthetic agent are required to obtain anesthesia in the mandibular canal itself.

CERVICAL BLOCK ANESTHESIA

The techniques to be discussed may be indicated for any procedure on the neck for which a contraindication to their use does not exist. The contraindications are local infection along the needle routes, lack of familiarity with the technique, unsuitable emotional status of the patient, and inability to properly position the patient.

Technique of Injection

The position of the patient is most important. The upper half of the table should be elevated 20 degrees from the horizontal. The head rest of the table should be lowered 10 degrees to extend the head. The chin should be elevated. These maneuvers should produce an arc of 30 degrees in the curvature of the neck. The chin should next be rotated to the side opposite the proposed block, some 45 degrees from the midline vertical plane.

The transverse process of the cervical vertebrae should now be palpable lateral and posterior to the posterior border of the sternocleidomastoid muscle. It is emphasized that the operator *must* be able to palpate these processes away from the muscle, so that the carotid artery and jugular vein are not in the needle routes. The transverse process of C2 may be found about one fingerbreadth inferior to the tip of the mastoid process, just posterior to the posterior border of the sternomastoid muscle. An intradermal wheal is made at this point.

At the posterior border of the muscle, at a point midway between the tip of the mastoid process and the upper border of the clavicle, the transverse process of C4 may be palpated.

Figure 8. Mental nerve block.

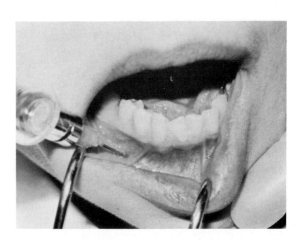

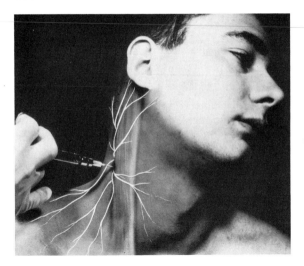

Figure 9. Block of cervical plexus. Superficial nerve distribution illustrated.

When the external jugular vein can be seen, the above point may be just superior to where the vein crosses the muscle. Another wheal is raised at this point. A 27-gauge needle, attached to a 3 ml. finger-control syringe is used. The anesthetic solution may be 2.0 ml. of 0.5 to 2.0 per cent lidocaine (Xylocaine) with epinephrine or the same amount of the solution of the operator's choice. Through this second wheal, 3 ml. of anesthetic may be injected just beneath the border of the muscle, thus blocking the superficial cervical plexus. One 2.5-inch, 25- or 27-gauge needle should now be attached to the syringe and the point advanced toward the palpated transverse process of C4 until the bone is contacted. If aspiration does not produce blood, 3 ml. of anesthetic is slowly injected (Fig. 9), the needle left in, the syringe refilled and reattached to the needle, the needle then withdrawn to just below the skin surface, and directed upward, backward and inward toward the palpated transverse process of C3 until the bone is contacted. Again, if aspiration reveals no blood, 3 ml. of the solution is deposited here. The needle is then completely withdrawn and reinserted through the wheal made over the transverse process of C2 and the same procedure repeated there.

It should again be noted that the operator *must* be able to palpate the transverse process, especially C2, since the solution should be deposited lateral and slightly posterior to the posterior tubercle of this transverse process. The anterior branches of the second cervical nerve, the superior cervical ganglion, the vagus, hypoglossal and glossopharyngeal nerves may be anesthetized with this injection by using 6 ml. of solution instead of the usual 3 ml. If a bilateral block is needed, the above procedures are repeated on the opposite side.

Specific procedures for which cervical block may be used are:

1. Tracheostomy: bilateral superficial cervical plexus block, combined with infiltration over the incision site.

2. Thryoglossal duct cyst and sinus: bilateral superficial and deep cervical block, possibly combined with block of the lingual and superior laryngeal nerves.

3. Branchial cleft cyst: unilateral superficial and deep cervical block, possibly combined with unilateral mandibular block.

4. Operation on the larynx, including laryngectomy: bilateral superficial and deep cervical block with 6 ml. of solution deposited at C2 transverse processes, combined with superior laryngeal nerve block and the addition of C5 to the deep cervical block.

5. Thyroidectomy: bilateral superficial and deep cervical block – as above.

6. Parotidectomy: combined with local infiltration anesthesia along the line of incision, and in minute amounts under the skin flap.

SUPERIOR LARYNGEAL NERVE BLOCK

The position is the same as for cervical block except that the chin need *not* be rotated a full 45 degrees off the midline vertical plane. The inferior border of the hyoid bone and the superior

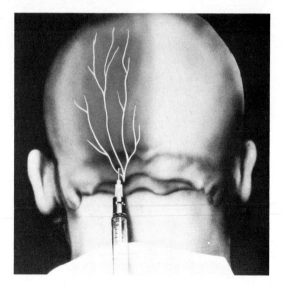

Figure 10.   Greater occipital block.

border of the thyroid cartilage are identified by palpation near their cornua. The solution (2 ml.) is deposited in this space. The anesthesia of the laryngeal mucosa should be satisfactory in five to six minutes. This block is a useful adjunct for minor laryngeal procedures such as direct laryngoscopy and certain difficult intubations in patients awake or under neuroleptanalgesia.

BLOCK OF THE GREATER AND LESSER OCCIPITAL NERVES

The greater occipital nerve innervates the largest part of the posterior scalp as high as the

vertex. It arises as the major portion of the posterior division of the second cervical nerve. The lesser occipital nerve, a branch of the superficial cervical plexus, contributes sensation to the posterolateral scalp.

Anesthetization of these trunks is frequently useful both in scalp surgery and in the diagnostic workup of occipital headache.

Technique of Injection

The greater occipital nerve is anesthetized with a fine gauge, 1-inch needle. A small wheal is raised one fingerbreadth below and one fin-

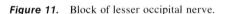

Figure 11.   Block of lesser occipital nerve.

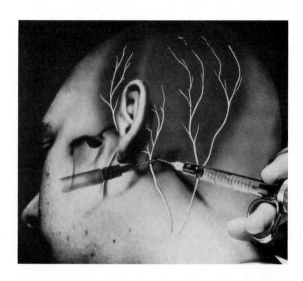

gerbreadth lateral to the external occipital protuberance. The needle is advanced through the
wheal until contact is made with the skull,
withdrawn 0.5 cm. and 2 to 3 ml. of anesthetic
deposited (Fig. 10).

The lesser occipital nerve is blocked on the
posterior aspect of the tip of the mastoid
process (Fig. 11).

REFERENCES

Eriksson, E.: Illustrated Handbook in Local Anaesthesia.
    Chicago, Year Book Medical Publishers, Inc., 1969.
Farr, R. E.: Practical Local Anesthesia. Philadelphia, Lea
    & Febiger, 1923.
Mead, S. V.: Anesthesia in Dental Surgery. St. Louis, The
    C. V. Mosby Co., 1951.
Pitkin's Conduction Anesthesia. Philadelphia, J. B. Lippin-
    cott Co., 1946.

Chapter 34

NEUROLOGY

by J. A. Resch, M.D., and A. B. Baker, M.D.

That there is considerable interrelationship between the disciplines of otolaryngology and neurology is generally well accepted and, as a matter of fact, this is the raison d'etre for this chapter. A certain amount of repetition of material presented elsewhere in the book is unavoidable, and there may be an attendant difference of opinion as well. This is not necessarily undesirable. On the contrary, it may tend to improve understanding of the subject.

SYMPTOMS OF COMMON INTEREST

Vertigo

This is a symptom which brings a large number of patients to the otolaryngologist or neurologist. Conditions of the middle and inner ear which cause this symptom will have been discussed elsewhere. The neurologist enters the picture when consideration is given to the eighth cranial nerve or more central structures.

The patient usually complains of dizziness. From the neurologists's point of view, *true vertigo* refers to a sense of movement, either of the subject or the environment To him the more common complaint of *dizziness* refers to a sense of "giddiness" or "light-headedness" in which no actual movement sensation occurs. In general, it can be said that vertigo usually indicates a lesion below the tentorium. It is often caused by a lesion of the vestibular apparatus. This may be *peripheral* (semicircular canals, vestibular nerve) or *central* (vestibular nuclei, tracts in the brain stem, cerebellum, or cerebrum). Each type of vertigo may have its own characteristics. The peripheral type is usually explosive in onset, episodic in nature, aggravated by change of posture, short in dura-

tion (a few minutes to hours), associated with tinnitus and deafness, and accompanied by horizontal nystagmus. The central type of vertigo is generally slow in onset, is not accompanied by tinnitus or deafness, is more continuous or prolonged, the associated nystagmus is often vertical as well as horizontal, and, finally, there is evidence of other central nervous system involvement.

Infants or children have vertigo primarily from infections or tumors of the brain stem. In the case of the brain stem the commonest tumor is the pontine glioma, which produces symptoms that are gradual in onset, are associated with other cranial nerve involvement, and have a progressive course even though the vertigo may improve temporarily. Cerebellar tumors may also produce vertigo and are a common childhood tumor. Usually they are astrocytomas or ependymomas, and the vertigo is associated with incoordination and signs of increased intracranial pressure, e.g., headache and papilledema. Adults, on the other hand, have vertigo primarily as a result of inner ear problems but, aside from these, multiple sclerosis, cerebellopontine angle tumor, trauma, thrombosis of the posterior inferior cerebellar artery, and toxins (chiefly drugs) assume increasing importance.

Labyrinthine disease per se will have been discussed in detail elsewhere in this text. From the neurologist's viewpoint certain characteristics are ascribed to it. These are acute onset, marked accentuation by head movement, marked nausea, paroxysmal occurrence, tinnitus and deafness, *absence* of central nervous system involvement, normal spinal fluid, and self-limited course but with recurrent attacks.

Multiple sclerosis is one of the more common causes of vertigo. The vertigo may be episodic since the disease is characterized by remissions and exacerbations. As a rule, however, one also finds other neurological complaints and scattered neurological findings; over a long period of time there will be a progressive downhill course.

An *acoustic neuroma* will often cause acute vertigo. The associated tinnitus and deafness, on the other hand, are slowly progressive. A decreased ipsilateral corneal reflex will appear as time goes on. Impaired caloric testing will be present on the involved side. A very high percentage of patients will have increased cerebral spinal fluid protein. A lesser, but still significant, number will have x-ray changes of the internal auditory meatus. In addition, evidence of cerebellar dysfunction will occur. Facial impairment is present rather late in the course.

In the case of *trauma* the resultant vertigo is characterized by a postural component, e.g., precipitation by stooping. There will also be associated headache and memory impairment. Although self-limited, the symptoms may persist for years.

Vertigo occurring in *thrombosis* of the *posterior inferior cerebellar* artery is very sudden in onset. Paraesthesia and hypesthesia are present on the ispilateral side of the face and the contralateral side of the body. In addition, there will be an ipsilateral Horner's syndrome and ipsilateral incoordination. Although the vertigo will eventually pass, it may be severe over a period of weeks.

Drugs are not infrequently associated with vertigo. Salicylates, quinine, and barbiturates are common offenders. Marked horizontal nystagmus will be present in drug-induced vertigo. There is no associated central nervous system deficit. This form of vertigo is also transient, disappearing in days.

In the older age group one is more likely to see ischemia due to basilar artery involvement, brain stem hemorrhage, and brain stem glioma as a background for this symptom. *Basilar artery ischemia* will produce intermittent vertigo, usually just hours in duration. Accompanying this will be intermittent ocular disturbance (diplopia), intermittent dysphagia or dysarthria, and intermittent motor or sensory disturbances. The latter may shift from one side of the body to the other. *Brain stem hemorrhage produces a vertigo* of quite acute onset. It is frequently associated with hypertension. The vertigo may be an isolated symptom and improve slowly over a period of weeks. *Brain stem gliomas*, on the other hand, produce vertigo

which is slow in onset and progressive in nature. There will be associated involvement of cranial nerve nuclei and long tract findings.

There are a number of remote causes of vertigo. In *carotid sinus syncope* the vertigo is often associated with loss of consciousness and convulsions. A fall in blood pressure and bradycardia will be present.

Hypotension secondary to drugs (tranquilizers), posture, sympathetic surgery, or diabetes may be manifested by vertigo only when the patient assumes the upright position. A fall in blood pressure will be in evidence and there often is loss of consciousness. The symptoms disappear when the patient lies down.

Psychogenic vertigo is an ill-defined condition. It is not a true vertigo. The patient appears tense, and there is evidence of psychoneurosis. Movement does not produce an exacerbation. *Vertiginous seizures* due to temporal lobe lesions must be considered in any differential diagnosis.

Tinnitus and Deafness

The neurologist often consults with the otolaryngologist and audiologist in his assessment of hearing deficits, and the technique of testing is described in another chapter.

In infants and children the symptom is associated with congenital causes (idiopathic, cretinism), infections (purulent meningitis, mumps, syphilis), diffuse sclerosis, and tumors of the brain stem. In adults it occurs in the classic Meniere's syndrome, after trauma (head injury with petrous fracture), acoustic neuroma, toxins, pontine glioma, nasopharyngeal carcinoma, as well as in other conditions.

Dysphagia

This symptom occurs in conjunction with bulbar palsies. In infancy and childhood (birth to 10 years) poliomyelitis and brain stem glioma are the more common causes.

Poliomyelitis is characterized by acute onset, fever, systemic involvement, tight neck musculature, decreased deep reflexes in involved limbs, scattered muscle weakness, and, usually, the presence of other cases in the community. The history will reveal that the patient has not been immunized for poliomyelitis. The cerebral spinal fluid will have pleocytosis.

A *brain stem glioma* will manifest itself by a

oculi reflex
outer aspect
glabella, or a
followed by
is muscle wi
is also know
or the *naso*
the site of st
normal indiv
in nuclear a
nerve, absei
exaggerated
palsy and py
of the seven
extrapyrami
response ma
It disappear
tent respons
sign.

The *palpe*
traction of t
ious stimuli
a loud nois
auro- or ac
or cochleo-
bilateral, the
the side of tl
in response
stimulus is
laris, optico
reflex in res
face or in th
trigeminofac
ino-orbicula
response to
as palatopal

The *ocul*
the retractic
of the heli
opposite di
auricles, m
gaze to one

The *palp*
one closes
ward. This
ing of the
associated
exaggeratio
Bell's phen
types of fa

The *orbi*
percussion
nose, whicl
lateral qua
muscles. If
lated, ther
protrusion

progressive course which, however, may at times show temporary improvement. It will be associated with cranial nerve involvement, ataxia, spasticity of limbs, and increase of protein in the cerebral spinal fluid.

In youth (11 to 30 years) poliomyelitis, Guillain-Barré syndrome, multiple sclerosis, and myasthenia gravis are responsible.

In *Guillain-Barré syndrome,* in contradistinction to poliomyelitis, the patient will be afebrile and without systemic symptomatology. The muscles will be tender and radicular pain present. There will often be limb weakness of a flaccid type. The cerebral spinal fluid protein will be increased, but the cell count will be normal (albumino-cytologic dissociation).

In *myasthenia gravis* the patient will have fatigability relieved by rest. The reflexes are normal. Ocular symptoms will be present early. A myasthenic reaction will be in evidence on electromyographic testing. Administration of edrophonium chloride (Tensilon) intravenously will temporarily ameliorate the symptoms.

Multiple sclerosis is a relatively infrequent cause of dysphagia. This disease is characterized by remissions and exacerbations and scattered neurological findings, among which will be incoordination and scanning speech.

In middle age (31 to 60 years) poliomyelitis, Guillain-Barré syndrome, brain stem glioma, cerebellopontine angle tumor, occlusion of the posterior inferior cerebellar artery, and syringobulbia are most frequently responsible.

Tetanus will be accompanied by a history of injury, trismus, rigid abdominal musculature, and marked perspiration. Hypersensitivity to mechanical irritation manifested by convulsions or muscle spasms is present. Local tetanus involving the head and neck is almost a separate form of the disease. It may be relatively chronic, and general symptoms may be mild or absent. On the other hand, dysphagia and laryngeal spasm may be present.

Occlusion of the posterior inferior cerebellar artery will be discussed elsewhere. Although dysphagia is present in this condition it is not a major problem.

Syringobulbia is manifested by a lower motor neuron involvement of the pharyngeal structures and tongue. It will often be accompanied by involvement of the shoulders and upper extremities so there should be no real problem in its diagnosis.

In old age amyotrophic lateral sclerosis, pseudobulbar palsy, and basilar artery insufficiency or occlusion predominate in the etiol-

ogy. *Amyotrophic lateral sclerosis* will produce fasciculation and atrophy of the tongue along with the dysphagia. Atrophy, weakness, and fasciculation of the hands will also be present. Dysarthria is an invariable accompaniment. Hyperactive tendon reflexes and positive toe signs are present as a rule, certainly if the disease has been present for some time. *Superior bulbar palsy* (pseudobulbar palsy), although producing dysarthria and dysphagia, will show no atrophy of the tongue. Neither will there be fasciculations or pyramidal tract findings. The dysphagia is more pronounced when the patient tries to swallow fluids. The face will be masklike. Some degree of intellectual impairment will be in evidence. Emotional incontinence will be manifested by precipitous crying and laughing, ordinarily without sufficient reason. *Basilar artery insufficiency* has been described in the section on vertigo. *Occlusion of the basilar artery* has an acute onset, and the patient will most certainly be confused if not in coma. If the patient is responsive, dysphagia, dysarthria, emotional lability, hemiplegia or quadriplegia, and pupillary changes (fixed, miotic) will be noted. The prognosis here is grave. Other causes of dysphagia include myopathy, dermatomyositis and polymyositis, peripheral nerve involvement, postdiphtheritic paralysis, and botulism.

The importance of early recognition of the acute signs of bulbar involvement merits considerable emphasis. The pooling of secretions will be an early symptom. The patient is often apprehensive. This is due in large measure to the central nervous system effect of hypoxia. The sagging pharyngeal structures tend to compromise the airway. Tracheostomy is a lifesaving procedure and should be done early before irreparable damage to the central nervous system, which is extraordinarily sensitive to oxygen deprivation. This is particularly the case in myasthenia gravis, poliomyelitis, Guillain-Barré syndrome and tetanus. Later in the course of the patient's management, feeding by nasal gavage and possibly gastrostomy will have to be introduced.

Disturbance of Speech

Speech disorders may exist on the basis of lesions interfering with the organs of speech and the immediate innervation of these organs, with consequent disturbance in phonation and articulation, or, on a basis of a hemispheral lesion, with disruption of the central mechanisms of the language process with resultant

aphasia.]
marily wi
Phonati
produced
intensity
the vibra
phonatior
Dysphe
vocal co
branch of
local pro
interferes
cords. Tl
cause is a
dysphoni
in its etic
clude pa
and ceret
Aphon
It is usua
ruption o
or laryng
still spea
call forci
Hysterica
Articula
sound pr
palate. T
sounds i
words ar
articulatic
ranging f
the organ
synthesis
turbances
neurologi
character
Nuclea
Paralys
in an inal
labials "
speech re
palsy as
syndrome
Paralys
weakness
nounce t
"NG." T
centuatec
in poliom
ritic para
Paralys
duces a
nounce li
linguopal
"R"). Th
ing. Thi

the cornea. Because of paralysis of the stylohyoid muscle and posterior belly of the digastricus type there may be weakness of deglutition, and the base of the tongue may be depressed. There is hyperacusis, especially for low tones, which sound louder and higher; this may result when the stapedius is paralyzed.

The patient may be able to close his eye but cannot do so against the resistance of the examiner's fingers. It may also be easier for the examiner to open the eye on the involved side against the patient's resistance than on the normal side. If the weakness is minimal, decreased or absent winking on the affected side may have diagnostic significance. The patient also may not be able to individually close the eye on the involved side. The *levator sign* of *Dutemps* and *Cestan* is brought out by having the patient look down and then slowly close the eyes. The upper lid on the paralyzed side moves upward slightly because of unopposed reaction of the levator palpebral superioris. In *Negro's sign* the eyeball on the paralyzed side deviates outward and elevates more than the normal one when the patient raises his eyes; this is due to overaction of the superior rectus and inferior oblique. In the *Bergara-Wartenberg sign* there is diminution or absence of palpebral vibrations in the orbicularis oculi as the examiner attempts to open the closed eyelids against resistance. This is an earlier and sensitive sign of facial palsy, both peripheral and central. In the *platysma sign of Babinski* there is failure of the platysma to contract on the involved side when the mouth is opened. The electromyogram is of value when analyzing the status of peripheral facial palsy or when there is definite peripheral central facial involvement. This will be discussed under the section on laboratory aids.

The site of involvement of the lesion resulting in peripheral facial paralysis determines the associated symptoms. The lesion may be nuclear or infranuclear. In nuclear or immediate infranuclear involvement there is usually preservation of sensation and secretory function. There may be, however, related symptoms because of proximity of the sixth and seventh nerves.

In the *Millard-Gubler syndrome* there is a lateral rectus paralysis accompanied by ipsilateral facial paralysis probably caused by a lesion of the root fibers and a contralateral hemiplegia because of involvement of the corticospinal pathway.

In the *Foville syndrome* a facial paralysis resulting from involvement of root fibers accompanies an ipsilateral paralysis of conjugate gaze caused by a lesion of the parabducens nucleus or the medial longitudinal fasciculus and a contralateral pyramidal hemiplegia. Involvement of the ascending afferent pathways may cause sensory changes. In infranuclear involvement just peripheral to the pons or between the pons and the facial canal, tinnitus, deafness, and vertigo will be added to the facial weakness. Because of involvement of the nervus intermedius there may be loss of taste on the anterior two thirds of the tongue and diminution of salivary and lacrimal secretion. If the lesion is large enough in the cerebellopontine angle it may extend to the fifth nerve, cerebellar peduncles and cerebellum and cause ipsilateral pain or sensory changes, ipsilateral ataxia, and nystagmus. If the nerve is involved in the facial canal between the internal auditory meatus and geniculate ganglion one has facial paralysis together with nervus intermedius involvement. There is often hyperacusis, with paralysis of the nerve to the stapedius. Lesions are not too common at this site.

Involvement at the geniculate ganglion produces complete facial paralysis, hyperacusis, loss of taste, impairment of secretory functions, and pain in the region of the ear drum. There may be a herpetic eruption; the vesicles are present on the ear drum and in the external auditory meatus. Geniculate neuralgia, with or without herpes, is called Hunt's neuralgia or the Ramsey Hunt syndrome. With involvement of the facial nerve peripheral to the geniculate ganglion but central to the departure of the nerve to the stapedius there is a peripheral facial paralysis accompanied by hyperacusis, loss of taste, and diminution of salivation. Lacrimation is not impaired. Involvement of the facial nerve within the facial canal subsequent to the departure of the nerve to the stapedius and proximal to the departure of the chorda tympani causes a facial paralysis, loss of taste on the anterior two thirds of the tongue, and diminution of salivary secretion. However, hearing and lacrimation are not affected. A lesion within the facial canal but peripheral to the departure of the chorda tympani results only in a peripheral type of facial paralysis, with no accompanying changes. A lesion in the parotid gland after the emergence of the nerve from the stylomastoid foramen causes only partial involvement, because only certain branches of the pes anserinus are affected, thereby paralyzing some of but not all the muscles of facial expression.

In Bell's palsy there is no involuntary facial movement on emotional stimulation, such as one will see in the central facial palsy.

Although Bell's palsy is often used as a synonym for the peripheral variety of facial paralysis, the term should be used only if the paralysis is the result of a lesion peripheral to the geniculate ganglion.

The patient may not be aware of the facial paralysis until he sees his face in the mirror. Occasionally there is a mild pain in the ear or some subjective numbness or stiffness of the face. There is sometimes history of exposure to cold or wind on the affected side or of a mild systemic infection prior to the onset of the paralysis. It is thought that the condition results from compression of the nerve by edema or periostitis of the facial canal, or from ischemia secondary to arteriolar spasm of the nutrient vessels. There is ample evidence to suggest that inflammatory involvement of the nerve (possibly viral) is responsible for a certain number of cases. The prognosis varies, but in the majority of patients healing is fairly prompt and complete. Electromyography will be useful in prognosis.

Melkersson's syndrome is characterized by recurring facial palsy, recurring facial edema, and a congenitally fissured tongue. It is sometimes familial.

Möbius syndrome consists of paralysis or weakness of the facial muscles in combination with a similar involvement of the extraocular movements, particularly the adbucens. The etiology is aplasia or hypoplasia of the nuclear centers in the brain stem.

Involvement of facial expression will also be seen in parkinsonism (masked facies), myasthenia gravis (myasthenic smile), and in muscle atrophy (myopathic facies). In severe hemiatrophy or in progressive facial atrophy there is underdevelopment of muscles on a congenital basis. The muscles of mastication may also be involved, together with the muscles of facial expression and trophic changes in the skin, subcutaneous fat, connective tissue, cartilage, and bone. There may be hemifacial hypertrophy, thought to have a central origin.

Irritative motor phenomena may occur in focal seizures (jacksonian seizure). Muscle disorders have been described elsewhere in this paragraph. There may be facial hemispasms with pyramidal involvement of the opposite side of the body (Brissaud's syndrome).

Faulty regeneration of the seventh nerve as a result of a peripheral type of palsy may result in abnormal associated or *synkinetic movements*. There may even be facial spasm or facial contracture. A true facial spasm is not a *tic*. Tremors of the face, particularly of the perioral type, are seen in general paresis and alcoholism. They may also be of psychogenic origin or occur as a result of hyperthyroidism. *Rosenbach's sign* is manifested by a fine tremor of the closed eyelids and is seen in both hyperthyroidism and hysteria. Fasciculations of the facial muscles may be present in progressive muscle atrophy or amyotrophic lateral sclerosis. Abnormal facial muscle activity will also be part of various movement disorders described in the next section. Faulty healing may also result in the syndrome of the *gustatory lacrimal reflex,* which is described elsewhere.

Movement Disorders

Dystonia involving tongue and lips as well as facial grimaces may be an expression of extrapyramidal disease or of drug intoxication (phenothiazines). Of interest here are dystonic movements (torsion spasm) which are similar in many aspects to those in athetosis but involve larger portions of the body. The disturbance results from excessive muscular tone in certain muscle groups. Movements are slow, bizarre, and grotesque in type, being undulant, writhing, twisting, and turning in nature. They may involve the entire body. Of importance here is the fact that the face, tongue, head, and neck may be solely involved. There will then be dysarthria, facial grimacing, and torticollis. The state of hypertonicity may be severe enough to produce pain. Although involuntary, these movements may be increased by voluntary activity and emotion. Movements of this type are usually manifestations of *dystonia musculorum deformans,* a rare heredofamilial disorder of progressive nature. There is an extrapyramidal type of involvement.

Dystonic movements can also occur in other degenerative diseases, vascular disease, or tumor involving the basal ganglia. A much more common cause is the side effect from certain drugs (phenothiazines). There is a *tardive dyskinesia* which occurs late in the use of these drugs even after they have been discontinued. Hence, the name and diagnostic dilemma. This form is fairly limited and involves the lips, tongue, and facial muscles. *Spasmodic torticollis* is another form of dystonic movement disorder affecting the head and neck and sometimes the shoulder. The movements may be intermittent at first or appear only in paroxysms. Later there is a persistent muscle contraction with resultant deviation of the head. Although it has not always been the case, most neurologists now feel that this is an extrapyramidal disorder. Torticollis may also be congenital or an acquired musculoskeletal or neuromuscular defect. Admittedly some cases may be psychogenic, but the majority, in all probability, are of organic nature. Another disorder which merits comment is that manifested by head tremor aggravated by intention, e.g., when the patient is performing the finger-to-nose test. This is an essential tremor which will almost invariably be associated with a similar tremor of the upper extremities and which frequently is familial.

Palatal myoclonus (palatal nystagmus) consists of involuntary movements of the soft palate and pharynx. Occasionally other areas, including the larynx, eye muscles, and diaphragm, may be involved. The affliction may be unilateral or bilateral. The frequency of movements is from 50 to 240 per minute. Although drugs and sleep have little influence on this abnormal movement, it may be suppressed by voluntary effort. Sound may also accompany the movements and there will be clicking or respiratory noises. Lesions of the olivodentorubrometencephalic pathways are involved. The etiology may be vascular, neoplastic, inflammatory, or degenerative, and the symptoms occur most frequently in later adult life.

Facial Pain and Sensory Disturbance

There are a host of neuralgias which are of common interest to the otolaryngologist and the neurologist. These include vidian nerve, geniculate, occipital (C_2–C_3), phrenic, superior laryngeal, sphenopalatine, tympanic, glossopharyngeal, and trigeminal neuralgia, and Sluder's and Costen's syndromes. Disturbance of sensation of the face may result from involvement of the trigeminal nerve, the brain stem, or the thalamus. In the case of peripheral impairment of the trigeminal, there should be no diagnostic difficulty. The brain stem sensory involvement will usually be accompanied by other neurological signs, including quite often diminished sensation in the opposite extremities. Involvement more rostrally, such as is seen in tumors or cerebral vascular disease of the thalamus, will produce a complete hemihypesthesia in which the face is perforce included.

A somewhat detailed discussion of various neuralgias is in order.

Sphenopalatine Neuralgia. Also known as Sluder's syndrome, this is a form of neuralgia resulting from involvement of the sphenopalatine ganglion. It is characterized by pain to the orbital area, cheeks, roof of the mouth, root of the nose, upper jaw, and teeth. It sometimes extends to the ear, occiput, neck, shoulders, and arms. It should be stated, however, that the existence of such a symptom complex is presently questioned.

Glossopharyngeal Neuralgia. This neuralgia produces paroxysms of pain originating on one side of the throat and extending to the ear drum. The patient is unable to chew or swallow. Cool drinks are particularly aggravating. The tonsillar fossa is the site of the "trigger zone," and the pain can be relieved by cocainizing this area.

Costen's Syndrome. Costen's syndrome is the result of disease or irritation of the temporomandibular joint. It may be seen in trismus. It can result from a blow on the chin, fracture of the jaw, ill-fitting dentures, impacted teeth, and malocclusion. Any one of these defects may produce pressure on the auriculotemporal branch of the mandibular nerve as it crosses the temporomandibular joint. Pain in and anterior to the ears as well as about the nose and eyes may occur. The pain is nonpulsating and nonparoxysmal. Crepitus within the mandibular joint may be in evidence. The joint may also be tender to palpation. Trismus may be secondary to the joint irritation.

Trigeminal Neuralgia. Tic douloureux, trifacial neuralgia, or Fothergill's neuralgia is due to involvement of the trigeminal ganglion. The maxillary and mandibular branches are most frequently involved.

"Trigger zones" may be present at the angle of the mouth or upper lip. Pain is often precipitated by washing the face, talking, chewing, shaving, or brushing the teeth as well as drafts of air. The patient will very likely protect the face at all times. There will be poor oral hygiene and loss of weight because of the inability to tolerate chewing or swallowing.

Headache

This is one of the most common neurologic complaints, and the cause may vary from such benign conditions as tension to such serious illness as brain tumor. Treatment will tax the skill and diagnostic ability of the physician.

There are a number of informative data that should be obtained in each case of headache:

Location

1. Generalized or focal; unilateral or bilateral; orbital or supraorbital; nuchal.

2. Headaches of eye, sinus, or scalp origin are often well localized to the area of stimulation.

3. Migraine is usually unilateral and involves the head or face.

4. Posterior fossa lesions are often localized to the occipital region.

5. Headaches secondary to neck strain or neck pathology remain localized to the nuchal region.

Nature or Intensity

1. Steady, constant pain (tension, muscle spasm, sinus headache).

2. Pulsating, throbbing (tumors, migraine, hypertension, meningitis, etc.).

3. Relieved by medication? If so, how much? Relief from sleep or rest?

4. Aggravated by sneezing, coughing, ingestion of alcohol, or posture. (Characteristically, those headaches resulting from displacement of pain-sensitive structures are aggravated by coughing, sneezing, or head movement.)

It must be kept in mind that the severity of the head pain is not always a measure of the seriousness of the illness. Psychogenic headaches may be very intense, while certain brain tumors may produce only a minimum of distress.

Duration. Intermittent; constant over weeks or months; present both day and night; related to periods of activity and rest, such as weekend headaches.

Precipitants. It is often instructive to elicit precipitating factors, which may include fatigue, tension, heavy work, allergy, noise, eye strain, sinusitis, drugs, alcohol, injections, trauma, vascular disease, and so forth.

Associated Findings. Visual disturbances, nausea, or vomiting, focal symptomatology, tightness and soreness of neck musculature and so forth.

A careful survey of the above factors will often suggest the possible etiology of the headache. To assist in the proper diagnosis, it may be well to describe briefly some of the more striking features of some of the more common headache types.

Ocular Headache

Causes. Refractive errors, glaucoma, infections of orbit, paralysis of ocular muscles. Seen in pianists, typists, bookkeepers, students.

Character. Frontal in location, often bilateral and circumocular; aggravated by use of eyes; absent on awakening; usually appears in afternoon; absent during weekends when eyes are not used.

Aural (Sinus) Headaches

Location. Frontal area in frontal sinus; root of nose and retro-orbital in the ethmoid sinuses; over cheek bones in maxillary sinuses.

Nature. Dull, nonpulsating quality, most severe in A.M. on awakening; increased by shaking head, coughing, or sneezing or by engorgement of mucosa (excitement, alcohol, head down position, menstruation).

Brain Tumors

Causes. Local traction on vessels; displacement of brain; distant traction; internal hydrocephalus (traction on meninges or basilar vessels).

Nature. Early intermittent, later severe, persistent, deep, steady, at times agonizing; often awakens patient at night; does not prevent sleep; increased by stooping, straining, or sudden turning of head; associated with diplopia, papilledema, focal findings.

Inflammation Headache

Nature. Throbbing, persistent pain localized to occipital region; aggravated by head movement or jugular compression; relieved by rest and quiet; often worse at night in chronic meningitis; associated with nuchal rigidity and spinal fluid pleocytosis.

Head Injury

Nature. Recurrent; periodic or throbbing; localized or diffuse; often disappears for months only to return; aggravated by posture (stooping), emotional factors, and fatigue; may be associated with vertigo, memory impairment.

Lumbar Puncture Headache

Nature. Postural headache accentuated by upright position; uninfluenced by drugs; may take weeks to disappear.

Vascular Distention Headache. There are a large number of headaches that are due to dilatation of some part of the cranial arterial tree. These headaches are all improved by procedures that lower the cranial arterial pressure.

Hangover headache. This is a familiar headache resulting from the vasodilatation produced by overindulgence in ethyl alcohol. It is a diffuse, throbbing pain aggravated by head movement and reduced by carotid pressure.

Caffeine withdrawal headache. This type is usually seen when caffeine is suddenly withheld after excessive administration or use. It is a deep, generalized occipital pain aggravated by coughing and sneezing and often associated with lethargy and rhinorrhea. It can be readily terminated by the administration of caffeine or amphetamine.

Postseizure headache. A moderately intense, generalized head pain lasting for hours and accompanied by lethargy; develops in many individuals after a convulsion.

Post-traumatic headache. In about 50 per cent of individuals, headache develops following an injury. (See Head Injury Headache).

Postspinal headache. In certain individuals intense headache may follow spinal puncture. It has been suggested that this headache is due to effect of traction upon various pain-sensitive structures as a result of prolonged leakage of spinal fluid through the puncture hole.

Hypertension headache. This is often a major complaint in hypertension. It is a very painful, throbbing pain localized either to the frontal or occipital areas. It occurs on awakening and is often relieved by sitting up or moving about. The frequency and severity are not related to the elevation of blood pressure. These headaches are not relieved by hypotensive drugs. They are improved by ergotamine tartate but respond best to analgesics.

Tension Headache. This occurs in a tense, apprehensive, ill-at-ease person. Not an isolated complaint but associated with a wide range of symptoms such as chest complaints (palpitation, pain), gastric trouble (anorexia, nausea, feeling of bloating, urinary frequency, diarrhea, hyperhydrosis. These patients are irritable, have crying spells, tremor, and hyperactive reflexes. The tension headache is characterized by a constant, dull pain; band about head; caplike quality; present for days or weeks without letup; continues during night; prevents sleep; generalized; associated with tightness and pain in neck muscles; *no prodromata*; chiefly *bilateral.*

Migraine. The exact cause of migraine is unknown. The headaches are produced by dilatation of branches of the external carotid artery. There is a strong familial tendency, with many members of a family suffering from the same type of disturbance. The role of allergy, toxins, or the endocrines has not been established, although the occurrence of these headaches around the menses suggests some associated endocrine factor. Psychological factors no doubt are extremely important as a precipitating mechanism.

Individual. People subject to migraine are frequently intense and driving, perfectionistic, compulsive, ambitious, and efficient, with excessive conscientiousness and marked rigidity. There may be a family history of similar headaches.

Prodromes. The following precede headaches by days: euphoria; increased appetite; very keen intellectually; increased sex drive; lassitude; fluid retention.

Aura. The most immediate sensations preceding the headache are: scintillating scotoma; visual disturbances (water over cornea, snow falling, cobwebs before eyes, known as teichopsia); numbness over half of body; paraesthesias; aphasia; ophthalmoplegia (ptosis, diplopia); hemianopsias.

Headache. The headaches themselves are recurrent; severe; usually *unilateral* but will shift from one side to another, although one side may predominate; last for hours or days; *do not interfere* with sleep; associated with nausea and vomiting.

Migraine equivalents. Occasionally there is a prodromal aura but no headache: abdominal migraine (periodic abdominal pain, nausea, and occasional headache); precordial migraine (pain in chest with radiation to axilla and left arm); pelvic migraine (pain in pelvis and genitalia); ophthalmic migraine (ocular disturbances); ophthalmoplegic migraine (ocular palsies).

Cluster Headaches. These are nasociliary headaches, Horton's headache, or histamine cephalgia.

Causes. Probably not a true entity; some are probably migraine, others may be allergy or tension headaches.

Nature. Pain in and around eye associated with reddening of eye, unilateral lacrimation, and running nostril on affected side; pain lasts a few hours; occur at intervals of hours or days and then disappear for months or years; grouping of attack with free interval has led to term of cluster headaches; in severe cases the patient may have edema of upper lip and ptosis.

Cervical Spine Headaches

Cause. Neck pathology: osteoarthritis; "whiplash" injuries; bony changes; meningeal changes; postural strain as seen in typists, draftsmen, or students.

Nature of headache. Constant; persists for months; diffuse and occipital in location; no interference with sleep as a rule; some relief from analgesics; soreness and tightness of neck and shoulder muscles; bony changes in cervical spine.

Temporal Arteritis

Cause. Probably a form of periarteritis nodosa.

Symptoms. Usually occurs in patients 60 to 80 years of age; intense pain and tenderness over temporal region of one or both sides; nodularity of temporal artery; systemic symptoms (malaise, fever, weakness); blindness in 50 per cent of patients; self-limited cause with partial or complete resolution in six to 12 months.

Leakage of Cerebral Spinal Fluid

Rhinorrhea and otorrhea are of common interest and should be noted here for sake of completeness. They are discussed elsewhere in the text.

Olfaction

Disturbances of olfaction are of considerable diagnostic value to the neurologist. In head trauma there is commonly a complete loss of olfaction because of shearing off of the olfactory filaments. Insofar as a central cause of olfactory loss is concerned, one would have to have bilateral cortical or tract lesions to produce this situation. Of great importance is the fact that an olfactory groove meningioma can cause unilateral loss of olfaction. This often occurs early and for a time may be the only symptom.

Secretory Disturbances

Abnormal dryness of the mouth is referred to as xerostomia and can be of central or peripheral origin. It may be functional in origin. In *Sjogren's syndrome* there is deficient secretion of the lacrimal and mucosal glands, keratoconjunctivitis, and dryness of the mouth and upper respiratory tract.

Reflexes

The *corneal reflex* is diminished when there is involvement of either the ophthalmic division of the fifth cranial nerve (peripheral) or of the descending sensory root of the fifth nerve (central). The latter is not infrequently compromised by cerebellopontine angle tumors. In the face of symptoms of tinnitus and vertigo, an ipsilateral decrease of the corneal reflex becomes quite significant.

The *gag reflex*, if depressed bilaterally, is not of particularly great significance unless one sees other evidence of involvement. It may be depressed bilaterally in hysterical individuals. However, when it is unilaterally involved it indicates interference with the ninth cranial nerve.

The *sternutatory reflex* is mediated through the trigeminal nerve and is elicited by tickling the nasal mucosa. Its absence would indicate interruption of the maxillary division of the trigeminal nerve.

There are a variety of *autonomic reflexes*, among which are included the pupillary, lacrimal, salivary, palatal, pharyngeal, sneezing, sucking, coughing, swallowing, vomiting, carotid sinus and oculocardiac reflexes. A number of these are part of the autonomic nervous system emotional reaction. They are not generally thought of as reflexes but should be. These consist of laughter, which is characterized by deep inspiration followed by a series of short, jerky expirations which may be accompanied by laryngeal sounds; weeping is a similar mechanism accompanied by sobs and usually by lacrimation. In supranuclear bulbar palsy there is emotional lability and consequent easy triggering of these emotional reflexes.

Reflexes associated with *bilateral supranuclear pyramidal tract involvement* are frequently accompanied by a snout reflex, jaw jerk, and palmomental sign.

Reflexes associated with both the *pyramidal and extrapyramidal* functions are manifested by hyperactivity of the orbicularis oris and oculi reflexes (Myerson's sign).

There are a number of *signs of tetany* which are of value. In Chvostek's sign, tapping over the point of emergence or division of the facial nerve anterior to the ear is followed by spasm or tetanic contraction of the ipsilateral facial muscles. Mechanical stimulation of the protruded tongue (by means of a percussion hammer) may be followed by transient depression or dimpling at the site of stimulation (Schultze's sign). It should be noted, however, that a similar phenomenon is present in patients with myotonia. Increased reaction to stimulation of the oral and lingual mucosa will be manifested by contractions of the lips, masseters, and tongue. It is usually elicited by percussion of the inner surface of the lips or of the tongue (Escherich's sign).

ETIOLOGIC CONSIDERATIONS

Infection

Organisms commonly involved in the infections of otolaryngologic-neurologic conditions are the pneumococcus, streptococcus, meningococcus, *Haemophilus influenzae,* staphylococcus, *Mycobacterium tuberculosis, Treponema pallidum, Corynebacterium diptheriae, Clostridium tetani,* and a variety of viruses. Meningitis is most often pneumococcal in type and is the result of extension through previous fracture or defects from local sepsis in the middle ear and paranasal sinuses. The infectious process may produce a simple meningitis, or it may cause brain abscess or lateral sinus thrombosis. In connection with the latter, the patients may have *otic hydrocephalus* complete with increased intracranial pressure and its attendant signs. Central sinus thrombosis and superior sagittal sinus thrombosis are also complications with which one must reckon.

Brain abscess is a focal area of encephalitis which initially consists of an area of purulent exudate surrounded by soft tissue. A capsule forms during a variable period of two to four or even six weeks. A number of mechanisms may be responsible for the formation of the abscess; it may be a direct extension from osteomyelitis of the skull, infectious pachymeningitis or leptomeningitis, infective mastoid cells or paranasal sinus, infections of the face or orbit, or infections of the venous sinuses in the skull. An abscess may also be metastatic from systemic infections, infection of the heart or lung, focal infectious processes and, occasionally, may occur in association with extraction of infected teeth. Abscesses may also be the result of direct implantation of head wounds. *Otogenous abscesses* (middle ear, mastoid cells, petrous pyramid) are found either in the temporal lobe or cerebellum. *Rhinogenous abscess* (nose, paranasal sinus) is usually found in the frontal lobe.

Clinical diagnosis of brain abscess is made on the evidence of systemic infection (e.g., fever), leukocytosis, together with a rapid increase of intracranial pressure and focal central nervous system signs. If the systemic aspects are minimal, the abscess is often difficult to differentiate from a neoplasm. It may also be confused with meningitis if it is near the surface and there is spread of infection to the subarachnoid space. Subdural and extradural abscesses are not difficult to diagnose. Exploration may be required. Diagnostic procedures which are of assistance in the diagnosis of brain abscess are the lumbar puncture, which may reveal pleocytosis as well as increased intracranial pressure; electroencephalogram, which may show a focal abnormality; and skull x-ray, which may show a shift of the pineal gland. The radioisotope brain scan, angiography, and pneumoencephalogram will also be of assistance in establishing the precise location of the abscess for the purpose of surgical management.

Diphtheria is seldom seen but is of interest because of postdiptheritic paralysis of the palate and other pharyngeal structures.

Tetanus is easily recognizable by the trismus when it is full blown, but it may be less evident in case of mild involvement. It may also produce disturbances in swallowing and respiration. Tracheostomy should be considered early in treatment even though the symptoms may still be mild.

Tumors

Tumors occur in the brain more frequently than in any other area. A fair number have relevance for the otolaryngologist and these will be discussed.

In Children. Cerebellar tumors are the most common type of childhood brain tumor. The cell types consist of the astrocytoma, ependymoma, and medulloblastoma. The *cerebellar tumor* produces unsteadiness, nystagmus, and headache, the latter as a result of increased intracranial pressure; early papilledema is common. *Pinealoma* accounts for 2 per cent of the gliomas in children and will cause extraocular muscle impairment, impaired upward gaze and ptosis (Parinaud's sign), and *bilateral hyperacusis.* Occasionally there will be sexual changes (macrogenitosomia praecox). The pineal gland may be enlarged and calcified on skull x-ray. Brain stem gliomas have been discussed previously. They are usually astrocytomas and follow a progressive (two to three years) slow course with cranial nerve palsy.

In Adults. In adults the pattern of tumors changes in that the supratentorial location is the more likely one. *Meningiomas* constitute 15 per cent of all intracranial tumors occurring in adults. As a rule, they originate in the sagittal sinus area, sphenoidal ridge, or olfactory groove. They are slow growing, and on x-ray one will see calcification of bony skull changes. Of greatest interest to the otolaryngologist are the sphenoidal ridge and olfactory groove meningiomas. In the case of the sphenoidal ridge types, there will be unilateral exophthalmus and oculomotor nerve involvement with resultant diplopia and unilateral visual loss.

The *olfactory groove meningioma* produces unilateral or bilateral anosmia, mental or personality change, and late optic atrophy. In the *Foster Kennedy syndrome* there is optic atrophy on the side of the tumor with papilledema on the opposite side.

Acoustic neuromas constitute 2 per cent of intracranial tumors. They originate in the vestibular nerve, and vertigo, therefore, may be the first symptom. Other findings consist of ipsilateral tinnitus and deafness, ipsilateral corneal hypesthesia, ipsilateral incoordination of cerebellar origin, and ipsilateral facial paresis late in the process. A skull x-ray may show petrous erosion. Spinal puncture will in many instances reveal increased spinal fluid protein.

Nasopharyngeal carcinoma may impair hearing. One may have metastatic extension from the central nervous system of meningiomas and other tumors into the nasopharynx and sinuses.

Extension of tumors of the nasopharynx may produce *Garcin's syndrome*, which is accompanied by paralysis of cranial nerves (third through tenth), usually on one side but occasionally on both. Although caused by infection of the retropharynx space, it can also be caused by invasion by neoplasm or granuloma and is most often the result of metastasis. Tumors of the glomus jugularis (chemodectoma) should be mentioned, but are discussed more fully elsewhere. In this tumor there may be involvement of the ninth, tenth, and eleventh nerves at the jugular foramen as well as evidence of seventh and eighth nerve dysfunction.

Vascular Disease

Vascular disease is a frequent source of symptoms occurring in the province of the otolaryngologist. Symptoms and signs such as vertigo, nystagmus, dysphasia, and dysarthria are a frequent accompaniment of the various brain stem vascular syndromes. Central and lateral sinus thrombosis have already been noted under infection. Vascular disease is by its very nature often a diffuse process. One of the difficulties occurring is a differentiation between disturbances of the anterior circulation (internal carotid, middle cerebral, and anterior cerebral arteries) and the posterior circulation (vertebral and basilar arteries). A vague symptom such as dizziness may be related to either vascular bed. Internal carotid artery insufficiency may produce light-headedness but is also accompanied by such symptoms as ipsilateral amaurosis and contralateral sensory and motor signs. On the other hand, the vertebral basilar insufficiency will more likely produce true vertigo and will also have diplopia and other evidence of brain stem involvement.

There are a number of ways in which disorders of cerebral circulation may arise:

Decrease in cardiac output. This may reduce cerebral blood flow: Stokes-Adams syndrome; hypotension (postural, postsurgery, drugs such as tranquilizers and barbiturates); vasodilatation; high spinal anesthetics.

Disorders of blood vessels. This would include narrowing or occlusion as seen in atherosclerosis, syphilis, or collagen diseases; emboli of different types (cardiac, fat, tumor, air parasites); alteration of vessel walls as in atherosclerosis, aneurysms, and toxic processes.

Changes in blood properties. These are caused by polycythemia; dehydration; anticoagulants; vitamin K administration; hemophilia.

CEREBRAL VASCULAR ACCIDENTS

There are three general types of cerebral vascular accidents, viz., hemorrhage, thrombosis, and embolus. *Hemorrhage* occurs fairly suddenly, usually during activity, and as a rule, is accompanied by profound effects such as unconsciousness and hemiplegia. The neck will be rigid and a lumbar puncture will reveal the presence of fresh blood. *Thrombosis*, the most common form of cerebral vascular accident, will be intermittent or gradual in onset, It may have been preceded by instances of transient neurological impairment. The event often is associated with the resting state. Cerebral spinal fluid examination is usually not particularly helpful other than to exclude the possibility of hemorrhage, which in milder form may simulate the thrombosis. *Embolus* has the most sudden onset of all. Even though the findings may be rather marked, there is a tendency to revert to a considerable degree. The cerebral spinal fluid may show the presence of both red and white cells, the latter in increased amount. There is an age factor in that the embolus occurs in the younger individual, hemorrhage is more common in the middle-aged individual, and thrombosis in older people.

Disturbances of some of the more common types of vascular involvement are:

Sinus Thrombosis. Sinus thrombosis is seen more frequently in childhood (three to five years) and involves primarily the longitudinal and straight sinuses; it complicates debilitating diseases; is accompanied by sudden loss of consciousness, edema of forehead, and distention of veins of the scalp. The cerebral spinal fluid will be blood-tinged. Spasticity of the lower limbs may be present, and the patient may have hemiplegia. Recovery will frequently occur. The patient, however, may have persistent convulsions. Although this form of cerebral vascular involvement would not be confused with any otolaryngological condition, it is included because of the association with infections of the ears and sinuses.

Embolization. In youth (six to sixteen years) one is most apt to encounter embolization to the central nervous system. This may result from valvulitis or acute infections of throat and teeth. There is often a long history of fever, malaise, weight loss, and joint pain. Symptoms occur with a sudden onset of lethargy or coma. Although focal symptoms are often present, there are also diffuse neurological findings; for example, bilateral positive toe signs. Laboratory examination will reveal leukocytosis, increased sedimentation rate, and pleocytosis. General physical examination may reveal a cardiac murmur and petechiae.

Subarachnoid Hemorrhage. Subarachnoid hemorrhage is the most common form of vascular accident in young adults (17 to 35 years). It is usually secondary to a ruptured aneurysm. It is accompaneid by excruciating nuchal pain, rigidity of the neck, and subhyaloid hemorrhages. The patient may have impairment of consciousness. There may be focal findings. The cerebral spinal fluid will be bloody.

The foregoing should offer very little in the way of diagnostic problems to the otolaryngologist. When one gets into the cerebral vascular disease of adults (35 to 65 years), the various forms of transient ischemic events, reversible ischemic neurological deficits, and completed strokes will often have symptoms of common interest, for example, vertigo and unsteadiness. Some of the more common syndromes are as follows.

Insufficiency of Internal Carotid and Middle Cerebral Arteries. *Transient unilateral muscular weakness* or sensory disturbances *always on same side*; speech disturbances if weakness is right-sided; permanent weakness if middle cerebral involved; bruit in neck; *intermittent or permanent disturbance of vision in ipsilateral eye.*

Thrombosis of Internal Carotid Artery. Depends on efficiency of collateral circulation (chiefly older individuals); *sudden unilateral motor weakness*; unilateral hemihypesthesia; aphasia if left internal carotid involved; rarely mental symptoms with little motor involvement; *decreased pulsation in neck*; bruit in neck and loss of vision in ipsilateral eye (pathognomonic).

Posterior Inferior Cerebellar Artery Thrombosis (Wallenberg Syndrome).

Vertigo; ipsilateral facial paresthesia and hypesthesia; dysphagia, ipsilateral Horner's syndrome; ipsilateral incoordination; contralateral hypesthesia over trunk and limbs.

Basilar Artery Insufficiency. *Recurrent vertigo* (minutes); transient visual dimness; diplopia; dysphagia and dysarthria; *transient hemiparesis which shifts from side to side*; transient episodes of confusional states or *even loss of consciousness* (falling or dropping spells).

Thrombosis of the Anterior Spinal Artery. Because it applies the pyramids and emerging hypoglossal fibers, thrombosis of the anterior spinal artery is usually followed by either an alternating hypoglossal hemiplegia or an alternating hypoglossal hemianesthetic hemiplegia. The former is also known as crossed hypoglossal paralysis or the syndrome of the pyramid and the hypoglossal nerve. It is accompanied by ipsilateral flaccid paralysis of the tongue with contralateral paresis of the arm and leg. In the case of the latter it is known as syndrome of the pyramid, the medial lemniscus, and the hypoglossal nerve. In addition, there is contralateral loss of proprioceptive sensibility and diminution of tactile sensation. There may be bilateral signs of the foregoing nature in varying degree in patients in whom circulation to both sides is cut off. Lesions of the anterior spinal artery may miss the hypoglossal nerve. They may also affect the medial longitudinal fasciculus. All the foregoing are sometimes referred to as *Dejerine's anterior bulbar syndromes.*

Hemiplegia cruciata (crossed hemiplegia or syndrome of the decussation) is a vascular lesion of the decussation of the pyramids. There is contralateral spastic paresis of the lower extremities as a result of pyramidal fiber involvement of the leg which has not yet decussated. There is an ipsilateral spastic paresis as a result of damage to those fibers already crossed. Of importance to the otolaryngologist is the fact that there may also be ipsilateral flaccid paresis and atrophy of the sternocleidomastoid and trapezius muscles and, occasionally, ipsilateral paralysis of the tongue.

Anterior Inferior Cerebellar Artery Thrombosis. Since this vessel supplies the lateral tegmentum of the upper medulla and lower pons, restiform body, lower portion of the cerebellar peduncle (brachium pontis), flocculus, and inferior surface of the cerebellar hemisphere, thrombosis is accompanied by ipsilateral cerebellar asynergia and incoordination, ipsilateral loss of facial pain, temperature, and light touch sensation; Horner's syndrome; ipsilateral deafness and ipsilateral type of facial palsy. Contralaterally there is incomplete loss of pain and temperature sensations in the limbs and body. *Postoperative thrombosis* of this artery may follow excision of an *acoustic neuroma*.

Superior Cerebellar Artery Thrombosis. This artery supplies the lateral part of the tegmentum of the pons and midbrain, upper portion of the brachium pontis, brachium conjunctivum (superior cerebellar peduncle), superior surface of the cerebellum, and cerebellar nuclei. Thrombosis of this artery produces ipsilateral cerebellar asynergia with hypotonus and involuntary movements, often choreiform or choreo-athetoid in type, together with ipsilateral Horner's syndrome. Contralaterally there is loss of pain and temperature sensation of the face and body, and there may be a central type of facial palsy as well as occasional *partial deafness*.

Thrombosis of the Vertebral Artery. This may cause a number of syndromes. The *syndrome of Avellis* is characterized by involvement of the spinothalamic tract and of the nucleus ambiguus, usually with an associated involvement of the bulbar nucleus of the accessory nerve. In some instances there is coincidental involvement of the medial lemniscus and the tract of the solitary fasciculus. As a result of the foregoing, there is ipsilateral paralysis of the soft palate, pharynx, and larynx, with contralateral loss of pain and temperature sensations on the trunk and extremities. In addition, there may be contralateral loss of proprioception of the body. There may also be ipsilateral anesthesia of the pharynx and larynx as well as loss of taste. Occasionally there is an ipsilateral Horner's syndrome and a contralateral pyramidal tract paralysis, which has also been described.

Cestan-Chenais Syndrome. The syndrome of Cestan-Chenais is caused by the occlusion of the vertebral artery below the point of origin of the posteroinferior cerebellar artery. This involves the nucleus ambiguus, restiform body, and descending sympathetic pathways. There will be paralysis of the soft palate, pharynx, and larynx, ipsilateral cerebellar asynergia, and a Horner's syndrome; there is contralateral hemiplegia together with diminished proprioception and tactile sensation. This differs from the Wallenberg syndrome, already described, primarily because of the addition of pyramidal signs and proprioception disturbance and the omission of pain and temperature disturbances.

Occasionally the Cestan-Chenais syndrome may be extensive and variable, including such things as involvement of the nuclei of the eleventh and twelfth nerves, ipsilateral paralysis of the sternocleidomastoid and trapezius muscles and of the tongue. There may be involvement of the descending root of the trigeminal nerve with ipsilateral loss of pain and temperature sensations on the face. There may be spinothalamic involvement with loss of pain and temperature sensations on the opposite half of the body.

Babinski-Nageotte Syndrome. The syndrome of Babinski-Nageotte resembles that of Cestan-Chenais but is believed to be caused by multiple or scattered lesions, chiefly in the distribution of the vertebral artery. There will be ipsilateral paralysis of the soft palate, larynx, and pharynx, and sometimes of the tongue. In addition, there will be ipsilateral loss of taste on the posterior third of the tongue, loss of pain and temperature around the face, cerebellar asynergia, and Horner's syndrome, in conjunction with contralateral spastic hemiplegia and loss of proprioceptive sensibility, and diminution of tactile sensation. There also may be loss of pain and temperature sensations of the limbs and trunk.

Basilar Artery Thrombosis. An occlusion of the basilar artery may have a gradual onset or even a fluctuating course but the symptoms can appear precipitously, in which case death will occur in a short time. There are bilateral cranial nerve and long tract findings. There may also be bilateral supranuclear fiber involvement to the bulbar nuclei as well as of the ascending sensory pathways. As a result, there is a clinical picture of pseudobulbar palsy, including disturbance of both deep and superficial sensations on the body and extremities and sometimes on the face. Usually there are miotic pupils, decerebrate rigidity, profound coma or akinetic mutism, and respiratory and circulatory difficulties. Similar brain stem symptoms may occur post-traumatically or after surgery because of sudden increase in intracranial pressure, subarachnoid hemorrhage, or a rapidly expanding supratentorial mass lesion. The symptoms then are the result of hemorrhage into and edema of the brain stem.

Thrombosis of Medial Pontine Branches. This may result in involvement of the nuclei of the sixth and seventh nerves or their emergent fibers, medial longitudinal fasciculus, pyramidal tract, and medial lemniscus; as a result, there will be ipsilateral facial paralysis and paralysis of the lateral rectus movement or of conjugate lateral gaze, together with contralateral hemiplegia, loss of proprioceptive sensibility, and diminution of tactile sensation.

Thrombosis of the Lateral Pontine Branches. This involves the middle cerebellar peduncle, superior olivary body, facial nucleus, vestibular and cochlear nuclei and, in part, the motor and sensory nuclei of the trigeminal nerve, medial longitudinal fasciculus, and spinothalamic tract. Symptoms consist of ipsilateral cerebellar asynergia plus signs of involvement of the fifth, seventh, and eighth cranial nerves. Often there are contralateral loss of pain and temperature sensations on the trunk and limbs and contralateral loss of tactile and proprioceptive sensations.

Thrombosis of the Upper Pontine Branches of the Basilar Artery. This thrombosis results in contralateral hemiplegia, including the face and tongue, contralateral loss of pain, temperature, and proprioceptive sensations on the face, trunk, and extremities as a result of involvement of the pyramidal tract, medial lemniscus, the spinothalamic tract and the ventral and dorsal secondary ascending tracts of the trigeminal nerve.

Thrombosis of the Internal Auditory Artery. This will produce ipsilateral deafness and loss of vestibular function. There are a number of other symptoms of intra- and extramedullary involvement, and although these may be of vascular origin and, hence, are included in this section, they are also found in association with other conditions such as syringobulbia, syringomyelia, multiple sclerosis, polioencephalitis, trauma, and neoplasms.

Jackson's Syndrome. The syndrome of Jackson, or vago-accessory-hypoglossal paralysis, is caused by a nuclear or radicular lesion of the tenth (nucleus ambiguus), eleventh, and twelfth nerves on one side and is manifested by ipsilateral flaccid paralysis of the soft palate, pharynx, and larynx, with flaccid weakness and atrophy of the sternocleidomastoid and trapezius muscles, and of the tongue.

Schmidt's Syndrome. The syndrome of Schmidt, or the vago-accessory syndrome, is the result of a lesion of the nucleus ambiguus and of the bulbar and spinal nuclei of the eleventh nerve and their radicular fibers and results in ipsilateral paralysis of the soft palate, pharynx, and larynx together with flaccid weakness and atrophy of the sternocleidomastoid and trapezius muscles.

Tapia's Syndrome. The syndrome of Tapia, or vago-hypoglossal palsy, occurs when there is ipsilateral paralysis of the soft palate, pharynx, and larynx, and paralysis and atrophy of the tongue. This results from a tegmental lesion in the lower third of the medulla and involves the ambiguus and hypoglossal nuclei. Schmidt's and Tapia's syndromes are actually more likely to result in extramedullary lesion with resultant involvement of the vagus and hypoglossal nerves high in the neck.

Vernet's Syndrome. The syndrome of Vernet is the result of a lesion at the jugular foramen and is characterized by ipsilateral paralysis of the ninth, tenth, and eleventh nerves. Although usually of traumatic origin (for example, basilar skull fracture), it is seen with vascular lesions, neoplasms, *thrombosis* of the jugular *bulb*, aneurysms of the internal carotid artery, syphilis, tuberculosis, and adenitis.

Villaret's Syndrome The syndrome of Villaret is the result of a lesion in the retropharyngeal or the retroparotid space. It is manifested by ipsilateral paralysis of the ninth, tenth, eleventh, and twelfth nerves along with cervical sympathetic fibers (Horner's syndrome).

Collet-Sicard Syndrome. The syndrome of Collet and Sicard is similar to that of Villaret with the exception of including Horner's syndrome. Some authorities feel that these syndromes of Villaret and Collet and Sicard are the same.

Garel-Gignoix Syndrome. In the syndrome of Garel and Gignoix there is involvement of the vagus and accessory nerves below the jugular foramen.

Trauma

Trauma is more appropriately discussed in other chapters of this book. Disturbances created by trauma include otorrhea, rhinorrhea, deafness, anosmia, or parosmia, post-traumatic seizures, among which are uncinate or olfactory seizures and vertiginous seizures, and post-traumatic headaches.

Degenerative Diseases

Diffuse Scleroses. There are a group of inflammatory-degenerative conditions which may or may not be familial and which produce diffuse demyelination of the brain. They occur in children and adolescents and are of interest to the otolaryngologist in that they may be associated with deafness along with other neurological symptoms, such as dementia, blindness, spasticity of extremities, and so forth.

Multiple Sclerosis. A most challenging

problem merits consideration in some detail. It is a very common disorder of young adults (17 to 35 years) and is characterized by remissions and exacerbations together with scattered neurological deficits. There are a number of clinical types, of which some are of common interest to the neurologist and otolaryngologist.

EARLY DIFFUSE TYPE. This type is characterized by varied and vague symptoms; for example, dizziness, weakness, paresthesias, lability of emotions, and ill-defined visual complaints. In addition, the objective neurological findings may often be rather minimal, e.g., absent abdominal reflex, brisk tendon reflexes, mild reflex asymmetry, a few beats of ankle clonus, and equivocal toe signs. These patients are often considered to be psychoneurotic until more solid findings occur.

CEREBELLAR TYPE. The cerebellar type is a very common form in the younger age group. There will be frequent remissions, incoordination of the limbs, intention tremor, unsteadiness of gait, scanning speech, as well as associated pyramidal tract and sensory changes. This condition must be differentiated from acoustic neuroma and cerebellar tumor. The prognosis is thought to be comparatively good.

MESENCEPHALIC TYPE. The mesencephalic type is manifested by retrobulbar neuritis, oculomotor palsy, and nystagmus. Pineal tumor must be considered in the differential diagnosis, as well as neurosyphilis. The prognosis is good; as a matter of fact, the patient invariably recovers from a particular episode.

SPINAL TYPE. The spinal type is manifested by spasticity, ataxia due to posterior column disease (impaired position sense) and sensory changes (sensory level, paresthesia), and bladder involvement. An older age group is primarily affected. The differential diagnosis must consider cord tumor and subacute combined degeneration. The prognosis is guarded, and this particular type has a slow, downhill course.

CEREBRAL TYPE. This type will occur in the form of hemiparesis and emotional lability and psychosis. The differential diagnosis includes psychosis of a functional type and brain tumor. The prognosis is usually good, with frequent remissions.

BULBAR TYPE. The bulbar type is of some interest to the otolaryngologist. It is frequently associated with vertigo, trigeminal pain, and dysarthria. The differential diagnosis includes trigeminal neuralgia and brain stem tumor.

Signs and symptoms. There are a number of presenting symptoms which should bring the

physician to suspect multiple sclerosis. Among these are transient sensory disturbance in a young person, electric paresthesias extending to limbs and trunk on flexion of the neck (Lhermitte's sign), *trifacial neuralgia* in the presence of associated vague findings, sudden loss of vision, usually unilateral (retrobulbar neuritis), impaired bladder function in a young person, impaired use of hand in writing due to incoordination of finer movements (Oppenheim's useless hand), and sudden onset of hemiplegia in a young person in the absence of evidence of other causes such as tumor or vascular disease.

The course is variable and in some patients is prolonged and benign and in others is more progressive, causing severe disabilities. Indications for a good prognosis are a complete recovery from the initial attack, mild relapses which show diminished frequency during the first five years of disease, a long intermission after the initial attack, and presenting symptoms confined to optic pathways, cranial nerves and sensory tracts.

Diagnosis. The diagnosis of multiple sclerosis should be made with some circumspection in individuals past the age of 40, in whom the deficit is that of a single lesion only, the course is progressive without any remissions, there is the presence of papilledema (occurs in less than 1 per cent of multiple sclerosis patients), and convulsions are present or there is mononeuritis.

SYRINGOBULBIA. Syringobulbia will produce brain stem symptomatology which the otolaryngologist will see as nuclear involvement of the bulbar structures. There often will be other evidence of the condition such as involvement of the shoulder girdle muscles; the diagnosis should not be a difficult one.

PROGRESSIVE MUSCULAR ATROPHY AND AMYOTROPHIC LATERAL SCLEROSIS. These may be bulbar in nature for a long period of time. This situation presents a problem since it must be differentiated from tumors of the nasopharynx as well as the brain stem. The onset is usually in middle age or later. Electromyography will be of assistance in diagnosis. Although bulbar involvement may be the initial manifestation, one usually will find later corroborative evidence in the general neurological examination.

MUSCULAR DYSTROPHY. Muscular dystrophy may give a rather characteristic myopathic facies. The family history will be of value. The patients are more often in the younger age group. Electromyographic and enzyme studies will give laboratory support to the diagnosis.

Intoxications

Intoxications may produce a *cerebral type* of *speech* disturbance. This is characterized by dysarthria as well as other signs described previously.

Of special interest are the various drugs which cause impairment of eighth cranial nerve function. These include quinine, salicylates, and streptomycin.

Movement disorders may also be caused by a variety of psychoactive drugs, especially the phenothiazides. Pseudoparkinsonism is a rather obvious disturbance. There are, however, distinct disturbances limited to the tongue and lips (tardive dyskinesia) which may not be so easily diagnosed. They can be confused with hysteria. The symptoms are manifested by protrusion of the tongue and various grimaces and lip movements.

Dilantin may produce cerebellar signs such as nystagmus, dysarthria, and ataxia.

Hysteria

Hysteria (conversion reaction) may be manifested by a variety of symptoms. Dysphonia and dysphagia are common. Dysphonia may cause quite a problem. There is a form of spastic dysphonia which may be organic in nature, although a psychological cause cannot always be excluded. Deafness may have a hysterical basis. Bilaterally depressed corneal or gag reflexes may also be seen in hysteria. Sensory disturbances involving the head and neck are a possibility. The ipsilateral extremities and trunk are often involved as well, and the sensory loss frequently comes to the exact midline. Hyperosmia is considered functional in origin. Hyperacusis and dizziness may be psychogenic complaints. A difficult differential diagnosis arises in the case of trauma involving the head and neck. The latter condition is the so-called whiplash injury. These patients may often complain of dizziness, by which they generally mean light-headedness. Headache is often present, along with difficulty in concentration. These symptoms, of course, could just as well be psychological in origin, and therein lies the diagnostic problem. Abnormal electroencephalograms, particularly if serial records indicate a lessening of severity or change in pattern, are of some value. Psychometric testing may show the presence of underlying organic brain disease, and this would tend to clarify the situation. Personality tests, on the other hand, can be of help in establishing a basis for the psychological cause of the symptoms.

Autonomic Disturbances

Horner's Syndrome. Horner's syndrome often occurs in conjunction with brain stem disease but may also be seen in lesions of the cervical sympathetic ganglia or in the upper spinal cord in approximately the second thoracic segment. In its classic form it is manifested by pseudoptosis, miosis, injection of the sclera, real or apparent enophthalmus, and ipsilateral dryness of the face.

Face-Hand Syndrome. This is a reflex sympathetic dystrophy which is seen as a residuum of stroke or myocardial infarction. There may be redness and edema of the involved parts together with persistent burning pain.

Decreased Salivation and Lacrimation. A lesion of the superior or inferior salivatory nuclei, their descending fibers, or the submaxillary, sphenopalatine, otic ganglia or their postganglionic fibers will cause a decrease in the amount of salivation and in the amount of mucous secretion in the nose, mouth, and pharynx, together with a decrease in lacrimation. Stimulation of these structures by an irritative process would, of course, increase these secretions. In general it can be said the disturbance of the sympathetic division causes little disturbance in these functions, although stimulation of the sympathetic is followed by formation of thick, viscid saliva. Salivation is stimulated reflexly by olfactory, gustatory, psychic, and other stimuli mediated through the hypothalamus and cortex. It may be inhibited centrally. Lacrimation may be either stimulated or inhibited centrally.

Crocodile Tear Syndrome. The syndrome of crocodile tears is characterized by lacrimation when food is taken into the mouth. This is an unusual residuum of a peripheral facial palsy and constitutes a paradoxic gustatory-lacrimal reflex. Tears appear when strongly flavored food is placed on the tongue. It is thought to be due to a faulty regeneration of the nerve fibers in which filaments having to do with salivary secretion have grown along the pathway to the lacrimal gland.

Chorda Tympani Syndrome. This consists of unilateral sweating and flushing in the submental region after eating.

Auriculotemporal Syndrome. A similar syndrome is the auriculotemporal syndrome, which is manifested by flushing, warmness, and excessive perspiration on one side following the ingestion of highly seasoned food. This is usually a sequela of trauma or infection of the parotid gland, with injury to the regional nerves. It may be associated with trigeminal sensory changes. In the regeneration of the severed auriculotemporal nerve, the secretory fibers to the parotid gland become misdirected to the sweat glands and the vasodilator endings, or there may be abnormal local irritability of cholinergic fibers.

Skin Changes. The skin changes secondary to autonomic disturbance will be manifested by loss of pilomotor responses, anhidrosis, and vasodilatation when the sympathetic pathways are interrupted. Stimulation, on the other hand, will have the opposite effect. Trophic changes to the skin, mucous membranes, and subcutaneous tissue occur in the presence of sympathetic interruption. The skin then becomes smooth, thin, pale, and glossy. However, there may be flushing, erythema, cyanosis and other types of discoloration. Seborrhea or oiliness is sometimes present. Changes in hair glands may occur. Lesions in the sensory ganglia may produce changes such as those seen in herpes zoster. Edema of the skin may result from autonomic nervous system involvement, for example, angioneurotic edema (Quincke's disease), myxedema, hemiedema. Various pigmentary changes can take place; vitiligo (leukoderma) consists of patchy loss of pigmentation.

Metabolic Disease

Myopathy, of various types, may be secondary to metabolic disturbances such as myxedema or hyperthyroidism.

Collagenoses

Dermatomyositis and polymyositis may begin initially with *dysphagia* and, for a time, this may be the only symptom. Diagnosis may be established by the assistance of electromyography because other evidence of neuropathy or myopathy may not be present. The examination of the blood for rheumatoid factor, lupus erythematosus cells, serum electrophoretic pattern, erythrocytes, and sedimentation rate may be of further assistance. Of importance is the fact that collagenoses, especially in older individuals, may be associated with malignancy. Collagenoses may also be instrumental in the production of brain stem symptoms secondary to vasculitis.

LABORATORY AIDS

The various auditory and labyrinthine tests, including electronystagmography, are discussed elsewhere in this text. There are a number of laboratory procedures which may be performed by the neurologist. These are cerebral spinal fluid examination, electroencephalogram, electromyogram, and neuroradiologic procedures (angiography, pneumoencephalography, myelography).

Cerebral Spinal Fluid

Method
General considerations. Lumbar puncture is the simplest method of gaining access to the subarachnoid space and is so frequently used that every practitioner should be capable of carrying it out. The spinal cord terminates at the lower border of the first lumbar vertebrae in the adult, and the subarachnoid space continues to the second sacral vertebrae. A needle can be introduced below the first lumbar vertebra without risk of injury to the cord. A lumbar puncture can be performed with the patient either sitting or lying on one side. In either position maximum flexion of the spine should be obtained. Landmarks, particularly the spinous processes, should be carefully determined. A line joining the highest points of the iliac crests passes between the third and fourth lumbar spines, and the puncture can be performed either at this point or at one level higher.

1. Care must be given to the proper preparation of the skin prior to the puncture. The skin is prepared with suitable antiseptics, and sterile drapes are placed around the puncture area. Sterile gloves should be worn by the physician, and only the hub of the needle should be touched. A sharp, 20 gauge needle is best suited for this procedure in order to avoid unnecessary injury to the meninges.

2. When the subarachnoid space is penetrated, the spinal fluid pressure should be measured with a water manometer; if the reading is elevated, the pressure should be observed for a few minutes and every effort made to obtain maximum relaxation of the patient.

3. Queckenstedt's test (jugular compression in the neck) should not be done routinely. It is indicated only if spinal block or lateral sinus thrombosis is suspected. As a rule, it is con-

traindicated when intracerebral pathology is present.

4. If the fluid is blood-tinged at first, it should be collected into several tubes after the pressure has been determined. If the fluid clears rapidly, the bleeding was probably produced by the puncture.

5. Three tubes of spinal fluid should be collected for the usual tests. If adequate studies are not carried out, a repetition of the spinal puncture may be necessary.

6. Cisternal puncture is a more complex procedure and should be done only by an experienced physician. It is done only if a spinal puncture cannot be carried out at the normal sites. The patient's neck is shaved as high as the external occipital protuberance and the entire area carefully prepared with antiseptics and draped. A midline point is selected about 2 inches below the external occipital protuberance for insertion of the needle. The needle is advanced slowly, pointing slightly upward so that the occipital bone is encountered at a depth of 3 to 4 cm. The tip of the needle is then depressed and moved along the base of the occiput. At intervals of a few millimeters the stylet should be removed in order to make sure that the cistern has not been entered. The cistern is usually encountered at a depth of 4 to 5 cm. If the needle is inserted too rapidly and too deeply, it will penetrate the medulla.

Indications for spinal puncture:

1. To obtain fluid for cytological, chemical, and other investigations such as pressure that might aid in the diagnosis of the illness (subarachnoid hemorrhage, meningitis, encephalitis, and so forth).

2. For relief of intracranial pressure (use caution).

3. To introduce therapeutic substances into the subarachnoid space (not commonly carried out).

4. To introduce radiographic material for diagnostic purposes (myelography and clivography).

5. To introduce air into subarachnoid spaces for diagnostic purposes (air encephalography).

6. For spinal anesthesia; it must be kept in mind that these anesthetic agents can be irritative and may result in the delayed onset of radicular pain.

Contraindications to spinal puncture

1. The most important contraindication is a high-grade, choked disc, especially when a subtentorial tumor is suspected. In such cases there is a danger of displacement of portions of the cerebellum into the foramen magnum with medullary compression. Before a spinal tap is done, a careful ophthalmoscopic examination must be made; if papilledema is present, the spinal puncture should be avoided.

2. Spinal puncture should be avoided in any patient suspected of having a subtentorial tumor, even in the absence of papilledema.

3. Spinal puncture is best avoided in cases of respiratory paresis caused by acutely developing central nervous system lesions.

4. Spinal tap should be performed with great caution in the presence of a possible spinal epidural abscess situated in the lumbar region. It is possible to introduce purulent material from the abscess into the subarachnoid space.

5. Spinal puncture should be performed with great caution in patients with evidence of a large extramedullary tumor. Sudden displacement of the tumor by removal of spinal fluid may result in complete cord compression with disastrous neurologic deficit.

6. In severely psychoneurotic patients, the spinal puncture is best avoided unless one strongly suspects concomitant disease for which the procedure is diagnostically indicated.

Complications of spinal puncture

1. Herniation of cerebellum with medullary compression in subtentorial tumors and in increased intracranial pressure.

2. Displacement of spinal cord tumor with acute cord compression.

3. Spinal headache, chiefly a postural headache and probably due to continued seepage through dural puncture area.

4. Meningitis, introduced from local abscess or poorly prepared puncture site.

Pressure. Normal pressure is 100 to 150 mm. water when patient is recumbent or 300 to 360 mm. of water when sitting up. It is increased in tumors, hydrocephalus, sinus thrombosis, and meningitis and decreased after repeated taps or in patients with spinal block. In Queckenstedt's test the jugular veins are compressed, with resultant immediate rise in pressure followed by a rapid fall when pressure is released. In a block at the foramen magnum or above the needle in the spinal canal, there will be an incomplete rise and fall of pressure on jugular compression. One should not do a spinal tap when a tumor is suspected, particularly if in the posterior fossa.

Appearance

1. Clear and colorless; unclean tubes or an increase of cells or protein alter the clarity of the fluid.

2. Turbid if it contains more than 1000 white blood cells.

3. Bloody fluid indicates subarachnoid bleeding or traumatic tap. The appearance is that of faint cloudiness if 500 to 1000 red cells are present, pink if there are 1000 to 3000 red cells, and red if over 5000 red cells per cu. mm. In the face of bloody fluid one should: (1) Take three consecutive spinal samples. Decreasing turbidity is evidence of a "traumatic tap." (2) Centrifuge spinal fluid. If supernatant fluid is yellow, bleeding has been present for some time. (3) Apply benzidine in glacial acetic acid. Heat, cool, and add 1 ml. hydrogen peroxide. A blue color indicates old bleeding and not a traumatic tap.

Cell Count. A normal cell count is 3 to 5 mononuclears per cu. mm.

1. If tap is bloody, count red and white cells and allow one white cell for each 700 red cells.

2. Polymorphonuclear increase occurs in acute infection, as pyogenic infections (bacterial meningitis, endocarditis, brain abscess).

3. Mononuclear increase is seen in viral infections and some tumors.

4. Check fluid for tumor cells, yeasts, parasites.

Protein. Normal protein is 15 to 40 mg. per 100 ml. The ratio of albumin to globulin is 8 to 1.

Protein increase. Protein increase occurs with diseases associated with venous stasis (meningeal tumors, vascular lesions such as thrombosis); inflammatory disease of meninges with leukocytes; metabolic disturbances (peripheral neuritis, myxedema).

Froin reaction. Very high protein (over 500 mg. per 100 ml.) results in xanthochromia; coagulation of spinal fluid; spinal subarachnoid block due to tumor compression or chronic inflammatory process.

Colloidal gold reaction. This is a test for increased globulin ratio in spinal fluid. The colloidal gold solution tends to precipitate out in different degrees, depending upon protein concentration of spinal fluid.

Pandy test. Carbolic acid is added to spinal fluid to check for increased globulin. Positive reaction varies from opalescence to milky turbidity.

Sugar. Normal sugar is 50 to 80 mg. per 100 ml. Increased sugar occurs in hyperglycemia and after intravenous glucose. Decreased sugar is found in bacterial infections of meninges and tuberculosis.

Chlorides. Normal chloride is 720 to 750 mg. per 100 ml. Chlorides are reduced to 650 mg. per 100 ml. in purulent meningitis and reduced below 650 mg. in tubercular meningitis.

SPINAL FLUID MANIFESTATIONS OF DISEASE

Purulent Meningitis. Cloudy fluid; increased pressure; markedly increased cells, chiefly polymorphonuclears, from 500 to 20,000; elevated protein from 100 to 500 mg. per 100 ml.; reduced sugar; organisms isolated from fluid.

Multiple Sclerosis. Normal pressure; high normal protein; increase in globulins (gamma globulin); no cell increase; first zone colloidal gold curve in 40 per cent of patients.

Cerebral Hemorrhage. Spinal fluid xanthochromic or blood-tinged; increased pressure.

Brain Abscess. Elevated spinal fluid pressure; increased polymorphonuclears in fluid. Same picture produced by extradural abscess or sinus thrombosis.

Viral Infections. Usually the spinal fluid reveals only a mild, nonspecific lymphocytic increase.

Brain Tumors. At best, the spinal fluid reveals only an increased pressure.

Brain Trauma. Blood-tinged fluid may occasionally be present.

Electroencephalogram

This procedure is of value in a number of instances. Olfactory, auditory, and vertiginous seizures are characterized by temporal lobe dysrhythmia. Although the records are often also diffusely abnormal, a focal involvement of a temporal lobe is frequently seen. The routine electroencephalogram may not always be positive. An electroencephalogram taken during sleep, particularly with nasopharyngeal leads, may uncover previously masked spike activity from the temporal lobes.

A more sophisticated electroencephalographic approach is that of the evoked potential study, which may be useful in analyzing hearing deficits in young children and infants.

The serial electroencephalogram, as has been noted before, may help to establish an organic basis for certain post-traumatic symptoms such as headache, dizziness, and difficulty in concentration.

Electromyography

The electromyographer is in a position of rendering valuable assistance in a number of diagnostic categories. In the case of bulbar palsy the electromyogram may assist in the differential diagnosis between a supranuclear and nuclear or peripheral type of involvement. A nuclear or lower motor neuron involvement will result in fibrillation potentials on needle electrode investigation. The tongue, because of the difficulty in controlling its movement, may be a source of artifacts; nevertheless, it is possible to establish nuclear or lower motor neuron involvement here. The facial and sternocleidomastoid muscles are much easier to study. Remote muscle assessment may be of assistance. In amyotrophic lateral sclerosis, for example, it is with rare exception that the limb muscles would be free of the abnormal potentials of this character disorder. In myasthenia gravis one finds a very definite pattern of electromyographic disturbance. There is a decline in amplitude in the motor unit response to repetitive stimuli. In nuclear or peripheral facial nerve involvement one may receive assistance from the electromyographer not only in diagnosis but also in prognosis. Both sides of the face are tested. Two modes of testing are used for this study: stimulation and needle electrode analysis. The technique is most useful in the first few days of the facial paralysis. If one tests the paralyzed side early, there may be a normal or slightly prolonged latency. This is a good prognostic sign, particularly if the motor unit response is normal in amplitude, or at worst slightly reduced. If there is no response to stimulus, the prognosis is considered poor, and the assumption has to be made that the nerve is fairly completely degenerated. The electromyographic response varies over the first several days of paralysis. Initially, in patients in whom the prognosis is favorable, the results of muscle stimulation are normal or almost so. By the third day the latency of response to stimulation is usually increased, and the muscle potential response is definitely decreased. This probably means that fewer muscle fibers are responding. If the response is progressive it would indicate that some nerve fibers are degenerating and, as a corollary, the condition is worsening. This would be fairly clear after the fourth day of onset. Changes of diagnostic import are usually not in evidence after the fifth day. The electromyogram taken in the first few days of paralysis should be of assistance to the surgeon who contemplates a surgical approach to the treatment of facial palsy.

Neuroradiology

Angiography in which the vertebral and basilar arteries are visualized along with the posterior cerebral vessels can be of value in clarifying lesions in the subtentorial region. It is most helpful in the diagnosis of tumors since displacement of the vessels will indicate the presence of such a lesion.

Pneumoencephalography with positioning of the patient so that air can be placed in the subtentorial region may be helpful in demonstrating the presence of a brain stem or a cerebellopontine angle tumor.

Myelography in which the clivus is visualized will give similar information.

In addition to the audiometric and spinal fluid testing for an acoustic neuroma, one, of course, would initially have had skull x-ray with special views of the internal auditory canals. There will be enlargement of the meatus and other changes which, in about two thirds of patients, will lead to an x-ray diagnosis.

TREATMENT

Infections

Intravenous penicillin remains the treatment of choice for pneumococcal meningitis and pyogenic brain abscess. Appropriate antibiotic agents should be utilized for various other pyogenic organisms. The important thing to remember is that the blood brain barrier is resistant to the passage of therapeutic agents, and intravenous antibiotics in large doses are usually required for effective therapy. In the case of pneumococcal meningitis one must be certain to treat the infection over a number of weeks after apparent recovery since there is a considerable risk of secondary abscess formation because of the fact that the purulent exudate has a tendency to seal off a pocket of infection in the sulci of the cerebrum. Syphilis of the central nervous system is also most amenable to intravenous penicillin therapy, again in large dosage.

Cerebrovascular Disease

In acute stroke, general medical care is of great importance. This involves attention to secretions of the nasopharynx, maintenance of a patent airway, support of general circulation, attention to the urinary bladder, and adequate nutrition. The serum electrolyte status, blood urea nitrogen level, and blood sugar level should be ascertained and corrective measures instituted when required. There is little specific treatment for infarction. One hesitates to use anticoagulant therapy, particularly when the cerebrum is involved for fear of hemorrhage in the softened areas. Inhalation therapy with carbon dioxide (95 per cent O_2, 5 per cent CO_2, or variation thereof) has definitely improved cerebral blood flow but is rather uncomfortable to tolerate after a few minutes. Papaverine, given intravenously by slow drip, has also been shown to improve cerebral blood flow. At the moment, however, there is some question concerning increase of perfusion to infarcted areas because of the fear of adding further damage by increasing edema. Surgery (endarterectomy) in the face of completed stroke is contraindicated. In the case of transient ischemic events or a progressive stroke there is place for definitive therapy. When not contraindicated medically, anticoagulant therapy is of use in transient ischemic attacks. In patients in whom it is contraindicated (for example, severe hypertensives), one can use vasodilators, the most useful of which (on an oral basis) would be papaverine. In a progressing stroke the patient is initially heparinized and this is then followed by oral anticoagulants.

Headache

In most instances a combination of analgesics and barbiturates is useful in the symptomatic control of headache. The vascular headaches, particularly migraine and the cluster headache, respond favorably in many instances to methysergide (Sansert—Sandoz Pharmaceuticals). However, there are a number of undesirable side effects, and this medication must be used with some caution. When an aura precedes migraine by a sufficient interval, ergot preparations will be of value either by injection, inhalation, or the oral route. Unfortunately this circumstance is not always present. Nevertheless, in some instances the patient with a vascular headache does respond to some extent to the ergot preparations at any time in the course. The so-called cluster headache, which is also known as histamine cephalgia or Horton's headache, is also treated by intravenous or subcutaneous histamine desensitization. This method should be considered when the simpler measures are ineffective.

Multiple Sclerosis

Steroid therapy is of definite value in the treatment of multiple sclerosis. It is most efficacious in the treatment of the initial attack or exacerbations. The course of treatment consists of intravenous administration of ACTH for a ten-day to two-week period. Forty to 60 units of ACTH are placed in 1000 ml. of diluent, usually 5 per cent dextrose in distilled water, and administered slowly by intravenous drip over a period of eight to ten hours. Subsequent to the initial intravenous course it is sometimes desirable to administer the ACTH indefinitely, usually 40 units every 48 to 72 hours. It is best to individualize the treatment, depending upon the patient's tendency to exacerbate. Oral steroids are used by some. We have found oral steroids to be of greatest use in the case of optic neuritis. Adjunctive treatment consists of parenteral and oral vitamin preparations.

Neuralgia

It is not the purpose of this chapter to discuss surgical treatment. However, its place in the management of the various neuralgias is well recognized. In recent years it has been possible to obviate surgery in some conditions, particularly in trigeminal neuralgia. Diphenylhydantoin (Dilantin—Parke, Davis & Co.) has had considerable impact on the treatment of this condition. It responds to dosages of 100 mg. three times daily. Initially, however, one may have to use much larger amounts, for example, 100 mg. five or six times per day. The patient may become ataxic at these levels. Dosage is gradually reduced to a maintenance level of 100 mg. two or three times daily. Carbemazepine (Tegretol—Geigy Pharmaceuticals) is a more recent addition to the drug treatment of trigeminal neuralgia. There are a number of adverse reactions involving the hepatic or the hemopoietic systems particularly. This drug, therefore, although definitely beneficial, must be used with care. The initial dosage is 100 mg. twice daily. It should then be gradually increased by 100 mg. increments every 12 hours until freedom from pain is reached. In most instances 400 to 800 mg. per day should suffice. The maintenance dose can be as little as 200 mg. per day.

Facial Nerve Palsy

The general care of the patient is in the opinion of many physicians still an essential.

Some place the patient at bed rest or at least on a modified rest regimen for the initial phase of the treatment. Steroids have been found useful and should be administered over the initial two or three weeks after diagnosis. Due attention must be paid to the status of the facial muscles during the time of nerve regeneration. This may consist of splinting with tape, together with light massage. More recently electric stimulation has been used several times daily in an effort to preserve tone and to avoid fibrosis of the facial muscles. Small portable stimulators are available, and the patient can be instructed in their use. Due protection must be given to the eyes, including suturing of the lids in some instances.

Dysphagia

Treatment has been considered under the discussion of the acute bulbar situation. It is worthwhile to emphasize the fact that tracheostomy should be done early. Nutrition should not be neglected and, although nasal gavage may suffice in some instances, a feeding gastrostomy may be necessary in others. A bulbar diet is satisfactory in many cases.

Tumors

The treatment is surgical and will be discussed elsewhere.

Rhinorrhea and Otorrhea

Although these conditions may at times respond favorably to conservative management, surgery may be required.

Movement Disorders

It is obvious when movement disorders are the result of drug intoxication (phenothiazines) that the offending medication should be withdrawn. Antihistamines have been tried but without appreciable success in the tardive dyskinesias. L-DOPA (1-diphenylalanine) has recently been used with some success in dystonias. Thalamotomy has also been employed in the various movement disorders. The various derivatives or sympathetic variations having similar reaction have been used with some success in parkinsonism. More recently L-DOPA has been shown to be a most effective remedy.

Vertigo and Dizziness

In vertigo of labyrinthine origin, niacin and one of the antimotion sickness preparations remain the most useful combination. We have had some success with intravenous procaine in patients who do not respond to the simpler remedies. Antihistamine preparations are often used as an adjunct to the niacine-antimotion sickness combinations. The dizziness or vertigo resulting from hypotension is symptomatically treated with the wearing of elastic hose and, in some instances, administration of ephedrine. Postural vertigo may respond to niacin and papaverine. When vertigo or dizziness is a result of cerebrovascular disease, treatment of the primary condition is required. When the symptom is occasioned by salicylates, propoxyphene, or barbiturates, discontinuation of the offending drug is obviously indicated. The effect of these drugs is transient, and the patient usually recovers in a few days. Vertiginous seizures are treated with appropriate anticonvulsant medication after exclusion of a causative surgical lesion.

REFERENCES

Baker, A. B.: An Outline of Clinical Neurology. Dubuque, Iowa, William C. Brown Book Company, 1958.
Baker, A. B.: Clinical Neurology. Vol. 3. New York, Harper & Brothers, 1962.
DeJong, R. N.: The Neurologic Examination. New York, Harper & Row, 1967.

Chapter 35

NEUROSURGERY

by Frank H. Mayfield, M.D., and John M. Tew, Jr., M.D.

Many responsibilities and problems are shared by the otolaryngologist and the neurosurgeon. Disorders that begin in the ear and its environs or in the paranasal sinuses commonly invade the intracranial cavity. Occasionally the reverse is true. Also, many lesions of the central nervous system refer or produce symptoms that lead patients and referring physicians to consult the otolaryngologist primarily.

From time to time the development of new medications, diagnostic methods, and improved instrumentation modify treatment and indications for operation. The utilization of chemotherapy and the development of microsurgical techniques in the treatment of lesions of the pituitary gland and the eighth nerve offer cases in point.

Space precludes a comprehensive presentation of the specialty of neurosurgery here; hence, the authors have elected to commit this chapter to consideration of those areas in which the responsibilities of the specialists more frequently overlap and in which, from personal experience and the literature, our own opinions appear to differ from our colleagues in otolaryngology, and to include in our material certain important exemplary examples of disorders that are both rare and sufficiently unusual that they might escape the reader's attention if not recorded here.

The material will be considered generally under the following categories: Tumors, Infections, Pain, and Trauma.

TUMORS

Tumors of the Nasopharynx, Nose, and Paranasal Sinuses

Mucocele

Mucocele is defined as the accumulation and retention of mucoid material within a sinus as a result of continuous or periodic obstruction of the ostium of the sinus (Hayes, 1964). The secretion is usually clear, thick, and tenacious unless invasion by bacteria has occurred and created a pyocele in which the color and consistency of the accumulated material varies with the infecting organisms (Krueger, 1965). Secondary erosion and distention of the sinus walls occurs as the intraluminal pressure increases.

Mucoceles are most frequently found in the frontal sinus (Mortada, 1968). Chronic in nature, a source of recurrent frontal headache, they may erode through either the anterior or posterior wall of the frontal sinus. In the former instance, a tender, fluctuant mass presents beneath the periosteum of the frontal bone, commonly known as a Pott's puffy tumor, and demands local drainage and exenteration of the sinus. If the posterior sinus wall is destroyed, epidural abscess, subdural empyema, meningitis, or brain abscess may develop. This complication will be covered in a separate section of this chapter.

Mucoceles of the ethmoid sinuses commonly destroy the adjacent thin lamina papyracea and displace the orbital contents laterally or downward, resulting in exophthalmus and diplopia. Compression of the superior orbital fissure produces ocular palsies and diminished sensation in the forehead.

Mucoceles of the maxillary sinus rarely lead to neurologic complications (Bloom, 1965; De, 1966); only a few well documented cases are recorded. Proptosis due to upward displacement of the orbital contents (Parker, 1961), exophthalmos caused by destruction of the floor of the orbit (Montgomery, 1964), diplopia due to displacement of orbital contents, and paresis of the oculomotor as well as the optic nerve as in the orbital apex syndrome (Pooley and Wilkinson, 1913; Lundgren and Olin, 1961) are documented features.

Less than 75 mucoceles of the sphenoid sinuses have been reported. However, this condition must always be suspected when one is confronted with an expanding mass in the sphenoid sinus and sella turcica. Recurrent headaches and visual disturbances (diplopia and visual deficits) are characteristic symptoms (Reinecke and Montgomery, 1964). Indeed, this condition may be confused with ophthalmoplegic migraine (Pincus and Daroff, 1964), a plausible error considering the chronic nature of both diseases (Fig. 1). Signs of chiasmal compression, ocular nerve palsies, exophthalmos, and intermittent cerebrospinal fluid rhinorrhea have been recorded. However, spontaneous intracranial infection is most unusual (Hayes and Creston, 1964).

The radiographic findings consist of: (1) opacification of the sphenoid sinus; (2) ballooning and rarefaction of the bony wall of the sphenoid sinus; (3) destruction of the interseptum of the sinus; (4) erosion of the floor and walls of the sella turcica; and (5) lateral and upward displacement of the carotid arteries (Figs. 2 to 6). Tomography and carotid angiography are essential in the investigation of this lesion (Norman and Yanagisawa, 1964; Bloom, 1965; Nevins and Leaver, 1967).

It is imperative that the correct diagnosis be reached prior to treatment (radiotherapy or surgical) of all masses in the sphenoid sinus and sella turcica. Although sphenoid mucoceles account for only a small portion of these lesions, they may always be cured by adequate endonasal drainage and exenteration of the sinus.

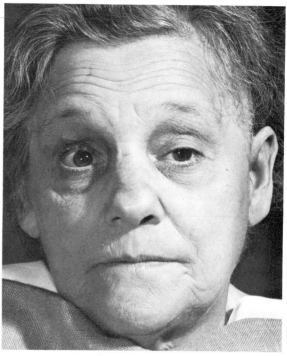

Figure 1. A 65 year old female with 10-year history of blindness in the left eye of rapid onset associated with severe headache and sinusitis. Nine years later recurrent bouts of headache in the retro-orbital and temporal regions were accompanied by partial third, fifth (first division) and sixth nerve palsies. Note ptosis and sparing of left pupil. Figures 2 through 6 show diagnostic procedures used in confirming the cause of the problem.

It should be emphasized that intracranial exploration of these lesions must be avoided, since spinal fluid rhinorrhea and meningitis are almost certain to follow.

Encephalomeningoceles and Nasal Gliomas

Encephalomeningoceles. Glial tumors in the nasal region vary from the encephalomeningocele, a developmental defect in which the basal meninges protrude through a bony defect creating a spinal fluid sac filled with cerebral tissue, to a solid mass of glial tissue, which may be entirely separate from the brain and unassociated with defects in the cranium. Regardless of the nature of the lesions, their growth potential is low and radical removal is seldom followed by recurrence (Black and Smith, 1950). Preoperative differentiation of these masses from others indigenous to the area is difficult but of great importance. Attention should be directed to the presence of a

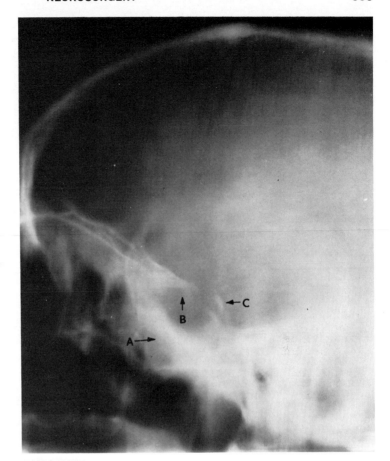

Figure 2. Lateral tomographic cut in the midsellar plane, showing (A) opacification of the sphenoid sinus; (B) erosion of the left anterior clinoid process; and (C) ballooning of the sella turcica and erosion of the posterior clinoid process.

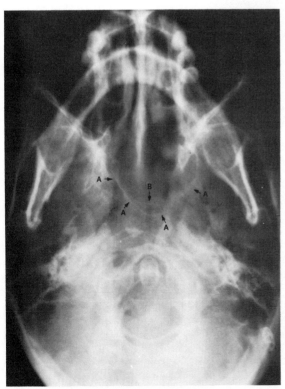

Figure 3. Base view of the skull demonstrating (A) marked ballooning of the walls of the sphenoid sinus and destruction of the interseptum of the sinus; and (B) thinning of the dorsum sella process.

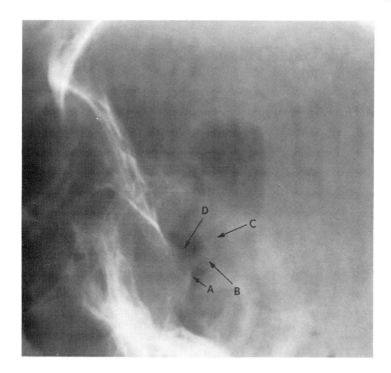

Figure 4. Pneumoencephalogram demonstrating (A) posterior displacement and marked thinning of the posterior clinoid process and dorsum sella; (B) shadow in the chiasmatic cistern which probably represents the pituitary stalk and optic chiasm; (C) air filling the anterior aspect of the third ventricle; and (D) bulging of the diaphragm sella, the dural covering of the pituitary gland and the chiasmatic cistern. There is no significant suprasellar mass.

Figure 5. The sphenoidal mucocele was opened via a transseptal approach and 30 cc. of emulsified Pantopaque was placed in the cavity. Anteroposterior and lateral radiographs demonstrated the boundaries of the cavity. In the lateral view A indicates the encroachment of the cyst on the superior orbital fissure; B the undersurface of the anterior clinoid and the optic foramen; and C shows the thinned posterior clinoid and dorsum sella. The floor of the pituitary fossa was completely destroyed and the dura covering the gland lay free in the mucocele cavity. (D) Transnasal drainage resulted in complete recovery except for longstanding optic atrophy.

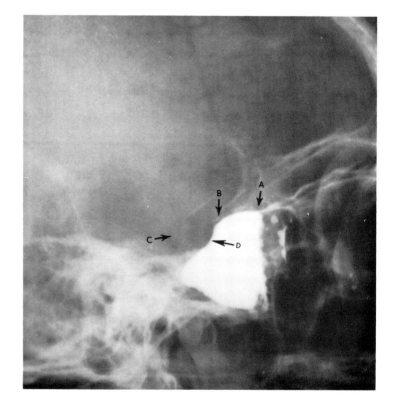

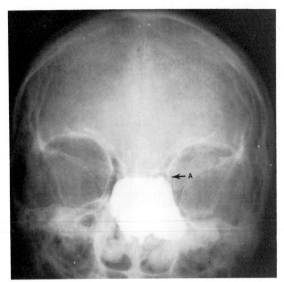

Figure 6. Anteroposterior radiograph showing (A) encroachment of cyst on the superior orbital fissure.

nasal or paranasal mass in early life, widening of the nasal bridge, separation of the upper margins of the nose resembling hypertelorism and, in the case of an intranasal mass, attachment between the middle turbinate and the nasal septum (an unlikely site for polyp, particularly in early life) (Davis and Alexander, 1959).

Encephalomeningoceles may be divided into the following types: occipital, sincipital, and basal (Blumenfeld and Skolnik, 1965). The ma-

jority occur in the occipital region (75 per cent). Of the 15 per cent presenting in the sincipital region, the following variations have been documented: (1) nasofrontal, in which the mass presents in the midline at the bridge of the nose; (2) naso-orbital, in which the mass presents in the anteromedian aspect of the orbit and causes proptosis; (3) naso-ethmoidal (Suwanwela and Horgsaprabhas, 1966), in which the mass distorts the side of the nose at the junction of the nasal and ethmoid bones.

The basal region accounts for only 10 per cent of encephalomeningoceles, but this group is of greatest interest and importance to this discussion since they commonly present in the nasal or pharyngeal region where they may be mistaken for less complex lesions indigenous to the area (Anderson, 1947; Finerman and Pick, 1953). Accurate preoperative definition is necessary to the proper surgical treatment in order to prevent recurrence and complications such as spinal fluid rhinorrhea, which frequently follows attempts at endonasal excision. The following types of basal encephalomeningoceles have been recognized: (1) spheno-orbital, in which the mass presents in the superior orbit via the superior orbital fissure and causes exophthalmos; (2) intranasal, when the lesion passes through the lamina cribrosa and presents between the middle turbinate and the nasal septum; (3) sphenopharyngeal, in which the mass escapes through the sphenoid bone and presents in the epipharynx; (4) sphenomax-

Figure 7. Photograph taken through the mouth of a six week old infant with partial cleft lip and cleft palate. Note the large basal intranasal encephalomeningocele protruding into the mouth through the palatal defect. (Matson, D. D.: Neurosurgery of Infancy and Childhood, Springfield, Ill., Charles C Thomas, 1969.)

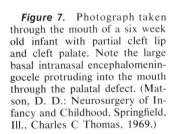

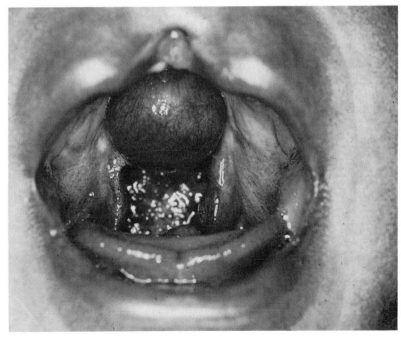

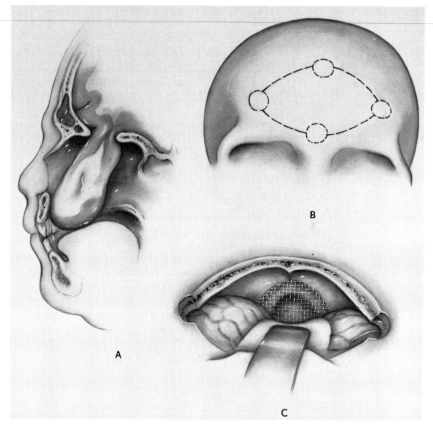

Figure 8. *A*, Semidiagrammatic view of a basal intranasal encephalomeningocele protruding into the mouth through a cleft palate. *B*, The bifrontal craniotomy flap used to expose the frontal fossa. *C*, The pedicle of herniated brain has been excised. A stainless steel mesh is used to close the defect in the floor of the frontal fossa in the cribriform region. The dural defect is closed with a graft of autogenous fascia.

illary, in which the lesion passes through the infraorbital fissure into the pterygomaxillary fossa and presents as a mass on the medial aspect of the maxilla.

Encephalomeningoceles demand an intracranial surgical approach (Matson, 1969), as illustrated by the following case of an infant with a basal (intranasal) encephalocele (Figs. 7 and 8).

Nasal Gliomas. Nasal gliomas which have no direct connection with the central nervous system may take their origin from embryonic nests which may have been isolated from the frontal lobe by closure of the cranial sutures during embryonic development, or may arise from the primitive olfactory membrane (Mood, 1938). In most instances they are neoplasms of low growth potential and can be eradicated by local excision (Black and Smith, 1950). However, the olfactory neuroblastoma, a highly malignant neoplasm which arises from the olfactory apparatus (Holland et al., 1959), erodes the floor of the frontal fossa, and may present

as a mass in the nose or cranial cavity (Robinson and Solitare, 1966), must be treated by radical excision and high voltage radiotherapy, to which it is highly sensitive. Despite this regimen, distant metastases and limited survival is the common result (Hutter et al., 1963), as illustrated by the case illustrated in Figures 9 to 12.

Craniopharyngiomas

Craniopharyngioma, a solid and cystic tumor which arises as a proliferation of the squamous cell nests in the superior region of the anterior lobe of the pituitary gland, has long been a fascinating lesion because of its unusual embryonic origin from the primitive stomodeum (Matson, 1969), its unique location susceptible to accurate clinical and radiographic diagnosis, and the tantalizing possibility of cure by radical excision. Despite its localized nature, the craniopharyngioma erodes bone and com-

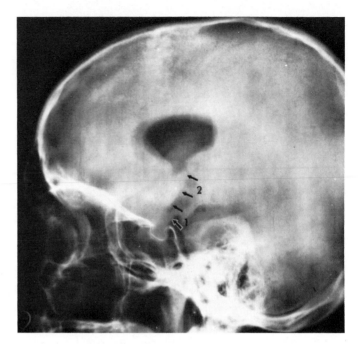

Figure 9. A 47 year old male presented with headaches, papilledema and bilateral anosmia. Plain skull films were normal. A pneumoencephalogram demonstrated a large subfrontal mass displacing the anterior portion of the third ventricle (arrows 1 and 2).

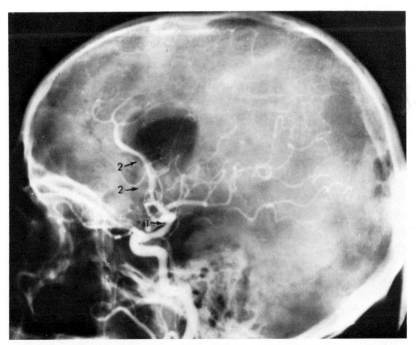

Figure 10. A left carotid angiogram of patient shown in Figure 9 confirmed the presence of a mass which was displacing the internal carotid artery laterally and posteriorly (1); 2 indicates displacement of the anterior cerebral and pericallosal arteries posteriorly and to the right of midline.

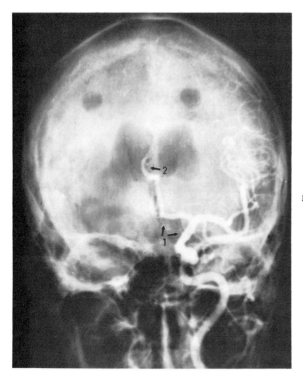

Figure 11. Anteroposterior view of left carotid angiogram of patient shown in Figure 9.

Figure 12. The patient shown in Figure 9 was explored through a frontal craniotomy, and a large subfrontal tumor was removed. The tumor arose from the dura in the cribriform area; however, the large defect in the dura and bone of the frontal fossa (A) was not recognized, and the patient expired as a result of postoperative meningitis. At necropsy a tumor was found extending into the nose. The cribriform area was completely destroyed. The optic nerve (B), carotid artery (C) and oculomotor nerve (D) were not involved.

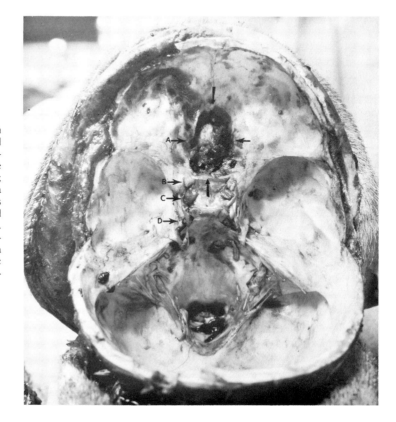

presses adjacent neural structures by progressive expansion. The se la turcica is eroded or enlarged in 60 per cent of patients, calcification is present in 60 to 90 per cent, depending on the age of the patient, and visual field defects are present in 60 per cent. Accordingly, it is essential to distinguish the craniopharyngioma from other lesions presenting in this manner. Matson (1960, 1969), Kahn (1969), and others (Sweet, 1968) have advocated a radical total excision through a right frontal craniotomy. However, others, dissatisfied with this maneuver, have advocated transfrontal biopsy, evacuation of the cyst, and supravoltage radiotherapy (Kramer et al., 1961). In addition, others (Hamberger et al., 1960) have proposed the transsphenoidal approach, an appealing suggestion for lesions primarily restricted to the sella turcica and recurrent cystic lesions in which previous intracranial excision has been unsuccessful. The long-term results of radiotherapy require further evaluation. Matson's statistics for radical primary excision in children are most commendable. There have been no deaths in the last 40 cases, and 38 patients are engaged in gainful activity (Matson, 1969).

Intracranial Aneurysms

The initial intracranial course of the internal carotid artery through the cavernous sinus places it adjacent to the sphenoid sinus and the anterior clinoid of the sella turcica. Therefore, aneurysms of the internal carotid artery, particularly those within the cavernous sinus where they are unlikely to produce subarachnoid hemorrhage, may present as a mass lesion indistinguishable from tumors of the parasellar region (Cushing, 1912). Because of the disastrous events which may follow failure to recognize aneurysms, bilateral carotid angiography should be completed prior to definitive therapy of all parasellar lesions in which the diagnosis is unclear. This concept is particularly relevant in patients undergoing radiotherapy and in exploration of the sella turcica via the transsphenoidal approach. It may be impossible to differentiate the progressively enlarging intrasellar aneurysm from tumors which produce a characteristic expansion and erosion of the sella turcica. Such a circumstance is well documented by the case history of Ellen O'B., a 61 year old woman whose radiographs were reproduced in a textbook of radiology edited by Holmes and Robbins (1955) as a typical example of erosion and expansion of the sella turcica by a pituitary adenoma (Fig. 13). Because of progressive deterioration in pituitary function and visual fields, the patient underwent a transsphenoidal approach to the sella turcica by Drs. Hirsch and Hamlin. However, when the floor of the eroded sella turcica was entered, a gush of arterial blood was controlled with difficulty, and subsequent angiography

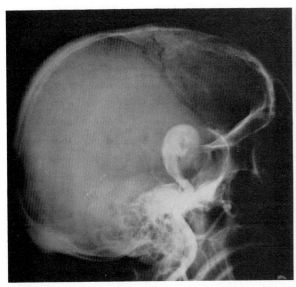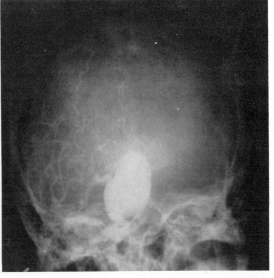

Figure 13. Radiographs of the sella turcica of a female patient were published in Holmes and Robbins (1955). "Enlargement of sella turcica due to pituitary tumor" was the caption. Subsequent carotid angiography demonstrated a 3.5 × 2.5 cm. aneurysm filling the sella turcica and extending above. (White, J. C., and Ballantine, H. T.: J. Neurosurg. *18*:34, 1961.)

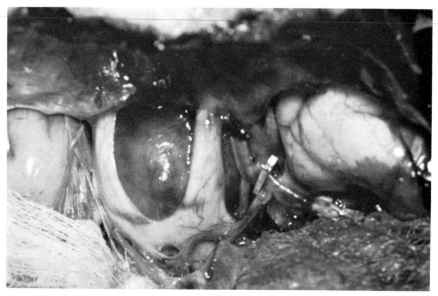

Figure 14. Operative photograph of patient shown in Figure 13 showing the aneurysm beneath the optic nerve and chiasm. (White, J. C., and Ballantine, H. T.: J. Neurosurg. *18*:34, 1961.)

demonstrated a 3 × 2.5 cm. aneurysm filling the sella turcica (Fig. 14).

In their outstanding report of the subject, White and Ballantine (1961) reported three personal cases and 22 communicated by their colleagues. They emphasized the importance of careful preoperative studies, particularly angiography, if the transsphenoidal approach is to be employed.

Aneurysm may be suspected by circular calcification in the aneurysmal wall (Zollinger and Cutler, 1932) and erosion of the outer wall of the optic foramen (Jefferson, 1955). However, even with angiography aneurysms may be overlooked because of thrombus in the lumen of the aneurysm (Rhonheimer, 1959). Clinical features of supraorbital pain, unilateral blindness, diminished sensation of the forehead, and ophthalmoplegia (cavernous sinus syndrome) suggest an infraclinoidal aneurysm.

It is important for the surgeon to recognize these aneurysms, since early treatment may reverse the neurologic deficit. Proper therapy in most cases requires common carotid ligation in the neck rather than direct surgical treatment (Jefferson, 1937; Gallagher et al., 1956).

Chordoma

The chordoma is a rare, invasive tumor which arises in the basal portion of the sphenoid and occipital bones. It originates from the nodochordal remnants in these bones or at the spheno-occipital synchondroses (Friedman et al., 1962; Falconer et al., 1968) and erodes the clivus and adjacent bone to present in the sphenoid sinus (Harrison, 1961) or nasopharynx (Ormerod, 1960; Batsakis and Kitt eson, 1963; Wright, 1967). Simultaneous intracranial spread usually occurs, so that invasion of the dura and distortion of strategic structures at the base of the brain interfere greatly with radical surgical removal. For those lesions presenting in the sphenoid and nasopharynx, the transsphenoidal approach offers certain advantages; biopsy and partial resection may be performed with ease (Wright, 1967; Guiot, 1967; Hardy, 1969). Similarly the transcervical-transclival approach to the ventral surface of the brain is of value in the radical attempt to extirpate the tumor (Stevenson et al., 1966). Although the ultimate outlook for patients with intracranial chordoma is poor, the tumors are slow-growing, and they create a bulky mass which is placed ventral to the brain stem and cranial nerves; thus, radical intracapsular removal may result in great symptomatic improvement and significant prolongation of the patient's life (Poppen and King, 1952; Falconer et al., 1968). High voltage radiotherapy and intracavitary radiation have been advised but are of unproved value (Zoltan and Fenyes, 1960; Wright, 1967; Falconer et al., 1968). A few instances of metastatic chordoma have been documented; however, the histologic appearance of these lesions has been benign (Russell and Rubinstein, 1963).

Fibrous Dysplasia

Fibrous dysplasia, an osseous hyperplasia of unknown etiology, may involve the craniofacial bones (Schlumberger, 1946). Characteristically monostatic in form, the frontal or sphenoid bone is involved in the majority of cases (Ramsey et al., 1968). The feminine sex preponderance, sexual precocity, and skin lesion associated with the polyostotic form (Turner's syndrome) are seldom encountered in association with this form. The disorder occurs during childhood and becomes inactive when skeletal growth is completed. The presenting findings are ptosis, exophthalmus, diminution in visual acuity, diminished hearing, and cosmetic deformity. The radiographic picture is that of marked thickening and increased density of the involved bone. In 50 cases reported by Sassin and Rosenberg (1968), the frontal and sphenoid bones were involved in 50 per cent of patients; the optic canal was involved in 20 per cent, most of whom had severe visual deficits secondary to optic nerve compression. Hearing loss and tinnitus secondary to temporal bone dysplasia have been reported (Basek, 1967). Occasionally dysplasia of the sphenoid and frontal bone produces an intracranial as well as an orbital mass. Increase in the serum alkaline phosphatase and increased radioactive uptake by the bony lesion (isotopic brain scan) are confirmatory laboratory findings.

Conservative treatment is indicated, namely, curettage and partial resection, unless complete resection can be achieved without creating a significant cosmetic and functional deficit. In the case of optic foramina encroachment, careful serial evaluation of visual acuity and fields is mandatory. If progressive deterioration occurs, surgical treatment consists of removal of the orbital roof and the medial wing of the sphenoid until the optic nerve is free in its canal (Matson, 1969). Similar but less extensive decompression may be required in cases of progressive exophthalmus. Surgical treatment for cosmetic reasons alone seldom has been necessary.

Aneurysmal Bone Cysts

Aneurysmal bone cysts, commonly found in long bones, are rare lesions which occasionally involve the bones of the cranium and base of the skull. The facial bones, mandible, and maxilla are more frequent hosts for this benign, though highly vascular, lesion which is characterized by destruction and expansion of the parent bone (Lichtenstein, 1957).

The radiographic picture consists of central rarefaction, expansion of the bone, and preservation of a cortical shell of bone outlining the mass lesion.

The lesion commonly presents as a cosmetic deformity of the face. However, we have recently seen one patient in whom a large mass expanded into the temporal fossa and produced a severe neurologic deficit. A similar case has been reported by Constantini et al. (1966). Therefore, in lesions of the cranial bones, careful preoperative study is indicated to exclude intracranial spread.

The surgical treatment consists of radical curettage and packing of the cavity with cancellous bone chips. The highly vascular nature of this tumor may make it a formidable surgical challenge (MacCarty et al., 1961).

Pituitary Adenomas

Adenomas of the pituitary are of three types: chromophobe, acidophil, and basophil (Russell and Rubinstein, 1963; Martins et al., 1965). The chromophobe, by far the commonest tumor, is said to be composed of nonsecretory cells, and thus the secondary disturbances of pituitary dysfunction are due to compression of adjacent normal tissue. Accord-

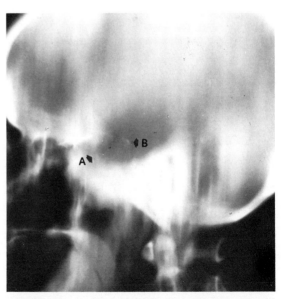

Figure 15. A 68 year old female with progressive bitemporal hemianopsia developed confusion, headaches, papilledema and obtusion. A midline tomogram of the sella turcica shows the typical ballooning of the sella and thinning of the anterior (*A*) and posterior (*B*) clinoids characteristic of pituitary adenomas. Opacification of the sphenoid sinus indicates that it is probably filled with tumor.

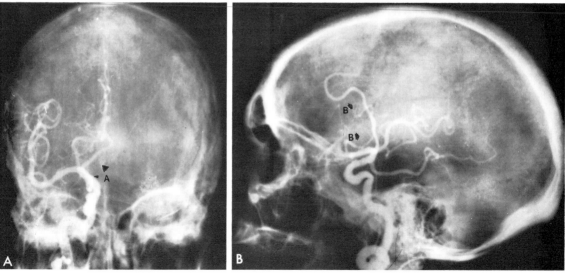

Figure 16. *A*, Carotid angiography of patient shown in Figure 15 shows marked displacement of the anterior cerebral artery laterally (A) and posteriorly (B, in right-hand figure, *B*). This case indicates the extraordinary intracranial extension which may occur in pituitary adenomas. In such cases, transcranial surgery is mandatory. *B*, Lateral view.

ingly, the lesion may go unrecognized until the optic pathways are severely compromised or a chance skull radiograph demonstrates the characteristic expanded sella turcica (Fig. 15). As the adenoma expands it will eventually burst the dural capsule and escape in one of several directions: (1) into the sphenoid sinus and occasionally through the base of the skull into the nasopharynx; (2) laterally into the temporal fossa; or (3) upward where it may compress optic pathways or third ventricle, hypothalamus, and frontal lobes. Any or all of the structures may be clinically involved (Fig. 16) (White and Warren, 1945).

In the early years of neurologic surgery, a large ballooned sella turcica was regarded as the classic sign of a pituitary tumor. Oscar Hirsch, pioneering Viennese otolaryngologist (1910), was quick to recognize that these lesions could be treated by transnasal intracapsular removal. Indeed, because of the initial high mortality associated with intracranial removal of pituitary tumors, Harvey Cushing (1912) employed a modification of this approach for many years until he accumulated experience which decreased the complications with the intracranial approach and he became convinced that greater return in visual function could be achieved with the transfrontal extirpation of these tumors.

Analysis of Cushing's large and beautifully documented series (Henderson, 1939) shows little difference between the mortality of the two approaches; however, the incidence of recurrence even with radiotherapy was considerably greater following transsphenoidal extirpation. Despite this disadvantage, others have continued to employ the transsphenoidal route (Guiot and Thibaut, 1959; Hamberger et al., 1961; Hamlin, 1962; Bateman, 1962; Montgomery, 1963; Svien and Litzow, 1965). In this regard, one must cite the tremendous contribution of Hirsh (1959), which has extended over a half century. With the advent of sophisticated contrast studies, improved radiotherapy techniques, and the unique contribution of the microsurgical techniques (Hardy and Wigser, 1965; Guiot et al., 1962) employing radiographic control, we again must look carefully at the individual values of these surgical techniques. Indeed, the indications for the transsphenoidal approach might be considered in (Ray and Patterson, 1962): (1) the aged or debilitated individual who tolerates intracranial surgery poorly; (2) those on the verge of blindness in whom manipulation of the optic nerve from the intracranial approach might increase the deficit; (3) cystic or acutely hemorrhagic tumors; (4) lesions confined to the sella turcica or sphenoid sinus; or (5) recurrent cystic or solid lesions causing compression of optic nerves or chiasm, in which decompression by the sphenoidal route can be safely achieved.

If the transsphenoidal approach to lesions of the sphenoid sinus, pituitary fossa, and environs is contemplated, it is imperative that preliminary contrast studies determine the degree of intracranial extension of the tumor and exclude anomalies of the intracranial vessels. Undoubtedly the measure of success resulting from renewed interest in this technique will depend greatly on the degree of cooperation between ophthalmologists, otolaryngologists and neurosurgeons.

Finally, in our enthusiasm for a seemingly simpler technique, we must be mindful of the superb record established by a host of Dr. Cushing's successors who have continued to improve on his admirable results with the

transcranial approach to pituitary tumors (Horrax, 1958; Ray and Patterson, 1962).

Malignant Tumors of the Nasopharynx and Paranasal Sinuses

Carcinoma of the nasopharynx and paranasal sinuses frequently presents with neurologic symptoms, particularly if early local symptoms such as obstruction of the eustachian tube and sinus ostia are overlooked. Focal invasion of the orbit, the superior orbital fissure, and the base of the skull may produce atypical facial

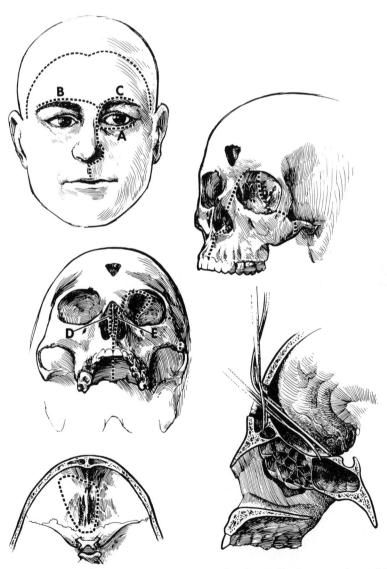

Figure 17. Skin incisions and lines of osteotomy. A, B and C refer to elective extensions of the basic paranasal incision. D and E indicate line of resection to avoid or include septum. Note the low frontal craniectomy, exenteration of the frontal sinus and reflection of the dural attachment from the floor of the frontal fossa to allow removal of the cribriform plate and orbital roof. (Van Buren, J. M.: J. Neurosurg. *28*:343, 1968.)

pain (see section on pain), proptosis, ocular palsies, and cranial nerve palsies. Twenty-five per cent of patients had one or more cranial nerve palsies; 12 per cent presented with persistent pain in the face (Lederman, 1966). Attention should be directed toward early signs, since the prognosis is extremely poor when the tumor has invaded the nervous system (Shedd et al., 1967). In addition, one must recognize the more benign nature of the nasopharyngeal fibroma, which is locally invasive but may be totally removed even if the orbit and base of the skull have been invaded (Hall and Wilkins, 1968).

Malignant tumors of the nose and paranasal sinuses offer a more favorable prognosis than those of the nasopharynx. Perhaps this is related to earlier recognition and more radical surgical treatment (Oliver, 1967). Smith et al. (1954), Ketcham et al. (1966) and Leffall and White, (1966) advocate radical resection of tumors of the sinuses; they propose that recurrence frequently is the result of invasion of the base of the frontal fossa in the region of the cribriform plate. Early attempts to achieve radical resections through a transfacial approach resulted in an extremely high incidence of complications and led to a combined craniofacial approach in which the entire cribriform plate, sphenoid, and ethmoid sinuses and orbit, if necessary, could be resected (Ketcham et al., 1966; Van Buren et al., 1968). The technique is illustrated in Figure 17. Seeking to avoid injury to the basal dura, the orbital surface of the frontal lobe, and the optic nerves, a neurosurgical team reflects the dura from the frontal fossa and cribriform plate, where it is extremely adherent. Through a small frontal craniectomy, the frontal sinus is exenterated, and osteotomy of the planum sphenoidale is extended until adequate resection is achieved. The procedure is then assumed by the maxillofacial team, who complete the radical maxillectomy and orbitectomy. Following this procedure, it is essential that any rents in the basal dura be closed with care to avoid cerebrospinal fluid fistula. Dural grafts are poorly tolerated in this situation, where vascularity is marginal and contamination is certain.

We have had experience with only two cases of malignant tumors arising from the sinuses in which surgery and radiotherapy failed to control the lesion. Radical sinusectomy and orbitectomy have resulted in an apparent cure in each instance. However, the follow-up period is one and three years only. The more extensive experiences of Van Buren et al (1968),

Ketcham et al. (1966) and Leffall and White (1966) indicate that this radical procedure has distinct value and may be performed with acceptable morbidity.

Tumors of the Posterior Cranial Fossa

The eighth cranial nerve is the site of tumor origin more frequently than any other cranial or spinal nerve. It arises from the sheath of the nerve and has been variously classified as a neuroma, a neurinoma, or a neurilemmoma. In addition, however, it has come to have a synonym which is incorrect, namely, tumor of the cerebellopontine angle (Fig. 18).

Although it has long been recognized that tumors of the acoustic nerve begin on the distal portion of the nerve and, hence, within the internal auditory canal, until recently it rarely was recognized until it had reached sufficient size to fill the cerebellopontine angle and press upon the pons and medulla, this despite the fact that the presenting symptoms in all patients were deafness and tinnitus in the affected ear, often for weeks, months, or years.

However, the term "cerebellopontine angle tumor" is, of course, not acceptable, since many other lesions occur in this location, notably the meningiomas, cholesteatomas, and certain gliomas, which must be differentiated from the acoustic nerve tumor.

From a surgical standpoint, the history of the acoustic neuroma falls into three definite periods: (1) Cushing, (2) Dandy, and (3) House.

Cushing, whose experience (dating from 1890 to 1933) and skill with brain tumors was both extensive and consummate, was convinced that the large tumors he was called upon to deal with could not be removed totally, even though they were known to be benign. This was based on an overwhelming mortality and morbidity when total removal was undertaken. Accordingly, he advised intracapsular enucleation of the lesion as a palliative measure.

Dandy followed this principle for a time, but early recurrence and an overwhelming mortality with secondary operation (55 per cent dead in five years) led him to undertake total removal in all cases, and he achieved a surgical mortality of 10 per cent.

After Dandy's (1925) epoch-making publications in this field, all neurosurgeons, including the senior author, began to undertake total removal as a primary procedure in tumors of this

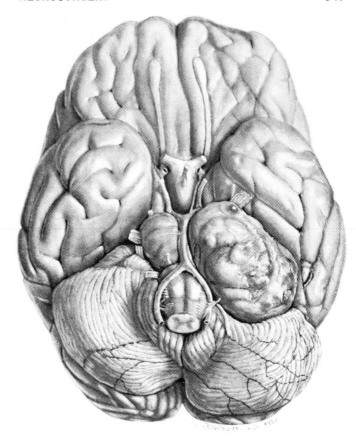

Figure 18. The typical appearance of a large cerebellopontine angle acoustic neuroma, as seen in a necropsy specimen. Note the distortion of the pons and the basilar artery. (Walters, W. (ed.): Lewis' Practice of Surgery. New York, Harper and Row, 1943.)

type, with a surgical mortality ranging from 5 to 15 per cent. Preservation of the facial nerve with this type of procedure was rare, but subsequent operations in which the facial nerve was replaced by graft with the hypoglossal nerve and the spinal accessory nerve usually provided an acceptable, if not totally satisfactory, result.

House (1968), already a master with the surgical microscope in the temporal bone, encountered and removed a small acoustic neuroma in the internal auditory canal in a patient who was being treated for Meniere's disease. Recognizing the probability that tumors of this type might be the cause of unilateral deafness (sensory neural deficit) and tinnitus, and with characteristic vigor and skill, he has confirmed that the lesion is indeed common and can be recognized in many instances while it is still small and removed through the ear totally and safely. The observations of House and his associates have stimulated many otolaryngologists and neurosurgeons to look anew at this problem; in a sense, a new specialty—neuro-otology—has developed. The problem of the most favorable method of approaching acous-

tic neuromas (transaural or transcranial) is one of the many they are attempting to solve.

Acoustic Nerve Tumors

The acoustic nerve tumor arises from the Schwann sheath, cells of which cover the axons from a point at which the latter penetrate the pia mater to their termination. It is recalled that the point of penetration of the leptomeninges varies greatly with different nerve roots and, in the case of the auditory and vestibular nerves, the distance may be as great as 1 cm. (Skinner, 1931). This fact may well account for the frequency with which acoustic tumors arise within the internal auditory canal (Henschen, 1910), where the nerve root usually acquires its reticulin and Schwann-cell components. In this location the expanding tumor causes erosion of the internal auditory meatus prior to escape of the mass into the cranial cavity. Indeed, we have designated these lesions as tumors of the ear and tumors of the brain. It is in the former category that the contributions of modern otology have been so valuable, allowing us to correctly diagnose

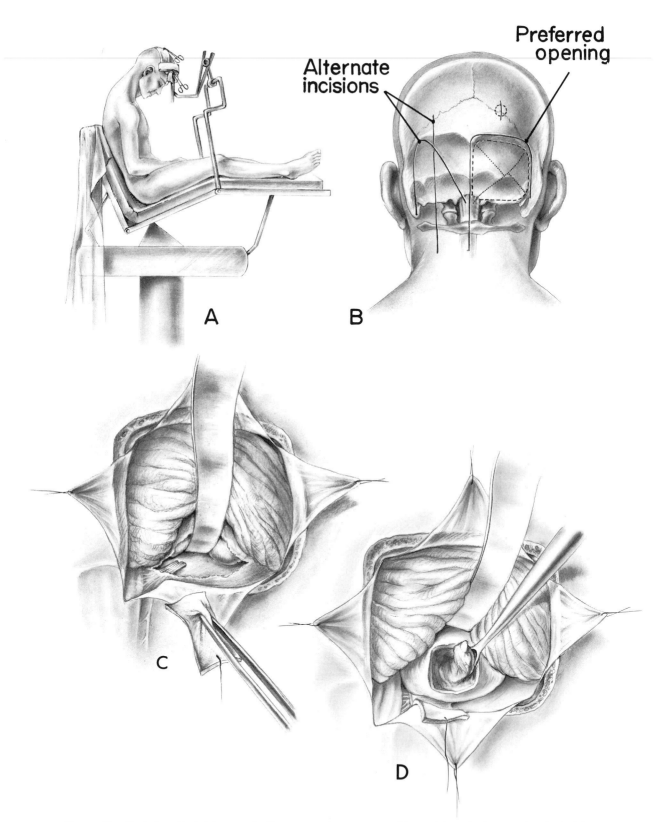

Figure 19. Technique for total removal of large acoustic neuromas, with special emphasis on saving the facial nerve. *A*, Operative sitting position. The legs are wrapped firmly with elastic bandages or encased in a pressure suit to avoid hypotension and air embolism. *B*, Operative exposure and dural opening. A separate burr hole is included to permit release of ventricular fluid. *C*, The arachnoid is opened over the tumor and the tumor retracted to isolate the lower cranial nerves (IX, X, XI). *D*, A self-retaining retractor is placed on the cerebellar hemisphere, which has been relaxed by removal of spinal fluid or administration of osmotic diuretics. Resection of the cerebellum is seldom necessary. A generous intracapsular removal of tumor is performed.

Illustration continued on opposite page.

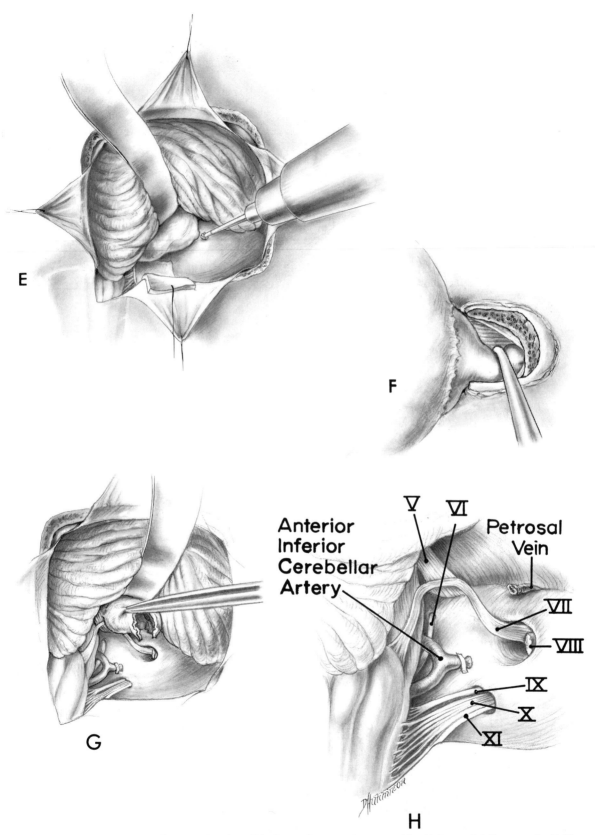

Figure 19. *Continued. E*, The posterior rim of the internal meatus is removed by high speed drill or punch. *F*, The tumor is separated from the porus acusticus and the facial nerve. *G*, Under direct vision, the collapsed tumor capsule is teased from the brain stem, anterior inferior cerebellar artery, and facial and trigeminal nerves. *H*, Final exposure of the structures in the cerebellopontine angle. Anastomosis of the severed facial nerve is possible if required. (Drake, C. G.: J. Neurosurg. *26*:554, 1967.)

these lesions on the basis of otologic and vestibular findings alone, thereby discovering the tumor while it is confined to the auditory canal. In this stage, total removal can be achieved without injuring the adjacent brain stem or subarachnoid pathways, and frequently allowing anatomical preservation of the facial, vestibular, and auditory nerves (House, 1961; Rand and Kurze, 1968).

Tinnitus, unilateral sensorineural hearing impairment, and mild unsteadiness are the acknowledged early and consistent symptoms in acoustic tumors. Although we have not had a patient with acoustic tumor complain of episodic bouts of true vertigo, such occurrences have been reported (Hitzelberger, 1967; Rand and Kurze, 1968; Sheehy, 1968). In addition, the vestibular responses may be normal in small acoustic tumors (60 per cent in House's series), therein creating a problem in differentiating tumor from Meniere's disorder or other lesions of the cochlea. The presence of neurologic symptoms and signs indicates expansion of tumor mass into the cerebellopontine angle. The earliest clinical sign is diminished sensation of the cornea or face, indicating compression of the sensory root of the trigeminal nerve. Facial nerve paresis is seldom recognized even in large brain tumors (Mack, 1968). However, sophisticated clinical tests may demonstrate alteration in taste, hearing, and sensation of the skin of the posterior wall of the external auditory canal (House, 1964). Further expansion of tumor compresses the cerebellum and lower brain stem and results in nystagmus, ataxia, spasticity of gait, and pyramidal tract signs. Obstruction of the aqueduct produces hydrocephalus and papilledema, a late finding. Posterior fossa myelography has, therefore, been of great value in differentiating functional from neoplastic lesions and, finally, in determing the precise size of angle tumors (Baker, 1963; Scanlan, 1964; Hitzelberger and House, 1968). This technique has greatly reduced the number of negative explorations and allowed proper selection of the operative approach.

In those tumors extending beyond the confines of the meatus to cause "neurologic signs" there is no proper alternative to the suboccipital approach, particularly in those patients with brain compression (Fig. 18). In this situation one is dealing with a lesion that has a high risk of death if treatment is inadequate. Experience has shown that they can be treated best by the neurosurgeon through the standard suboccipital approach (Fig. 19, *A* to *H*). Therefore, any approach which places emphasis on partial removal of the tumor and salvage of the facial nerve is not warranted. In those cases in which it is necessary to sacrifice a facial nerve in order to excise a large tumor completely (Fig. 20), this seems a small price to pay for the cure of a disease that otherwise would be fatal, particularly in view of the excellent results which have been achieved with various anastomotic techniques for restoration of facial nerve function (Coleman and Walker, 1950; Dott, 1958; Drake, 1967).

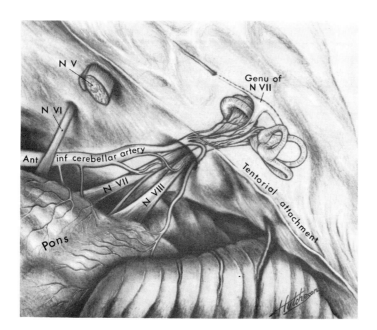

Figure 20. Semidiagrammatic view of the cerebellopontine angle, demonstrating the arterial supply of the seventh and eighth nerves and the labyrinth. Note that arterial branches may take a recurrent course to supply the brain stem. Care must be exercised in preserving the anterior inferior cerebellar artery, since occlusion may result in a disastrous brain stem infarction. (Atkinson, 1949.) (Rhotan, A. L., Jr.: *In* Rand, R. W.: Microneurosurgery. St. Louis, The C. V. Mosby Co., 1969.)

In conclusion, we believe that by applying the new data which have been made available to us by the otologists and adhering to the fundamental surgical principles which are not a matter of conjecture it is reasonable to hope that the overwhelming majority of acoustic neurinomas can be recognized and dealt with while they are still within the auditory canal. It would seem inevitable that some will still present themselves when the tumor has become large. In this event there is no doubt in our minds that the morbidity and mortality will be held at the lowest possible level by a skilled neurosurgeon who has an adequate exposure of the lesion. For all but the very small tumors complete removal is best accomplished by the conventional method (Dandy, 1925; McKissock, 1965; Drake, 1967; Olivecrona, 1967; Rand and Kurze, 1968). However, preservation of the facial nerve may be facilitated by using a temporal approach (Fig. 20) according to House and colleagues (1961).

Other Posterior Fossa Tumors

Meningioma. Although the acoustic nerve tumors account for 85 to 90 per cent of neoplastic lesions arising in the area of the cerebellopontine angle, tumors of diverse origins occur in this location. In his original monograph on meningiomas, Cushing (1938) recognized that meningiomas arose in the angle; in several instances he was unable to distinguish the clinical picture from that of the acoustic nerve tumor. Indeed, in their recent monograph in which 200 acoustic nerve tumors were reported, House and colleagues (1968) found 13 meningiomas. It is difficult to distinguish meningiomas clinically from tumors of the eighth nerve. It is important to note, however, that the plain radiographs of the skull may show an osteoblastic reaction in the petrous portion of the temporal bone, a feature characteristic of intratemporal meningioma. However, marked destruction of bone may occur as well (Nager, 1964). Although contrast studies usually are not helpful in distinguishing angle tumors, the meningioma may be recognized by an angiographic stain and positive isotopic scan, indicating its vascular character.

Congenital Cholesteatoma. Congenital cholesteatoma is a benign tumor which arises from embryonic rests of epidermal tissue in the petrous bones. Not to be confused with secondary cholesteatoma resulting from chronic mastoid infection, this lesion usually presents with progressive sensorineural deafness and facial paralysis (Olivecrona, 1949; Cawthorne and Griffin, 1961). However, facial tic and episodic facial paralysis have been observed (Jefferson, 1937). Marked erosion of the petrous bone and a scalloped mass are the characteristic myelographic findings.

Metastatic tumors of the base of the skull, malignant tumors of the nasopharynx, neuromas of the trigeminal and glossopharyngeal nerves (Jefferson, 1955a), glomus jugulare tumors (Rosenwasser, 1968), astrocytomas (Matson, 1969), aneurysms of the anterior inferior cerebellar artery (Drake, 1968), and arachnoid cysts (Bengochea and Blanco, 1955; Nichols and Blanco, 1953; Tew, 1967) are lesions which must be considered when a mass is discovered in the cerebellopontine angle or environs. Therefore, one should be aware of the possibilities and prepared to deal with the lesion appropriately.

INFECTIONS

Neurologic Complications of Sinus and Ear Infections

The neurologic complications of infections of the ear and paranasal sinus are extracranial and intracranial in location. The sinuses are mucosal-lined cavities within bone, the apertures of which are readily obstructed by inflammatory changes within the lumina. As the intraluminal pressure increases, pain occurs which may be localized over the sinus as well as referred to other sites about the face. The intracranial complications of mastoid and paranasal sinus infections occur as a result of extension through a fistula or the oval or round windows (Fig. 21). However, facial nerve paralysis and labyrinthitis are more commonly complications of osteomyelitis of the temporal bone. Diplopia due to abducent nerve palsy, exophthalmus, oculomotor nerve palsy, and diminished sensation of the forehead are features of the superior orbital fissure syndrome which in partial or complete form may result from paranasal sinusitis. Venous thrombosis of the retro-orbital veins is an early manifestation of orbital cellulitis, which may lead to chemosis, exophthalmus, diplopia, and immobility of the globe. Necrotizing orbital cellulitis and sinusitis may be seen in debilitated individuals as a result of mucormycosis (Green et al., 1967) and Wegner's granulomatosis. Extensive bone destruction and cranial nerve palsies are common.

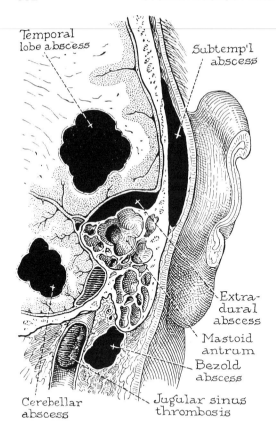

Temporal lobe abscess

Subtemp'l abscess

Extra-dural abscess

Mastoid antrum

Bezold abscess

Cerebellar abscess

Jugular sinus thrombosis

Figure 21. A frontal section through the mastoid antrum, showing the various locations which abscesses springing from the mastoid and middle ear may occupy. A thrombus in the sigmoid sinus is also shown. (From Cushing, H.: Diseases of the brain. *In* Homans, J.: Textbook of Surgery. Springfield, Ill., Charles C Thomas, 1935.)

In each of these conditions early recognition, prompt antibiotic therapy, and drainage when indicated are the therapeutic methods of proved value and undoubtedly are responsible for the continuing low incidence of neurologic complications of ear and sinus infections.

As noted in the section on mucoceles, pyoceles develop in the sinuses. Similar to chronic cholesteatoma found in the mastoid, the lesions require drainage and radical resection lest persistent destruction of bone lead to compression of the cranial nerves confined in the bone adjacent to the cavities.

Osteomyelitis and Epidural Abscess

Osteomyelitis of the bone of the calvarium occurs by direct extension of infection from the mastoid and nasal sinuses (French and Chou, 1969) spread through the haversian canal by thrombosis of intraosseous vessels. The spread of the process is facilitated on reaching the diploë because of the absence of valves in diploic veins. The frontal, parietal, and temporal bones are most commonly involved. Rup-

ture of the suppurative lesion into the subperiosteal space gives rise to a localized collection beneath the skin or so-called "Pott's puffy tumor," facilitating recognition and external drainage. However, if the lesion ruptures into the epidural space and remains unrecognized, serious neurologic complications may develop. Osteomyelitis and epidural abscess are to be suspected if there are local and systemic signs of sepsis—pain, fluctuance, tenderness, erythema, fever, and malaise. Rarely is there nuchal rigidity or any other sign of meningeal irritation. Radiographic evidence of osteomyelitis may develop slowly and appear as only small areas of rarefaction of the bone. However, confirmatory findings of opacification of the adjacent sinus and clouding of the mastoids are early radiographic signs.

Obviously early recognition requires direct exploration; there is no role for delay in this disorder. Drainage of the sinus and extensive removal of the infected bone is desirable. It should be noted that the bone usually regenerates quickly and readily because of the retention of the periosteum. If the suppuration has extended to the epidural space, this must be debrided with care in a manner that will allow removal of granulation tissue and pus but maintain the dura mater.

Subdural Empyema

Subdural infection (empyema) in the absence of direct implantation of a foreign body is a result of extension from adjacent areas of infection, commonly in the sinuses and ears. The infection probably reaches the subdural space by extension through the dura mater via small arterial and venous channels or by direct extension in thrombi propagated in the dural sinuses or emissary veins. The latter has been documented in a number of patients in whom osteomyelitis and epidural abscess have been absent.

The clinical features should distinguish subdural empyema from other forms of intracranial infection. The illness usually begins with localized headache and focal signs of infection in the diseased mastoid or sinus. Development of systemic signs of infection—fever and malaise—are followed shortly by alterations in consciousness which may progress to stupor or coma. As the process of spread through the subdural space continues, seizures are a frequent occurrence and progressive neurologic deficits may develop. Nuchal rigidity, hemiparesis, aphasia, diminished sensation, and visual field deficits have all been recorded in a majority of patients. Skull radiography will demonstrate the focus of mastoiditis or sinusitis and perhaps an area of osteomyelitis. Carotid angiography may show displacement of the intracranial vessels from the inner table of the skull, indicating a peripheral extracerebral mass. Spinal fluid examination usually shows elevated pressure, mild pleocytosis (less than 1000 cells), normal sugar and chloride, and absence of any organisms on gross stain or culture.

Treatment of subdural empyema consists of effective drainage of the infected sinus; there is no reason to delay this maneuver pending treatment of the intracranial sepsis, since further delay serves only to propagate infection into the subdural space. Botterell and Drake (1952) stressed the mode of spread of infection in the subdural space: From the paranasal sinuses it spreads along the interhemispheric fissure, over the frontal convexity, and under the orbital surfaces of the frontal lobes; from the mastoid purulent material spreads underneath the temporal and occipital lobes, over the cerebellum, over the convexity, and along the posterior interhemispheric fissure. Loculation of pus may occur in any of the areas; however, it is more likely to be concealed between the hemispheres, underneath the cerebral lobes, and over the cerebellum. Appropriate placement of cranial burr holes is facilitated by this knowledge. Rather than placing multiple burr holes as advocated by Botterell and Drake (1952), McLaurin (1969), and others, we prefer to use a two-inch trephine craniotomy in the frontal and occipital regions. This technique provides ample room for inspection and exploration of the subdural space. Catheters are placed in situ for repeated irrigation and instillation of antibiotics. In addition, it is important to change the patient's position frequently in order that loculation in the occipital region may be diminished.

Despite these vigorous maneuvers and massive intravenous and local antibiotics, the mortality for this disease remains exceedingly high, in the range of 50 to 60 per cent.

Meningitis

Meningitis, the commonest intracranial infection, is a pyogenic infection of the pia arachnoid of the brain and spinal cord. In the preantibiotic era meningitis was a common and deadly complication of middle ear and sinus suppuration. Fortunately recognition of the mechanism of spread to the subarachnoid space (Shambaugh, 1967) and the institution of proper antibiotic therapy have decreased the incidence of mortality with this condition greatly. It should be noted that meningitis accounts for about 95 per cent of all intracranial infections associated with sinus and mastoid disease (Beekhuis and Taylor, 1969). Septic thrombophlebitis, direct extension through the subdural space, and hematogenous spread are the modes of seeding the subarachnoid space from sinus and mastoid infection (Alpers, 1958). The mortality remains high in meningitis associated with spread from both these foci, particularly in sinus suppuration: 31 per cent as compared to 7 per cent for otitic meningitis (Beekhuis and Taylor, 1969). This unfortunate figure is perhaps related to late recognition of meningeal spread from sinus disease because of masking of the signs by the local process, inadequate treatment of sinus suppuration, and a generally higher index of suspicion of meningitis when ear infection is concerned.

Accordingly it is important to watch carefully for the symptoms and signs of meningitis. Headache, lethargy, and irritability are the early symptoms of meningeal infection and should lead the physician to elicit signs of meningeal irritation (nuchal rigidity, limited flexion of the legs, fever, and alterations in the mental status). Ultimately the diagnosis rests with the analysis of the spinal fluid. Certainly a spinal puncture must be performed as soon as meningitis is suspected, except, of course, when there is elevated intracranial pressure and focal signs indicating a mass lesion (brain abscess), in which case other diagnost c procedures are safer. Bacterial meningitis usually is accompanied by elevated spinal fluid pressure, pleocytosis (greater than 1000, predominantly polymorphonuclear leukocytes), elevated protein, decreased sugar (less than 50 per cent of blood sugar value; simultaneous blood sugar always should be obtained), and decreased chloride content (Alpers, 1958). The cloudy appearance of the fluid is related to the degree of pleocytosis and protein content. The value of meticulous cytologic, chemical, and bacteriologic analysis of the spinal fluid cannot be overemphasized. Broad-spectrum antibiotic coverage should be initiated as soon as spinal puncture has been completed. Specific antimicrobic therapy then may be instituted in accordance with the results of culture and antibiotic sensitivities. In some severe cases systemic corticosteroids may be of benefit (Toole et al., 1969; Eisen et al., 1969). Of course, prompt attention to the local infection in the sinus or ear is necessary to prevent continued seeding of the subarachnoid space.

Brain Abscess

Brain abscess is a localized collection of pus in a cavity created by the necrosis of cerebral tissue and encapsulated by deposition of inflammatory cells from the blood and glial reaction of the adjacent cerebral tissue. Despite the reduced incidence of brain abscess attributable to antibiotics and early recognition of extracranial suppuration, mastoid and paranasal sinus infection remains the leading cause of brain abscess, except in centers where a large population of patients with cardiac defects are encountered (Matson and Salom, 1961; Beekhuis and Taylor, 1969). The mechanisms of propagation from sinus and mastoid suppuration include: (1) direct extension, (2) vascular

extension via septic thrombophlebitis and perivasculitis, and (3) extension through preformed pathways as in congenital defects, tumors, or traumatic fistulas.

The brain abscess begins as an inflammatory process (cerebritis), which consists of leukocytic infiltration and microscopic necrosis. At this stage clinical and diagnostic efforts usually fail to localize the focus of infection. However, in seven to ten days, a capsule is initiated about the necrotic core by the deposition of a granulomatous layer and the proliferation of glial and fibrous tissue elements from the adjacent blood vessels. Enlargement of the mass and provocation of edema in the adjacent cerebral tissue usually produce focal neurologic abnormalities unless the mass is located in the frontal lobe, where it may produce only signs of increased intracranial pressure. The isotopic brain scan (Fig. 22) has proved to be a most valuable tool in distinguishing conversion of cerebritis to abscess and in localizing the mass lesion created by an abscess (Wang and Rosen, 1965; Tefft et al., 1966). However, cerebral angiography remains the safest and is generally regarded as the most reliable procedure in localizing brain abscess; in some instances specific angiographic features may indicate abscess rather than some other intracerebral mass (Chou et al., 1966).

Otogenic sources probably account for 40 to 50 per cent of all brain abscesses, while sinus infection causes 10 to 15 per cent. This feature accounts for the greater incidence of abscesses in temporal and cerebellar locations. The symptoms of brain abscess are general and focal in nature. The former consists of mental dullness, lethargy, headache and, occasionally, fever. The symptoms may be masked or confused with those related to the condition in the sinus and mastoid. Fever and meningeal signs usually are not present in the absence of coincidental meningitis. Focal signs — hemiparesis, hemisensory deficit, and hemianopsia — frequently accompany temporal and parietal abscesses, a most common site for otitic propagation of infection. Ataxia, vertigo, cranial nerve palsies, and increased intracranial pressure (due to obstruction of the aqueduct of Sylvius or fourth ventricle outlet) are signs of cerebellar hemisphere abscess, also a favorite site for spread from the infected middle ear. Frontal lobe abscesses are almost always the result of sinus infection and seldom have consistent localizing neurologic features. Increased intracranial pressure, papilledema, and stupor are features which precede the onset of

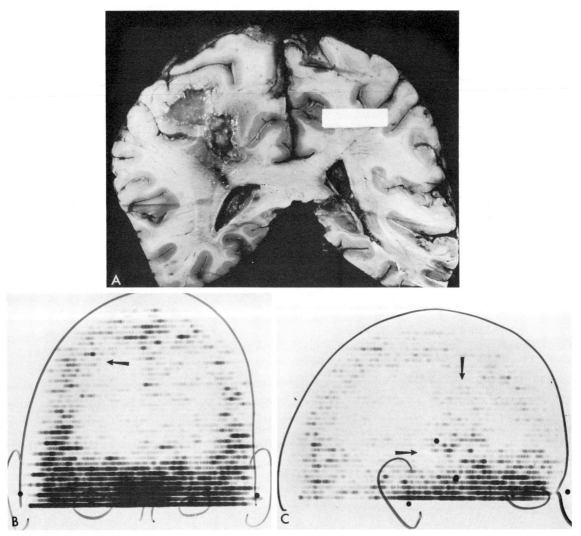

Figure 22. Multilocular abscess located in the frontoparietal region correctly localized by isotopic brain scan. *B* and *C*, Technetium-99 radioactive brain scan, showing distinct areas of uptake (arrows) corresponding to the lesions found at postmortem examination of the brain.

fatal brain stem herniation or rupture of the abscess into the ventricular system.

Lumbar puncture and air encephalography must be done with great care in suspected brain abscess and only when brain scan and angiography have failed to sufficiently localize the lesion. Such a circumstance seldom occurs except in cerebellar abscess. In this situation, positive contrast ventriculography may be the preferable procedure (Siquera et al., 1968; Wilkinson, 1969).

The treatment of brain abscess consists of broad-spectrum antibiotic coverage and systemic corticosteroids to reduce brain swelling, and surgical evacuation of the abscess. It is our opinion that delay of definitive surgical treatment to obliterate meningitis or local infection in the sinuses is ill advised. In this regard it must be emphasized that the cause of death in brain abscess is brain stem compression secondary to herniation of the medial temporal lobe, cerebellar tonsils, or rupture of the abscess into the ventricular system (Ballantine, 1969).

The surgical treatment of brain abscess is disputed, since some surgeons feel strongly that the mass should be excised completely via craniotomy and direct vision as soon as the diagnosis is reached (Ballantine, 1969; Matson, 1969), while others prefer needling the abscess through a burr hole, aspirating the purulent material and instilling a radiopaque material (Kahn and Arbor, 1939; Maxwell and DeLong, 1968), either Thorotrast or micropaque barium. In such instances repeated taps or catheter drainage may be performed on the basis of serial studies of the size of the cavity. Others have instilled opaque material to outline the abscess cavity as a means of improving localization preparatory to open craniotomy and excision. It is our opinion that each of these maneuvers has distinct value according to the clinical situation. Obviously the ideal treatment is complete excision of the abscess, but this may be a dangerous and unwise step in individuals who are extremely ill with the systemic toxicity of local infection and meningitis. In those individuals with lesions located beneath vital neurologic structures, as in the left motor and speech areas, total excision may produce a profound neurologic deficit. Accordingly we are prepared in such circumstances to tap the abscess, repeatedly if necessary, and we rely on systemic antibiotics and brain shrinking agents to control the cerebral edema. In addition, prompt treatment of the local infection is imperative.

PAINFUL DISORDERS OF THE HEAD AND NECK

Pain in the head and neck is probably one of the most complex and difficult disorders encountered by the otolaryngologist and neurosurgeon. How does one distinguish the various neuralgias of the cranial and upper cervical nerves (Fig. 23), a condition in which severe paroxysms of pain radiate into the distribution of a nerve in which there is no structural evidence of disease, from the symptomatic head and neck pain in which distinct pathological lesions involve the peripheral nerve, ganglion, posterior rootlet or the brain stem and upper spinal cord?

Fortunately we possess a large armamentarium of successful techniques for relieving pain in the region of the head and neck. Accordingly it is important to reach the correct diagnosis prior to alleviating pain, which may be the only alerting feature of an underlying pathological disorder. In order to achieve this goal, precise definition of the clinical features of the facial and cervical neuralgias is important. In this regard we shall review the classic features which have been so carefully documented by numerous observers.

Neuralgias

Trigeminal Neuralgia

Trigeminal neuralgia or "tic douloureaux," a common disorder in which the possessor is so miserable it has been recognized since the earliest days of medical history (Crawford and Walker, 1951), is characterized by: (1) paroxysms of intense pain lasting seconds to minutes and separated by intervals of freedom from pain; (2) provocation of the paroxysms of pain by peripheral stimuli to the face and mouth as in chewing, swallowing, shaving, touching or, at times, even a whiff of air striking the face; (3) radiation of pain into the distribution of the trigeminal nerve, usually the second or third division; (4) restriction of pain to a single side of the face; and (5) no neurologic defect in the region of the trigeminal nerve—that is, no diminution of sensation or weakness of the masticatory muscles.

Departure from these features may occur but must be considered with care. Slight sensory deficit of the face or cornea, persistence of a dull, aching pain between the paroxysms of pain, flight of pain beyond the trigeminal distri-

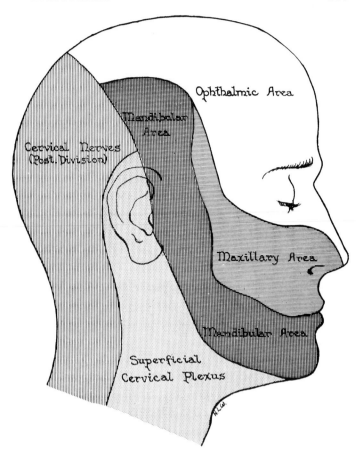

Figure 23. Sensory distribution of divisions of the trigeminal nerve and the cervical nerves to the occiput and neck. The overlap, variation and sensory invasion which may occur as a result of anastomosis between these nerves must be recognized in the management of painful conditions. (Spurling, G. R.: Practical Neurological Diagnosis. 2nd ed. Springfield, Ill., Charles C Thomas, 1940.)

bution or across the midline of the face are features which should suggest the possibility of multiple sclerosis, brain stem vascular anomaly, syringomyelia, or posterior fossa tumors. It has been noted that facial pain is more likely to occur in association with lesions involving the gasserian ganglion than in those affecting the posterior root (White and Sweet, 1969). Acoustic neuromas, neuromas of the trigeminal nerve, and meningiomas are rarely associated with trigeminal neura gia. However, congenital cholesteatoma causes ticlike pain in a high percentage of patients (Revilla, 1947; Taarnhoj, 1952), particularly when the tumor compresses the ganglion in the middle fossa (Krayenbühl, 1936).

Tumors invading the nerve divisions of the trigeminal nerve may produce facial pain. Malignant tumors of the sinus and nasopharynx frequently invade the cranial nerve, but generally the associated pain is accompanied by neurologic deficit. Cranial nerve palsies are common, as in the superior orbital fissure and jugular foramen syndromes.

If symptomatic causes for trigeminal neuralgia can be exacted by the careful details of history-taking and neurologic examination, few diagnostic procedures will be necessary. However, in doubtful cases the previously noted lesions may be excluded by intracranial angiography, pneumoencephalography, and posterior fossa myelography.

The initial treatment of trigeminal neuralgia is medical. Carbamazepine (Tegretol) is proving to be extremely beneficial in relieving severe bouts of tic pain. Loss of effectiveness appears in some persons, and others have relapse shortly after cessation of the drug. Toxicity poses another hazard; indeed, some find the nausea, ataxia, and vertigo too troublesome. Severe complications, including agranulocytosis and renal and hepatic injury have not been excessive but require careful monitoring of appropriate laboratory values. Tegretol is of particular value in the patient with severe pain in need of relief, and for treatment of mild protracted pain and of recurrent pain following operative procedures.

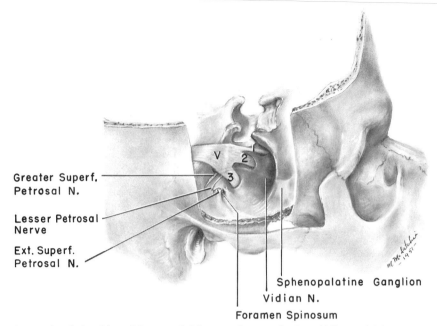

Greater Superf. Petrosal N.

Lesser Petrosal Nerve

Ext. Superf. Petrosal N.

Sphenopalatine Ganglion

Vidian N.

Foramen Spinosum

Figure 24. Anatomic relationships of the superficial petrosal nerves in the middle cranial fossa. Although the vidian nerve and the sphenopalatine ganglion cannot be seen from the middle fossa, their course beneath the floor of the fossa is indicated in outline.

This illustration also serves to point out the lamination of the divisions of the trigeminal rootlets in Meckel's cave and to elucidate the technique for placing isolated coagulation lesions in this ganglion for the treatment of trigeminal neuralgia. (White, J. C., and Sweet, W. H.: Pain: Its Mechanisms and Neurosurgical Control. Springfield, Ill., Charles C Thomas, 1969.)

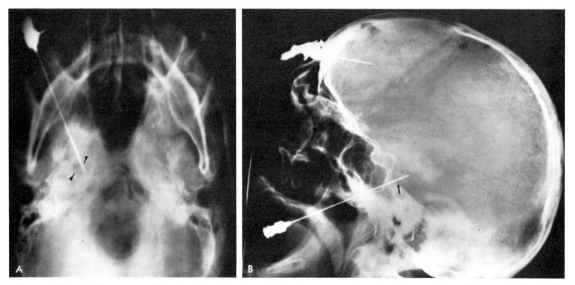

Figure 25. *A,* Placement of insulated needle through the foramen ovale, according to the technique of Härtel. The arrows indicate the margins of the foramen ovale as seen in the basal view of the sinus. *B,* This shows the extension of the needle tip well past the plane of the clivus, where it lies in the spinal fluid bathing the gasserian ganglion.

The various operative procedures which have been developed to alleviate the pain of trigeminal neuralgia are numerous, and all have some unique value. In particular, differential section of the posterior root in the middle fossa has found great favor with neurologic surgeons (Frazier, 1925; Stookey, 1955). However, attempting to avoid loss of touch perception over the face, Dandy (1929) sectioned the posterior root in the posterior fossa where he was apparently able, with great ability, to identify a small group of intermediate fibers which relayed proprioceptive sensation from the face. Recently, with the aid of the operating microscope, Jannetta (1967) has confirmed Dandy's impression that preservation of the fibers leaves light touch intact while abolishing pain in the same area. A number of less complicated and hazardous procedures fortunately have been developed. Injection of various nerve trunks with neurotoxic agents has been and remains a highly effective and simple procedure for the temporary relief of pain. Injection of alcohol or phenol into the gasserian ganglion, designed to produce destruction of the ganglion and thus permanent relief of tic (Harris, 1940), has been associated with high incidence of complications (nonparalytic keratitis and anesthesia dolorosa). Seeking to avoid such an occurrence, Jaeger (1959) injected 0.5-ml. increments of boiling water into the gasserian ganglion. This maneuver achieved a significant lowering of the complications but has not gained favor with other surgeons.

In 1931 Kirschner introduced a technique of coagulation of the gasserian ganglion. Large series of patients have been treated by this tactic over the past four decades in Europe, where it has enjoyed considerable attention (Kirschner, 1942). However, despite continued improvement in technique and results, it only recently has been employed in this country. Sweet (1968b) and Wepsic (1969) have been responsible for bringing this technique to our attention (Fig. 24). Their results to date in nearly 100 cases have been extremely favorable. We recently have begun to evaluate the features of this technique and have found it extremely desirable because it is capable of relieving trigeminal neuralgia while sparing proprioceptive sensation over the face and cornea and avoiding injury to the other cranial nerves, including the motor root of the trigeminal nerve. Furthermore, it is simple in principle and execution and has no significant morbidity (Fig. 25); therefore, it can be performed on people who are not candidates for more drastic surgical procedures. We have not, of course, had ample time to evaluate the incidence of recurrence following this procedure. However, since repeat coagulation is so simple and safe, recurrence can be handled with ease. The technique has been particularly beneficial in the aged patient with bilateral trigeminal neuralgia who already has had a posterior rhizotomy and in whom contralateral anesthesia would be a great handicap.

Nervus Intermedius Neuralgia

There is substantial anatomic evidence that pain fibers from the geniculate ganglion innervate a portion of the ear, the deep structures of the head and neck, and the facial muscles (Fig. 26). Ramsey Hunt (1915) determined the cutaneous and mucosal distribution of the facial nerve, largely on the basis of the location of vesicular eruption in herpes zoster of the geniculate ganglion (Fig. 27). Additional evidence comes in the form of paresthesias, which have been noted to radiate into the medial surface of the auricle and anterior two thirds of the tongue in patients with Bell's palsy. Other pain fibers pass in the greater superficial petrosal nerve, branches of the facial nerve to the expressive muscles, and perhaps with the taste fibers of the chorda tympanic nerve. Anatomic dissections in man have shown great variation in anastomosis between facial, vagus, and trigeminal nerves, a finding which undoubtedly accounts for the confusion surrounding the clinical features of painful disorders affecting these nerves.

The typical pain referred over the nervus intermedius is usually continuous rather than paroxysmal; it is dull to aching in character, although severe episodes of sharp, burning pain radiating deep into the ear and mouth have been recorded; the pain usually radiates into the depth of the ear and external canal, which may be sensitive to manipulation. The conclusive diagnosis depends on reproduction of the pain by stimulation of the nervus intermedius at the pons; long-term relief of pain is obtained by section of the fibers of the nerve. Such a delicate maneuver requires an awake, cooperative patient and the visualization provided by the operating microscope. The anatomy and operative approach to the nervus intermedius have recently been described by Rhoton (1968) and Sachs (1968).

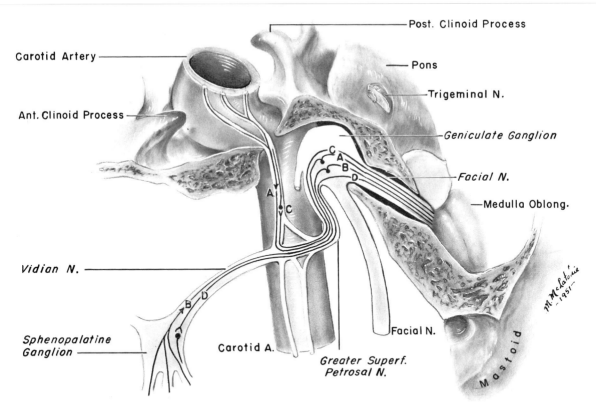

Figure 26. Afferent and efferent fibers in the greater superficial petrosal nerve and nervus intermedius. Afferent impulses may pass from the internal carotid artery (A) and from the vidian nerve (B) via the greater superficial petrosal nerve to the cell bodies in the geniculate ganglion. Efferent vasodilator and secretory fibers pass from the brain through the geniculate ganglion without synapse to terminate around cells on the internal carotid (C) or in the sphenopalatine ganglion (D). (White, J. D., and Sweet, W. H.: Pain: Its Mechanisms and Neurosurgical Control. Springfield, Ill., Charles C Thomas, 1961.)

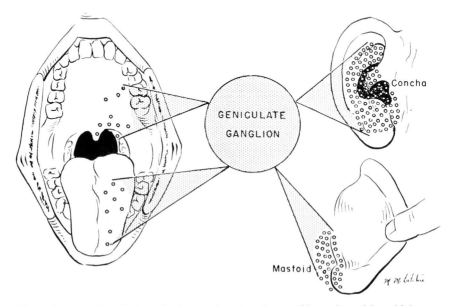

Figure 27. These diagrams show the locus in the mouth and on the ear of herpetic vesicles which apparently occur in the sensory distribution of the geniculate ganglion. Sensory fibers pass via the nervus intermedius to the geniculate ganglion. White, J. C., and Sweet, W. H.: Pain: Its Mechanisms and Neurosurgical Control. Springfield, Ill., Charles C Thomas, 1969.

Vagoglossopharyngeal Neuralgia

Although the ninth and tenth nerves individually may conduct paroxysms of pain in the throat, tongue, ear, and jaw, or any combination of these areas, it frequently is impossible to distinguish the characteristics of this disorder into two separate clinical categories; therefore, White and Sweet (1969) have suggested the term "vagoglossopharyngeal neuralgia" as a more realistic title. Recognition depends on the following features: (1) unilateral paroxysms of pain in the region of the tongue, throat, ear, and larynx; (2) the pain seldom confined to the area from which it initially arose and frequently involving all the above area; (3) pain usually brief in duration and sharp in character, although prolonged bouts of constant dull or burning pain may occur; (4) paroxysms of pain which may be induced by swallowing, stroking the skin of the ear, mucous membrane of the tonsillar and pharyngeal regions; (5) attacks of pain sometimes accompanied by anatomic and cardiovascular responses, namely salivation, bradycardia, hypotension, and syncope. If these features are prominent, one must consider hypersensitivity of the carotid sinus (Ray and Stewart, 1948). However, bradycardia, syncope, and hypotension may be associated with severe episodes of pain in the throat and ear (Riley et al., 1942).

In view of the considerable variation in the character of neuralgias of the vagoglossopharyngeal nerve, astute otolaryngolic and neurologic evaluation is essential to exclude symptomatic lesions such as tumors of the nasopharynx, paranasal sinuses, larynx, local infection, and tumors compressing the ganglia or posterior rootlets of these nerves in the posterior fossa.

Tegretol has been effective in the therapy of this disorder as in trigeminal neuralgia. Removal of the styloid process has been noted to relieve a painful condition of the throat attributed to elongation of the styloid process or ossified extensions which may irritate the lateral pharyngeal wall as the stylopharyngeal muscles pull it across the anomaly during the act of deglutition (O'Brien, 1962). Superior laryngeal neurectomy may be successful in relieving pain which radiates outside the confines of the larynx (Echols and Maxwell, 1934; Ballantine, 1966). If the simple methods fail, rhizotomy of the ninth and tenth rootlets in the posterior fossa is an advisable procedure (Dandy, 1927; White and Sweet, 1969). Care must be taken to exclude radiation of pain through the fibers of the nervus intermedius. For this reason, some surgeons cut the fibers routinely rather than relying on stimulation data. Care should be taken to avoid cutting the lower rootlets of the vagus lest undue hoarseness occur (Walker, 1966).

Periodic Migrainous Neuralgia

Periodic migrainous neuralgia is a conspicuous syndrome distinguished by a bevy of eponyms and descriptive titles: Horton's syndrome, histamine cephalalgia, autonomic faciocephalalgia, petrosal neuralgia, cluster headaches, and erythromelalgia.

Clinical features of the syndrome resemble both migraine cephalalgia and trigeminal neuralgia. Unilateral paroxysms of constant severe burning pain, beginning in the eye or forehead and radiating into the face, temple, and neck, constitute the nature of this condition. The episodes of pain occur in clusters during the day or, more characteristically, awake the patient from his sleep. An episode of pain usually builds to a peak intensity in a crescendo fashion in a period of 30 to 45 minutes then promptly ends. Although rarely preceded by visual or sensory aura, the paroxysms of pain are commonly accompanied by autonomic disturbance in the form of tearing, rhinorrhea, salivation, ptosis, myosis, injection of conjunctiva, and dilatation of facial and scalp vessels. All these features are unilateral in occurrence and are not provoked by external stimuli; however, a number of our patients have noted that ingestion of even modest amounts of alcohol will precipitate an attack. Although sinusitis and other nasal disorders have been implicated in the pathogenesis of this condition, Schiller (1960) and others have been singularly unimpressed by this association.

The medical treatment is similar to that effective for migraine cephalalgia, namely, ergotomine tartrate (Schiller, 1960) and methysergide (Graham, 1964). However, the undesirable and occasionally disabling side effects of the latter drug necessitate careful evaluation and surveillance of those being so treated. Corticosteroids have been beneficial in the control of severe and protracted bouts of pain (Graham, 1964).

Surgical procedures vary from simp e to complex and are generally designed to attack anatomical components of the disorders at various sites. Sphenopalatine ganglionectomy, vidian neurectomy, and stellate ganglionectomy are procedures which have been largely abandoned because of lack of value. Resection of the superficial temporal artery has provided striking relief in occasional cases; however, there is no method for se ecting those who might benefit from this simple procedure (White and Sweet, 1969). Greater superficial petrosal neurectomy has been of distinct value in 50 to 75 per cent of patients in the experience of Gardner et al. (1947). The recurrence of pain following petrosal neurectomy has led to section of the nervus intermedius in the posterior fossa (Sachs, 1968). (See Fig. 26.)

Atypical Face Pain

This final group contains the painful disorders which are poorly characterized and therefore deviate from the commonly occurring features of other neuralgias. Radiation of pain into deep structures beyond individual cranial nerve zones; lack of restriction to hemicranial location; pain which is constant, dull, and aching in character; and tendency of patients to drug addiction and personality disorders are features which may indicate atypical facial pain. Obviously this is not a very gratifying diagnosis. Thus, one must search carefully for obscure conditions which might be the basis of these symptoms.

Symptomatic Pain of Head and Neck

Costen's Syndrome

Temporomandibular neuralgia was described by Costen (1934) and said to consist of medial movement of the condyle, leading to pressure against the auriculotemporal and chorda tympanic nerves. Headache and burning in the throat, tongue, and nose are characteristic complaints. Diminished salivation has been noted. Relief is said to be obtained by repositioning the jaw with dental prostheses (Smolik and Hempstead, 1952). We have not seen any successful cases treated in this fashion, although most patients with facial pain have been treated by dentists or orthodontists prior to neurosurgical consultation.

Dental Disease

Dental infection, pulpitis, apical abscess, and impacted teeth must be considered in the evaluation of atypical facial pain which may even be diffuse in nature.

Tumors, Infections, and Trauma

Deep-seated neoplasms, infection, and traumatic lesions frequently give rise to atypical head and neck pain. The features of each condition have been covered in the appropriate section.

CRANIAL TRAUMA

Skull Fractures

In the course of the evaluation and treatment of closed head injuries, one is rarely influenced greatly by the presence or absence of a skull fracture. Therefore, classification of fractures based on description of the line or bone involved is of little value. It is important, however, to determine if the fracture is compound (open), or if the fragments are depressed against or into the brain, a situation in which dural laceration is likely to occur. It is, of course, important to determine if paranasal sinuses are involved, particularly in the case of depressed fractures. Similarly, basal fractures and fractures involving the frontal and sphenoid bones and the petrous portion of the temporal bone deserve special consideration.

For the most part, brain injury is more severe when the force applied to the head is sufficient to fracture the skull, The fracture per se, however, is rarely responsible for the injury. In fact, some of the severest brain injuries occur without any evidence of skull fracture.

The vault of the adult skull is composed of dense, strong, laminated, and resilient membranous bone. The base of the skull is composed of relatively inelastic cartilaginous bone. The base is not subject to direct force and, hence, can be fractured only when the vault undergoes considerable deformation. Since the base of the skull is fragile and houses such important structures as the carotid arteries, cranial nerves, and brain stem, fractures in this region may assume particular importance. Fractures of the base are frequently difficult to visualize radiographically, particularly by routine techniques. There are certain clinical signs that identify a fracture of the base of the skull which otherwise might not be apparent. Bleeding from the auditory canal or from the nose or mouth without evidence of direct injury to the part usually is an expression of basal fracture.

At times ecchymosis may appear over the mastoid (Battle's sign) several days after head injury. This occurs, presumably, as a result of bleeding into the tissue about the base of the skull adjacent to a fracture site. The same is true of ecchymosis about the orbits, which appears as a result of extravasation of blood into the facial tissues after fractures that traverse the anterior fossa. It is, of course, understood that leakage of cerebrospinal fluid from the nose, eustachian tube, or external auditory canal is indicative of a basal fracture either in the frontal or posterior cranial fossae.

The cranial nerves are often injured in fractures of the base which involve their foramina. Anosmia occurs secondary to disruption of the olfactory nerve filaments as they traverse the cribriform plate. Indeed, the olfactory nerve is the most commonly injured cranial nerve in craniocerebral trauma (Turner, 1943). The optic nerve is rarely injured in basilar fractures; but any injury is seldom recognized early because of the difficulty in test ng vision in the severely injured patient with depressed consciousness and facial swelling (Hughes, 1962). Oculomotor palsy is uncommon in the absence of orbital fracture; however, abducens palsy is frequent but has little or no localizing value in the head-injured patient.

Cranial Nerve Injuries in Skull Fractures

Facial Nerve Injuries

Peripheral facial paralysis is a common occurrence following fracture of the temporal bone. The site of injury to the nerve appears to be related more to the structure of the temporal bone than to the nature of the head injury producing the fracture (McHugh, 1963). The most frequent site of injury to the nerve is within the middle ear, where it is crushed against the underlying labyrinthine capsule or contused and compressed by the shattered fragments of the tegmen tympani and the thin bone overlying the facial canal (McHugh, 1959). In transverse fractures of the temporal bone, the facial nerve is frequently lacerated or severed, and facial paralysis is immediate in onset; whereas in longitudinal fractures, by far the more common type, the nerve is more likely to be contused, compressed, or stretched and, accordingly, the paralysis of the facial muscles may be delayed in onset. In the case of transverse fractures in which the nerve is severely injured and paralysis immediate in on-

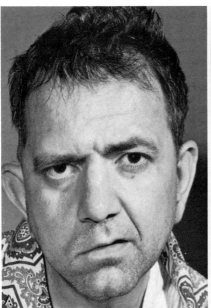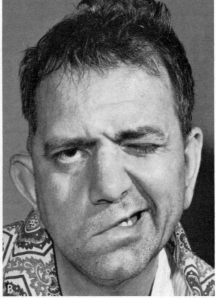

Figure 28. A 47 year old male with a convulsive disorder fell and struck the right occiput. Shortly thereafter blood drained from the right ear and a right facial paresis was noted. There was a complete facial paralysis, peripheral in type, with loss of taste and diminished tearing. Hearing was normal, except for hyperacusis on the right. Facial electromyogram showed complete denervation eight days postinjury. Maximal stimulation of the facial nerve produced no response. Decompression of the longitudinal portion of the facial nerve was performed. Evidence for recovery is absent three months later. *A*, Repose; *B*, maximal voluntary facial contraction.

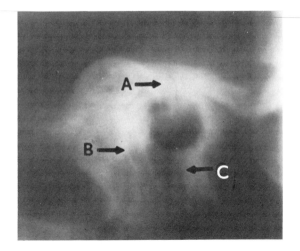

Figure 29. Radiographic view of petrous fracture. A points to transverse fracture across the facial canal; B, longitudinal portion of the facial canal (fallopian canal), and C, fracture extending through the middle ear.

set, recovery is unlikely in the absence of operative decompression and intrapetrous anastomosis, as advocated by Ballance and Duel (1932) (Figs. 28 and 29). However, in the case of longitudinal fracture, spontaneous recovery of paralysis occurs in the majority of patients (McHugh, 1959). Signs of recovery should appear within 21 days. Facial electromyography and other electrodiagnostic steps provide a controlled basis upon which to determine need for surgical exploration (Collier, 1963).

Auditory Nerve Injuries

Transverse fractures of the temporal bone are associated with a high incidence of permanent hearing loss due to contusion or transection of the auditory nerve (McHugh, 1963). Such fractures are frequently accompanied by irreversible facial paralysis, as was previously noted. However, longitudinal fractures are more likely to involve the middle ear, spare the labyrinth, and give rise to a conduction type hearing loss. Thus, if there is a unilateral conductive hearing loss with a marked air-bone gap in the face of an intact tympanic membrane, disruption in the ossicular chain has occurred (Kossner, 1961; Jackson and Magi, 1966). Successful techniques for the repair of this disturbance have been developed (Kossner, 1961; Perri, 1962; Gunderson, 1964). Recognition of this condition has been greatly facilitated by techniques for temporal bone laminography, which provide precise identification of the fracture sites and the position of the ossicles (Fig. 30).

Vascular Injuries in Skull Fractures

Pulsating Exophthalmos

Fractures and penetrating wounds of the base of the skull may result in injury to the cranial vessels (Cairns, 1942). Traumatic occlusion of carotid or vertebral arteries is, however, a rare circumstance. More commonly, the lumen of the carotid artery is lacerated by the sharp fragments of bone lining the carotid canal, and because of the unique location of the artery in the cavernous sinus, the blood remains within the vascular system. Accordingly, signs of intracranial hemorrhage do not occur. Moreover, the development of the ocular and neurologic symptoms secondary to elevation of pressure within the veins draining the cavernous sinus may be delayed several days, a feature attributable to secondary enlargement of the fistula and dilatation of orbital venous channels. Pulsating exophthalmos, failing visual acuity, diplopia, retro-ocular pain, and a continuous bruit constitute the characteristic findings of this disorder (Hamby, 1966; Mayfield and Wilson, 1967).

Surgical treatment is indicated as early as the patient's general condition will allow (Dandy, 1937). Failure to lower the arterial pressure leading to the fistula results in progressive enlargement of venous drainage from the sinus and diminishes the likelihood of success with subsequent simple surgical maneuvers. Ligation of the common and external carotid arteries in the neck occasionally succeeds in reducing the bruit and orbital pathology, although additional maneuvers, such as intracra-

PURE TONE AUDIOGRAM

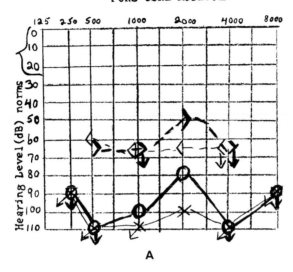

A

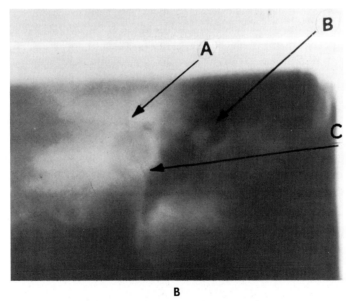

B

Figure 30. A 44 year old male who struck his occiput in a fall developed sudden onset bilateral deafness and bleeding from right ear. *A*, Audiologic evaluation showed a profound neural sensory deficit in both ears and a slight conductive component in the right ear, as indicated by the pure tone audiograms. *B*, Note the distinct linear fracture extending through the cochlea (A) and (C). An intact ossicle (B) is demonstrated.

nial ligation of the carotid and exophthalmic arteries and embolization of the cavernous carotid artery, are necessary to completely control the fistula. Parkinson (1965) has made an extensive study of this condition and has demonstrated several intracavernous branches of the normal carotid artery which account for persistence of the fistula even though all apparent inflow has been obliterated.

Epistaxis

Massive epistaxis may result from blunt or penetrating injuries of the internal carotid artery (Hamilton, 1953; Petty, 1969). We have recently had two such cases, one of which was secondary to a missile injury to the carotid artery two months prior to the epistaxis. In dealing with epistaxis of such magnitude, the ordinary maneuvers may not be satisfactory. In this regard, we have devised a technique in which a 30-cc. Folety catheter balloon is placed in each nasopharynx and posterior choana. With each bag inflated and the nostrils manually occluded, it is possible to control the hemorrhage until surgical treatment can be instituted (Moore, 1969).

Cerebrospinal Fluid Fistula

Prevention of intracranial infection is the primary goal in the treatment of basal skull fracture and other conditions associated with cerebrospinal fluid fistula. The high incidence of mortality prior to advent of antibiotic therapy has been attributed to fulminant or recurrent meningitis (Munro, 1935; Cairns, 1937; Calvert and Cairns, 1942). However, others have advocated early closure of the fistula as a means of preventing morbidity due to this complication (Teachenor, 1927; Lewin, 1954). Presently most neurologic surgeons advocate closure of spinal fluid fistula only in persistent cases and rely on systemic antibiotics to prevent meningitis during the period of active leakage (Coleman, 1937; Adson, 1941; Gurdjian and Webster, 1944; Morley and Hetherington, 1957; Ray and Bergland, 1969).

Other than spinal fluid rhinorrhea and otorrhea secondary to traumatic disruptions in the basilar dura and leptomeninges associated with skull fractures, there are numerous other lesions which lead to this condition: tumors of the pituitary fossa (Norsa, 1953); tumors of the nose, nasopharynx, and paranasal sinuses; infections of the paranasal sinuses; congenital defects in the dura (Rockett et al., 1964); nasal

encephalomeningoceles (Suwanwela and Horgsaprabhas, 1966); arachnoid cysts of the sella turcica (Brisman et al., 1969); spontaneous rhinorrhea resulting from lesions obstructing cerebrospinal fluid circulation and causing increased intracranial pressure (hydrocephalus) (Ommaya et al., 1968; Rovit et al., 1969); and surgical procedures in the region of the paranasal sinuses and mastoid. The high incidence of cerebrospinal fistula and meningitis secondary to stereotaxic implantation of yittrium in the pituitary fossa has led to the virtual abandonment of this procedure (Sweet, 1969). With other stereotaxic and open procedures, special precautions must be exercised to prevent persistent spinal fluid fistula. This precaution is particularly important in view of the current popularity of transnasal and translabyrinthine surgical approaches to the cranial cavity (House and Hitzelberger, 1964).

Fortunately the majority of spinal fluid fistulae close spontaneously and require only short-term supportive therapy. In our experience the following regimen has been successful: (1) immediate institution of parenteral antibiotics, and continuation until one week following cessation of spinal fluid drainage. Ampicillin, a synthetic penicillin effective against gram-positive and most gram-negative pathogens, is commonly employed. It can be administered orally after cessation of the fluid leak. (2) The patient is kept quiet, with the head of the bed elevated 30 degrees. (3) Daily lumar spinal puncture and drainage of spinal fluid is performed. (4) Nose and throat cultures are obtained to determine the nature of bacterial flora. (5) Radiographic laminography is scheduled and performed as early as the patient's condition permits, provided the drainage persists beyond the period at which cessation might have been expected (eight to ten days). The value of this study has been well documented in that the site, nature, and extent of the bony defect can be demonstrated. In addition, herniation of cerebral tissue or meninges through the defect may be uncovered. In such situations early surgical repair is indicated, since spontaneous closure is unlikely (Jefferson and Lewtas, 1963; Brawley and Kelly, 1967).

We have not seen any cases of otorrhea secondary to basilar skull fracture that failed to close spontaneously. However, several fistulae secondary to congenital defects in the dura (Ecker, 1947) and postoperative transaural operative procedures have required operative closure (House and Hitzelberger, 1964). Spinal fluid leak associated with fracture through the paranasal sinuses is much more likely to persist, particularly if there is comminution or depression of the fracture and if there is tissue interposed between the fracture lines. In the conditions in which there is increased intracranial pressure and hydrocephalus, the fistula should close spontaneously if the intracranial pressure is lowered by removal of the obstruction to the flow of spinal fluid. However, in some circumstances, the fistula has been so well developed that secondary surgical closure has been required as well (Ommaya et al., 1968; Rovit et al., 1969).

Correct location of spinal fluid fistula is essential if it is to be successfully closed by surgical maneuvers. The following methods have been advocated in the more difficult cases: (1) Injection of fluorescein into the lumbar subarachnoid space and observation for fluorescence from pledgets of cotton placed at strategic sites in the nostrils, eustachian tubes, and external auditory canals (Kirchner and Proud, 1960). Caution must be exercised in this procedure lest the fluorescein cause aseptic meningitis (Mahaley and Odom, 1966). In this regard we recommend cautious in ection of not greater than 1 ml. of 5 per cent sodium fluorescein mixed with 20 ml. of spinal fluid. (2) Injection of radioiodinated serum albumin (RISA) into the subarachnoid spaces has been advocated by DiChiro et al. (1964) but has not proved valuable, in our experience, unless the leakage of fluid is brisk. Montgomery (1968) has used a modification of this technique, namely, collecting the accumulated radioactivity in pledgets placed in the cavities of the sinuses overnight following injection of intrathecal RISA. However, results with this technique have been difficult to interpret because of the unbound RISA which is freely secreted in tears and mucus. (3) Pantopaque cisternography has been advocated and found particularly helpful in spinal fluid leak through the internal auditory meatus (Teng and Edalatpour, 1963; Rockett et al., 1964).

The surgical technique for closure of spinal fluid fistula developed by Dandy (1926, 1944) consists of a transcranial intradural exposure of the dural defect and its closure with a patch of autogenous fascia. Few refinements have been made since this procedure was devised. The extradural approach proposed by Adson (1941) has gained few advocates. However, all have recognized that at times it may be extremely difficult to localize the fistula once one is in the cranial cavity. In this regard it is important to have excluded a fistula through the internal auditory canal or mastoid prior to craniotomy. Morley and Wortzman (1965) directed our attention to the significance of lateral extensions of the sphenoid sinus into the greater w ngs of the sphenoid in 25 per cent of normal skulls, creating a situation in which the fistula may originate in the middle rather than the anterior cranial fossa. Similarly, Ray and Bergland (1969) have proposed that the sphenoid be opened and packed with muscle in patients in whom the fistula cannot be identified at operation. Hirsch (1952) has successfully closed fistulas extending through the sphenoid sinus by the endonasal approach, and Montgomery (1963) has popularized the transethmoidal approach, in which the sphenoid is packed with fat and a septal mucosal flap is rotated to cover the defect in the floor of the anterior fossa. Observed success with this simple technique justifies its further use, particularly in these situations: recurrence following transcranial procedures; fistulas that can be defined as traversing the sphenoid sinus; and fistulas following transsphenoidal operative procedures.

REFERENCES

Adson, A. W.: Cerebrospinal rhinorrhea: Surgical repair of fistula. Proc. Staff Meet. Mayo Clin. 16:385, 1941.

Alpers, B. J.: Diseases of the Meninges. Clinical Neurology. Philadelphia, F. A. Davis Co., 1958.

Anderson, F. M.: Intranasal (sphenopharyngeal) encephalocele: A report of a case with intracranial repair and review of the subject. Arch. Otolaryng. (Chicago) 46:644, 1947.

Atkinson, J. R., and Foltz, E. L.: Intraventricular "RISA" as a diagnostic aid in pre- and post-operative hydrocephalus. J. Neurosurg. 19:159, 1962.

Baker, H. L.: Myelographic examination of the posterior fossa with positive contrast medium. Radiology 81:791, 1963.

Ballance, C., and Duel, A. B.: Operative treatment of facial palsy by the introduction of nerve grafts into the fallopian canal, and by other intratemporal methods. Arch. Otolaryng. 15:1, 1932.

Ballantine, H. T.: Superior laryngeal neurectomy in the relief of vagal neuralgia. Personal communication, 1966.

Ballantine, H. T.: Brain abscess. In Gurdjian, E. S. (ed.): Cranial and Intracranial Suppuration. Springfield, Ill., Charles C Thomas, 1969, p. 89.

Basek, M.: Fibrous dysplasia of the middle ear. Arch. Otolaryng. 85:4, 1967.

Bateman, G. H.: Transsphenoidal hypophysectomy: A review of 70 cases treated in the past two years. Trans. Amer. Acad. Ophthal. Otolaryng. 66:103, 1962.

Batsakis, J. G., and Kittleson, A. C: Nasopharyngeal chordoma. Arch. Otolaryng. 78:168, 1963.

Beekhuis, G. J., and Taylor, M.: Ear and sinus aspects of intracranial suppurative disease. In Gurdjian, E. S.

(ed.): Cranial and Intracranial Suppuration. Springfield, Ill., Charles C Thomas, 1969.

Bengochea, F. G., and Blanco, F. L.: Arachnoid cysts of the cerebellopontine angle. J. Neurosurg. *12*:66, 1955.

Birnbaum, L. M., and Owsley, J. Q., Jr.: Frontonasal tumors of neurogenic origin. Plastic Reconstr. Surg. *41*:462, 1968.

Black, B. K., and Smith, D. E.: Nasal glioma. A.M.A. Arch. Neurol. Psychiat. *64*:614, 1950.

Blom, S.: Tic douloureux treated with a new anticonvulsant. Arch. Neurol. *9*:285, 1963.

Bloom, D. L.: Mucoceles of the maxillary and sphenoid sinuses. Radiology *85*:1103, 1965.

Blumenfeld, R., and Skolnik, E. M.: Intranasal encephaloceles. Arch. Otolaryng. *82*:527, 1965.

Botterell, E. H., and Drake, C. G.: Localized encephalitis, brain abscess and subdural empyema. J. Neurosurg. *9*:348, 1952.

Brawley, B. W., and Kelly, W. A.: Treatment of basal skull fractures with and without cerebrospinal fluid fistulae. J. Neurosurg. *26*:57, 1967.

Brisman, R., Hughes, J., and Mount, L.: Cerebrospinal fluid rhinorrhea and the empty sella. J. Neurosurg. *31*:538, 1969.

Burns-Cox, C. J., and Higgins, A. T.: Aneurysmal bone cyst of the frontal bone. J. Bone Joint Surg. *51*:344, 1969.

Cairns, H.: Injuries of frontal and ethmoidal sinuses with special reference to cerebrospinal rhinorrhea and aeroceles. J. Laryng. Otol. *52*:589, 1937.

Cairns, H.: The vascular aspects of head injury. Lisbon Med. *19*:375, 1942.

Calvert, C. A., and Ca rns, H.: Discussion on injuries of the frontal and ethmoid sinuses. Proc. Roy. Soc. Med. *35*:805, 1942.

Cawthorne, T., and Griffin, A.: Primary cholesteatoma of the temporal bone. Arch. Otolaryng. *73*:252, 1961.

Chou, S. N., Story, J. L., French, L. A., and Peterson, H. O.: Some angiographic features of brain abscess. J. Neurosurg. *24*:693, 1966.

Coleman, C. C.: Fracture of skull involving paranasal sinuses and mastoids. J.A.M.A. *109*:1613, 1937.

Coleman, C. C., and Walker, J. C.: Technique of anastomosis of the branches of the facial nerve to the spinal accessory for facial paralysis. Ann. Surg. *131*:960, 1950.

Collier, S.: Electrodiagnosis and surgical indications in facial palsy. Arch. Otol. *78*:421, 1963.

Costantini, F. E., Iraci, G., Bene Detti, A., and Melanotte, P. L.: Aneurysmal bone cyst as an intracranial space-occupying lesion. J. Neurosurg. *25*:205, 1966.

Costen, J. B.: A syndrome of ear and sinus symptoms dependent upon disturbed function of the temporomandibular joint. Ann. Otol. *43*:1, 1934.

Courville, C. B., and Rosenwald, L. K.: Intracranial complications of infections of nasal cavities and accessory sinuses. Arch. Otolaryng. *27*:692, 1938.

Crawford, J. V., and Walker, A. E.: Surgery for Pain: A History of Neurologic Surgery. Baltimore, The Williams & Wilkins Co., 1951.

Cushing, H.: The Pituitary Body and Its Disorders. Philadelphia, J. B. Lippincott Co., 1912.

Cushing, H.: Tumors of the Nervus Acusticus. Philadelphia, W. B. Saunders Company, 1917.

Dandy, W. E.: Operation for total removal of cerebellopontine (acoustic) tumors. Surg. Gynec. Obstet. *41*:129, 1925.

Dandy, W. E.: Pneumocephalus (intracranial pneumatocele or aerocele). Arch. Surg. *12*:949, 1926.

Dandy, W. E.: Glossopharyngeal neuralgia (tic douloureux): Its diagnosis and treatment. Arch. Surg. *18*:687, 1927.

Dandy, W. E.: An operation for the cure of tic douloureux: Partial section of the sensory root at the pons. Arch. Surg. *18*:687, 1929.

Dandy, W. E.: Carotid-cavernous aneurysms (pulsating exophtha mos). Zbl. Neurochir. *2*:77, 1937.

Dandy, W. E.: Treatment of rhinorrhea and otorrhea. Arch. Surg. *49*:75, 1944.

Danoff, D., Serbu, J., and French, L. A.: Encephalocoele extending into the sphenoid sinus. J. Neurosurg. *24*:684, 1966.

Davis, C., and Alexander, E.: Congenital nasofrontal encephalomeningoceles and teratomas: Review of 7 cases. J. Neurosurg. *16*:365, 1959.

De, S. K.: A case of muco-pyocele of the maxillary antrum simulating malignant neoplasm. J. Laryng. *80*:548, 1966.

Diamant, M.: Hypophysectomy in a non-pneumatized sphenoid. Arch. Otolaryng. *74*:29, 1961.

DiChiro, G., Reames, P. M., and Matthews, W. B.: RISA-ventriculography and RISA cisternography. Neurology *14*:185, 1964.

Dott, N. M.: Facial paralysis: Restitution by extra petrous nerve graft. Proc. Roy. Soc. Med. *57*:900, 1958.

Drake, C. G.: Surgical treatment of acoustic neuroma with preservation or reconstitution of the facial nerve. J. Neurosurg. *26*:459, 1967.

Drake, C. G.: Further experience with surgical treatment of aneurysms of the basilar artery. J. Neurosurg. *29*:372, 1968.

Eagleton, W. P.: Meningitis: Result of disease of the petrous apex and sphenoidal basis. Surg. Gynec. Obstet. *60*:586, 1935.

Echols, D. H., and Maxwell, J. H.: Superior laryngeal neuralgia relieved by operation. J.A.M.A. *103*:2027, 1934.

Ecker, A.: Cerebrospinal rhinorrhea by way of the eustachian tube: Report of cases with dural defect in middle or posterior fossa. J. Neurosurg. *4*:177, 1947.

Eisen, A. A., et al.: Adrenal steroid therapy in neurologic disease. Canad. Med. Ass. J. *100*:66, 1969.

Ekbom, K. A., and Westerberg, C. E.: Carbamazepine in glossopharyngeal neuralgia. Arch. Neurol. (Chicago) *14*:595, 1966.

Falconer, M. A., Ian, C. B., and Duchess, L. W.: Surgical treatment of chordoma and chondroma of the skull base. J. Neurosurg. *29*:261, 1968.

Feinmesser, N.: Facial paralysis following a fracture of skull. J. Laryng. *71*:838, 1957.

Finerman, W. B., and Pick, E. I.: Intranasal encephalomeningocele. Ann. Otol. (St. Louis) *62*:114, 1953.

Frazier, C. H.: Subtotal resection of sensory root for relief of major trigeminal neuralgia. Arch. Neurol. Psychiat. *13*:318, 1925.

French, L. A., and Chou, S. N.: Osteomyelitis of the skull and epidural abscess. *In* Gurdjian, E. S. (ed.): Cranial and Intracranial Suppuration. Springfield, Ill., Charles C Thomas, 1969.

Friedman, I., Harrison, D. F. N., and Bird, E. S.: The fine structures of chordoma with particular reference to the physaliferous cell. J. Clin. Path. *15*:116, 1962.

Furlow, L. T.: Tic douloureux of the nervus intermedius. J. Neurosurg. *15*:299, 1958.

Gallagher, P. G., et al.: Large intracranial aneurysm producing panhypopituitarism and frontal lake syndrome. Neurology *6*:829, 1956.

Gardner, W. J., Stowell, A., and Duttinger, R.: Resection

of the greater superficial petrosal nerve in treatment of unilateral headache. J. Neurosurg. *4*:105, 1947.

Graham, J.: Corticosteroids. Personal communication, 1967.

Graham, J. R.: Methysergide for prevention of headache: Experience in five hundred patients over three years. New Eng. J. Med. *270*:67, 1964.

Green, W. H., Goldberg, H. I., and Wohl, G. T.: Mucormycosis infections of the craniofacial structures. Amer. J. Roentgen. *101*:802, 1967.

Guiot, G.: Personal communication, 1967.

Guiot, G., and Thibaut, B.: L'exterpation des adénomes hypophysaires par voie trans-sphenoidale. Neurocherurgia *1*:133, 1959.

Guiot, G., et al.: Two atypical forms of hypophyseal adenomas: Ideal indications for transsphenoidal approach. Gag. Méd. (France) *69*:13, 1962.

Gunderson, T.: Reconstruction of the ossicular chain by incus prosthesis. Acta Otolaryng. (Stockh.) *58*:227, 1964.

Gurdjian, E. S., and Webster, J. E.: Surgical management of compound depressed fracture of frontal sinus, cerebrospinal rhinorrhea and pneumocephalus. Arch. Otolaryng. *39*:287, 1944.

Hall, L. J., and Wilkins, S. A., Jr.: Nasopharyngeal fibroma. Amer. J. Surg. *116*:530, 1968.

Hamberger, C. A., et al.: Surgical treatment of carniopharyngioma: Radical removal by the transantrosphenoidal approach. Acta Otolaryng. *52*:285, 1960.

Hamberger, C. A., et al.: Transantrosphenoidal hypophysectomy. Arch. Otolaryng. *74*:2, 1961.

Hamby, W. B.: Carotid-Cavernous Fistula. Springfield, Ill., Charles C Thomas, 1966.

Hamilton, J. G.: Massive epistaxis following closed head injuries. Guy's Hosp. Rep. *102*:360, 1953.

Hamlin, H.: The case for transsphenoidal approach to hypophysial tumors. J Neurosurg. *19*:1000, 1962.

Hardy, J.: Microneurosurgery of the hypophysis. *In* Rand, R. W.: Microneurosurgery. St. Louis, The C. V. Mosby Co., 1969.

Hardy, J., and Wigser, S. M.: Trans-sphenoidal surgery of pituitary fossa with radiofluoroscopic control. J. Neurosurg. *23*:612, 1965.

Harris, W.: An analysis of 1,433 cases of paroxysmal trigeminal neuralgia and the end results of gasserian alcohol injection. Brain *63*:209, 1940.

Harrison, D. F. N.: A case of primary chordoma of the sphenoid sinus. J. Laryng. *75*:429, 1961.

Hayes, G. J., and Creston, J. E.: Mucocele of the sphenoid sinus. Arch. Otolaryng. *79*:653, 1964.

Henderson, W. R.: The pituitary adenomata: A follow-up study of the surgical results in 338 cases (Dr. Harvey Cushing's series). Brit. J. Surg. *26*:811, 1939.

Henschen, F.: Quoted in Russell, D. S., and Rubinstein, L. J., p. 244.

Hirsch, O.: Über methoden der operations Behandlung von hypophysentumoren auf endonasalem Wege. Arch. Laryng. Rhin. *24*:129, 1910.

Hirsch, O.: Successful closure of cerebrospinal fluid rhinorrhea by endonasal surgery. A.M.A. Arch. Otolaryng. *56*:1, 1952.

Hirsch, O.: Life-long cure and improvements after transphenoidal operation of pituitary tumors. Acta Ophthal. Kbh., (Suppl.) *56*, 1959.

Hitzelberger, W. E.: Tumors of the cerebellopontine angle in relation to vertigo. Arch. Otolaryng. *85*:539, 1967.

Hitzelberger, W. E., and House, W. F.: Polytome-pantopaque: A technique for the diagnosis of small acoustic tumors. J. Neurosurg. *29*:214, 1968.

Holland, F. D., et al.: Olfactory neuro-epithelioma (neuroblastoma). A.M.A. Arch. Otolaryng. *69*:724, 1959.

Holmes, G. W., and Robbins, L. L.: Roentgen Interpretations. Philadelphia, Lea & Febiger, 1955.

Horraz, G.: Treatment of pituitary adenomas: Surgery versus radiation. A.M.A. Arch. Neurol. Psychiat. *79*:1, 1958.

House, W. F.: Surgical exposure of the internal auditory canal and its contents through the middle cranial fossa. Laryngoscope *71*:1363, 1961.

House, W. F. (ed.): (Monograph) Transtemporal bone microsurgical removal of acoustic neuromas. Arch. Otolaryng. (Chicago) *80*:597, 1964.

House, W. F. (ed.): (Monograph) II. Acoustic neuroma. Arch. Otolaryng. *88*:575, 1968.

House, W. F., and Hitzelberger, W. E.: Postoperative cerebrospinal fluid leak. (In monograph: Transtemporal bone microsurgical removal of acoustic neuromas.) Arch. Otolaryng. *80*:749, 1964.

Hughes, B.: Indirect injury of the optic nerve and chiasma. Bull. Johns Hopkins Hosp. *111*:98, 1962.

Hunt, J. R.: The sensory field of the facial nerve: A further contribution to the symptomology of the geniculate ganglion. Brain *38*:418, 1915.

Hunter, C. R., and Mayfield, F. H.: Role of the upper cervical roots in the production of pain in the head. Amer. J. Surg. *78*:743, 1949.

Hutter, R. V. P., et al.: Esthesioneuroblastomas: A clinical and pathological study. Amer. J. Surg. *106*:748, 1963.

Jackson, F. E., and Magi, M.: Traumatic dislocation of the incus associated with basilar skull fracture. J. Neurosurg. *24*:570, 1966.

Jaeger, R.: The results of injecting hot water into the gasserian ganglion for relief of tic douloureux. J. Neurosurg. *16*:656, 1959.

Jannetta, P. S.: Gross description of the human trigeminal nerve and ganglion. J. Neurosurg. *26*:109, 1967.

Jefferson, G.: Glosso-pharyngeal neuralgia. Lancet *2*:397, 1931.

Jefferson, G.: Compression of the chiasm, optic nerves, and optic tracts by intracranial aneurysms. Brain *60*:444, 1937.

Jefferson, G.: The trigeminal neuromas with some remarks on malignant invasion of the gasserian ganglion. Clin. Neurosurg. *1*:11, 1955a.

Jefferson, G.: Further remarks concerning compression of the optic pathways by intracranial aneurysms. Proc. Congr. Neurol. Surg. *1*:55, 1955b.

Jefferson, A., and Lewtas, N.: Value of tomography and subdural pneumonography in subfrontal fractures. Acta Radiol. Diag. *1*:118, 1963.

Jefferson, G., and Smalley, A. A.: Progressive facial palsy produced by intratemporal epidermoids. J. Laryng. *53*:417, 1938.

Kahn, E. A., and Arbor, S.: Treatment of encapsulated abscess of the brain: Visualization by colloidal thorium dioxide. Arch. Neurol. Psychiat., *41*:158, 1939.

Kahn, E. A.: Correlative Neurosurgery. Springfield, Ill. Charles C Thomas, 1969.

Ketcham, A. S., et al.: Complications of intracranial facial resection for tumors of the paranasal sinuses. Amer. J. Surg. *112*:591, 1966.

Killian, J. M., et al.: Carbamazepine in treatment of neuralgia. Arch. Neurol. (Chicago) *19*:129, 1968.

Kirchner, F. R., and Proud, G. O.: Method for the identification and localization of cerebrospinal fluid rhinorrhea and otorrhea. Laryngoscope *70*:921, 1960.

Kirschner, M.: Die Behondlung der trigeminus Neuralgia. Muenchen Med. Wschr. *89*:461, 1942.

Kossner, H. K.: Repair of traumatic interruption of ossicular chain. Arch. Otolaryng. *74*:347, 1961.

Kramer, S., McKissack, W., and Concannon, J. P.: Craniopharyngiomas: Treatment by combined surgery and radiation therapy. J. Neurosurg. *18*:217–226, 1961.

Krayenbühl, H.: Primary tumours of the root of the fifth cranial nerve: Their distinction from tumours of the gasserian ganglion. Brain *59*:337, 1936.

Krueger, T., McFarland, J., and Ommaya, A.: Pyocele of the sphenoid sinus. J. Neurosurg. *22*:616, 1965.

Kune, Z.: Treatment of essential neuralgia of the ninth nerve by selective tractotomy. J. Neurosurg. *23*:494, 1965.

Lederman, M.: Cancer of the Nasopharynx. Springfield, Ill., Charles C Thomas, 1961.

Lederman, M.: Carcinoma of the nasopharynx. Lancet *2*:1455, 1966.

Leffall, L., Jr., and White, J. E.: Cancer of the nasal cavity and paranasal sinuses. Amer. J. Surg. *112*:436, 1966.

Lewin, W.: Cerebrospinal fluid rhinorrhea in closed head injury. Brit. J. Surg. *42*:1, 1954.

Lichtenstein, L.: Aneurysmal bone cyst. J. Bone Joint Surg. *39-A*:873, 1957.

Lundgren, A., and Olin, T.: Muco-pyocele of the sphenoidal sinus or posterior ethmoidal cells with special reference to the apex orbital syndrome. Acta Otolaryng. *53*:61, 1961.

McHugh, H. E.: Surgical treatment of facial paralysis and traumatic conductive deafness in fractures of the temporal bone. Ann. Otol. *68*:855, 1959.

McHugh, H. E.: Facial paralysis in birth injury and skull fracture. Arch. Otolaryng. *78*:443, 1963.

McKenzie, K. G., and Alexander, E.: Post-fossa tumors. Clin. Neurosurg. *2*:22, 1955.

McKissock, W.: Acoustic tumors. Proc. Roy Soc. Med. *58*:1078, 1965.

McLaurin, R. L.: Subdural infections. *In* Gurdjian, E. S. (ed.): Cranial and Intracranial Suppuration. Springfield, Ill., Charles C Thomas, 1969, p. 73.

MacCarty, C. S., et al.: Aneurysmal bone cyst of the neural axis. J. Neurosurg. *18*:671, 1961.

Mack, E. W.: EMG of facial musculature as an aid in early diagnosis of acoustic neuroma. J. Neurosurg. *29*:565, 1968.

Mahaley, M. S., and Odom, G. L.: Complication following intrathecal injection of fluorescein. J. Neurosurg. *25*:298, 1966.

Martins, A. N., Hayes, G. J., and Kempe, L. A.: Invasive pituitary adenomas. J. Neurosurg. *22*:268, 1965.

Matson, D. D.: Neurosurgery of Infancy and Childhood. Springfield, Ill., Charles C Thomas, 1969.

Matson, D. D., and Crigler, J. F.: Radical treatment of craniopharyngioma. Ann. Surg. *152*:699, 1960.

Matson, D. D., and Crigler, J. F.: Management of craniopharyngioma in childhood. J. Neurosurg. *30*:377, 1969.

Matson, D. D., and Salom, M.: Brain abscess in congenital heart disease. Pediatrics *27*:772, 1961.

Maxwell, J. A., and DeLong, W. B.: Use of micropaque barium in radiographic visualization of brain abscesses. J. Neurosurg. *28*:280, 1968.

Mayfield, F. H., and Wilson, C. B.: The pathological basis for postural (intermittent) exophthalmos. J. Neurosurg. *26*:619, 1967.

Montgomery, W. W.: Transethmoid sphenoidal hypophysectomy with septal mucosal flap. Arch. Otolaryng. *78*:68, 1963.

Montgomery, W. W.: Mucocele of the maxillary sinus causing exophthalmos. E.E.N.T. Monthly *43*:41, 1964.

Montgomery, W. W.: Location cerebrospinal fluid fistula with radio-isotopes. Personal communication, 1968.

Mood, G. F.: Congenital anterior herniation of brain. Ann. Otol. *47*:391, 1938.

Moore, D., et al.: Massive epistaxis from aneurysm of the carotid artery, In press.

Morelli, R. J.: Intracranial neurilemmoma of the hypoglossal nerve. Neurology *16*:709, 1966.

Morley, T. P., and Hetherington, R. F.: Traumatic cerebrospinal fluid rhinorrhea and otorrhea, pneumocephalus and meningitis. Surg. Gynec. Obstet. *104*:88, 1957.

Morley, T. P., and Wortzman, G.: The importance of the lateral extensions of the sphenoidal sinus in post-traumatic cerebrospinal rhinorrhea and meningitis: Clinical and radiological aspects. J. Neurosurg. *22*:326, 1965.

Mortada, A.: Pulsating frontocele and exophthalmos. Amer. J. Ophthal. *65*:425, 1968.

Munro, D.: The modern treatment of craniocerebral injuries with special reference to the maximum permissible mortality and morbidity. New Eng. J. Med. *213*:893, 1935.

Nager, G. T.: Meningiomas Involving the Temporal Bone. Springfield, Ill., Charles C Thomas, 1964.

Nevins, M. A., and Leaver, R. C.: Sphenoid musocele: An unusual mimic of pituitary neoplasm. Arch. Intern. Med. (Chicago) *120*:607–609, 1967.

Ney, K. W.: Facial paralysis and surgical repair of the facial nerve. Laryngoscope *32*:322, 1922.

Nichols, P., and Blanco, F. L.: Traumatic arachnoid cyst simulating acoustic neurinoma. J. Neurosurg. *10*:538, 1953.

Norman, P. S., and Yanagisawa, E.: Mucocele of the sphenoid sinus. Arch. Otol. (Chicago) *79*:646, 1964.

Norsa, L.: Cerebrospinal rhinorrhea with pituitary tumors. Neurology (Minneapolis) *3*:864, 1953.

O'Brien, M. A.: Neuralgias in otolaryngology. Irish J. Med. Sci. *442*:439, 1962.

Olivecrona, H.: Cholesteatoma of the cerebellopontine angle. Acta Psychiat. Neurol. *24*:639, 1949.

Olivecrona, H.: Acoustic tumors. J. Neurosurg. *26*:6, 1967.

Oliver, P.: Cancer of the nose and paranasal sinuses. Surg. Clin. N. Amer. *47*:595, 1967.

Ommaya, A. K., et al.: Non-traumatic cerebrospinal fluid rhinorrhea. J. Neurol. Neurosurg. Psychiat. *31*:245, 1968.

Ormerod, R.: A case of chordoma presenting in the nasopharynx. J. Laryng. *74*:540, 1960.

Parker, L. S.: Mucocele of the right maxillary sinus with proptosis of the right eye. J. Laryng. *75*:507, 1961.

Parkinson, D.: A surgical approach to the cavernous portion of the carotid artery: Anatomical studies and case report. J. Neurosurg. *23*:474, 1965.

Perri, F. A.: Reconstruction of hearing by surgical procedures. J. Occup. Med. *4*:518, 1962.

Petty, J. M.: Epistaxis from aneurysms of the internal carotid artery due to a gunshot wound. J. Neurosurg. *30*:741, 1969.

Pincus, J. H., and Daroff, R. B.: Sphenoid sinus mucocele: A curable cause of ophthalmoplegic migraine syndrome. J.A.M.A. *187*:459, 1964.

Pooley, G. H., and Wilkinson, G.: A case of temporary total blindness of the left eye due to pressure of cystic distention of the left maxillary antrum on the optic nerve. Ophthal. Rev. *32*:130, 1913.

Poppen, S. L., and King, A. B.: Chordomas: Experiences with 13 cases. J. Neurosurg. *9*:139, 1952.

Ramsey, H. E., Strong, E. W., and Frazell, E. L.: Fibrous

dysplasia of the craniofacial bones. Amer. J. Surg. *116*:542, 1968.

Rand, R. W., and Kurze, T.: Preservation of vestibular, cochlear, and facial nerves during microsurgical removal of acoustic tumors. J. Neurosurg. *28*:158, 1968.

Ray, B. S., and Bergland, R. M.: Cerebrospinal fluid fistula: Clinical aspects, techniques of localization, and methods of closure. J. Neurosurg., *30*:399, 1969.

Ray, B. S., and Patterson, R. H.: Surgical treatment of pituitary adenomas. J. Neurosurg. *19*:1, 1962.

Ray, B. S., and Stewart, H. J.: Role of the glossopharyngeal nerve in the carotid sinus reflex in man: Relief of carotid sinus syndrome by intracranial section of the glossopharyngeal nerve. Surgery *23*:411, 1948.

Reinecke, R. D., and Montgomery, W. W.: Oculomotor nerve palsy associated with mucocele of the sphenoid sinus. Arch. Ophthal. *71*:50, 1964.

Revilla, A. G.: Tic douloureux and its relationship to tumors of the posterior fossa: Analysis of twenty-four cases. J. Neurosurg. *4*:233, 1947.

Rhonheimer, C.: Zur Symptomatologie der sellaren Aneurysmen: Ein beitrag zur differential Diagnose der chiasma Syndrome. Klin. Mbl. Augenheilk. *134*:1, 1959.

Rhoton, A. L., Kobayashi, A., and Hollinshead, W. H.: Nervus intermedius. J. Neurosurg. *29*:609, 1968.

Riley, H. A., et al.: Glossopharyngeal neuralgia initiating or associated with cardiac arrest. Trans. Amer. Neurol. Ass. *68*:28, 1942.

Robinson, F., and Solitare, G.: Olfactory neuroblastoma. J. Neurosurg. *25*:133, 1966.

Rockett, F. X., Wittenborg, M. H., Shillito, J., and Matson, D. D.: Pantopaque visualization of a congenital dural defect of the internal auditory meatus: A report of a case. Amer. J. Roentgen. *91*:640, 1964.

Rosenwasser, H.: Glomus jugulare tumors. Arch. Otolaryng. *88*:29, 1968.

Rovit, R. L., Schlecter, M. M., and Nelson, K.: Spontaneous "high-pressure cerebrospinal rhinorrhea" due to lesions obstructing flow of cerebrospinal fluid. J. Neurosurg. *30*:406, 1969.

Rushton, J. G., Gibilisco, J. A., and Goldstein, N. P.: Atypical face pain. J.A.M.A. *171*:545, 1959.

Russell, D. S., and Rubinstein, L. J.: Pathology of Tumors of the Nervous System. Baltimore, The Williams & Wilkins Co., 1963.

Sachs, E.: The role of the nervus intermedius in facial neuralgia. J. Neurosurg. *28*:54, 1968.

Sassin, J. F., and Rosenberg, R. N.: Neurological complications of fibrous dysplasia of the skull. Arch. Neurol. *18*:363, 1968.

Scanlan, R. L.: Positive contrast medium (iophindylate) in diagnosis of acoustic neuroma. Arch. Otol. *80*:698, 1964.

Schiller, F.: Prophylactic and other treatment for "histaminic," cluster, or limited variant of migraine: Comparative study, therapeutic recommendation and discussion of the nature of the syndrome. J.A.M.A. *173*:1907, 1960.

Schlumberger, H. G.: Fibrous dysplasia of single bones (monostatic fusions dysplasia). Milit. Surg. *99*:504, 1946.

Schoenrock, L., and Mayfield, F. H.: Rhinorrhea and Otorrhea. Read before the Ohio State Neurosurgical Society, May 16, 1969. (Submitted for publication by the Ohio State Medical Journal.)

Shambaugh, G. E.: Meningeal complications of otitis media. *In* Surgery of the Ear. Philadelphia, W. B. Saunders Company, 1967, p. 306.

Shedd, D. P., von Essen, C. F., and Eisenberg, H.: Cancer of the nasopharynx in Connecticut. Cancer, *20*:508, 1967.

Sheehy, J. L.: The neuro-otologic evaluation. (Monograph II.) Arch Otolaryng. *88*:44, 1968.

Siquera, E. B., et al.: Positive contrast ventriculography, cisternography and myelography. Amer. J. Roentgen. *104*:123, 1968.

Skinner, H. A.: Quoted in Russell, D. S., and Rubinstein, L. J., p. 243.

Smith, R. R., Klopp, C. T., and Williams, J. M.: Surgical treatment of the frontal sinus and adjacent areas. Cancer *7*:991, 1954.

Smolik, E. A., and Hempstead, E. J.: Trigeminal neuralgia and mandibular joint dysfunction. Postgrad. Med. *12*:419, 1952.

Sperti, L., et al.: Effects of selective intracranial section and stimulation of vago-accessory roots. Arch. Sci. Biol. (Bologna) *48*:103, 1964.

Stevenson, G. C., et al.: A transcervical approach to the ventral surface of the brain stem for removal of a clivus chordoma. J. Neurosurg. *24*:544, 1966.

Stookey, B.: Differential dorsal root section in the treatment of bilateral trigeminal neuralgia. J. Neurosurg. *12*:501, 1955.

Suwanwela, C., and Horgsaprabhas, C.: Fronto-ethmoidal encephalomeningocele. J. Neurosurg. *25*:172, 1966.

Svien, H., and Litzow, T. S.: Removal of certain hypophyseal tumors by the transantral-sphenoid route. J. Neurosurg. *23*:603, 1965.

Sweet, W. H.: Personal communication, 1968a.

Sweet, W. H.: Radiofrequency Coagulation of the Gasserian Ganglion and Rootlets for Idiopathic Trigeminal Neuralgia. Presented at Society of Neurological Surgery, April, 1968b.

Sweet, W. H.: Summary of surgical aspects of papers on pituitary ablation in treatment of diabetic retinopathy. *In* Goldberg, M. F., and Fine, S. (eds.). Washington, D.C., Public Health Service Publication, No. 1890. 1969, p. 415.

Symonds, C.: A particular variety of headache. Brain *79*:217, 1956.

Taarnhoj, P.: Decompression of the trigeminal root and the posterior part of the ganglion as a treatment in trigeminal neuralgia. J. Neurosurg. *9*:288, 1952.

Teachenor, F. R.: Intracranial complications of fracture of skull involving frontal sinus. J.A.M.A. *88*:987, 1927.

Tefft, M., Matson, D. D., and Neuhauser, E. B. D.: Brain abscess in children: Radiologic methods for early recognition. Amer. J. Roentgen. *93*:675, 1966.

Teng, P., and Edalatpour, N.: Cerebrospinal fluid rhinorrhea with demonstration of cranionasal fistula with pantopaque. Radiology *81*:802, 1963.

Tew, J. M.: Arachnoid Cysts of the Cerebellopontine Angle. Presented at New England Neurosurgical Society, April, 1967.

Thiry, S.: Expérience personnelle basée sur 225 cas de neuralgie essentielle du ners trijumeau traitée par electrocoagulation stereotaxique du ganglion de gasser entré 1950 et 1960. Neurochirurgie *8*:86, 1962.

Toole, J. F., et al.: Brain inflammation and steroids: Two double-edged swords. Ann. Intern. Med. *70*:221, 1969.

Turner, J. W. A.: Indirect injuries of the optic nerve. Brain *66*:140, 1943.

Van Buren, J. M., Ommaya, A. K., and Ketcham, A. S.: Ten years' experience with radical combined craniofacial resection of malignant tumors of the paranasal sinuses. J. Neurosurg. *28*:341, 1968.

Walker, A. E.: Neuralgias of the glossopharyngeal, vagus and intermedius nerves, *In* Knighton, R. S., and

Dumke, P. R. (eds.): Pain. (Henry Ford Hospital International Symposium.) Boston, Little, Brown and Company, 1966, p. 421.

Wang, Y., and Rosen, J. A.: Positive brain scans in nonspace occupying lesions. Amer. J. Roentgen. *93*:816, 1965.

Wepsic, J.: Evaluation of Selective Radiofrequency Lesions of Gasserian Ganglion for Facial Pain. Presented at Society of University Neurosurgeons, May, 1969.

White, J. C., and Ballantine, H. T.: Intrasellar aneurysms simulating hypophyseal tumors. J. Neurosurg. *18*:34, 1961.

White, J. C., and Sweet, W. H.: Pain and the Neurosurgeon. Springfield, Ill., Charles C Thomas, 1969.

White, J. C., and Warren, S.: Unusual size and extension of a pituitary adenoma: Case report of a chromophobe tumor with unusually extensive compression of the base of the brain, and a review of the literature on the pathways of extension of these tumors. J. Neurosurg. *2*:126, 1945.

Wilkinson, H. A.: Selective third ventricular catheterization for pantopaque ventriculography. Amer. J. Roentgen. *105*:348, 1969.

Wright, D.: Nasopharyngeal and cervical chordoma: Some aspects of their development and treatment. J. Laryng. *81*:1337, 1967.

Zollinger, R., and Cutler, E. C.: Aneurysm of the internal carotid artery: Report of a case simulating tumor of the pituitary. Arch. Neurol. Psychiat. *30*:607, 1933.

Zoltán, L., and Fenyes, I.: Stereotactic diagnosis and radioactive treatment in a case of spheno-occipital chordoma. J. Neurosurg. *17*:888, 1960.

Chapter 36

OPHTHALMOLOGY AS IT RELATES TO OTOLARYNGOLOGY

by Kenneth W. Rowe, Jr., M.D.

Both because of the eye's relationship to otolaryngology and because of its anatomic relationship to the sinuses, the nose, and the bones of the face, no textbook on otolaryngology would be complete without a chapter on the eye. Although relatively small, the eye is an extremely important sensory receptor and contributes significantly to the general appearance of the patient. Injury or loss of an eye or of an eyelid produces not only a significant cosmetic defect, but may also result in severe emotional disturbance. It is in this area of trauma that the relationship between ophthalmology and otolaryngology is most clearly evidenced. Let us, therefore, consider some of the ophthalmologic conditions which might be encountered in a patient who has sustained injury to the head and neck.

TRAUMA

General Considerations

In the initial examination of the injured patient it is most important from an eye standpoint to ascertain that the globe is intact. Incidental injury to the eyelids or to the extraocular muscles can be diagnosed and treated later. However, if there has been a perforation of the cornea or sclera, squeezing on the part of the patient or pressure on the eye by a nurse or physician may cause further damage. One of the best clues to indicate an ocular perforation is an irregularity of the pupil. Most lacerations or perforations of the globe occur anteriorly and are accompanied by an outflow of the aqueous humor found in that segment of the eye. Since the iris is extremely thin and fragile, it is carried along by a wave of escaping aqueous and becomes prolapsed or at least incarcerated in the wound edges. This traction, even on a peripheral part of the iris, results in pupillary distortion. The pupil is generally pear-shaped, with the stem of the pear pointing toward the area of perforation.

An intact eye has an intraocular pressure of about 15 to 20 mm. of mercury. This intraocular pressure maintains the curves and optics of the normal cornea. Whenever there is a perforation of the globe, the eye immediately becomes soft. This leads to a distortion of the fine optical properties of the eye, and the patient, if conscious, is unable to see clearly. The examining physician will have difficulty in obtaining a clear view of the fundus even if the remaining ocular media are perfectly clear. If the patient is able to read a Snellen Eye Chart or the print on a prescription pad, magazine, or newspaper there is little likelihood that he has suffered a perforated globe. If, in addition, the examiner can obtain a clear view of the fundus, one can be further reassured that the globe is intact. Should an ocular perforation be suspected, a metal shield of the type used after cataract surgery should be taped over the eye. This shield rests on the cheek and brow, thereby preventing pressure from accidentally being applied to the globe itself.

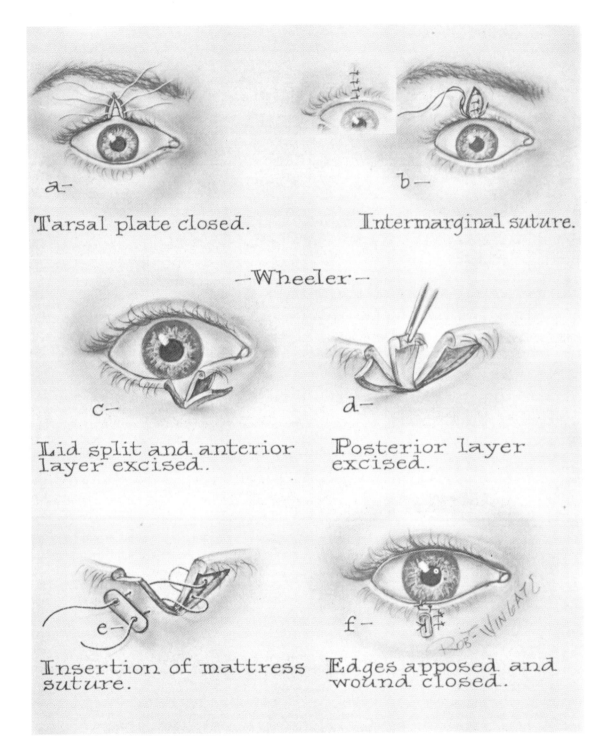

a—

Tarsal plate closed.

b—

Intermarginal suture.

—Wheeler—

c—

Lid split and anterior layer excised.

d—

Posterior layer excised.

e—

Insertion of mattress suture.

f—

Edges apposed and wound closed.

Figure 1. Repair of a simple lid laceration. (Berens and King: An Atlas of Ophthalmic Surgery. Philadelphia, J. B. Lippincott Co., 1961.)

Lid Lacerations

The closure of simple lid lacerations represents no particular problem for the surgeon accustomed to working on the face. Lacerations parallel to the margin of the lid lie in the normal skin folds and heal extremely well. It is important to remember when dealing with lacerations of this type which involve the upper lid that the levator of the lid inserts into the tarsal plate about 1 cm. above the lid margin. A through-and-through laceration in this area will disinsert the levator. Unless it is resutured to the tarsus, a permanent ptosis or drooped eyelid will result.

Lacerations which are perpendicular to the lid margins and which involve the margin itself require a bit more care in their closure. Since there is a normal and natural tendency for scar tissue to contract, such a laceration may lead to a notch's being formed in the lid margin. Even when these are quite small, they are cosmetically quite noticeable. Successful management of these lacerations depends upon extremely careful closure of the eyelid in two layers. A deep layer, which includes the conjunctiva and tarsal plate, must be closed separately from the overlying skin and orbicularis muscle (Fig. 1). If the wound edges have been crushed or are dirty, they should be debrided prior to attempting any closure.

Lacerations which involve the medial canthal area may sever either the upper or lower lacrimal canaliculus. Failure to recognize and to repair such an injury will lead to persistent tearing. Since the lower canaliculus drains 80 to 90 per cent of the total lacrimal gland secretion, repair of a severed lower duct is particularly important. Reapproximation of a severed canaliculus is difficult even in an ideal case and should be performed at the time of the original injury. Several different techniques have been described, but all utilize some sort of stent to maintain the continuity of the sutured ends of the canaliculus. Such a stent is generally left in place for at least six weeks following surgical repair (Fig. 2).

Conjunctival Injuries

Small conjunctival scratches and lacerations are often seen in facial trauma. When such an injury lies within 5 mm. of the limbus it does not expose an underlying extraocular muscle and requires no suturing. When examining conjunctival lacerations it is important to remember that the medial rectus inserts approximately 5 mm. from the limbus; the inferior rectus inserts at approximately 6 mm.; the lateral is found 7 mm. from the limbus; and the superior rectus, 8 mm. The tendon of each of these extraocular muscles is about 1 cm. wide. More extensive conjunctival lacerations, particularly if they involve the areas of insertion of the recti muscles, ought to be sutured.

Some of the worst ocular injuries occur from chemical burns of the cornea and conjunctiva, especially when by strong acids and alkalies. In automobile accidents involving foreign made cars in which the battery is carried within the passenger compartment, sulfuric acid burns of the skin and eyes are frequently seen. Whenever a patient complains of getting some irritating and possible caustic chemical into his eye, prompt and copious irrigation may make the difference between vision in the weeks or months to come. If contamination with an acid or alkali is even remotely possible, steps should be carried out immediately to irrigate the eye and no time wasted trying to determine

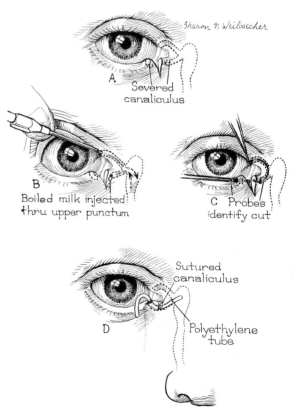

Figure 2. In all medial lid lacerations, canaliculus damage should be suspected. Techniques of identifying transected ends of lacrimal canaliculi are shown in B and C; one method of repair is shown in D. (Paton, D., and Goldberg, M. F.: Injuries of the Eye, the Lids and the Orbit.)

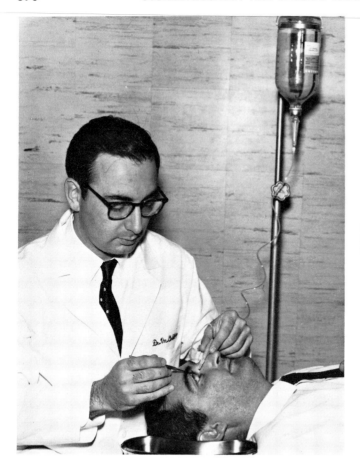

Figure 3. Technique for copious irrigation of the eye. Note the use of a lid retractor. (Paton, D., and Goldberg, M. F.: Injuries of the Eye, the Lids and the Orbit.)

which chemical is the contaminant. In order to overcome the blepharospasm which is always present, some form of topical anesthetic should be applied. With the aid of a lid speculum and a standard intravenous setup (Fig. 3), irrigation should be continued until a minimum of 2 L. of fluid has been used. An isotonic solution is best for such irrigation, since the cornea is normally bathed by tears which are somewhat hypertonic. However, in the event that only distilled water or tapwater is available, it is better to use one of these than to delay the irrigation. Even with prompt and copious irrigation, both acid and alkali burns tend to form adhesions between the lids and to produce marked corneal scarring (Fig. 4).

Extraocular Muscles

Unless the trauma to the orbit is extremely severe, laceration of an extraocular muscle practically never occurs. More often an extraocular muscle is injured either by contusion to the muscle directly or to its nerve supply. The resulting paresis of any of the extraocular muscles leads to diplopia. This may well be masked if the eyelid is either swollen shut or if injury to the levator palpebrae muscle prevents raising the upper lid. As part of the examination of an injured patient, the eyelids should be opened and the patient questioned regarding double vision. When diplopia is pres-

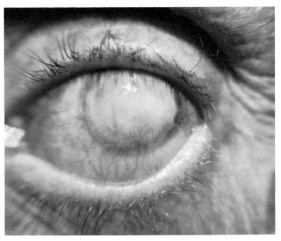

Figure 4. Old alkali burn of the cornea.

ent, the involved extraocular muscle can be easily determined. First the patient is asked whether the separation of images occurs only in the horizontal direction. If this is the case, the medial or lateral recti are incriminated. When any of the vertical extraocular muscles are involved, there is usually a combination of vertical and horizontal displacement of the diplopia images. The extraocular muscles are so arranged that a pair of them (one from each eye) is primarily responsible for rotation of the eyes into each of the six cardinal directions of gaze. The six cardinal directions of gaze and the muscles responsible for rotating the eye into each of these positions are listed in table form below:

Cardinal Direction	Muscles Responsible
1. Eyes right	Right lateral rectus and left medial rectus
2. Eyes left	Right medial rectus and left lateral rectus
3. Eyes up right	Right superior rectus and left inferior oblique
4. Eyes down right	Right inferior rectus and left superior oblique
5. Eyes up left	Right inferior oblique and left superior rectus
6. Eyes down left	Right superior oblique and left inferior rectus

Since these pairs of muscles are the only ones responsible for the coordinate binocular excursion of the eyes into each of the six cardinal directions of gaze, a paralysis of any one of them will lead to maximum diplopia in that field of gaze. Instructing the patient to look into each of the cardinal directions of gaze and to report in which area the separation of images is greatest will lead to the diagnosis of a pair of muscles, one of which has to be responsible for the diplopia. In the case of trauma it is usually easy to determine which eye is involved. When it is not immediately obvious which is the lagging eye and which, therefore, has the paretic muscle, an examining physician should cover one eye and see which image disappears. Because of the reversal of the retinal image, the lagging eye sees the more peripheral image.

An orbital fracture, particularly one which involves the floor of the orbit, may permit herniation of some of the retrobulbar fat and extraocular muscles. These may become trapped in the fracture site. This is often seen in the so-called blowout fracture of the orbital floor. Such a patient will have difficulty in looking up, not because there is paralysis of the elevators of the eye but because there is trapping of the inferior oblique and inferior rectus. In or-

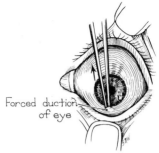

Figure 5. *A* The forced duction test. Under topical anesthesia the limbal conjunctiva and Tenon's capsule are firmly grasped with a toothed forceps and are tugged superiorly. Resistance to this supraduction is often encountered when orbital tissue is incarcerated in a blowout fracture of the orbital floor. (Paton, D., and Goldberg, M. F.: Injuries of the Eye, the Lids and the Orbit.)

der to differentiate true paralysis from that which results from trapping, it is necessary to perform a forced duction test. This may be done in some cooperative patients under topical anesthesia, but it can always be done in a patient under general anesthesia. The globe is grasped adjacent to the limbus with small toothed forceps and is rotated up, down, in, and out. Under normal circumstances no restriction or limitation or motion is encountered (Fig. 5). If there is trapping of any of the extraocular muscles, the amount of forced duction possible will be limited. Muscles which have been trapped need to be freed promptly in order to minimize the amount of scarring which may occur and which may lead to permanent diplopia. In the case of contusion injuries the prognosis for return of normal muscle function is usually excellent, although it may require six months.

Corneal Scleral Lacerations

These injuries carry a grave prognosis for vision, not so much because of the injury to the cornea or sclera, but because of the injury to the underlying iris, lens, vitreous, and retina. When these structures are not damaged, there can be very dramatic and excellent visual results obtained from suturing corneal-scleral lacerations. In order to obtain the best results, suture placement in the cornea is critical. If the suture passes through the full thickness of the cornea it will act as a wick and allow aqueous to leak back out of the anterior chamber. This may cause a delay in the reformation of the anterior chamber of the eye. The risk of infection also increases because bacteria may travel in a retrograde fashion along the suture tract into the eye. It is also extremely important to place the suture at the same depth on both sides of a corneal wound. If this is not done properly, one edge of the corneal wound will ride higher than the other. This will cause a marked amount of astigmatism, which often is not correctable with ordinary spectacle lenses. Most ophthalmic surgeons today prefer to use 10-0 or smaller suture material and to repair corneal lacerations with the use of an operating microscope in order to insure the most accurate placement of these sutures.

Intraocular Hemorrhages

Blunt trauma not leading to perforation may cause hemorrhage in the anterior chamber, which is called hyphema. Blood in the anterior chamber generally absorbs without incident. Occasionally it may block the trabecular meshwork in the angle of the anterior chamber and cause a secondary glaucoma. For this reason, patients with hyphema are generally hospitalized for observation. When glaucoma does develop, it is necessary to irrigate the blood out of the anterior chamber. With more extensive injury there may be bleeding back into the vitreous humor. This carries a more serious prognosis because blood absorbs much more slowly from the vitreous. As it does absorb it may lead to the development of contraction bands in the vitreous which can subsequently detach the retina. Retinal hemorrhages of all varieties may occur in cases of blunt trauma to an eye (Fig. 6).

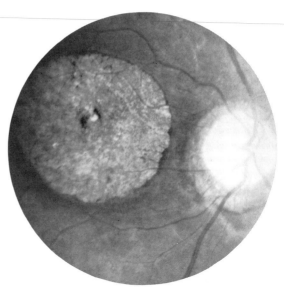

Figure 7.   Macular hole resulting from blunt ocular trauma.

Macular Edema

Macular edema is another retinal complication of blunt trauma to an eye. This is caused by a shock wave which is transmitted from the front of the eye to its posterior pole via the fluid media of the intraocular contents. Whenever present, macular edema produces a profound loss of vision. This edema results in a very subtle increase in the retinal sheen in the macular area. Unless the examining physician is familiar with these subtle changes, the patient's complaints will seem out of proportion to the apparent injury. As the macular edema subsides, the retina may atrophy, producing a macular hole and permanent visual loss (Fig. 7). There is no satisfactory treatment for this particular condition, although there are reports that systemic steroids may be somewhat helpful in preventing degeneration from occurring following an episode of macular edema.

Choroidal Rupture

The same mechanism that produces the edema discussed previously may also cause a rupture in the underlying choroid. The retina is relatively elastic and withstands a shock wave transmitted through the fluid media of the eye. However, the underlying choroid is much less elastic and, when stretched, will break. Such breaks or tears are generally crescent-shaped, with the concave side pointed toward the disc.

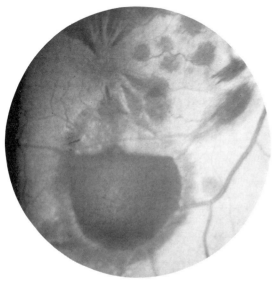

Figure 6. Retinal hemorrhage as a result of blunt injury to the globe.

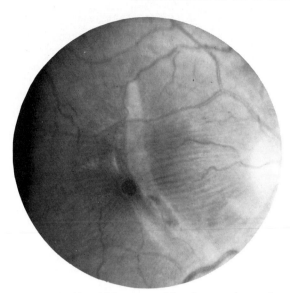

Figure 8. Choroidal tear resulting from ocular contusion injury.

When they lie outside the macula area there is little or no effect on vision. Unfortunately a large percentage of them tend to occur within the macula itself (Fig. 8). Since the rods and cones depend for their blood supply upon the capillaries of the underlying choroid, its rupture will lead to death and atrophy of the involved visual receptors of the retina. Immediately after a choroidal break has occurred it is filled with bright red blood, which may be the same color as the surrounding choroid. For this reason it may go unrecognized for several days. With the passage of time the blood in this torn area will become clotted and deoxygenated. The crescent will then become dark brown or even black in appearance. Even later the blood elements will be resorbed, leaving a pale yellow or white crescent in the area where the choroid is totally absent. Again, there is no known treatment, but such fundal disease should be looked for whenever one is dealing with patients with facial trauma.

Optic Nerve

The orbital area of the optic nerve is almost never injured, even with extensive facial trauma. The section of the optic nerve which passes through the optic foramen is very firmly fixed by its meningeal covering to the periosteum of the foramen. With head and neck trauma, especially when there has been a basal skull fracture, there may be tearing of or hemorrhage into the optic nerve at the foramen.

Such an injury leads to a prompt and profound decrease in visual acuity and has a very poor prognosis for the return of any vision. Since the optic foramen lies well behind the entrance of the central retinal artery and vein into the nerve, there is no immediately visible funduscopic change. Whenever a patient who has sustained head or neck injury complains of profound loss of vision without any significant ophthalmic findings, one must suspect that there has been damage to the optic nerve. Within a matter of two or three weeks the optic nerve will show increasing pallor as a result of the retrograde degeneration of its nerve fibers; within months these nerve heads will become white and atrophic. The optic nerve is similar to tracts of the central nervous system and shows no regeneration following such an injury.

In cases of skull fracture in which the diagnosis of a subdural hematoma is being entertained, an ophthalmologist is frequently consulted to determine the presence of papilledema. Some recent work has been done using balloons implanted in monkey skulls in order to produce rapid increases in intracranial pressures. These studies indicate that 12 to 24 hours must elapse from the onset of increased intracranial pressure before papilledema becomes obvious ophthalmoloscopically; therefore, it is to be regarded as a late sign of developing subdural hematoma, but its absence most definitely does not rule out the possibility of increasing intracranial pressure.

LACRIMAL SYSTEM

Because the lacrimal duct connects the eye with the nose, this system is of interest to the otolaryngologist as well as the ophthalmologist.

Lacrimal Gland

The lacrimal gland is located in the upper outer quadrant of the orbit just behind the supraorbital ridge in a fossa of the frontal bone. The tears are secreted from this gland into the upper fornix of the conjunctiva through 17 or more separate openings. The gland does not begin to secrete tears until ten days to two weeks after birth. It is for that reason that children with obstruction of the nasal lacrimal duct generally do not develop symptoms until two weeks of age or older. The lacrimal gland is parasympathetically innervated. Infections and tumors of the lacrimal gland are exceedingly rare. Occasionally in a child dacryoadenitis may be seen accompanying measles, mumps, or influenza. Dacryoadenitis almost never occurs in an adult. In his book on tumors of the eye, Reese (1963) has published 115 consecutive cases of expanding lesions in the lacrimal gland fossa. These are listed in the table at the bottom of this page.

It can be seen from this table that approximately 50 per cent of the lesions of the lacrimal gland fossa do not require surgical therapy. In the case of the benign mixed tumors, dermoids, and adenomas, simple excision is sufficient. In primary malignant tumors of the lacrimal gland, exenteration of the orbital contents is indicated. In addition, in malignant disease, the lacrimal fossa and the frontal bones surrounding it are also removed even if there is no gross or x-ray evidence of bony involvement. This makes it extremely important to know the tissue diagnosis of a lacrimal gland tumor prior to definitive surgery. On the other hand, cutting into an encapsulated tumor mass which may be malignant and running the risk of spreading the malignant cells is seldom wise surgical policy. Perhaps the best compromise is to remove the gland in toto if the expanding lesion is relatively confined to the lacrimal fossa and then to plan more definitive surgery, if necessary, after obtaining adequate histologic diagnosis. If an extremely large tumor has spread well beyond the lacrimal fossa, a small biopsy may be taken and then definitive surgery planned.

The tears pass normally from the superior temporal fornix down across the cornea by a combination of gravity and by the blink action of the lid. Continuous tear production and blinking are necessary in order to prevent the cornea from drying out. When there is deficient tear production, as in Sjögren's syndrome or when the blink reflex is interfered with as in Bell's palsy, care must be taken to prevent drying of the cornea. When the cornea does become dry, the epithelium becomes sticky and will be abraided when the eyelids do close over the dry area. Once the integrity of the corneal epithelium has been interfered with there is a much greater likelihood of the development of a bacterial corneal ulcer. This will result in a permanent corneal scar and could possibly lead to the complete destruction of an eye. The exposure and drying of a cornea always begins in the inferior part of the cornea toward six o'clock. For this reason, this is the area of the eye to examine most closely whenever one is dealing with a patient with Bell's palsy. Should injection begin to develop in this area, it can often be eliminated and the exposure controlled simply by using some kind of artificial tear such as 0.5 per cent methylcellulose drops. Should this not suffice, and particularly should the Bell's palsy become permanent, thought must be given to suturing the eyelids together. Sometimes producing a small adhesion at the lateral canthus, which is called a lateral tarsorrhaphy, will suffice. At other times more extensive intramarginal adhesions of the eyelid are necessary (Fig. 9).

Nasolacrimal Duct

Although some differences of opinion exist as to the exact development of the nasolacrimal duct embryologically, it is agreed that it begins as a solid cord of cells which subsequently canalize. This canalization generally is complete at birth or soon afterward. By two weeks of age, when an infant begins to manufacture tears, the duct is generally capable of handling them. Each time the orbicularis muscle closes the eyelids, pressure is applied on the nasolacrimal sac. This forces tears downward toward the nose and empties the sac. With relaxation of the blink, a slight amount of negative pressure is created in the sac. This sucks additional tears into the punctum and sac. Under normal circumstances the tear sac is empty of tears, and pressure over the lacrimal fossa will not cause any significant retrograde flow of tears through the canaliculi and out of the puncta.

If a part of the nasolacrimal duct fails to develop its normal patency, a child will begin to tear excessively from the involved eye some time after two weeks of age. The majority of these congenital obstructions are found distal to the nasolacrimal sac. In these children, pressure over the sack will cause mucus and tears to flow back out of the superior and inferior puncta. In time the blocked tear secretions will

Granuloma	31		(26%)
Nonspecific dacryoadenitis		26	
Sarcoid		5	
Malignant lymphoma	28		(25%)
Carcinoma	27		(24%)
Mixed tumor	25		(21%)
Dermoid cyst	2		(2%)
Adenomas	2		(2%)
Total	115		

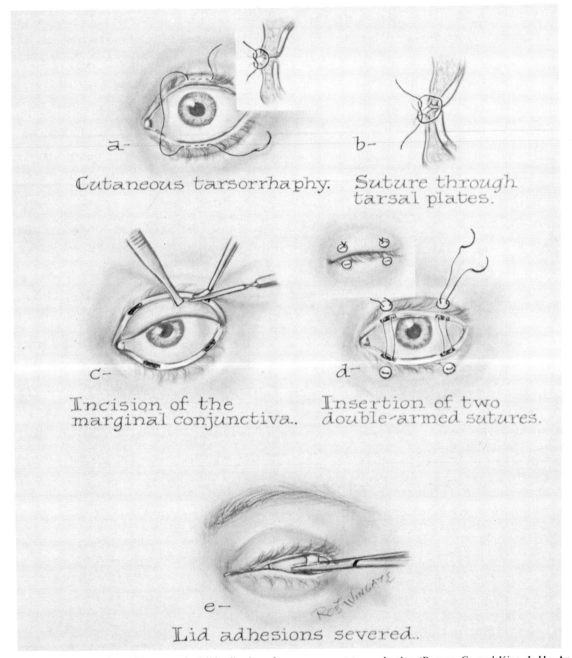

Figure 9.   Formation of intramarginal lid adhesions for a permanent tarsorrhaphy. (Berens, C., and King, J. H.: An Atlas of Ophthalmic Surgery. Philadelphia, J. B. Lippincott, 1961.)

become infected. Such infection will produce further scarring and contraction of the duct.

Since a great many of these obstructions will open spontaneously if given sufficient time, the initial therapy for infantile obstruction of the tear duct consists of the use of a topical antibiotic combined with massage of the lacrimal fossa in order to keep the tear sac emptied of secretion as much of the time as possible. Should the duct fail to open after two weeks of this sort of conservative treatment, probing should be carried out under general anesthesia. Although somewhat hazardous in a small infant, general anesthesia is justified in order to prevent making false passages with the probes. Another advantage of general anesthesia is that with an infant perfectly still it is much easier to determine the exact level at which the obstruction occurs. Following induction of satisfactory anesthesia, the punctum must be dilated slightly in order to accept even the smallest Bowman probe. After dilatation of the

punctum, the Bowman probe is introduced into the punctum opening. It is passed directly inferiorly for a distance of 1 to 2 mm. and then turned at a right angle and passed horizontally toward the nose. If the canaliculus is patent, the probe will slip easily over into the sac, and the tip of the probe can be felt resting against the lacrimal bone. When the lacrimal bone has thus been encountered, the probe is rotated once again into the vertical position and passed down the duct into the nose (Fig. 10). Approximately 90 per cent of infants with nasolacrimal obstruction are cured with a single probing. Those which do not respond to a first probing should have the benefit of a second one, because approximately half of those not cured by a first probing will be by a second. The remaining patients will have to have a dacryocystorhinostomy.

Acute dacryocystitis is rarely seen in adults. When it occurs spontaneously it is more common in females and is generally the result of

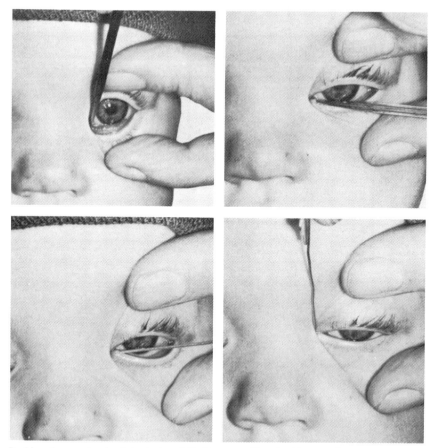

Figure 10.   Probing the nasolacrimal duct. *A* and *B*, Punctum dilated with a regular punctum dilator. *C*, Bowman's probe (usually No. 1 size) passed downward for 2 mm., then rotated into horizontal position and passed medially. *D*, When contact is made with nasal bone, upper end of probe is rotated into vertical position, so that lower end of probe is directed toward first molar tooth. (The Eye in Childhood. Chicago, Year Book Medical Publishers, 1967.)

infection by Streptothrix. The other common cause in adults is obstruction of the tear duct secondary to facial fractures. Such patients nearly always require a dacryocystorhinostomy in order to be rid of the persistent tearing.

Dacryocrystorhinostomy

There are many variations of this surgical procedure (Fig. 11). Basically it consists of making a curvilinear incision over the infraorbital rim beginning at the lower end of the medial canthal ligament and extending the incision for at least 15 to 20 mm. Bleeding in this area is generally brisk, particularly when the angular vein or its large branches are interrupted. These vessels are clamped and tied or cauterized by diathermy. As the orbital rim is encountered, the periosteum is incised and with periosteum elevators is raised off the anterior lacrimal crest and removed from the lacrimal fossa. This serves to displace the lacrimal sac laterally. A Bowman probe is then introduced through the lower caniculus and is used to indent the lacrimal sac from within. An osteotomy is made in the lacrimal bone opposite the area where the probe presents on the medial wall of the sac. This bony window may be made with either a circular Stryker saw or with a bone chisel and Kerrison forceps. Care is taken when enlarging the bony window not to destroy the underlying nasal mucosa. Vertical incisions are made in the nasal mucosa and in the medial wall of the lacrimal sac. The top and bottom of these incisions are extended in order to provide posterior and anterior flaps of lacrimal sac and nasal mucosa.

An attempt is then made to suture separately both the posterior and anterior flaps in order to provide continuity between the medial wall of the sac and the nasal mucosa. Generally this proves more difficult than most drawings on the subject would suggest. An alternative method of establishing continuity between the sac and the nose is to place a small piece of rubber tubing such as a small diameter French catheter from the sac down into the nose. The end of the tubing resting in the sac can be secured by a suture which passes through the upper fundus of the sac and out onto the skin. This suture is tied over a button and can be freed postoperatively when it is desired to remove the rubber stent. The end of the rubber tubing which passes down into the nose can also be secured to a long piece of heavy silk suture which can be brought out through the nose and

used subsequently to extract the tubing once it has been freed from above. There is generally more success in closing the anterior than the posterior flaps of this anastomosis. Following this the subcutaneous tissue is reapproximated with buried catgut sutures. The skin is then closed separately, and a pressure dressing is applied over the wound. In the postoperative care of such patients, early irrigation of the dacryocystorhinostomy is extremely important. If this is not done, the blood clots which fill the sac and bony ostium may provide a matrix into which scar tissue and eventually new bone will grow.

TUMORS

As the otolaryngologist becomes more and more interested in head and neck tumors he will of necessity have to consider those of the eye and the orbit. Fortunately intraocular tumors are generally diagnosed while they are still confined within the globe, and simple enucleation suffices for the treatment of them.

Intraocular Tumors

The commonest intraocular tumor found in children is the retinoblastoma. This is a particularly interesting tumor because of its potential for genetic transmission. The first retinoblastoma within any family occurs as a spontaneous mutation in an autosomal chromosome. Enucleation, which sometimes must be bilateral, plus radiation has produced enough cures from this tumor that we are now seeing second and third generations with this disorder. The mutation which causes the tumor is unfortunately passed along in an autosomal dominant fasion; therefore, 50 per cent of the offspring of a patient who has had a retinoblastoma cure can be expected to have the tumor. Early in its growth this tumor tends to extend locally through the retina and optic nerve. By this pathway it may reach the orbit and central nervous system. When it does metastasize it spreads preferentially to the skull and other bones.

The commonest intracular tumor in adults is malignant melanoma of the choroid. Like melanoma elsewhere it tends to metastasize early to widely scattered areas of the body. Fortunately ocular symptoms also occur early. If the eye is removed while the tumor is still small, the chance of a cure is much better than when a large lesion fills the entire globe. Un-

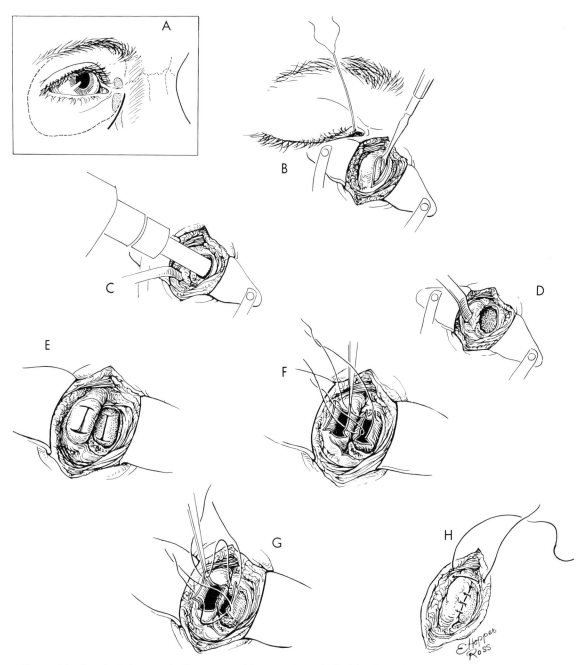

Figure 11.   Lacrimal duct repair (dacryocystorhinostomy). *A*, An incision is made 6 – mm. medial to, and extending down over, the orbital rim for 20 mm. Lacrimal probe is passed through the upper canaliculus into the sac to aid in identification. *B*, Periosteum is incised along the anterior lacrimal crest and pushed laterally with the sac. *C*, A window is made through the lacrimal bone and crest with the Iliff trephine and Stryker saw. *D*, The nasal mucosa is seen through the hole in the bone. *E*, I-shaped incisions are made in the sac and nasal mucosa. *F*, The posterior flaps are sutured together with two or three interrupted 4-0 chromic catgut sutures. *G*, The anterior flaps are sutured together. *H*, The subcutaneous tissues are approximated with two or three interrupted plain catgut sutures and the skin wound closed with Dermalon. (The Eye in Childhood. Chicago, Year Book Medical Publishers, 1967.) Page 142.

fortunately, however, even very small choroidal melanomas have been found extending through the sclera along vessels.

The treatment of both these tumors consists of removing the eye while the tumor remains within it. Efforts to produce cures from these tumors need to be directed to their early diagnosis. In nearly all cases the tumors are easily seen ophthalmologically through a widely dilated pupil.

Orbital Tumors

Orbital tumors most commonly present by causing exophthalmos or forward displacement of an eye. The amount of displacement and its direction depend upon where the tumor originates. Very small tumors in the muscle cone will cause pressure directly forward on the globe and produce exophthalmos. Tumors which lie anterior to the equator of the globe may cause eccentricity of the eye and fullness of an eyelid long before there is actual forward displacement of the eye itself.

Several things must be kept in mind when making a diagnosis of exophthalmos. First, there may be a rather marked asymmetry of the bony orbits bilaterally. This may give the appearance of exophthalmos when it is really not present. If such bony asymmetry is not obvious externally, it should show on careful x-ray examination of the orbits. Myopia or nearsightedness, particularly of the axial type in which there is an overall elongation of the eye, may give the appearance of unilateral exophthalmos. This can easily be determined by refraction of the eyes. Since all the recti muscles are retractors of the globe, paralysis of one or more of these extraocular muscles may allow some forward displacement of the globe when there is actually no tumor present within the orbit. It is important, therefore, to determine that all the extraocular muscles are intact and functioning before considering minimal exophthalmos to be tumor produced. Finally, it should never be forgotten that the commonest cause of exophthalmos, whether unilateral or bilateral, is thyroid in origin, and the differential diagnosis of exophthalmos must include this entity.

The ten most common causes of exophthalmos, in order of their frequency, are thyroid, hemangioma, malignant lymphoma, chronic granulomas (pseudotumor), lacrimal gland tumor, meningioma, lymphangioma, glioma of the optic nerve, metastatic malignant tumors, and peripheral nerve tumors.

X-rays provide the most help in the diagnosis of an expanding orbital lesion. Calcium deposition or bone formation is seen in osteomas and occasionally in the wall of a mucocele. Phleboliths are sometimes seen in cavernous hemangiomas. Bony erosion or destruction is generally seen in sinusal as well as in metastatic carcinomas. Lacrimal gland tumors, multiple myeloma, and the histiocytoses are all associated with erosion of the orbital bones. A unilateral enlargement of the optic foramen is diagnostic of a tumor of that nerve. Most commonly this turns out to be a glioma. Orbital air injection helps in outlining a tumor mass, but will not be diagnostic of the tumor type.

With very large orbital tumors, biopsy serves to provide a specific diagnosis. Smaller tumors may be removed through the lateral wall of the orbit by a Krönlein approach.

Nasopharyngeal Tumors

Approximately one third of primary tumors arising in the nasopharynx will produce ocular signs or symptoms at some time. Such tumors reach the orbit by extention through the foramen lacerum. From there they extend along the internal carotid artery to the superior orbital fissure. As they extend into the orbit they may cause exophthalmos or a paralysis of any of the extraocular muscles. In addition, they may cause pressure on the optic nerve, resulting in decrease in vision or the visual field. Since the primary site is difficult to examine, the patient may concult an ophthalmologist initially because of the eye symptoms rather than because of any nasopharyngeal symptoms. Sinus neoplasms also produce exophthalmos by direct extention into the orbit. The antrum has been the commonest primary site of such tumors in several reported series.

MISCELLANEOUS OPHTHALMOLOGIC CONDITIONS OF INTEREST TO THE OTOLARYNGOLOGIST

Glaucoma

Glaucoma is a disease that affects approximately 2 per cent of the population over the age of 40. It is characterized by an increase in the normal intraocular pressure. In a normal eye there is a constant production of aqueous humor by the ciliary body epithelial processes. Aqueous humor then percolates between the border of the pupil and the lens into the anterior chamber. From there it drains to the angle between the root of the iris and the anterior surface of the cornea. In this angle it travels through the trabecular meshwork which separates the anterior chamber from the canal of Schlemm. From the canal of Schlemm aqueous drains via collector channels into the episcleral veins. The regulation between the production of aqueous and its outflow from the eye maintains a normal intraocular pressure of approximately 20 mm. of mercury. Pressures above this level, particularly for any length of time, are associated with progressive cupping of the optic nerve head and loss of visual field. The vast majority of patients with glaucoma have glaucoma of the open angle type. This disease presents with an insidious slow onset and little in the way of visual symptoms. By the time the patient is aware of visual field loss there has already been extensive damage to the eye. The treatment for this particular disease is medical. The intraocular pressure is lowered by the use of miotic drugs such as pilocarpine. In addition, acetazolamide (Diamox) is used to reduce by almost 50 per cent the production of aqueous humor, and epinephrine topical drops are used both to reduce the production of aqueous and to increase its outflow from the eye. The patient with open angle glaucoma has adequate space between his iris and cornea to allow for dilatation of his pupil without an increase in intraocular pressure.

Narrow angle glaucoma results when the root of the iris forms a very narrow angle with the back of the cornea. In such a patient, moderate dilatation of the pupil may cause the iris to roll up into the angle and cause mechanical obstruction of the trabecular meshwork and a sudden dramatic rise in intraocular pressure. This sudden increase in intraocular pressure is accompanied by pain, blurred vision, and marked injection of the eye. The treatment of this particular condition is surgical and the intraocular pressure is normalized following the production of a peripheral iridectomy. Since this disease occurs when the pupil dilates slightly, it often occurs after the patient has been watching a long movie in a dark theater or some similar activity in subdued lighting. It may also come on at a time of severe emotional crisis, and often occurs during hospitalization for some other reason. It must enter into the differential diagnosis of any red painful eye with blurred vision.

The ophthalmologist is frequently asked whether a patient with open angle glaucoma can safely be given atropine or some similar parasympathetic blocker. The answer is that as long as the patient continues his antiglaucomatous medication he should be able to tolerate easily any normal preoperative dose of atrophine or related drug.

REFERENCES

Berens, C., and King, J. H.: An Atlas of Ophthalmic Surgery. Philadelphia, J. B. Lippincott Company, 1961.

Fasanella, R. M. (Ed.): Management of Complications of Eye Surgery. Philadelphia, W. B. Saunders Company, 1957.

Hartmann, E., and Gilles, E.: Roentgenologic Diagnosis in Ophthalmology. (G. Z. Carter, (trans.); C. Berens, (ed.). Philadelphia, J. B. Lippincott Company, 1959.

Hogan, M. J., and Zimmerman, L. E.: Ophthalmic Pathology. 2nd ed. Philadelphia, W. B. Saunders Company, 1962.

Paton, D., and Goldberg, M. F.: Injuries of the Eye, the Lids, and the Orbit. Philadelphia, W. B. Saunders Company, 1968.

Reese, A. B.: Tumors of the Eye. 2nd ed. New York, Hoeber Medical Division, Harper and Row, 1963.

Vaughn, D., Cook, R., and Asbury, T.: General Ophthalmology. 5th ed. Los Altos, Calif., Lange Medical Publications, 1968.

The Ophthalmologic Staff of The Hospital for Sick Children, Toronto: The Eye in Childhood. Chicago, Year Book Medical Publishers, Inc., 1967.

Chapter 37

AEROSPACE MEDICINE

By Kent Gillingham, M.D.

In addition to the upper respiratory infections and other otolaryngologic diseases of mundane origin that a flight surgeon sees, he is regularly required to evaluate, treat, and prevent conditions arising in the domain of the otolaryngologist that are directly caused by the hostile environment of aerospace. By far the most prevalent and troublesome of those conditions are the ones caused by (1) extensive changes in atmospheric pressure, and (2) abnormal static and kinetic environments.

PATHOLOGIC CONDITIONS RELATED TO CHANGES IN ATMOSPHERIC PRESSURE

Boyle's Law

At constant temperature the volume, V, of a given mass of gas is inversely proportional to the pressure, P, or:

$$PV = a \text{ constant.}$$

This equation, known as Boyle's Law, declares

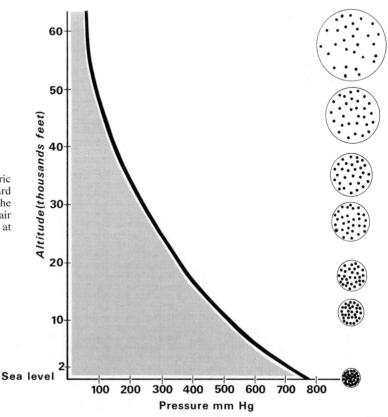

Figure 1. Relationship of barometric pressure to altitude (U. S. Standard Atmosphere, 1962). At the right are the relative volumes that a given mass of air at constant temperature would occupy at various altitudes.

that if one decreases the pressure on a gas without changing its temperature, the gas will expand; and if one increases the pressure, the gas will contract.

In Figure 1 standard barometric pressure is plotted on the horizontal axis, while altitude, from sea level to 60,000 feet, is plotted vertically. At 18,000 feet, which is at one half of an atmosphere (380 mm. Hg) of pressure, the same number of particles of air that would occupy 1 L. at sea level will occupy 2 L., providing the temperature of the air is kept at, for example,

body temperature. Conversely, a quantity of air that was 2 L. at 18,000 feet would be one 1 L. at sea level. Incidentally, Figure 1 also shows that the absolute rate of change of atmospheric pressure is greater at the lower altitudes: the pressure drops about 150 mm. Hg as we ascend from sea level to 6000 feet; but from 20,000 feet, we must ascend to over 32,000 feet to establish a similar difference in pressure.

Figure 2 depicts what normally happens to the air in a rigid or semirigid body cavity that communicates with the environment, during as-

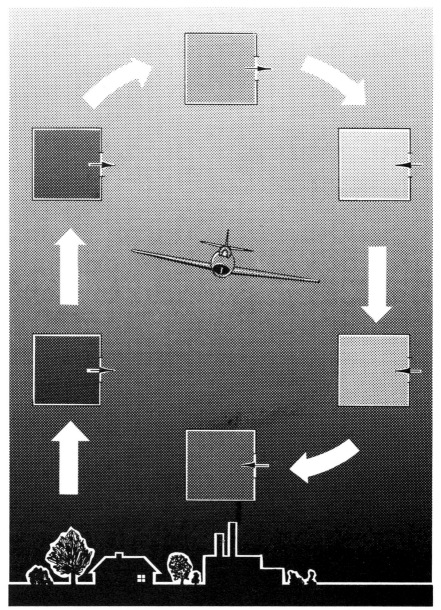

Figure 2.   Mechanism of equalization of barometric pressures between the inside and outside of a rigid body cavity communicating with the atmosphere. During ascent, air moves out of the cavity; during descent, it re-enters.

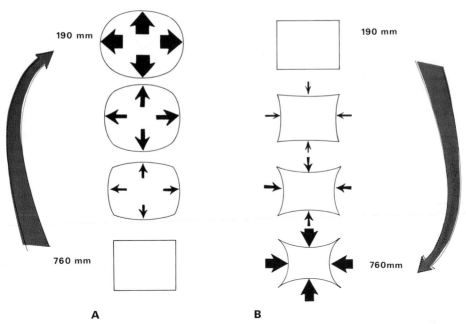

Figure 3. Mechanism of acute barotrauma to the walls of a body cavity having less than continuous communication with the outside atmosphere: *A*, barotrauma on ascent; *B*, on descent.

cent and descent through the atmosphere. As we ascend, the air expands and leaves the cavity, so that the pressure within the cavity comes to equal that of the surrounding atmosphere. During descent, the atmospheric air enters the cavity until equality of internal and external pressures is again established.

Suppose, however, that free passage of air into and out of the cavity is for one reason or another impossible. Figure 3 *a* shows what would happen if a noncommunicating body cavity were to ascend to 34,000 feet: the pressure within the cavity would be four times the pressure without. What more frequently happens is that air is able to move out of the cavity during ascent, but because of structural complexities at the orifice, air cannot re-enter the cavity during descent. In the hypothetical situation shown in Figure 3 *b* the block occurs at 34,000 feet and results, after descent to sea level, in four times the pressure outside the cavity as in. The net difference in pressure across the walls of the cavity would be, in this extreme example, 570 mm. Hg (760 minus 190), or three fourths of an atmosphere.

Acute Barotitis Media

Acute barotitis media (acute aerotitis media, acute otitic barotrauma) is a traumatic inflammation of the middle ear caused by a difference in pressure between the middle-ear space and the surrounding atmosphere, and characterized by the symptoms of otalgia, tinnitus, deafness and, occasionally, vertigo. The true incidence of acute barotitis media is extremely difficult to assess, because symptoms are often relatively mild and tolerable, and because members of air crews tend to be reluctant to report symptoms that might cause them to be removed from flying status. King in Gillies (1965) relates that in one study 8.9 per cent of 1000 cadets examined in a decompression chamber during World War II had both subjective and objective evidence of acute barotitis media; another 32.5 per cent, however, had injected tympanic membranes, either with no symptoms or with mild symptoms relieved at once by autoinflation. Recent evidence suggests that the number of cases of severe acute barotitis media has increased, and that the increase is related to the high rate of descent commonly employed in jet aircraft.

Mechanism. The key to understanding the cause of acute barotitis media lies in an appreciation of the fact that the membranocartilaginous proximal part of the auditory (eustachian) tube acts as a "flutter" valve, allowing air to pass easily out of the middle-ear space into the nasopharynx, but collapsing when a greater pressure exists in the nasopharynx than in the middle ear. Only by muscular action, as in yawning, swallowing, or Valsalva's maneuver, can the proximal auditory tube be opened in the face of a relatively negative pressure in the middle ear, and only by such action can the negative pressure be equalized.

Now let us consider what happens in the middle ear and eustachian tube during ascent and descent. When one has ascended to about 150 feet above ground level, the pressure in the middle ear is about 5 mm. Hg above that of the surrounding atmosphere; a feeling of fullness in the ear is present and the tympanic membrane bulges slightly. At 500 feet above ground the pressure difference becomes about 15 mm. Hg, whereupon the auditory tube is forced open and air leaves the middle ear, resulting in a clicking or popping sound as the tympanic membrane returns to its normal position (Fig. 4 *a*). The auditory tube remains open until the pressure in the middle ear drops to about 4 mm. above that in the nasopharynx, and then it closes, 4 mm. not being a sufficient pressure difference to maintain the patency of the tube at lower altitudes. As ascent continues, a similar sequence of events recurs about every 500 feet, except that the pressure difference required to open and keep open the auditory tube becomes less as altitude increases. (Only 3.5 mm. Hg of pressure difference is needed to force open the tube at 35,000 feet.)

Descent is another story (Fig. 4 *b*). Because air cannot passively enter the auditory tube and middle ear from the nasopharynx when a higher pressure exists in the nasopharynx, one must voluntarily open the tube to ventilate the middle ear during descent. If this is not done, and the pressure difference between the atmosphere and the middle ear is allowed to build up, it becomes more and more difficult to open the auditory tube until, finally, it is impossible. Under that circumstance the tube is said to be "locked." It has been stated that locking occurs

when atmospheric pressure is approximately 80 to 90 mm. Hg greater than that in the middle ear, but there is considerable variability between individuals, and between events in a given individual, with respect to the value of locking pressure. Once locking has occurred, one must ascend again to an altitude at which he can actively ventilate his middle ear, or with certainty he will develop acute barotitis media. Moreover, the reader should appreciate the fact that, with a steady rate of descent, the risk of barotitis increases as altitude decreases because of the greater rates of pressure change encountered at lower altitudes.

In addition to the primary cause of barotitis–a significant change in air pressure–certain other factors seem to contribute to the development of the disease. Temporary pathologic changes in the auditory tube, such as might be caused by an upper respiratory infection or allergy, undoubtedly predispose one to an attack of barotitis media. Also, an unresolved recent attack of barotitis media can increase the likelihood of another attack. Chronic pathologic changes in the eustachian tube, tonsils, and adenoids are also supposed to increase the risk of acute barotitis media. Dental malocclusion has been suggested, but not confirmed, as a factor. Finally, preoccupation with aerial combat or some other demanding task, or just plain ignorance of the necessity and the technique for achieving autoinflation, can result in the development of acute barotitis media.

Symptoms. The onset of pain during descent may be gradual or sudden, and it may involve one or both ears. At a pressure difference of 60 mm. Hg between the atmosphere and the middle ear, the pain usually is as severe as that of acute suppurative otitis media. With further increases in differential pressure, the pain in the ear becomes more intense and radiates to structures adjacent to the involved ear. If the differential pressure exceeds a certain critical value, usually between 100 and 200 mm. Hg, the tympanic membrane ruptures; thereupon the agonizing pain subsides, leaving in its place a dull ache which may persist for several days. A conductive deafness generally accompanies the acute otalgia and persists to a varying degree until the ensuing pathologic changes in the middle ear are resolved. Perceptive deafness, tending to be a more permanent sequela to acute barotitis media, has also been reported, but the exact cause of it is not understood. Tinnitus and vertigo may accompany the acute episode of barotrauma, and tinnitus may persist beyond the acute episode in conjunction

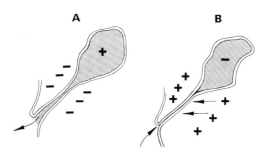

Figure 4. Middle ear, auditory tube, and nasopharynx (*A*) during ascent, and (*B*) during descent. Air cannot passively enter the middle ear when a greater pressure exists in the nasopharynx; hence, one must voluntarily open the auditory tube to ventilate the middle ear during descent.

with either a conductive or a perceptive deafness.

Signs. The common signs associated with acute barotitis media are, in order of increasing severity, retracted tympanic membrane; inflamed, congested tympanic membrane; solitary or multiple hemorrhages into the drumhead; amber-colored effusion in the middle ear, which can be noted at any time from immediately after landing to 12 hours after onset of symptoms; hemotympanum, with its characteristic bluish black appearance behind the drumhead; and, finally, rupture of the tympanic membrane, which usually occurs in the anterior portion of the pars tensa and is generally accompanied by bleeding into the external acoustic meatus.

Treatment. During the descending part of a flight, one should swallow, yawn, perform Valsalva's maneuver, or the like, as vigorously and as frequently as is necessary to insure the equalization of pressure between the middle ear and the atmospheric environment. If those measures fail after a refractory "ear block" has been recognized, reascent and a more gradual descent should be accomplished, if possible. As acute barotitis media frequently results from nasopharyngeal and tubal congestion associated with an upper respiratory infection or allergy, decongesting nasal sprays which reach the nasopharynx are often effective in opening the auditory tube when applied during or shortly after descent and can prevent the further development of barotitis. Autoinflation of the middle ear should always be tried by patients with early acute barotitis media. If this fails, politzerization should be done. If politzerization is unsuccessful, direct eustachian tube catheterization is indicated. Myringotomy should be done in the event the above measures fail, if inflammatory changes in the middle ear are marked, or if the patient presents several days after the onset of symptoms.

In addition to the foregoing, the treatment of acute barotitis media in all its degrees of severity is according to conventional otolaryngologic procedures. The relief of pain is of particular importance in this condition, and it is accomplished through the use of oral, not aural, analgesics. The treatment of predisposing diseases of the nose and nasopharynx, such as acute viral rhinitis, pharyngitis, or suppurative sinusitis, should accompany treatment of the involved ear. The average case of barotitis media will resolve in a week or ten days, after which the patient can safely fly again. If he must or strongly desires to fly sooner, intubation of the tympanic membrane is a relatively simple procedure that provides the patient's recuperating ear with a reasonable degree of safety during flight. Those few individuals in whom an acute barotitis media does not resolve quickly, or in whom recurrent bouts of barotitis are a problem, should be subjected to a thorough search for underlying chronic pathologic conditions (sinusitis, nasal polyposis, septal deviation) that are causally related to the development of barotitis media.

DELAYED BAROTITIS MEDIA

Delayed barotitis media is a condition akin to acute barotitis media in that a pressure gradient between the middle ear and the environment is the cause; and the symptoms and signs, although less severe, are similar in character. Delayed barotitis media occurs after the air crew member has breathed 100 per cent oxygen for a time and has had no significant difficulty in "clearing his ears" during descent. The victim of this condition typically has terminated his flight at night, has gone to sleep asymptomatic, and is awakened in the early morning hours with pain and a "stopped-up" feeling in one or both ears. Examination at this time will reveal retraction and hyperemia of the tympanic membrane and, possibly, serous fluid in the middle ear.

The mechanism of development of delayed barotitis media probably involves some degree of irritation of the auditory tube and its orifice as well as nasopharyngeal drying by the prolonged breathing of 100 per cent oxygen. The irritation is supposedly sufficient to prevent adequate ventilation of the middle ear during sleep (when active inflation of the middle ear is at a minimum), and aural atelectasis occurs. Of specific importance in the case of delayed barotitis media is that the absorption of the nearly pure oxygen from the middle ear is considerably faster than would be the case if air occupied the space, under the condition of a non-ventilated ear. The treatment of delayed barotitis media is not essentially different from that of acute barotitis media.

Barosinusitis

Barosinusitis (aerosinusitis, sinus barotrauma) is an acute or chronic inflammation of one or more of the paranasal sinuses, resulting from a difference in air pressure between the atmosphere and the air within the sinus cavity.

Barosinusitis of the frontal sinus is by far the most common by virtue of the length and narrowness of the nasofrontal duct. Maxillary barosinusitis is less common; and barotrauma to the ethmoid labyrinth is a rare event for obvious anatomic reasons. Referring to the relative incidence of barosinusitis, King in Gillies (1965) states that in a study of 328 patients suffering barotrauma, 250 had barotitis and 100 had barosinusitis, both conditions being present in 22 of the patients. In those patients with barosinusitis, the frontal sinus alone was involved in 70 per cent, the maxillary sinus alone was involved in 19 per cent, the frontal and maxillary sinuses together were affected in 10 per cent, and the ethmoid sinuses were affected in 1 per cent.

Mechanism. When the air within a sinus can communicate freely through its ostium into the nasal passage, the events depicted in Figure 2 occur upon ascent and descent through the atmospheric pressure gradient. When free communication does not exist, events like those shown in Figure 3 are the result; the vast majority of "sinus blocks," in fact, are associated with the conditions shown in Figure 3 b, wherein air can leave but not enter the sinus cavity. In such a case the peak absolute pressure (approximately equal to systolic blood pressure plus local barometric pressure) within the mucosa and submucosa of the sinus walls is considerably greater than the pressure (somewhat less than local barometric pressure) within the interior of the sinus. In the case of sinus barotrauma that occurs on ascent, the relatively high pressure within the interior of the blocked sinus causes ischemia of the mucosa and submucosa and thereby initiates pain. The degree of severity of the barosinusitis developed during either ascent or descent depends on the net difference in pressure between the sinus walls and the interior, and the rate at which the difference was achieved.

The actual blockage of a sinus ostium that results in barosinusitis can be caused by one or several underlying pathologic conditions of the nose and sinuses:

Developmental. Valvular folds of mucous membrane; narrow or stenotic ducts.

Traumatic. Old fractures of the maxilla, resulting in scarring of the ducts with stenosis, surgical scarring, mucocele, or pyocele.

Allergic. Edema of nasal or sinus mucosa; polyposis; drug reaction.

Infectious. Acute or chronic rhinitis, sinusitis, or nasopharyngitis (viral or bacterial); chronic specific granulomata (lethal midline granuloma, sarcoidosis, lues).

Neoplastic. Benign or malignant tumor causing obstruction.

Chemical. Rhinitis medicamentosa (topical); antihypertensive therapy; dehydration hypertrophy.

The action of a polyp or fold of swollen mucosa in the development of maxillary antral barotrauma during ascent and descent is shown diagrammatically in Figure 5. Note that the configuration of the tissue about the ostium in the two examples is such as to create a flap-valve at the ostium, permitting flow of air only into (Fig. 5 a) or out of (Fig. 5 b) the sinus. Any pathologic condition resulting in a flap- or ball-valve type of obstruction can have the same effect.

Occasionally a flyer develops delayed barosinusitis, a condition analogous to delayed barotitis media. In this condition the pain occurs several hours after a long flight during which 100 per cent oxygen has been used. It is probable that occlusion of an ostium, followed by rapid absorption of the oxygen within the cavity, is responsible for a relatively rapid decrease in pressure within the sinus, with consequent barotrauma and pain.

A point of distinction between barosinusitis and barotitis media is that, whereas the susceptibility of an air crew member or passenger to acute barotitis media is more or less inversely proportional to the amount of his flying experience, no such relation is present with respect to his susceptibility to barosinusitis. That is because with experience one learns the various techniques of voluntarily ventilating the middle ear during flight, but since one cannot voluntarily ventilate a sinus, flying experience cannot appreciably aid one in learning to avoid barosinusitis.

Symptoms and Signs. Pain is the predominant symptom, and often the only one. It is almost always severe; in fact, it can be so severe as to cause syncope. The pain is referred to the location characteristic of pain arising in the involved sinus, and the rather high incidence of frontal pain attests to the high frequency of

A 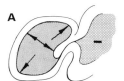 **B**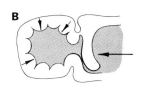

Figure 5. Mechanism of development of maxillary antral barotrauma (*A*) during ascent, or (*B*) during descent. In these examples, a flap-valve of abnormal mucosa at the ostium permits flow of air in one direction only.

barosinusitis involving the frontal sinuses. Tenderness to percussion over the affected sinus is usual and diagnostic. Lacrimation and epistaxis can be additional symptoms. A sucking noise high up in the nose has been described by some patients and is thought to be associated with submucosal hemorrhage.

Roentgenograms provide the most reliable information in the investigation of the patient's condition: there is roentgenographic evidence of pathologic changes in one or more sinuses in the majority of cases of barosinusitis; the later the study is done, the more likely it is to reveal the changes. The appearance of an air-fluid level in the affected sinus is of the greatest diagnostic significance; to demonstrate this, one must be sure to have the radiograph taken with the patient in the upright position. Finally, of course, one must be aware of the fact that the radiologic examination does not always distinguish between underlying pathologic conditions contributing to the development of barosinusitis, and changes resulting directly from the barotrauma.

Treatment. Equalization of pressure in the sinus with that of the atmosphere and relief of pain are the prime, immediate considerations in the treatment of acute barosinusitis. If conditions permit, the patient should reascend and then descend more slowly in the hope that the barotrauma will not recur with the slower rate of descent. Of absolute necessity in the treatment of barosinusitis is nasal decongestion, preferably by the application of 10 per cent cocaine on a cotton pledget directly to the ostium of the affected sinus. When such direct treatment is unavailable, the use of a decongestant nasal spray is better than no treatment. In fact, so important is nasal decongestion in the immediate treatment of barosinusitis that "flights" in decompression chambers are never taken without a readily available bottle of decongestant spray for application by the patient or chamber technician. Systemic vasoconstrictors are useful adjuncts in the management of acute barosinusitis when systemic factors have contributed to the development of the disease.

The treatment of predisposing pathologic conditions according to conventional otorhinolaryngologic practices must be accomplished in patients with a history of oft-repeated episodes of barosinusitis, and in patients with barosinusitis that does not resolve within a length of time in line with the severity of the acute injury.

To prevent the development of barosinusitis, the grounding of an air crew member with an upper respiratory infection is considered necessary during the course of his disease. If grounding is not practical in such a case, it is advisable to administer nasal decongestants prior to flight. Allergic conditions, polyps, chronic infections, septal deviation, and other conditions that might affect the patency of sinus ostia during exposure to the changing barometric pressure of flight should be corrected prior to exposure, if possible and practical.

POSTEXTRACTION MAXILLARY BAROSINUSITIS

A type of barosinusitis occurring in patients with recent extraction of maxillary posterior teeth has been described. Such a procedure often deprives of rigid support a portion of the floor of the maxillary antrum. Theoretically, at least, the decrease in atmospheric pressure during flight, coupled with compromised patency of the antral ostium and the defect in the alveolar bone, can result in herniation and perforation of the antral membrane at the extraction site. It is for this reason that patients who have recently undergone oral surgical procedures in the proximity of a maxillary antrum are cautioned not only against sneezing and blowing the nose, but also against air travel. (A far more common reason for grounding an air crew member after any dental extraction, however, is the possibility of hemorrhage from the extraction site.)

Barodontalgia

Barodontalgia (aerodontalgia) is a toothache produced by lowered barometric pressure, appearing during flight or during decompression in an altitude chamber. The only significant symptom is pain, but the pain can be sufficient to render an air crew member incapable of performing his duties.

The precise mechanism of development of barodontalgia is not known, but it is clearly evident that it is related to a pre-existing pathologic dental condition. The common concept of barodontalgia is that gas trapped in or near a defective tooth expands with exposure to the decreased barometric pressure and causes pain by compromising part of the blood supply to the tooth or by exerting direct pressure on exposed nerve endings.

Several generalities seem to bear up after three decades of experience with high-altitude military flying. One is that the offending tooth is likely to be one with a recently inserted filling. Another is that the pulp of the involved tooth is usually vital if the pain occurs during ascent; but if the pain begins during descent and persists on the ground, pulpal degeneration and periapical periodontitis are the causal factors. One should remember, however, that maxillary barosinusitis often results in pain referred to the upper premolars and molars, and that when barosinusitis develops, it is much more likely to do so during descent.

The treatment of barodontalgia is to prescribe an analgesic and provide appropriate dental care for the diseased tooth, with particular emphasis on careful clinical and radiographic diagnosis.

Alternobaric Vertigo

A true, whirling vertigo, experienced by air crew members, divers, caisson workers, and others exposed to large, rapid variations in barometric pressure, has been most recently studied by Lundgren and Malm (1966). They chose to retain the term *alternobaric vertigo* to describe the phenomenon, the term more suitably reflecting the nature of the causal events than does the more simple "pressure vertigo," also in current use. In any case, a clear distinction must be made in the reader's mind between alternobaric vertigo, caused by pressure changes, and pilot's vertigo (spatial disorientation in flight), to be discussed in the next few pages.

A typical case of alternobaric vertigo occurs during or immediately after an attempt by the victim to equalize the pressure in his middle ear by Valsalva's maneuver. He may hear a hissing sound as air suddenly enters a partially collapsed middle ear, and he then experiences a few seconds to a minute of intense whirling vertigo and ataxia. Sometimes the vertigo appears during the build-up of a pressure difference between the middle ear and the atmosphere and is terminated by the sudden equalization of pressures.

The exact causal mechanism of alternobaric vertigo is not understood. It is probably safe to assume that the effect of the changing barometric pressure is transmitted to the inner ear through the oval or round window, or both, with consequent distortion of the membranous non-auditory labyrinth in such a way as to stimulate one of the vestibular end-organs. It has been proposed by Benson (Gillies, 1966), moreover,

that in the ear of the person susceptible to alternobaric vertigo the bony wall over the lateral semicircular canal is very thin, and a condition similar to a pathologic fistula exists. However, most otologic surgeons consider such a possibility to be extremely remote. Certainly one pathologic condition is nearly always present in the involved ear of the susceptible person, and that is that the auditory tube is not normally patent and does not allow equalization of air pressure between the atmosphere and the middle ear at a normal rate. For that reason an upper respiratory infection is reasonably considered cause for grounding an air crew member, not only because the condition is conducive to the development of barotitis media and barosinusitis, but also because it could result in a fatal case of alternobaric vertigo should the attack occur in a critical phase of flight.

EFFECTS OF ABNORMAL STATIC AND KINETIC ENVIRONMENTS

Spatial Disorientation

The Problem. Spatial disorientation, or "pilot's vertigo" as it is sometimes called, is a condition in which an air crew member is unable to determine accurately his spatial attitude in relation to the surface of the earth. In other words, spatial disorientation is not knowing which way is up. The pilot who is disoriented, but is unaware of that fact and flies his aircraft accordingly, is said to have *primary spatial disorientation; secondary spatial disorientation* implies awareness of a confusion or conflict between sensory modalities subserving spatial orientation, with vacillation on the part of the pilot and, very often, subsequent deterioration of control of the aircraft. Be aware that the term "vertigo," as used by pilots, is synonymous with spatial disorientation, whereas vertigo in conventional medical usage generally refers to a sensation of rotation that is present when no such actual motion exists.

The cost of spatial disorientation is greater than one might expect. The classic figures on this subject are those of Nuttall and Sanford (1959), who studied the problem of spatial disorientation for two years in an overseas command of the U.S. Air Force during peacetime. They found that 4 per cent of all major aircraft accidents and 14 per cent of the fatal aircraft accidents in that command were caused by spatial disorientation. Current Air Force-wide estimates of the contribution of disorientation to the accident rate reveal similar percentages. The additional determination has been made that, in the Air Force, disorientation is involved in over 25 per cent of those accidents in which a physical, physiologic, or pathologic condition of the pilot is implicated as causal. The U.S. Navy has established that, from 1958 to 1966, losses of 395 Navy aircraft were ostensibly due to spatial disorientation, at an estimated cost of $150,000,000. It appears, therefore, that the problem of pilot's vertigo is a significant one from the standpoint of military economics, especially when the combined losses of all three services are estimated. Although very few data are available on the incidence of spatial disorientation in commerical air transport operations, we do know that the commonest cause of fatal general aviation accidents is "continuation of VFR (Visual Flight Rules) flight into IFR (Instrument Flight Rules) weather conditions, with subsequent loss of aircraft control"—most likely a result of disorientation.

At this point the reader should review the chapter "Vestibular Physiology" that he may fully understand the normal mechanisms of spatial orientation before undertaking to understand why those mechanisms fail in abnormal static and kinetic environments. In the follow-ing discussion the principle of visual dominance over the vestibular system must be remembered; the fact that the various vestibular illusions cannot exist when the pilot has good visual reference to the real horizon is a foregone conclusion. Only during conditions of poor visibility (IFR weather, night) or when vision is otherwise restricted (as in formation flight) can there occur vestibular illusions of a magnitude that can compromise flight safety.

Conditions Caused by Inadequacies of the Semicircular Duct System

Graveyard Spin. The graveyard spin was probably the first hazardous condition of flight recognized to be caused by a vestibular illusion. It involves (Fig. 6) the production of a sensation of spinning as the aircraft angularly accelerates into a spin, the cessation of the perception of the spin as the cupulae return to their neutral positions during the relatively constant angular velocity of the spin, the false sensation of spinning in the opposite direction during the initial phase of recovery (angular deceleration) from the spin, and the pilot's elimination of the false sensation by putting the aircraft back into an ofttimes fatal spin in the original direction. In the current age of relative sophistication on the part of pilots about the mechanisms of the vestibular illusions in flight, the graveyard spin is thought not to be the hazard it was during the

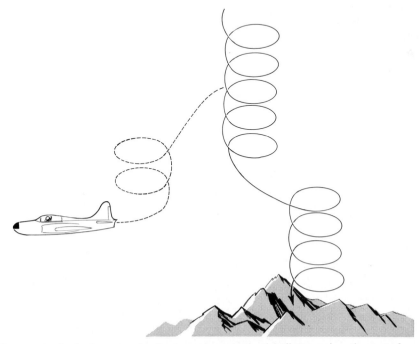

Figure 6. The graveyard spin. In recovering from a prolonged spin, the pilot perceives the start of a spin in the opposite direction. (The dotted line indicates perceived motion; the solid line shows actual motion.) Correcting for this false impression, the pilot enters another spin in the original direction.

days of the development of all-weather flight; in those days pilots failed to understand why they should not trust their own sensations, which had never lied to them before, before trusting a handful of panel instruments which, like all things mechanical, seemed always to malfunction just when they were needed the most.

Graveyard spiral. The graveyard spiral is similar to the graveyard spin in that it involves the restoration of the cupulae to their neutral positions during a protracted constant angular velocity. The difference is that, in the graveyard spiral, the aircraft is in a coordinated, banked turn, rather than in a spin. Because the net gravitoinertial force on an aircraft and its contents in a coordinated turn is always perpendicular to the floor of the aircraft (not toward the center of the earth), a novice pilot can easily become confused about the direction of the true vertical after flying for a while in a turn. As the airplane in a bank cannot maintain altitude with the same stick position and power setting used for level flight, the pilot will usually add power and pull back on the stick to make up the lost altitude. Failing to recognize that his aircraft is banked and turning, his maneuvering serves to tighten the turn, which only makes matters worse. The pilot who can be convinced by his instruments to level the wings (stop the turn) will survive; the unfortunate condition that exists, however, is that stopping the turn causes endolymph to flow and deviate the cupulae, so as to create in the pilot the perception of turning

when there is no turn. Unless the pilot ignores the false sensation of turning and brings the aircraft to a level altitude, and keeps it there long enough for the false sensation to dissipate, he will continue tightening his graveyard spiral until he either gets a visual fix on the horizon or makes abrupt contact with the ground.

Leans. The leans is by far the most common vestibular illusion in flight (Fig. 7). It consists of a very compelling impression that the aircraft is banked in one direction, even though the pilot knows he is flying with wings level. In an attempt to compensate for the false impression, the pilot often leans in the direction opposite that of the perceived bank, whence the name. Two possible causes of the illusion have been proposed. The first considers that a subthreshold (i.e., unperceived) rate of roll in one direction is followed by a suprathreshold roll rate back to the upright position, which leaves the pilot with only half of a true perception, the half generated during the return roll. The net impression, then, would be one of having rolled away from the level position in the direction opposite that of the original, unperceived roll. The other explanation of the leans is that the perception of bank resulting from a perceived roll out of the level position fatigues after a number of seconds, the absence in the aircraft of the accustomed earth-vertical gravitational force being contributory. When the pilot rolls back out of his banked turn, he then suffers the illusion of banking away from the level position,

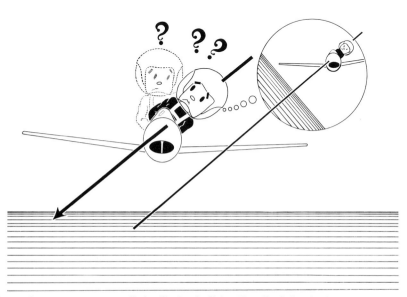

Figure 7.   The leans, the most common vestibular illusion in flight. The pilot is leaning in an attempt to align himself with the falsely perceived vertical.

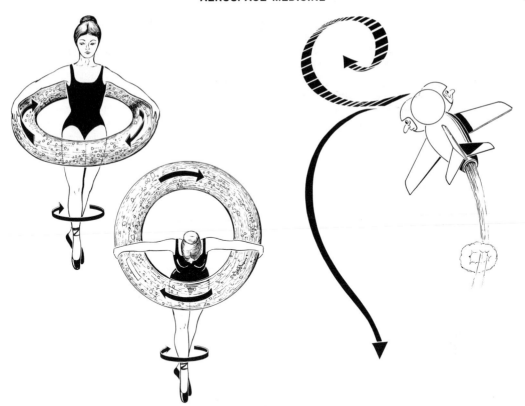

Figure 8. The Coriolis illusion. Because endolymph gains or loses angular momentum more slowly than do the semicircular ducts when the latter are brought, respectively, into or out of a plane of constant angular velocity, a flow of endolymph occurs in those ducts. Erroneous sensations of angular motion are the result.

because his perceptual processes have "forgotten" that he was actually banked in the other direction initially. Whatever the mechanism of the illusion, nearly every pilot who has flown solely by reference to instruments has experienced the leans at least once, but most instrument-rated pilots can maintain control of their aircraft in spite of that particular type of disorientation.

Coriolis illusion. The leans is the commonest vestibular illusion in flight, but the Coriolis illusion is much more deadly. This type of disorientation strikes as the aircraft is in a turn and the pilot rotates his head to look for something in a more or less obscure portion of the cockpit. The feeling that results is one of sudden, pronounced spinning, rolling, or pitching of the aircraft, occurring simultaneously with the head movement. To explain the development of the illusion, we must invoke the principle of conservation of angular momentum (Fig. 8). As one rotates at a constant angular velocity in a given spatial plane, the endolymph in the semicircular ducts has a certain amount of angular momentum in that plane, after the speed of the endolymph has had a chance to

come up to the speed of the ducts. When the head is rotated in a spatial plane that cuts across the plane of the constant angular velocity, angular momentum is suddenly taken away from the seimicircular ducts that were in the plane of the constant rotation. The endolymph in those ducts, however, continues to rotate in the new spatial plane of the ducts, thus deviating the associated cupulae, until its angular momentum is dissipated by friction and the cupular restoring force. The sensation of angular motion resulting from the described cupular deviation will be in the new plane of the semicircular ducts, which is neither in the plane of the original, constant angular velocity nor in the plane of the head movement.

Similarly, a set of semicircular ducts which was not in the plane of the constant angular velocity, but is thrust into it by the head movement, immediately gains angular momentum in the plane of the constant velocity. The endolymph within, not being attached to the duct walls, does not gain angular momentum in that plane until frictional and other forces have time to accelerate the endolymph; in the meantime there is a net difference in angular velocity between the ducts and the endolymph, which results in deflection of the cupulae in the ampullae of the ducts. Again the resulting sensation originating in these ducts will not be in the plane of the head movement. In general the combined action of all six semicircular ducts during a head movement in a plane that cuts across a plane of constant angular velocity is such that a sensation of rotation is generated in a plane more or less perpendicular to the planes of the other rotations. Thus, if one pitches his head downward during a constant yaw to the left, for example, he will perceive a roll in the counterclockwise direction.

The Coriolis illusion is so often fatal because it tends to occur at a very critical phase of flight several minutes prior to landing, when air speed is still relatively high and altitude is disappearing rapidly, and the pilot is quite busy with calculations and communications. In a high-performance aircraft, there is little margin for error so close to the ground, and the pilot who turns his airplane upside down in response to a Coriolis illusion may not recover in time to avoid disaster.

Conditions Caused by Inadequacies of the Otolith-organ System. In flight the force of gravity, which is always directed toward the center of the earth (i.e., vertically downward), combines vectorially with any inertial force resulting from linear acceleration to form a resultant force which cannot be qualitatively distinguished from either gravity or inertial force. The importance of this fact is that the direction of the resultant force is often erroneously perceived as vertical by the pilot deprived of outside visual reference.

Oculogravic Illusion. Figure 9 shows a pilot in an aircraft undergoing a substantial forward linear acceleration; unable to resolve the inertial force (opposite the acceleration) from the force of gravity, he is interpreting the direction

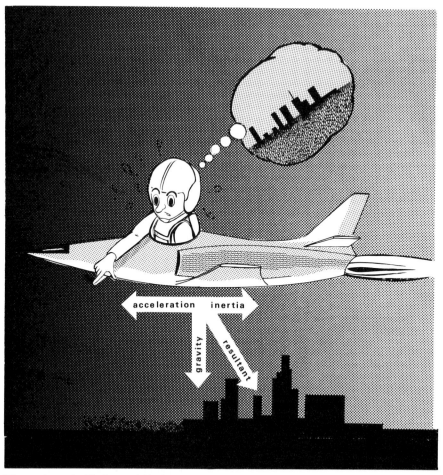

Figure 9. The oculogravic illusion. In this illustration the pilot falsely senses a nose-up attitude of the accelerating aircraft because his inner ears and somatosensory proprioceptors are causing him to interpret the direction of the resultant gravitoinertial force as downward.

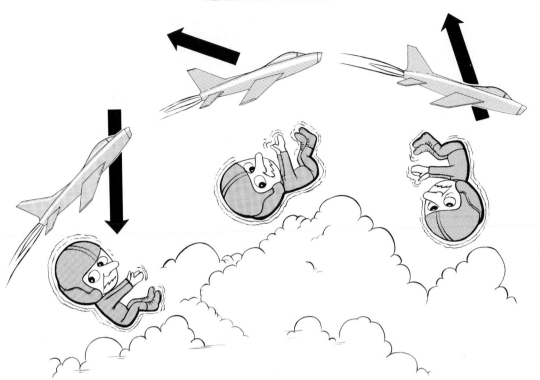

Figure 10. The inversion illusion, a variety of oculogravic illusion resulting from a backward-and-upward-rotating resultant gravitoinertial force vector.

of the resultant gravitoinertial force as "downward." The pilot senses a nose-up attitude of the aircraft because the positions of the otolithic membranes on their respective maculae are nearly identical to what they would be in unaccelerated flight if the pilot were to tilt backward through the angle between the gravitoinertial resultant force and the true vertical. The erroneous localization of the vertical under such circumstances is referred to as the oculogravic illusion (also, posturogravic illusion). The imminent danger to the pilot in the illustration is that, in trying to "level off" from his falsely perceived nose-high attitude, he will dive the airplane into the ground. As can no doubt be appreciated, the oculogravic illusion ranks with the Coriolis illusion in deadliness: it commonly occurs shortly after takeoff in high-performance aircraft, at an altitude too low to allow any margin for erratic aircraft control occasioned by spatial disorientation of the pilot.

Inversion Illusion. A special form of oculogravic illusion is the inversion illusion. It has been known to occur during level-off from a rapid climb, as the centrifugal force (resulting from nosing the aircraft over) and the inertial force (resulting from the tangential acceleration associated with the diminishing angle of climb)

combine to counteract the force of gravity in such a way that the resultant gravitoinertial force vector actually rotates backward through 180 degrees or so and ends up directed vertically upward rather than downward (Fig. 10). One would expect that the feeling of inversion which results would be modified or negated by more accurate sensations originating in the semicircular ducts, but such does not appear to be the case. Pilots have reported having extreme difficulty in maintaing control of their aircraft in the presence of the inversion illusion, because the tendency is to pitch the aircraft down to compensate for the feeling of inversion, which maneuver only aggravates the situation by intensifying the illusion.

Elevator Illusion. The elevator reflex has been mentioned in the chapter on vestibular physiology. The elevator illusion is said to occur in turbulent weather conditions, when vertical linear accelerations cause vestibulo-ocular (elevator) reflexes in which the eyes move up or down, resulting in temporary displacements of the perceived horizontal. The significance of the elevator illusion from the standpoint of aerospace safety has not been established.

The otolith organ system contributes indirectly to another type of spatial disorientation in flight by virtue of the fact that it is inadequate to correct for certain visual and somatosensory proprioceptive illusions. A pilot flying over a sloping cloud formation can become convinced that the cloud deck is horizontal and fly with wings parallel to the surface of the clouds rather than truly horizontal. On a dark night, ground lights and stars may blend in the pilot's eye so as to cause him to lose track of the horizon, with occasionally serious consequences. Sometimes a dark sky and a lake or ocean will not be visually separable, and the pilot will perceive the shoreline as the horizon—an equally dangerous situation.

The otolith-organ system is completely useless in correcting for illusions incurred through the somatosensory proprioceptive system during so-called "seat-of-the-pants" flying. Obviously the same gravitoinertial forces act on the otolith organs as act on the other proprioceptors, and when a centrifugal or other inertial force combines with the force of gravity to yield a resultant force, neither the somatosensory proprioceptors nor the otolith organs can discern the direction of action of gravity from the direction of the resultant gravitoinertial force vector; in fact, the one organ system actually reinforces the oft-fatal errors of the other.

Such errors in spatial orientation as have been mentioned in these pages exemplify two important principles of aerospace vestibular physiology: first, that the visual system will dominate the vestibular system whenever it has a reasonable chance of providing a sense of a structural spatial environment; second, that while the vestibular system is remarkably sensitive and reliable in a terrestrial statokinetic environment, on a flying platform it is grossly inadequate.

Prevention of Spatial Disorientation. All pilots are susceptible to spatial disorientation, some more than others. In general the more experience in instrument flying a pilot gets, the more resistant he becomes to disorientation, although the pilot with recent experience will fare far better in resisting disorientation than one whose experience is in the distant past. When a pilot practices flying solely dependent on instruments for maintaining spatial orientation, he develops the capacity for substituting accurate visual (instrument panel) information for erroneous vestibular information; i.e., he practices asserting visual dominance, which can be accomplished at either an unconscious or a conscious level. If visual dominance is maintained unconsciously, which is the ideal situa-

tion, spatial disorientation does not exist for the pilot in spite of the presence of patterns of motion that render the vestibular sense completely inaccurate. If visual dominance is maintained only at a conscious level, then the pilot is fighting his spatial disorientation, and struggling to maintain control of his aircraft according to information he thinks is right, to the exclusion of that which he feels is right.

In addition to providing pilots with appropriate flying experience to decrease the effects of spatial disorientation, pilot training programs thoroughly indoctrinate the trainees in the mechanisms and hazards of "pilot's vertigo." This is done to minimize the number of those unfortunate pilots who do not realize that their human senses are fallible, and do not recognize spatial disorientation when it appears.

Motion Sickness*

Definition and Importance. Seasickness, airsickness, carsickness, train sickness, amusement-park-ride sickness, camel sickness, and the like are collectively called motion sickness. The symptoms are apathy, headache, stomach awareness, pallor, perspiration, salivation, nausea, vomiting, and prostration, in roughly that temporal order, and usually with the affected individual undergoing either actual or perceived motion, although there are exceptions to the latter generalization.

The principal importance of motion sickness is military. Armstrong (1961) states that in World War II, 10 to 11 per cent of all pilot trainees became airsick during their first ten flights, and 1 to 2 per cent were eliminated from training for intractable motion sickness. The incidence of motion sickness among trainees for other air crew positions (navigators, gunners) was much higher. A particularly serious situation was found among air-borne assault troops: under "unfavorable" conditions as many as 70 per cent of these troops became airsick during delivery into combat. Amphibious assault troops were similarly affected. Current estimates of the number of pilot trainees who get motion sickness run at about 18 per cent, with about 40 per cent of all air crew trainees becoming motion sick during some phase of their training. Between 0.5 and 1.5 per cent of air crew trainees have refractory motion sickness and must discontinue training.

---

*The reader is referred to Money (1970) for the most recent review of the subject at this writing.

In the exploration of space, the most important vestibular problem anticipated is motion sickness. Although some of the Russian cosmonauts have developed motion sickness during their flights, the astronauts of the United States have been remarkably free of motion sickness during flight, even though some have been seasick after splashdown. Some scientists believe that motion sickness will have to be reckoned with if a manned satellite is rotated to provide artificial gravity. Extremely nauseating Coriolis effects are incumbent in such a system, and the evidence indicates that careful selection and training of space crews will be necessary to prevent critical performance decrements as a result of "space sickness" generated by the rotating environment.

Etiology. In identifying the factors related to the development of motion sickness, we find that vestibular stimulation is the prime suspect. Repetitive, prolonged, or otherwise abnormal stimulation of the semicircular ducts, as occurs during testing on a rotating chair or during caloric testing, can certainly cause motion sickness. As already mentioned, Coriolis stimulation of the semicircular ducts is an extremely effective producer of motion sickness. Likewise, abnormal stimulation of the otolith organs, as on a four-pole swing, an elevator, or a heaving ship deck, can result in motion sickness. Human centrifuges, aircraft during aerobatics, life rafts bobbing on the ocean, and ordinary two-pole swings stimulate both the semicircular ducts and the otolith organs; and motion sickness does occur in response to such stimulation. A fact of extreme significance with regard to the pathogenesis of motion sickness is that bilateral loss of vestibular end-organs gives the deprived individual complete immunity to motion sickness.

Visual stimulation can also result in motion sickness. People who become sick while watching movies of roller coasters or ships on rough seas, or while scanning microscope slides, are good examples of the phenomenon of a moving visual environment causing motion sickness without direct vestibular stimulation. In fact, one can become motion sick in the absence of even visually perceived motion: "antigravity" houses in amusement parks (constructed on a slant so that the force of gravity is not perpendicular to the floor) can cause motion sickness in particularly susceptible individuals who enter those structures. But the visual system can prevent as well as produce motion sickness. It has long been appreciated that when outside visual reference is denied to a person undergoing extraordinary motion, such as is the case with a sailor below deck in a storm, he is more likely to become motion sick than he would be if he could view the horizon.

Motion sickness can result in the absence of unusual vestibular *or* visual stimulation; some individuals can be made sick while sitting in a special room with sequentially activated speakers presenting a revolving sound source to the subject. It appears, moreover, that any sensory system capable of transmitting information about spatial orientation can be implicated in the pathogenesis of motion sickness. Finally, a state of fear or insecurity about one's spatial orientation has long been recognized as a potentiator of actual motion in the production of airsickness and seasickness.

The foregoing observations relating to the vestibular, visual, and other factors in the development of motion sickness strongly suggest to this author that the common denominator in each episode of motion sickness is an unusual conscious or unconscious concern over spatial orientation, frequently caused by conflict of spatial orientation information from separate sensory systems in a person with at least a partially functional vestibular system.

The actual mechanism of production of motion sickness continues to elude satisfactory conceptualization, let alone verification. One hypothesis that has been proposed is that the sensory incongruity causes the cerebellum—the orientation computer of the body, so to speak—to work at a greater than normal activity level in its effort to resolve the conflict, with the result that excessive amounts of some neurohumor are produced by the hyperactive cerebellum, and the neurohumor stimulates an area of the adjacent brain stem that initiates the progression of symptoms; this is referred to as the "cerebellar sweating" hypothesis. I personally prefer a modification of the above hypothesis that takes into consideration both a proposed function of the vestibular efferent system and the known proximity of the vestibular nuclei to autonomic centers in the brain stem (Gillingham, 1966), as follows: The unusual concern over spatial orientation, whether generated by fear of falling or by sensory incongruity, results in a need for the organism to obtain and process more information about its spatial orientation; the additional information is sought through an increase in the sensitivity of the vestibular end-organs, brought about by the functioning of the vestibular efferent system. The increased sensitivity of the end-organs then causes action potentials to flow into the vestibular nuclei in greater than normal abundance, even during the unaccelerated, resting state. The greater neural activity in the medial vestibular nuclei then "spills over" into the juxtaposed dorsal motor nuclei of the vagus, and motion sickness is the result. Such speculation awaits neurophysiologic support, but begins to rationalize some of the more difficult to explain aspects of the etiology of motion sickness.

Management.   First, ascertain that the cause of the symptoms is really motion sickness and not something of more serious nature.

Once symptoms have developed, treatment generally tends to be ineffective. One obviously should try to limit the offending motion, if possible. Supplying the patient with an outside visual reference will often stop the progression of symptoms; if that fails or cannot be accomplished, the patient should be instructed to lie down and keep movements of his head at a minimum. Oral medications are useless once the symptoms of motion sickness have appeared. Various antihistaminic suppositories and injections, scopolamine nasal spray (or nose drops) and injections, barbiturate injections, and even morphine, have been used to control motion sickness in desperate situations.

From the standpoint of prophylaxis the most effective oral antimotion-sickness medication is scopolamine, 0.5 to 1.0 mg. 30 or more minutes prior to exposure to motion. The side effects of scopolamine are such as to preclude its use in air crews, although it can be employed practically in air-borne and amphibious troops. Less effective than scopolamine but more acceptable in terms of having minimal side effects are meclizine (Bonine) and cyclizine (Marezine) in oral doses of 50 mg. 30 or more minutes before exposure.

Although questionnaires and special vestibular tests have been developed to indicate the probability that one will develop motion sickness during air-crew training, there is no justification for preventing a man's undertaking the training on the basis of a history of susceptibility to motion sickness or on the basis of results of vestibular testing. The reason for this is that the great majority of susceptible trainees habituate to motion sickness-producing stimuli to the point where they can effectively carry out required military tasks.

REFERENCES

Armstrong, H. G. (ed.): Aerospace Medicine. Baltimore, The Williams & Wilkins Company, 1961.

Flight Surgeon's Guide. Air Force Pamphlet 161–18. Washington, D. C., Department of the Air Force, 1968.

Gillies, J. A. (ed.): A Textbook of Aviation Physiology. London, Pergamon Press, 1965.

Gillingham, K.: A Primer of Vestibular Function, Spatial Disorientation, and Motion Sickness. Aeromedical Review 4–66. Texas, USAF School of Aerospace Medicine, Brooks Air Force Base, 1966.

Lundgren, C., and Malm, L.: Alternobaric vertigo among pilots. Aerospace Med. 37:178, 1966.

Money, K.: Motion sickness. Physiol. Rev. 50:1–39, 1970.

Nuttall, J., and Sanford, W.: Spatial disorientation in operational flight. In Medical Aspects of Flight Safety. London, Pergamon Press, 1959, pp. 73–92.

Section Ten

PHYSICAL DIAGNOSIS
(METHODS OF
EXAMINATION)

Chapter 38

THE PHYSICAL EXAMINATION

by William H. Saunders, M.D.

Most parts of the ears, nose, and throat can be examined directly by inspection or palpation. A few parts such as the paranasal sinuses or the mastoid air cells require additional techniques for adequate examination. Even there, however, the appearances of adjacent mucous membranes often enable the examiner to infer a great deal about their condition.

GENERAL COMMENTS

Position for Examination. There are two methods of approaching the otolaryngic patient for examination. In the first both the patient and the examiner are seated. In the second the patient is seated, but the examiner stands. Both methods have their advantages and their adherents. I prefer to sit when examining the patient.

It is important to position the patient properly. His back should be straight, both feet should be on the floor with the knees together, and he should be leaning forward just a little. Patients tend to slump and often must be repositioned during the examination. The examiner may position himself with both of his legs alongside the patient or he may sit directly in front of the patient's knees (Fig. 1). The latter position seems more direct and requires less shifting of position.

Proper positioning of the patient's head is important. This is done by a hand placed firmly on top of the head to tip and rotate the head as required. Constant repositioning of the head is a key to most examining procedures.

Bracing the Hands. In all examinations steadiness is essential. To hold instruments

without a tremor yet firmly, the examiner must constantly brace his hands on the patient's cheek. If this is not done there is apt to be instability.

Importance of Palpation. The importance of palpation when examining the pharynx,

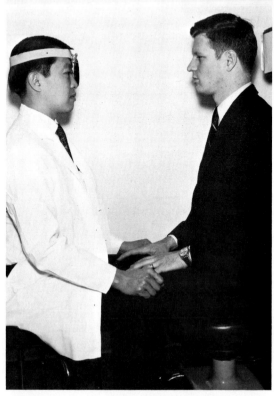

Figure 1. Note upright position of patient. Head is forward, not against headrest. Examiner straddles patient.

905

tongue, tonsils, and hypopharynx cannot be stressed too strongly. This is not to say that palpation is expected to be a part of every routine examination, but it always should be used when the patient's symptoms cannot be explained adequately by inspection (Fig. 2). Tumors developing beneath folds of mucous membrane or situated deep in the body of the tongue may go unrecognized if palpation is not used.

Gagging. Gagging is a reflex which often defeats the inexperienced examiner. To avoid gagging the patient, movements must be deft and certain and the posterior third of the tongue avoided. The patient should "pant like a dog" during the laryngeal examination, not hold his breath.

Excessive gagging seems to be a combination of sensory and psychic elements. Topical anesthetization of the pharynx will eliminate gagging in most patients, but some patients still gag, even before the mirror touches the throat. The rare patient who cannot or will not cooperate can be given an adequate dose of morphine or Demerol or Seconal. An hour later even the patient with the easiest gag is relaxed, obviating the necessity for a general anesthesia. Fortunately patients requiring this much sedation are rare.

The Head Mirror or Head Light. The best light for the physician to use in examination of the ears, nose, and throat is a head mirror

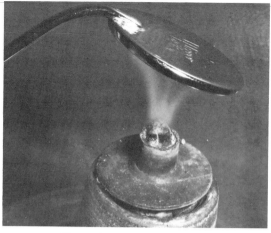

Figure 3. Warming the mirror.

reflecting light from a bright 150-watt clear bulb. Sometimes a "spotlight" bulb is used. One great advantage of the mirror over the head lamp is that it is possible to focus a reflected light more sharply than a direct light. A sharp focal point is of particular importance in examining the posterior nose and the tympanic membrane.

The mirror should focus at about 10 to 12 inches for effective work. Mirrors with too long a focal length are commonly found. Since the focal distance of the mirror is fixed, the examiner must constantly adjust his head position to keep his light bright.

Warming the mirror. The laryngeal or nasopharyngeal mirror is best warmed by holding the glass surface directly above the flame of an alcohol lamp (Fig. 3). The back of the mirror is always tested for warmth on the back of the examiner's hand just before use. Other methods such as dipping the mirror in hot water or storing it in an electrically heated container are also used but are generally not so efficient as direct warming over an alcohol flame.

Preparation of Cotton Applicator. Applicators used for cleaning or for applying medication to the ear canal should be wound specially (Fig. 4). The usual commercial applicator is too thick and too firm. What is needed is a wisp of cotton on the end of a triangular wire applicator. The triangular-shaped applicator is better than the twisted applicator since the latter holds the cotton so tightly that it cannot be removed quickly. The tip of the applicator is placed in the center of the cotton and the cotton twisted onto the applicator so as to leave a small tuft at the end.

The Myringotomy Knife. Although not a routine part of the physical examination, it

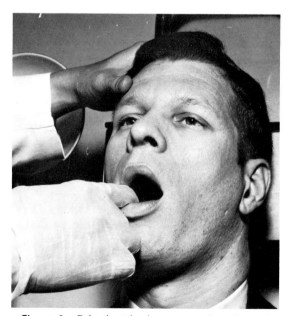

Figure 2. Palpation is important when inspection alone does not provide a ready explanation of the patient's symptoms.

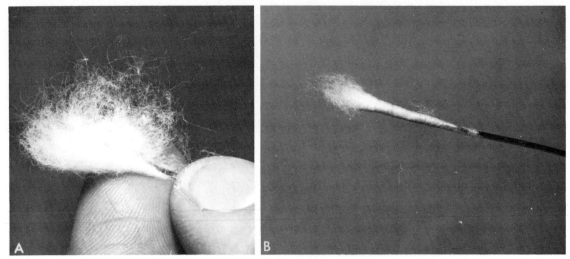

Figure 4. Winding of a cotton applicator with tuft at tip that can be firmed as needed.

sometimes is necessary to use a myringotomy knife as an adjunct to the examination. Of utmost importance is a carefully sharpened blade. Sharpness can be tested by inspecting the knife under the operating microscope and by pulling the blade through a piece of cotton. A small myringotomy made with a sharp, barbless blade is almost painless.

Tongue Depressor. To depress the tongue some physicians prefer an angulated metal instrument but most use simple wooden depressors (Fig. 5). The tongue, being a strong muscular organ, cannot be controlled unless the patient is willing to cooperate. Gagging occurs when the posterior half of the tongue is touched; therefore, the depressor should be applied to the middle third of the tongue and the tongue pressed firmly downward and scooped forward at the same time. If it seems easier, half of the tongue can be depressed at a time rather than the entire tongue. Often in using the wooden tongue blade, enough pressure must be exerted to cause the blade to bend. Occasionally two wooden depressors are

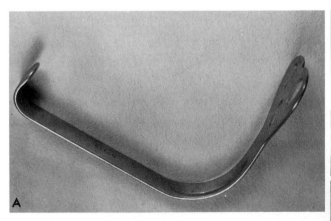

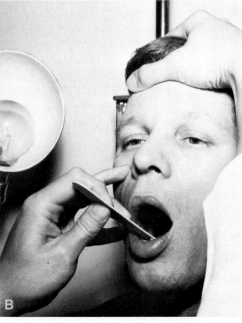

Figure 5. *A,* Metal tongue depressor. *B,* Note how fingers brace on cheek for steadiness. Tongue blade actually bends, often more strongly than shown here. Hand on head tilts and turns head repeatedly.

needed, back to back. During all intraoral examinations the examiner must be careful not to press the patient's lower lip against his teeth.

The Nasopharyngoscope. This instrument is employed occasionally but as compared to the nasopharyngeal mirror its usefulness is sharply limited. It does give an end-on view of the eustachian tube, but the need for this particular view is limited. It may also show some of the superior meatus that is otherwise not visible. Although its use is worth mastering, the nasopharyngoscope is no substitute for the mirror.

Soft Palate Retractor. Ordinarily the nasopharynx can be examined without retraction of the soft palate, but sometimes the uvula and soft palate simply will not relax or separate enough from the posterior pharyngeal wall to afford adequate visualization with the small nasopharyngeal mirror. In this situation, after preliminary topical anesthesia of the mucosa of both the oral and nasal surfaces of the soft palate, a special retractor can be inserted to hold the palate forward (Fig. 6). Then the examiner can look into the nasopharynx with a mirror of almost any size. Sometimes a rubber catheter passed through the nose and out the mouth is used as a retractor, but this is less effective than the special metal retractor.

Examination of the Oropharynx

The examination of the oropharynx is the easiest of the several parts of the otolaryngic examination. The beginner likes to use a flash light or otoscope and a tongue blade, and if such a system of lighting is ever of any use it would be here. It is highly recommended, however, that the head mirror or a bright head lamp be used just as in all other parts of the otolaryngic examination. If the tongue blade is in the left hand, the right hand is free for palpation or use of another instrument.

In dealing with patients who complain of a "sore throat," remember that there are three distinct parts of the pharynx, each of which requires a different examining technique: (1) the nasopharynx or oropharynx, which can be inspected using only a tongue blade and a bright light; (2) the epipharynx or nasopharynx, the examination of which requires a tongue blade and small mirror; and, (3) the hypopharynx, for which is needed a large mirror. Patients often cannot tell which part of their pharynx is affected, and to inspect only the oropharynx may be to overlook disease in the other two thirds of the pharyngeal space.

The Tongue. In examination of the tongue both inspection and palpation are important. Without use of palpation it is entirely possible, for example, to overlook a neoplastic lesion deep in the muscular substance of the tongue, since not all lesions of this type produce surface ulceration. With paralysis of the hypoglossal nerve the tongue deviates toward the weak side because the muscle of the normal side pushes it there. Before paralysis is manifest, however, there may be fasciculation of the tongue. Later there is atrophy.

There are three lingual papillae: filiform,

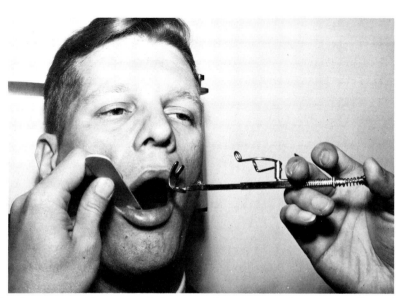

Figure 6. Soft palate retractor. The two small rings brace the retractor against the upper lip; as the spring is slowly released, the palate is drawn forward.

fungiform, and circumvallate. The filiform papillae may become greatly elongated in the condition known as lingua nigrans. The circumvallate papillae, arranged in an inverted V shape at the base of the tongue are sometimes mistaken by the patient for tumors. Absence of lingual papillae causes a slick tongue suggestive of pernicious anemia.

Palatine Tonsils. The palatine or faucial tonsils are said to be of normal size when they do not present beyond the level of the tonsillar pillars, but this is only a rough guide. Greatly enlarged at the time of infection, the tonsils regress rapidly once infection is cleared and return to a normal appearance.

There are crypts in the tonsils lined by squamous epithelium. When crypts are deep, epithelial debris collects and extrudes from the tonsil as a cheesy white plug. In examination a pillar retractor may be used to withdraw the anterior pillar for better inspection. Palpation is also important in some instances.

Waldeyer's ring. This is a name given to the lymphoid elements of the pharynx made of the adenoid, lateral pharyngeal bands, faucial tonsils, and lingual tonsils. Also present in many patients are scattered bits of lymphoid tissue on the posterior pharyngeal wall. These pink nodules are of great concern to certain patients who make a habit of inspecting their oral cavities.

Buccal Mucosa. The buccal mucosa contains sebaceous glands which in the adult can be seen as yellowish spots beneath the mucosa. These have been called Fordyce spots

and are of no significance. They are not clearly seen in children.

The Teeth. The examiner should note the condition of the patient's teeth and gums. Caries are frequently present and unnoticed. Soft gums are common, and bleeding from the gums is a common cause of expectorated blood. Gingivitis of this sort is a precursor of pyorrhea, a serious dental disorder.

Wharton's Ducts. The orifices of the submandibular salivary glands are situated on a papilla directly behind the lower central incisor teeth, one minute opening on each side of the frenum of the tongue (Fig. 7). Although not easy to see, one usually can detect the orifice with the unaided eye as a tiny, dark slit from which clear saliva oozes or spurts when the gland is massaged toward its duct. The operating microscope is a great aid in seeing the orifice clearly.

Stenson's Duct. The orifice of the parotid gland is situated opposite the upper second molar tooth (Fig. 8). Ordinarily it is readily visible and easy to probe when probing is indicated. Massaging the parotid gland toward its orifice will express secretions.

Examination of the Nasopharynx

The best method of examining the nasopharynx is with the No. 0 nasopharyngeal mirror (Fig. 9). Ordinarily in children of five years and over and in most adults the nasopharynx can be inspected successfully with the mirror. This

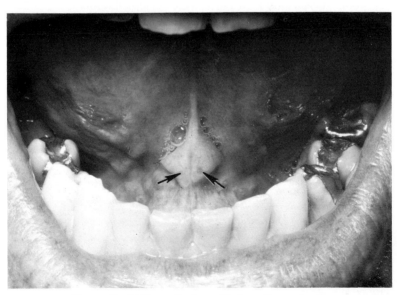

Figure 7. Orifices of submandibular salivary glands.

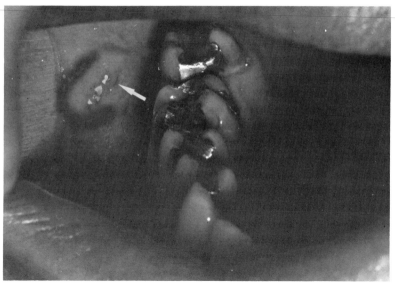

Figure 8. Orifice of parotid duct.

mirror, warmed and placed alongside and just posterior to the uvula, is rotated slowly so as to give a panoramic view of the structures of the nasopharynx. Not all the nasopharynx can be seen at one time in this small mirror, and a slow rotation of the mirror is needed to bring one section after another into view. The trick of the technique is to depress the tongue sufficiently, so that there is adequate space in which to position the mirror. Depression of only half the tongue often works better than trying to depress the entire tongue. Also, the patient should be asked to breathe or "sniff in" through his nose. This causes the soft palate to relax and is in contrast to the laryngeal examination during which the patient should breathe through his mouth.

The nasopharynx can also be seen by looking directly through the anterior nares. First, vasoconstrictors are applied. Then by sighting along the floor of the nose a surprisingly good view of the nasopharynx is often obtained in both children and adults. This route, in fact, may become the one of choice in making a biopsy of the nasopharynx, since the view is direct.

The practice of palpating the nasopharynx is to be discouraged, especially in children. Better and less distressing methods of examination are usually possible.

The Choanae. Separated by the sharp midline ridge of the vomer are the two posterior nasal choanae. The posterior tips of the three lower turbinates are seen in each choana. The supreme turbinate often is not seen. Under each turbinate is the corresponding nasal meatus. The posterior aspect of the middle meatus is of particular importance because it is here that the maxillary sinus drains. Pus from the maxillary sinus characteristically trickles over the posterior tip of the inferior turbinate after escaping from the middle meatus. The sphenoid and posterior ethmoid sinuses drain into the superior meatus or the sphenoethmoid recess, high in the posterior choana (Fig. 10).

Often the posterior tip of the inferior turbinate is large, either pale or bluish, and sometimes pitted. The condition may be mistaken for a nasal polyp or tumor. Vasoconstriction with topical ephedrine will shrink the swollen

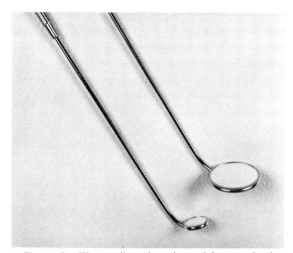

Figure 9. The smaller mirror is used for examination of the nasopharynx; the larger is a laryngeal mirror.

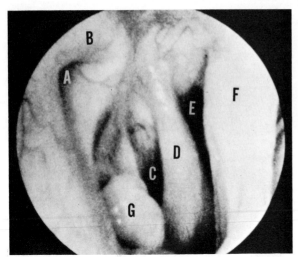

Figure 10. *A*, Eustachian tube; *B*, torus; *C*, middle meatus; *D*, middle turbinate; *E*, superior meatus; *F*, septum; and *G*, inferior turbinate.

mucosa and help to identify the true nature of the tissue.

The Eustachian Tube. To either side of the posterior choana, on a level with the inferior turbinate, is the pharyngeal orifice of the eustachian tube. One should not expect to see into the tube but simply to identify it in relation to the adjacent structures. If one cannot see the orifice of the eustachian tube then he must consider what abnormality hides it in that particular patient.

Above the tube is the *torus tubarius*, a cartilaginous cushion. The *fossa of Rosenmüller* is above the torus. In the adult without lymphoid tissue, these structures are clearly identified. In a child in whom the adenoid is apt to be prominent, the eustachian tube and its associated structures may not be identified clearly.

The *adenoid* or pharyngeal tonsil is an important structure in the nasopharynx. Large in children and swelling with upper respiratory infections, the adenoid regresses in adolescence until, in most adults, only remnants remain. When the adenoid is large, scarcely any other nasopharyngeal structure can be identified.

Examination of the Larynx

Usually the laryngeal examination is not difficult if conducted properly. The approach to the patient is important. The examiner should first explain what he is going to do and then proceed with a reassuring yet firm attitude. The patient's position is often of great impor-

tance. He should be erect, with the jaw protruded forward a little. The head is never allowed to fall back against the headrest but is forward.

As the patient protrudes his tongue it is wrapped with gauze and held firmly. Enough pull is exerted to hold the tongue forward. If the patient does not pull back on his tongue, little forward traction is needed. Care is used not to cut the frenum on the lower incisor teeth. The gauze should not be mounded up on the top of the tongue as this obstructs the examiner's view of his mirror. With the tongue held firmly the patient is asked to breathe gently through his mouth or to "pant like a dog."

Bracing is of paramount importance to achieve steadiness. The fingers of both hands brace on the patient's cheeks (sometimes on the upper lip or teeth) (Fig. 11). The No. 5 laryngeal mirror is held rather close to the glass end to increase steadiness.

After warming the glass surface of the No. 5 laryngeal mirror (Fig. 9), it is introduced edgewise over the tongue to the level of the uvula. The back of the mirror *touches* and *elevates* the uvula and the adjacent soft palate in one steady motion. After the mirror is positioned and the beam of light focused sharply on the mirror, the examination begins. The beginner is apt to let the light wander and then, even though the mirror is positioned correctly, he sees nothing of the larynx because his lighting is faulty.

The first structures noted in the mirror are those of the hypopharynx and base of the tongue. The *circumvallate papillae* and *lingual*

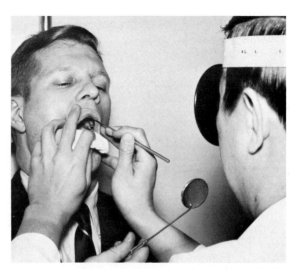

Figure 11. How patient may see his own larynx, if this ever seems indicated. Note how the examiner's hand are both braced firmly.

tonsils can be seen well with the laryngeal mirror. In some adults the lingual tonsils are small or may seem to be absent altogether; in others they are prominent. When they are large there is a median furrow between them. Occasionally the lingual tonsils are so large as to occlude the valleculae. Leading from the base of the tongue to the epiglottis is the *median glossoepiglottic fold*. Laterally on each side of the pharynx are the two *lateral pharyngoepiglottic folds*. These structures serve as useful landmarks in describing the exact position of tumors and other abnormalities of the hypopharynx.

The valleculae, two cup-shaped depressions where the base of the tongue joins the epiglottis, are separated in the midline by the median glossoepiglottic fold. Frequently there are large veins seen in the valleculae, and mucous retention cysts may be present.

The *epiglottis* is a fanlike cartilaginous structure attached to the base of the tongue overhanging the larynx. Its upper or free margin is ordinarily thin. It tends to thicken a little along its lateral and inferior margin where it is attached to the pharyngoepiglottic and *aryepiglottic folds*. The latter folds connect the epiglottis to the arytenoid cartilages.

The anterior or lingual surface of the epiglottis ordinarily is readily seen, but the posterior surface, even in the most cooperative of patients, is apt to be obscure. For complete inspection one must see all the way to the tubercle of the epiglottis, situated low on its posterior surface just above the anterior commissure of the larynx.

As an aid to inspecting the epiglottis and in getting the epiglottis withdrawn for a better look at the larynx, the examiner must insist on having the patient phonate repeatedly with a *high pitched* "he-e-e," or "a-a-a." Most patients will not do this correctly unless the examiner demonstrates. In effect, the two should sing a duet. Even then, some patients phonate with a low sound, thinking a high-pitched one silly.

At this point, if the larynx is not coming into view as expected, the examiner should check the patient's position. Many will have slumped and must be pulled upright and their chins drawn forward in order to give the best possible view with the mirror (Fig. 12).

The True Vocal Cords. The true vocal cords because of their striking appearance and motion claim most attention of the inexperienced examiner, but their inspection certainly is only part of the complete examination. The true cords are attached anteriorly to the mid-

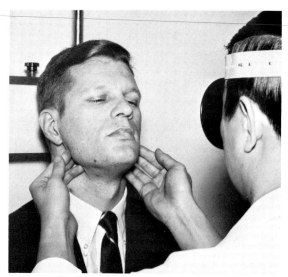

Figure 12. Drawing the chin forward is of assistance in viewing the larynx.

line of the thyroid cartilage, a fixed position. Posteriorly they attach to the vocal processes of the mobile arytenoid cartilages. As the vocal processes move they carry the posterior attachments of the true vocal cords with them and thus open the glottic chink during inspiration and close it during phonation (Fig. 13).

Viewed in the reflected light of the laryngeal mirror the true cords look white and their free edges appear almost sharp. Through the laryngoscope the cords are more pink or flesh colored than white, with distinctly rounded edges.

The anterior commissure is often difficult to see because of the overhang of the epiglottis. No examination of the larynx, however, can be considered complete until the anterior commissure is studied. Having the patient phonate with a high pitched "e-e-e" withdraws the epiglottis in most instances; rarely an epiglottis retractor may be needed.

The *laryngeal ventricle* is the space between the false and true vocal cords. Although one cannot see into the ventricle by indirect laryngoscopy, some hint as to its presence can be gained. Tilting the patient's head to one side will give a little better view of the ventricle.

The *arytenoid* (pitcher- or jug-shaped) cartilages form the posterior attachments for the vocal cords. They are mobile and articulate with the cricoid, and by a rotating motion they swing the posterior aspects of the vocal cords in and out during phonation and respiration. Rarely the joints may become immobile as a result of cricoarytenoid anklylosis. The vocal process of the arytenoid near the posterior ex-

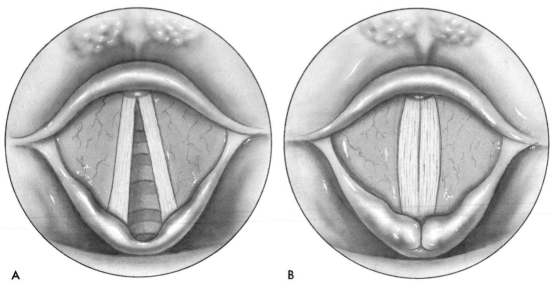

A   **B**

Figure 13. *A*, Mirror view of larynx on inspiration. *B*, Larynx in phonation.

tremity of each vocal cord appears as a pale, slightly depressed area. This is the site of contact ulcers and laryngeal granulomas. Between the arytenoids is the *posterior commissure* of the larynx and behind and lateral are the pyriform recesses.

The arytenoids also attach to the epiglottis via the aryepiglottic folds, in which are found the *cuneiform* and *corniculate* cartilages. These folds along with the false cords and the true cords serve as the sphincters of the larynx to protect the trachea and bronchi from aspiration of foreign bodies, and to help to build up intrathoracic pressure for cough and other functions.

Examination of the subglottic space with the mirror is not so effective as with the laryngoscope since with the latter instrument the true cords can be displaced and the immediate subglottic space inspected. Nevertheless, some of the subglottic area is visible by mirror technique and this important part of the larynx should always be noted. The upper several rings of the *trachea* are usually visible in the laryngeal mirror, and if the patient and examiner are properly positioned it may be possible to see the tracheal bifurcation and even into the mainstem bronchi. To do this the patient must lean forward more than usual while the examiner kneels on the floor in order to look up into the mirror.

The two *pyriform recesses* are located lateral and posterior to the arytenoid cartilages. Broad above, they taper down like a funnel inferiorly. Having the patient phonate with a *low* pitched "a-a-a" opens the pyriform recess and provides a better view of its deepest parts. If there is a collection of secretions in the pyriform recess the patient should be asked to swallow. Normally this action clears the secretions. If mucus remains, the patient is said to have a positive "pooling" sign, indicating possible obstruction to the upper esophagus such as tumor, foreign body, or paralysis would produce.

The *false cords.* The false vocal cords lie directly above the true cords. During phonation they are almost immobile. Occasionally, however, the examiner may see the false cords close above the true cords—a condition known as dysphonia plica ventricularis. Cysts in the laryngeal ventricle (under the false cord) may cause an upward bulging of the false cord.

Examination of the Neck

The otolaryngologist is concerned with the external neck chiefly because it is the site of primary and metastatic tumors, congenital lesions and cysts, infections, and paralyses. Trauma to the neck is also important. Landmarks must be appreciated if diagnosis is to be accurate.

The *hyoid* (upsilonlike) bone is suspended superiorly from the mandible by muscles and ligaments and joined inferiorly to the thyroid cartilage by the thyrohyoid ligament. It is a key landmark in the neck. Its greater cornua points directly to the first part of the external carotid artery. The hyoid can be identified best

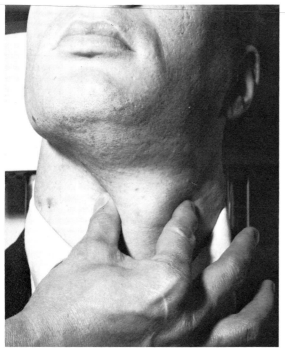

Figure 14. Testing for laryngeal crepitation by sharp rocking motion of the thyroid cartilage.

by grasping it between the thumb and index finger and then moving it from side to side.

Above the hyoid are the submaxillary triangles where there are lymph nodes (ordinarily not palpable) and the submandibular salivary glands. In young patients these glands are well supported, but in the aged they tend to drop and become prominent because of lack of fascial support. They have been mistaken for tumors in the elderly.

The area directly beneath the hyoid and just above the notch of the thyroid cartilage is known as the thyrohyoid space. This is the commonest site for the thyroglossal cyst.

Palpation of the *thyroid* (shieldlike) cartilage is important. In cervical trauma it may be fractured; in laryngeal cancer it may be expanded. The superior thyroid notch provides ready identification. Sharp rocking of the cartilage from side to side tests for normal laryngeal crepitation (Fig. 14). This occurs as the thyroid cartilage crosses back and forth across the cervical spine, and the sign is absent when a tumor of the postcricoid area serves as a rubbery cushion between larynx and spine.

The *cricothyroid space* is almost immediately subcutaneous and is the preferred site for emergency tracheostomy. It is here that the so-called delphian node appears. Classically this node, when enlarged, is taken to indicate tu-

mor of the thyroid gland, but metastatic disease of the larynx may also spread to this node.

The *cricoid* (ring-shaped) cartilage is the only complete ring of cartilage in the neck. It may be fractured when there is a crushing trauma to the anterior neck. This cartilage usually can be identified even in fat necks and serves as a ready guide to the structures above and below.

The *tracheal* rings may be palpated directly below the cricoid. Ordinarily from four to six rings are palpable between cricoid and sternum, but sometimes in a patient with a short neck the cricoid rests directly at the level of the sternum. In such a patient tracheostomy is most difficult.

The isthmus of the thyroid crosses the midline of the neck at the level of the cricoid and upper tracheal rings. It can be palpated in most necks and traced to where it blends with the two lateral lobes of the gland. Tenderness may represent thyroiditis, a frequently overlooked condition.

The anterolateral neck is the location of most metastatic nodes. These nodes are located under the deep fascia, and the examiner must feel deep to the sternocleidomastoid muscle along the course of the carotid sheath to detect them (Fig. 15). The bifurcation of the

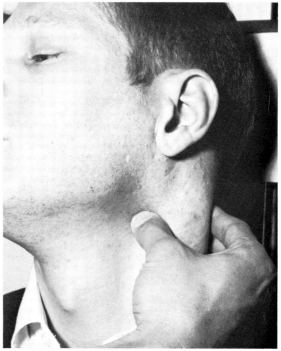

Figure 15. Palpation of the neck must include the tissue deep to the sternocleidomastoid muscle.

common carotid causes an enlargement in the artery which is easy to confuse with a lymph node. Tenderness of the carotid bifurcation which may extend down along the common carotid is caused by an overlooked condition called "carotodynia" or "carotid arteritis."

To test the sternocleidomastoid muscle the examiner asks the patient to press his head forward against resistance (Fig. 16). This makes the two muscles stand out clearly unless there is paresis of the eleventh cranial nerve. Weakness of the trapezius muscle, also supplied by the eleventh nerve, is demonstrated by having the patient attempt to hold both arms over his head. The examiner will be able to depress the weaker arm but not the stronger (Fig. 17).

Examination of the Ear

External Ear. In examination of the auricle one must give attention to its size, shape, and position on the head. Some patients have no auricle; some are abnormally small (microtia); in other patients the auricle stands out promi-

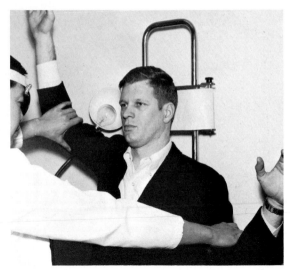

Figure 17. How to test for function of the trapezius muscle. One arm can be depressed, the other cannot.

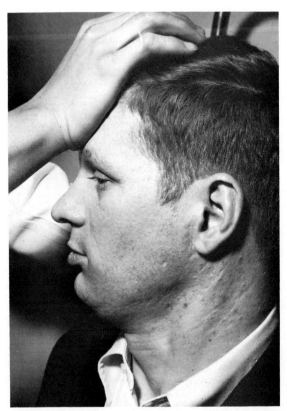

Figure 16. Demonstrating tensing of the sternocleido-mastoid muscle against the examiner's restraining hand.

nently from the head. Thickening and twisting of the cartilage may indicate old injury, as in cauliflower ear.

Tophi (uric acid crystals from gout) may be found along the rim of the auricle. Rarely the auricle becomes calcified and completely inflexible. A small dimple or tract just in front of the tragus is common and is a remnant of the first branchial apparatus.

Ordinarily the *external auditory canal* is sufficiently large that by drawing the tragus anteriorly and the auricle upward the meatus is spread enough to afford at least a partial view of the ear canal and the tympanic membrane. This preliminary maneuver also permits selection of the correct size speculum. An ear speculum is used to dilate and straighten the outer or cartilaginous aspect of the external auditory canal; the largest speculum that will fit is chosen (Fig. 18). Oval specula fit better than round ones. The speculum is inserted only into the cartilaginous canal since this is the only part that can be stretched. The inner half of the ear canal is bony, and pressure here is painful. The hand that holds the speculum also grasps the auricle and stretches it upward and posteriorly (Fig. 19). This leaves the examiner's other hand free to use a second instrument. In children the auricle is retracted downward.

The position of the patient's head is of great importance in the aural examination. The head must not be directly upright but tilted toward the opposite shoulder to compensate for the normal inclination of the ear canal (Fig. 20). The beginner usually fails to tilt the head sufficiently and, as a result, finds that he is looking

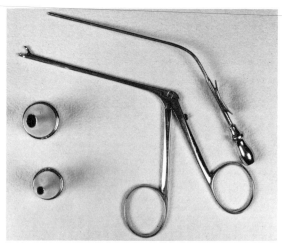

Figure 18. Two ear specula (always use the largest that will fit); an aural forceps and a small angulated sucker.

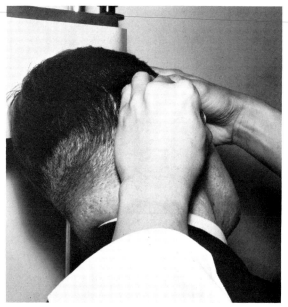

Figure 20. The head must be tilted toward the opposite shoulder in most cases if all the tympanic membrane is to be seen.

not at the drumhead but at the wall of the canal.

Cleaning of the ear canal is an essential step before examination is complete. Most patients do not have excessive wax or debris in their ear canals and nothing needs to be done to prepare them for examination.

In others, however, wax may fill most of the canal or there may be dead skin, fungal growth, pus, or even a foreign body blocking the canal. To clean the ear canal one can irrigate it with warm (body temperature) tapwater

(Fig. 21) or remove cerumen by use of a metal spoon. The latter technique requires a delicate touch since even the slightest abrasion of the epithelium of the inner half of the ear canal (osseous portion) may result in pain and hematoma. The outer half of the canal is much less sensitive and less subject to injury. Almost

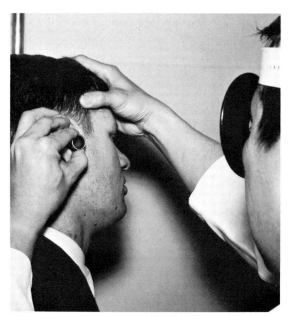

Figure 19. Note how one hand holds aural speculum and also draws auricle upward and backward. The second hand positions the head.

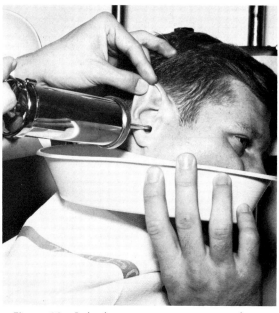

Figure 21. Irrigation to remove cerumen or other material in the ear canal blocking a view of the tympanic membrane. Be certain water is at approximate body temperature or vertigo may develop.

always there is a small slit superiorly where an instrument can be inserted. A suction tip also may be useful in cleaning the ear canal of soft wax, pus, and flakes of dead skin.

Commercially available cotton applicators have no place in cleaning the ear canal since they are too large. The proper applicator must be prepared by the examiner himself (Fig. 4). It consists of a *wisp* of cotton wound firmly around a triangular-tipped metal applicator with a small tuft left at the end. The tuft can be firmed as necessary. Several new tips may be needed for cleaning as the cotton soaks up pus or soft wax. Sometimes debris in the canal cannot be removed readily with a dry cotton applicator; wetting the cotton with a drop of metacresylacetate (Cresatin) helps to pick up dead skin and wax more readily.

By pressing on the tragus and pulling upward on the auricle one can test for tenderness in the external auditory canal—a sign of acute external otitis (Fig. 22). In acute otitis media movements of the external ear do not cause pain. There is a noticeable difference in the manner in which different patients respond to cleaning of the ear canal. The normal patient does not like to have his ear canal cleaned but will tolerate it; the patient with acute external otitis may not permit any manipulations because of exquisite tenderness; the patient with chronic external otitis has an itching ear and enjoys the cleaning procedure.

In some patients the entire drumhead cannot be seen because of the overhanging wall of a prominent anterior ear canal. In almost every patient it is necessary to tilt and turn the head to see all of the drumhead.

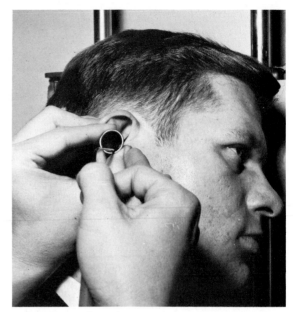

Figure 23. Use of aural sucker to clean debris from ear canal or from the surface of the drumhead. The same instrument serves well as a probe.

The squamous epithelium of the tympanic membrane actually is less sensitive than that of the adjacent bony ear canal, and one may wipe or suck gently on the drumhead if necessary.

Palpation of the drumhead with a firm-tipped cotton applicator wound by the examiner is helpful in manipulating an aural polyp or in testing the consistency of a bulging mass behind the membrane. A small sucker tip is a most useful instrument (Fig. 23). It serves additionally as a palpating instrument.

The Siegle or pneumatic otoscope is useful both for the magnification it provides and because it can create positive and negative pressure in the ear canal (Fig. 24). Alternating changes in pressure move the drumhead and give the examiner an idea as to its mobility. If there is serum or pus in the middle ear, for example, the tympanic membrane moves sluggishly. An atrophic area in the drumhead moves in and out with exceptional excursions. Sometimes a secondary membrane which has healed across an earlier perforation is so thin as to be transparent and it cannot be seen without magnification and alternating pressure. Suction with the Siegle otoscope may also pull down pus from an attic perforation.

A rubber tip may be fitted onto the customary speculum used with the Siegle otoscope if needed for a tight fit in the ear canal. This is of particular importance in performing the fistula test. There is no better way to be certain

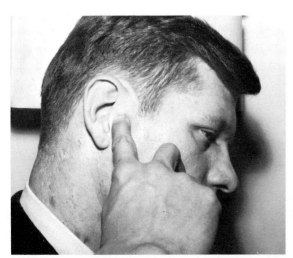

Figure 22. Pressure on the tragus causes exquisite tenderness in the presence of acute external otitis.

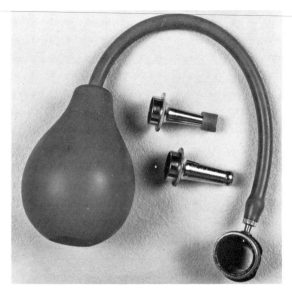

Figure 24. The Siegle or pneumatic otoscope. One of the specula can be fitted with a rubber tip if the special metal tip itself does not provide an airtight seal.

of a tight fit than to look through the Siegle otoscope and observe the epithelium of the ear canal or middle ear blanch under positive pressure.

The operating microscope has great merit in the diagnostic setting as well as in the operating room (Fig. 25). The instrument should be included in every office. It provides a *binocular* system in addition to a brilliant light and magnification. Meticulous and painless manipulations in the ear canal and in the middle ear itself are essential to accurate diagnosis. Binocular vision is of great help in this respect.

The landmarks of the tympanic membrane are shown in Figure 26. Not all are seen in every drumhead because of the wide latitude of normal variations. A good way to begin the examination is to search out the entire annulus to make certain that all the drumhead is seen. Sometimes the anterior and inferior aspects of the annulus cannot be seen because of an overhang of the anterior ear canal wall.

The primary landmarks, the manubrium and short process of the malleus, are actually imbedded in the eardrum. In disease the malleus may be rotated from its normal vertical to a somewhat horizontal position. The malleus stands out prominently, especially its short process, when there is a negative pressure in the middle ear pulling the drumhead inward. The opposite is true in purulent otitis media when elevated intratympanic pressures bulge the drumhead outward.

Color changes in the tympanic membrane are of importance. Normally it is shiny gray and resembles oiled paper. When serum collects in the tympanic cavity the color becomes amber; with blood, it is blue; with pus, white. Dense white plaques (tympanosclerosis) in the membrane are the residual of healed otitis media. Exceptionally thin atrophic areas represent secondary membranes which have closed a perforation but without the middle fibrous layer. Sometimes these areas are so transparent that one is apt to mistake them for perforations. The use of a Siegle otoscope to move the membrane will obviate that error.

In many normal ears the incus is seen shining through the posterosuperior quadrant of

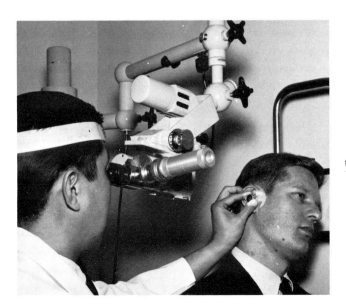

Figure 25. Operating microscope in use. The tube leading to one side is for a second observer.

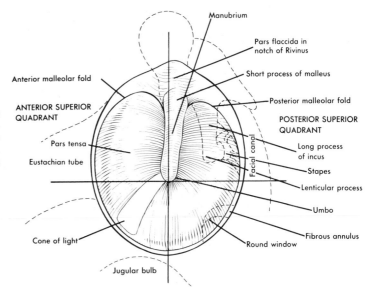

Figure 26. Landmarks of the tympanic membrane. Not all are seen in every normal drumhead. (Saunders, W. H. and Paparella, M. M.: Atlas of Ear Surgery. St. Louis, The C. V. Mosby Company, 1968.)

the drumhead. It is behind the drumhead and is not imbedded in it as is the malleus; therefore, its image is less distinct. In the same quadrant the chorda tympani nerve sometimes is seen as it curves across the upper part of the eardrum.

The niche of the round window occasionally may be seen in the posteroinferior quadrant. The cone of light, always present in the normal drumhead, may be broken up or even missing in abnormal drumheads.

The Temporomandibular Joint. Patients with ear pain of undisclosed origin may have a temporomandibular joint disorder. When the patient opens his jaws widely and the examiner presses his index fingers into the joints, there should be no pain on closing (Fig. 27). In some types of temporomandibular joint disease, however, this maneuver causes distinct discomfort and the patient may wince with pain. Even when there is no tenderness there may be an

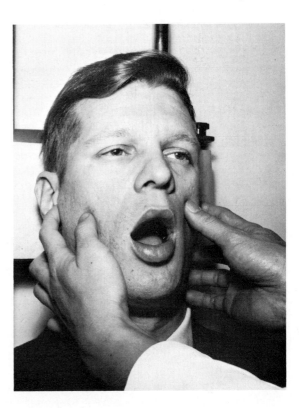

Figure 27. Testing for tenderness in the temporomandibular joint, a common cause of referred otalgia.

unequal opening of the two joints or a grating sensation.

Tympanic Membrane. The greater part of the tympanic membrane consists of the pars tensa—two layers of epithelium (outer squamous and inner cuboidal) with a middle layer of fibrous tissue. Superiorly, between the anterior and posterior malleolar folds and just above the short process of the malleus, is the much smaller flaccid portion, also called Shrapnell's membrane. It has no fibrous layer.

Examination of the Nose

External Nose. In the recently injured nose there may be crepitation of the nasal bones or obvious displacement of the bony or cartilaginous aspects. The external nasal contour is of importance. Just by looking at the nose one can learn many times about the patient's symptoms. A thin, narrow nose which looks attractive often functions poorly. The patient cannot inhale adequately, especially when there is slight additional interference. A depressed dorsum may indicate old injury, septal destruction by syphilis, or weakening of the septum from an earlier submucous resection operation.

Internal Nose. The internal nose is examined with the nasal speculum. The speculum is held in the left hand and opened vertically so that one blade does not impinge painfully on the nasal septum. It must be opened as widely as the nostril will permit (Fig. 28). The upper blade is fixed against the ala by the index finger and the blades introduced only into the nasal vestibule. The speculum is held in the left hand while the right hand tilts and turns the head so that all aspects of the internal nose are seen. There is a tendency for the beginner to hold the hand and wrist "cocked up" so that the hand gets in the way of the light source. This error can be avoided by depressing the wrist.

Nasal vestibule. The nasal vestibule is that part of the nose which is skin lined. It is necessary to tilt the head back strongly in order to look carefully into the dome of the vestibule.

Nasal septum. The nasal septum is inspected to see if it is perforated, ulcerated, or deformed. A straight nasal septum is the rule in the infant and young child but it is the exception in the adult. The caudal or anterior end of the nasal cartilage may be dislocated and protrude prominently into one vestibule. Anteriorly on the septum just posterior to the mucocutaneous junction is a plexus of blood vessels known as Kiesselbach's plexus. Minor trauma here may precipitate a nosebleed.

Lateral wall. The lateral wall of the nose is important since it contains the openings of the nasolacrimal duct and the paranasal sinuses. The nasolacrimal duct opens into the inferior meatus (under the inferior turbinate) rather anteriorly. It is not seen during the routine examination. The middle meatus is under the middle turbinate and affords openings for the anterior ethmoid and frontal sinuses. The sphenoid and posterior ethmoid sinuses open into the sphenoethmoid recess or superior meatus, a cleft between the septum and middle turbinate high in the nose. None of the sinal orifices, with the occasional exception of the sphenoid, is seen by direct inspection.

Vasoconstrictors are of great importance in intranasal examination because by shrinking the mucosa, especially that of the inferior turbinate, they provide a better look into the nose than could otherwise be had. A topical anesthetic such as Pontocaine, 1 per cent, or cocaine, 4 per cent, is valuable if there is to be any manipulation. Either vasoconstrictors or anesthetics may be introduced from a spray bottle or on cotton wet with the solution. A word of caution should be offered concerning anesthetic solutions: They are potentially hazardous, and no excess should be used. The solution should be sprayed from a hand sprayer rather than from a compressed air sprayer because the latter disperses too great a dose.

The value of transillumination as a method of examination is somewhat unsettled. A sinus filled with pus or blood usually fails to transilluminate, whereas a normal sinus usually transilluminates clearly. Yet there do appear to be exceptions, and transillumination is used less than it formerly was.

The sinal areas, frontal and maxillary especially, can be percussed and palpated for tenderness (Fig. 30). Another way to palpate the maxillary area is with a finger under the upper lip. Sometimes a swelling will present here before one can detect it through the thickness of the cheek. The floor of the frontal sinus is thin, so that pressure here may elicit tenderness before it is found over the thicker anterior wall. Mucoceles of the frontal sinuses characteristically present as a bulging mass in the floor of the sinus that can be indented with the finger, much like a Ping-Pong ball.

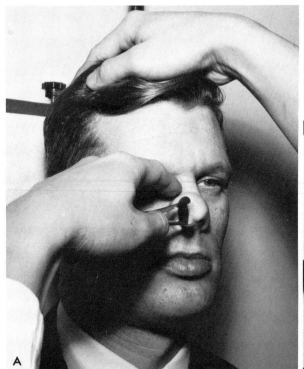

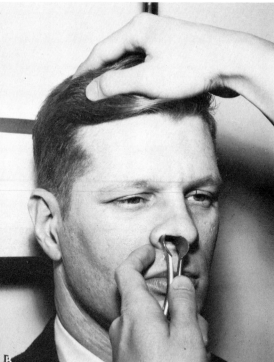

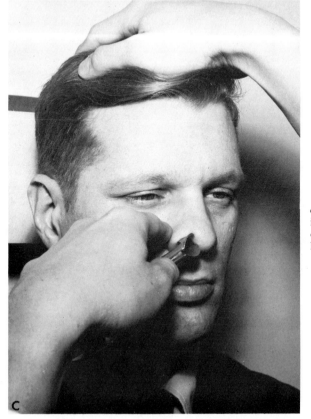

Figure 28. *A*, Note how widely the nasal speculum can be opened without discomfort. The hand on the head is the real key to the examination. In *B*, the blades are opened transversely. *C*, Improper use of the nasal speculum; the speculum is not opened fully.

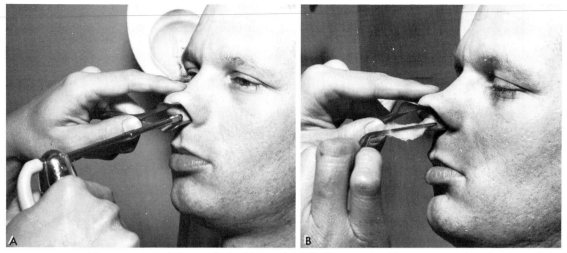

Figure 29. *A,* Vasoconstrictor being applied with atomizer. *B,* Cotton wet with a vasoconstrictor being applied to nasal mucosa.

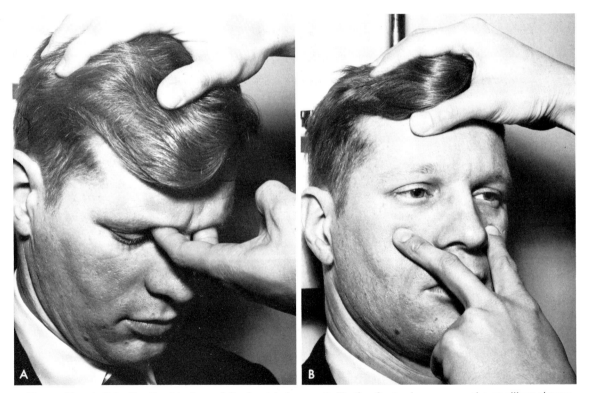

Figure 30. *A,* Palpating the thin floor of the frontal sinuses. *B,* Testing for tenderness over the maxillary sinuses.

REFERENCES

Saunders, W. H.: Physical Diagnosis of the Ear, Nose and Throat. (A 30-minute color-sound motion picture.) The Ohio State University, Departments of Photography and Otolaryngology, revised 1969.

Saunders, W. H., and Paparella, M. M: Atlas of Ear Surgery. St. Louis, The C. V. Mosby Company, 1968.

The Ears. 18-minute, color, 16 mm., sound film (National Medical Audiovisual Center Production) (Consultant).

The Nose. 14-minute, color, 16 mm., sound film (National Medical Audiovisual Center Production) (Consultant).

Chapter 39

VESTIBULAR FUNCTION TESTING

VESTIBULAR TESTS

by
G. O. Proud, M.D.

Whenever the symptoms of dizziness, ataxia, unilateral tinnitus aurium or sensorineural hearing loss call for an assessment of the vestibulocerebellar complex, a number of spontaneous and evoked phenomena should be observed, recorded, and evaluated in an effort to determine whether the difficulty is of central or peripheral origin. Time-saving, combined tests should be employed if it is feasible to do so without imposing a penalty upon the patient; however, in some instances only isolated tests are available for determining pinpoint localization of a lesion. In the sections that follow, the various methods by which investigation of the integrity of the vestibulocerebellar complex may be accomplished will be presented, and examples of combined testing techniques will be described.

Audiological Tests

Even though the patient may not present with the complaint of hearing loss, a complete audiological assessment (including speech discrimination, tonal decay, SISI, SAL, and loudness balance tests) is indicated. The reason for this philosophy is apparent when one recalls that the nervus acusticus, like the other eleven cranial nerves, is subject to peripheral as well as central damage. The various techniques by means of which the auditory division is evaluated are discussed elsewhere in this volume.

Gait Tests

The patient is instructed to walk in easy fashion, first with eyes open and then with eyes closed or with blindfold applied. Wandering with eyes closed is to be expected in the normal subject, but a tendency to fall to one side consistently may indicate a recent peripheral vestibular lesion. The reason lies in the fact that the muscle tonicity on each side of the body is dependent upon a constant barrage of neural impulses (resting discharge) passing from the static labyrinth to the central nervous system, thereby keeping it informed and oriented as to the position of the body relative to the environment. The brain responds by sending information along peripheral nerves to the postural muscles to provide an increase or decrease in tonicity as the occasion demands. Thus, a right vestibular lesion may cause diminution or alteration in the resting discharge with subsequent loss of muscle tonus on the same side. The patient, then, has a tendency to fall, or feels as if he is pushed to the right. This condition, however, is only temporary; after a period of days or weeks the labyrinth heals and a steady gait is resumed. On the other hand, the static labyrinth may be destroyed, in which case the vestibular nuclei take over the resting discharge, and rehabilitation ensues (McCabe, 1970). The test may be "sharpened" by requesting the patient to walk a chalk line heel to toe, imposing a more severe balancing task. The direction of fall in a lesion of the cerebellar hemisphere is not localizing, but unsteadiness and/or atypical gait is to be expected in most cerebellar lesions. This is an example of a combined test.

Heath Rails Test

This method of investigation consists of requiring the patient to walk a series of three wooden rails, each of which bears transverse marks at one-foot intervals and is three inches high. Rail one is nine feet long and four inches wide; rail two is nine feet long and two inches wide; and rail three is six feet long and one inch wide. The barefoot patient walks the entire length of the first rail three times in any fashion that he may choose in order to "get the feel of it." The actual test is performed by walking the entire rail length heel to toe three times; the distance walked each time is recorded. The identical process is repeated on rails two and three. After all scores are obtained, added, and averaged they are compared with the norms established by Heath and Goetzinger (1961). The test is a refinement of the gait test and is of particular value in the evaluation of children who may be frightened by the prospect of caloric or rotational tests.

Romberg Test

This test is performed by asking the patient to stand erect with eyes closed, feet together, and arms hanging comfortably at the sides. Consistent swaying or falling to one side indicates recent peripheral (end-organ) involvement on the same side for the same reasons as those described in the section on gait tests. Here, again, the direction of the fall is not localizing in the instance of a cerebellar lesion, but unsteadiness is to be expected. The test may be sharpened by making the subject extend his hands and stand with feet in tandem fashion. It is interesting to note that exertion of constant effort to achieve balance is fatiguing which is, in turn, irritating. Consequently, patients with cerebellar disease are frequently fussy and are reluctant to cooperate in testing.

Bárány Pelvic Girdle Response

The positioning of the patient is the same as that described under the Romberg test. Gentle but firm pressure is applied first to one shoulder then the other. Pressure is then applied to the sternum and lastly to the intrascapular area. The normal subject keeps his balance by shifting the pelvic girdle toward the area where pressure is applied. The inability to do so, according to Bárány, suggests the presence of a lesion in the cerebellar vermis. Consistent lack of girdle shift when pressure is applied to one shoulder only points to peripheral involvement on the opposite side.

Extended Arm Test

In this instance the patient sits on the examination table with eyes closed, arms extended straight ahead, and fingers spread wide apart for 15 seconds. Drift of the arms to one side may be seen in the event of an end-organ lesion on the same side. Patients with cerebellar disease tend to exhibit asthenia of the arm on the same side as the lesion but do not show arm drift. The widespread fingers enable the observer to look for tremor of cerebellar origin at the same time.

Past-pointing

This examination is performed with patient and examiner seated. Each extends an arm toward the other with index finger outstretched. The subject, with eyes closed, is asked to bring his finger to the top of the examiner's finger, raise his extended arm to full height and return it to the original position. The same procedure is carried out three times with each arm. The test is a variation of the extended arm test, and again drift and asthenia are the phenomena to be evaluated.

Tests for Cerebellar Function

A number of methods have been proposed for assessment of cerebellar function alone. Among them are the alternate, fine movement test and the water-filled tumbler test. The former requires the patient first to bring the tip of the index finger, then in rapid succession middle, ring, and small fingertips into contact with his own thumb tip on the same side. The identical procedure is repeated with the other hand. The tumbler test is performed by having the subject twirl a half-filled tumbler of water above his head, holding the bottom of the glass in his fingers and palm. The patient with a cerebellar lesion may perform these acts awkwardly with the hand on the side of the lesion. It is to be recalled that no muscular activity actually stems from the cerebellum, but the effects of smoothness and inhibition arise largely in this center.

Spontaneous Nystagmus

Further otoneurologic assessment calls for an evaluation of spontaneous nystagmus, of which there are two basic types. The first, pendular nystagmus, is of ocular origin and lacks a quick component. Pendular nystagmus is usually congenital, but some cases of multiple sclerosis exhibit this type of oscillatory eye movement. It may be present only in the primary position of gaze and may convert to jerk nystagmus on lateral gaze. Wariness is called for on the part of the examiner, for the pendular component may be so subtle and fine in the primary position that it may be missed. In any case of jerk nystagmus the examiner is well advised to examine for pendular nystagmus in the primary position with an otologic microscope or an ophthalmoscope which gives 13-power magnification so that pendular nystagmus, when present, will not be overlooked.

As a rule, it may be said that nystagmus of labyrinthine origin is usually horizontal and unidirectional in character, with the quick component toward the healthy side. It is also transient, since it disappears when the labyrinthine function is restored or when compensation occurs incident to total labyrinthine destruction. Nystagmus of central origin ordinarily is multidirectional; but if it is unidirectional, the quick component beats toward the side of involvement. Nystagmus of central origin may be produced by disease almost anywhere in the central nervous system, since the entire vestibulocerebellar complex is under control of the corticopontinocerebellar fibers which have genesis in the frontal, temporal, and parietal lobes of the brain and end in the cerebellar hemisphere of the opposite side. However, nystagmus of central origin usually indicates posterior fossa disease, for the bulk of the vestibulocerebellar complex is located in this area.

The postcaloric response usually is diminished or lacking in the presence of spontaneous vestibular nystagmus, while it may be normal in the case of nystagmus of central origin. On occasions one sees mystagmus which is senseless, wandering, nonrhythmical, and lacking in quick component. This is known as oculomotor asthenia and is seen in cerebellar hemisphere disease.

Optokinetic Nystagmus

This type of eye movement has also been named railroad, picket fence or train nystagmus (Scala and Spiegel, 1938), and its presence is normal; its absence abnormal. A passenger in a speeding automobile watches an object until it passes beyond his lateral field of vision, then his eyes "jerk" back to the primary position and follow another object until it, in turn, disappears. The test is performed by turning a drum, with vertical stripes upon its surface, first to the left then to the right. This test is useful in distinguishing between a central or peripheral origin of spontaneous nystagmus. A spontaneous nystagmus of labyrinthine origin will convert to a normal optokinetic response, whereas a central spontaneous nystagmus will not be changed. A directional preponderance of optokinetic nystagmus may indicate a lesion of the parietal lobe.

Positional Nystagmus

The significance of positional nystagmus is quite different from that of spontaneous nystagmus. The term refers to an eye movement which occurs or is altered in its form or intensity upon assumption of certain positions of the head. The test is performed by having the patient sit on the side of the examination table. He is then commanded to lie in the supine position with his head hanging over the end of the table and turned to the right. After 20 seconds he sits up, and 20 seconds later he returns to the supine, head-hanging position and turns head and eyes to the left.

Two types of positional nystagmus may be seen. The first appears after a lateral period of 5 or 10 seconds, is associated with vertigo, and disappears after 15 to 20 seconds. If, after the nystagmus has disappeared, the patient is allowed to sit up, the nystagmus (and vertigo) may recur. If this procedure is repeated several times, the reaction will be eliminated altogether, but can be elicited again after a period of rest. Such a patient is suffering from benign, paroxysmal, postural vertigo, the cause of which is unknown; it is assumed to be of peripheral origin. In such an instance the other otoneurological findings are not abnormal and the prognosis is usually favorable.

The second type of positional nystagmus is not associated with a latent period or vertigo, nor is it fatigable; it is suggestive of a central lesion. If persistent positional nystagmus is observed, a complete neurological examination should be done. An irritative lesion of the vestibular nuclei is to be suspected.

Galvanic Current Tests

Stimulation of the labyrinth via electrical current can be accompanied by applying a current of 2 to 7 ma. between an electrode placed on the mastoid and another electrode located somewhere else on the body. This procedure is seldom used because it is impossible to predict the course of the current. Hence, it is difficult to say which structures are being tested. However, in the absence of the labyrinth, the current will stimuate the vestibular nerve, so that the function of this nerve may be tested under these conditions.

Rotational Tests

This method of examination does not test one labyrinth to the exclusion of the other, and the physical equipment necessary for its performance takes considerable space. However, rotatory tests may be applied, if available, when caloric irrigation is contraindicated.

Caloric Tests

This method offers the advantage of testing each labyrinth individually. The subject is placed in the supine position with the head upon a headrest so that the tragus of the ear and the outer canthus of the same eye are on a line vertical to the ceiling, thus placing the horizontal canal in the vertical plane.

After ensuring that no tympanic membrane perforation exists, and that the water can flow freely, a measured amount of hot or cold water of known temperature is brought into contact with the drum membrane over a measured period of time. If cold water is used, a downward convection current is set up in the otic fluid, producing a nystagmus with the quick component away from the stimulus. The direction of nystagmus is reversed when warm water is used for douching. The duration, direction, and amplitude of the nystagmus (all of which vary with the stimulus intensity) are noted and recorded. Some otologists place Frenzel's glasses on the patient to prevent fixation and to facilitate observation by superior illumination and magnification. Very effective evaluation of nystagmus may be carried out by means of observation through a Zeiss surgical microscope with a microruler incorporated in the lens so that the amplitude of maximum excursion may be measured with accuracy. After nystagmus has ceased the same procedure is repeated on the opposite ear after a resting period of at least four minutes. Some examiners use ice water in varying amounts (between 3 and 5 ml.) and others use water of 30 or 44° C. (usually between 250 and 400 ml.). Regardless of the technique employed, the basic phenomena to be observed are hypoactivity, prolonged erratic response, perversion of nystagmus, hot-cold dissociation, and directional preponderance.

Unilateral hypoactivity may be caused by a lesion existing anywhere from the labyrinth to the brain stem. Examples are surgical damage of the static labyrinth, viral labyrinthitis, endolymphatic hydrops, purulent labyrinthitis, vestibular neuronitis, and tumors of the cerebellopontine angle. Drug toxicity, notably from streptomycin, is to be suspected when bilateral hypoactivity is encountered.

Although simple prolongation of postcaloric response had been reported in very early endolymphatic hydrops, confirmation is lacking; and the difficulty in differentiating between it and contralateral hypoactivity creates an imbroglio. If, on the other hand, the caloric response on one side lasts the expected time of one and a half to two minutes and persists for three minutes or longer on the other side with repeated alterations in intensity and speed, such a response is considered to be prolonged and erratic. The fastigial nucleus in the roof of the fourth ventricle exerts, through the hook bundle, an inhibitory effect upon the vestibular nuclei of the opposite side and a facilitatory influence upon those of the same side. Hence, a prolonged, erratic, postcaloric response on one side could be produced by a lesion of the fastigial nucleus on the opposite side.

When one stimulates the horizontal canal and sees vertical nystagmus (sometimes referred to as "perversion of" nystagmus) one should suspect a posterior fossa lesion or a cerebellopontine angle lesion. In the former case the lesion is usually localized to the side of the abnormality; in the latter there is usually a loss of function on the affected side with the perverted response present on stimulation of the opposite side.

Hot-cold dissociation is seen in streptomycin ototoxicity. The persistence of response to stimulation by warm water when the cold response is absent supposedly indicates a favorable prognosis for the return of static labyrinth function if the medication is discontinued.

The phenomenon of postcaloric directional preponderance was reported by Hallpike (1956). This observer douched the two ears in tandem fashion, first with water at 30 then at 44° C. He noted that some subjects exhibited a prolongation of nystagmus to one side whether the same side was stimuated with hot or the opposite side with cold water. He concluded that such directional preponderance indicated involvement of the posterior portion of the temporal lobe on the side to which the preponderance was directed. Others feel that directional preponderance represents an occult spontaneous nystagmus of central origin.

If the use of water as a stimulus is contraindicated, the caloric reaction may be elicited by using the cold air apparatus of Dundas Grant. This device cools the air by means of ethyl chloride evaporation and will usually produce a response after 15 seconds of stimulation.

Tests for Cranial Nerve Function

When an otoneurological examination is carried out, combined tests again become possible while the usual tests for integrity of cranial nerves are being done. Only the olfactory, optic, trigeminal, and spinal accessory nerves are checked by isolated tests. Olfaction is tested by asking the patient to identify common odors such as oil of peppermint. A test of vision is frequently unnecessary since the patient usually volunteers a description of difficulty with vision. The fifth cranial nerve is tested by comparing the corneal and facial sensitivity on the two sides by touching these areas lightly with a wisp of cotton. The eleventh nerve is checked by shoulder shrugging and head turning against the resistance of pressure exerted by the examiner's hands.

The integrity of cranial nerves III, IV, and VI may be investigated while the examiner is looking for spontaneous nystagmus as the subject gazes in all directions. Facial nerve functions may be evaluated during the interview with the patient, and the sensitivity of the ear canal may be tested during the routine ear examination. The eighth nerve is checked by audiological testing and by the postcaloric response which was discussed earlier.

The usual complete otorhinolaryngologic examination is, of course, carried out. While the pharynx and nasopharynx are being checked, the gag reflex may be evaluated; thus, any ninth nerve weakness may be revealed. Nerve ten paresis may be noted when a paralyzed cord is seen during the laryngeal examination, and when the tongue is protruded for the same examination a twelfth nerve weakness may be noted.

SUMMARY

The examiner should not be dogmatic in drawing conclusions from the data which he has assembled. One should not make a diagnosis or localization on the basis of one finding, but the correlation of an accurate history and all findings should be accomplished in order to arrive at the diagnosis.

REFERENCES

Goetzinger, C. P., Ortiz, J. D., Rousey, C. L., and Dirks, D. D.: A re-evaluation of the Health Railwalking Test. J. Educ. Res. *54*:3; 187–191, 1961.

Hallpike, C. S.: The caloric tests. J. Laryng. *70*:15–28, 1956.

Heath, S. R.: Railwalking performance as related to mental age and etiological type among the mentally retarded. Amer. J. Psychol. 55:240–247.

McCabe, B. F., and Ryu, J. H.: Experiments on vestibular compensation. Laryngoscope *79*:1728–1736, 1969.

Scala, N. P., and Spiegel, E. A.: The mechanism of optokinetic nystagmus. Trans. Amer. Acad. Ophthal. *43*:277–299, 1938.

Smith, J. L., and Cogan, D. G.: Optokinetic nystagmus: A test for parietal lobe lesions. Amer. J. Ophthal. *48*:187–193, 1959.

ELECTRONYSTAGMOGRAPHY
by
Hugh O. Barber, M.D.

Electronystagmography (ENG) (or electro-oculography [EOG]) is a process by which a record of eyeball position and movement is made through identification of changes in the electrical field around the eye with changing eye-position. The permanent record so obtained is termed an electronystagmogram.

The eye acts as an electrical dipole, the cor-

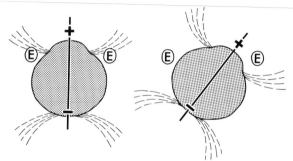

Figure 1. The electrical dipole of the eye forms the basis for the ENG record. See text.

nea carrying a positive charge and the retina, a negative. This corneoretinal potential varies from about 300 to 1200 microvolts in different individuals under different conditions and averages about 1 millivolt. Electrodes near the eyes (Fig. 1) detect increasing positivity or negativity during eyeball movement. These electrical changes are amplified and displayed on a recorder, usually a pen writer on a band of paper moving from the observer's right to left.

Photoelectric nystagmography (PENG) (Torok et al., 1951; Pfaltz and Richter, 1956) employs the principle of detection of reflection of infrared light from the corneoscleral region onto a nearby photocell and consequent alterations in the electrical charge generated by the photocell corresponding to different eye positions. Although reliance on the corneoretinal potential may be avoided by this method, PENG has not been so widely used as conventional electronystagmography.

HISTORICAL BACKGROUND

The advantages of having a permanent record of eye movements have been recognized for many years. As early as 1881 Hogyes (Torok et al., 1951) inserted a light metal rod into the eyes of experimental animals. According to Aschan et al. (1956), various mechanical methods of recording movements of the human eye were employed from 1891 to 1925, some with considerable success.

Schott (1922) and Meyers (1929) first recorded nystagmus by detection of the electrical field around the eye. Meyers mistakenly thought that the currents represented action potentials of the extraocular muscles. The corneoretinal potential was first clearly identified as the source of the electrical charge by Mowrer et al. in 1936, and Fenn and Hursh showed in 1937 that changes in corneoretinal potential difference detected at the electrodes near the eye are proportional to the angle of deviation of the eyes. These facts form the basis for modern electronystagmography.

More detailed information on the electrical charges of the eye may be obtained from Marg's (1951) excellent review.

ELECTRONIC CONSIDERATIONS

The electronic detection, amplification, and recording of eye movements is achieved by means of a differential amplifier; a basic diagram of the system is shown in Figure 2. The tiny electrical potential at the eye (V EYE) must be amplified some 400,000 times by the amplifiers. RES refers to the electrical resistance (impedance) between electrode and tissue, and RI represents input resistors of the "black box." Note that RES must be very much less than RI, otherwise the voltage produced by the eye, being divided between RES and RI, appears at reduced amplitude across the amplifier input. RI in modern amplifiers is at least 1,000,000 ohms, and it is important to minimize electrode-skin impedance to at most 10,000 ohms. The electrode impedance should be measured more than once during the conduct of the

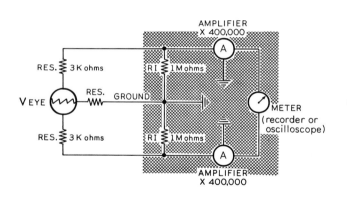

Figure 2. Diagram of a differential amplifier. The shaded area is the "black box." See text.

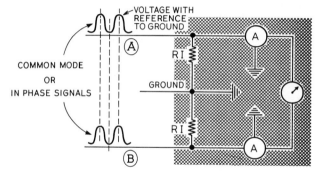

Figure 3. Diagram of system by which unwanted electrical interference is rejected. See text.

examination to detect variations; care to achieve low electrode-skin impedance is especially important in direct current (DC) systems of the type illustrated in Figure 2.

The "double amplifier" feature of a differential amplification system is designed to suppress unwanted electrical interference or "noise," especially 60 cycle noise (Fig. 3). Sixty cycle interference is usually common mode or in phase on the two inputs to the two amplifiers. This is especially true if the two active patient leads are kept close together (unshielded) or entwined, as is usually the case in practice. Measuring between the two active patient leads A and B in Figure 3, there will be no voltage if the common mode signals are equal in amplitude.

Analogy. If acoustic energy reached both round and oval windows of the cochlea precisely in phase, displacement of the basement membrane could not occur.

Thus, the ENG recorder registers nothing for in phase signals. However, the eye gives a signal which is positive with respect to ground in A while negative with respect to ground in B. The recorder then measures the difference between A and B.

We thus refer to the "common mode rejection" of unwanted signals (chiefly 60 cycle) in a differential amplifier. A single amplifier system would be swamped by ambient electrical noise unless extreme shielding precautions were taken. The common mode rejection of a good differential amplifier is often 10^4; that is, 1 volt in phase on A and B will produce an output of only 0.1 millivolt on the recorder.

It should be noted that if the in phase signal is great, say 1 volt, the amplifiers may be saturated and the eye signal distorted at the recorder.

The 60 cycle interference signal increases as RES increases (Fig. 2), and this is a further reason for making RES as low as possible. Sixty cycle interference appearing in the recorder output may therefore indicate high electrode-skin impedance.

Practical Point. If 60 cycle noise persists after checks for broken leads, separation of leads and verification of low electrode impedance, the cause is likely to be unbalanced amplifiers.

Refer now to Figure 4. The patient is instructed to maintain gaze to right for a prolonged period.

A illustrates a direct current (DC) system, as in Figure 2, whereby the recorder pen faithfully indicates the deflection of the eyes to the right as long as it is maintained. B, C, and D illustrate the pen movement produced by alternating current (AC) systems while the eyes are maintained in right deviation. At B, despite maintenance of eye deflection, the recorder pen returns gradually to the baseline.

Points X-Y in B, C, and D indicate the varying times in which this return takes place and is designated as the "time constant" of the ampli-

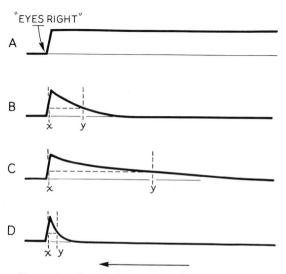

Figure 4. The ENG record resulting from persistent deviation of eyes to right. See text.

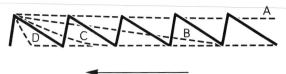

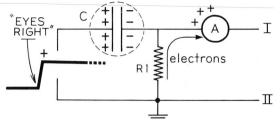

Figure 5. The time constant may influence recording of vestibular nystagmus. See text.

Figure 6. An AC system with capacitor. See text.

fier. B, C, and D illustrate the chief characteristic of an AC system of amplification, its obligation to return the recorder pen to baseline within a certain period of time measured in seconds.

Now consider the possible effect of the time constant on vestibular nystagmus (Fig. 5). Time constants B and C are sufficiently long so as not to distort a faithful record of the nystagmus by electronic intrusion. Time constant D, however, is so short as to force the recorder pen to return to baseline well before the eye returns to "baseline" in the slow component of the nystagmic beat. This results in a grossly distorted record of the nystagmus. While time constants of 0.1 to 0.5 second are suitable for such examinations as electroencephalography, they are unsuited to record nystagmus accurately. A time constant of 2 seconds in an AC system might be considered a minimum period, and many workers use instruments with time constants ranging from about 3 to 10 seconds.

One might reasonably ask: "Why not use a DC system exclusively if it indicates eyeball position accurately and AC does not?" The problem with DC systems is their common tendency to baseline drift, which may make their clinical use difficult. AC systems are relatively tolerant of such electronic shortcomings as unstable electrodes or electrode impedance values that are rather high. A more stable recording system results. This has been achieved through introduction of a capacitor in the circuit (Fig. 6).

With eye movement, a positive charge is placed on one side of the capacitor C. Electrons rush immediately to the other side of C from the amplifier A and are strongly bound in C. This leaves a positive charge at A, corresponding to the positive charge on the eye electrode. Electrons from Side II of the circuit are attracted to A, but their passage is impeded by resistor RI. Within a certain time, however (depending on the degree of resistance offered by RI), enough electrons reach A to neutralize its charge; during this period the pen of the recorder gradually returns to the baseline, which corresponds to electrical neutrality.

Figure 7 represents a simple analogy which may clarify this arrangement. Imagine that water is poured quickly from container A into tank B; unfortunately there is a leak (C) in the tank so that receptacle D is required. E is the time variation of water level in B. In electronic terms, A is the electrode, B the capacitor, C the resistor (actually a conductance), D the ground, and E the resulting ENG record. The capacitor is simply a store for the electrical charge. If leak C is small, the water will move slowly from B to D. In our AC recorder this corresponds to high impedance in resistor RI and, hence, a relatively long time constant. If C is large (RI low), electronic "water" leaks quickly to the amplifier and this corresponds to a short time constant.

Although AC systems of amplification are

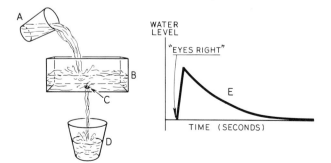

Figure 7. Mechanical analogy to explain varying time constants. See text.

Duration

Duration of induced nystag
relation to (at least, peripheral
ity that its measurement is r
(Stahle, 1958; Aschan et al., 1
1956).

ENG recording of vestibul:
vides a record of biologica
usually easy to analyze ma
analog data may be converted
computer storage and retrieva
1968). There can be no dou
nique will be extended for cli
purposes in the years ahead.

INFLUENCE OF
CONDITION

The ENG record of nystag:
susceptible to variations in
which the patient is examine
ences, apart from disease, are
tions, visual fixation, state c
and drug intake.

Electronic Conditions

See comments given ear
tronic Considerations.''

Electrodes. Skin-electr
should be measured. Sufficien
application should be taken
is reduced to a minimum, c
10,000 ohms and preferabl
ohms. If a DC recording sy
advisable to wait at least fiv
application of the electrod:
allow the electrode pickup to

perhaps most suitable for routine clinical use by virtue of their stability and lower cost, DC amplification must be employed where knowledge of eyeball position is required. To be fair, it must be stated that modern DC amplifiers are available that produce acceptably stable records. This is achieved by various means; one system uses a chopper-stabilized amplifier, another uses the patient's signal to amplitude modulate a high frequency carrier signal which is amplified through a conventional AC amplifier, then demodulated to reconstruct the original signal.

There are many other important details to the electronic basis for electronystagmography, and a full account is beyond the scope of this work. For further information on desirable electronic features of recording apparatus the reader is referred to Rubin's paper (1968).

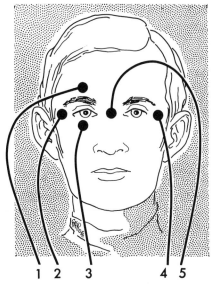

Figure 9. Electrode placement near eyes. See text.

THE ELECTRONYSTAGMOGRAM

All forms of linear eye movement may be recorded, including pendular or swinging eye movements, rapidly alternating movements in the horizontal axis, and other ocular movements. Vestibular or jerk nystagmus is characterized by a deflection of the eyes in one direction as the primary movement or slow beat, followed by a quick return of the eyes to the axis of central gaze (quick beat). Such nystagmus, if recorded by electronystagmography on a band of paper moving from right to left, has the configuration displayed in Figure 8. Points a-b represent the slow beat and b-c, the quick beat.

Refer now to Figure 9. Paired electrodes 2 and 4 identify nystagmus in the horizontal axis, and 1 and 3 in the vertical axis. Electrode 5 is the ground. By convention, pen movements upward in the horizontal leads indicate eyeball movement to the right and vice versa. For the vertical leads, pen deflection upward indicates eyeball displacement upward and vice versa. By common agreement the direction of nystagmus is determined by the direction of the quick beat; the nystagmus shown in Figure 8

would thus beat to the left for the horizontal leads (Fig. 9, electrodes 2–4) and toward the lower lid for vertically placed leads (Fig. 9, electrodes 1–3).

Vestibular nystagmus may be spontaneous, often as an indication of vestibular disease, or induced, as by rotational or caloric stimulation. Parameters of observation of induced nystagmus consist of its duration and intensity; the intensity is accepted as the more sensitive index of the vestibular reaction. Intensity may be judged by the velocity of the slow component, frequency of beats, amplitude, or a combination of these. Measurements are usually made at the peak of the reaction. The slow phase velocity or vestibular eye speed (VES) reflects cupular displacement most reliably and is the most accurate single parameter of observation of induced nystagmus (Dohlman, 1925; Henriksson, 1956). The intensity of spontaneous and positional nystagmus may be calculated in the same way.

CALCULATION OF NYSTAGMUS
RESPONSE

Calibration (Fig. 10)

Instruct the patient to gaze back and forth between two spots subtending accurately a known angle at the nasion, frequently 20 degrees. This calibrates pen movement, a certain pen excursion in millimeters corresponding to

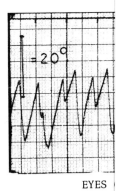

EYES
Figure 12. ENG record of n

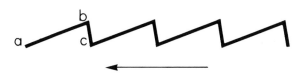

Figure 8. The ENG record of vestibular nystagmus. See text.

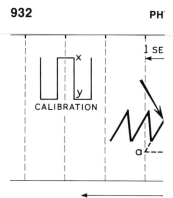

Figure 10. Calculation of V[
nent).
Paper speed: a–b = 1 second
Calibration of eye movement:
　　　XY = 20° = 22 mm
Slow phase of nystagmus shown
Dustance b–c = 30 mm. (measu[
$$\text{Velocity (speed)} = \frac{\text{Distance}}{\text{Time}} = \frac{\text{D}}{\text{T}}$$

If the paper were stationary a
move at the same rate for a meas
example 1 second), the slow beat

b–c. The speed of eye moveme[

From calibration, distance xy
xy mm. on the paper strip. Thus,
moves during the slow phase of
$$\frac{b\text{–}c \text{ mm.}}{a\text{–}b \text{ sec.}} \times \frac{xy}{xy}$$

in degrees per second.

In our example: $\frac{30 \text{ mm.}}{1 \text{ sec.}} \times \frac{20}{22}$

(say) 20 degrees of eye mo
izontal or vertical axes. Th
recorder should be adjuste
cursion approximates 20 r

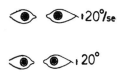

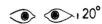

Figure 11. Caloric irrigation
is conventional nystagmus. The

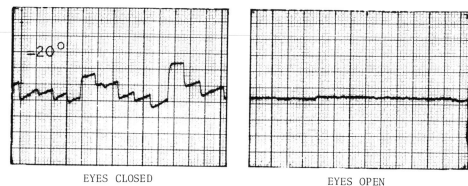

EYES CLOSED　　　　　　　　　　　EYES OPEN

Figure 13. Patient had had right labyrinthectomy 10 months before. Nystagmus absent with eyes open, obvious with eyes closed.

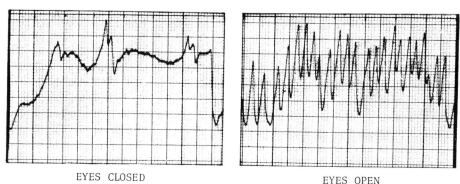

EYES CLOSED　　　　　　　　　　　EYES OPEN

Figure 14. Ocular fixation nystagmus. Nystagmus marked with eyes open, abolished by eye closure.

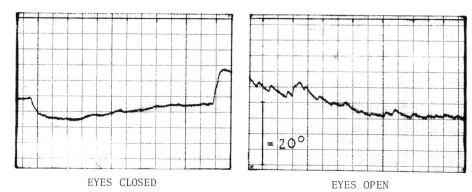

EYES CLOSED　　　　　　　　　　　EYES OPEN

Figure 15. Medullary infarction. Nystagmus with eyes open, abolished with eye closure.

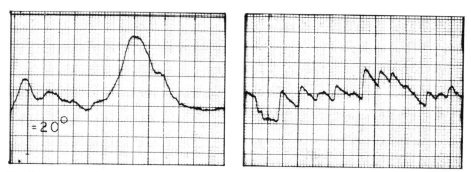

Figure 16. Spontaneous nystagmus (eyes closed) in vestibular neuronitis. At left, patient is sleepy; nystagmus appears only when patient alerted (right).

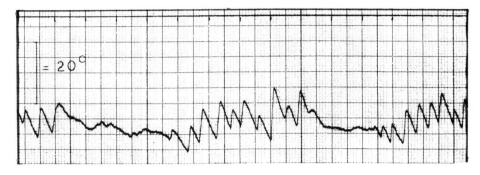

L - 30°

Figure 17. Caloric response in normal subject (eyes closed). Periods of absence of nystagmus (suppression) apparent during the expected nystagmus response.

tagmus (Figs. 16 and 17). Conversely, mental alertness enhances nystagmic activity. It is advisable to keep the patient alerted by a routine method such as with tasks of mental arithmetic suited to intellectual capacity or by answering a series of questions (Barber and Wright, 1967). Some examples of "dysrhythmic" (beats of varying amplitude and frequency) postcaloric nystagmus are clearly due to lack of alerting in the subject, at least during examination with closed eyes (Fig. 18).

Clinical Analogy. A sluggish knee jerk may become active if the patient is instructed to interlock the fingers of the two hands and try to pull the hands apart. Sluggish nystagmus may become obvious if the mind "pulls" on a diverting mental task.

Drug Intake

Certain drugs may cause important alterations in the electronystagmogram. Alcohol and barbiturates especially may produce changing direction positional nystagmus through their central nervous system effect (Fig. 19). Phenothiazines may have a similar influence, and antihistamines (e.g., dimenhydrinate) may suppress the level of vestibular reactivity to caloric stimulation. The combination of droperidol and fentanyl (Innovar) is a potent nystagmus suppressant (Dowdy et al., 1965; Vancil et al., 1969). It is reasonable to suspect that other agents whose site of action is the central nervous system, e.g., amphetamines, have a significant influence on nystagmus formation. For these reasons it is advisable to instruct the patient to avoid intake of any but essential medications for at least 48 hours before testing, and for longer periods when such drugs as phenobarbital have been ingested.

Advantages and Disadvantages of Electronystagmography

Advantages

1. Ocular nystagmus is the cardinal physical sign in otoneurological diagnosis. With elec-

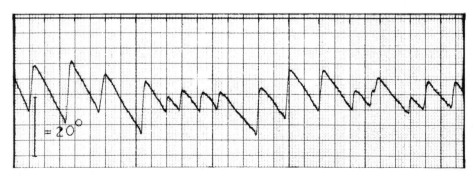

L - 30°

Figure 18. Postcaloric dysrhythmia in normal subject (eyes closed). Beats of varying amplitude and frequency.

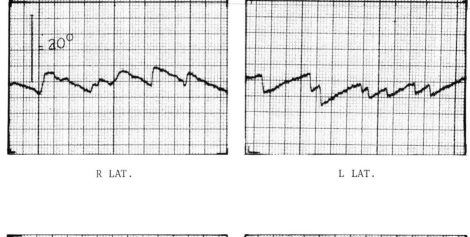

R LAT.   L LAT.

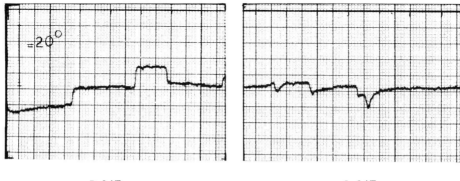

R LAT.   L LAT.

Figure 19. Positional alcohol nystagmus. Horizontal leads, eyes closed. Top two tracings made one hour after alcohol taken at lunch. Bottom two tracings of same patient five days later, no alcohol in interval.

tronystagmography the yield of nystagmus is greatly increased, to the order of about ten times over observation by direct inspection of the eyes (Aschan, 1964). Nystagmus may be recorded with eyes open or closed, in dark or light, and with the enhancing effect of mental alerting.

2. A permanent record of the nystagmus is made and is available for discussion, review, and comparison to subsequent records.

3. It is only by electronystagmography that the most important feature of vestibular nystagmus, its intensity, may be accurately calculated.

4. The intensity of nystagmus induced by caloric or rotational stimulation may be determined with precision in the presence of spontaneous nystagmus. This is notoriously difficult or impossible when duration of nystagmus is the sole measurable parameter (Fig. 20).

5. By means of electronystagmography all parameters of nystagmus may be recorded on magnetic tape. A system of analog-digital conversion may then prepare these data for computer analysis, an obvious attraction to the researcher and clinician.

6. Manipulation of eyes open/eyes closed conditions of recording nystagmus may clarify the type of nystagmus, i.e., whether it is vestibular, ocular, or "oculomotor." (See Figures 13, 14, and 21.)

7. Nystagmus induced by motion may be transmitted via slip ring connections or telemetry to an ENG recorder located at some distance. This may be a considerable convenience to the examiner.

8. The electronystagmographic examination is one part of the scrutiny of the patient with dizziness, and it is lengthy. Vestibular function tests with ENG recording may be reliably made by a technician, thus releasing the doctor for those important parts of the investigation that only he is qualified to undertake. Much "medical" time is thereby saved.

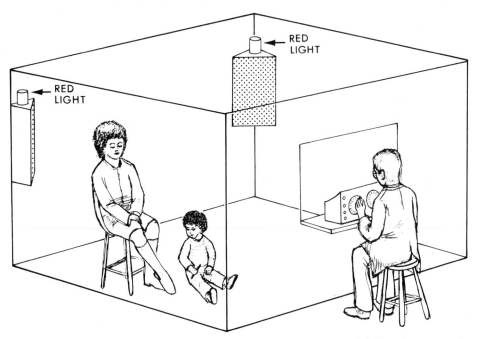

Figure 1. The sound field utilized for gross sound audiometry, pure tone sound field audiometry, and conditioned orientation response audiometry.

Response behavior includes all those previously observed in gross sound audiometry: attention diversion, looking at the examiner or parent, laughing, crying, searching for the sound, pointing to the loudspeakers, and so forth.

Unlike play audiometry, there is very little intrinsic reward to the response behaviors in sound field audiometry. For this reason, babies tend to adapt or habituate rather rapidly. Spradlin (1965) seems overly pessimistic about this problem in clinical audiometry, since he assumes repeated signal presentation as in a descending threshold procedure. An ascending threshold procedure is preferred by the author for this reason. An interval of at least 30 seconds between signals works better for most children.

Taylor's (1964) concern for a state of maximum attention or response readiness achieved by visual stimuli is empirically as valid for pure tone sound field measurements as in the use of gross sounds. It may require a second person in the room or a cooperative parent, and watchful waiting by the examiner for appropriate moments of optimal outgoing attention. This philosophy in testing may not be essential to the measurement, but it has seemed to improve concurrent validity with standard pure tone audiometry accomplished in follow-up years.

Conditioned Orientation Response (COR)

Suzuki and Ogiba (1960, 1961) condition the child to look toward one of two loudspeakers in front of him. A small window framing a doll is illuminated immediately following the pure tone signal. Davis and Goldstein (1970) pay well deserved respect to this method with their comment: "Orienting reflexes are probably the best single method of reflex audiometry, and...they are at their best in the critical period from 6 to 12 months of age." Further testimony to its effectiveness is the number of adoptions of this method with minor modifications (MacPherson, 1960; Houston Speech and Hearing Center, 1964; Kimball, 1964; Reddell and Calvert, 1967). In many clinics (including the author's) a single light is frequently used as a reinforcer without utilizing the opportunity for localization information.

SPEECH AUDIOMETRY

The use of speech for the measurement of hearing has impressive face validity. If the child can repeat what is said to him or respond appropriately to a command, the examiner has accomplished an assessment of a major segment of the nervous system. Conversely, the pure tone audiogram alone represents the integrity of only a portion of the auditory system. It is no wonder that speech audiometry has become popular as a diagnostic tool.

Speech audiometry for children must consider the age of the child, his familiarity with words, the cultural norms for language, and the response mode. The hearing impairment imposes its own peculiar restrictions. There is often delayed language development, including sparse vocabulary and disordered syntax and grammar. The child's speech may be so unintelligible that the discrimination score may represent a test of examiner listening if a talkback response is used.

Yet speech audiometry has developed for hearing-impaired children. A picture-identification multiple-choice model has been used by many, especially for threshold purposes. This has managed the response question at the cost of introducing another problem: the closed set. A small number of possible alternatives represented by pictures reduces the discriminating precision of the speech material while increasing its reliability. The closed set condition may thus have less negative impact on speech threshold than on speech discrimination measurement.

Speech Reception Threshold

Replicating adult audiometry, the late 40's saw speech reception threshold procedures utilizing sentences (Keaster, 1947) and spondaic words (Meyerson, 1947). Siegenthaler et al. (1954) used monosyllabic words to obtain speech thresholds. The children were to act on Keaster's simple request, and pointed to pictures for Meyerson and Siegenthaler et al. Objects were selected by the child from a tray as Sortini and Flake (1953) and Monsees (1953) invited the child to sample specific toys.

Screening

A recorded screening test using the picture-identification design was developed by Griffing, Simonton and Hedgecock (1967). The VASC, for "Verbal Auditory Screening for Children," has been used with many four and five year old children and also with mentally retarded children (Dansinger, 1966), as well as those from low income areas (Hartman, 1965).

A tape recording of spondee words is played through receivers at progressively attenuated levels until the child passes an arbitrarily determined screening level (e.g., 25dB Hearing Level) by pointing to appropriate pictures. Two children can be tested at one time.

Although its inventors claim a 90 per cent accurate classification by VASC, the test has been criticized for yielding too many false negatives, i.e., children with true hearing impairment who pass the test. This seems to have resulted from the closed set condition which favors guessing and the intrinsic nature of spondaic words which will "pass" high frequency impairments. The latter problem has been partly resolved by the inclusion of a birdlike higher frequency sound. Nevertheless, such studies as reported by Horowitz, Sullivan and Mazor (1970) suggest that validation against threshold and ENT findings leaves something to be desired.

The VASC was used much sooner than validation studies could be accomplished. But the basic idea is a good one, with simplicity and standardization as its virtues. Further studies of validation and application need to be done.

Auditory Discrimination Testing

The early adult word lists for tests of auditory discrimination (PB-50 and W-22) were modified by Haskins (1949) to balance word lists for children as to familiarity and phonetic structure. This was not an easy task, but was an important objective. Watson (1957) has noted the absence of many of the W-22 and PB-50 words from the recognition vocabulary of children. Schlanger (1961) related scores on the Peabody Picture Vocabulary test and speech reception threshold. A number of investigators (Howes, 1957; Rosenzweig and Postman, 1957; Oyer and Doudna, 1960; Owens, 1961; Fulton, 1967; and Epstein, Giolas and Owens, 1968) have shown in different ways the dependence of adult discrimination scores on familiarity; the generalization should apply to children.

Haskins' (1949) lists, known as the PBK-50 for "Phonetically Balanced Kindergarten," have been very popular despite an almost total lack of systematic research on their use. The requirement of a spoken repetition response has led to informal modification of the PBK-50 administration. Frustrations with younger children have produced several multiple-choice picture-identification tests by Myatt and Landes (1963) and by Siegenthaler and Haspiel

(1966). Ross and Lerman (1968) have further refined Myatt and Landes' test.

Applications

Applications of the speech threshold and discrimination measurement of children have taken interesting routes. Grey and associates (1965) found no effects of congenital brain injury alone, or in combination with sensorineural hearing impairment, upon figure-ground thresholds (selected spondees—white noise) in children pointing at pictures. Perhaps the discrimination of spondee words is an overly simple task. A similar experiment is needed to examine the effects upon the discrimination of monosyllables at soft intensities in a background of differing noises.

The Collaborative Research Project of the Perinatal Research Branch, National Institute of Neurological Diseases and Stroke, has been studying children longitudinally. The hearing of three year old children has been screened in 12 separate hospitals, by use of spondaic words at a "high" and "low" fence. These findings are beginning to be analyzed and should be worth studying when they become available.

"Triplet Audiometry," developed by Huizing and associates (1958, 1960) tests discrimination with the information contained in three filtered frequency bands: below 900 Hz, between 900 and 1800 Hz, and above 1800 Hz. The developers argue for application of these three measures to hearing aid, auditory training, and rehabilitation decisions.

But some of the problems inherent in discrimination measurements of children have limited their diagnostic applications. Filtered speech tests, popular in adult audiology, have had little or no application to children. Use of conditioned GSR speech audiometry, successful with adults (Ruhm and Carhart, 1958; Chaiklin, 1959), has not been reported with children.

More research is needed on speech audiometry with children. A discrimination test is needed that is culture free, that respects word familiarity and phonemic power. Designs along the lines of the Fairbanks Rhyme Test (1958) deserve further study.

HEART RATE AUDIOMETRY

Although the human heart rate response to acoustic stimulation has not been firmly established as a clinical test of hearing, several investigators have suggested such a possibility (Zeaman and Wegner, 1956; Beadle and Crowell, 1962; Murphy and Smyth, 1962; Johansson et al., 1964; Jasienska et al., 1967). Alterations in magnitude, duration, and latency of heart rate when humans are presented with an acoustic signal have been shown to be a function of the nature of the stimulus and the state of the subject (Fig. 2). Further, the direction of this alteration, i.e., acceleration or deceleration, has been shown to be sensitively dependent upon the maturing state of the subject. Investigators of such heart rate changes in children have been mainly concerned with the nature of the response over the first six months of life and the effects of stimulus repetition and various stimulus characteristics.

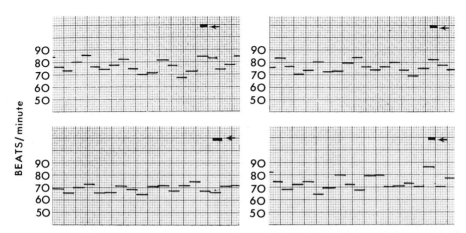

Figure 2. Heart rate changes (beats per minute) in an adult following stimulation by a 40 dB sensation level 500 Hz (upper left) and 2000 Hz (upper right) 800 msec. tone compared to control nonstimulus condition (lower left and right). All data were obtained with a Waters Cardiotachometer.

Developmental Considerations

Heart rate response to auditory signals during the first five days of life has been consistently reported to be characterized by a monophasic acceleration (Bridger, 1961; Bartoshuk, 1962a and b; 1964; Graham et al., 1968). Several investigators treat this "immature" response as one of alerting or startle (Keen et al., 1965; Gray and Crowell, 1968; Schulman, 1969). Gray and Crowell (1968) suggest that this acceleration of heart rate reflects sympathetic nervous system activity. Murphy and Smyth (1962) noted increased heart rate after a 100 dB pure tone was applied to the mother's abdomen at 30 weeks postconception in 235 fetal subjects out of 290. When the stimulus is kept constant, the acceleratory response has been shown to increase in magnitude over the first five days of life (Bartoshuk, 1962a and b; Graham et al., 1968). They attribute this finding to an increased state of wakefulness over that period. This has obvious implications for the design of any clinical test of hearing concerned with neonatal assessment.

In Schulman's (1969) provocative study with low- and high-risk infants, she found that all her subjects, age one to seven weeks, demonstrated an acceleratory monophasic response during natural sleep. However, during wakefulness the low-risk subjects exhibited a deceleratory response, whereas the high-risk subjects continued to demonstrate an acceleratory response. Dr. Schulman suggests that the acceleratory heart rate response is a more primitive response characteristic of (1) all sleeping infants, (2) young awake premature infants, and (3) infants with high probability of CNS damage.

It has been suggested that the more mature decelerative response of infants represents active attention to the stimulus and may therefore involve a larger segment of the auditory system (Lewis and Spaulding, 1967; Gray and Crowell, 1968; Schulman, 1969). In a cross-sectional study, Gray and Crowell (1968) reported a monophasic acceleration for two day old infants, sometimes acceleration and sometimes deceleration for six week old infants, and a consistent deceleration in 11 week old subjects (Fig. 3).

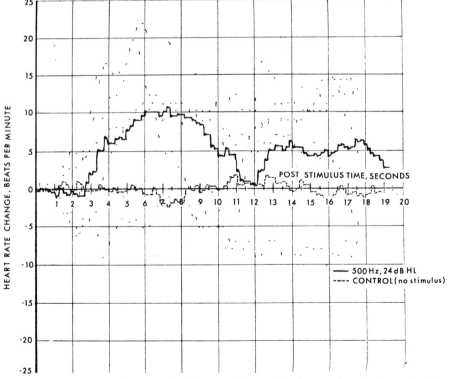

Figure 3. Heart rate changes of a three month old sleeping infant following a series of 500 Hz signals at 24 dB HL. The responses have been averaged through a digital computer; dots are raw, unaveraged responses. (From Schulman, C. A., and Fontana, V. J.: A clinical technique for the evaluation of hearing levels in infants.)

Stimulus Effects

The effect of various stimulus parameters on heart rate has been the subject of several investigations (Beadle and Crowell, 1962; Bartoshuk, 1962a and b, 1964; Keen et al., 1965; Steinschneider et al., 1966; Jasienska et al., 1967; Clifton et al., 1968, 1969). Steinschneider et al. (1966) observed progressive increments in response size and duration and shorter latencies with progressive increases of white noise intensity, i.e., 50, 70, 85 and 100 dB (SPL). Bartoshuk (1962a and b) was the first to report this in neonates, finding an increase in response magnitude with an increase of stimulus intensity from 80 dB (HL) to 91 dB (HL). In a later paper Bartoshuk (1964) demonstrated an approximately linear relationship between heart rate response and stimulus intensity in infants 24 to 100 hours old. This relationship is shown in Figure 4.

The effects of stimulus duration have also been studied (Keen et al., 1965; Clifton et al., 1968). Comparing stimuli with durations of two and ten seconds, Keen and his associates reported that a 10-second stimulus evoked its peak response at 16.5 beats after the onset of the stimulus; the response to the two-second stimulus reached a peak at 8.4 beats post-stimulus onset. With stimuli of two-, six-, 10-, 18- and 30-second duration, Clifton's group continued to find a maximal amplitude response for the 10-second stimulus.

Frequency- or pitch-dependent response patterns either have not been discernible (Beadle and Crowell, 1962) or responses have been similar across frequency (Jasienska et al. 1967; Bridger, 1961).

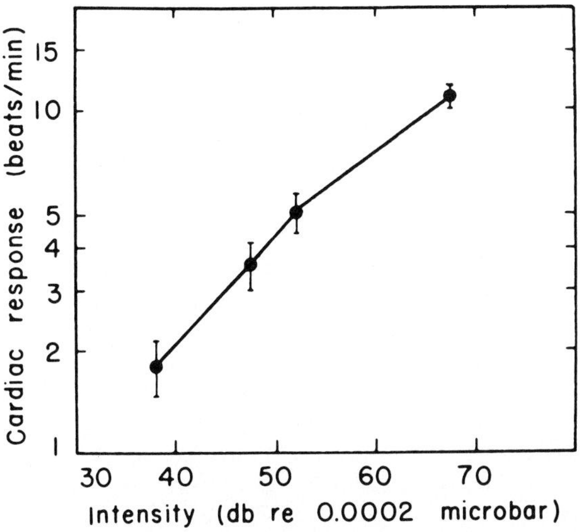

In a study of four month old subjects Clifton and Meyers (1969) observed that response magnitude was significantly greater for a pulsed tone than for a continuous one. In addition, a reliable heart rate deceleration to stimulus offset was observed for the continuous but not for the pulsed signal. The increased response magnitude under pulsed conditions was attributed to stimulus complexity.

Threshold Audiometry

Three groups have made some attempt to measure a threshold of sensitivity in the neonate, utilizing the heart rate response (Beadle and Crowell, 1962; Bartoshuk, 1964; Steinschneider et al., 1966). Beadle and Crowell described responses from one infant to 80 per cent of signals varying in frequency at 40 dB HL. Bartoshuk suggested threshold between 38 and 48 dB SPL for a 1000 cps tone. Responses were obtained at intensities as low as 55 dB SPL by Steinschneider et al. Bartoshuk reported a mean "response" of 1.2 beats per minute on control (nonsignal) trials, with responses for 38 dB SPL trials greater than on control trials in 67 per cent of the subjects; but these differences were not statistically significant.

Habituation

Heart rate response decrement to repeated auditory stimulation has been reported by Bridger (1961). By presenting neonates one to five days old with a tone of 40-second duration and an intersignal interval (ISI) of one half second, complete habituation was effected after 18 stimulus presentations. Although not all subjects demonstrated habituation, for those who did, a stimulus of long duration with a short ISI was most effective. Employing 120 subjects aged one to four days old, Bartoshuk (1962a) also reported response decrement across trials, with no difference observed between 15 and 60 second ISI or between the age or sex of the subjects. In a later study, Bartoshuk (1962b) did observe greater response decrement with a six-second ISI as compared to a 60-second ISI.

Keen and his associates (1965) demonstrated that the prolonged response to a stimulus of 10-second duration was habituated after six

Figure 4. Relationship between heart rate and stimulus intensity in neonates (From Bartoshuk, A. K.: Psychon. Sci. *1*:151–152, 1964.)

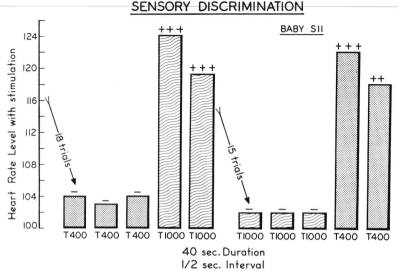

Figure 5. Recovery with change in frequency after habituation. (From Bridger, W. H. Reprinted from *The American Journal of Psychiatry*, Volume 117, pages 991–996, 1961. Copyright 1961, the American Psychiatric Association.)

trials to equal the response obtained with a two-second stimulus. There was no intertrial habituation to the two-second stimulus and no further response decrement to the 10-second stimulus across later trials. Graham et al. (1968) reported rather slow intrasession habituation with little or no intersession habituation. They concluded that the immature acceleratory response might be more resistant to habituation than the more deceleratory.

Dishabituation and Discrimination

After achieving habituation with stimulus repetition or prolongation, alteration of the stimulus in some parameter has been observed to result in dishabituation (Bridger, 1961; Bartoshuk, 1962a). Figure 5 shows the results of Bridger's (1961) classic study. Bridger presented a 400 Hz tone to neonates one to five days old for 21 trials, effecting complete habituation. On the 22nd trial, he changed to a 1000 Hz tone and observed a 20 beat per minute increase in response. After this response had been habituated over the next 17 trials, he reintroduced the 400 Hz tone and again observed an increase in the magnitude of response. Fifteen of his 50 subjects were able to make such a discrimination. He reported that one subject could discriminate between tones of 200 and 250 cps when this method was used.

Bartoshuk (1962a) presented his two to four day old subjects with 17 trials of an 80 dB (HL) 500 Hz signal to effect habituation. On the eighteenth trial the signal was increased to 91 dB (HL) and a corresponding increase in response magnitude was obtained.

These demonstrations by Bridger and Bartoshuk open the way for investigating difference limen for frequency (DLF) and intensity (DLI) in children, with possible applications of the latter for indirect measurement of loudness recruitment in neonates.

General Comments

The reader may now wish to consider the amount of time and study that has been given to the description of heart rate changes following acoustic stimuli. Yet efficient, standardized methods of application to the clinical audiometry of infants and children remain to be accomplished. The EKG equipment for heart-rate audiometry is less expensive and easier to manipulate than that presently utilized in electric response audiometry (to be discussed later). Some parameter studies suggest a potential application to loudness threshold, loudness recruitment and adaptation, loudness, pitch, and phonemic discrimination, and to localization. Further work in this area may be fruitful.

PERIPHERAL VASCULAR RESPONSE (PVR) AUDIOMETRY

A relative of heart rate response that measures pulse volume at the periphery is peripheral vascular response audiometry. For the reader interested in cardiovascular dynamics, the autonomic mechanism of vasoconstriction following a sound is described succinctly by Hogan (1969). This peripheral vasospastic reaction has been known since at least 1955 when Lehmann reported it following a 90 phon white noise. Some observers agreed that noises of 70 dB HL intensity or greater were necessary before responses could be obtained (Stranco et al., 1962; Jensen et al., 1964). But Kottmeyer (1961) was able to obtain responses to "floating tones" at sensation levels of only 10, 20, and 30 dB above threshold. Apart from Lehmann, who studied the forehead, the others used a finger plethysmograph to study pulse volumetric changes.

In an especially encouraging report, Daly (1965) obtained PVRs from 80 per cent of his adult sleeping subjects at 5 dB above volunteered thresholds with only 4 per cent "false-positive" judgments. Success with this method was judged to result from the relative stability in the ongoing pulse volume.

On the other hand, Drettner (1967) found disappointing results with children when he used a method of thermal conductivity (Hensel and Bender, 1956). The median threshold was 85 to 90 dB HL with large variability. False positives seemed to result when child had cold and pale extremities, indicating prestimulus peripheral vasoconstriction.

Hogan (1969) reported a comparison of heart rate, respiration, and finger-pulse volume in 20 normal subjects, age 15 to 25 years. He found pulse volume to demonstrate responses at least as well as the others. Unfortunately an intensity of 80 dB SPL was the only one used. Incidentally, when all three physiologic measures were used, all 20 of the subjects were judged to have yielded responses. This is one of the few suggestions that a multivariate approach might yield more clinical power.

Generally the PVR shows enough promise to deserve further investigation. Some effort should be made to replicate Daly's sleep study, but with young subjects.

RESPIRATION AUDIOMETRY

Alterations in the depth and rate of respiration following acoustic signals have been studied by a few workers over the last decade (Goldie and Green, 1961). Rosenau (1962) observed a difference of 30 to 40 dB between the altered respiration thresholds of sleeping children and behavioral thresholds (awake), favoring the behavioral. But the size of the difference increased to 55 and 60 dB in normal hearing and experimentally induced hearing-impaired children. The reader may note that the same direction for this comparison between hearing-impaired and normal listeners has been displayed previously in Heart Rate Audiometry.

Teel (1966) found a difference of only 15 dB between respiratory and volunteered thresholds in hearing-impaired children, ages seven to 11. Two to four year old normal hearing children were reported by Bradford et al. (1970) to yield respiration thresholds within 10 dB of behavioral. A yet-to-be published study of children ages four to 16 by the same authors found continued good agreement under awake conditions, but greater variability in the sleep respiration responses, possibly related to depth of sleep.

NON-NUTRITIVE SUCKING RESPONSE (NSR) AUDIOMETRY

The sucking response has a long history in newborn research since Jensen demonstrated (in 1932) discrimination among various tastes and temperatures. There seems to be some difference of opinion regarding its application for hearing measurement. Bronschtein and Petrowa (1952) reported sucking inhibition in newborns after 60 to 70 dB HL acoustic signals. But Kaye and Levin (1963) found as much sucking suppression in a nonstimulated control group as in the experimental group. In fact, Kaye (1966) found that repeated tonal stimulation would lead to sucking arousal. Keen (1964) found more sucking reduction after a 10-second tone than after a two-second tone.

Figure 6 shows the apparatus used by Levin and Kaye (1963) to study non-nutritive sucking responses. It is a standard rubber nipple containing a lever-action device which activates a microswitch controlling a polygraph pen. Another method (Sameroff, 1967) uses a blind Evenflo nipple connected by polyethylene tubing to a pressure transducer and finally to an amplifier and oscillograph unit.

Sameroff's study of sucking bursts in the neonate did not support Bronschtein and Petrowa's observations of sucking inhibition. On

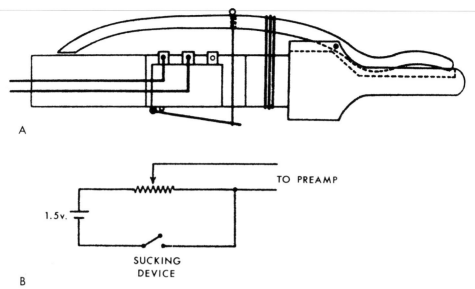

Figure 6. A microswitch-activating rubber nipple used by Levin and Kaye to study sucking changes to acoustic stimulation.

the contrary, an increase in signal level increased the number of sucking bursts. More accurately, as Sameroff points out, whatever was going out at the time of signal level was lengthened. If the infant was sucking, the burst was lengthened; if the infant was between bursts, the interval was lengthened.

Butterfield and Siperstein's (in press) paper on contingent auditory stimulation is a fascinating report on how the infant appears by sucking to actively manipulate the presence or absence of background music (Clancy Brothers). Figure 7 shows one of their subjects with nipple (to

pressure transducer) and headphones in place, similar to the method described by Sameroff. Figure 8 demonstrates how Butterfield and Siperstein's infants increased sucking duration (median) "on music" and reduced sucking when music was not played during sucking but was played in the interval between sucking periods. These are compared to the average of the silence and noncontingent control conditions. One of the remarkable findings was that music averaging 40 dB SPL "resulted in clearly different suck durations to the During and Between contingencies," suggesting that these dis-

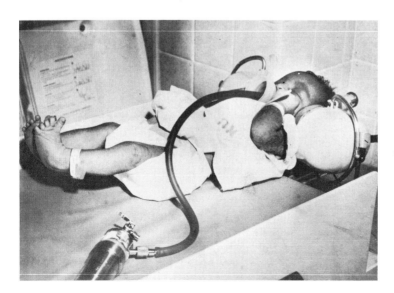

Figure 7. Infant with pressure transducer for sucking experiment. (From Butterfield and Siperstein.)

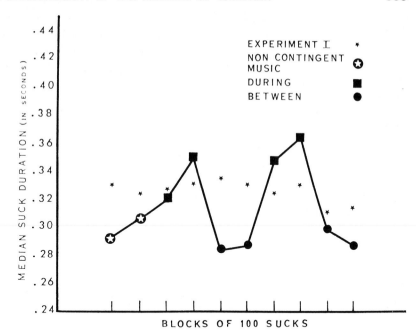

Figure 8. Changes in sucking with and without music compared to silent (star) and non-contingent music conditions.

criminations were also accomplished at very soft levels.

It was not Butterfield and Siperstein's intention to develop an audiometric technique. They have ably demonstrated a dynamic interaction between the newborn and his auditory environment in which the newborn is an active participant rather than a passive receptor. But their design offers another approach into the use of non-nutritive sucking for discriminative as well as threshold measurements.

ACOUSTIC IMPEDANCE AUDIOMETRY

The ear's physical properties of acoustic resistance and compliance will vary with changes in its physiological properties. Fill the ear with fluid, thicken the tympanic membrane, tighten or immobilize the ossicular chain, or disarticulate the ossicles and you will affect the amount of energy absorbed through the middle ear or reflected back out the external canal. It follows that absolute or relative measures of acoustic impedance ought to be available without any requirement other than sitting or lying. The possible application to children is inviting.

Metz (1946) is usually credited with the first contemporary effort to measure absolute acoustic impedance of the ear, using the mechanical acoustic bridge. Zwislocki (1963) adapted the bridge for clinical application and, in a series of

papers (1963, 1964, 1967a and b, 1969), Feldman demonstrated the differential impedance values obtained with the variety of middle ear conditions.

The measures using Zwislocki's bridge appear to be reliable enough with adults (Nixon and Glorig, 1964; Tillman et al., 1964; Feldman, 1967a and b). However, there appears to be as much as 20 per cent overlap between measures for otosclerotic and for normal ears (Feldman, 1967a and b), as well as less well defined amounts of overlap between normals and patients with other pathological conditions. In addition, precise measures with the mechanical acoustic bridge require a quiet patient with a reasonable-diameter auditory meatus so that the bridge-to-meatus seal may be maintained. The mechanical acoustic bridge has not had popular application to the measurement of children.

The electro-acoustic variety of impedance bridge has earned much more attention and popularity for testing children. The present models (Madsen and Grason-Stadler) permit much more movement of the patient and fit very small meatuses. In addition to measurements of resistance, tympanometry, a measure of eardrum compliance under artificial pressure variations in the meatus, may be carried out. Relative impedance audiometry, measuring impedance changes after stapedial reflex arousal, is an added and popular procedure with electro-acoustic impedance equipment as a "ballpark" measure of hearing sensitivity.

Brooks (1971) studied more than 1000 British schoolchildren, ages four to 11. Average time necessary to measure middle ear pressure, compliance, and the effect of stapedial reflex of one ear was five minutes. All the children completed the examination. Brooks found "normal" middle ear pressures for children from zero to a negative 170 mm. of waterpressure and a reflex to signals up to 100 dB hearing level. There were no sex differences. In the "abnormal" group, compliance and pressure tended to lower with age (reduction in fluid?), although a small group had a compliance shift upward with age (increased scarring?), and reflex thresholds were either unavailable or required more than 100 dB signal level.

One year to three year old children were studied by Robertson et al. (1968). Reflexes were observed in most of the children, ages 18 months or more, usually in both ears, and to mean signal levels between 75 dB and 85 dB Hearing Level (ASA, 1951). Similar results were obtained by Lamb and Norris (1969) with children ages four and a half to almost 12. In addition, they found only slightly poorer measures for mentally retarded children. The variability was greater for the latter group, probably reflecting more movement and talking by the children. But Lamb and Norris caution against using reflex thresholds in the absence of other measures of hearing with children. Although test-retest means were close, within-subject variability was considerable, sometimes as large as 26 to 30 dB. It is possible that this problem could be resolved by averaging two or even three separate reflex thresholds, since test time seems so short (Robertson, 1966; Brooks, 1971).

Diagnostic elaboration with relative impedance audiometry depends on (1) an expected range between reflex threshold and hearing threshold of between 70 and 85 dB, and (2) a loudness-dependent reflex threshold. The absence of reflex threshold has been related to conductive hearing problems (Metz, 1946; Terkildsen and Nielsen, 1960; Klockhoff, 1961), whereas a range less than 60 dB between reflex and hearing threshold strongly suggests the loudness recruitment cochlear sign (Kristensen and Jepsen, 1952; Metz, 1952; Thomsen, 1955; Ewertsen et al., 1958; Lamb et al., 1968; Terkildsen, 1960).

Terkildsen (1960) found reflex thresholds 60 dB or less above auditory thresholds in almost two thirds of a group of 127 congenitally hearing-impaired children. He interpreted the absence of a reflex threshold in most of the remainder as lack of sufficient signal intensity above hearing levels greater than 70 dB. Brooks' (1971) study of middle ear diseases in British schoolchildren has been described earlier in this section.

It would appear that relative impedance audiometry is gaining in popularity as increasing skill is obtained in its use. Efforts to sharpen diagnostic measures have led to the comparison of reflex thresholds generated by acoustic (stapedial) vs. nonacoustic (tensor tympanic) signals (Klockhoff and Anderson, 1960; Klockhoff, 1961; Holst et al., 1962). The relative impedance and tympanometric methods are likely to become a part of the standard battery of special acoustic tests with adults and perhaps with children.

ELECTRIC RESPONSE AUDIOMETRY

Study of the electrical responses of the child's auditory system has been accomplished in two major ways: (1) the changes in the brain wave evoked by an acoustical signal, and (2) the evoked cochlear microphonic and action potential. The first has been given considerable attention; the second has just recently earned small but renewed interest.

Early Period

That an acoustic signal could alter the size and shape of the raw brain wave has been known since at least 1939 (Davis, P.A., 1939; Davis et al., 1939). But it was almost immediately recognized that the response to sound was not always identifiable in the background of ongoing EEG activity. Ten years later Marcus and associates (1949) reported using EEG to assess the hearing of children. Marcus reported on 71 children in 1951, one as young as 10 months. Gidoll (1952) reported a readable response from an 18 month old sleeping child.

This early work was concerned with the problem of identifying changes in the raw brain wave. It established the application to children and its use with the instantly cooperative sleeping child. The method was not adopted widely, partly because of difficulties in reading the brain wave, the inaccessibility of equipment, and the relative success with behavioral audiometry.

Standardization Period

The 1950's were a period of standardization primarily stimulated by the work of Arthur

Derbyshire. Derbyshire and his associates (1956) identified three major components in a readable response: an on-effect, a continued response, and an off-effect. Responses were rated on a scale which took note of the number of different criteria met and the number of different channels in which these criteria were seen simultaneously. Some no-stimulus control trials were interspersed, replicating all conditions with the exception of the acoustic signal, and response was rated "blind," i.e., without knowledge of intensity level or frequency or whether the acoustic signal had actually been delivered (Derbyshire, 1956; Derbyshire and Farley, 1959; Withrow and Goldstein, 1958; Goldstein, 1960).

Their efforts met with some modest success. The Derbyshire group found an 18 dB average difference between behavioral audiograms and raw EEG responses during sleep. Variations in the sample were wide. The Goldstein team reported a tighter relationship ($\pm$ 10 dB) between EEG audiometry and behavioral thresholds for hearing-impaired schoolchildren.

Clinical applications began to be reported. Children with peripheral hearing impairments gave slightly "better" EEG responses than those suspected to have some central component (Goldstein et al., 1963; Taylor, 1963a and b). But the method was reported to fail in the task of screening the mentally retarded (Webb et al., 1964).

At this point, EEG audiometry seemed difficult, requiring great care in reading the waves, a tedious process at best, and restricted to a few laboratories.

The Averaging Computer

Dawson (1947, 1950, 1951, 1953, 1954) was responsible for developing the superimposition technique which was a conceptual breakthrough for the signal-to-noise problem in reading acoustically evoked responses. It exploits the randomness of the ongoing background electrical activity contrasted with the relatively regular "signature" nature of an acoustically evoked response. A train of short acoustic signals is introduced, and responses, time-locked to the signal, are superimposed upon each other. The background random activity tends to average out, whereas the superimposed evoked responses tend to stand out clearly from the background.

The concept was translatable into computer technology with Clark's (1958) development of the average response computer and the use of the computer by Rosenblith (1967) and others (Geisler et al., 1958; Siebert, 1959) for the averaging of EEG responses.

Electroencephalic Audiometry

Use of an averaging or summing computer has stimulated and broadened interest in studying the acoustically evoked responses of children. Electrodes are attached to the scalp to tap the voltage potential between the vertex and the mastoid or earlobe. Three types of responses have been identified: (1) early component: 18 to 50 msec.; (2) slow component: approximately 80 to 300 msec.; and (3) very late component: about 275 msec. and beyond. Initial interest in the early component centered mainly on separation of the acoustic response from a muscle potential (Bickford et al., 1964). But more recent work by Horwitz et al., (1966), Ruhm and his associates (1967), Goldstein and Rodman (1967), and Yoshie and Okudaira (1969) presents convincing arguments for auditory neurogenesis of the early component. The timing constants of the auditory nervous system, cochlea-to-cortex, lend further theoretical weight to these arguments.

The major interest of clinician and researcher up to the present time has been the so-called late component. Attempts to describe a characteristic wave form include a positive peak (P_1) at 50 to 80 msec., a negative peak (N_1) between 70 and 150 msec., a second positive peak (P_2) at 170 to 225 msec. A second negative peak (N_2) at 275 to 325 msec. either completes the slow components or is considered the initial landmark of the "very late" wave.

The time constants noted above are relative. They will be influenced by the state of the subject, the intensity of the signal, age and maturation, rise time of the signal, intersignal interval, attention, and many other factors. In a study of infants age one to 12 months, Lentz and McCandless (1971) describe two additional characteristics seen frequently: a positive-going wave form without a preceding N_1 negative peak, and a phase reversal, especially during quiet sleep, for the youngest subjects. There is considerable variability within the child's responses, which seems to lessen as he grows older; relatively stable responses are seen after age four in a normal nervous system. This variability makes reading the waves more difficult at the time that the need for valid interpretation of a response is greatest.

A major advantage to EEG studies is the opportunity to explore hearing adequacy while the child is asleep. But sleep tends to wash out the N_1 response and enhances the N_2 component.

Sedation is often necessary if natural sleep cannot be accomplished. Chloral hydrate (Cody et al., 1967), chlorpromazine (Rapin and Graziani, 1967), Nembutal (Price and Goldstein, 1966; Suzuki and Taguchi, 1968), and Valium (Burian, 1970) do not produce sedative-dependent distortions in the wave form. But Pentothal seems to cause high voltage, fast activity, affecting P_2 and N_2 and sometimes N_1 (Price and Goldstein, 1966; Rapin and Graziani, 1967), and should be avoided.

ERA and Behavioral Threshold

There is considerable question whether evoked vertex responses and behavioral thresholds are necessarily measures of the same physiological system. Davis and Zerlin (1966) emphasized that the vertex potential is simply reporting a change in nervous state. Abe (1954) and Rose and Malone (1965) observed that on-effects and off-effects look the same in the EEG although they sound very different. Rapin (1964) adopted a very conservative view of the sound of the brain wave. Derbyshire et al. (1964) implicated the reticular system as a primary route for different sensory modalities when they yield nonspecific responses. But Vaughan and Ritter (1970), Stohr and Goldring (1970), and Williamson et al. (1970) argue rather convincingly that the vertex potential results from the primary projection area of each modality and each lemniscal pathway.

Considerable effort has been spent relating the evoked responses of children and their behavioral thresholds. Davis (1964, 1965, 1966) and his associates (1967) reported close relationship between EEA and behavioral thresholds in hearing-impaired children, whereas a large average difference was noted for normal-hearing adults. Suzuki and Taguchi (1965) failed to obtain EEA responses from 42 per cent of normal-hearing children at a sensation level 20 dB above volunteered threshold. These results would obtain if the size of the evoked late component were loudness-dependent rather than intensity-dependent. Loudness recruitment close to threshold would explain good threshold relationships between EEA and behavioral thresholds for the hearing impaired with poor correlation for the normal hearing.

On the other hand, Price and Goldstein (1966) were able to obtain good agreement with behavioral thresholds for both normal-hearing and hearing-impaired children.

EEA with younger children appeared in its earlier history to yield more ambiguous findings, more difficult to interpret. Davis et al. (1967) endorsed EEA for school-age children down to age four, but observed "that the same children who have been 'enigmas' in the hearing clinic have also proved to be difficult to assess by evoked response audiometry." McCandless (1967) reported considerable difficulty obtaining readable responses from children below age two. It should be emphasized that Davis and McCandless were both referring to threshold derivation. They, along with many others (Lowell, 1960; Goodman, Appleby and Scott, 1964; Barnett and Goodwin, 1965; Morrell, 1965; Weitzman et al., 1965; Suzuki et al., 1966; Schulte et al., 1967; Ferriss et al., 1967), had studied and described the evoked responses above threshold.

Lentz and McCandless' (1971) findings on infants one, three, six and twelve months old represent a sobering yet stimulating commentary on the problem. At age one month, two thirds of the infants gave no EEA responses at all to signals below 60 dB HL; at three months, almost half did not "respond" below 60 dB HL; at six months, one third. On the other hand, eleven premature or high-risk infants who did not respond to 100 dB SPL noisemakers gave readable EEA response at 20 or 60 dB HL. Another two premature infants who failed to respond to EEA, did respond to 20 or 60 dB HL noises. For infants who were awake, telemetry of responses was employed to provide greater physical freedom (Reneau and Mast, 1968). Although the children were less restricted, movement artifacts were still observed.

But an equally impressive study by Suzuki and Origuchi (1969) compared the EEA responses during sedated sleep with conditioned orienting reflex (COR) thresholds from 47 normal hearing children (four months through four years) and from 133 hearing-impaired children (one year through five years). COR was 10 dB (mean) lower than EEA in normal hearing children, and 6 dB lower in mild to moderately impaired children. Children with severe losses showed EEA slightly (0.43 dB mean) more sensitive.

Suzuki and Origuchi (1969) showed improving thresholds for both COR and EEA responses when neonates were compared to infants. Davis and Onishi (1969) obtained similar EEA findings.

Very Late Components

The very late components (P_{300} and beyond) relate to perception, meaning, attention, association, or preparation for a contingent response. Abe (1954) considered the late component relatively passive cortical response, with the very late response an active cortical response. Walter (1964a, 1965a and b, 1966) and his associates (1964, 1965a, b, and c) have led the way in studying the contingent negative variation (CNV) or expectancy wave (E-Wave). Some of the early applications of study of the slowly developing CNV is in speech audiometry (Derbyshire et al., 1964; Burian et al., 1969). But as yet the CNV has not been explored in infants and children relative to speech signals.

Electrocochleogram

The study of human cochlear potentials was reported as early as 1935 by Fromm, Nylen and Zotterman, but there was only moderate interest until 1960 (Andreyev et al., 1939; Perlman and Case, 1941; Lempert et al., 1947). The Johns Hopkins group (Ruben et al., 1961) revived this approach and explored its application to pediatric hearing measurement (Ruben et al., 1962).

The method used was similar to that with experimental animals: the use of a platinum electrode against the round window membrane after tympanotomy. Ruben and his associates did observe, in addition to cochlear microphonics, the eighth nerve action potentials of some of the children examined. They claimed no more than a qualitative indication for their method. Its general applicability to pediatric studies seemed limited to a few patients in whom surgery might be needed or in whom other approaches were unsatisfactory.

A nonsurgical method employing an extratympanic electrode in the external meatus has been developed by Yoshie and his associates for the measurement of cochlear microphonics (Yoshie and Yamaura, 1969) and averaged action potentials (Yoshie and Ohashi, 1969). Applications to children's audiometry have not yet been reported but will probably be available before this chapter is published. The program of the Electric Response Audiometry Study Group annual meeting in 1971, held in Vienna, contained a number of presentations on electrocochleography.

General Comments

Is there light glimmering at the end of the tunnel? It is obvious that clinical EEA presently is a difficult, technical, expensive task that requires (1) close study and a long period of calibration and practice; (2) team (division of labor) operation with emphasis on making the child comfortable; (3) rapid, efficient execution and completion in limited, sedated time; (4) close monitoring of sleep levels; (5) special efforts to control equipment and movement artifacts; and (6) a critical, sober, ongoing process of correlation with COR and perhaps one other physiological measure. The reader should observe at this point that some of these clinical laboratories have had more than 10 to 15 years of experience in EEA.

Taguchi et al. (1969) and Davis and Onishie (1969) seem to have learned that large, readable signals (S/N) yielding more sensitive thresholds are obtained from the high voltage, slow waves showing sleep spindles as contrasted with low voltage, fast REM sleep or very light sleep. Signal averagers have also learned to look elsewhere, at N_{300} away from the more mature N_{100} typical of adults.

Where next? A fetal elecroencephalic response was reported by Barden et al., (1968) from one fetal subject following induction of labor; but five other subjects did not respond. Sakabe and his associates (1969) carried the banner of early identification to the zenith, reporting auditory evoked responses from the abdomen of an eight month pregnant woman.

No! The immediate present will see more concern with the very early vertex response, electrocochleography, and the diagnostic integration of all the electrical responses from the auditory system. Any soothsayer of the next decade in EEA would examine the clinical questions of attention, active listening as distinguished from passive hearing, phonemic discrimination, and speech EEA. Despite most severe research difficulties, the main area of study will eventually shift to the very late (300 msec. and beyond) wave and the CNV, partly because of the compelling nature of these questions and partly because orienting thresholds are available through other less expensive and potentially just as reliable physiological measures, e.g., EKG, respiration, and plethysmography.

ELECTRODERMAL AUDIOMETRY

An acoustic signal perceived by the listener will lower the resistance of the skin to a small externally introduced current or reduce the electrical potential between two points on the skin. Known as the Feré and Tarchanow effects, respectively, these physiological responses can be monitored by electrodes and be read out by appropriate recording apparatus. But these effects also adapt out or extinguish readily after repeated stimuli; thus, a stronger associated signal or even a noxious agent such as mild faradic shock may be used to reinforce the response. Hence, the conditioning procedure utilizing shock for audiometry has been referred to as conditioned galvanic skin response audiometry or conditioned electrodermal audiometry.

Electrodermal audiometry (EDA) or galvanic skin response audiometry (GSR) enjoyed considerable notoriety in the 1950's for medico-legal considerations and, in some laboratories, for measuring the hearing of children. Developed from the research and environment of the psychological laboratory, it is surprising and sobering now to discover how little research was actually done on EDA itself.

The procedures for testing children are well described by Hardy and Pauls (1952) and by O'Neill and Oyer (1966). A two-man team is preferred, with one occupying the child while the second controls the stimulus and monitors responses. Pickup electrodes are usually placed on the sole of one foot with shock electrodes on the other leg, thus permitting the hands to be free for the manipulation of toys. Extraneous movements are kept to a minimum. Partial reinforcement of tone by shock, a 40 to 60 per cent reinforcement schedule, is usually preferred. Response criteria usually include a resistance drop between 2 and 4 seconds after tonal onset (Goldstein, 1963; Stewart et al., 1961).

But EDA has not always been successful, and often with children who had not been successfully evaluated by other means. A number of investigators have reported difficulty in conditioning aphasic and other brain-injured children (Goldstein et al., 1954, 1955; Goodhill et al., 1954; Hardy and Pauls, 1959). The Goldstein group (1955) observed that difficult-to-condition children often had lower skin resistance.

EDA under sedation has also been disappointing. Irwin et al. (1957) report poor conditioning of mentally retarded children after sedation, and other workers (Lienert and Traxel, 1959; Uhr and Miller, 1960) report reduction in the response itself with the use of tranquilizers. EDA is additionally limited in that children cannot be tested while asleep (Davis and Goldstein, 1970).

Many examiners have not favored EDA because of its use of shock. This is unfortunate since shocks levels can be controlled and conditioning could be established with other agents, e.g., bright light.

Recently EDA has not been among the most popular procedures with children. Clinically it is evident that a failure to respond on EDA may not represent a failure to hear, but rather a failure to condition, or extinction, or some other artifact. The author is impressed with the lack of an impressive body of research on EDA; work in this area will be necessary for the procedure to be rejuvenated.

SUMMARY

There are currently several popular methods of testing hearing in children. Behavioral and conditioning procedures remain the methods of choice for most children by the majority of audiologists. But "objective" procedures, especially heart rate, respiratory rate, relative impedance, and EEG are increasingly important. Electrodermal audiometry seems out of favor, with EEG in favor and in danger of the same overselling given the GSR. Diagnostic procedures seem very promising, especially the integration possible within impedance audiometry and within electric response audiometry.

The consumer, be he professional or layman, must be cautious of being overawed by glittering technology and the magic of the computer. The quality of an audiology clinic or an otologic practice is only in a limited sense represented by its hardware. The refinement of method is critical when it enables a specific audiologist the freedom to investigate to the maximum. The goal is competent judgment and only competent judgment, whether it ensue from subjective or objective procedures.

ACKNOWLEDGMENTS

The author wishes to acknowledge gratefully the assistance of Richard Brown and Richard Seewald, who helped review the literature of electric response and heart rate audiometry. Special thanks is also due Elaine Engelbart, who read the manuscript critically and offered helpful suggestions for its accomplishment.

REFERENCES

Abe, M.: Electrical responses of the human brain to acoustic stimulus. Tohoku J. Exp. Med. *60*:47, 1954.

Andreyev, A. M., Arapova, A. A., and Gershuni, G. V.: [Electrical cochlear potentials in man.] Fiziol. Zh. USSR *26*:205, 1939.

Barden, T. P., Peltzman, P., and Graham, J. T.: Human fetal electroencephalographic response to intrauterine acoustic signals. Amer. J. Obst. Gynec. *100*:1128, 1968.

Barnet, A. B., and Goodwin, R. S.: Averaged evoked electroencephalographic responses to clocks in the human newborn. Electroenceph. Clin. Neurophysiol. *18*:441, 1965.

Barr, B.: Pure tone audiometry for preschool children. Acta Otolaryng. Suppl. 121, 1955.

Bartoshuk, A. K.: Human neonatal cardiac acceleration to sound: Habituation and dishabituation. Percept. Motor Skills *15*:15, 1962a.

Bartoshuk, A. K.: Response decrement with repeated elicitation of human neonatal cardiac acceleration to sound. J. Comp. Physiol. Psych. *55*:9, 1962b.

Bartoshuk, A. K.: Human neonatal cardiac responses to sound: A power function. Psychon. Sci. *1*:151, 1964.

Beadle, K. R., and Crowell, D. H.: Neonatal electrocardiographic responses to sound. J. Speech Hear. Res. *5*:112, 1962.

Bench, J.: The law of initial value: A neglected source of variance in infant audiometry. Int. Audiol. *9*:314, 1970.

Bickford, R., Jacobsen, I., and Coy, D.: Nature of averaged evoked potentials to sound and other stimuli in man. Ann. N.Y. Acad. Sci. *112*:204, 1964.

Bloomer, H.: A simple method for testing the hearing of small children. J. Speech Dis. *7*:311, 1942.

Bradford, L. J., Rousey, C. L., and Bradford, M. A.: Respiration audiometry with the pre-school child. Laryngoscope. *82*:28, 1972.

Bridger, W.: Sensory habituation and discrimination in the human neonate. Amer. J. Psychiat. *117*:991, 1961.

Bronschtein, A. L., and Petrowa, J. P.: Die Erforschung des akustischen Analysators bei Neugeborenen und Kinder im frühen Sauglingsalter. Pawlow-Z. Hohere Nerventatigkeit *2*:441, 1952.

Brooks, D. N.: Electroacoustic impedance bridge studies on normal ears of children. J. Speech Hear. Res. *14*:247, 1971.

Burian, K.: Discrepancies between subjective and ERA threshold. ERA *7*:18, 1970 (Abstract).

Burian, K., Gestring, G. F., and Haider, M.: Objective speech audiometry. Int. Audiol. *8*:387, 1969.

Butterfield, E. C., and Siperstein, G. N.: Influence of contingent auditory stimulation upon non-nutritional suckle. Presented at the Third Symposium on Oral Sensation and Perception: The Mouth of the Infant. Will appear in the proceedings of the conference to be published by Charles C Thomas.

Carhart, R.: Questions and speculations, *In* McConnell, F., and Ward, P. H. (eds.): Deafness in Childhood. Nashville, Vanderbilt University Press, 1967, Chapter 15, p. 229.

Chaiklin, J. B.: The conditioned GSR auditory speech threshold. J. Speech Hear. Res. *2*:229, 1959.

Clark, W. A., Jr.: Average response computer (ARC-1). Quart. Rep. Electronics Mass. Inst. Tech., 1958, pp. 114–117.

Clifton, R. K., Graham, F. K., and Hatton, H. M.: Newborn heartrate response and response habituation as a function of stimulus duration. J. Exp. Child Psych. *6*:256, 1968.

Clifton, R. K., and Meyers, W. J.: The heart-rate response of four-month-old infants to auditory stimuli. J. Exp. Child Psychol. *7*:122, 1969.

Cody, D., Klass, D., and Bickford, R.: Cortical audiometry: An objective method of evaluating auditory function in awake and sleeping man. Trans. Amer. Acad. Ophthal. Otolaryng. *19*:81, 1967.

Cotton, J. C., and Hall, J.: Administration of the 6-A audiometer test to kindergarten and first grade children. Volta Rev. *41*:291, 1939.

Curry, E. T., and Kurtzrock, G. H.: A preliminary investigation of the ear-choice technique in threshold audiometry. J. Speech Hear. Dis. *16*:340, 1951.

Daly, R. L.: Peripheral vasoconstriction and electroencephalography as estimators of hearing threshold. ASHA *7*:419, 1965 (Abstract).

Dansinger, S.: Verbal auditory screening with the mentally retarded. Amer. J. Ment. Defic. *71*:387, 1966.

Davis, H.: Some properties of the slow cortical evoked response in humans. Science *146*:434, 1964.

Davis, H.: Slow cortical responses evoked by acoustic stimuli. Acta Otolaryng. *59*:179, 1965.

Davis, H.: Validation of evoked response audiometry (ERA) in deaf children. Int. Audiol. *2*:77, 1966.

Davis, H., Davis, P., Loomis, A., Harvey, E., and Hobart, G.: Electrical reaction of the human brain to auditory stimulation during sleep. J. Neurophysiol. *2*:500, 1939.

Davis, H., and Goldstein, R.: Audiometry: Other auditory tests. *In* Davis, H., and Silverman, S. R.: Hearing and Deafness. 3rd ed. New York, Holt, Rinehart and Winston, 1970, p. 221.

Davis, H., Hirsh, S., Shelnutt, J., and Bowers, C.: Further validation of evoked response audiometry (ERA). J. Speech Hear. Res. *10*:717, 1967.

Davis, H., and Onishie, S.: Maturation of auditory evoked potentials. Int. Audiol. *8*:24, 1969.

Davis, H., and Zerlin, S.: Acoustic relations of the human vertex potential. J. Acoust. Soc. Amer. *39*:109, 1966.

Davis, P. A.: Effects of acoustic stimulation on the waking human brain. J. Neurophysiol. *2*:494, 1939.

Dawson, G. D.: Cerebral responses to electrical stimulation of peripheral nerve in man. J. Neurol. Neurosurg. Psychiat. *10*:134, 1947.

Dawson, G. D.: Cerebral responses to nerve stimulation in man. Brit. Med. Bull. *6*:326, 1950.

Dawson, G. D.: A summation technique for detecting small signals in a large irregular background. J. Physiol. *115*:2, 1951.

Dawson, G. D.: Autocorrelation and automatic integration. Electroenceph. Clin. Neurophysiol. *4*:26, 1953.

Dawson, G. D.: A summation technique for the detection of small evoked potentials. Electroenceph. Clin. Neurophysiol. *6*:65, 1954.

Derbyshire, A. J.: Personal communication, 1956.

Derbyshire, A. J., and Farley, J. C.: Sampling auditory responses at the cortical level. Ann. Otol. *68*:675, 1959.

Derbyshire, A., Fraser, A., McDermott, M., and Bridge, A.: Audiometric measurements by electroencephalography. Electroenceph. Clin. Neurophysiol. *8*:467, 1956.

Derbyshire, A., McDermott, M., Fraser, A. B., Farley, J. S., Dhruvanajan, P. S., Oppfelt, R., Palmer, C. W., and Elliot, C.: Auditory function evaluated by direct observation of EEG responses. Proceedings of a conference held in Toronto, Canada, Oct. 8–9, 1964. Acta. Otolaryng. (Suppl.) *206*:106, 1965.

Derbyshire, A. J., Palmer, C. W., Elliot, C. R., Cassidy, R., and Kapple, H.: EEG responses to words. ASHA *6*:392, 1964.

Dix, M. R., and Hallpike, C. S.: The peep-show: A new technique for pure-tone audiometry in young children. Brit. Med. J. *2*:719, 1947.

Donnelly, K. G.: The vibro-tactile technique of conditioning young children for hearing tests. In Lloyd, L. L., and Frising, D. R. (eds.): The Audiologic Assessment of the Mentally Retarded. Proceedings of a National Conference, Parsons, Kansas, 1965, pp. 59–70.

Drettner, B.: The peripheral vascular response in audiometric testing. Acta Otolaryng. *64*:5, 1967.

Eisenberg, R. B.: Auditory behavior in the human neonate: I. Methodologic problems and the logical design of research procedures. J. Aud. Res. *5*:159, 1963.

Eisenberg, R. B., Coursin, D. B., and Rupp, N. R.: Habituation to an acoustic pattern as an index of differences among human neonates. J. Aud. Res. *6*:239, 1966.

Epstein, A., Golas, T. G., and Owens, E.: Familiarity and intelligibility of monosyllabic word lists. J. Speech Hear. Res. *11*:435, 1968.

Ewertsen, H. W.: Teddy-bear screening audiometry for babies. Acta Otolaryng. *61*:279, 1966.

Ewertsen, H., Filling, S., Terkildsen, K. and Thomsen, R.: Comparative recruitment testing. Acta Otolaryng. (Suppl.) *140*:116, 1958.

Ewing, A. W. G.: Aphasia in Children. London, Oxford Medical Pub., 1930.

Ewing, I. R.: Deafness in infancy and early childhood. J. Laryng. *58*:279, 1943.

Ewing, I. R., and Ewing, A. W. G.: The ascertainment of deafness in infancy and early childhood. J. Laryng. *59*:309, 1944.

Ewing, I. R., and Ewing, A. W. G.: Opportunity and the Deaf Child. London, University of London Press, 1947.

Fairbanks, G.: Test of phonemic differentiation: The rhyme test. J. Acoust. Soc. Amer. *30*:596, 1958.

Feldman, A.: Impedance measurements at the eardrum as an aid in diagnosis. J. Speech Hear. Res. *6*:315, 1963.

Feldman, A.: Acoustic impedance measurement as a clinical procedure. Int. Audiol. *3*:156, 1964.

Feldman, A.: A report of further impedance studies of the acoustic reflex. J. Speech Hear. Res. *10*:616, 1967a.

Feldman, A.: Acoustic impedance studies of the normal ear. J. Speech Hear. Res. *10*:165, 1967b.

Feldman, A.: Acoustic impedance measurement of post-stepedectomized ears. Laryngoscope *79*:1132, 1969.

Ferriss, G. S., Davis, G. D., Dorsen, M., and Hackett, E. R.: Maturation of the evoked response to auditory stimuli in human infants. Electroenceph. Clin. Neurophysiol. *23*:83, 1967.

Field, H., Copack, P., Derbyshire, A. J., Dressen, G. J., and Marcus, R. E.: Responses of newborns to auditory stimulation. J. Aud. Res. *7*:271, 1967.

Frisina, D. R.: Audiometric evaluation and its relation to habilitation and rehabilitation of the deaf. Amer. Ann. Deaf *107*:478, 1962.

Frisina, R.: Measurement of hearing in children. In Jerger, J. (ed.): Modern Developments in Audiology. New York, Academic Press, 1963, pp. 126–166.

Fromm, B., Nylen, C. O., and Zotterman, Y.: Studies in the mechanism of the Wever-Bray effect. Acta Otolaryng. *22*:477, 1935.

Fulton, R. T.: Task adaptation and word familiarity of W-22 discrimination lists with retarded children. J. Aud. Res. *7*:353, 1967.

Geisler, C., Freshkopf, L., and Rosenblith, W.: Extracranial responses to acoustic clicks in man. Science *128*:1210, 1958.

Giddoll, A.: Quantitative determination for hearing to audiometric frequencies in the electroencephalogram; Preliminary report. Arch. Otolaryng. *55*:597, 1952.

Goldie, L., and Green, J.: Changes in mode of respiration as an indicator of level of awareness. Nature *189*:581, 1961.

Goldstein, R.: Comparison of methods for evaluating electroencephalic responses to tones. J. Speech Hear. Dis. *25*:303, 1960.

Goldstein, R.: Electrophysiologic audiometry. In Jerger, J. (ed.): Modern Developments in Audiology. New York, Academic Press, 1963.

Goldstein, R., Kendall, D., and Arick, B. E.: Electroencephalographic audiometry in young children. J. Speech Hear. Dis. *28*:331, 1963.

Goldstein, R., Ludwig, H., and Naunton, R. F.: Difficulty in conditioning galvanic skin responses: Its possible significance in clinical audiometry. Acta Otolaryng. *44*:67, 1954.

Goldstein, R., Polito-Castro, S. B., and Daniels, J. T.: Difficulty in conditioning electrodermal response to tone in normally hearing children. J. Speech Hear. Dis. *20*:27, 1955.

Goldstein, R., and Rodman, L. B.: Early components of averaged evoked responses to rapidly repeated auditory stimuli. J. Speech Hear. Res. *10*:697, 1967.

Goodhill, V., Rehman, I., and Brockman, S.: Objective skin resistance audiometry. Ann. Otol. *63*:22, 1954.

Goodman, W. S., Appleby, S. V., and Scott, J. W.: Audiometry in newborn children by electroencephalography. Laryngoscope *74*:1316, 1964.

Graham, F. K., Clifton, R. K., and Hatton, H. M.: Habituation of heartrate response to repeated auditory stimulation during the first five days of life. Child Dev. *39*:35, 1968.

Gray, M. L., and Crowell, D. H.: Heart rate changes to sudden peripheral stimuli in the human during early infancy. J. Pediat. *72*:807, 1968.

Grey, H. A., D'Asaro, M. J., and Sklar, M.: Auditory perceptual thresholds in brain-injured children. J. Speech Hear. Res. *8*:49, 1965.

Griffing, T., Simonton, K., and Hedgecock, L. D.: Verbal auditory screening for preschool children. Trans. Amer. Acad. Ophthol. Otolaryng. *1*:105, 1967.

Guilford, R., and Haug, O.: Diagnosis of deafness in the very young child. Arch. Otolaryng. *55*:101, 1952.

Hardy, W. G., and Pauls, M. D.: The test situation in PGSR audiometry. J. Speech Hear. Dis. *17*:13, 1952.

Hardy, W. G., and Pauls, M. D.: Significance of problems of conditioning in GSR audiometry. J. Speech Hear. Dis. *24*:123, 1959.

Haskins, H. L.: A Phonetically Balanced Test of Speech Discrimination for Children. Unpublished master's thesis, Northwestern University, Chicago, 1949.

Hensel, H., and Bender, F.: Fortlaufende Besteimmung Der Hautdurchblutung am Menschen mit einem elektrischen Warmeleitmesser. Pfluger Arch. Ges. Physiol. *263*:603, 1956.

Hirsh, I. J.: Conditioning in audiometry. In The Measurement of Hearing. New York, McGraw-Hill Book Co., 1952, Chapter 10, p. 271.

Hirsh, I. J.: Auditory training. In Davis, H., and Silverman, S. R. (eds.): Hearing and Deafness. 3rd ed. New York, Holt, Rinehart, and Winston, 1970, Chapter 13, p. 347.

Hogan, D. D.: Autonomic responses as supplementary

hearing measures. *In* Fulton, R. T., and Lloyd, L. L.: Audiometry for the Retarded. Baltimore, The Williams & Wilkins Co., 1969, Chapter 8, pp. 248–250.

Holst, H., Ingelstedt, S., and Ortegren, V.: Eardrum movements following stimulation of the middle ear muscles. Acta Otolaryng. *182:*73, 1962.

Horowitz, L. S., Sullivan, R. F., and Mazor, M.: A field comparison of pure tone and verbal auditory screening (VASC) methods as applied to preschool children. ASHA *12:*450, 1970 (Abstract).

Horwitz, S. F., Larson, S. J., and Sances, A., Jr.: Evoked potentials as an adjunct to the auditory evaluation of patients. *In* Proceedings of the Symposium on Biomedical Engineering, Milwaukee, 1966, *1:*49.

Houston Speech and Hearing Center: Audiometric assessment technique. ASHA *6:*261, 1964.

Howes, D.: On the relation between the intelligibility and frequency of occurrences of English words. J. Acoust. Soc. Amer. *29:*296, 1957.

Huizing, H. D., Kruisinga, R. H. H., and Taselaar, M.: Triplet audiometry: An analysis of band discrimination in speech reception. Acta Otolaryng. *51:*256, 1960.

Huizing, H. D., and Taselaar, M.: Triplet testing and training—an approach to band discrimination and its monaural summation. Laryngoscope *68:*535, 1958.

Irwin, J. V., Hind, J. E., and Aronson, A. E.: Experience with conditioned GSR audiometry in a group of mentally deficient individuals. Train. Sch. Bull. *54:*26, 1957.

Ishisawa, H.: A study on play audiometry. Otologia Fukuoka (Suppl. 7) *6:*397, 1960.

Jasienska, A., Dwornicka, B., Norska, I., and Smolarz, W.: Examination of hearing in newborns by ECG. Arch. Otolaryng. *86:*68, 1967.

Jensen, K.: Differential reactions to taste and temperature stimuli in new born infants. Psych. Monogr. *12:*365, 1932.

Johansson, B., Wedenberg, E., and Westin, B.: Measurements of tone response by the human foetus. A preliminary report. Acta Otolaryng. *57:*188, 1964.

Kaye, H.: The effect of feeding and tonal stimulation on non-nutritive sucking in the human newborn. J. Exp. Child Psych. *3:*131, 1966.

Kaye, H., and Levin, G. R.: Two attempts to demonstrate tonal suppression of non-nutritive sucking in neonates. Percept. Motor Skills *17:*521, 1963.

Keaster, J. A.: A quantitative method of testing the hearing of young children. J. Speech Hear. Dis. *12:*159, 1947.

Keaster, M. J.: A Pure Tone Audiometric Test for Preschool Children. Unpublished master's thesis, University of Wisconsin, 1951.

Keen, R.: Effects of auditory stimulation on sucking behavior in the human neonate. J. Exp. Child Psych. *1:*348, 1964.

Keen, R. E., Chase, H. H., and Graham, F. K.: Twenty-four hour retention by neonates of an habituated heart rate response. Psychon. Sci. *2:*265, 1965.

Kimball, B. D.: Addendum to previous article. ASHA *6:*500, 1964.

Klockhoff, I.: Middle-ear muscle reflexes in man. Acta. Otolaryng. *Suppl. 164,* 1961.

Klockhoff, I., and Anderson, H.: Reflex activity in the tensor tympani muscle recorded in man: A preliminary report. Acta Otolaryng. *51:*184, 1960.

Knox, E. C.: A method of obtaining puretone audiograms in young children. J. Laryng. *74:*475, 1960.

Kottmeyer, G.: Plethysmographische Untersuchungen nach schwellennahen sensorischen und sensiblen Reizen. Arch. Ohr. Nas. Kehlkopfheilk. *177:*297, 1961.

Kristensen, H., and Jepsen, O.: Recruitment in otoneurological diagnostics. Acta Otolaryng. *42:*553, 1952.

LaCrosse, E. L., and Bidlake, H.: A method to test the hearing of mentally retarded children. Volta Rev. *66:*27, 1964.

Lamb, L. E., and Norris, T. W.: Acoustic impedance measurement. *In* Fulton, R. T. and Lloyd, L. L. (eds.): Audiometry for the Retarded, with Implications for the Difficult-to-Test. Baltimore, The Williams & Wilkins Co., 1969.

Lamb, L., Peterson, J., and Hansen, S.: Application of stapedius muscle reflex measures to diagnosis of auditory problems. Int. Audiol. *7:*188, 1968.

Lassman, F. M.: Audiology. Bull. Univ. Minn. Hosp. and Minn. Med. Found. *24:*281, 1953.

Lehmann, G.: Untersuchungen zur Frage der nervosen Larmbelastung. Karl Arnold Festschrift. Koln and Opladen, Westdeutscher Verlag, 1955.

Lempert, J., Wever, E. G., and Lawrence, M.: The cochleogram and its clinical application. Arch. Otolaryng. *45:*61, 1947.

Lentz, W., and McCandless, G. A.: Averaged electroencephalic audiometry in infants. J. Speech Hear. Dis. *36:*19, 1971.

Leventhal, A. S., and Lipsitt, L. P. Adaptation, pitch discrimination and sound localization in the neonate. Child Dev. *35:*759, 1964.

Lewis, M., and Spaulding, S. J.: Differential cardiac response to visual and auditory stimulation in the young child. Psychophysiology *3:*229, 1967.

Lienert, G. A., and Traxel, W.: The effects of meprobamate and alcohol on galvanic skin response. J. Psych. *48:*329, 1959.

Ling, D., Ling, A. H., and Doehring, D. G.: Stimulus response and observer variables in the auditory screening of newborn infants. J. Speech Hear. Res. *13:*9, 1970.

Lipsitt, L. P., and DeLucia, C. A.: An apparatus for the measurement of specific response and general activity of the human neonate. Amer. J. Psychiat. *73:*630, 1960.

Lloyd, L. L.: A Comparison of Selected Auditory Measures on Normal Hearing Mentally Retarded Children. Unpublished doctoral dissertation, University of Iowa, 1965.

Lloyd, L. L., Spradlin, J. E., and Reid, M. J.: An operant audiometric procedure for difficult-to-test patients. J. Speech Hear. Dis. *33:*236, 1968.

Lloyd, L. L., and Young, C. E.: Pure tone audiometry. *In* Fulton, R. T., and Lloyd, L. L. (eds.): Audiometry for the Retarded, With Implications for the Difficult-to-Test. Baltimore, The Williams & Wilkins Co., 1969, p. 164.

Lowell, E. L.: Some fundamental problems in the use of electroencephalography in the assessment of hearing. *In* Ewing, A. (ed.): The Modern Educational Treatment of Deafness. Manchester, England, Manchester University Press, 1960.

Lowell, E., Rushford, G., Hoversten, G., and Stoner, M.: Evaluation of pure tone audiometry with preschool age children. J. Speech Hear. Dis. *21:*292, 1956.

Lowell, E. L., Troffer, C. I., Warburton, E. A., and Rushford, G. M.: Temporal evannation: A new approach in diagnostic audiology. J. Speech Hear. Dis. *25:*340, 1960.

MacPherson, J. R.: The Evaluation and Development of Techniques for Testing the Auditory Acuity of Trainable Mentally Retarded Children. Unpublished doctoral dissertation, University of Texas, Austin, Texas, 1960.

Marcus, R. E.: Hearing and speech problems in children. Observation and use of EEG. Arch. Otolaryng. 53:134, 1951.

Marcus R., Gibbs, E., and Gibbs, F.: Electroencephalography in the diagnosis of hearing loss in the very young child. Dis. Nerv. Syst. 10:170, 1949.

McCandless, G.: Clinical application of evoked response audiometry. J. Speech Hear. Res. 10:468, 1967.

Metz, O.: The acoustic impedance measured in normal and pathological ears. Acta Otolaryng. Suppl. 63:1946.

Metz, O. Threshold of reflex contraction of muscles of middle ear and recruitment of loudness. Arch. Otolaryng. 55:536, 1952.

Meyerson, L.: A verbal audiometric test for young children. Amer. Psychol. 2:291, 1947.

Meyerson, L., and Michael, J. L.: The Measurement of Sensory Thresholds in Exceptional Children: An Experimental Approach to Some Problems of Differential Diagnosis and Education with Special Reference to Hearing. Cooperative Research Project No. 418, United States Office of Education, Department of Health, Education, and Welfare. Houston, Texas, University of Houston, 1960.

Miller, A. L.: The use of reward techniques in testing young children's hearing. Hear. News 30:5, 1962.

Moffitt, A. R.: Speech Perception by Infants. Ph.D. dissertation. Minneapolis, University of Minnesota, August, 1968.

Monsees, E. K.: Children's auditory test. Volta Rev. 55:446, 1953.

Morrell, F.: Clinical neurology: Some applications of scanning by computer. Calif. Med. 103:406, 1965.

Murphy, K. P.: Development of hearing in babies—a diagnostic system for detecting early signs of deafness in infants. Child and Family 1:16, 1962.

Murphy, K. P., and Smyth, C. H.: Responses of foetus to auditory stimulation. Lancet 1:972, 1962.

Myatt, B. D., and Landes, B.: Assessing discrimination loss in children. Arch. Otolaryng. 77:359, 1963.

Nixon, J. C., and Glorig, A.: Reliability of acoustic impedance measures of the eardrum. J. Aud. Res., 4:261, 1964.

O'Neill, J. J., and Oyer, H. J.: Applied Audiometry. New York, Dodd, Mead and Co., Inc., 1966.

O'Neill, J. J., Oyer, H. J., and Hillis, J. W.: Audiometric procedures used with children. J. Speech Hear. Dis. 26:61, 1961.

Owens, E.: Intelligibility of words varying in familiarity. J. Speech Hear. Res. 4:113, 1961.

Oyer, H. J., and Doudna, M.: Word familiarity as a factor in testing discrimination of hard-of-hearing subjects. Arch. Otolaryng. 72:351, 1960.

Perlman, H. B., and Case, T. J.: Electrical phenomena of the cochlea in man. Arch. Otolaryng. 34:710, 1941.

Price, L.: Evoked response audiometry: Some considerations. J. Speech Hear. Dis. 34:137, 1969.

Price, L., and Goldstein, R.: Averaged evoked responses for measuring auditory sensitivity in children. J. Speech Hear. Dis. 31:248, 1966.

Rapin, I.: Evoked responses to clicks in a group of children with communication disorders. Ann. N. Y. Acad. Sci. 112:182, 1964.

Rapin, I., and Graziani, L.: Auditory-evoked responses in normal, brain-damaged and deaf infants. Neurology 17:881, 1967.

Rapin, I., and Steinberg, P.: Reaction time for pediatric audiometry. J. Speech Hear. Res. 13:203, 1970.

Reddell, R. C., and Calvert, D. R.: Conditioned audiovisual response audiometry. International Conference on Oral Education of the Deaf, 1967, p. 502.

Reneau, J., and Mast, R.: Telemetric EEG audiometry instrumentation for use with the profoundly retarded. Amer. J. Ment. Defic. 72:506, 1968.

Richmond, J. G., Grossman, H. J., and Lustman, S. L.: Hearing test for newborn infants. Pediatrics 11:634, 1953.

Ritter, W., and Vaughan, H. G., Jr.: Averaged evoked responses in vigilance and discrimination: A reassessment. Science 164:326, 1969.

Robertson, E.: An Investigation of Relative Impedance Measurements in Infants and Young Children. Unpublished master's thesis, Louisiana State University, Baton Rouge, Louisiana, 1966.

Robertson, E., Peterson, J., and Lamb, L.: Relative impedance measurements in young children. Arch. Otolaryng. 88:162, 1968.

Rose, D. E., and Malone, J. C.: Some aspects of the acoustically evoked response to the cessation of stimulus. J. Aud. Res. 5:27, 1965.

Rosenau, H.: Die Schlafbeschallung: eine Methode der Horprufung beim Kleinstkind. Z. Laryng. Rhinol. Otol. 41:194, 1962.

Rosenblith, W.: Some quantifiable aspects of the electrical activity of the nervous system. Rev. Mod. Physics 31:532, 1967.

Rosenzweig, M. R., and Postman, L.: Intelligibility as a function of frequency of usage. J. Exper. Psych. 54:412, 1957.

Ross, M. E., and Lerman, J.: A Picture Identification Test for Hearing Impaired Children. Final report, Project No. 7–8038, United States Office of Education, 1968.

Rousey, C., Snyder, C., and Rousey, C.: Change in respiration as a function of auditory stimuli. J. Aud. Res. 4:107, 1964.

Ruben, R. J., Bordley, J. E., and Lieberman, A. T.: Cochlear potentials in man. Laryngoscope 71:1141, 1961.

Ruben, R. J., Lieberman, A. T., and Bordley, J. E.: Some observations on cochlear potentials and nerve action potentials in children. Laryngoscope 72:545, 1962.

Ruhm, H. B., and Carhart, R.: Objective speech audiometry: A new method based on electrodermal response. J. Speech Hear. Res. 1:169, 1958.

Ruhm, H., Walker, E., and Flanigin, H.: Acoustically-evoked potentials in man; mediation of early components. Laryngoscope 77:806, 1967.

Sakabe, N., Arayama, T., and Suzuki, T.: Human fetal evoked response to acoustic stimulation. Acta Otolaryng. (Suppl.) 252:29, 1969.

Sameroff, A.: Nonnutritive sucking in newborns under visual and auditory stimulation. Child. Dev. 38:443, 1967.

Sanders, J. W., and Josey, M. F.: Narrow-band noise audiometry for hard-to-test patients. J. Speech Hear. Res. 13:74, 1970.

Schlanger, B. B.: Effects of listening training on auditory thresholds of mentally retarded children. ASHA 8:273, 1962.

Schulman, C. A.: Effects of auditory stimulation on heart rate in premature infants as a function of level of arousal, probability of CNS damage, and conceptional age. Dev. Psychobiol. 2:172, 1969.

Schulte, F. J., Akiyama, Y., and Parmelee, A. H.: Auditory evoked responses during sleep in premature and full term newborn infants. Electroenceph. Clin. Neurophysiol. 23:97, 1967.

Siebert, W. M.: Processing Neuroelectric Data. Technical Report 351, Communications Biophysics Groups of the Research Laboratory of Electronics, Massachusetts Institute of Technology, Cambridge, Mass., 1959.

Siegenthaler, B., and Haspiel, G.: Development of two standardized measures of hearing for speech by children. Cooperative Research Program, Project No. 2372, United States Office of Education, 1966.

Siegenthaler, B., Pearson, J., and LeZak, R. J.: A speech reception threshold test for children. J. Speech Hear. Dis. *19*:360, 1954.

Sortini, A., and Flake C.: Speech audiometry for pre-school children. Laryngoscope *63*:991, 1953.

Spradlin, J. E.: Operant principles applied to audiometry with severely retarded children. *In* Lloyd, L. L. and Frisina, D. R. (eds.): The Audiologic Assessment of the Mentally Retarded: Proceedings of a National Conference, Parsons, Kansas, 1965, pp. 33–44.

Spradlin, J. E., and Lloyd, L. L.: Operant conditioning audiometry (OCA) with low level retardates: A preliminary report. In Lloyd, L. L. and Frisina, D. R. (eds.): The Audiologic Assessment of the Mentally Retarded: Proceedings of a National Conference, Parsons, Kansas, 1965, p. 45.

Spradlin, J. E., Lloyd, L. L., Hom, G. L., and Reid, M. J.: Establishing tone control and evaluating the hearing of severely retarded children. In Jervis, G. A. (ed.): Expanding Concepts in Mental Retardation. A symposium for the Joseph P. Kennedy, Jr., Foundation, 1968, p. 170.

Steinschneider, A., Lipton, E. L., and Richmond, J. B.: Auditory sensitivity in the infant: Effect of intensity on cardiac and motor responsivity. Child Dev. *37*:233, 1966.

Stewart, M. A., Stern, J. A., Winokur, G., and Fredman, S.: An analysis of GSR conditioning. Psych. Rev. *68*:60, 1961.

Stohr, P. E., and Goldring, S.: Origin of somatosensory evoked scalp responses recorded from the human scalp. Electroenceph. Clin. Neurophysiol. *28*:360, 1970.

Stranco, G., Galioto, G. B., and Seghizzi, P.: La resposta pletismografica allo stimolo sonora possibilita della sua applicazione nella simulazione della sordita. Boll. Mal. Orech. *80*:191, 1962.

Sullivan, R., Miller, M. H., and Polisar, I. A.: The portable peep-show: A further modification of the peep-show. Arch. Otolaryng. *76*:49, 1962.

Suzuki, T., Kamijo, Y., and Kiuchi, S.: Auditory test of newborn infants. Ann. Otol. *73*:914, 1964.

Suzuki, T., and Ogiba, Y.: A technique of pure tone audiometry for children under three years of age: Conditioned orientation reflex (C.O.R.) audiometry. Rev. Laryng. *1*:33, 1960.

Suzuki, T., and Ogiba, Y.: Conditioned orientation reflex audiometry. Arch. Otolaryng. *74*:192, 1961.

Suzuki, T., and Origuchi, K.: Averaged evoked response audiometry (ERA) in young children during sleep. Acta Otolaryng. (Suppl.) *252*:19, 1969.

Suzuki, T., and Sato, I.: Free field startle response audiometry. Ann. Otol. *70*:997, 1961.

Suzuki, T., and Taguchi, K.: Cerebral evoked response to auditory stimuli in waking man. Ann. Otol. *74*:128, 1965.

Suzuki, T., and Taguchi, K.: Cerebral evoked response to auditory stimuli in children during sleep. Ann. Otol. *77*:103, 1968.

Suzuki, T., Tonaka, Y., and Arayama, T.: Detection of hearing disorders in children under three years of age. Int. Audiol. *5*(2):74, 1966.

Taguchi, L., Picton, T. W., and Orpin, J. A.: Evoked response audiometry in newborn infants. Acta Otolaryng. (Suppl.) *252*:5, 1969.

Taylor, I. G.: The techniques of auditory testing by EEG during sleep. Proc. Roy. Soc. Med. *56*:995, 1963a.

Taylor, I. G.: The use of the electroencephalogram in the diagnosis of auditory problems. Int. Audiol. *2*:100, 1963b.

Taylor, I. G.: The Neurological Mechanisms of Hearing and Speech in Children. Manchester, England, Manchester University Press, 1964.

Teel, J. R.: Respiratory Audiometric Thresholds for Children Ages Seven to Eleven. Unpublished master's thesis, University of Kansas, 1966.

Terkildsen, K.: Acoustic reflexes of the human musculus tensor tympani. Acta Otolaryng. Suppl. *158*:230, 1960.

Terkildsen, K., and Nielsen, S.: An electroacoustic impedance measuring bridge for clinical use. Arch. Otolaryng. *72*:339, 1960.

Thomsen, K.: The Metz recruitment test and a comparison with the Fowler method. Acta Otolaryng. *45*:544, 1955.

Tillman, T. W., Dallos, P. J., and Kuruvilla, T.: Reliability of measures obtained with the Zwislocki acoustic bridge. J. Acoust. Soc. Amer. *36*:582, 1964.

Tokay, F. H., and Hardick, E. J.: Validity and reliability of Békésy audiometry with preschool age children. J. Speech Hear. Res. *14*:205, 1971.

Turkewitz, G., Birch, H. G., Moreau, T., and Cornwell, A. C.: Effect of intensity of auditory stimulation on directional eye movements in the human neonate. Anim. Behav. *14*:93, 1966.

Uhr, L., and Miller, J. G. (eds.): Drugs and Behavior. New York, John Wiley & Sons, Inc., 1960.

Utley, J.: Suggestive procedures for determining auditory acuity in very young acoustically handicapped children. Eye, Ear, Nose, Throat Monthly *228*:590, 1949.

Vaughan, H. G., Jr., and Ritter, W.: The sources of auditory evoked response recorded from the human scalp. Electroenceph. Clin. Neurophysiol. *28*:360, 1970.

Waldrop, W. A.: A puppet show hearing test. Volta Rev. *55*:488, 1953.

Walter, W. G.: The convergence and interaction of visual, auditory and tactile responses in human non-specific cortex. Ann. N. Y. Acad. Sci. *112*:320, 1964a.

Walter, W. G.: Slow potential waves in the human brain associated with expectancy, attention, and decision. Arch. Psychiat. und Nervenkrankheiten vereingt mit Zeitschrift Gesgonte Neurol. und Psychiat. *206*:309, 1964b.

Walter, W. G.: Effects on anterior brain responses of an expected association between stimuli. J. Psychosom. Res. *9*:45, 1965a.

Walter, W. G.: Brain responses to semantic stimuli. J. Psychosom. Res. *9*:51, 1965b.

Walter, W. G.: Expectancy waves and intention waves in the human brain and their application to the direct cerebral control of machines. Electroenceph. Clin. Neurophysiol. *21*:616, 1966.

Walter, W. G., Aldrich, V. J., Cooper, R., McCallum, C., and Cohen, J.: Responses to semantic stimuli in the human brain. Electroenceph. Clin. Neurophysiol. *19*:314, 1965a.

Walter, W. G., Aldrich, V. J., Cooper, R., McCallum, C., and Cohen, J.: The interaction of responses to semantic stimuli in the human brain. Electroenceph. Clin. Neurophysiol. *18*:514, 1965b.

Walter, W. G., Cooper, R., McCallum, C., and Cohen, J.: The origin and significance of the contingent negative variation or "expectancy wave." Electroenceph. Clin. Neurophysiol. *18*:720, 1965c.

Walter, W. G., Cooper, R., Aldrich, V. J., McCallum, C.,

and Winter, A. L.: Contingent negative variation: An electric sign of sensori-motor association and expectancy in the human brain. Nature 203:380, 1964.

Watson, T. J.: Speech audiometry for children. In Ewing, A.W.G. (ed.): Educational Guidance and the Deaf Child. Manchester, England, University of Manchester Press, 1957, p. 278.

Webb, C., Kinde, S., Weber, B., and Beedle, R.: Procedures for Evaluating the Hearing of the Mentally Retarded. Mt. Pleasant, Michigan, Central Michigan University Press, 1964, p. 73.

Weitzman, E. D., Remond, A., and Lesevre, N.: Chrontopographic study of auditory evoked potentials recorded on the scalp in normal humans during sleep and the awake state. Rev. Neurol. (Paris) 113:253, 1965.

Wilder, J.: The law of initial values. Psychosom. Med. 12:393, 1950.

Williamson, P. D., Goff, W. R., and Allison, T.: Somato-sensory evoked responses in patients with unilateral cerebral lesions. Electroenceph. Clin. Neurophysiol. 28:566, 1970.

Withrow, F., and Goldstein, R.: Electrophysiologic procedures for determination of threshold in children. Laryngoscope 68:1674, 1958.

Wolfe, W. G., and MacPherson, J. R.: The Evaluation and Development of Techniques for Testing the Auditory Acuity of Trainable Mentally Retarded Children. Cooperative Research Project No. 172, United States Office of Education. Austin, University of Texas, 1959.

Yoshie, N., and Ohashie, T.: Clinical use of cochlear nerve action potential responses in man for differential diagnosis of hearing losses. Acta Orolaryng. (Suppl.) 252:71, 1969.

Yoshie, N., and Okadaira, T.: Myogenic evoked potential responses to clicks in man. Acta Otolaryng. (Suppl.) 252:89, 1969.

Yoshie, N., and Yamaura, K.: Cochlear microphonic responses to pure tones in man recorded by a non-surgical method. Acta Otolaryng. (Suppl.) 252:37, 1969.

Zeaman, D., and Wegner, N.: Cardiac reflex to tones of threshold intensity. J. Speech Hear. Dis. 21:71, 1956.

Zwislocki, J.: An acoustic method for clinical examination of the ear. J. Speech Hear. Res. 6:303, 1963.

Chapter 41

MEASUREMENT OF HEARING IN ADULTS

by Raymond Carhart, Ph.D.

The audiological methods for exploring the hearing of adults include pure tone audiometry, speech audiometry, and various special auditory tests. The information gained through these procedures serves the clinician in two ways: First, this information contributes to the differential diagnosis of ear diseases. Second, it allows the clinician to judge his patients' practical needs and capabilities in hearing.

PURE TONE AUDIOMETRY

Methodology

The classic method for determining hearing loss across the major portion of the range of audible frequencies is to measure the patient's thresholds for pure tones. The test sound is generated by an audiometer conforming to strict specifications (ASA-Z24.5-1951 or ANSI-S3.6/1969). This device produces one frequency (or pure tone) at a time. The pure tone is presented to the patient's test ear either by air conduction (via a monaural earphone) or by bone conduction (through a vibrator placed on the skull). The intensity of this stimulus is varied in 5 decibel (dB) steps until the tester has found the faintest level at which the patient can hear the tone. This level is the patient's threshold for that particular sound. The frequencies ordinarily employed during air conduction testing are 125, 250, 500, 1000, 2000, 4000 and 8000 Hz. Sometimes 125 Hz is dropped, and sometimes 3000 Hz is added. Bone conduction responses are usually obtained only at frequencies from 250 through 4000 Hz.

Several methods for presenting stimulus sequences have been advocated, but the Hughson-Westlake technique is clinically preferable (Carhart and Jerger, 1959). This procedure is simple. One first presents to the patient a clearly audible tone that lasts about a second. This sound is usually 1000 Hz. As soon as the patient hears the tone, he signals to the tester by raising his finger or pressing a light switch. Once it is clear that the patient understands his task, the tester reduces the tone to an intensity so small that it will be inaudible to the patient. The tester then starts a series of one second tonal presentations which are successively increased in 5 dB steps until the patient again responds. This response is the clue to the tester to drop the intensity 10 to 15 dB and begin a new ascent; thereafter the entire procedure is repeated until the clinical threshold is determined. Technically this threshold is the minimum level at which perception is achieved in half or more of the ascents. A practical criterion is to accept three responses at a single intensity as indicating this level. The usual practice is to measure all air conduction thresholds in one ear before starting on the other ear. The preferred sequence of tones is to ascend from 1000 through 8000 Hz before descending from 500 through 125 Hz, with 1000 Hz being repeated at the end as a check on the patient's reliability. Whenever both air and bone conduction responses are explored, all thresholds by air are obtained first.

Air conduction testing reveals the patient's sensitivity for sounds entering his external auditory canal and traversing the middle ear system to his inner ear. An obstruction or lesion anywhere along this path will reduce his responsiveness and cause a loss in his reception of air-borne sounds. His efficiency at any test frequency is expressed in terms of the hearing level at which his threshold for that tone lies. This hearing level, in turn, is defined as the number of decibels separating it from a standard reference value, designated as the 0 dB hearing level. This reference value varies physically from one test tone to another. The contemporary criteria are international. They are designated as the ISO 1964 standard (ISO-R389-1964). These criteria, which are incorporated in the 1969 American standard (ANSI-S3.6-1969), approximate the average sensitivity to be expected of normal young adults.

Prior to the adoption of the ISO 1964 reference levels, the ASA 1951 values (ASA-Z24.5-1951) were used in the United States. This earlier standard specifies zero hearing levels that are 6 to 15 dB higher in intensity than those of ISO 1964. The clinician must remember this fact when he compares different sets of test results. A patient whose hearing has remained stationary will appear to have greater hearing loss according to ISO 1964 than according to ASA 1951 by the amount of the discrepancies between the two sets of reference levels.

Bone conduction stimuli are not channeled through the external and middle ear mechanisms because they are initiated by a calibrated vibrator placed on the skull at either the mastoid process or the midline of the forehead; consequently bone conduction audiometry essentially measures sensitivity from the cochlea inward. When hearing loss is revealed by this method, it indicates the approximate amount and pattern of sensorineural involvement. At the time of this writing, the American National Standards Institute defines the reference threshold for audibility for bone-conducted sound as "the median value of threshold determinations on a large number of individuals between 18 and 30 years of age" (ANSI-S3.6-1969), whereas the Hearing Aid Industry Conference has adopted numerical values (Lybarger, 1966). These specifications do not parallel perfectly the ISO 1964 standard for air conduction, but they yield bone conduction norms in sufficiently good agreement with it to be clinically useful.

One critical requirement of acceptable pure tone audiometry is that measurements be made in a quiet room (ASA-S3.1-1960) by a skilled tester. Another is that the audiometer be maintained in good calibration. A third requirement is that the ear not under test be properly masked by a competing sound, so that the patient will not give a false response because his nontest ear is inadvertently stimulated by the test tone. The masking sound should be either a broad-spectrum white noise or a narrow band of noise centered at the test frequency (Lidén et al., 1959). In either event this sound must be variable in intensity and must be calibrated so that its masking efficiency can be modified as needed. A good clinician adjusts his procedure not only to the type of masking sound he is using but also to the peculiarities of his patient's hearing loss. Among his guidelines there are two rules that are particularly important: First, the nontest ear should be masked routinely during bone conduction audiometry. Second, masking is mandatory during air conduction audiometry whenever the nontest ear exhibits thresholds that are at least 40 dB better than those of the test ear. Moreover, if a strong masker must be used, there is danger that the masking sound will cross the head from the nontest ear and interfere with hearing in the test ear. This danger can be somewhat lessened by using only as much masking as the circumstance requires (Hood, 1960) and by supplying this sound via an earphone that inserts directly into the external auditory meatus (Gyllencreutz and Lidén, 1967).

Interpretation of Results

A pure tone threshold that has been carefully obtained from a patient whose responses are reliable is usually accurate to within 5 to 10 dB (Witting and Hughson, 1940; Carhart and Jerger, 1959). The clinician must therefore allow for this margin of uncertainty when he is evaluating single thresholds; but even so, the total trend of a patient's hearing pattern may be judged with high confidence. For example, a useful guideline in evaluating results of treatment or assessing progression of impairment since an earlier test is to consider a systematic change averaging 10 or more dB at two or three adjacent frequencies as representing a real shift in sensitivity.

The threshold relationships a patient exhibits have important practical and diagnostic significances. These relationships are easily seen when test results are plotted in audiogram form, as is done in Figure 1. Here the graph for the left ear depicts results from a patient with stapedial otosclerosis, while the right ear audiogram illustrates findings on a patient with cochlear otosclerosis.

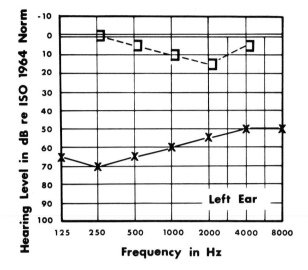

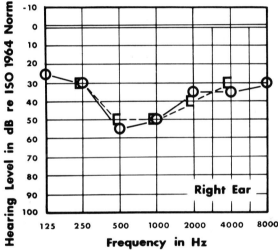

Figure 1. Illustrative audiograms of stapedial otosclerosis (left ear) and cochlear otosclerosis (right ear). Key: Air conduction, left = x———x and right = o———o; bone conduction, left =]------], right = [------[.

Consider first the problem of judging the handicap depicted by each audiogram. It is the air conduction curves which furnish clues to the degree and nature of each patient's everyday auditory handicap. The hearing levels at which this curve courses across the chart indicate the pattern of hearing loss for air-borne tones and, hence, for environmental sounds. Moreover, responsiveness in the frequency range from 500 through 2000 Hz is sufficiently linked to reception of connected speech so that a rough estimate of the work-a-day handicap is possible by averaging the air conduction thresholds in this range. Davis (1965) has developed a classification for estimating this handicap from such an average (Table 1). Observe

that the audiogram for the left ear shown in Figure 1 may be judged to represent a rather marked handicap because its 500 to 2000 Hz average is 60 dB, whereas the 47 dB average for the other audiogram in the figure indicates a milder handicap.

An audiogram is extremely helpful in several phases of diagnosis, most notably in distinguishing a conductive from a sensorineural impairment. Here the basic principle is that a lesion or anomaly in the external or middle ear which interferes with sound transmission causes a loss for air-borne sound but not for bone-conducted tones, whereas a sensorineural lesion causes losses for both types of stimulation (Carhart, 1950). The rationale for this difference is obvious. Air-conducted tones will be attenuated by such a transmissional obstruction before they reach the inner ear. Hence, thresholds for air conduction will show hearing loss. By contrast, tones presented via the bone vibrator reach the inner ear by an alternate path which does not include the obstruction; consequently their thresholds are not comparably impaired. The audiogram depicting this relationship reveals an air-bone gap (poorer hearing by air than bone) that bespeaks pathology peripheral to the inner ear. This situation is illustrated by the record of the left ear in Figure 1. Remember that this ear possessed stapes fixation. Here the air conduction curve centers at 60 dB of loss, and it rises slightly from low to high frequencies. The bone conduction curve is near zero hearing level. Without a knowledge of the diagnosis, these relations tell us that the patient has a conductive impairment. Conversely the results shown in Figure 1 for the right ear exemplify an interweaving of air and bone conduction curves that is the hallmark of pure sensorineural hearing impairment. In this case the loss was due to cochlear otosclerosis. The superimposition of threshold curves resulted because now the auditory deficit was caused by dysfunction in the inner ear, a region which both types of stimulus must traverse. The end result is reduced sensitivity for both.

Another aid to diagnosis is found in the minor audiometric distortions that conductive impairments impose on the bone curve (Huizing, 1964; Tonndorf, 1966). These distortions do not alter the general level of this curve, but they do modify its shape in distinctive manners. These effects are due to physical changes in the sound transmission system; they are caused by abnormalities in the external or middle ear rather than in the inner ear. They

TABLE 1. Classes of Hearing Handicap ISO — 1964

dB	CLASS	DEGREE OF HANDICAP	AVERAGE HEARING THRESHOLD LEVEL FOR 500, 1000 and 2000 IN THE BETTER EAR*		ABILITY TO UNDERSTAND SPEECH
			More Than	*Not More Than*	
	A	Not significant		25 dB (ISO)	No significant difficulty with faint speech
25					
	B	Slight handicap	25 dB (ISO)	40 dB	Difficulty only with faint speech
40					
55	C	Mild handicap	40 dB	55 dB	Frequent difficulty with normal speech
	D	Marked handicap	55 dB	70 dB	Frequent difficulty with loud speech
70					
	E	Severe handicap	70 dB	90 dB	Can understand only shouted or amplified speech
90					
	F	Extreme handicap	90 dB		Usually cannot understand even amplified speech

*Whenever the average for the poorer ear is 25 dB or more greater than that of the better ear in this frequency range, 5 dB are added to the average for the better ear. This adjusted average determines the degree and class of handicap. For example, if a person's average hearing threshold level for 500, 1000, and 2000 c./s is 37 dB in one ear and 62 dB or more in the other, his adjusted average hearing threshold level is 42 dB and his handicap is Class C instead of Class B. (Davis, H.: Trans. Amer. Acad. Ophthal. Otolaryng. 69:740, 1965.)

produce minor threshold shifts that are of mechanical origin. These shifts are as yet only partially cataloged. The clearest example is the modest notching of the bone curve caused by stapes fixation (Carhart, 1962). (See left ear, Figure 1.) An audiogram that indicates conductive impairment and includes approximately this patterning of bone thresholds alerts the diagnostician to consider stapedial otosclerosis as a very probable cause of loss. Conversely, when a patient is known to have stapes fixation, one's estimate of this patient's cochlear sensitivity can ordinarily be improved by removing this notching from the bone curve. Of course, one must remember that the patterns of mechanical distortion exhibited by the bone curve can be changed by middle ear surgery (Holmgren, 1957). Moreover, other kinds of conductive lesion produce their own distinctive reshaping of the bone conduction audiogram. For example, chronic supprative otitis media often causes a 5 to 10 dB improvement in threshold at 250 and 500 Hz accompanied by 10 to 15 dB poorer response at 2000 and 4000 Hz (Carhart, 1962).

Although the patterns of hearing loss caused by sensorineural maladies are extremely varied, a third aid to diagnosis results from the fact that particular diseases tend to produce distinctive audiometric configurations. To be sure, considerable variation exists within each category, but the clinician who is familiar with the contours characterizing different types of sensorineural involvement is aided by this knowledge in reaching a differential diagnosis. Examples of these distinctions are found in Volume II, where the various sensorineural diseases are discussed in detail. Suffice it here to give a quick résumé of a few trends. Meniere's disease usually causes more low frequency than high frequency loss during its initial stages, although later on the degree of high frequency loss tends to increase variably (Lindsay, 1960). Exposure to intense sounds such as gunfire and industrial noise can cause permanent threshold shifts usually characterized by notched high frequency losses (Bunch, 1970). In older individuals this impairment is enhanced and its configuration is somewhat obscured by the addition of sociocusic and presbycusic components (Ward, 1969). Meningitis leaves its victims with extreme deafness wherein responsiveness, if it remains at all, is commonly restricted to low frequencies (Bordley and Hardy, 1951). The typical audiogram of maternal rubella is flat, but sometimes it is gently sloping or rising (Barr and Lundström, 1961). Several conditions ordinarily induce losses with gradual to marked high frequency increases. Examples are progressive hereditary losses (Huizing et al. 1966), presbycusis (Schmidt, 1967), and toxic deafness resulting from acute disease or the use of various drugs (Shambaugh, 1967). Some patterns of high frequency loss are relatively distinctive, as with the sloping but sigmoid configuration resulting from Rh incompatibility (Carhart, 1967a). There are a few conditions which usually produce hearing losses that become greater with higher frequency, but which also cause trough-shaped or bizarre configurations. Noteworthy in this regard are cochlear otosclerosis (Carhart, 1963), auditory nerve tumors (Johnson, 1965), and hereditary deafness (Konigsmark et al. 1970).

Another diagnostic clue is found in the degree of hearing loss for air-borne sounds. There is an upper limit to the deficit which conductive lesions, either alone or in combination, can produce. The reason for this phenomenon is that very strong sounds in the air surrounding the patient's head cause direct vibration of his skull. When this happens he begins to hear by bone, and his conductive lesion is overridden. The limit imposed in audiometry by this situation is about 75 dB for the lower frequencies and 55 dB for the higher ones. Thus, an air conduction loss that exceeds this limit either results from a combination of a conductive and a sensorineural cause or is due entirely to sensorineural damage.

Air conduction losses arising from coexistent pathologies sometimes add to one another, while at other times they do not. The general rule is that such losses cumulate when the abnormalities causing them are located at different points within the auditory system, but the losses do not sum when the underlying abnormalities involve the identical structures. For example, the hearing deficit due to a conductive impairment superimposes upon the deficit due to a sensorineural one. In this instance the patient's cumulative handicap is revealed by his air conduction audiogram, while the magnitude of his sensorineural loss is shown by the depression in his bone curve after correction is made for the minor mechanical distortion that his conductive impairment produces. Bearing the same proviso in mind, the portion of loss resulting from this latter impairment is disclosed by the air-bone gap. By contrast, acoustic trauma (a cochlear lesion) will obscure the high frequency portions of loss due to Meniere's disease (cochlear pathology) if the former, considered alone, would produce more loss at these frequencies than the latter would. Conversely the acoustic trauma notch will not appear in the audiogram of such a patient provided it is smaller than the high frequency impairment due to Meniere's disease.

SPEECH AUDIOMETRY

Methodology

The ability to understand speech is measured with standardized test materials presented to the patient at calibrated levels. The equipment used must conform to the specifications that have been established for speech audiometers (ASA-Z24.13-1953; ANSI-S3.6-1969). The acoustic characteristics of the test room must also be adequate.

A special procedure is needed to designate the level of the speech materials that are used as the test stimuli, since these materials are not steady-state sounds. The standard method is to adjust the speech so that the average deflection of its peaks as read on the audiometer's VU meter equal the deflections produced by a 1000 Hz signal. The speech is then described as having the same sound pressure level as the 1000 Hz tone possesses when it is emitted from the audiometer's test earphone. Sometimes the speech materials are generated from a loudspeaker, in which case their level at the site of the patient's head must be analogously specified. Here it is better to use a speech spectrum noise rather than a 1000 Hz tone as the calibration signal (Tillman et al., 1966).

Two kinds of clinical measurement can be obtained. In either instance the usual clinical procedure is to have the patient repeat aloud what he hears. Each has a unique usefulness (Carhart, 1951). One is the speech reception threshold or SRT; the other is the discrimination score. When discrimination scores are obtained at several levels, the results may be graphed to yield an articulation curve (Davis and Silverman, 1970).

Measurement of the SRT. The patient's speech reception threshold (SRT) is the hearing level at which the patient can reproduce half the test items. The material most commonly used in the United States is a list of 36 spondaic words selected by Hirsh et al., (1952). These words are bisyllables of equal stress, such as "baseball." They were recorded according to two plans. The spondees are in stairstep sequences of descending intensity in the version known as CID W-2. When using this version the tester sets the beginning of the recording at a level at which the initial words are audible but are near the patient's SRT. The clinical threshold is defined as the starting level minus the number of words he can repeat. The other version is the CID W-1 Test. Here, all spondees are recorded at the same level, and the tester can make up and down adjustments in intensity until he has bracketed the SRT, which is defined as the point of 50 per cent intelligibility. However, a particularly good technique is to use exactly the same descending sequence as employed with the CID W-2 recording; Hirsh et al. recommend this method. Moreover, if a patient has difficulty with recorded spondees, these same words may be spoken in slower tempo at the moment of test (monitored live-voice method). Here, of course, a trained talker is required so that test items will be said at properly controlled intensities.

The SRT is resistant to minor variations in the test material and in the reproducing equipment. Hence, clinically valid measures can be obtained with other materials provided standardized procedures and appropriate precautions have been observed. Consequently many clinicians are now using spondee words recorded on magnetic tape, in which event they have either prepared their own tapes or have obtained tapes from professional colleagues.

In those rare instances in which the patient cannot understand spondees readily, the SRT can be obtained using simple sentences or connected conversation as the test material. Provided even this fails, the level at which the patient detects the presence of speech can usually be determined. This latter level constitutes the speech awareness threshold (SAT). It is not analogous to the SRT, which is the threshold for actual understanding of the test items, but the SAT supplies an estimate of a more limited type of responsiveness.

Measurement of Discrimination Scores. These scores are ordinarily obtained with materials designed to determine the patient's ability to decipher the fine details of articulated speech. Lists of monosyllabic words are the preferred clinical tool. Each word is preceded by a standard carrier phrase (such as, "You will say") in order to maintain the natural relationships among words of different inherent strengths.

An entire list is administered at a single intensity level, and the discrimination score for that level is the percentage of items which the patient understands precisely. It is necessary to use a second list if a discrimination score for another presentation level is desired.

The first widely used discrimination test consisted of 20 lists of 50 words each. Each list was composed so as to approximate the phonetic balance of spoken English. These materials are known as PB 50 lists (Egan, 1948). Much of our early information on discrimination for monosyllables was obtained with the Rush Hughes version of these lists, which was recorded in the mid 1940's (Davis, 1948). This version had peculiarities that made it a difficult test, and at that time many clinicians preferred presenting the PB 50 lists by monitored live voice. In 1952 Hirsh and his associates made available four phonetically balanced lists, each consisting of 50 relatively familiar monosyllables. These lists, in various randomizations, were recorded phonographically as the CID W-22 Test. Soon thereafter, the W-22 Test was adopted by the Veterans Administration for adjudication purposes, and it has subsequently come into very wide clinical use. Concurrently a number of newer tests, notably the Peterson-Lehiste CNC Lists (1962); The Fairbanks Rhyme Test (1958) and the modified Rhyme Test (Kreul et al., 1968) have enjoyed some popularity along with the old PB 50 lists.

The discrimination score, unlike the SRT, is highly susceptible to variations in the test material, the test procedure, the talker, the method of reproduction, and the physical characteristics of the speech audiometer; consequently each clinician must establish norms for his own test situation. Thereafter he must maintain continuous surveillance to guarantee against a change in any critical variable. For example, the advantage of using test materials that have been previously recorded can be nullified if phonograph records are allowed to become too worn or if tape reproducing heads are not cared for properly. Finally, some clinicians are satisfied with discrimination scores based on administering 25 words (half-lists), but there are many instances in which whole lists give more definitive results (Carhart, 1965).

The discrimination score also varies with the level of presentation. This fact has led to two different procedures. One of these is to plot the patient's intelligibility curve, or articulation function (Davis, 1948). This method is popular abroad where shorter lists are often used, and is valuable when extensive clinical data are desired (Fournier, 1951; Hahlbrock, 1957). It requires that a separate discrimination test be administered at each of several audible levels. These levels are chosen so that the patient's discrimination is measured from an intensity so low that scores are poor to one high enough so that the score is either at its best or where presentation is limited by the patient's tolerance or by the output of the test equipment.

Figure 2 plots four kinds of intelligibility curve to illustrate the important differences that may exist between patients. Curve A shows the normal circumstance wherein the discrimination score improves with increased presentation until essentially 100 per cent intelligibility is achieved and then maintained. Curve B is similar in slope but it is displaced to the right, indicating that greater intensities are needed for equivalent performance but that responses are not otherwise abnormal. Curve C is not only displaced to the right; it also has a more gradual slope, indicating that once the initial handicap is overcome by the necessary increase in signal strength, the rate of improvement in intelligibility with further increase in intensity is slower than normal. Moreover, the plateau of maximum discrimination is here reached at less than 100 per cent, showing that a deficit in crispness of reception will remain even at optimal presentation levels. Curve D also fails to reach 100 per cent, but its most distinctive feature is a peak in intelligibility which is not retained as intensity is increased further. This configuration indicates that discrimination deteriorates when speech levels are either too high or too low, so that there is only a small range of intensities where precision in distinguishing the fine details of speech is at its best.

The administration of several tests so as to obtain an intelligibility curve is too time-consuming for many clinical situations. Here the practical alternative is to measure discrimination at a key intensity level. The usual goal is to obtain a score that will be on the patient's plateau of best discrimination, i.e., so that one may measure any deficit in crispness of intelligibility that he retains when the listening conditions are optimal for him. The problem facing the clinician is to choose the proper intensity at which to present the single test. Differences in hearing loss can be counteracted by selecting an appropriate sensation level (e.g., at a specified intensity above the patient's SRT), but we observe from Figure 2 that other difficulties are present. Intelligibility curves rise at different rates and not all of them exhibit plateauing, so that no single sensation level can lead to the maximum discrimination score for all patients. The problem is complicated by the fact that, even for normals, plateauing occurs at different levels for different sets of test material (Carhart, 1965). The most widely accepted expedient today is to administer the test material at 40 dB above the patient's SRT, since most patients whose curves possess a plateau will have reached the plateau at or below this sensation level. Of course, one cannot be sure on the basis of one measurement that such is the case for any specific patient. Moreover, there are instances in which the patient cannot tolerate the 40 dB sensation level or in which his loss is so great that the speech audiometer cannot produce a signal of the required strength. In such cases a lower sensation level (preferably 26 to 30 dB) must be employed, but one is less certain of obtaining maximum discrimination scores. Finally, in

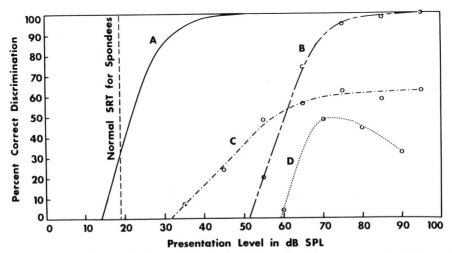

Figure 2. Types of intelligibility function. A = normal response; B = normal except for displacement to right; C = displaced to the right, altered slope and lowered plateau; D = displaced to the right, altered slope, lowered maximum score and decreasing discrimination losses at levels higher than the one evoking maximum score.

view of all these considerations, there obviously are times when the clinician must obtain discrimination scores on two or more levels before he can be satisfied that he has gathered the minimum information on discrimination that is necessary to evaluate the patient.

The foregoing discussion has centered on clinical speech audiometry as it has evolved in in the United States. Of course, the general principles apply everywhere, but specifics vary from country to country. Test materials have had to be developed for each language (for example, Ferrer, 1960; Fournier, 1951; Hahlbrock, 1957; Lidén, 1954), and tests have even had to be modified from one English-speaking country to another (Fry, 1961; Macrae et al., 1963). Moreover, structural differences between languages have modified the types of material which proved reasonable in various native tongues (Ferrer, 1960).

Interpretation of Results

The Threshold for Speech. The usual expectation is that the SRT will approximately equal the average of the patient's two best thresholds in the 500 to 2000 Hz range (Fletcher, 1950). This Fletcher average is particularly useful when the pure tone thresholds differ substantially from one another, but a number of other estimates are almost as accurate and are often used. These include the three frequency averages across the 500 to 2000 Hz range, the average of 500 and 1000 Hz, and the single threshold at 1000 Hz. Moreover, in those instances in which hearing improves sharply for the high frequencies, the SRT is often better than the foregoing guidelines would predict. These relations apply not only monaurally, but they also apply binaurally provided one averages in the better threshold at each frequency regardless of ear.

One value of the SRT is that it allows the clinician to estimate the patient's work-a-day handicap in receiving connected conversation. Here the criteria for evaluating the practical significance of average loss for 500 to 2000 Hz that are presented in Table 1 apply also to the SRT.

Another application employs comparison of the SRT and the pure tone average. When the two scores of a patient are in close agreement one can have more confidence in each type of measurement (Carhart, 1952). Conversely, any marked discrepancy calls for further exploration in order to discover the reason. This rea-

son may be in one of several realms: First, errors sometimes occur because of faulty equipment, failure of the patient to understand instructions, and the like. Second, the patient may exhibit true variability in his responses. Third, he may have extra trouble interpreting speech, so that the SRT does not coincide with the pure tone average. This difficulty can arise from causes as dissimilar as (1) failure to acquire adequate understanding of English because of foreign background or a very early hearing loss, or (2) aphasia resulting from cortical insult. Finally, the patient who is simulating a hearing loss often gives notably better thresholds for speech than for pure tones.

Intelligibility for Speech. The patient's maximum discrimination score and the contour of his intelligibility curve supply information that has several kinds of clinical application. However, the clinician must have experience with the particular test he is using before he can judge when a discrimination defect is attributable to the configuration of the patient's pure tone loss and when additional factors are operating.

For one thing, the clarity of detail the patient may be expected to hear in everyday life may be judged from his discrimination scores (Davis, 1948). Here applications include assessing his ability either unaided in quiet, with hearing aids (Niemeyer, 1966), against competing sounds (Carhart and Tillman, 1970), after ear surgery (Silverman et al., 1948), after a regimen of medical treatment, or following a program of auditory training.

Secondly, discrimination scores also assist in differentiating among auditory disorders. Here the basic question is whether the patient's performance is as good as the acoustic features of his impairment would lead one to anticipate. Some types of patients conform to expectation and others do not.

On an acoustical basis patients with a nearly flat audiogram should achieve excellent scores provided the signal is made strong enough to override their deficits in sensitivity (Fletcher, 1952). Such performance is realized when the hearing loss is caused by middle ear abnormalities (Huizing and Reyntjes, 1952) or by cochlear otosclerosis (Sanders, 1965). Patients whose audiograms show moderate increased loss for high frequencies still get enough acoustic information so that they should get good discrimination scores when speech is sufficiently intense. Otosclerotics with sensorineural involvement furnish an example. Patients with sharply dropping high frequency loss will show discrimination deficits because they are deprived of receiving some of the acoustic elements needed to distinguish phonetic details of speech. This deprivation is slight if the patient can still receive 3000 Hz nearly as well as he can lower frequencies. It increases progressively as the drop-off shifts downward in frequency, becoming marked when the break in the audiogram is at 500 Hz (Lidén, 1967).

Some types of patients do not yield discrimination scores that are as good as their audiograms would lead one to predict. Patients with Meniere's disease (Schuknecht, 1963), some clinical presbycusics (Pestalozza and Shore, 1955), and persons suffering hearing loss due to certain ototoxic drugs exhibit an extra discrimination problem despite ample speech intensity. Other conditions have relatively unpredictable but often extremely disruptive effects on understanding of speech. One example is congenital lues. However, the most important instances from the diagnostic point of view are tumors on the eighth cranial nerve or within the cerebellopontine angle (Johnson, 1968), because an unusually poor discrimination score can be one of the first symptoms of such a tumor.

SPECIAL AUDITORY TESTS

A large number of other hearing tests have been developed as aids to differential diagnosis. Some of the more widely used of these tests are described below, following which their interpretations are discussed.

Methodologies

Impedance Audiometry. The impedance of the middle ear can be determined by an acoustic bridge inserted into the external auditory canal. This device generates a pure tone which is reflected from the eardrum. Adjustments are made so that the reflected sound is balanced within the bridge. Thereafter, any change in impedance that occurs may be noted by its effect on this balance.

Change in acoustic impedance may be used to measure the reflex activity of the tympanic muscles (Jepsen, 1963). The procedure is to connect the acoustic bridge to one ear and use the impedance change in this ear to determine the response through the second ear to another pure tone. This latter stimulus is progressively increased in intensity until the level in this second ear is sufficient to cause the middle ear

muscles to contract. Since this contraction is bilateral, the reflex also manifests itself in the first ear, where it is measured. The intensity in the other ear that produced this contraction is the threshold of the reflex in that ear. Normally a hearing level of 80 to 90 dB is required to reach this threshold. The person with a hearing loss who responds by yielding a reflex at this same level is evidencing recruitment, while the person without recruitment will require an increase in stimulus level corresponding to his hearing loss (Lamb et al., 1968).

The acoustic bridge may also be used to assess the status of the ear into which it is inserted. This type of measurement has its primary application in evaluation of conductive losses (Klockhoff, 1961). One technique employed is known as tympanometry (Terkildsen and Thomsen, 1959). Here the procedure is to measure, preferably graphically, the changes in impedance that are caused when the air pressure in the external auditory canal is progressively varied from substantially negative to substantially positive. Distinctive patterns of change in impedance with change in pressure differentiate among conditions such as those in which the middle ear is normal, in which pressure is pathologically negative, in which fluid is in the middle ear, or in which the ossicular chain is disrupted.

Békésy Audiometry. Békésy (1947) developed an instrument that allowed the patient automatically to trace his monaural thresholds for pure tones. The patient controlled stimulus intensity by pressing a signal button as long as he heard the stimulus. The intensity of the pure tone decreased as long as he did so, while its level increased whenever the button was released. The resulting variations in intensity, representing the patient's tracking between his boundary of inaudibility and audibility, were recorded on a chart by a moving pen. The midpoint between extremes in the tracing was designated as threshold.

This principle has since been used in a number of ways. Jerger (1960b) employed a method which compared the tracings for two different types of stimulus with one another. One stimulus was pulsed. It consisted of 200-msec. beeps of pure tone interrupted by 200-msec. intervals of tonelessness. The other stimulus was a continuous tone. Of course, neither stimulus was audible to the listener except during those times when he allowed it to be by his manipulation of the signal button.

Jerger defines five major categories of patient response on the basis of the relations between the tracings for the interrupted and the continuous stimuli. He calls the relation where the two tracings interweave the Type I pattern. Type II pattern exhibits a separation between the two tracings that starts at about 1000 Hz (or higher), with the response to the continuous stimulus being the poorer and with the separation between tracings limited to 20 dB or less. Also, the tracing for the continuous stimulus often but not invariably narrows after the separation occurs. Jerger's Type III pattern consists of a separation wherein the tracing for the continuous mode decays very sharply, often to the point at which response to it ceases entirely. The Type IV pattern is much like the Type II except that the separation between tracings now appears across all or almost all of the frequency range. The Type V pattern is unique in that here the response for the pulsed tone is the poorer of the two (Jerger and Herer, 1961). The frequency range over which this condition manifests itself varies from patient to patient.

Threshold Tone Decay Tests. These tests use an ordinary pure tone audiometer to search for abnormal auditory adaptation. Several variations in procedure are employed in the United States. Carhart's method (1957) consists of presenting the test tone to the patient for one minute at threshold level, provided the patient continues to hear the stimulus that long. If he does not do so, the tone is immediately increased by 5 dB and a new minute of timing is begun. The same process is repeated until the patient holds the tone in awareness for a full minute, at which point the test for that frequency is over. The amount of adaptation, or tone decay, is the span in dB between the initial threshold and the terminal level. Sørensen's method (1962) is similar except that the listening period is 90 seconds instead of a minute. Owens (1964) modified a procedure originally described by Hood (1955). In Owens' test a 20-second rest period is allowed after the stimulus has decayed at one level before presentation is made at the next higher level. The process is started 5 dB above threshold and is continued either until the tone is heard for a minute or until at least four increments in intensity have been given.

The SISI Test. This test supplies a quick measure of the patient's responsiveness to small changes in the intensity of a pure tone (Jerger et al., 1959). This tone is presented continuously, usually at 20 dB above the patient's threshold for it; and every five seconds a 1 dB pip of this same tone is added momen-

tarily. The SISI score is the percentage of 20 such increments that the patient hears. Scores lower than 35 per cent are classified as negative and those over 70 per cent as positive. The test may be given at octave intervals, but a more limited sampling of frequencies is usually adequate. Another way of shortening the test is to compute the SISI score after the first 10 increments, provided the patient either hears at least nine of them or misses all but one. Two variations in the basic procedure are useful when one wishes to discover whether the patient is particularly insensitive to brief changes in tone intensity. One variation is to use increments of either 2 dB or even 5 dB rather than of 1 dB. The other variation is to retain the 1 dB increments but to superimpose them on a tone which is maintained for all patients at a single high intensity, i.e., about 85 dB ISO hearing level (Thompson, 1963).

Loudness Balance Tests. These tests investigate whether the experience of loudness rises normally with progressive increases in the intensity of a pure tone. One abnormal condition, known as recruitment, occurs when loudness grows more quickly than normal (Hirsh, 1952). An example is the patient whose threshold is at the 40 dB hearing level but who has no deficit in loudness by the time the tone is raised to the 80 dB hearing level. The reverse abnormality, in which loudness grows too slowly, is decruitment.

Since loudness is an inner experience, there is no direct way of comparing the patient's perception of it with that of another listener. Hence, this perception can be measured only by having him compare, or balance, the loudnesses of two tones that are presented to him. One of these must be a tone for which his hearing is normal, while the other is the tone for which loudness experience is being explored. Two procedures for doing so are available.

One technique is the alternate binaural loudness balance (ABLB) test (Fowler, 1937, 1950). It can be used when the patient has normal hearing in one ear at the test frequency. Response through this ear can then serve as the standard against which loudness experience for the same tone via the other ear is judged. The method for doing so is simple. The test tone is alternated back and forth between the ears at one-second intervals. This stimulus is fixed at a predetermined intensity in one ear, and its level is varied on the other side until the patient reports that its loudnesses in the two ears are equal. This balancing ordinarily does not need to be done at more than two frequencies for any patient. Hood (1969) advises fixing the intensity in the good ear and achieving balance by varying the signal to the impaired side. He suggests that this be done at 20 dB intervals (in the good ear) up to a hearing level of 100 dB. An alternative clinical procedure, proposed by Jerger (1962), is to fix the intensity of the tone at 10 or 20 dB above threshold in the ear with the hearing loss. Recruitment is judged to be absent by either procedure if the patient experiences equivalent loudnesses when the two stimuli are about the same number of decibels above their respective thresholds in the two ears. Conversely, if the intensity in the good ear must now be elevated to essentially the same hearing level as in the poor ear, recruitment is classified as complete. Recruitment is partial provided the outcome lies between these two extremes. When testing for decruitment, the better clinical procedure is to use a relatively high sensation level in the ear suspected of abnormal response. Decruitment may be found when thresholds are near normal in both ears, in which event the alternating tone may be fixed in either ear. The reaction is here judged normal if approximately the same level is required in the other ear for balance. Otherwise, decruitment is assigned to the ear that required the greater hearing level.

The other loudness balancing technique is Reger's test (1936). Here only one ear is stimulated. The patient balances loudness for a frequency at which his hearing is normal against the loudness evoked by a frequency for which he has a loss. These two stimuli, each lasting about a second, are alternated. The intensity of tone for which there is loss is maintained constant at 10 or 20 dB sensation level, and the level of the other tone is varied until the two are equally loud. This task is difficult for those patients who are confused by the unavoidable disparity in the pitches of the two stimuli. When the test can be used, one can estimate the amount of recruitment present at the frequency for which there is impaired sensitivity. This estimate is based on the degree to which the disparity in thresholds for the two frequencies is eliminated by their loudness balance, but allowance must be made for those peculiarities between frequencies inherent in the normal phon relationships, or equal loudness contours (Fletcher, 1953).

Neither of the foregoing tests can be used with precision when the patient has a bilateral hearing loss across the entire frequency range.

In such a patient no stimulus can serve as the referent for normal loudness experience. A number of qualitative estimates of recruitment can still be made. One of the most useful of these is based on the spans in dB between the patient's threshold for a stimulus (tone or speech), his most comfortable listening level, and his uncomfortable listening level for it (Newby, 1964; Dix, 1968). Provided the patient is judging on loudness experience alone, recruitment is indicated by spans that are clearly narrower than normal.

Localizational Audiometry. A number of European clinicians are employing directional audiometry. This technique measures the patient's capacity to locate the source of a pure tone which is received binaurally in a sound field (Nordlund, 1964). This tone is generated by a loudspeaker that is out of sight. Sometimes the loudspeaker is moved from one azimuth position to another, and sometimes several loudspeakers are arranged around the patient.

Breakdown in localizational capacity may also be demonstrated with the Simultaneous Binaural Median Plane Localization test, which was once erroneously thought to be a method of achieving ABLB (Jerger and Harford, 1960). The principle of this test is simple. Bursts of a pure tone that are about a second in length are presented binaurally by earphone. Stimulus level is maintained constant on one side and is varied in intensity on the other. These signals ordinarily form a fused image which shifts in its apparent position as the relative intensities of its two components vary. The patient's assignment is to find the intensity relationship which leads the image to be centered in the midline.

Monaural Distorted Speech Tests. Speech materials have been modified in various ways in order to produce tests of unusual difficulty with which to explore for subtle unilateral disturbances in the central auditory pathways (Bocca and Calearo, 1963). One approach is to remove some frequencies by filtering. Bocca et al. (1954) introduced this procedure with Italian sentences that were filtered above 500 Hz. Interestingly, the Rush-Hughes recordings of PB-50 words function as though mildly filtered (Goldstein et al., 1956). A second form of distortion that is popular with the Italian school is to accelerate the test material radically (Calearo and Lazzaroni, 1957). A third procedure is to interrupt speech at various rates (Bocca and Calearo, 1963). The foregoing tests may be administered at only one suprathreshold level, or entire intelligibility curves may be obtained with them.

Binaural Distorted Speech Tests. These tests explore the capacity of the central nervous system to coordinate two incoming speech patterns, each of which is incomplete. The incoming patterns are chosen in such a way that a person with normal interpretative capacity achieves much better performance when receiving both messages than when receiving either one alone. One test of this type was proposed by Bocca (1955) and adapted to English by Jerger (1960c). Test material which has had low-pass filtering at 500 Hz is fed to one ear at 40 dB sensation level while the same material is presented to the other ear in unfiltered form at only 5 dB sensation level. Matzger (1959) devised a somewhat analogous test in which a narrow band of high frequencies from a speech sample go to one ear, while a restricted band of low frequencies from the same sample go to the other ear. Several variations on Matzger's test have since been proposed in attempts to find an optimal combination of filtering, presentation level, and kind of speech material (Palva, 1965).

A different approach is available in the alternated speech test advocated by the Italians (Bocca and Calearo, 1963). In this case the test material is both interrupted and staggered so that the silent intervals on one side are filled by bits of speech to the other ear, and vice versa. Performance is measured at several alternation rates between one and ten cyclings per second.

Binaural Competing Speech Tests. Here the purpose is to ascertain whether the listener possesses the normal ability to keep a train of speech received via one ear separated from a second train reaching the other ear. One version of this type of test employs competing words, such as sets of digits (Kimura, 1963). Another version consists of spondees that are so timed that the second syllable of one spondee coincides with the first syllable of the other spondee (Katz, 1968). A third approach is to administer monosyllabic words to one ear concurrently with whole sentences being administered contralaterally (Jerger et al., 1961).

Electrodermal Audiometry. This technique measures the occurrence of transient changes in the electrical resistance of the skin. The patient is attached to an instrument which records these changes along with information as to when each test stimulus is administered (Goldstein, 1963). Before starting the test proper, the patient is given a series of pure tones which he can hear clearly. Immediately following at least some of these stimuli he receives an unpleasant but harmless electric shock. Through this conditioning procedure he comes to anticipate the shock whenever he hears the tone, and this expectation triggers a brief electrodermal response (EDR). Following the preliminary conditioning, the intensity of the tone is varied. The lowest intensity at which the EDR persists is taken as the patient's threshold. This method is relatively definitive with many adults, but it requires skillful manipulation of tone and shock sequences to keep the EDR from weakening as the test proceeds.

EEG Audiometry. Electroencephalography has been adapted to the measurement of responses to sound. There currently is a great deal of interest in EEG audiometry, and the technique of obtaining averaged evoked potentials has proved useful with children (Goldstein, 1967). However, much more must be learned before we may expect EEG audiometry to reach its full level of clinical usefulness.

Delayed Auditory Feedback Tests. Two tests employ a system for delaying sound that disrupts the patient's coordination in performing an assigned task. These tests are designed to cause the patient to demonstrate involuntarily that he is hearing a sound. The first test uses the patient's own speech to disturb his capacity to read a standard passage aloud (Winchester and Gibbons, 1957). His normal reading rate while listening to himself through earphones is first determined. The reading is then repeated while a special circuit delays the earphone signal by about 0.2 second. This produces an unnatural way of hearing himself talk that disturbs the patient's speech production. Now he hesitates and repeats himself often enough to substantially increase the time required to re-read the passage. The most severe interference occurs for a normal hearer when the delayed speech is returning to the patient about 40 dB above his SRT. The second test requires the patient to tap simple rhythms by hand (Ruhm and Cooper, 1964). The patient hears his tapping pattern as a set of pure tone beeps coming through an earphone. When this pattern is delayed to the earphone, disruption of the tapping rhythm is evidence that the pattern of beeps is being heard. This phenomenon persists very close to the threshold for the test tone, so that one may estimate this threshold fairly well by noting the faintest intensity at which the delayed feedback disturbs the tapping sequence.

Stenger Test. This test is designed to discover the individual who is simulating a unilateral hearing loss, particularly a severe one. A single signal (either a pure tone or speech) is transmitted through separate channels to the two ears. When pure tones are used, an air conduction audiogram for each ear is first obtained in the regular manner except that masking is not used at any time. The patient with a true unilateral loss is likely to exhibit a shadow curve in the poor ear, whereas the person simulating a loss will not do so but instead will feign a very severe loss. The crucial procedure comes next. The test stimulus is now pulsed simultaneously to both ears. Its intensity is made a few dB stronger than threshold in the "good" ear, while it is presented at a substantially higher level in the "poor" ear. Because the simulator is really responding through both ears, the patient will hear a single image localized to the side receiving the more intense excitation, namely, the poor side. Successive presentations of the tone follow, with the signal to the poor ear made progressively weaker. A point is soon reached at which the simulator must deny hearing the tone because it has become fainter than his admitted threshold on the poor side, and he is unaware that the tone is simultaneously occurring above his threshold on the good side. This procedure is continued until the signal is so weak on the poor ear that the sound image experienced by the patient begins to shift to his good ear because of the stimulus that is also present there. The patient begins to respond again as soon he can identify a stimulus in the good ear. The tester knows from this occurrence that the stimulus level in the poor ear is close to the true threshold for that ear. If the patient becomes suspicious of what is happening, the skilled clinician alters his technique so as to catch the patient in other ways.

Other Tests. The foregoing catalog of special auditory tests has reviewed some of the major audiological techniques which have been devised as aids to differential diagnosis. Many variations on these several procedures have been advocated, and other kinds of tests have been developed. Thus, the foregoing discussion merely illustrates the diversity of audiological approaches which can be taken and mentions some of the methodologies that have won recognized usefulness.

Interpretation of Results

Combinations of the special auditory tests described previously assist in exploring specific diagnostic problems. A general summary of the six major applications of thest tests is given in Table 2. The discussion which follows expands these applications by recounting in general terms the test findings that are most commonly encountered.

Conductive Abnormalities. The hallmark of a conductive loss, as pointed out earlier, is an essentially normal level of hearing for pure tones by bone conduction with a substantial air-bone gap because sensitivity by air conduction is impaired. The speech reception threshold is in good agreement with the hearing loss by air conduction, and discrimination for speech is excellent. The hearing loss would also be manifest by electrodermal and electroencephalographic exploration, but these techniques are redundant. Other results to be expected are a Type I Békésy tracing, no appreciable threshold tone decay, negative SISI scores, and lack of recruitment. Finally, measurements of acoustic impedance and tympanometry yield results which supply information that helps to differentiate among conductive lesions. The results of these tests vary uniquely when the middle ear cavity contains fluid, when it is under abnormal pressure, and when there is abnormal function of the ossicular system (Klockhoff, 1961; Zwislocki and Feldman, 1969).

Inner Ear Abnormalities. Hearing losses resulting from disorders and lesions of the cochlea ordinarily exhibit equal impairment by air and bone conduction plus speech reception thresholds that are equivalent to the pure tone deficit in the midfrequencies. As described earlier, audiometric configurations are diverse in pattern and tend to be somewhat characteristic for particular etiologies. Likewise, speech discrimination varies from very good to only fair, again somewhat systematically with the cause of the loss. Recruitment ordinarily appears when sought by loudness balancing or acoustic reflex tests (Hallpike and Hood, 1959; Lamb et al., 1968). Békésy tracings are usually Type II (Jerger, 1962), and SISI scores for higher frequencies are ordinarily positive (Harford, 1967). Threshold tone decay is often evident at higher frequencies, but it reaches maximum values of only about 25 dB, and there are many instances in which it is minimal. Electrodermal and electroencephalographic audiometry reveal about the same hearing loss as encountered with voluntary tests, and interaural threshold disparities largely or completely disappear when tests such as the Simultaneous Binaural Median Plane Localization test are given (Jerger and Harford, 1960).

TABLE 2. Configurations of Responses Most Commonly Obtained From Adults Exhibiting Six Major Types of Auditory Problems

	TYPE OF AUDITORY PROBLEM					
TYPE OF HEARING TEST	Conductive	Sensori-neural: Cochlear	Sensori-neural: Retrocochlear	Auditory CNS: Brain Stem	Auditory CNS: Temporal Lobe	Simulated Hearing Loss
Pure tone: air	HL	HL	HL	N or HL	N	HL
bone	N	HL	HL	N or HL	N	HL
Speech: reception	HL	HL	HL	N or HL	N	HL—
discrimination	E	VG to F	G to VP	G to P	E to F	Var
Acoustic reflex	Abs	R	VC	?	?	N
Tympanometry	VC	N	N	N	N	N
Békésy: I vs. C	I	II	III or IV	I	I	V
Threshold tone decay	0	0 to 25	>25	0 to >25	0	–
SISI	Neg	Pos	Neg+	Neg	Neg	Neg+
Binaural loudness balance	Q	R	Q or D	Q,R or D	D	–
Monaural loudness balance	–	R	Q	–	–	–
Localizational	VC	Dis	VC	Abn	N	–
Monaural distorted speech	–	–	–	PDT	PDT	–
Binaural distorted speech	–	–	–	PDT	PDT	–
Binaural competing speech	–	–	–	PDT	Pos	–
Electrodermal	HL	HL	HL	N or HL	N	N
Electroencephalographic	HL	HL	HL	?	?	N
Delayed auditory feedback	HL	Var HL	HL	–	–	N
Stenger	HL	HL	HL	–	–	N

KEY: N = normal; HL = hearing loss; HL– = HL less for speech than tones; E = excellent; VG = very good; G = good; F = fair; P = poor; VP = very poor; Var = varied; I, II, III, IV and V = type of Békésy tracing; 0 to >25 = dB tone decay; Neg = low score; Pos = high score; VC = varies with condition; Neg+ = low score with large increments; Q = no recruitment; R = recruitment; D = decruitment; ? = awaits clarification; Dis = image displaced; Abn = grossly abnormal; PDT = positive depending on test; – = test not applicable.

The most useful audiological clues to differentiation among inner ear disorders are to be found in the configurations of pure tone loss and the relative clarity of discrimination for speech (see earlier discussion). There also tends to be some clustering of other test results. For example, patients with Meniere's disease more often exhibit reduction in amplitude of Békésy tracings for continuous tone than do persons with cochlear otosclerosis (Sanders, 1965). Again, threshold tone decay tends to be more strictly concentrated to higher frequencies in Meniere's disease than in presbycusis (Willeford, 1960); while recruitment is particularly strong in acoustic trauma and in Meniere's disease (Dix et al., 1948; Schuknecht, 1963). However, a great deal of further analyses must be done before these latter kinds of clues are well enough understood to be major aids in diagnosing among cochlear pathologies. The important thing is that such clues may come to have great future usefulness. Consider, for example, the hypothesis by Harbert and Young (1964) that narrowing of a continuous Békésy tracing is evidence of rapid adaptation resulting from pathological functioning of the dendritic network within the inner ear.

Retrochochlear Abnormalities. A major application of special auditory tests has been their use in the discovery of tumors within the internal auditory meatus and the cerebellopontine angle. Highly distinctive auditory symptomatology often results from these space-occupying lesions. Patients with such problems usually will exhibit hearing loss unless the tumor is very small. Their pure tone audiograms will be of the sensorineural variety, and their speech reception thresholds will usually coincide with their sensitivity for midfrequencies.

The basic loss in auditory sensitivity will also be revealed when the acoustic reflex is tested and during both electrodermal and electroencephalographic audiometry, but these tests add no differential information. The most distinctive finding includes the fact that, although speech discrimination may sometimes be fairly good, it much more commonly is very severely disturbed (Johnson, 1968), even to the point at which understanding of spondees and simple sentences is disrupted. Again, the Type III Békésy tracing, which is frequently found in such conditions, is an impelling clue of an active retrocochlear condition (Jerger, 1960b; Johnson, 1968). The Type IV tracing also is often encountered here. Another very strong indication is extreme and very rapid threshold tone decay (Tillman, 1969). Concurrently, SISI scores are usually low (Harford, 1967). Recruitment is ordinarily but not invariably absent (Dix et al., 1948; Johnson 1968), decruitment sometimes occurs, and directional audiometry may show some deterioration in localizational ability (Nordlund, 1964).

Some sudden sensorineural deafnesses replicate the symptomatology described above. These may be assumed to be the result of acute involvement of the eighth nerve (Jerger et al., 1961a).

By contrast, chronic degeneration of the nerve such as characterizes neural presbycusis (Schuknecht, 1964) ordinarily produces only a portion of the aforementioned symptomatology (Schmidt, 1967). Type III and Type IV Békésy tracings are not to be expected. Here threshold tone decay tends to occur over a wider frequency range, to be more variable, and to be more extreme than found with inner ear lesions; but dramatically rapid and complete abnormal adaptation is not common. Speech discrimination may be poorer than the audiogram would suggest (Gaeth, 1948), but the drastic disruption of intelligibility sometimes caused by other retrocochlear conditions is not common. Ordinarily SISI scores are low and recruitment is usually absent. Of course, interpretation of findings is complicated by the fact that neural presbycusis often appears in combination with epithelial (or cochlear) presbycusis.

Disorders of the Central Auditory Nervous System. With the probable exception of some conditions involving the brain stem (Carhart, 1967a; Calearo and Antonelli, 1968), lesions and malfunctions within the central auditory nervous system do not ordinarily produce gross and easily observed disruptions in hearing. Auditory behavior here is almost always equivalent to that of normal hearers when measured by pure tone audiometry, conventional speech audiometry, or any of the other pure tone tests mentioned here except binaural loudness balancing and localizational audiometry. It is necessary to employ tests that impose particularly difficult listening tasks when seeking out disorders of the central auditory nervous system (Jerger, 1960a). Distorted and competing speech tests have proved especially useful in this regard.

Of course, the sites, natures, and extents of central auditory lesions vary substantially; consequently, the resultant subtle breakdowns in response differ from one patient to the next. We are still in the process of learning how to interpret these breakdowns, but major guidelines have emerged which give some help in distinguishing brain stem lesions from those involving the temporal lobe and cerebral areas.

Brain stem disorders tend to manifest themselves in two major ways. For one thing, there may still remain residues of abnormality in processing relatively simple stimuli. As mentioned previously, losses for pure tones are sometimes present. Calearo and Antonelli (1968) report the patterns to be of the sensorineural variety without recruitment, while Davis and Goodman (1966) have observed decruitment. Carhart (1967b) has suggested that some lesions of the cochlear nuclei may mimic inner ear lesions in their loudness functions, Békésy tracings, and SISI scores; whereas Parker et al. (1968) have observed patients with brain stem involvement in whom relatively good pure tone thresholds appeared concurrently with recruitment and severe tone decay. The Simultaneous Binaural Median Plane Localization test may pose an impossible obstacle for such a patient, while the task of performing alternate binaural loudness balancing remains easy irrespective of whether recruitment is present.

Secondly, intelligibility for high fidelity speech varies substantially when there is brain stem involvement, but this discrimination is often very good. When such is the case and pure tone sensitivity is not impaired, appropriate distorted speech tests can be used to investigate whether integration of auditory stimuli is disrupted in one of several ways (Bocca and Calearo, 1963). First, the intelligibility of interrupted speech may be reduced when presentation is via the contralateral ear. Second, tasks involving bilateral interaction are often adversely affected. Thus, blending two filtered segments of a speech message, or fusing speech that is alternated between ears, or coping with time compressed speech may become difficult.

Temporal lobe disorders will ordinarily yield poorer scores for monaurally distorted speech or for faint unfiltered speech when the material is presented via the ear contralateral to lesion than when it is received via the ipsilateral ear (Bocca et al., 1955). Similarly, breakdown on competing message tests is greater when the primary message enters the system contralaterally (Jerger, 1964). Mixed speech stimuli, such as Bocca's filtered speech to one ear and faint speech to the other, do not show a binaural improvement over the score that is achieved monaurally when only the ipsilateral fraction of the combined test is administered. The Simultaneous Binaural Median Plane Localization task can now be performed with ease; decruitment often appears for the stimulus entering the contralateral ear.

Finally, diffuse cortical involvements sometimes reduce efficiency during difficult speech tests. One example involves time compressed speech, while another is alternated speech (Bocca and Calearo, 1963).

Simulated Hearing Loss. The audiological procedures for identifying simulated hearing loss (pseudohypacusis) and for estimating the true level of hearing efficiency are well developed. Typically the pseudohypacusic yields a pure tone audiogram with approximately equal loss by air and by bone. His responses may be somewhat variable on retest, and a sophisticated examiner can often manipulate the situation so as to produce appreciable shift in the patient's avowed thresholds. A fairly common finding is that the hearing loss for pure tones is substantially greater than for speech (Fournier, 1958). Responses to both the speech reception and the speech discrimination test are often bizarre. Acoustic reflexes and tympanometric responses are normal. During the SISI test the pseudohypacusic frequently refuses to admit awareness of even large increments; i.e., his score is grossly on the negative side.

Four tests yield particularly definitive information. The Békésy tracing shows a hearing loss as would be expected, but it often takes on the unique Type V pattern (Rintelmann and Harford, 1967). Electrodermal audiometry can be used successfully in almost all instances to reveal approximately the patient's true thresholds for both pure tones and speech (Chaiklin and Ventry, 1963). These thresholds will either be normal or, if the patient is simulating an

overlay on a true hearing loss, they will be greatly improved over his voluntary responses. Again the patient will usually show breakdown on the delayed auditory feedback test at levels fainter than his admitted threshold, and with the Ruhm-Cooper (1964) technique it is possible to discover approximately his threshold sensitivity. Finally, the Stenger test may often be used to plot the true hearing level in the avowedly impaired ear provided a unilateral hearing loss is being feigned (Fournier, 1958; Chaiklin and Ventry, 1963).

SUMMARY

Conventional pure tone audiometry indicates the patient's level and configuration of hearing loss by both air and bone conduction. Speech audiometry yields measures of both the patient's threshold for speech and his capacity to discriminate its finer details. Several other auditory tests are also clinically useful. The patient's performance on such tests not only indicates his practical hearing efficiency; it also assists in the differential diagnosis of disorders of the conductive mechanism, the inner ear, the retrocochlear neural pathway, and the auditory central nervous system. In addition, auditory tests can be used to penetrate simulated hearing loss.

REFERENCES

ANSI–S3.6–1969: USA Standard Specifications for Audiometers. New York, American National Standards Institute, 1970.

ASA–S3.1–1960: American Standard Criteria for Background Noise in Audiometer Rooms. New York, American Standards Association (now American National Standards Institute), 1960.

ASA–Z24.5–1951: Specification for Audiometers for General Diagnostic Purposes. New York, American Standards Association (now American National Standards Institute), 1951.

ASA–Z24.13–1953: Specification for Speech Audiometers. New York, American Standards Association (now American National Standards Institute), 1953.

Barr, B., and Lundström, R.: Deafness following maternal rubella. Acta Otolaryng. 53:413, 1961.

Békésy, G. v.: A new audiometer. Acta Otolaryng. 35:411, 1947.

Bocca, E.: Binaural hearing: Another approach. Laryngoscope 65:1164, 1955.

Bocca, E., and Calearo, C.: Central hearing processes. In Jerger, J. (ed.): Modern Developments in Audiology New York, Academic Press, 1963, Chapter 9, p. 337.

Bocca, E., Calearo, C., and Cassinari, V.: A new method for testing hearing in temporal lobe tumors. Acta Otolaryng. 44:219, 1954.

Bocca, E., Calearo, C., Cassinari, V., and Migliavacca, F.: Testing "cortical" hearing in temporal lobe tumors. Acta Otolaryng. 45:289, 1955.

Bordley, J. E., and Hardy, W.: The etiology of deafness in young children. Acta Otolaryng. 40:72, 1951.

Bunch, C. C.: Traumatic deafness. Beltone Translation Series, No. 23, 1970.

Calearo, C., and Antonelli, A. R.: Audiometric findings in brainstem lesions. Acta Otolaryng. 66:305, 1968.

Calearo, C., and Lazzaroni, A.: Speech intelligibility in relation to the speed of the message. Laryngoscope 67:410, 1957.

Carhart, R.: Clinical application of bone conduction audiometry. Arch. Otolaryng. 51:798, 1950.

Carhart, R.: Basic principles of speech audiometry. Acta Otolaryng. 40:62, 1951.

Carhart, R.: Speech audiometry in clinical evaluation. Acta Otolaryng. 41:18, 1952.

Carhart, R.: Clinical determination of abnormal auditory adaptation. Arch. Otolaryng. 65:32, 1957.

Carhart, R.: Effect of stapes fixation on bone conduction response. In Schuknecht, H. (ed.): Otosclerosis. Boston, Little, Brown and Company, 1962, Chapter 14, p. 175.

Carhart, R.: Labyrinthine otosclerosis. Arch. Otolaryng. 78:477, 1963.

Carhart, R.: Problems in the measurement of speech discrimination. Arch Otolaryng. 82:253, 1965.

Carhart, R.: Probable mechanisms underlying kernicteric hearing loss. Acta Otolaryng. (Suppl.) 221:6, 1967a.

Carhart, R.: Questions and speculations. In McConnell, F. and Ward, P. H. (eds.): Deafness in Childhood. Nashville, Vanderbilt University Press, 1967b, Chapter 15, p. 229.

Carhart, R., and Jerger, J. F.: Preferred method for clinical determination of pure tone thresholds. J. Speech Hear. Dis. 24:330. 1959.

Carhart, R., and Tillman, T. W.: Interaction of competing speech signals with hearing loss. Arch Otolaryng. 91:273, 1970.

Chaiklin, J. B., and Ventry, I.: Functional hearing loss. In Jerger, J. (ed.): Modern Developments in Audiology. New York, Academic Press, 1963, Chapter 3, p. 76.

Davis, H.: The articulation area and the social adequacy index for hearing. Laryngoscope 58:761, 1948.

Davis, H.: Guide for the classification and evaluation of hearing handicap in relation to the international audiometric zero. Trans. Amer. Acad. Ophthal. Otolaryng. 69:740, 1965.

Davis, H., and Goodman, A. C.: Subtractive hearing loss, loudness recruitment and decruitment. Ann. Otol. 75:87, 1966.

Davis, H., and Silverman, S. R.: Hearing and Deafness. New York, Holt, Rinehart and Winston, Inc., 1970.

Dix, M. R.: Loudness recruitment and its measurement with especial reference to the loudness discomfort level test and its value in diagnosis. Ann. Otol. 77:1131, 1968.

Dix, M. R., Hallpike, C. S., and Hood, J. D.: Observations upon the loudness recruitment phenomenon, with especial reference to the differential diagnosis of disorders of the internal ear and the VIIIth nerve. J. Laryng. Otol. 62:671, 1948.

Egan, J. P.: Articulation testing methods. Laryngoscope 58:955, 1948.

Fairbanks, G.: Test of phonemic differentiation: The rhyme test. J. Acoust. Soc. Amer. 30:596, 1958.

Ferrer, O.: Speech audiometry: A discrimination test for Spanish language. Laryngoscope 70:1541, 1960.

Fletcher, H.: A method for calculating hearing loss for speech from an audiogram. Acta Otolaryng. (Suppl.) 90:26, 1950. (See also J. Acoust. Soc. Amer. 22:1, 1950.)

Fletcher, H.: The perception of speech sounds by deafened persons. J. Acoust. Soc. Amer. 24:490, 1952.

Fletcher, H.: Loudness. In Speech and Hearing in Communication. Princeton, New Jersey, D. Van Nostrand Company, 1953, Chapter 11, p. 176.

Fournier, J. E.: Audiometrie Vocale. Paris, Libraire S. A. Maloine, 1951.

Fournier, J. E.: The detection of auditory malingering. Beltone Translation Series. No. 8, 1958.

Fowler, E. P.: The diagnosis of diseases of the neural mechanism of hearing by the aid of sounds well above threshold. Laryngoscope 47:289, 1937.

Fowler, E. P.: The recruitment of loudness phenomenon. Laryngoscope 60:680, 1950.

Fry, D. B.: Word and sentence tests for use in speech audiometry. Lancet 22:197, 1961.

Gaeth, J. H.: Study of Phonemic Regression Associated with Hearing Loss. Doctoral Dissertation, Northwestern University, Evanston, Ill., 1948.

Goldstein, R.: Electrophysiologic audiometry. In Jerger, J. (ed.): Modern Developments in Audiology. New York, Academic Press, 1963, Chapter 5, p. 167.

Goldstein, R.: Electrophysiologic evaluation of hearing. In McConnell, F., and Ward, P. (eds.): Deafness in Childhood. Nashville, Vanderbilt University Press, 1967, Chapter 5, p. 48.

Goldstein, R., Goodman, A. C., and King, R. B.: Hearing and speech in infantile hemiplegia before and after left hemispherectomy. Neurology 6:869, 1956.

Gyllencreutz, T., and Lidén, G.: Improved methods in bone conduction audiometry. Acta Otolaryng. (Suppl.) 224:229, 1967.

Hahlbrock, K. H.: Sprach audiometrie. Grundlagen und praktische Anwendung einer Sprachaudiometrie für das Deutsche Sprachgebiet. Stuttgart, Georg Thieme, 1957 (Revised 1970).

Hallpike, C. S., and Hood, J. D.: Observations upon the neurological mechanism of the loudness recruitment phenomenon. Acta Otolaryng. 50:472, 1959.

Harbert, F., and Young, I. M.: Threshold auditory adaptation measured by tone decay test and Békésy audiometry. Ann. Otol. 73:48, 1964.

Harford, E. R.: Clinical application and significance of the SISI test. In Graham, A. B. (ed.): Sensorineural Hearing Processes and Disorders. Boston, Little, Brown and Company, 1967, Chapter 18, p. 223.

Hirsh, I. J.: Loudness and recruitment. In The Measurement of Hearing. New York, McGraw-Hill Book Co., 1952, Chapter 8, p. 203.

Hirsh, I. J., Davis, H., Silverman, S. R., Reynolds, E. G., Eldert, E., and Benson, R.: Development of materials for speech audiometry. J. Speech Hear. Dis. 17:321, 1952.

Holmgren, L.: Acoustical evaluation of factors involved in stapes mobilization. Acta Otolaryng. 48:124, 1957.

Hood, J. D.: Auditory fatigue and adaptation in the differential diagnosis of end-organ disease. Ann. Otol. 64:507, 1955.

Hood, J. D.: The principles and practice of bone conduction audiometry. Laryngoscope 70:1211, 1960.

Hood, J. D.: Basic audiological requirements in neuro-otology. J. Laryng. Otol. 83:695, 1969.

Huizing, E. H.: Bone conduction loss due to middle ear pathology —pseudoperceptive deafness. Int. Audiol. 3:89, 1964.

Huizing, E. H., van Bolhuis, A. H., and Odenthal, D. W.:

Studies on progressive hereditary perceptive deafness in a family of 335 members. Acta Otolaryng. 61:35, 1966.

Huizing, H. C., and Reyntjes, J. A.: Recruitment and speech discrimination loss. Laryngoscope 62:521, 1952.

ISO–R389–1964: Standard Reference Zero for the Calibration of Pure Tone Audiometers: International Standards Organization (procure through American National Standards Institute, New York, N.Y.), 1964.

Jepsen, O.: Middle-ear muscle reflexes in man. In Jerger, J. (ed.): Modern Developments in Audiology. New York, Academic Press, 1963, Chapter 6, p. 194.

Jerger, J.: Audiological manifestations of lesions in the auditory nervous system. Laryngoscope 70:417, 1960a.

Jerger, J.: Békésy audiometry in analysis of auditory disorders. J. Speech Hear. Res. 3:275, 1960b.

Jerger, J.: Observations on auditory behavior in lesions of the central auditory pathways. Arch. Otolaryng. 71:797, 1960c.

Jerger, J.: Hearing tests in otologic diagnosis. Asha 4:139, 1962.

Jerger, J.: Auditory tests for disorders of the central auditory mechanism. In Fields, W. S. and Alford, B. R. (eds.): Neurological Aspects of Auditory and Vestibular Disorders. Springfield, Charles C Thomas, 1964, Chapter 5, p. 77.

Jerger, J., Allen, G., Robertson, D., and Harford, E.: Hearing loss of sudden onset. Arch. Otolaryng. 73:350, 1961a.

Jerger, J., Carhart, R., and Dirks, D.: Binaural hearing aids and speech intelligibility. J. Speech Hear. Res. 4:137, 1961b.

Jerger, J., and Harford, E.: Alternate and simultaneous balance of pure tones. J. Speech Hear. Res. 3:15, 1960.

Jerger, J., and Herer, G.: An unexpected dividend in Békésy audiometry. J. Speech Hear. Dis. 26:390, 1961.

Jerger, J., Shedd, J. L., and Harford, E.: On the detection of extremely small changes in sound intensity. Arch. Otolaryng. 69:200, 1959.

Johnson, E. W.: Auditory test results in 110 surgically confirmed retrocochlear lesions. J. Speech Hear. Dis. 30:307, 1965.

Johnson, E. W.: Auditory findings on 200 cases of acoustic neuroma. Arch. Otolaryng. 88:598, 1968.

Katz, J.: The SSW test: An interim report. J. Speech Hear. Dis. 33:132, 1968.

Kimura, D.: A note on cerebral dominance in hearing. Acta Otolaryng. 56:617, 1963.

Klockhoff, I.: Middle ear muscle reflexes in man. Acta Otolaryng. (Suppl.) 164:1, 1961.

Konigsmark, B. W., Salman, S., Haskins, H., and Mengel, M.: Dominant midfrequency hearing loss. Ann. Otol. 79:42, 1970.

Kreul, E. J., Nixon, J. C., Kryter, K. D., Bell, D. W., and Lang, J. S.: A proposed clinical test of speech discrimination. J. Speech Hear. Res. 11:536, 1968.

Lamb, L., Peterson, J., and Hansen, S.: Application of stapedius muscle reflex measures to diagnosis of auditory problems. Int. Audiol. 7:188, 1968.

Lidén, G.: Speech audiometry, an experimental and clinical study with Swedish language material. Acta Otolaryng. (Suppl.) 114, 1954.

Lidén, G.: Undistorted speech audiometry. In Graham, A. B. (ed.): Sensorineural Hearing Processes and Disorders. Boston, Little, Brown and Company, 1967, Chapter 26, p. 339.

Lidén, G., Nilsson, G., and Anderson, H.: Narrow-band masking with white noise. Acta Otolaryng. 50:116, 1959.

Lindsay, J.: Hydrops of the labyrinth. Arch. Otolaryng. 71:500, 1960.

Lybarger, S. F.: Interim bone-conduction thresholds for audiometry. J. Acoust. Soc. Amer. 40:1189, 1966.

Macrae, J. H., Woodruff, P., and Farrant, R. H.: Standardization of the Commonwealth Acoustic Laboratories' recordings of phonetically balanced monosyllabic test words. J. Otolaryng. Soc. Austral. 1:197, 1963.

Matzger, J.: Two new methods for assessment of central auditory functions in cases of brain disease. Ann. Otol. 68:1185, 1959.

Newby, H. A.: Audiology. New York, Appleton-Century-Crofts, Inc., 1964, p. 169.

Niemeyer, W. von: Anpassung von Hörapparaten. Hals-Nasen-Ohren-Heilkunde Stuttgart, Zöllner, F. (ed.). Stuttgart, Georg Thieme Verlag, Band III, Teil 3: 1873, 1966.

Nordlund, B.: Directional audiometry. Acta Otolaryng. 57:1, 1964.

Owens, E.: Tone decay in VIIIth nerve and cochlear lesions. J. Speech Hear. Dis. 29:14, 1964.

Palva, A.: Filtered speech audiometry. Acta Otolaryng. (Suppl.) 210:1, 1965.

Parker, W., Decker, R. L., and Richards, N. G.: Auditory function and lesions of the pons. Arch. Otolaryng. 87:228, 1968.

Pestalozza, G., and Shore, I., Clinical evaluation of presbycusis on the basis of different tests of auditory function. Laryngoscope 65:1136, 1955.

Peterson, G., and Lehiste, I.: Revised CNC lists for auditory tests. J. Speech Hear. Dis. 27:62, 1962.

Reger, S.: Differences in loudness response of the normal and hard-of-hearing ear at intensity levels slightly above the threshold. Ann. Otol. 45:1029, 1936.

Rintelmann, W. F., and Harford, E. R.: Type V Békésy pattern: Interpretation and clinical utility. J. Speech Hear. Res. 10:733, 1967.

Ruhm, H. B., and Cooper, W. A., Jr.: Delayed feedback audiometry. J. Speech Hear. Dis. 29:448, 1964.

Sanders, J. W.: Labyrinthine otosclerosis. Arch. Otolaryng. 81:553, 1965.

Schmidt, P. H.: Presbycusis. Int. Audiol. (Suppl.) 1:4, 1967.

Schuknecht, H. F.: Meniere's disease: A correlation of symptomatology and pathology. Laryngoscope 73:651, 1963.

Schuknecht, H. F.: Further observations on the pathology of presbycusis. Arch. Otolaryng. 80:369, 1964.

Shambaugh, G. E., Jr.: Surgery of the Ear. Philadelphia, W. B. Saunders Company, 1967.

Silverman, S. R., Thurlow, W. R., Walsh, T. E., and Davis, H.: Improvement in the social adequacy of hearing following the fenestration operation. Laryngoscope 58:607, 1948.

Sørensen, H.: Clinical application of continuous threshold recording. Acta Otolaryng. 54:403, 1962.

Terkildsen, K., and Thomsen, K. A.: The influence of pressure variations on the impedance of the human ear drum. J. Laryng. Otol. 73:409, 1959.

Thompson, G.: A modified SISI technique for selected cases with suspected acoustic neurinoma. J. Speech Hear. Dis. 28:299, 1963.

Tillman, T. W.: Special hearing tests in otoneurologic diagnosis. Arch. Otolaryng. 89:25, 1969.

Tillman, T. W., Johnson, R. M., and Olsen, W. O.: Earphone versus sound-field threshold sound-pressure levels for spondee words. J. Acoust. Soc. Amer. *39*:125, 1966.

Tonndorf, J.: Bone conduction, studies in experimental animals. Acta Otolaryng. (Suppl.) *213*:3, 1966.

Ward. W. D.: Effects of noise on hearing thresholds. *In* Ward, W. D. (ed.): Noise as a Public Health Hazard. ASHA Rep. *4*:40, 1969.

Willeford, J. A.: The Association of Abnormalities in Auditory Adaptation to Other Auditory Phenomena. Doctoral dissertation, Northwestern University, Evanston, Ill., 1960.

Winchester, R., and Gibbons, E. W.: Relative effectiveness of three modes of delayed sidetone presentation. Arch. Otolaryng. *65*:275, 1957.

Witting, E. G., and Hughson, W.: Inherent accuracy of a series of repeated clinical audiograms. Laryngoscope *50*:259, 1940.

Zwislocki, J. J., and Feldman, A. S.: Acoustic impedance of pathological ears. ASHA Monographs *15*:1, 1970.

Chapter 42

HEARING AIDS

by Robert C. Cody, M.A.

Any instrument that brings sound to a listener's ear more efficiently may be called a hearing aid. This may be done in a number of ways; by nonelectrical devices which collect sound energy from the air and direct it into the ear, by various prostheses or audiosurgical procedures involving the external and middle ear, or by the electroacoustical instruments which introduce amplified sounds into the external auditory meatus. This chapter is concerned with the latter, which we commonly call hearing aids.

HISTORICAL DEVELOPMENT OF THE HEARING AID

The cupped hand was undoubtedly the first and most natural aid for those with impaired hearing. The effectiveness of this device is due to the palm of the hand collecting more sound energy than the auricle alone and directing it into the external meatus. It is not known whether it was by accident or the product of some inventive mind that an ear trumpet was found to do this task more effectively. The ear trumpet was popular for centuries and led to many ingenious adaptations, including acoustic chairs, fans, pipes, hats, vases, and speaking tubes. Although these devices met with varying degrees of success, they should not be discredited because they provided from 10 to 20 decibels (dB) increase in sounds received by the hearing impaired, and also alerted the speaker to the fact that the listener had a hearing loss and he should speak louder.

Alexander Graham Bell is usually credited with the invention of the electrical hearing aid about 1900; this was an outgrowth of his scientific and educational background, interest in telegraphy, and desire to bring better hearing to the deaf. This crude device consisted of a carbon microphone, batteries, and an earphone, all connected with wires. The electronic hearing aid was a major breakthrough that has led to undreamed of results in communication for the deaf and severely hard of hearing. In general, however, the amplification obtained from these early aids was far from satisfactory though speech was louder and many people who could not hear with an ear trumpet could hear with these aids. Later a carbon amplifier was added to give even greater amplification.

Some of the disadvantages of early hearing aids included crackling, hissing, and rattling noises generated by the carbon granules used in the microphone and amplifier. They were first produced in table or desk models and were not easily portable. Eventually the size was reduced sufficiently to be worn in a special harness on the body. Heavy wires connected the microphone, amplifier, and receiver with a large battery pack. These aids were not only heavy but quite uncomfortable and daily wear required a determined individual.

By the early 1920's, with the invention of the electronic vacuum tube, the carbon amplifier became obsolete. The first vacuum tubes were rather large, so early vacuum tube aids were either desk size or too heavy to be readily portable. In the mid 1930's, with the reduction in tube size, hearing aids were reduced to models that could be worn on the person. Batteries for these aids were still quite large and needed to be strapped to the body. During the 1940's batteries were so reduced in size they could be incorporated into the same case which held the microphone and amplifier; thin electrical cords connected to the receiver on the ear. Some of these aids were less than the size of a cigarette package. This was not only a great convenience, but it was now possible for even small children to benefit from wearable amplification.

A dramatic breakthrough in hearing aid size came in the early 1950's with the development of the transistor, which replaced the vacuum tube and required only one small battery to operate. More recently, microminiature circuits have enabled further reduction in size to the point that aids are available which will fit within the concha of the auricle.

Since the advent of the first electrical model in the early 1900's, the size and wearability of hearing aids has not only been reduced tremendously, but the clarity and fidelity of the amplified sounds have improved. This has had a profound effect on providing education and communication to the deaf and severely hard of hearing, enabling them to participate more meaningfully in a hearing world.

MODERN HEARING AIDS

Some 300 to 400 different hearing aid models are now offered for sale in the United States. For the most part they can be classified under three general categories: group, portable, and wearable hearing aids.

Group Hearing Aids

These consist of one or more microphones, an amplifier, and several earphones (receivers). These aids are generally used in classrooms for the deaf or hard of hearing, but some have been installed in churches, auditoriums, and theaters. A recent innovation with group hearing aids has been the use of an inductance loop which creates an electromagnetic field around the room. Each listener receives the sound signals via a magnetic pickup coil in their wearable type hearing aid.

The inductance loop group hearing aid frees the listener from being wired to a fixed amplifier and allows normal movement about the room. This is ideal for educational systems and can be adapted for use in the home.

Portable (Desk Type) Hearing Aids

These hearing aids consist of a microphone, amplifier, and battery in a relatively small case connected to an earphone headset designed for individual use. A portable hearing aid can be used by a hearing impaired child in a classroom of normal hearing children. These instruments are most widely used in classrooms where only one or two children have sufficient hearing impairment to warrant amplification but need better fidelity than is offered by wearable hearing aids. Some physicians find these units helpful for communicating with hard of hearing patients in the office or examining room. Speech and hearing clinicians often use portable amplifiers while working with clients needing auditory training. These units may be obtained with either monaural or binaural amplification (two complete microphone-amplifier-receiver systems in the same case) and with large earphones or small insert type receivers.

Wearable Hearing Aids

There are a variety of different models of hearing aids that can be worn on the person. The following are commercially available:

Torso Models. Microphone, amplifier, and battery for the torso models are within one case worn in a pocket or specially designed pouch on the chest. Thin wires run to a small receiver attached to a plastic earmold which is inserted into the external auditory meatus. Available with either air conduction or bone conduction receivers, these aids can be worn monaurally, binaurally, or with a Y-cord (pseudobinaural). Binaural fittings would involve the purchase of two monaural aids—one for each ear—but some binaural models have two complete aids within the same case. Y-cord fittings involve a monaural hearing aid with a bifurcated cord running to a receiver in each ear.

Postauricular Models. Microphone, amplifier, battery and receiver are housed in a small case which fits behind the ear with a short length of plastic tubing connecting the receiver to an earmold fitted in the external auditory meatus. These aids are available in air conduction models only but can be worn monaurally or binaurally (a complete aid on each ear).

Eyeglass Models. Microphone, amplifier, battery and receiver are within the temple bow of eyeglasses with plastic tubing connecting the receiver to the earmold in the ear. These instruments are comparable (in some cases identical) to the postauricular models. Though a few bone conduction models are available, the torso model bone conduction aid is better suited for this kind of amplification because it offers greater gain than the eyeglass models.

Many of the torso, postauricular and eyeglass

hearing aids are equipped with an electromagnetic telephone pickup coil that enables the listener to enjoy amplified telephone conversations with the exclusion of environmental and room noises. These aids can also be used in conjunction with an inductance loop system.

CROS Model. In the early 1960's, Harford (1969) carried out investigations of a special type of hearing aid designed for severe unilateral deafness. This developed into what is now called the CROS (contralateral routing of signal) and the BICROS hearing aids.

This utilizes either a postauricular or an eyeglass hearing aid. The microphone is mounted on the side of the impaired "unaidable" ear with wires routed to the amplifier and receiver on the side of the normal or near normal ear. A length of tubing connects the receiver with a special nonoccluding earmold fitted in the concha. This special earmold allows the amplified sounds from the hearing aid to enter the ear canal without preventing normal sound transmission to the good ear. Use of the CROS led to the development of the BICROS hearing aid.

BICROS Model. This is similar to the CROS, with the addition of a microphone on the better ear side. This was found useful for those persons with one unaidable ear and a significant but aidable hearing loss in the other ear.

Auricular Model. The culmination of efforts to miniaturize hearing aids and to satisfy the wearer's desire to conceal his impairment has led to the smallest of hearing aids, the auricular model.

The microphone, amplifier, battery, and receiver are contained within either a standard earmold or are held in place with a grommet which occupies the concha and part of the external auditory meatus. At the present time these aids are very limited in usable gain and are impractical for persons with more than mild hearing loss.

In general, the larger the hearing aid components, the greater the power and amplification characteristics. Therefore, persons with severe hearing loss will usually require a torso model aid; mild to moderately severe losses might gain ample benefit from ear level aids.

AMPLIFICATION CHARACTERISTICS OF HEARING AIDS

There are many terms used to describe the electrical and acoustic characteristics of hearing aids. Knowledge of certain of these terms, such as gain, maximum power output, and frequency response are necessary for understanding a discussion of the amplification characteristics. Although USA Standards Institute (formerly American Standards Association) has published standard methods for the measurement of the electroacoustical properties of hearing aids (ASA S 3.3–1960), they did not specify a precise method for reporting these measurements. As a result, five or six different ways of stating gain, power, and frequency response have been used, making it difficult to determine a hearing aid's performance from reading advertisements and manufacturers' specifications.

About 1960 the Hearing Aid Industry Conference (HAIC) developed a standard method of reporting hearing aid performance (Lybarger, 1961). Some manufacturers do not adhere to HAIC recommendations so it is still difficult to evaluate the specifications of their instruments. The following descriptions of terms are a brief summary of the USASI and HAIC methods recommendations:

Gain. Gain is the difference in decibels (dB) between the input sound pressure level (SPL) to the microphone and the output SPL from the receiver. HAIC gain is expressed as a single value taken from the average amplification at 500, 1000, and 2000 Hz with the input SPL of 60 dB and the hearing aid's volume control turned full on.

Frequency Response. Frequency response is usually expressed in graphic form, with the relative acoustic gain of an aid expressed as a function of frequency. The basic frequency response is the acoustic gain produced over a frequency range from 200 to 5000 Hz with an input SPL of 60 dB and the volume control turned to full on. HAIC frequency range is derived by drawing a line across the frequency scale at a level 15 dB below the HAIC gain. The two points at which the –15 dB line intersects the frequency-response-curve define the HAIC frequency response of the aid.

The range of frequencies which an aid will amplify is affected by the microphone and the receiver characteristics. In general, microphones are ineffective at low frequencies and receivers cut off the high frequencies, resulting in maximal amplification in the middle frequency range which is important for the reception and understanding of speech (300 to 3000 Hz).

Maximum Power Output. This is sometimes called the saturation sound pressure level and is the maximum SPL a hearing aid is capable of producing with the volume control full on and the input signal increased until the output of the aid can no longer increase. HAIC defines output as the average (in dB) of the saturation level 500, 1000, and 2000 Hz.

Most hearing aids have external or internal controls which can be adjusted so as to cause variations in the electrical gain, power, or frequency response characteristics to compensate for a number of different types of hearing loss. Further acoustical variations are possible in the length and size of tubing connecting the hearing aid receiver with the earmold, the insertion of acoustic filtering devices in the tubing or receiver, and in the shape and design of the earmold itself. Because of the adjustments that can be made in hearing aid characteristics, it is possible for many of those with impaired hearing to benefit from amplification which is somewhat "tailored" to meet their acoustical needs.

AUDIOLOGY AND HEARING AID EVALUATION

Audiology is a professional discipline devoted to the science of hearing, its measurement, and rehabilitation. The basic qualifications for an audiologist have been established by the American Speech and Hearing Association (9030 Old Georgetown Road, Washington, D.C.) and include the completion of work for a master's degree. ASHA further recognizes the completion of academic and experience requirements for clinical competency by awarding a certificate attesting to the professional qualifications of the holder. Under the most desirable conditions, a hearing aid evaluation should be given by an audiologist either following or in conjunction with an otological examination. Otologic clearance for a hearing aid evaluation is of the utmost importance to assure there is nothing which can be done medically or surgically to improve the person's hearing.

Hearing tests are taken as an aid to diagnosis, for determining the amount and type of hearing impairment, and to determine the patient's rehabilitation needs. Testing should include, as a minimum, the following measurements of hearing acuity:

1. Pure tone tests of both air and bone conduction thresholds throughout the test frequencies of 250 to 8000 Hz. The pure tone audiogram alone should not be used for determining the need for amplification, but it does yield useful information pertaining to the extent of loss as a function of frequency and to the type of hearing loss (conductive, sensorineural, or mixed).

2. Speech audiometry to ascertain the speech reception threshold (SRT), discrimination loss for speech (PB DISCRIM), and dynamic range.

SRT is defined as the level (in dB) at which a listener can correctly repeat 50 per cent of the test material presented. Thresholds will vary, depending on the type of speech material used; simple sentences will differ from monosyllabic words, and both will differ from the thresholds of two-syllable spondaic words. Spondee words (such as "hot dog," "baseball," "eardrum," etc.) are the most widely used to determine a listener's SRT. The SRT will usually approximate the average pure tone air conduction threshold for the "speech frequencies" (500, 1000, and 2000 Hz).

The discrimination loss for speech is the per cent of the phonetically balanced (PB) monosyllabic words a listener repeats correctly at a level that is sufficiently high so that a further increase in intensity will not result in a higher score (called PB MAX). These word lists are usually presented at a level of *SRT plus 40 dB* or the most comfortable loudness level (MCL) for the listener.

Pure conductive hearing loss will usually produce normal or near normal discrimination scores (90 to 100 per cent). Sensorineural loss, especially severe high frequency loss, will usually show diminished scores (less than 90 per cent). Sensorineural loss accompanied with auditory recruitment (i.e., Meniere's) will show drastically reduced discrimination ability. As a general rule, the poorer the speech discrimination score, the less likely the listener will benefit from a hearing aid.

Dynamic range is the difference between the SRT and the level at which speech becomes uncomfortably loud to the listener. The dynamic range gives us the limits within which amplification can be tolerated. A very restricted dynamic range would contraindicate the successful use of a hearing aid.

There are a number of other tests the audiologist or otologist might administer in a differential diagnosis, but the aforementioned should be prerequisite to an evaluation for consideration of amplification. With these test results, it is possible to determine the amount and type of hearing loss as well as its effect on the patient's communication with others. An audiological evaluation should answer the following questions: Does a hearing problem exist and, if so, is it medically or surgically remediable? If not remediable, is a hearing aid indicated?

When a hearing aid evaluation is indicated, additional testing is done which allows a determination of the patient's hearing ability with and without an aid. Speech audiometry is administered through a loudspeaker in quiet and with a background of competing noise. A hearing aid evaluation should determine: Can the patient benefit from amplification? If he can, what characteristics should the hearing aid have? Should it be worn on the torso or at ear level? What settings and adjustments are necessary for the aid? Whether or not a hearing aid is recommended, are other rehabilitation procedures necessary and where can they be obtained?

Another objective of a hearing aid evaluation is to determine whether one particular instrument will benefit the patient more than another. Recommendation of a particular aid will depend on its ability to produce the best SRT, highest tolerance level, and the best speech discrimination scores. Other factors which must be taken into consideration by the audiologist include its "ruggedness of design, availability of service, initial cost, and its attractiveness (size, appearance, and so forth). In the eyes of the purchaser, too often the first consideration is given to the factor of attractiveness" (Newby, 1964).

Some audiologists do not actually try hearing aids on a patient but, rather, recommend an instrument which—according to the manufacturer's specifications—best compensates for the hearing loss insofar as frequency response, gain, and power are concerned. Most audiologists believe that hearing aids should be tried on the person to best predict the benefits of amplification. The Research Subcommittee on Hearing Aid Evaluation Procedures of the American Speech and Hearing Association (1967) recommends that a "hearing aid evaluation must include testing with wearable hearing aids." In addition, the audiologist should "adhere to a policy of referring patients about to purchase hearing aids only to recognized organizations and individuals (hearing aid dealers) who have demonstrated their competence in dealing with hard of hearing persons, and the adequacy of their facilities and service."

Certain follow-up procedures are necessary when the patient has purchased a hearing aid.

Although these will be discussed thoroughly in the chapter, Rehabilitative Audiology, they might include hearing aid orientation and recheck, counseling, aural rehabilitation (speech reading, auditory training, speech conservation, and therapy), and periodic re-evaluation of the patient's hearing.

HEARING LOSS AND AMPLIFICATION

A hearing aid is basically a miniature electrical public address system; it make sounds louder. It is not a "high fidelity" instrument because it does not amplify sounds much above 3500 to 4000 Hz, but it does help many hearing impaired persons toward better communication. The purpose of a hearing aid is to make it easier for the listener to hear and to understand speech. Any aid that fails to do this will be considered unsatisfactory by its wearer.

In the early days of wearable hearing aids, it was felt that only those patients with pure conductive loss could benefit from a hearing aid. Most persons with a conductive loss need only to have speech made louder in order to hear and to understand well, making them ideal candidates for amplification. On the other hand, because of their reduced speech discrimination ability, persons with sensorineural loss were advised against amplification because it was thought it would not help them. It is true that a hearing aid will usually not improve the discrimination score and will sometimes have an adverse affect on intelligibility, but in the great majority of cases, discrimination is not noticeably affected by amplification and these patients do benefit from hearing speech at a louder level. This is fortunate because persons with sensorineural loss account for the majority of patients seen in audiology clinics for hearing aid evaluation. The use of amplification has proved to be beneficial for most or these patients.

Until recently it was considered a general rule that a person did not need amplification unless his loss for speech was greater than 30 to 40 dB in the better ear. This is no longer true. There are too many exceptions to the "rule." Many people with only minimal hearing loss benefit from amplification and, in fact, aids have even been found to be helpful for persons with one normal or near normal ear. The CROS and BICROS hearing aids have benefited persons who had previously been advised against amplification.

In summary, the person with a flat, conductive loss will receive the most benefit from a hearing aid because he can tolerate higher levels of amplification, has good speech discrimination ability, and does not have a problem of auditory recruitment. The person with a sensorineural loss who displays good hearing for low frequencies but rapidly diminishing acuity for the higher frequencies of the speech range is the least likely to benefit. But with patients in whom irreversible, sensorineural hearing loss exists, the possibility of beneficial amplification should not be ruled out.

Any person with a hearing loss is a potential hearing aid user. There are many borderline cases, but minimal, high frequency, sensorineural, unilateral, or profound hearing loss does not automatically disqualify a person from consideration for amplification. The best "rule" to follow is that a person is a candidate for amplification if he can perform better with a hearing aid than without it.

There are many other factors which should be considered regarding a person's need for amplification of sound. They include age, occupation, socioeconomic status, intelligence, personality, attitudes toward hearing loss and hearing aids, other physical disabilities, and the need for better communication. Any one of these factors might determine whether a person may benefit from wearing a hearing aid. It is the responsibility of the audiologist and otologist to weigh these factors and to provide the patient with guidance in overcoming them if they stand in the way of beneficial use of amplification.

REFERENCES

Conference on Hearing Aid Evaluation Procedures. ASHA Reports, No. 2, September, 1967.

Davis, H., and Silverman, S. R.: Hearing and Deafness. Rev ed. New York, Holt, Rinehart and Winston, Inc., 1960.

Harford, E.: Is a hearing aid ever justified in unilateral hearing loss? Otolaryng. Clin. N. Amer. February, 1969.

Hearing Loss, Hearing Aids, and the Elderly. Hearings before the Subcommittee on Consumer Interests of the Elderly of the Special Committee on Aging, United States Senate. Washington, D.C., U.S. Government Printing Office, July, 1968.

Lybarger, S. F.: A new standard for measuring hearing aid performance. ASHA 3:121, 1961.

Newby, H. A.: Audiology. 2nd ed. New York, Appleton-Century-Crofts, Inc., 1964.

Chapter 43

COMMUNICATION DISORDERS OF SPEECH

by Jay Melrose, Ph.D.

In the third edition of the book *Speech Handicapped School Children*, (1967) the late Professor Wendell Johnson set forth the concept that when a child or an adult has a communication problem, then everyone who relates to that child or adult becomes "A Member of the Problem." This concept would seem to hold true for the other family members, for friends, for teachers, for clinicians, and certainly for the general practitioner, the pediatrician, and the otolaryngologist. The physician often becomes the earliest professional "Member of the Problem" as a result of the family's seeking help for a child with a possible speech, hearing, or language disorder. For the otolaryngologist this might be a direct contact in his private practice, a referral from another physician, consultation in a Community Speech and Hearing Center, service on a cleft palate team, staff responsibilities in a hospital or rehabilitation center, or duties as a member of the professional group working with an agency such as State Services for Handicapped Children.

Professor Johnson also offered a very useful definition of a speech problem that might serve as a guide to the otolaryngologist. Although he referred to a child's speech, there can be no question of appropriate application to the adult. He stated, "A straightforward general answer to the question of what is a speech problem or impairment or disorder is that a child's speech presents a problem for himself and for others when his listeners pay critical or anxious, or disapproving attention to how he speaks, or are distracted from what he is saying by his way of saying it."

The demands upon the otolaryngologist, then, would seem to dictate an awareness and knowledge of the various speech problems and their possible causes. After appropriate examination, he should be able to arrive at a tentative diagnosis. When necessary, he should seek consultation from colleagues in other specialties since final management decisions will usually involve various combinations of medicosurgical intervention, referral to speech, hearing and language clinicians, and referral for counseling or psychotherapy for the patient and/or his family.

It is extremely important during this early stage of the otolaryngologist's involvement as a "Member of the Problem" for him to be able to counsel the patient and his family carefully, clearly, thoroughly, and directly concerning his findings and the rationale behind his suggestions. Such good counseling can often prevent a minor speech deviation from becoming a serious major communication problem.

OBSERVATION, ANALYSIS, AND IDENTIFICATION OF SPEECH PROBLEM BEHAVIOR

Often the statements made in person or in writing by the adult patient, or by the parents of

In keeping with the decision to fo
tion of the presentation on symp
than causesn a study of current tex
ing with voice problems indicates
that such problems fall into the foll
ings:

1. Problems of intensity (loudn
2. Problems of pitch.
3. Problems of voice quality.
4. Problems of flexibility (varia

It is not unusual for combinatio
problems to coexist. Once again th
physician's first impressions can
against his built-in criteria based up
spectrum of voice production he ha
experienced. Curtis (1967) pointed
requirements for an adequate vo
that (1) the voice must be appropria
the speaking situation; (2) the pitc
be adequate in terms of the age an
speaker; (3) the voice quality must
bly pleasant; and (4) flexibility of bo
loudness must be adequate. Care
tion of the patient's vocal output du
formance of a few speaking and r
should help to pinpoint the areas in
problems exist.

Problems of Intensity (Loudness
most part, problems of loudness oc
the speaker does not speak loudly
often the case that a speaker does
have the ability to change the inte
voice as the size of the room in
speaking increases or as the noi
creases. In relatively few instance
seems to maintain an overly loud
when it is inappropriate for the spe
tion. Variety in the use of loudness
will be discussed in the section
flexibility.

Problems of Pitch. It should be
that a variety of pitches are emp
given speaker during the voiced po
utterance. These pitches range
below a pitch that is central. Fairb
1960) described these pitches as
follow a normal distribution about
pitch. This central pitch can be thou
pitch level habitually used by the
terms of vocal adequacy, then, the
can be perceived as being too high
for the age and sex of the speak
problem exists when the speaker us
pitches above and below his habitua
and seems to be producing voice th
tially a monotone. Finally, some sp

a child, are of little help in yielding precise information about the exact nature of the speech problem. Remarks like "He doesn't talk like other kids his age" or "We don't have any problem understanding her, but other people say they can't always get what she's saying" are more explanatory of the reasons behind the request for an appointment than they are descriptive of the deviant speech behavior. Careful observation and analysis of the patient's speech must be accomplished before decisions can be made concerning the presence or absence of a disorder. Is the problem one of misarticulation of speech sounds, of rate control, of disfluency, or voice deviation, or of lack of appropriate language development and usage? What are some of the observations that can be made, and how are such observations then analyzed to afford meaningful descriptions of the patient's speech behavior? It should be understood that the focus here is on the study of the speech output and not on any of the reasons for the performance.

Errors of Articulation

After listening to a patient's connected speech, the use of even an unrefined measure such as comparison with others of similar age might indicate that the speaker's output is relatively unintelligible. More careful analysis might show that this lack of intelligibility was the result of certain sounds of speech being omitted, or some sounds being substituted for other sounds, or distortion of some sounds. To use a visual analogy, suppose that each sound of a correctly articulated utterance were painted in an appropriate sequence on consecutive slats of a picket fence, with unmarked slats indicating word separation. This statement should be easy to read and understand. If, however, some of the slats were knocked out of the fence, or wrong letters were accidentally painted on, or some of the letters were distorted by the artistic efforts of passers-by, then it might be very difficult to comprehend the original message. A listener might receive a similarly distorted message if the sequence of sounds needed to transmit a spoken message from the speaker to the listener was interfered with through errors of articulation.

Errors of Omission. A child might wish to say, "I go to his house to play with his toys." If his speech was characterized by the omission of all /s/ and /z/ sounds, this utterance might then

be heard as, "I go to hi____ hou____ to play with hi____ toy____."

Errors of Substitution. Using the same sentence as before, if the speaker habitually substituted the voiceless /th/ for /s/, and voiced /th/ for /z/, he would say, "I go to hi*th* hou*th* to play with hi*th* toy*th*."

Errors of Distortion. Once again, if the speaker employed a lateral emission for the /s/ and /z/, which resulted in an utterance that sounded as if there were an excess of saliva in the mouth, the distorted sounds of the test sentence would undoubtedly interfere with easy communication: "I go to his hou*s*e to play with hi*s* toy*s*."

It is not atypical for combinations of errors to exist in the same speaker. Also, whereas only the /s/ and /z/ sounds were used as examples, such errors of articulation can be found in all speech sounds. The number and severity of the speaker's errors would thus dictate the estimate of intelligibility that would be made by the listener.

Problems of Rate

Rate is usually defined as the number of events per unit of time. In speech, the problem confronting the examiner is whether there is justification in the complaint that the patient's speech is too slow or too fast. A first impression can be gained by listening to the spontaneous speech of the child or adult as he responds to your questions. It must be noted that each speaker's rate varies tremendously, depending upon such factors as emotional state, familiarity with the listeners, complexity of the subject matter, and level of formality of the speaking situation. A fruitful approach might be to consider the research that has been done pertaining to rate problems of adults and then to suggest the use of reasonable parallels in the problems of children.

Although there is not an exact 1:1 ratio for rates that are used in oral reading and rates used in speaking, research on oral reading rates, and listener judgments of such reading tasks, have yielded information that is pertinent to clinical decisions. The report by Fairbanks (1960) indicated that the median oral reading rate for male college students who read a representative 300-word passage was 170 words per minute. Of course, there was a distribution above and below this point. Listener judgments indicated

that 160 to 170 words per minu
excellent. Moving toward the sl
to 160 w.p.m. was rated as satis
151 w.p.m. was too slow. For th
the continuum, 170 to 182 w.p.m
tory, 182 to 192 w.p.m. was dou
thing above 192 w.p.m. was too

Although this was a special p
forming a carefully controlled ta
might be of particular use to the
tried to read at various oral re
order to get a better feel for thes
resultant judgments.

In a special note on rate, Fa
pointed out that two oral readers
same overall rate and yet yield
listener judgments. In one case
would divide his articulation time
time in about a 2:1 or 3:1 ratio
elapsed time, and would be judg
tory or excellent. The second s
employ long pauses and rapid sp
speech pattern would most likely
rapid and stacatto in delivery, an
fast, despite the fact that the
between bursts limited the total
same overall rate.

Conversational speech and c
reading tasks can be observed ar
determine whether rate is indeed
"too fast" and also whether there
rapid-fire delivery which is difficu
hend.

Disfluency

It can readily be shown that
regardless of age, go through perio
speech is characterized by relativ
A child's parents will show conc
fact that their youngster, who was
fluent, is now engaging in spe
which is typified by many repetitic
syllables, words, and even who
These repetitions are usually
fortlessly, with no "struggle" beha
either not noticed by the child, or
ticular concern to him. In a candid
parents will admit that they ar
about the possibility that this obs
ior might be a forerunner of stutte

Johnson, Darley and Spriester
classify the disfluencies into the
tegories:

1. Interjections of sounds, syll
or phrases.

As points of self-reference, the examiner might recall his own voice quality following a bout of laryngitis, or after spending an afternoon cheering for a football team.

Problems of Flexibility (Variability). Up to this point the focus of the examiner has been directed toward evaluating the adequacy of loudness, pitch and voice quality. The factor of flexibility must now be considered in terms of its role in the estimate of vocal adequacy. In the previous discussion of pitch level, the explanation was given that there was a tendency for an individual to use a small cluster of contiguous pitches for most of the vocal output. However, other pitches that range above and below the central pitches are usually employed to produce an intonation or melodic pattern that is appropriate to the intended meaning or the expressed emotionality of the utterance. An obvious parallel can be drawn in the case of loudness. A speaker tends to use an overall loudness level, but employs increased or decreased intensity according to the dictates of emphasis and stress.

It becomes evident, then, that a speaker might have adequate voice quality, overall loudness level and pitch level, and still demonstrate a problem because he does not employ sufficient variability of pitch and loudness.

Language Problems

The physician's involvement with decision-making concerning language problems would be centered about three areas: the child who has not begun to use language, the child whose language usage does not seem to be up to the level of other children his age, and the adult who has lost the ability to use language at an expected and appropriate level.

It must be understood that we are not talking about speech production, but rather the stringing together of the sounds of speech into a symbolic code. Eisenson (1947) stated: "Language is any system of recognized symbols used to produce or prevent specific responses of thoughts, or feelings, or actions. . . . A symbol stands for something else. It implies that a connection of some sort has been made between a word and an idea. The connection must be formed in such a way that the name of the object or idea recalls the object or the idea." He then defined speech as "that form of language which man produces without resorting to agencies outside of his own organism."

A child of between two and five years of age may be brought in for evaluation because he seems to have mastered the sounds of speech, but has not evidenced any ability to use these sounds in the production of language. He may employ some limited gestures and may even seem to use a few grunts and shouts in a meaningful way. Another five year old may be using language, but may be limited to one- or two-word utterances. Bangs (1968) has presented some thoughts that might be useful to the examiner. She wrote, "Children who do not follow an orderly pattern when learning the language code may be referred to as *language disordered;* those who do follow an orderly pattern but one not commensurate with chronological age may be referred to as *language delayed."* The physician's previous experience with children, plus the norms for language development that will be presented in a following section, should prove useful in the final determination of the presence or absence of disordered or delayed language.

The majority of the adults who are referred for language problems will usually evidence psychological or neuropathological disturbances. For example, Berry and Eisenson (1945) stated, "Dysphasia represents a disorder of symbolic formulation and expression." The extent of the language problem in such cases, then, will best be determined through information supplied by the patient's family and friends relevant to the quantity and quality of premorbid language usage.

UNDERLYING CAUSES OF SPEECH PROBLEMS

In the last section the attention of the examiner was directed toward the observation, analysis, and identification of speech problem behavior. The problems that were considered were those of articulation, rate, disfluency and stuttering, voice, and language. For individual cases in each of these areas, evidence can be cited for etiologies that are organic or functional, or both. It is felt that the otolaryngologist would be in the best position to identify all the organic causes that could logically result in a speech problem. For each problem area, then, a few examples will be given of typical organic and functional etiologies. Generalization from such points of departure could then be accomplished readily and appropriately.

Articulation

Disorders such as cleft palate, cerebral palsy, dental anomalies, and hearing loss are all contributory to articulation problems. Since speech is learned behavior, mental retardation can readily be understood to be a factor in faulty and delayed articulatory proficiency.

Curtis (1967) cites faulty learning as a major nonorganic cause of disorders of articulation. As examples he includes poor speech models, as in the case where other members of the family have impaired speech, and also lack of stimulation and motivation. In this latter case, he refers to a child whose parents and siblings interpret his jargon and respond to his needs in such a way that there is no need for him to practice and learn better speech.

Emotional problems must also be considered as contributing factors. If, for example, there is a condition in the home in which infantile behavior yields some reward, then an infantile speech pattern might be retained. In the case of a home situation in which there are many loud and upsetting arguments, it has often been found that a child will have delayed speech development, as if he has made a judgment to attempt to avoid joining in the activities of an unpleasant adult world.

Rate

In the case of disorders of rate, there may be an organic problem in which there is a biochemical imbalance that causes overall hypo- or hyperactivity which is reflected in a speech rate that is too slow or too fast. Imitation of faulty models must also be considered. Finally, as an example, people who exhibit the emotional states of depression or agitation might also display slow or rapid rates of speech.

Disfluency and Stuttering

The research of Wendell Johnson (1963, 1967) reveals that there are periods in the development of most children during which they engage in considerable disfluent speech. Such disfluency might be the result of some specific excitement or the inability of the neurological mechanism to support all the complex activities that the young child is trying to master at the same time. This behavior is often noticed at a time when there are large spurts of language acquisition. There are also reports of increased disfluency when the child begins to attend school. In this instance the possibilities exist that the speech behavior might be reflecting a response to the demands of the school situation or might be indicative of an emotional reaction to being "pushed out" of the protective home environment.

For stuttering, three major theories of causation tend to be espoused by the various researchers in this area: stuttering as a reflection of neurosis; stuttering as a result of physiological predisposition; and stuttering as learned behavior. As is the case in the creation of strong theoretical formulations, the proponents of the various theories have carefully organized the existing data to fit their different frames of reference. The physician should attempt to learn more about these theories of causation since they tend to dictate differing approaches to therapy which might have a bearing on referrals for therapeutic management.

Voice

Since hypernasality and hyponasality are more problems of resonance than of voice quality, a fruitful approach might be the study of the structure and function of the oral and nasal mechanism. In hypernasality, some organic causes are cleft palate, palatal insufficiency, and neuromuscular involvement of the soft palate. In terms of functional causes, simple imitation cannot be ruled out. It should also be noted that nasality in speech might be typical of certain subcultures or geographical regions. Hyponasality is often the result of such organic etiologies as enlarged tonsils and adenoids, a deviated septum, or a broken nose. A child or adult who suffers from various allergies also evidences this denasal voice.

Laryngeal disorders account for the majority of the problems of voice quality. Representative examples would include incomplete closure of the vocal cords as the prime cause of breathiness; excessive laryngeal tension as the main source of the problems in harshness; and such problems as chronic laryngitis, vocal nodes, thickening of the cords, and laryngeal cancer as causes of hoarseness. Improper pitch placement and excessive loudness must also be considered as contributing factors.

TABLE 1. Per Cent Distribution of Speech Impairments by Age (U.S.A.) July 1959—June 1961

	ALL AGES	UNDER 25	25–44	45–64	65–74	OVER 75
Speech Defects: Percent of all impairments	4.6	18.3	2.7	1.7	1.8	1.0

Language

In the child some organic etiologies for language problems are congenital aphasia, other neuropathological disturbances, and hearing loss. Mental retardation is also usually a cause for retardation in language acquisition. Functional causes could be delayed language resulting from the confusion caused by bilingualism, emotional problems leading to withdrawal and refusal to learn and use language, and insufficient learning opportunities because of language deprivation in and about the home.

For the adult who previously had language skills, the primary cause of language difficulty is aphasia resulting from a stroke. Adults may also have been victims throughout their lives of language deprivation as a result of environmental conditions. Finally, emotional problems might tend to limit the quantity and quality of language usage.

STATISTICS CONCERNING INCIDENCE OF OCCURRENCE

In the last 30 or 40 years various surveys have been conducted in the United States in an attempt to determine the prevalence of speech (and hearing) defects in terms of the percentage of the entire population that have such communication problems. A wide range is reported, from about 3 to 13 per cent. For the most part the criteria for inclusion are not carefully spelled out. Those that seem to have a sound basis for estimation report about a 5 per cent incidence figure. Table 1 is a portion of Health Statistics from the U.S. National Health Survey (1965). They report a 4.6 per cent incidence as the figure for all impairments of speech for all ages. Of particular interest is their further breakdown by age groups, which shows that for those under 25 years of age the incidence is slightly over 18 per cent.

TABLE 2. Estimated Prevalence of Speech Defects in the United States (1950)*

TYPE OF SPEECH PROBLEM	AGES 5–21 YEARS		ALL AGES	
	PER CENT	NUMBER	PER CENT	NUMBER
Functional articulatory	3.0	1,500,000	3.0	6,000,000
Stuttering	.7	350,000	.7	1,400,000
Voice	.2	100,000	.2	400,000
Cleft palate speech	.1	50,000	.1	200,000
Cerebral palsy speech	.2	100,000	.2	400,000
Retarded speech development	.3	150,000	.3	600,000
Impaired hearing (with speech defect)	.5	250,000	.5	1,000,000
Total	5.0	2,500,000	5.0	10,000,000

*Figures given here are estimated in terms of 50,000,000 between the ages of five and 21 years and in terms of 200,000,000 total population.

TABLE 3. *Normal Development of Speech*

AGE LEVEL	ACTIVITY	DESCRIPTION OF BEHAVIOR
Birth–8 weeks	Reflexive vocalization	Crying, whimpering, production of vowel sounds; use of variations of consonants such as /k/, /l/, /g/, and /h/
8 weeks–6 months	Babbling	Awareness of sound production; differentiated crying; much sound repetition; addition of consonants such as /p/, /b/, /m/, /n/, /ng/, and /th/
6 months–12 months	Vocal play	Imitates and echoes his own vocal output; increased use of pitch and inflection; responds to outside vocal stimulation; decreases crying and increases speech sound production; addition of more consonants such as /t/ and /d/
12 months–18 months	True speech	Intentional use of some single words; much speechlike jargon; imitation of parental speech; use of gestures along with speech output; development of greater articulatory proficiency

TABLE 4. *Age of Articulatory Efficiency of 23 Consonant Sounds*

AGE	SOUNDS MASTERED
By 3½	/b/, /p/, /m/, /w/, /h/
4½	/d/, /t/, /n/, /g/, /k/, /ng/, /y/
5½	/f/
6½	/v/, /voiced th/, /zh/, /sh/, /l/
7½	/s/, /z/, /r/, /voiceless th/, /hw/

TABLE 5. *Normal Development of Language*

AGE LEVEL	DESCRIPTION OF LANGUAGE SKILLS
One year	Use of first real words; words are used as single words; the words are nouns; very limited vocabulary—one to three words
Two years	Increases vocabulary to 200–300 words; uses nouns and verbs; combines words; typical sentence length is two words
Three years	Vocabulary level is 600–1000 words; mean sentence length is 3.5 words; uses nouns, verbs, and personal pronouns
Four years	Vocabulary is now 1500–1600 words; sentence length is between four and six words; adds more pronouns, adjectives, adverbs, prepositions, and conjunctions
Five years*	Vocabulary increases to over 2000 words; sentence length is close to six words; all parts of speech are included

*From five years on, the main factors in language development are increased vocabulary, increased sentence length, and increased complexity of sentence structure.

Table 2 presents a breakdown of specific types of speech problems according to age groups. These data come from the American Speech and Hearing Association Committee on the Midcentury Conference (1952).

The source of these data (in their up-dated form) was the publication, *Human Communication and Its Disorders—An Overview*, which is a report that was prepared by the Subcommittee on Human Communication and Its Disorders of the National Advisory Neurological Diseases and Stroke Council (1969).

The startling fact is that even with the conservative estimate of 5 per cent of the total population (in 1970), there are an estimated 10 million people with clinical-level communication disorders of speech. Certainly the otolaryngologist must consider, as a vital part of his training, the securing of information that will help him meet the needs of this special population.

NORMAL DEVELOPMENT OF SPEECH AND LANGUAGE

It can be assumed that the study and use of normative data is an integral part of the training and practice of the medical specialist. Therefore, only two sets of normative data are presented in this section. These are for the normal development of speech and the normal development of language. Experts in these fields whose writings were studied differed slightly in the timetables they established, or in their names for the different stages or phases. Table 3 represents a consensus of specialists such as Berry and Eisenson (1945), Van Riper (1963), and Irwin (1947, 1948).

Following the initiation of true speech, the child would be expected to continue his mastery of individual speech sounds as well as to show rapid growth in language acquisition. Data adapted from Poole (1934) provide some useful guidelines for the evaluation of speech development (Table 4).

As in the case of the chart for the normal development of speech, Table 5, Normal Development of Language, is a summary of the researches of various experts such as Smith (1926), Gesell (1952), Lillywhite (1958), and Berry (1969).

As Lillywhite pointed out, the comprehension vocabulary, responses to commands, and understanding of grammatical forms always give indication of being further advanced than could be measured only by the language performance of the child.

The materials presented in Table 5 dealing with the normal development of speech and language, along with other norms that have been interspersed where relevant throughout the chapter, are particularly pertinent when employed with the subject matter of the next two sections: Diagnostic Techniques and Differential Diagnosis.

DIAGNOSTIC TECHNIQUES

The well trained otolaryngologist is accustomed to following certain specific procedures in his evaluation of a new patient. From the adult, or from the parents of a child, he will learn the chief complaint and then will attempt to secure as accurate and complete a case history as possible, with special attention being paid to items that are particularly pertinent to the problem. Next, he will perform the thorough examination that is routine in otolaryngology. It is expected that the information in the case history, along with the results obtained directly from his examination, and indirectly through reports from the laboratory and from radiology, will permit the physician to make an accurate diagnosis which would then lead to appropriate treatment.

In the case of communication disorders, however, the otolaryngologist must make some further decisions. If there is an active organic pathologic disorder, such as vocal nodes, it might require a surgical procedure, followed by a referral to a speech pathologist, to help the patient to avoid further vocal abuse. If the problem is one of faulty articulation, with no organic etiology, then a direct referral might be made to the speech pathologist.

In general, those working in the field of communication disorders would follow procedures similar to those undertaken by the otolaryngologist. That is, a case history would be taken which would be followed by various tests and examinations in order to arrive at a specific diagnosis. Then decisions would be made concerning a plan of therapy.

It is to be expected that different disciplines would be interested in having different questions answered in the taking of a case history and that different tests and examinations would be performed. In order to help the otolaryngologist to understand more about the professional practices of the speech pathologist, this section will describe very briefly some special case history formats that are typically employed, and also will outline some usual procedures that are followed in the diagnostic evaluation of a patient with a communication disorder.

Specialized Case Histories for Speech Problems

The book *Diagnostic Methods in Speech Pathology* by Johnson, Darley and Spriestersbach (1963), contains a basic clinical speech case history outline of the type that has proved to be extremely effective. The major headings include such items as the complaint, the source of referral, the history of the speech problem, developmental history, medical history, school history, social history, family history, and the examiner's comments on the interview. The format is designed so that under each major heading there are included many specific questions to enable the questioner to secure maximum information. This differs from the case history that the physician might take in that the emphasis here is on speech and speech-related items. For example, under the general heading, History of Speech Problem, are such items as the identification of the problem, parental attitudes concerning the faulty speech, attempts at correction, estimates of severity, siblings or relatives with similar problems, patient's attitude toward the problem, and detailed questions concerning speech development. Supplementary outlines are also included for communication disorders that are related to specific problems such as cleft palate, dysphasia, postlaryngectomy, and stuttering. The otolaryngologist might well refer to this book for the extensive case history outlines that are included.

Tests and Examinations

If a seven year old boy were referred for a diagnostic evaluation of his severe articulation problem, the following schedule would be typical: First, a complete case history would be obtained from his parents. Often this is accomplished while the child is in the sound-treated suite for an audiometric evaluation. Next, an attempt would be made to secure some samples of speech from the child in order to make a judgment of overall intelligibility of his speech, without attention being given to specific sound errors. An examination of the oral mechanism would follow. Here, there might be

a referral report from the otolaryngologist concerning some structural deviation. However, the speech pathologist would ordinarily check for gross anomalies. The child would then be asked to attempt various tasks in order to check the function of the articulators. For example, he might be asked to repeat some nonsense syllables as rapidly as possible, or to wag his tongue from side to side. The rate at which such tasks were accomplished might indicate normal function or the possibility of neuromuscular involvement.

Various tests have been developed to check articulatory proficiency, and this would be the next procedure. The tests are usually designed to enable the examiner to elicit a response to a picture in order to obtain a record of those speech sounds that the child has not mastered, to detect the particular type of error he makes, to note the consistency or inconsistency of the errors, to test the sounds in various phonetic contexts, and to determine whether the child can duplicate a sound that is made by the examiner, even though he might not have produced the sound correctly without sound stimulation. Finally, the child would be tested in order to estimate his level of language development. Many different tests are available to indicate overall language levels, problems in the expression of language, and problems in language reception.

Naturally when the patient is being seen for problems other than articulation disorders, appropriate substitution of special procedures would be made. Thus, a man with a harsh or hoarse voice might require a test of his habitual pitch level to see if it varies considerably from an estimated level of his natural pitch. There are special tests for dysphasia, and a whole battery of tasks is employed in the evaluation of stuttering. Similarly, many procedures have been devised to help specifically in the determination of the extent of the communication problem that is associated with cleft palate. There is the possibility that the speech pathologist might feel that referrals were in order to a psychologist, a dentist, or a neurologist. Eventually, however, all the tests, measurements, examinations, and referrals to outside sources would be completed, and the next steps would be to arrive at a diagnosis and to make any necessary plans for therapy.

DIFFERENTIAL DIAGNOSIS

The previous sections of this chapter have been placed into a sequence that was designed to highlight this section on differential diagnosis. The attempt was made to follow a natural and logical progression. It should make no difference whether the diagnostician is the otolaryngologist or the speech pathologist. The intent was to describe deviant speech behavior so that it could be observed, analyzed, and identified. Having decided upon the general nature of the problem, the diagnostician would then be able to employ the data on the incidence of occurrence, and the information on underlying causes, to help bring the problem into sharper focus. Next, norms could be studied pertaining to the development of speech and language skills. Finally, there is a presentation of the specialized case histories, and the tests and examinations that are typically used during the diagnostic evaluation of the child or adult who presents a communication disorder of speech.

The task of differential diagnosis is to recall all this general information on the mythical "average" child or adult, to couple it with the clinical findings for a specific patient, and then to arrive at a diagnosis that can be followed by an appropriate management decision.

Some illustrations might afford an operational definition of differential diagnosis in communication disorders. Suppose that two five year old boys were brought in for evaluation and that they were closely matched in most of the physical, emotional, and intellectual traits that could be measured and compared. Suppose, too, that they both evidenced moderate-to-severe articulation disorders along with a low rating of overall intelligibility. If all that was considered was the objective data from the tests, examinations, observations, and comparisons with norms, the decision might be made to advise immediate therapy for both. However, if the parents of one boy reported that three other older male siblings had all followed exactly the same speech and language developmental pattern, and that the brothers had all "caught up" to their peers by seven years of age and were currently free of their former problems, then the decision might be made to have the boy check in every six months and to delay any consideration of therapy. For the second boy, assume that there were no positive medical or psychological findings, and that the parental interview revealed other male siblings who evidenced no problems of speech development. For this child, the recommendation would be for immediate referral for therapy.

In another situation two boys might be showing a similar level of disfluency. Careful evaluation of existing differences in the two boys' level of awareness and concern, and evidence of avoidance mechanisms being initiated by one of the boys, would lead to the decision to have this boy seen for therapy. For both boys' parents, appointments would be made for counseling sessions.

Many examples might be fashioned to cover each of the disorders, but it is felt that the two instances are sufficient to illustrate the concept of response by the examiner to small, but highly significant, differences.

Although the otolaryngologist might be involved with the accomplishment of complete differential diagnoses in some patients with communication disorders, higher priorities for his time and skills would usually dictate his referral of such patients to the speech pathologist to complete the nonmedical aspects of diagnostic examination.

THERAPY

Speech is behavior that is unique to human communication, and when disorders of speech exist, therapy must be thought of as the use of skills, techniques, and methodologies that can effectively bring about desired changes in behavior. The otolaryngologist should know about the background and training of the speech pathologists to whom he refers his patients for therapy.

The speech pathologist's background in speech and hearing science usually includes courses in phonetics, anatomy and physiology, physics, acoustics, and linguistics. Required studies in psychology supply information on child development, learning, motivation, attention, perception, and cognition. Considerable study is also made of the various psychopathologies. The clinical program in speech disorders contains didactic courses for the study of each. Typical courses would be those in articulation, voice, stuttering, neuropathology, cleft palate, hearing loss, and language.

Clinical practicum is accomplished under careful staff supervision in a clinical facility that is located in or near the academic training center. It is in these supervised clinical sessions that the future speech pathologist learns the art of bringing about behavior change. What are some of the problems that might be encountered? A child with delayed speech must be stimulated to acquire new sounds. A stutterer must be shown how to rid himself of tics and grimaces and how to attempt to bring his stuttering under control. An aphasic must be helped to reconstruct the building blocks of language so that he can use speech to make his needs known. A child with a repaired cleft palate must learn to articulate more carefully so that his speech will be more intelligible. Skill in taking complete case histories and in writing reports must be developed. Counseling techniques to be used with children, young adults, and parents must be perfected.

It is during this clinical training period that the student clinician learns the "tools of the trade" such as the electronic devices, the materials, toys, games, and activities that will help a child or adult to change his speech behavior.

The formal training of the speech pathologist includes completion of an academic program to at least the Masters level and many hours of supervised clinical practicum and supervised early work experience.

The otolaryngologist can be assured that when he refers a patient for therapy, all the speech pathologist's clinical skills will be devoted to the mutual goal of overcoming the disastrous effects of communication disorders of speech.

OTHER RELATED PROFESSIONS

The complexity of the problems presented by those with communication disorders, and the deep level of involvement of all the "Members of the Problem," often dictates the advisability of the otolaryngologist's consultation with other related professionals. It would be expected that he would have established lines of referral with other medical specialists and with dentists, orthodontists and prosthodontists. Contact with workers in three other professions — social work, psychology, and speech pathology and audiology — might prove extremely valuable in the successful carrying out of management decisions.

Often a social worker's services are required for family counseling or perhaps for help with financial problems. Lists of local agencies and the names of certified social workers can be obtained from the National Association of Social Workers, 2 Park Avenue, New york, N.Y. 10016.

The American Board of Examiners in Profes-

sional Psychology will supply the names of local psychologists who have passed Board Examinations in such areas as clinical psychology, counseling psychology and school psychology. This information can be secured by writing the American Psychological Association, 1200 17th Street, N.W., Washington, D.C. 20036.

Lists of speech and hearing clinics that are registered with the Professional Services Board of the American Board of Examiners in Speech Pathology and Audiology, and the names of individuals who hold the Certificate of Clinical Competence in Speech Pathology and/or Audiology are available from the American Speech and Hearing Association, 9030 Old Georgetown Road, Washington, D.C. 20014.

REFERENCES

Bangs, T. E.: Language and Learning Disorders of the Pre-Academic Child. New York, Appleton-Century-Crofts, 1968.

Berry, M. F.: Language Disorders of Children. New York, Appleton-Century-Crofts, 1969.

Berry, M. F., and Eisenson, J.: The Defective in Speech. New York, F.S. Crofts and Co., 1945.

Curtis, J. F.: *In* Johnson, W., et al: Speech Handicapped School Children. 3rd ed. New York, Harper and Row, 1967.

Eisenson, J.: The Psychology of Speech. New York, F.S. Crofts and Co., 1947.

Fairbanks, G.: Voice and Articulation Drillbook. New York, Harper and Brothers, 1940.

Fairbanks, G.: Voice and Articulation Drillbook. 2nd ed. New York, Harper and Row, 1960.

Gesell, A.: Infant Development. New York, Harper and Brothers, 1952.

Human Communications: The Public Health Aspects of Hearing, Language and Speech Disorders. Washington, D.C., NINDB, Monograph 7:6, 1968.

Irwin, O. C.: Development of speech during infancy: Curve of phonemic frequencies. J. Exp. Psychol. *37*:187–193, 1947.

Irwin, O. C.: Infant speech: Development of vowel sounds. J. Speech Hear. Dis. *13*:31–34, 1948.

Johnson, W., Darley, F. L., and Spriestersbach, D.C.: Diagnostic Methods in Speech Pathology. New York, Harper and Row, 1963.

Johnson, W., et al: Speech Handicapped School Children. 3rd ed. New York, Harper and Row, 1967.

Lillywhite, H.: Doctors manual of speech disorders. J.A.M.A., *167*:850–858, 1958.

Poole, I.: Genetic development of articulation of consonant sounds in speech. Element. Eng. Rev., *22*:159–161, 1934.

Smith, M. E.: An investigation of the development of the sentence and the extent of vocabulary in young children. University of Iowa Studies in Child Welfare, 3, 1926.

Spahr, F. T.: 1971 White House Conference on Aging. Amer. Speech Hear. Ass., *13*:14–17, 1971.

Subcommittee on Human Communication and Its Disorders: Human Communication and Its Disorders—An Overview. Washington, D.C., National Advisory Neurological Diseases and Stroke Council, 15, 1969.

Van Riper, C.: Speech Correction. 4th ed. Englewood Cliffs, New Jersey, Prentice-Hall, Inc., 1963.

Chapter 44

REHABILITATIVE AUDIOLOGY

by S. Richard Silverman, Ph.D.

The evolution of Western man's attitudes toward deafness is perhaps most significantly reflected by his creation of arrangements and systems for the education of deaf persons. The history of our culture is marked by man's slow, faltering, and at times haphazard, frustrating, and irrational struggle toward enlightenment; and the history of the education of the deaf is no exception to this general rule.

The notion that deafness and muteness depend upon a common abnormality and that the deaf were poor if not impossible educational risks persisted through medieval times. The Justinian Code (sixth century) classified the deaf and dumb as mentally incompetent, and the Rabbis of the Talmud classified the deaf with fools and children (second century, B.C.). Cardano of Padua in the sixteenth century asserted that the deaf could be taught to comprehend written symbols or combinations of symbols by associating these with the object, or picture of the object, they were intended to represent. Dalgarno, in 1680, suggested the possibility of preschool education, and de L'Épée of France and Heinicke of Germany argued the merits of the language of signs and speech for the intellectual development of the deaf. Edward Miner Gallaudet brought the French (language of signs) system to the United States, and Alexander Graham Bell applied a science of speech to teaching the deaf. Itard in France, and later Urbantschitsch of the Vienna Polyclinic and his student Goldstein of the United States, both otolaryngologists, suggested the values and techniques in training every residuum of hearing. Universality of educational opportunity for deaf children of school age has now become a reality in our country. The deaf, although beset by problems of the changes in economic opportunity brought on by the changing technology, have, by and large, become economically and socially productive men and women. This is an absorbing story that has been set down in many contexts by many writers and need not be elaborated here.

In the past three decades many factors, not wholly unrelated, have stimulated interest in education and rehabilitation of persons with impaired hearing. As we have seen elsewhere in this publication, they include development of refined electroacoustic instruments, particularly audiometers, to measure hearing loss; improvement of hearing aids; evolution of surgery for otosclerosis and of reconstructive surgical procedures for the middle ear; development of promising investigative techniques in psychoacoustics, auditory biophysics, physiology, and microanatomy; recognition of the problem of noise-induced hearing loss in industry and the armed forces and the growing issue of noise as a pollutant; awareness of hazards to hearing such as heredity, unfavorable prenatal conditions, or perinatal stress or injury; and a growing public appreciation of the rehabilitative needs and the economic and social potential of handicapped persons.

Forward looking management of persons with impaired hearing requires (1) dissemination of information about hearing impairment and acoustic hygiene; (2) early identification through a "high-risk register," screening programs in clinics for babies and in schools, and thorough audiologic examinations prior to employment; (3) complete diagnosis; (4) appropriate medical and surgical treatment; (5) thorough assessment of hearing after completion of all indicated medical and surgical procedures, with particular attention to educational and rehabilitative needs; and (6) appropriate measures such as hearing aids, speech reading, speech correction and conservation, special education, vocational planning, and psychological guidance.

This simple statement of the important facets of the management of deafness should not cause us to underestimate its complexity, particularly when normal hearing is medically or surgically unattainable. We realize this when we ask the question, "What really is deafness?" Is it a number on a decibel scale that describes the severity of hearing impairment? Is it a disease like mumps or measles or meningitis? Is it an ankylosed stapes? Is it a piece of tissue in the auditory system that would be judged to be abnormal if viewed under a microscope? Is it an affliction to be conquered by the ingenious scientist? Is it the burden of a child whose parent hopes persistently and fervently that the scientist will be successful, and soon? Is it a special mode of communication? Is it something that is encountered occasionally in the man or woman whose fingers fly and whose utterances are arrhythmic and strident? Is it a cause to which diligent, skillful, and patient teachers have committed themselves for generations? Is it the agony of isolation from a piece of the real world? Is it the joy of accomplishment that mocks the handicap? Is it the bright mind and the potentially capable hands for which the economy has no use because they are uncultivated? Is it a crystallization of attitudes of a distinctive group whose deafness, modes of communication, and other associated attributes such as previous education, that they have in common, cause them to band together to achieve social and economic self-realization? Of course, it is all of these and more, depending on who asks the question and why.

In seeking the answer to the question, each one of us has his own motives, his own purposes, and his own responsibilities. The public official is concerned with the magnitude and severity of the problem, ways of organizing to solve it, legislative needs, and costs; the physician and the investigator study the causes and pathology of deafness, its "psychology" and its management; the educator considers the physical plant, personnel requirements, and methods of instruction and communication; the rehabilitator is sensitive to training and job opportunities; and the deaf person himself and those close to him seek the opportunity for him to be all he can and wants to be. As in the legend of the three blind men, it is difficult to perceive and comprehend the whole elephant. The focus of this chapter is on rehabilitative audiology, the management of irreversible deafness.

CLASSES OF HEARING HANDICAP

Many persons, both children and adults, suffer from impaired hearing. The handicaps that arise from this are economic, educational and, above all, social. These persons need help, both medical and educational.

In order to plan facilities for the medical treatment, for the rehabilitation, and for the special education required by those with impaired hearing, we must know how many persons with hearing problems there are in various age groups and in various communities. In addition, we must know the severity of their handicaps. Those who are profoundly deaf or have a severe handicap must be distinguished from those who are moderately hard of hearing, and these must all be distinguished from those who suffer only from the inconvenience of a minor handicap.

The first step in making such distinctions is to divide hearing impairment into categories of handicap. The Committee on Conservation of Hearing of the American Academy of Ophthalmology and Otolaryngology recommends the division of the handicap of hearing into classes or grades, according to Table 1. The overall handicap of impaired hearing is best estimated in terms of ability to hear everyday speech well enough to understand it, but for statistical purposes the more precise measurements of pure-tone audiometry are preferable. This table defines each category in terms of pure-tone audiometric measurements such as are regularly made in surveys and tests of hearing, since it is possible to estimate a person's threshold of hearing for speech reasonably well from pure-tone measurements.

Specifically, each class in the table is defined in terms of the average hearing threshold level for three audiometric frequencies that are important for the understanding of speech. The numbers represent the simple average of the hearing threshold levels in decibels (dB) at the frequencies 500, 1000, and 2000 Hz, obtained with an audiometer that is calibrated according to the 1964 recommendation of the International Organization for Standardization (ISO).

TABLE 1. *Classes of Hearing Handicap*

HEARING THRESHOLD LEVEL dB (ISO)	CLASS	DEGREE OF HANDICAP	AVERAGE HEARING THRESHOLD LEVEL FOR 500, 1000 AND 2000 Hz IN THE BETTER EAR*		ABILITY TO UNDERSTAND SPEECH
			More Than	*Not More Than*	
	A	Not significant		25 dB (ISO)	No significant difficulty with faint speech
25					
	B	Slight handicap	25 dB (ISO)	40 dB	Difficulty only with faint speech
40					
	C	Mild handicap	40 dB	55 dB	Frequent difficulty with normal speech
55					
	D	Marked handicap	55 dB	70 dB	Frequent difficulty with loud speech
70					
	E	Severe handicap	70 dB	90 dB	Can understand only shouted or amplified speech
90					
	F	Extreme handicap	90 dB		Usually cannot understand even amplified speech

*Whenever the average for the poorer ear is 25 or more dB greater than that of the better ear in this frequency range, 5 dB are added to the average for the better ear. This adjusted average determines the degree and class of handicap. For example, if a person's average hearing threshold level for 500, 1000, and 2000 Hz is 37 dB in one ear and 62 or more dB in the other, his adjusted average hearing threshold level is 42 dB and his handicap is Class C instead of Class B. (From Davis, H.: Guide for the classification and evaluation of hearing handicap in relation to the International audiometric zero." Trans. Amer. Acad. Ophthal. Otolaryng. *69:*740–751, 1965.)

With a given audiometric hearing threshold level some persons will understand speech more easily and accurately, and others less easily and accurately, than is indicated in the table. Intelligence, quickness of perception, special training, general education, language background, motivation, ability to understand, and time of hearing impairment onset all contribute to the degree of an actual handicap. Any impairment of the central nervous system may greatly complicate the situation. Any one of several of these various factors may be vital in determining a person's overall economic or educational potentialities.

DEFINITIONS OF HEARING DISORDERS

It is important here to clarify the definitions of deaf and hard of hearing children as they are discussed in this chapter.

A great deal of unnecessary confusion among the laity and well-intentioned professional workers alike has surrounded the precise classification of hard of hearing and deaf children and, unfortunately, has frequently obfuscated discussions of their problems. The confusion seems to grow out of the differences in frameworks of reference to which classification and nomenclature are related. For example, some workers classify the child who develops speech and language prior to onset of deafness as "hard of hearing" even though he may not be able to hear pure tones or speech at any intensity. This child, it is argued, unlike the congenitally profoundly deaf child who has not acquired speech naturally, behaves as a hard of hearing child in that his speech is relatively natural or "normal" and, therefore, he should be classified as "hard of hearing." It is obvious that a not too precise educational standard has guided the labeling if not the definition of the child. If, however, we consider the same child from a purely physiological standpoint, it is grossly misleading to term him "hard of hearing" when for all practical purposes he hears nothing at all.

The situation is complicated further by the use of terms that suggest not only physiological, communication, and educational factors but also gradations of hearing level and time of onset. To this category belong such terms as *deaf and dumb, mute, deaf-mute, semideaf, semimute, deafened, partially deaf,* and others. These terms are of little value from the physiological, communicative, or educational points of view, and it would be well to eliminate them from general usage.

Of course, the time of onset of deafness affects the psychological and educational developmental patterns and should be borne in mind in labeling and classifying a child. In 1937 the Committee on Nomenclature of the Conference of Executives of American Schools for the Deaf recognized the importance of the ability to speak, the ability to hear (as shown by their use of the word "functional"), and the time of onset of deafness in proposing the following classification and definitions.

The Deaf

Those in whom the sense of hearing is nonfunctional for the ordinary purposes of life. This general group is made up of two distinct classes based entirely on the time of the loss of hearing: (1) *The congenitally deaf,* those who are born deaf; (2) *the adventitiously deaf,* those who were born with normal hearing but in whom the sense of hearing becomes nonfunctional later through illness or accident.

The Hard of Hearing

Those in whom the sense of hearing, although defective, is functional with or without a hearing aid.

Some object vigorously to the restricting influence of the definitions and classifications of impaired hearing contained in these proposals of the Conference of Executives and others. They maintain that the continuing increase of fundamental clinical and therapeutic audiological knowledge precludes any "static categorization." For example, study of the thresholds of tolerance for speech and for pure tones has suggested that there is a useful portion of the auditory area even beyond the range of classic audiometry. Some individuals who have heretofore been termed "totally deaf" as a result of audiometric tests may be reached by auditory stimulation using proper amplification. And it may prove to be more fruitful to classify the person with a physical disability on some psychological scale of behavior that expresses how he lives with his disability.

We are aware that delimiting definitions are hazardous, and we recognize that each child's capabilities must be assessed individually by the best methods available to us so that we are not restricted by the tyranny of classification.

PREVALENCE OF HEARING DISORDERS

In general, disorders of hearing which are socially and economically handicapping are of three varieties: (1) loss of acuity so severe as to be classified as deafness; (2) loss of acuity which imposes only a partial handicap so that the patient is classified as hard of hearing; and (3) dysacusic disturbances in which garbled hearing is the primary symptom.

Analysis of numerous surveys, particularly those of the United States Public Health Service, suggests the following main points:

1. There are approximately 236,000 deaf individuals of all ages and both sexes in the United States today.

2. Approximately 6,000,000 Americans have partial hearing impairments of handicapping degree that are bilateral.

3. An additional 2,500,000 or so have significant unilateral losses.

4. Among school-age children there are about 38,000 in schools for the deaf, about 100,000 more requiring intensive special management, and circa 250,000 more who are auditorily handicapped to an important degree in the school environment.

5. About 700,000 persons suffer a combination of at least some degree of handicapping hearing deficit and some degree of handicapping visual problem.

6. Handicapping hearing losses are particularly prevalent in the older age group, and here they are more frequently combined with visual disabilities.

7. No reliable general data are available on the prevalence of hearing losses by cause, on the distribution or the patterns of losses, or on the incidence of dysacusis.

REHABILITATION AND EDUCATION

The most helpful and generally acceptable measures for hard of hearing persons are hearing aids, including auditory training; instruction in speechreading; speech conservation and correction; and educational, vocational, and psychological guidance.

Hearing Aids

The evolution, description, and selection of hearing aids are discussed in another chapter. It is important here to stress the need for training in the use of hearing aids. It is not likely that the hard of hearing adult or older child needs to be taught again to be aware of sound. On the other hand, gradual loss of hearing will be accompanied by a failure to attend to those aspects of sound that become more difficult to hear. Such patients, newly equipped with hearing aids, must not be sent out to unscramble for themselves the new buzzing confusion that is now with them. Attention to weak, not recently heard sounds must be focused, and gross discriminations must be carefully retrained. With higher frequencies again available, the telephone bell and the doorbell can be distinguished, but such discriminations may not be immediately obvious and therefore must be made part of a training program.

With respect to speech perception, several goals must be kept in view. Through audiometric testing, the clinician knows something of the character of a loss. This information plus the results of ingenious analysis by master teachers will show which auditory cues are available to the listener, which can be made available through training, and which are not likely to be available at all. The emphasis here, of course, is on the individualization of the program.

Drills and exercises are particularly useful for adults, especially when the items contain contrasting elements based on cues that the patient is to learn. Recognition based on such cases must be carefully trained through several stages. At first the cue may be used in isolation and slowly enough that the listener can succeed. Then speed becomes important, especially as the cue is introduced into syllable and word contexts, such as *b*ed and *r*ed. Finally, the availability of the cue must be demonstrated and trained as it occurs in the rapid exchanges of conversation. Teachers in many fields find that proceeding from easy, rewarded steps to the finer, more difficult ones will produce better learning with less frustration than when the most difficult and challenging aspects of auditory perception are introduced early.

All too frequently the promotional literature on hearing aids emphasizes the concealment of hearing loss. From the standpoint of rehabilitation, this may be one of the major abuses in the field of hearing impairment. A cardinal principle of good mental health is recognition of reality and adjustment to it. It is a disservice to handicapped persons to encourage them to evade reality. Some dealers are to be commended for emphasizing that the wearing of a hearing aid is a demonstration of courtesy, since it spares the wearer's associates and family from having to shout or repeat.

Speechreading

Speechreading, sometimes called lip reading, is the process through which a person understands speech by carefully watching the speaker. For hard of hearing persons it is an essential supporting skill. The eye and the ear together apparently are better than either one alone, and for this reason there has been emphasis in recent years on associating speechreading instruction with hearing and with auditory training.

The factors that contribute to speechreading ability have been suggested by experienced teachers, by investigators, and by speechreaders themselves. Jeffers, in a thoughtful overview, has organized the factors and analyzed the research relating to them. She emphasized three primary factors. One is *perceptual efficiency,* which includes the ability to identify speech sounds or elements and to perceive them rapidly, and also the ability to gain information from the face when the focus is on the mouth. Associated with these processes are visual acuity and attention and speed of focusing and peripheral vision. The second factor is *synthetic ability,* which includes the ability to identify parts and patterns (words and phrases) and the gist of a message. The third primary factor is *flexibility,* which fosters the ability to revise tentative identification of a message. Among major secondary factors are the amount and kind of training, language proficiency, motivation, and reaction to frustration and failure.

Associated with language proficiency is intelligence and also the extent and pattern of the subject's impairment of hearing, its duration, and his age at its onset. In general, investigations confirm the importance of visual perception, the ability to fill in missing words, and training. Language proficiency, as might be expected, is important for the speechreading skill of deaf children, but it seems not to be important for the adult population who already possessed language when their hearing failed. Duration of hearing impairment seems to be important, but the influence of hearing level is not clearly established.

Spoken language is a rapid succession of

utterances that are composed of some forty-odd meaningful sounds of varying degrees of visibility. The speechreader must be able to recognize all the visible movements, and he must fill in those that are invisible. Fortunately, sounds like "f" and "th" that are relatively difficult to hear are easy to see on the lips. Likewise, the sounds that are more difficult to see (like the short vowels) are easier to hear because they have more energy in the low and midfrequency range where the majority of hard of hearing people have useful residual hearing. The forty-odd sounds are produced by changing the shape of the mouth and the relative position of the tongue, teeth, lips, and jaw. It is these rapidly changing movements that the speechreader must observe and interpret. To help him to fill in the gaps in what he hears and sees, since only about one third of speech sounds are clearly visible, the speechreader can learn to use the sensations that he imagines or actually feels in his own speech muscles as he watches the speaker. Note what even an expert speechreader does when puzzled. He silently imitates the movements he sees. This imitation helps him to translate a visual image into a motor speech image, and usually gives him a valuable clue. This use of the muscle-feeling sense is a valuable training device.

Spoken language is not entirely visible. Sounds like "f" and "th" are rather easy to see on the lips but sounds like "k" and "g" are not. Furthermore, some sounds look alike such as "p" and "b" so that "pan" and "ban" would be confused. But just as we do in listening we must make use of contextual clues. The speechreader needs to do more of it.

Hardy, in *Hearing and Deafness*, makes the following practical suggestions to the speechreader:

1. Remember that hearing is the natural and normal way to understand speech. Therefore, be fitted with, and get instruction in the use of, the best possible hearing aid for *your* particular impairment.

2. Be determined to develop good speechreading skills. Don't forget that it can help you in every conversation.

3. Do not strain either to hear or to see speech. A combination of looking and listening enables you to understand most speakers readily. Actually, how you get it doesn't matter, just as long as you understand.

4. Keep relaxed, but remain alert and tuned in. Anticipate what may be said, but be ready to shift as the ideas develop.

5. Do not expect to get every word. Follow along with the speaker, and as you become familiar with the rhythm of his speech, key words will emerge to enable you to put two and two together.

6. Try to stage-manage the situation to your advantage. Since lighting is important, avoid facing a bright light, and try not to allow the speaker's face to be shadowed. Keep about six feet distance between you and the speaker, so that you can more readily observe the entire situation.

7. Try to determine the topic under discussion. Friends can be coached to give an unobtrusive lead, such as, "We are discussing the housing problem." This is particularly helpful in large conversational groups.

8. Maintain an active interest in people and events. Being abreast of national and world affairs, as well as of those of your community and intimate social circle, enables you to follow any discussions more readily.

9. Remember that conversation is a two-way affair. Do not monopolize it in an attempt to direct and control it.

10. Pay particular attention to your speech. A long-term hearing loss or a sudden profound loss may cause a marked deterioration of voice and articulation. This requires professional help, for a pleasant, well modulated voice and intelligible speech are a great asset.

11. Cultivate those subtle traits of personality that do so much to win friends and influence people. A sincere, ready smile, an even disposition, and a genuine sympathetic interest in other people can do much to smooth your path.

12. Remember that the education of *your* public is your responsibility. Many people are embarrassed because they have no idea of how to talk with the wearer of a hearing aid or with a speechreader. Put them at ease, and assure them that quiet, natural speech is their greatest favor to you.

Speech Correction and Conservation

The major speech problem with hard of hearing persons is correction and conservation of speech. They do not hear speech and speech patterns clearly and therefore have a poor model for imitation. Depending on its kind and severity, and time of onset, hearing impairment can affect the articulation, loudness, voice quality, and patterning.

Articulation is concerned with the production of phonetic elements and transitions between them. In the case of sensorineural deafness, for example, such sounds as "s" are difficult to perceive and, because there is little motor-kinesthetic feedback, the sound is frequently omitted or distorted. Loudness of speech is often affected in cases of conductive impairment. His own speech sounds abnormally loud to the talker and, hence, he drops his voice and can hardly be heard under conditions of listening stress. In the cases of long-standing sensorineural impairment voice is poorly modulated and is generally characterized by abnormal fluctuations in loudness and by harshness and stridency. Patterning, which refers to intonation, accent, and stress, can also be distorted. Even if these deviations in speech are not present when hearing impairment is first observed, it is helpful to begin speech work to conserve normal speech.

Educational, Vocational, and Psychological Guidance

We need to know the interests, aspirations, aptitudes, abilities, and limitations of the individual. To provide guidance for hard of hearing children and adults, one should be aware of the possibilities of education and rehabilitation to reduce the limiting effects of the hearing handicap.

Two paradoxes soon become evident to the counselor working in guidance with congenitally hard of hearing persons. One is that as a group they often have much more in common with the deaf than one would have thought prior to having actual experience with them. This is particularly true in terms of educational achievement, language skills, general knowledge, and certain behavioral patterns. Second, the hard of hearing seem to reflect more psychological disturbance than the deaf. They frequently share the problem of marginal people in any group, that of identification. The person born hard of hearing may not be able to find full acceptance among the normal hearing or the deaf. Whereas association with the hearing ideally offers a wider range of friends and interests, it may be at the price of frequent rejection or a subservient role. Association with the deaf is sometimes perceived as psychologically threatening in the sense that deafness is a magnification of their own real or perceived deficiencies. Furthermore, the small number of totally deaf people restricts the opportunities for identification with them.

The problems of vocational guidance with the hard of hearing that are different from those encountered with the normal hearing or the deaf are most often manifestations of the identity conflict. Effective guidance and counseling is, therefore, often a long-term process aimed at fundamental changes in the self-image. Rarely is such service provided hard of hearing persons. Consequently, it is common to see them go through life overcompensating for their hearing loss or magnifying its significance, both of which lead to vocational and personal dissatisfaction.

Educational guidance for hard of hearing children should recognize the particular needs listed in Table 2. With proper recognition of the difficulties and with appropriate auxiliary

TABLE 2. *Educational Needs of Children with Impaired Hearing**

GROUP	AMOUNT OF HEARING LOSS	EDUCATIONAL NEEDS
1	Less than 40 dB	Speechreading and favorable seating.
2	41 to 55 dB	Speechreading, hearing aid (if suitable) and auditory training, speech correction, and conservation, and favorable seating.
3	56 to 70 dB	Lip reading, hearing aid and auditory training, special language work, and favorable seating or special class.
4	71 to 90 dB	Probably special educational procedures for deaf children with special emphasis on speech, auditory training and language, with the possibility that the child may enter regular classes.
5	More than 90 dB	Special class or school for the deaf. Some of these children eventually enter regular high schools.

*Adapted from Silverman, S. R.: The hearing handicapped: Their education and rehabilitation. Postgrad Med. *23*:321–330, March, 1958.

aid, children whose hearing impairment is from less than 40 dB loss to a 70 dB loss (groups 1, 2, and 3 in Table 2) and some in group 4 may be placed in a special class for the hard of hearing within a public school system or in a regular classroom. Where the child is placed depends on the amount and time of identification of his hearing loss and the availability of special help. The latter includes special classes, itinerant teacher, and speech and hearing clinics in a university or hospital or provided by a community service for the hard of hearing.

There is no agreement as to the existence of a set personality structure for hard of hearing children, but in general, as already stated, they need to be made aware of their handicaps, and as Ramsdell suggested in *Hearing and Deafness,* "The most successful adjustment is the one that overrides and submerges the handicap in normal activities centering outside one's self."

DEAF CHILDREN AND ADULTS

Early Management of Deaf Children and Parental Guidance

When we consider deaf children, we must realize that special techniques are necessary to build the skills of communication. The essential and primary channel for receiving the acoustic symbols we call speech is either absent or severely restricted. All the skills of communication that depend on learning over this channel are adversely affected. From infancy to early school age, the chief mode of communication for the normal hearing child is auditory. The child hears and learns to talk from what he hears. Furthermore, he not only learns how to communicate, he also learns what to communicate.

The encouraging progress in the assessment of young children with hearing impairment has emphasized the value of early management. The period from birth to the age of five is particularly critical for the learning and development of children, whether hearing or deaf. Since the young child with hearing impairment is denied many of the normal experiences that lead to adequate development of communication, it is essential that he be given help and opportunity to reach his potential as early as possible. This means not only a program for the development of the skills of communication, but also a regimen that removes, wherever possible, the barrier which isolates the child from the world about him. Formal and informal intercommunications (by whatever means) tend to lessen the child's feeling of apartness and to make him feel wanted and significant. The child is thus motivated to communicate and it is the task of the parent and the teacher to show him the usefulness of speech and other means as tools of communication.

The increase in efforts for early identification and the growing confidence in its validity have resulted in the development of many programs of parent guidance particularly related to infants and young children. There appear to be no universally accepted specific aims or procedures in guiding parents; the emphases vary. For some the primary aim is to create realistic "acceptance" of the child's condition, and the counseling is weighted in the direction of psychotherapy. For others the stress is on conveying information in order to create an understanding of sensory deprivation and its effect on the total development of the child in general and of his communicative deficit in particular.

When parents become aware that their child is deaf, their initial reaction is usually one of profound grief. It is not pleasant to learn that one's child is deaf and that it is hopeless to expect a restoration of his hearing. Unfortunately some parents refuse to face this fact and begin a pilgrimage from one doctor to another, always hoping for a miracle and not heeding advice about the necessity for special education.

Other parents surround the deaf child with an overwhelming, protective "love" to compensate for his deprivation; they dress him, feed him, amuse him, and shield him from contacts with other children. He is thereby deprived of opportunities for normal development and his education is delayed.

Sooner or later all parents realize that special education is necessary; but here they are bewildered: "My child is deaf, but what do I do next?" Pediatricians, otologists, educators, and audiologists can help them to make the educational arrangements best suited to the child's needs. Children, schools, and communities differ, and no single answer is correct for all deaf children in all places. The actual choice of a particular school is often a difficult problem.

Perhaps the most significant fact about the education of the deaf in the United States is that it is universally available to all deaf children of school age. Of course, the quality of education may vary, but it is important that no child need be denied an opportunity for it. Where are these opportunities available?

Of 38,391 children enrolled in schools for the deaf in the academic year 1967-1968, 18,926 attended public residential schools for the deaf. These schools, open to qualified children without charge, are supported either directly or indirectly by state tax funds. Most of the public residential schools are supported by legislative appropriation and, hence, come under the control of the state authorities. The educational services of the remaining schools are purchased by the states on a per diem or per capita basis and are controlled by their own boards. Examples of the first group are the Indiana and Illinois schools for the deaf; in the second group we find such schools as the Lexington (New York) and the Clarke (Massachusetts) schools for the deaf.

Other tax-supported institutions for the deaf are public day schools and classes. A school is usually large enough to be a separate entity; for example, Horace Mann School, Roxbury, Massachusetts. Day classes are usually groups within a larger school unit, and there may be as few as one in a school or as many as ten; for example in La Crosse, Wisconsin. In 1967-1968, 2300 children were being educated in public day schools, and 13,070 were in public day classes. The remaining children were being educated in denominational or private schools, such as Lutheran School (Detroit) and Central Institute for the Deaf (St. Louis). Such schools may be either day or residential. There were 409 children in schools and classes for the multiply handicapped. The number of children in each class ranges generally from five to ten. Some deaf children have been absorbed into classes for the hearing. Deaf individuals attend high schools and colleges for the hearing. Most public residential schools provide education at the secondary level, and higher liberal arts education exclusively for the deaf is available at Gallaudet College, Washington, D.C. Technical postsecondary education is provided at the National Technical Institute for the Deaf, which is an integral part of a larger technical institute for the hearing, the Rochester Institute of Technology, Rochester, New York.

Until we have more evidence to support the point of view of either the day or the residential school, we must study each child's situation thoroughly to determine what educational placement is likely to be most fruitful for him.

Once a school for the deaf child is selected the "long pull" begins for the parents, the extended period of learning how to work most effectively with the school throughout their child's educational career. Parents are more apt to enter willingly into this important period if they feel that their earlier grief and bewilderment have been recognized, sympathetically understood, and met with kind and clear counsel. Here a heavy responsibility lies upon the school: First, to recognize the nature of the strong emotions that surround the relationship of the parents with their deaf child. Second, to develop home cooperation through constructive and informative reports and by encouraging frequent visits to the classroom

Parents must create every opportunity for the child to employ and practice at home the communication that he has learned at school. They can assist materially in developing the child's speech, in enriching his vocabulary, and in translating his experiences into meaningful language. If the child is at a residential school, contacts with home should be maintained by letters and photographs; news from home is very essential to the deaf child's happiness. Reports from the teachers must keep the parents informed concerning the child's progress.

As the deaf child reaches adolescence, his basic needs are the same as those of other children. He must soon be ready to earn money, to make decisions, to associate with the opposite sex, and to compete with the hearing. The schools and the home must prepare him for this broader environment.

Teachers, parents, and school executives must also cooperate in the selection of a school for further education or for vocational training. Many variables affect these decisions: the age of the child, his intelligence, his academic record, his interests and skills, the schools available, and the vocational opportunities in his community.

When the parents are able to observe the fruits of their long labors, they experience the comforting satisfaction that their efforts have played a tremendously significant role in the hoped for adjustment of their child. Parents should not overlook their debt to the teachers, whose wisdom, patience, and understanding have made possible the deaf child's development and growth.

EDUCATION OF DEAF CHILDREN

Goals of Education of the Deaf

Although there is little disagreement about the management and education of hard of hearing children, there is a controversy about the formal education of deaf children.

How one attempts to educate deaf children depends upon the goals which are set for them; these goals are, in turn, determined by what is considered the overall potential of the deaf child—educational, psychological, and social. From views and practices of those concerned with education of deaf children three schools of thought emerge.

One group stresses the limitations imposed by deafness, such as exclusion from certain types of employment, the implication of a minority status in education and social contexts, the difficulties of learning speech and speechreading, and the misunderstandings concerning the abilities and aspirations of deaf persons. The following statement best summarizes their viewpoint: "The aim of the education of the deaf child should be to make him a well-integrated, happy deaf individual, and not a pale imitation of a hearing person; to produce happy, well-adjusted deaf individuals, each different from the other, each with his own personality."

A second school emphasizes the great potential for deaf persons for education and participation in a world of hearing people. This group stresses the importance of early education and of auditory training and emphasizes the objective of "normalization—deviating only insignificantly from persons with normal hearing." In essence there is "one world" in which the deaf person must function—a world of hearing and speaking people.

A third group points to the economic, academic, and social achievements of deaf persons among the deaf and the hearing as evidence that proper and early training enables the deaf child to realize his potentialities. It is apparent, however, that there are situations in which deaf people may always be marginal and that the approach to them should be influenced accordingly. Realism demands that parents, and the child himself, be spared the psychological distress that stems from failure to achieve an unattainable goal of "normalcy."

Until more facts are available, a rational attitude seems to point to a recognition that deafness imposes certain limitations that must be accepted, while at the same time proper education in its broadest sense strives to couple the deaf person to the world about him in a psychologically satisfying way.

Educators agree universally that every deaf child should have an opportunity to communicate by oral speech. Some educators advocate supplementing oral instruction with other forms of communication such as the manual alphabet or the language of signs. The manual alphabet, fingerspelling, is a method of forming letters from A to Z by certain fixed positions of the fingers of one hand. This is a form of "writing" in the air and, obviously, requires knowledge of the language that is being communicated. The language of signs is another form of communication. This is a system of conventional gestures of the hands and arms that by and large are suggestive of the shape, form, or thought which they represent. The combined method, which attempts to make available speech communication, the manual alphabet and, sometimes, the language of signs depends upon the aptitude of the child and the context of the communication. For example, the language of signs and the manual alphabet are frequently employed in public assemblies.

The "oral-manual" controversy is not yet settled. It is encouraging, however, that numerous investigations are under way to study not only the linguistic, conceptual, and intellectual effects of modes of communication but also their influence on features of personality as emotional maturity and self-identity.

Development of Speech in a Deaf Child

Speech for the deaf child generally is learned by a multisensory approach that utilizes visual, tactile, and kinesthetic, as well as auditory stimulation. The emphasis on the use of a particular sense modality or combination varies with the amount of residual hearing and the age of child at time of instruction. The following factors are important in the attempt to develop oral speech:

1. An environment must be created for the child in which speech is experienced as a vitally significant means of communication. Oralism is as much an atmosphere, and an attitude, as it is a "method" of teaching.

2. Spontaneity of speech is encouraged, but formal instruction is necessary at the appropriate stage in development. Good speech in deaf children does not come of itself.

3. The proper combination of visual, auditory, tactile, and kinesthetic pathways should be exploited rationally and vigorously.

4. Judicious correction of poor articulation, and of undesirable rhythm and voice quality, is necessary. The acceptance of poor speech encourages its use.

5. Periodic evaluations of the social effec-

tiveness of the child's speech is necessary for long-range educational planning.

Auditory Training

Auditory training, with hearing aids, supplements other sensory experiences to improve the child's speech and his perception of others' speech. Out of experience grow the following guides for auditory training.

1. Most deaf children have a small, but useful, portion of residual hearing, and many who have been termed "totally deaf" can respond to amplified sound. Audiograms may not tell the whole story of a child's ability to appreciate speech through hearing. Formal auditory training, in addition to the use of a hearing aid, is essential to teach the deaf child to make use of this remnant of hearing.

2. Auditory training, even with a hearing aid, should be instituted as soon as it is determined that the child is deaf and should be geared to his auditory capabilities. Deaf children can be taught to discriminate various environmental sounds, even though grossly; within limits, they can be made aware of speech sounds. The combination of auditory training and amplification creates experiences with sound which are meaningful and which make the hearing aid more acceptable.

3. Children should be taught as early as possible the use and management of their own aids.

Speechreading

In the oral method of instruction, speechreading supplemented by amplified sound becomes the chief means of understanding spoken words. The following are aids to development of this skill in deaf children.

1. An atmosphere of oral communication must be created and speechreading must be shown to serve a purpose.

2. Even if the child is not expected to understand every word of a spoken message, he should be talked to and should be encouraged to take advantage of situational clues. Some educators suggest combining speechreading with fingerspelling.

3. Speechreading should be reinforced by other sensory clues whenever practical.

Development of Language

One of the most formidable tasks in the education of deaf persons is development of the understanding and expression of language. By ingenious techniques, teachers have been able to develop language in deaf children. Instruction recognizes the problems presented by needs for vocabulary, multiple meanings, verbalization of abstract ideas, and syntactical complexity. The subtle relation between the acquisition of concepts and the language used to express them is undergoing intensive study by psychologists interested in the education of deaf children. The following guides are helpful in efforts to develop language ability in deaf children.

1. Language teaching should be related to significant and meaningful experiences of children. Teachers and parents must be alert to the ideas that are developing in the children so that they may provide the children with language with which to express them.

2. Language must constantly be made to serve a purpose for the child.

3. All sensory channels should be used to teach language.

4. Deaf children need formal, systematic aids to the acquisition of language. Many shun language when they feel insecure in its use.

5. Schools and homes should create an atmosphere where language is used and where books are read regularly.

In summary, the fundamental task of the teacher of children with hearing impairment is to analyze the information she wishes to convey, be it speech, a word, or an idea, and to select the sensory channels best suited to transmit the information to the child.

VOCATIONAL REHABILITATION SERVICES

Each of the 50 states, the District of Columbia, Guam, Puerto Rico, and the Virgin Islands have vocational rehabilitation programs that serve eligible deaf clients.

The determination of eligibility and the actual extension of services are functions of the state vocational rehabilitation agencies. Eligibility rests upon the presence of a physical or mental impairment, the existence of a substantial handicap to employment as a result of the impairment, and reasonable expectation that vocational rehabilitation services will render the individual able to engage in a remunerative occupation or in an occupation more in keeping with his total characteristics. Eligibility also is ordinarily limited to disabled persons of working age, or nearly so.

Rehabilitation services are provided in accordance with a plan worked out by the client and his counselor, assisted by the vocational guidance team that is available. They may include in any appropriate combination:

1. Thorough physical, mental, and aural examinations.

2. Extended evaluation, up to 18 months for a severely handicapped deaf person, to determine employment potential.

3. Communication development, including hearing aids, speechreading, speech correction and conservation, auditory training, reading, writing, the manual alphabet, and the language of signs.

4. Individual counseling and guidance including attention to problems of personal adjustment as they influence employment.

5. Training for jobs — in school, on the job, by correspondence, or by tutor.

6. Maintenance and transportation during rehabilitation.

7. Necessary tools, licenses, and equipment.

8. Placement in the right job.

9. Follow-up to make sure that the rehabilitated worker and the job are properly matched.

This writer cannot improve on a previous contribution as an appropriate conclusion to this discussion.

"Although man has traveled a long tortuous road from pre-Christian era in evolving an enlightened understanding of the social problems of deafness, a large portion of society still looks upon the deaf and hard of hearing as queer, dependent, and, sometimes, ridiculous. We are all familiar with the cheap humor of which they are often the target. Since their handicap is not as visible as that of the blind and crippled, the deaf often find themselves in embarrassing and humiliating situations because others do not understand their special problems.

"The answer of the deaf to such misunderstanding is to continue their social and economic achievements as self-respecting and productive individuals. Our social action for the deaf, therefore, should not aim for special privileges for them, but should constantly strive to provide opportunity without discrimination for the deaf to help themselves.

"The achievements of the deaf in the United States since the founding of the first school for the deaf in Hartford in 1817 have been good, but the record can be improved. This is the conjoint task of the teacher, the parent, the scientist, the physician, and of course, the deaf person himself" (from *Hearing and Deafness*, Chapter 15).

SUGGESTED READINGS AND REFERENCES

Altshuler, K. Z. (ed.): Education of the Deaf: The Challenge and the Charge. Washington, U.S. Government Printing Office, Superintendent of Documents, 1967.

A report of a National Conference on Education of the Deaf arranged by the National Advisory Committee on the Education of the Deaf at the request of the Secretary of the Department of Health, Education, and Welfare of the United States in April, 1967. The conference brought together educators, audiologists, physicians, legislators, psychologists, social workers, leaders of the deaf community, deaf students, and others to discuss the needs of deaf persons. The conference was organized around the special needs of particular age groups, 0 to 5, 6 to 16, 17 to 22, and 22 plus. Recommendations for action to meet these needs are contained in the report.

American Annals of the Deaf. Published at Gallaudet College, Washington, D.C.

The January issue each year is a statistical compilation of the hearing-impaired. It also contains a directory of personnel and services.

Babbidge, H. D.: Education of the Deaf: A Report to the Secretary of Health, Education, and Welfare by his Advisory Committee on the Education of the Deaf. Washington, D.C., U.S. Department of Health, Education, and Welfare, 1965.

An assessment of the status and needs for the education of the deaf from preschool through adult levels. Recommendations for involvement of the federal government are included.

Carhart, R. (ed.): Human Communication and Its Disorders — An Overview. Bethesda, Maryland, National Institute of Neurological Diseases and Stroke, National Institutes of Health, Public Health Service, 1969.

A report (155 pages) prepared and published by the Subcommittee on Human Communication and Its Disorders devoted to definitions and current support status of human communication and its disorders and delineation of the research and training needs in hearing, central processes, and speech production.

Darley, F. (ed.): Identification Audiometry. Monograph Supplement No. 9. Journal of Speech and Hearing Disorders, 1961.

Report of a conference dealing with definition, objectives, and program responsibility for identification audiometry from preschool through adult age.

Davis, H. (ed.): The Young Deaf Child: Identification and Management. Proceedings of a Conference, Toronto, Canada. Acta Otolaryng. (Stockholm), (Suppl.) 206, 1964.

Report of a conference of American, Canadian, and European specialists dealing with the High Risk Register, prevention of deafness in very young children, identification, definitive tests of hearing of young children, differential diagnosis, medical and nonmedical management, parent training, biology of sensory deprivation, use of amplification, development of language, and improvements in electroacoustic instrumentation.

Davis, H., and Silverman, S. R. (eds.): Hearing and Deafness. New York, Holt, Rinehart and Winston, 1970.

A comprehensive introductory textbook in audiology covering hearing and hearing loss, auditory tests and hearing aids, rehabilitation for hearing loss, education and psychology, and social and economic problems. Varied specialists have contributed to it. The writer, one of the editors, has drawn extensively from *Hearing and Deafness* in writing this chapter. He cites especially the following chapters and authors:

    9. H. Davis
  12. M. Hardy
  13. I. J. Hirsh
  15. S. R. Silverman
  16. S. R. Silverman and H. S. Lane
  17. S. R. Silverman and H. Davis
  18. D. H. Ramsdell
  20. M. Vernon and B. Williams

He is grateful to these authors and to Holt, Rinehart and Winston.

Deland, F.: The Story of Lipreading, Washington, D.C., Volta Bureau, 1968.

Denes, P. B., and Pinson, E. N.: The Speech Chain: The Physics and Biology of Spoken Language. Baltimore, The Williams & Wilkins Company, 1963.

A popular but accurate treatment of our knowledge of communication by speech by workers at the Bell Telephone Laboratories.

Doctor, P. V. (ed.): Report of the Proceedings of the International Congress on the Education of the Deaf and of the Forty-first Meeting of the Convention of American Instructors of the Deaf. U.S. Document, No. 106. Washington, D.C., U.S. Government Printing Office, 1964.

A volume of 1269 pages reporting the presentations at an International Congress on the education of the deaf attended by more than 2000 persons from about 50 countries. The papers proceed sequentially from description and assessment of children through their educational experiences to their economic, psychological, and social accommodation to the world about them. The progression is from otological, audiological, psychological, and educational assessment, through expressive and receptive communication (including speech, speechreading, hearing, and manual methods) to learning that involves language, reading, concept formation, and the content of the curriculum including vocational preparation. The final portion deals with organization and administration.

Eagles, E. E., Hardy, W. G., and Catlin, F. I.: Human Communication: The Public Health Aspects of Hearing, Language, and Speech Disorders. Public Health Service Publication No. 1754. Washington, D.C., U.S. Government Printing Office, 1968.

A concise (28 pages) document from the National Institute of Neurological Diseases and Blindness dealing with definitions, prevalence, effects, prevention, and management of children with communicative disorders. There are also sections on services and goals for adults and essentials for community health programs.

Fellendorf, G. (ed.): Proceedings of International Conference on Oral Education of the Deaf. Washington, D.C., The Alexander Graham Bell Association for the Deaf, 1967.

Report in two volumes (2211 pages) of a conference observing the centennial of oral education of the deaf in the United States. It includes papers by world experts on identification of deafness, organization and administration of services, speech, auditory training, preparation of professional personnel, instruction in language, curriculum development, and educational trends.

Furth, H. G.: Thinking Without Language: Psychological Implications of Deafness. New York, The Free Press, 1966.

Hirsh, I. J.: Audition in relation to the perception of speech. *In* Carterette, E. C. (ed.): Brain Function III: Speech Language and Communication. Los Angeles, UCLA Press, 1966. pp. 93–115.

House, A. S. (ed.): Communicating by Language: The Speech Process. Proceedings of a conference, Princeton, New Jersey, 1964. Bethesda, Maryland, U.S. Department of Health, Education, and Welfare, National Institute of Child Health and Development.

Report of a conference of investigators and clinicians dealing with the perception of speech, speech behavior, and the structure of the linguistic code, development and deficits in language skills, production of speech, disorders of speech production and perception, neural mechanisms and models, man-machine communication, and machine analogies of human communication.

Jeffers, J.: The process of speechreading viewed with respect to a theoretical construct. *In* Proceedings of International Conference on Oral Education of the Deaf. Washington, D.C., Alexander Graham Bell Association for the Deaf, 1967, pp. 1530–1561.

Ott, J. T. (ed.): Proceedings of a National Workshop on Improved Opportunities for the Deaf, Knoxville, Tenn., 1964. Washington, D.C., U.S. Department of Health, Education, and Welfare, Vocational Rehabilitation Administration, 1965.

Report of a workshop emphasizing the needs and opportunities for deaf people in the world of work.

Silverman, S. R.: Education of deaf children. *In* Travis, L. E. (ed.): Handbook of Speech Pathology. New York, Appleton-Century-Crofts, Inc., 1969, Chapter 10.

A comprehensive exposition of the education of the deaf in the United States. Contains an extensive bibliography.

Whetnall, E., and Fry, D. B.: The Deaf Child. London, William Heinemann, Ltd., 1964.

An exposition of the development of communication in deaf children emphasizing an early auditory approach.

Section Twelve

RADIOLOGY AND RADIOTHERAPY

Chapter 45

RADIOGRAPHY OF THE TEMPORAL BONE

by Galdino E. Valvassori, M.D.

The study of the temporal bone has always been a challenge to the radiologist. On the one hand, because of the different density of its bony components and the air and fluid spaces around and within them, the temporal bone lends itself to accurate radiographic visualization. On the other hand, the concentration in a small volume of many important structures and the minuteness of those structures make the radiographic investigation quite difficult.

The study of the temporal bone can be achieved either by conventional radiography or by tomography. Conventional radiography has the advantage of being a simpler, less time-consuming study which can be accomplished with standard radiographic equipment available in most departments. It has, however, the intrinsic defect of offering a picture which is the summation on a single plane of multiple structures located in different planes, so that the small structures under investigation are often more or less obscured. These limitations are overcome by tomography, which is the method for examining tissue structures by blurring out objects above and below the desired plane. In order to obtain satisfactory results, a modern tomographic apparatus allowing a multidirectional scanning movement and a good coefficient of distinctness should be used. It is my belief that tomography bears the same relationship to radiography of the temporal bone as the oto-microscope bears to surgery of the ear. By the use of the oto-microscope, surgical procedures that were beyond the limits of accomplishment by naked eye observation are now performed. In the same way, by tomography it is possible to visualize struc-

tures and pathological changes that are beyond the limits of conventional radiography.

NORMAL RADIOGRAPHIC ANATOMY

The knowledge of the normal radiographic anatomy in the various projections is indispensible for the recognition and evaluation of the pathological conditions.

CONVENTIONAL RADIOGRAPHY

The projections to be discussed in this chapter include only those specifically used for the study of the mastoid and petrous pyramid. Standard views of the skull including the Towne and base views will not be included in this presentation, although they may add information of the utmost importance, especially when the lesion extends to or from adjacent structures.

Three basic views are used for the study of the mastoid and middle ear; Schüller's, Owen's, and Chausse III; and two projections for the study of the petrous pyramid and inner ear structures: transorbital, and Stenvers'.

The Schüller's or Rungstrom's projection is a lateral view of the mastoid obtained with the sagittal plane of the skull parallel to the film and with a 30 degree cephalocaudad angulation of the x-ray beam. It allows an excellent visualization of the extent of the pneumatization of the mastoid, of the distribution and degree of aeration of the air cells, of the status of the trabecular pattern, and of the position of the vertical portion of the sigmoid sinus (Fig. 1). Of the middle ear cavity only the upper portion

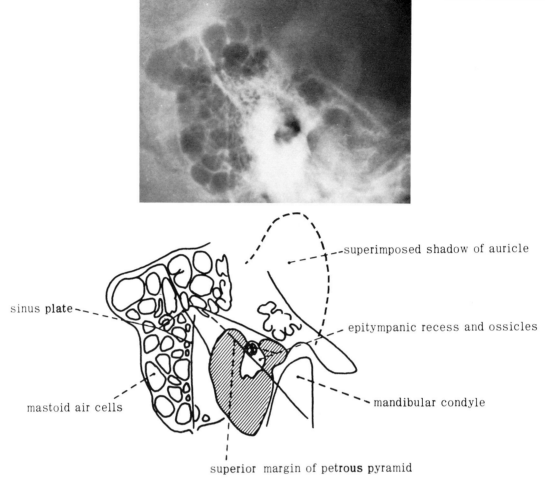

Figure 1.   Normal mastoid, Schüller's projection.

of the attic is usually visible, the remainder of the middle ear cavity being obscured by the superimposition of the petrous pyramid.

The Owen's projection resembles the Mayer's view but offers the advantage of less distortion. The patient's head is first positioned as for a Schüller's projection, and it is then rotated with the face away from the film for an angle of approximately 30 degrees. The x-ray beam is directed cephalocaudad with an angle of 35 degrees. By the rotation of the patient's head, the petrous pyramid, which in the Schüller's view was obscuring most of the middle ear cavity, is displaced downward and posteriorly. A well defined oval radiolucency is now outlined because of the superimposition of the attic and upper portion of the tympanic cavity upon the external auditory canal. Within the radiolucency the entire malleus and a portion of the incus are usually easily detectable (Fig. 2).

The Third Projection of Chausse is obtained by positioning the patient with the occiput on the film, the head rotated approximately 10 to 15 degrees toward the side opposite to the one under examination, and the chin flexed on the chest. There is no angulation of the x-ray beam. The purpose of this projection is the study of the attic, aditus, mastoid antrum and especially of the anterior two thirds of the lateral wall of the attic. One should remember that this wall from front to back runs first slightly inward, forming an average angle of 12 degrees with the sagittal plane of the skull, then turns outward to form the lateral margin of the aditus. The Chausse view is therefore complementary to the Owen's projection since it shows the anterior portion of the lateral wall of the attic, whereas the Owen's shows the posterior or aditus portion of it (Fig. 3).

The transorbital projection is obtained with the patient's back to the film in order to mag-

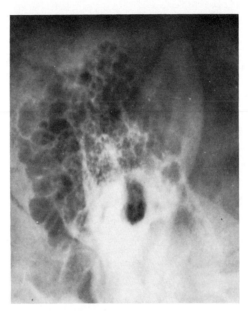

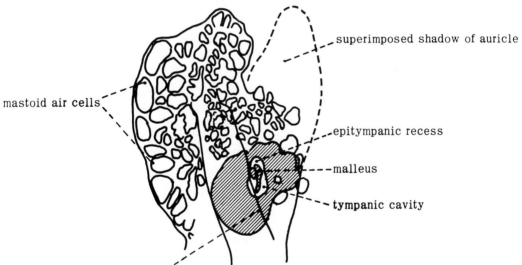

superimposed shadow of auricle

mastoid air cells

epitympanic recess

malleus

tympanic cavity

superior margin of petrous pyramid

Figure 2. Normal mastoid, Owen's projection.

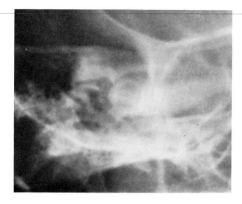

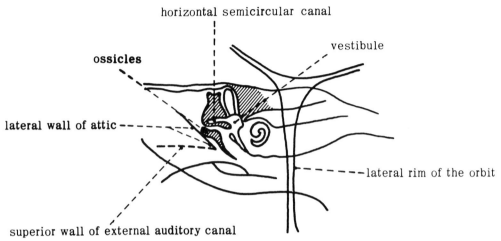

Figure 3. Normal mastoid, III projection of Chausse.

nify the orbit, the chin slightly flexed until the orbitomeatal line is perpendicular to the table top. In this view the petrous pyramid is clearly visualized through the radiolucency of the orbit (Fig. 4). In particular, the internal auditory canal is outlined in its full length from the medial wall of the vestibule to the well defined and smooth margin, concave medially, formed by the free margin of the posterior wall of the canal. In addition, the cochlea, vestibule, and semicircular canals are easily recognizable.

The Stenvers' projection is obtained with the patient facing the film with the head slightly flexed and rotated 45 degrees toward the side opposite to the side under examination. The x-ray beam is angulated 14 degrees caudad. Because of the rotation, the long axis of the petrous pyramid becomes parallel to the plane of the film and the entire pyramid is well visualized, including its apex (Fig. 5). The porus or medial opening of the internal auditory canal seen on face appears as an oval-shaped radiolucency open medially. Lateral to the porus the

internal auditory canal is seen quite foreshortened because of the rotation. The remainder of the inner ear structures are usually recognizable, especially the posterior semicircular canal which now lies in a plane parallel to the film.

TOMOGRAPHY

The use of special projections with various angulations of the x-ray beam or of the patient's head, which are indispensible in conventional radiography in order to visualize certain structures, is not required in tomography. The selection of the projections for the study of the temporal bone has been based on the following principles: it should be simple and easily reproducible, it should visualize the ear structures whenever it is possible under the same angle of surgical approach, it should follow the same plane as used in histological sections, it should cut certain structures at right angle to their axis.

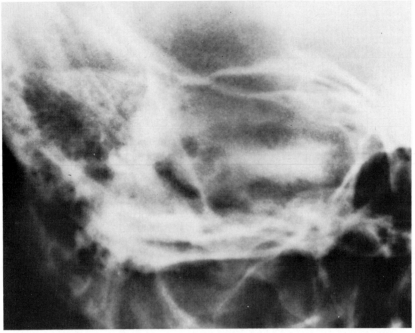

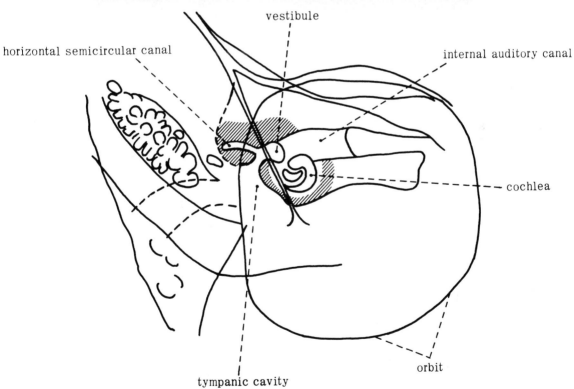

Figure 4. Normal mastoid and petrous pyramid, transorbital projection.

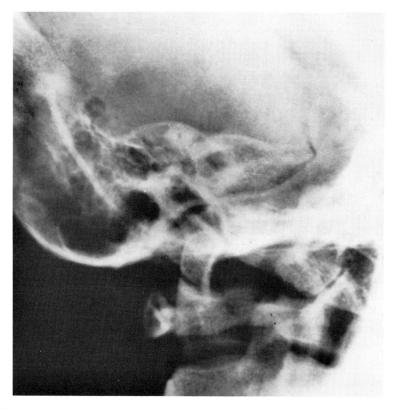

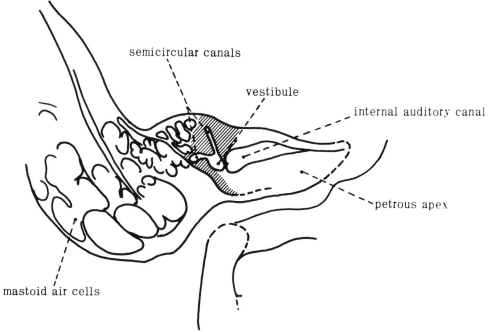

Figure 5. Normal mastoid and petrous pyramid, Stenvers' projection.

Five projections have been used. Two of them, frontal and lateral, are considered as basic; the other three, semiaxial, horizontal and Stenvers', are complementary according to the area and pathology under investigation.

In the frontal projection the patient may lie either prone or supine with the line from the tragus to the external canthus perpendicular to the table top. All three portions of the ear are clearly shown in this projection at different levels. Because of the impossibility of showing in this chapter the entire series of sections, we have selected two representative sections, one obtained at the level of the anterior portion of the attic and cochlea (Fig. 6) and the second at the level of the oval window and internal auditory canal (Fig. 7). In the lateral projection the patient lies prone, with the sagittal plane of the skull parallel to the table top. The side away from the table is examined in order to facilitate the centering, particularly when the skull is asymmetric. This projection is particularly useful for the study of the following structures from outside inward: external auditory canal, attic, ossicles, vertical portion of the facial nerve canal, vestibular aqueduct, and internal auditory canal, which is seen in cross-section. Again only two representative sections will be shown here, one at the level of the middle ear cavity (Fig. 8) and the following across the internal auditory canal (Fig. 9).

The oblique or semiaxial projection is obtained by rotating the head of the patient who lies supine on the table, 20 degrees toward the side under examination. In this way the medial or labyrinthine wall of the middle ear cavity, which usually forms an angle of approximately 15 to 25 degrees with the sagit-

(*Text continued on page 1031.*)

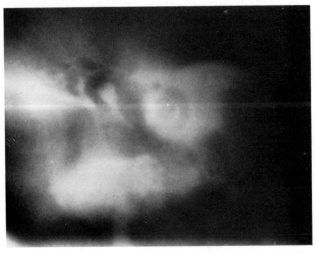

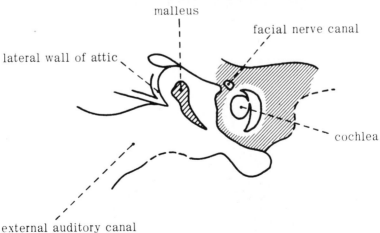

Figure 6. Frontal tomogram of a normal right ear.

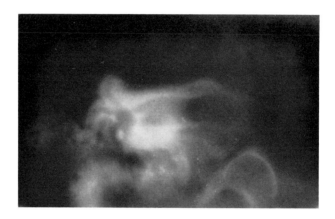

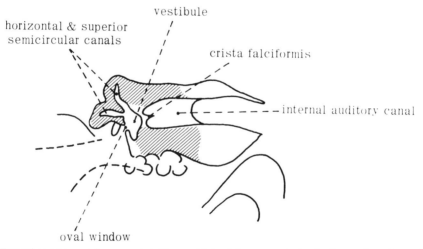

Figure 7. Frontal tomogram of a normal right ear obtained 5 mm. posterior to the section shown in Figure 6.

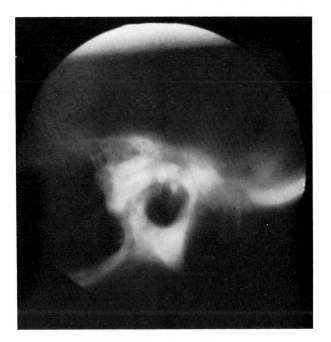

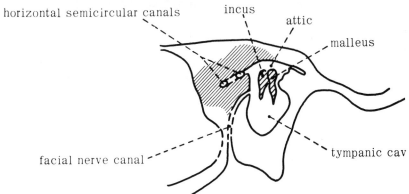

Figure 8. Lateral tomogram of a normal right ear obtained at 2.5 cm. from the patient's skin.

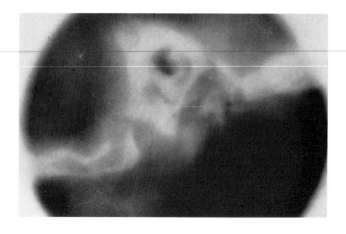

Figure 9. Lateral tomogram of a normal right ear obtained at 4 cm. from the patient's skin.

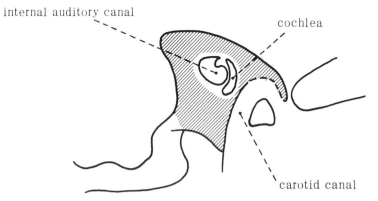

internal auditory canal

cochlea

carotid canal

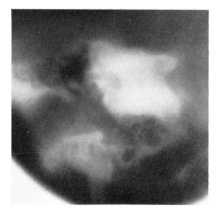

Figure 10. Semiaxial tomogram of a normal right ear.

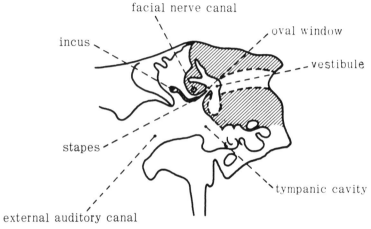

facial nerve canal

oval window

incus

vestibule

stapes

tympanic cavity

external auditory canal

tal plane of the skull, becomes perpendicular to the plane of the film and, therefore, to the plane of the sections. This projection is indispensible for the study of the oval window but also quite useful in the examination of the middle ear cavity. Figure 10 shows a representative section obtained at the level of the oval window.

Horizontal sections are obtained by a submentovertex direction of the x-ray beam and the plane running from the tragus to the external canthus parallel to the table top. A 15 degree flexion of the head is advisable, however, whenever the jugular fossa and the adjacent posteromedial aspect of the petrous pyr-

amid are under investigation. This projection has the unique advantage of following the same plane of the histological sections, thereby allowing a direct comparison between the two sections, but it has the inconvenience of being hard on the patient; it is usually impossible for elderly people to assume the necessary position. It furnishes information extremely valuable for the study of congenital malformations, fractures and tumors, especially glomus jugularis tumors. Figure 11 shows a representative horizontal section.

The Stenvers' sections are obtained with the patient either supine or prone and the head rotated 45 degrees so that the long axis of the

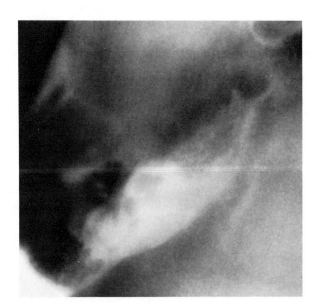

Figure 11. Horizontal tomogram of a normal right ear.

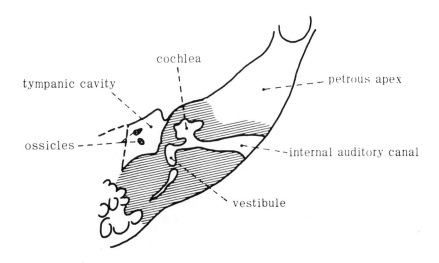

petrous pyramid under investigation becomes parallel to the table top. This projection is particularly useful for the study of the round window, posterior semicircular canal and carotid canal.

PATHOLOGICAL CONDITIONS

The major categories of pathological conditions involving the ear are congenital malformations, traumatic effects, inflammatory processes, neoplasms, and otodystrophies. Cholesteatomas and tympanosclerosis will be included under inflammatory processes since they usually occur in association with or as a complication of them.

It is of great advantage to the otolaryngologist to know the nature and extent of the pathological process in deciding whether corrective surgery could be attempted. In addition, whenever surgery can be performed, tomography may furnish important information leading to the selection of the most suitable surgical approach.

Congenital Malformations

Conventional radiography is of limited value in congenital malformations, except in the evaluation of the degree of development of the mastoid, because of the frequent absence of the normal radiolucencies of the mastoid air cells, external auditory canal, and middle ear cavity, the presence of a dense atretic block obscuring the superimposed structures and, finally, the distortion in axis and location of some of the structures. All these factors make the interpretation of a conventional radiogram extremely difficult or impossible. Tomography should be performed in at least two projections, frontal and lateral, with sections 1 or 2 mm. apart. Semiaxial sections for the study of the oval window and horizontal sections are added when necessary. Our clinical material includes a series of over 200 cases of congenital malformations of the ear divided as follows: 55 per cent of patients with anomalies of the sound conducting systems, and 25 per cent of patients with anomalies of the inner ear structures; the remaining 20 per cent represented a group of patients with combined external, middle, and inner ear anomalies.

Malformations of the Sound Conducting System. The impossibility of a direct otoscopic examination in most of these conditions resulting from a complete or partial atresia of the

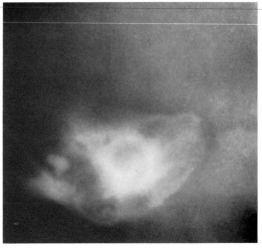

Figure 12. Atresia of the right external auditory canal. This frontal tomographic section shows complete agenesis of the external auditory canal with a thick atretic plate closing laterally a slightly hypoplastic but well aerated middle ear cavity. The ossicular chain is normal except for the handle of the malleus, which is fused to the atretic plate. The inner ear structures are normal.

external auditory canal makes the tomographic study more essential than in any other pathological process. In addition, this group is unquestionably the most important of the congenital anomalies not only because it is the most frequently encountered but above all because a functional surgical repair can often be successfully performed. The branchial origin of the middle ear cavity and ossicles explains the frequent association of abnormalities of other structures of the same embryological derivation; a typical example of this association is the mandibulofacial dysostosis also known as Treacher-Collins or Franceschetti syndrome.

A proper tomographic study can provide the surgeon with the following information, which is of basic importance in the decision of whether and how to perform corrective surgery:

1. Degree and type of abnormality of the tympanic bone, which may range from a minor deformity of the external auditory canal to a complete agenesis (Fig. 12).

2. Degree and localization of development of the mastoid cells and mastoid antrum.

3. Position of the sigmoid sinus and jugular bulb. It is not uncommon to demonstrate a deep jugular fossa protruding from below into the hypotympanic or tympanic cavity. Usually the jugular bulb remains covered by a thin shell of bone, but occasionally it may bulge without covering bone in the hypotympanum.

4. Degree of development of the middle ear cavity and ossicular chain (Fig. 13).

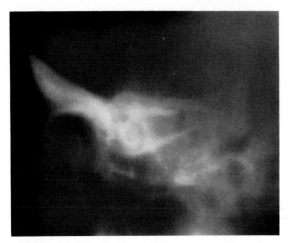

Figure 13. Atresia of the right external auditory canal. This frontal tomographic section shows complete agenesis of the right external auditory canal and middle ear cavity. The inner ear structures are normal. Notice the temporomandibular fossa lateral to the atretic plate taking the place of the missing external auditory canal.

5. Status of the labyrinthine windows.

6. Route of the facial nerve canal. A more anterior position than usual of the vertical or mastoid portion of the facial nerve canal is quite common in cases of aplasia or hypoplasia of the external auditory canal and middle ear cavity. In less frequent, but not rare, occasions the third portion of the facial nerve canal may be grossly ectopic and run horizontally outward.

7. Relationship of the meninges to the mastoid and petrous ridge. A low lying dura is frequently encountered as the middle cranial fossa deepens to form a large groove lateral to the labyrinth. Occasionally a dehiscency may be demonstrated in the tegmen with a soft tissue mass protruding into the middle ear cavity from above, indicative of a meningocele or a meningoencephalocele.

Malformations of the Inner Ear Structures. Congenital sensorineural deafness and vestibular loss may be the result of abnormalities involving the membranous portion of the labyrinth only (and therefore not radiographically demonstrable) or of anomalies involving both the membranous labyrinth and the otic capsule (and therefore roentgenographically visible). Congenital anomalies of the inner ear structures range from a complete agenesis or aplasia of the Michel type to hypoplasia of one or more of the structures (Fig. 14 *A* and *B*). Hypertrophy of the vestibule was observed in three patients and of the internal auditory canal in one patient and therefore appears to be a rarer type of anomaly. Of interest was the observation in our series that anomalies of the inner ear were combined with abnormalities of the sound conducting system in almost 20 per cent of the patients, a figure certainly far in excess of that pertaining to the general population. This high rate of occurrence may be explained by the general tendency of congenital anomalies to be multiple rather than single, or by the fact that both the external meatus and the membranous labyrinth are ectodermal in origin. The possible significance of this common embryological origin is, however, reduced by the recognition that the otic capsule is mesodermal in origin.

The recognition by tomography of inner ear anomalies is of no advantage so far as corrective surgery is concerned, but it has allowed the diagnosis during life of conditions which in the past were recognized only at autopsy.

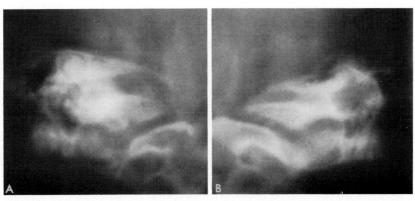

Figure 14. Malformation of the left inner ear structures (*B*) with comparison view of the normal right ear (*A*). This frontal tomographic section shows a large cavity in the area normally occupied by the labyrinth. Notice the rudimentary superior and horizontal semicircular canals and the hypoplastic internal auditory canal.

Traumatic Effects

The petrous pyramid, mastoid, and tympanic bone are unquestionably much more often involved in a fracture following trauma to the skull than demonstrated by standard radiographic examinations. They form, in fact, the commonest fractures of the base of the skull. The demonstration of a fracture is important from the therapeutic approach and from the medicolegal aspect.

One should be aware that whereas fractures with separation or displacement of the fragments can be easily demonstrated by conventional radiography or tomography, small fracture lines without displacement and separation of the fragments can be detected only by tomography if the plane of the fracture lies in, or close to, the direction of the x-ray beam. For this reason, multiple projections are indispensable. We have selected four projections of the petrous pyramids at about 45 degrees apart, namely frontal, lateral, Stenvers', and semiaxial. In addition, horizontal sections should be obtained whenever possible.

One or more of the three following clinical findings are present in the patients referred for radiographic studies:

1. Cerebrospinal fluid otorrhea, due usually to a fracture extending from the superior wall of the external auditory canal to the floor of the middle cranial fossa or to fracture of the tegmen, when a tear of the tympanic membrane is present.

2. Paralysis of the facial nerve, due to the involvement of the facial nerve canal with consequent simple compression or complete tear of the nerve. The commonest site of involvement is, in our experience, at the distal genu of the canal as it turns from the tympanic into the vertical segment.

3. Hearing loss. Conductive hearing loss is the result of disruption of the ossicular chain most often encountered in fracture involving the attic (Fig. 15). The commonest type of dislocation involves the incus, whose fixation by ligaments is looser than that of the malleus. A rarer interruption of the ossicular chain is due to fracture of the crura of the stapes or separation at the incudostapedial joint. The diagnosis of this type of interruption can be made radiographically by direct visualization of the fragments or by detection of an abnormal rotation of the long process of the incus which has lost its normal relationship to the oval window.

Fractures involving the labyrinth, large enough to be radiographically demonstrable, usually produce a complete nerve and/or vestibular loss. Longitudinal fractures of the petrous pyramid may involve one or more inner ear structures but often skip the labyrinth by running just in front or back of it. Transverse fractures of the petrous pyramid may occur at any level, although they tend to follow the plane of least resistance. This plane usually runs from the dome of the jugular fossa, to the petrous ridge medial, to the arcuate eminence, across the vestibule and basilar turn of the cochlea (Fig. 16).

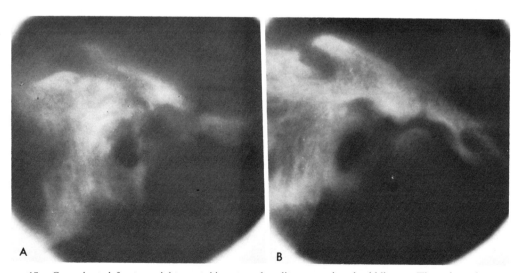

Figure 15. Comminuted fracture right mastoid, external auditory canal and middle ear. These lateral tomographic sections obtained at 2.5 cm. (*A*) and 2 cm. (*B*) from the patient's skin show complete detachment and elevation of a large fragment extending from the temporomandibular fossa to the tegmen antri and fragmentation of the anterior wall of the external auditory canal and middle ear cavity. Notice the encroachment of the fragments upon the ossicles in the attic.

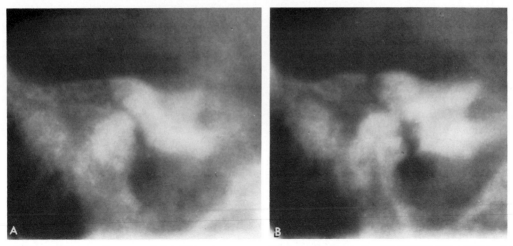

Figure 16. Transverse fracture of the right petrous pyramid. *A* and *B,* These frontal tomographic sections show the fracture line running from the arcuate eminence to the jugular fossa across the labyrinth.

Inflammatory Processes and Cholesteatomas

Acute Mastoiditis. This usually occurs in well pneumatized temporal bones in patients with acute suppurative otitis media. The typical radiographic finding consists of a diffuse haziness or clouding of the mastoid air cells. In the initial stage of the process the trabecular pattern is intact, although it appears less clear than usual because of the lack of the normal air-bone interface, as a result of the edema of the mucosa and/or collection of fluid in the air cells. A similar involvement is, of course, present in the air cells that have developed in the petrosa. Whenever the infection is not arrested by proper therapy, necrosis of the cell walls develops, which may lead to the formation of abscesses. Conventional lateral views such as the Schüller's and Owen's are usually satisfactory for the study of the mastoid (Fig. 17), but tomographic sections should be added whenever further information concerning the middle ear cavity and ossicular chain are requested. In

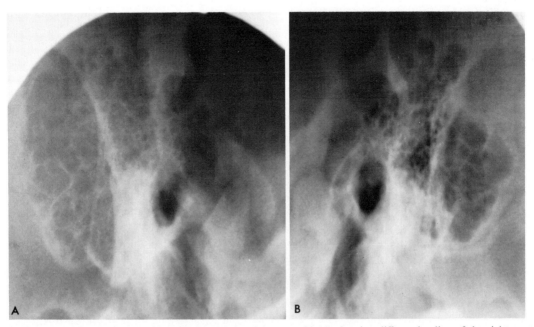

Figure 17. Acute mastoiditis. Owen's view of the right mastoid (*A*) showing diffuse clouding of the right mastoid cells without evidence of cell wall destruction. *B*, Owen's view of the normal left mastoid for comparison.

the differential diagnosis one should remember that reticuloendothelioses (in particular, eosinophilic granuloma) produce changes which are quite similar to acute mastoiditis and petrositis with areas of coalescence. However, the clinical course and the otoscopic findings are usually helpful in the differential diagnosis.

Chronic Mastoiditis. This is the result of longstanding or recurrent infectious processes. The typical radiographic findings consist of diffuse sclerosis of the trabecular pattern and diffuse clouding of the air cells and, if no perforation is present, of the middle ear cavity. Because of the thickening of the trabeculae, the air cells become constricted at first, and later, completely obliterated. The lumen of the residual air cells, the mastoid antrum, and the middle ear cavity are usually filled with granulation tissue and therefore appear cloudy. Erosion of the long process of the incus is not an unusual finding.

Tympanosclerotic plaques are occasionally demonstrated by tomography in the middle ear cavity and attic as irregular calcifications. Ankylosis of the ossicles, especially the head of the malleus, is best diagnosed in lateral tomographic sections by the filling in of the space between the anterior aspect of the head of the malleus and the attic wall.

Cholesteatoma. Microscopic otoscopy usually provides a qualitative diagnosis of cholesteatoma but gives no concept of the size of the lesion. The main purpose of the radiographic study is therefore to determine the degree and extent of the pathology of the cholesteatoma. This can be accomplished best by tomography. The pathognomonic findings of cholesteatomas are: (1) erosion of the anterior portion of the lateral wall of the attic and of the anterior tympanic spine in cases of attic perforation (Fig. 18); and (2) erosion of the posterior canal wall and of the posterior portion of the lateral wall of the attic in cases of posterosuperior marginal perforation (Fig. 19). Erosion of the ossicular chain, widening of the aditus, and enlargement of the mastoid antrum by destruction of the adjacent trabecular pattern with formation of a well defined cavity are other typical findings as the lesion progresses. If the cholesteatoma lies free in the middle ear or mastoid and it is not surrounded by granulation tissue or serous fluid it is possible to visualize the actual cholesteatoma sac as a soft tissue mass. However, when the cholesteatoma is surrounded by granulation tissue it is difficult or impossible to discern radiographically where the actual cholesteatoma ends and the granulation tissue begins, since both soft tissues have the same radiographic density.

An interesting observation was made in a group of patients referred for so-called congenital cholesteatoma or cholesteatoma developing behind an intact tympanic membrane. In these cases the inferior margin of the lateral wall of the attic, which is the first site of involvement in acquired cholesteatoma, is intact, but often the erosion involves the lateral attic wall from within, above the inferior margin. This produces a typical scooped-out appearance of the lateral wall of the attic which has become concave inward rather than straight as usual.

Neoplastic Conditions. The commonest of the benign tumors is certainly the osteoma, which can be found not only in the external auditory canal but often in the middle ear cav-

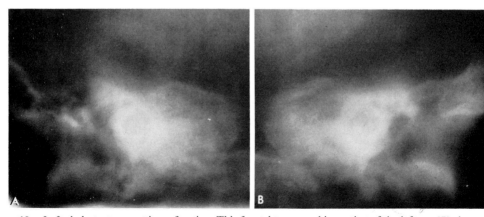

Figure 18. Left cholesteatoma, attic perforation. This frontal tomographic section of the left ear (*B*) shows erosion of the lateral wall of the attic by a soft tissue mass lateral to the ossicles, which appear displaced medially. *A*, Corresponding frontal tomographic section of the normal right ear for comparison.

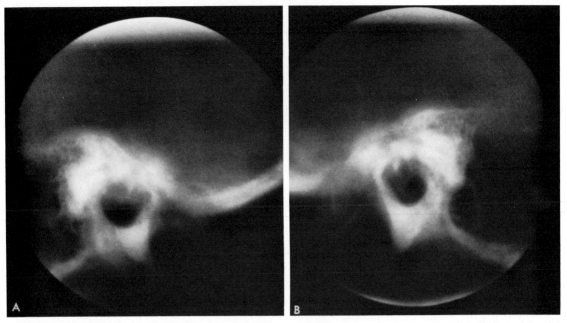

Figure 19. Right cholesteatoma, posterosuperior marginal perforation. This lateral tomographic section of the right ear (*A*) shows a soft tissue mass in the posterosuperior quadrant of the tympanic cavity and attic with erosion of the long process of the incus. *B*, Corresponding section of the normal left ear for comparison.

ity, especially in the attic. The use of radiography in osteomas is usually limited to cases obstructing the external auditory canal in order to find out whether any other disease is present behind the obstruction.

Malignant tumors of the ear are rare; among them, carcinoma occurs most frequently. The carcinoma is usually squamous cell type, originating in the external auditory canal and then extending into the middle ear, mastoid, and petrosa. The typical radiographic finding consists of destruction of the outline of the external auditory canal and middle ear, with a moth-eaten appearance of the mastoid as a result of

tendency of the neoplasm to infiltrate rather than erode bone.

Two lesions deserve special attention not only because of their relative frequency but, above all, because of the fundamental role played by radiology in their diagnosis; glomus jugularis tumors and acoustic neuromas. Both tumors are usually histologically benign but often follow a malignant clinical course because of the large destruction produced in the base of the skull and of the involvement of the adjacent cranial nerves and central nervous system by the growing tumor mass.

Glomus tumors. Glomus tumors arising in

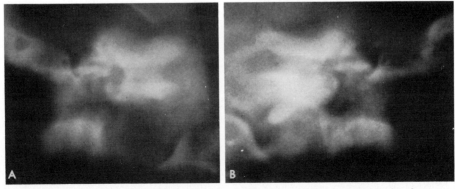

Figure 20. Right glomus jugularis tumor. Frontal tomographic section of the right ear (*A*) showing gross enlargement of the jugular fossa with destruction of the inferior wall of the tympanic cavity and erosion of the inferior aspect of the petrous pyramid and adjacent portion of the occipital condyle. *B*, Corresponding frontal tomographic section of the normal left ear for comparison.

the tympanic cavity (glomus tympanicum) produce a soft tissue mass, usually well outlined in tomographic sections, in the lower portion of the middle ear cavity with possible thinning and destruction of the inferior wall of the hypotympanum. In such cases the differential diagnosis between a glomus and an ectopic or a high jugular bulb protruding into the middle ear cavity may be difficult without a jugular venogram. Glomus jugularis tumors arising in the jugular fossa extend also into the middle ear cavity through a destruction of its floor (Fig. 20); however, in these cases the erosion of the cortical outline of the jugular fossa, the undermining of the petrous pyramid, and the involvement of the adjacent portion of the occipital bone (including the hypoglossal canal) are typical findings leading to the diagnosis. The radiographic evaluation should always include a tomographic study in various projections, including horizontal sections (Fig. 21) and, whenever necessary, a retrograde jugular venogram. This study is usually successfully performed by percutaneous puncture of the vein with a Seldinger needle. The stylet is then withdrawn and a guide wire is advanced through the lumen of the needle into the internal jugular vein until the bony roof of the jugular fossa is felt. The needle is then removed and an opaque polyethylene catheter is threaded into the jugular vein over the guide wire which is, in turn, removed. Twenty to 30 cc. of contrast material are injected and several

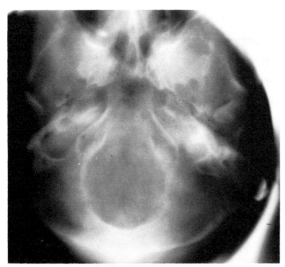

Figure 21. Right glomus jugularis tumor, same patient as Figure 20. Horizontal section of the base of the skull showing enlargement of the right jugular fossa and erosion of the posteroinferior aspect of the right petrous pyramid.

films obtained with a rapid cassette changer during and right after the injection. By this technique the position of the jugular bulb is clearly demonstrated as well as the presence of defects, narrowing, or complete obstruction of its lumen.

Acoustic neuromas. Acoustic neuromas account for approximately 10 per cent of unilateral sensorineural hearing loss and vestibular loss of unknown origin. They normally originate within the internal auditory canal and therefore produce osseous changes detectable by a proper radiographic study. Whenever conventional radiography is used, two projections are indispensable for the study of the internal auditory canal: the transorbital, which shows the canal in its full length; and the Stenvers' view for the study of the opening or porus of the canal, which is seen in this projection on face, whereas the canal is quite foreshortened. A more precise study of the internal auditory canals can of course, be obtained by tomography. This is particularly true whenever the petrous pyramids are extensively or asymmetrically pneumatized. Tomography should always be performed in two planes. The frontal sections are the most satisfactory for the study of the shape and size of the internal auditory canal and for the length of tis posterior wall, whereas the lateral sections add details of utmost importance concerning the status of the cortex and porus of the canal. In addition, both sides should always be examined for comparison purposes. In fact, while there are slight variations in size and shape in the internal auditory canals of one person, these variations are small when compared with the difference between various subjects.

The following four parameters should always be examined for the detection of changes indicative of an acoustic neuroma (all figures have been corrected for magnification):

VERTICAL DIAMETER. It normally ranges between 2 and 9 mm., with an average of 4.5 mm. An enlargement of 1 to 2 mm. of any portion of the internal auditory canal under investigation in comparison to the corresponding segment of the opposite side should be considered questionable, and an enlargement of 2 or more mm. as definitely abnormal (Fig. 22).

LENGTH OF THE POSTERIOR WALL. This normally ranges between 4 to 12 mm., with an average of 8 mm. Shortening of the posterior wall of one canal between 2 to 3 mm. should be considered as questionable, shortening by 3 or more mm. as definitely abnormal.

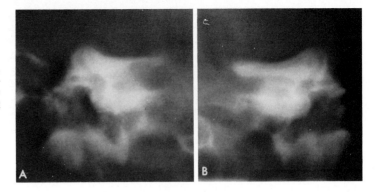

Figure 22. Right acoustic neuroma. Frontal tomographic sections showing enlargement of the right internal auditory canal (*A*) in comparison to the normal left side (*B*).

OUTLINE OF THE CANAL. The lumen of the normal internal auditory canal is surrounded by a well defined white line made up by cortical bone, denser than the surrounding bone of the petrosa. Destruction or demineralization of this cortical outline is, respectively, a positive or suggestive indication for a space-occupying lesion within the canal.

CRISTA FALCIFORMIS. It divides the canal into two compartments but is always located at, or above, the midpoint of the vertical diameter of the internal auditory canal. A reverse of this ratio or an asymmetry by at least 2 mm. in the position of the crista are strongly suggestive of an intracanalicular mass.

At this point the results of the tomographic study are correlated with the results of the audiometric, vestibular, and neurological tests in order to select the group of patients who should undergo an opaque cisternogram. This study is, of course, performed in all positive cases in order to confirm the diagnosis and to establish the size of the tumor mass. The questionable group is divided into two subgroups as follows: (1) If the other tests are suggestive of a retrocochlear lesion, an opaque cisternogram is performed without further delay. (2) If the other tests are more equivocal, the patient is kept under observation for one year and, at that time, if any worsening in the symptomatology or of radiographic findings has occurred, a cisternogram is performed. Finally, a cisternogram is decided upon whenever the audiometric and vestibular tests are consistently indicative of a retrocochlear lesion in spite of a negative tomographic study in order to rule out the presence of a tumor limited to the cistern, or a tumor that is too small to produce changes in the bony outline of the canal.

Opaque cisternography constitutes the final and most conclusive of the diagnostic tests. Two to 3 cc. of Pantopaque are injected in the subarachnoid space by lumbar puncture. Prior to the injection of the contrast material the intracranial pressure is measured and a few cubic centimeters of cerebrospinal fluid are withdrawn for chemical testing. Under fluoroscopic control the contrast material is then moved, by tilting the table into Trendelenburg position, into the posterior cranial fossa. The patient is kept in the lateral decubitus during this maneuver so that the contrast material will collect in the dependent cerebellopontine cistern. The patient's head is then progressively rotated to an oblique Stenvers'-like projection and finally to a full face down view. This latter projection is extremely important for the visualization of the entire internal auditory canal without superimposition of the contrast material collected in the cistern. During the study, multiple spot films are obtained at different angulations of the patient's head. Whenever the spot films show a very small or questionable intracanalicular defect the patient is

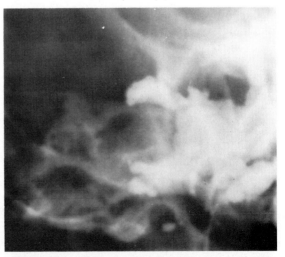

Figure 23. Right acoustic neuroma, same patient as Figure 22. The opaque cisternogram shows the presence of a tumor filling the internal acoustic canal and extending 1.5 cm. into the cerebellopontine angle.

moved to a tomographic table, and multiple lateral and frontal tomographic sections are obtained. The absence of filling of the internal auditory canal and the demonstration of a filling defect in the cerebellopontine cistern are positive evidence for a space-occupying lesion (Fig. 23).

Otodystrophies

Under the classification of otodystrophies we include two type of processes: (1) a localized disease of the ear, the otosclerosis; and (2) a group of diffuse processes such as Paget's disease, osteogenesis imperfecta and fibrous dysplasia, in which the involvement of the ear could be one of the pathological manifestations.

Both groups of diseases may produce, (1) conductive hearing loss by involvement of the ossicular chain and especially by the ankylosis of the stapes in the oval window; (2) sensorineural hearing loss by involvement of the inner ear structures; or (3) a mixed type of hearing loss by combination of the two types of involvement.

Tomography is essential for the study of the labyrinthine windows and of the labyrinthine capsule. Two views are used routinely for the demonstration of the oval window, frontal and semiaxial of the petrous pyramid. In the frontal view the oval window forms a well defined bony dehiscence in the inferolateral wall of the vestibule below the opening of the ampullar limb of the lateral semicircular canal. The normal footplate of the stapes, which measures 0.1 to 0.4 mm. in thickness, does not cast a shadow because of its obliquity to the x-ray beam. Six cuts are obtained in this projection,

1 mm. apart, and the oval window should be clearly detectable in at least two adjacent sections. In the oblique or semiaxial view the footplate of the stapes, which is now seen on end, casts a fine line extending across the oval window opening between the prominent borders of the oval window niche formed by the facial nerve canal superiorly and the promontory inferiorly. Again, six sections are obtained 1 mm. apart; the oval window is usually visible in three adjacent sections. The round window is best demonstrated in the Stenvers' projection.

In fenestral otosclerosis one observes narrowing or complete obliteration of the oval window by a bony plate of variable thickness produced by the involved footplate of the stapes (Fig. 24). Otosclerosis involving the cochlea produces a more or less severe disruption of the normal cochlear capsule, which usually appears as a sharply defined, homogeneously dense, although not homogeneously thick, bony shell outlining the lumen (Fig. 25). We categorized the observed radiographic changes according to the extension, degree, and type of the process. As far as the extension, three groups are recognized: (1) changes limited to the capsule of the basilar turn of the cochlea; (2) changes which diffuse to other portions of the cochlear capsule; and (3) changes widespread throughout the labyrinthine capsule. The degree is classified as minimal, moderate, or severe according to the size of the foci of involvement. The type of involvement depends upon the maturation of the process. Demineralizing or spongiotic changes correspond to the actively enlarging vascular otosclerotic foci. Sclerotic changes are the result of mature or maturing foci and they are formed by the opposition of mature otosclerotic bone. Such foci

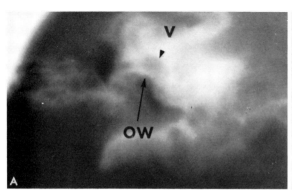
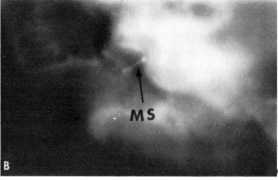

Figure 24.   Fenestral otosclerosis. *A*, Frontal section showing complete obliteration of the oval window by a thick footplate of the stapes. *B*, Frontal section of the same patient, obtained after stapedectomy and insertion of a metallic prosthesis, shows the oval window fully reopened and the metallic strut in good position. OW=oval window; V=vestibule; MS=metallic strut.

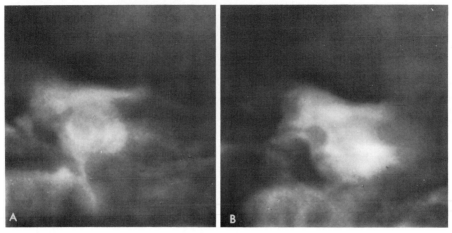

Figure 25. Cochlear otosclerosis. Frontal tomographic sections of the right ear showing diffuse (*A*) and severe (*B*) demineralization of the entire cochlear capsule with formation of a double ring effect about the middle coil. This type of involvement is typical for an active process.

appear in the portion of the capsule seen "on end" as areas of capsular thickening producing roughening or scalloping of the outer and inner aspects, and in the portions of the capsule seen "on face" as areas of increased density superimposed upon the radiolucency of the lumen.

The importance of tomography in otosclerosis can be summarized in the following points:

1. Diagnostic test in questionable cases.

2. Evaluation of the degree, type, and extent of the process.

3. Selection of side for corrective surgery.

4. Demonstration of possible abnormalities of the structures adjacent to the oval window with special attention to the course of the facial nerve canal.

5. Evaluation of the postsurgical status, especially in relation to two points: recurrence of the process, and position of the strut or prosthesis when radiopaque material is used.

6. Demonstration in patients with sensorineural deafness of foci of otosclerosis in the cochlea and in other areas of the otic capsule.

In Paget's disease the haversian bone of the pars petrosa is affected first, and because of its demineralization the cochlear capsule and the ossicles become at first more prominent than usual. Then the otic capsule itself becomes involved, producing an irregular and fuzzy appearance and, finally, a complete disappearance of the outline of the inner ear structures (Fig. 26). The progression of the involvement follows a path from the apex to the base of the petrous pyramid. The internal auditory canal is involved first, followed by the cochlea and the vestibular system. Obliteration of the oval window is often demonstrated.

Osteogenesis imperfecta involves the labyrinthine capsule, producing changes which are indistinguishable from the changes of otoscle-

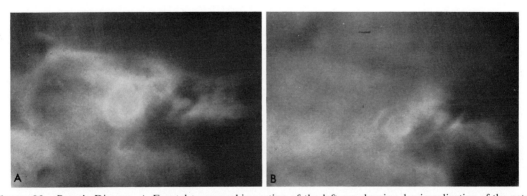

Figure 26. Paget's Disease. *A*, Frontal tomographic section of the left ear showing demineralization of the petrous apex but intact cochlear capsule. *B*, Frontal tomographic section of the same patient three years later. Notice the further demineralization of the petrous pyramid, the outline of which is completely washed out, and the involvement of the cochlear capsule.

rosis, although usually more widespread to the entire labyrinthine capsule. However, the appearance of the long bones, which are abnormally thin with the presence of multiple fractures often leading to a gross distortion, and the blue color of the sclera are unmistakable findings leading to the diagnosis.

The involvement of the skull by fibrous dysplasia is quite characteristic. Whereas the involvement of the calvarium and mandible consists of expansion of the affected portion by cystic lesions, the changes in the base of the skull including the temporal bone are almost always of the proliferative type. The affected petrous pyramid becomes extremely dense and thick with consequent asymmetry between the two sides. The outline of the labyrinthine capsule becomes, first, poorly distinguishable from the surrounding bone and, finally, may disappear as the lumen of the inner ear structures becomes partially or totally obliterated.

Involvement of the otic capsule, similar to the types described, has also been found in other rarer conditions such as osteopetrosis or Albers-Schönberg disease, cleidocranial dysostosis, Hurler's syndrome or dysostosis multiplex, and Pyle's syndrome or craniometaphyseal dysplasia.

REFERENCES

Agazzi, C., Cova, P. L., and Senaldi, M.: Semeiotica stratigrafica dell' osso temporale. Relazione al XVI, Radumo del gruppo Otorinolaringologico dell' Alta Italla, Dic., 1958.

Brunner, S., Petersen, O., and Sandberg, E.: Tomography in cholesteatoma of the temporal bone. Amer. J. Roentgen. 97:588–596, 1966.

Buckingham, R., and Valvassori, G.: Correlation of surgical and tomographic findings in cholesteatoma of the middle ear and mastoid. Transactions, July-August, 1967.

Compere, W.: Radiographic Atlas of the Temporal Bone. Book I. Amer. Acad. Ophthal. Otol., 1964.

Frey, K.: Diagnosis of traumas of the temporal bone. *In* Thin Section Tomography. Springfield, Ill., Charles C Thomas, 1972.

Jensen, J.: Malformations of the inner ear in deaf children. (Suppl.) Acta Radiol., 1969.

Mundnich, K., and Frey, K.: Das Rontgenschichtbild des Orhes. Stuttgart, Georg Thieme, 1959.

Naunton, R., and Valvassori, G.: Inner ear anomalies: Their association with atresia. Laryngoscope 78:1041–1049, 1968.

Portmann, M., and Guillen, G.: Radiodiagnostic en Otologie. Paris, Masson & Cie, 1959.

Reisner, K.: Tomography of the inner and middle ear malformations. Radiology 92:11–23, 1969.

Rosenwasser, H.: Glomus jugulare tumors. Arch. Otolaryng. 88:29–66, 1968.

Valvassori, G.: Radiographic Atlas of the Temporal Bone. Book II. Amer. Acad. Ophthal. Otol., 1964.

Valvassori, G.: Laminagraphy of the ear: Normal roentgenographic anatomy. Amer. J. Roentgen. 89:1155–1167, 1963.

Valvassori, G.: Laminagraphy of the ear: Pathologic conditions. Amer. J. Roentgen. 89:1168–1178, 1963.

Valvassori, G., and Pierce, R.: The normal internal auditory canal. Amer. J. Roentgen. 92:1233–1241, 1964.

Valvassori, G.: The abnormal internal auditory canal: The diagnosis of acoustic neuroma. Radiology 92:449–459, 1969.

Valvassori, G.: The interpretation of the radiographic findings in cochlear otosclerosis. Ann. Otol. 75:572–578, 1966.

Valvassori, G.: Radiologic diagnosis of cochlear otosclerosis. Laryngoscope 75:1563–1571, 1965.

Valvassori, G., Naunton, R., and Lindsay, J.: Inner ear anomalies: Clinical and histopathological considerations. Ann. Otol. 78:929, 1969.

Chapter 46

RADIOLOGY OF THE NOSE AND PARANASAL SINUSES

by Judah Zizmor, M.D., and Arnold M. Noyek, M.D.

The radiologic examination of the nose and paranasal sinuses is of primary importance in the diagnosis and treatment of rhinologic disease. Familiarity with the clinical and pathological evolution of diseases of the nose and paranasal sinuses adds wisdom to radiographic interpretation. Appropriate radiographic films of high quality enhance the radiologist's vision and the clinician's acumen and are essential for accurate diagnosis.

In this chapter the routine views for radiography of the nose and paranasal sinuses will be illustrated with appropriate radiographs of the normal adult. Additional views and special roentgen procedures and techniques will also be alluded to. The development of the nose and paranasal sinuses from the neonate to the adult will be outlined briefly. The abnormal radiographic signs of disease in the nose and paranasal sinuses will be described and illustrated, and the diseases causing them listed.

The following are the routine radiographic views for visualizing the paranasal sinuses, nasal cavities, nasopharynx and orbits (Merrill, 1967): (1) the posteroanterior Caldwell view; (2) the Waters view, (3) the lateral view, (4) the submental vertex base view, and (5) the right and left oblique orbital views.

CALDWELL POSTEROANTERIOR VIEW

The Caldwell (1908) posteroanterior view is of primary value in visualizing disease in the frontal and ethmoidal sinuses, nasal cavities, and orbits, and also contributes to the diagnosis of disease in the maxillary sinuses. The petrous ridges should be at the level between the lower and middle thirds of the orbits (Fig. 1).

Anatomy Revealed on Caldwell View

1. **Frontal Sinuses**
   A. Intersinus septum
   B. Compartmental septum
   C. Mucoperiosteal white line
2. **Ethmoid Sinuses**
   A. Supraorbital ethmoid
   B. Orbital plate of ethmoids
   C. Ethmoidal cells
   D. Crista galli
3. **Maxillary Sinuses**
   A. Nasoantral wall
   B. Lateral wall
4. **Orbits**
   A. Orbital floor
   B. Orbital roof
   C. Lateral orbital wall
   D. Sphenoidal ridge
   E. Lesser wing of sphenoid
   F. Greater wing of sphenoid
   G. Sphenoidal fissure
   H. Zygomaticofrontal suture
   I. Petrous ridge
5. **Nasal Cavities**
   A. Middle turbinate
   B. Inferior turbinate
   C. Bony nasal septum
   D. Cribriform plate
   E. Floor of nose

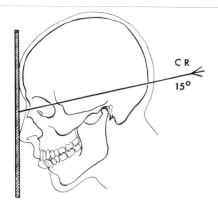

Diagram 1. Caldwell projection. C R = central ray.

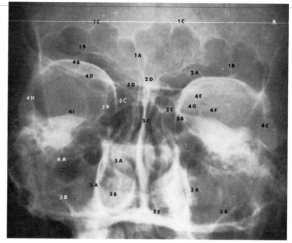

Figure 1. Normal Caldwell view.

WATERS POSTEROANTERIOR VIEW

This is the prime view for visualizing the maxillary antra (Waters and Waldron, 1915; Merrell and Yanagisawa, 1968). The feature inherent in the 15 degree caudad tilt of the x-ray tube in this view is the depression of the petrous portion of the temporal bones below the level of the maxillary sinuses, so that the antra can be visualized with clarity. The orbits, infraorbital foramina, nasal cavities, and zygomatic arches are well visualized. This view is well suited for the demonstration of pathological changes within the maxillary sinuses and fractures of the midfacial bony skeleton, such as blowout and tripod fractures of the orbits (Fig. 2).

Anatomy Revealed on Waters View

1. **Maxillary Antrum**
   A. Lateral wall
   B. Nasoantral wall
   C. Antral roof and floor of orbit
   D. Infraorbital foramen
   E. Superior orbital fissure
2. **Orbit**
   A. Inferior orbital rim

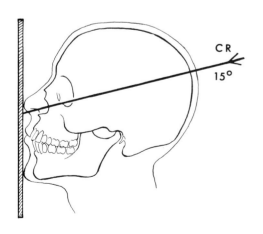

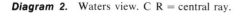

Diagram 2. Waters view. C R = central ray.

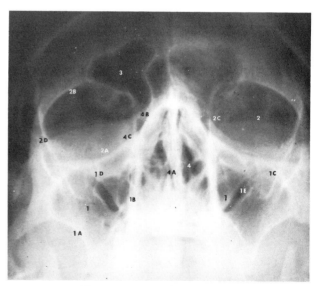

Figure 2. Normal Waters view.

B. Superior orbital rim
C. Medial orbital wall
D. Lateral orbital wall
3. **Frontal Sinus**
4. **Nasal Cavity**
    A. Bony nasal septum
    B. Nasal bone
    C. Frontal process of maxilla

LATERAL VIEW OF THE SINUSES

The lateral view indicates the anteroposterior development of the frontal, sphenoidal, and maxillary sinuses, and the sella turcica (Merrill, 1967; Merrell and Yanagisawa, 1968). The thickness of the bony walls, and the presence or absence of thinning, expansion, osteolysis, or osteoblastosis of these bony structures may be evaluated (Fig. 3).

Air profiles the nasopharynx and the soft palate and serves as a good contrast medium for outlining choanal polypi, adenoidal hypertrophy, and nasopharyngeal tumors.

Cysts or polyps of the antra may be detected if profiled with air despite the superimposition of the right and left antra.

In the plane of the superimposed right and left ethmoidal labyrinths and nasal cavities, the opacification of the air spaces and decalcification of ethmoidal bony septa is well shown in chronic hypertrophic polypoid sinusitis.

Anatomy Revealed on Lateral View of the Sinuses

1. **Frontal Sinuses**
    A. Anterior wall
    B. Posterior wall
    C. Roof of orbit and floor of anterior fossa
2. **Sphenoid Sinuses**
    A. Anterior wall
    B. Floor of sphenoid
    C. Roof of sphenoid
    D. Posterior wall of sphenoid
3. **Maxillary Sinuses**
    A. Anterior wall
    B. Posterior wall
    C. Floor
    D. Roof
    E. V-shaped shadow of body of zygoma
4. **Sella Turcica**
    A. Anterior clinoid process
    B. Posterior clinoid process
5. **Nasopharynx**
    A. Posterior wall
    B. Vault
    C. Soft palate

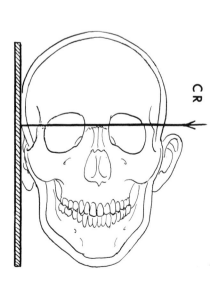

Diagram 3. Lateral projection.

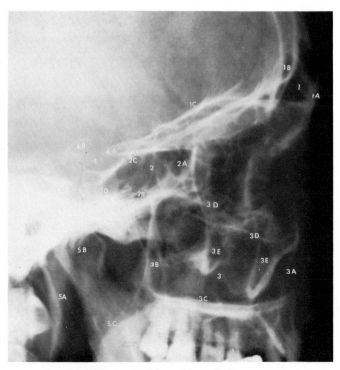

Figure 3. Normal lateral view.

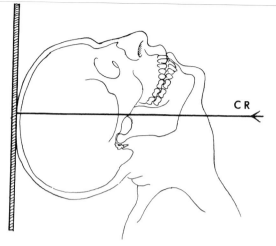

Diagram 4. Submental vertex projection.

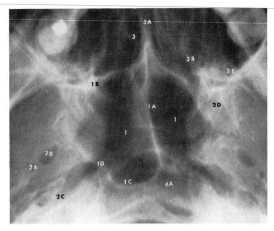

Figure 4. Submental vertex view.

SUBMENTAL VERTEX BASE VIEW

The submental vertex view surveys the sphenoidal sinuses, the nasopharynx, the nasal cavities, the bony floor of the middle fossa, the pterygoid hamuli and fossae, the posterior walls of the antra and orbits, the sphenoidal ridges, and the petrous bones (Merrill, 1967).

Soft tissue masses in the sphenoids, nasopharynx, and nasal cavities can be outlined in their midline or more lateral positions. Osteolysis or osteoblastosis of bony structures may indicate the presence of intracranial or nasopharyngeal tumors or bony dysplasias (Fig. 4).

Anatomy Revealed on Submental Vertex Base View

1. Sphenoid Sinus
   A. Intersinus septum
   B. Anterior wall
   C. Posterior wall
   D. Lateral wall
2. Base of Skull
   A. Foramen spinosum
   B. Foramen ovale
   C. Petrous apex
   D. Pterygoid fossa
   E. Posterior wall of antrum
3. Nasal Cavity
   A. Bony nasal septum
   B. Posterior ethmoidal cells
4. Nasopharynx
   A. Pharyngeal air shadow

RIGHT AND LEFT OBLIQUE ORBITAL VIEWS

The oblique orbital view provides excellent visualization of the superior ethmoid cells, frontal sinus, and optic foramen (Fuchs, 1932; Merrill, 1967). This view is often decisive in the diagnosis of ethmoidal and frontal mucoceles by revealing the characteristic smooth, round, or oval area of bony dehiscence, which may not have been evident in the Caldwell or Waters views. Inflammatory or neoplastic changes in the superior ethmoid, frontal, and sphenoid sinuses, as well as the optic foramen, may also be well shown (Fig. 5).

A radiographic examination of the paranasal sinuses is not complete without the oblique orbital view.

Anatomy Revealed on the Right and Left Oblique Orbital Views

A. Superior ethmoid cells
B. Frontal sinus
C. Optic foramen
D. Line of lesser wing of sphenoid
E. Sphenoidal fissure
F. Supraorbital ethmoid

ROUTINE RADIOGRAPHIC VIEWS FOR THE NASAL BONES AND NASAL SOFT TISSUES

The right and left lateral views, nonscreen films; the superoinferior axial occlusal view,

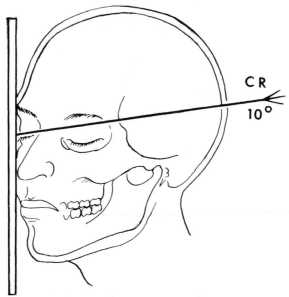

Diagram 5. Oblique orbital view.

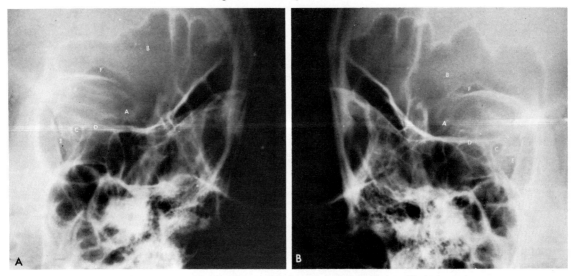

Figure 5. *A*, Right oblique orbital view; *B*, left oblique orbital view.

nonscreen film; and the Waters posteroanterior view, screen film (Fig. 2) visualize the nasal pyramid and its supporting septum (Merrill, 1967). Fractures and lesions producing bone destruction may be well shown. Lateral views of the nasal bones reveal depression or elevation of nasal bone fragments, whereas superoinferior axial views show medial or lateral displacement of nasal fractures.

Anatomy Revealed by Lateral View of Nasal Bones (Fig. 6 A and B)

A. Nasal bones
C. Anterior nasal spine of maxilla

Anatomy Revealed by Superoinferior Axial View (Fig. 6 C)

A. Right nasal bone
B. Left nasal bone
S. Septum

SPECIAL VIEWS AND RADIOGRAPHIC PROCEDURES

Special Views

Several views may be included in radiographic examination of the nose and paranasal sinuses that are not ordinarily requested but may be indicated in certain instances (Merrill, 1967). The open mouth view is good for visualizing the sphenoid sinuses but fails to survey the middle fossa adequately. In patients with facial injury the zygomatic arches can be well profiled by underexposed submental vertex views to show medial displacement of bone fragments (Fig. 7). Dental radiography may also be indicated in the investigation of sinus disease related to dental infection.

Tomography

Tomography, or planigraphy, is a radiologic technique which permits clear visualization of a layer of tissue at a predetermined depth (Moore, 1938; Merrill, 1967; Valvassori and Hord, 1968). All intermediate tissue layers are blurred out except for the plane under study by the opposing synchronous motion of the x-ray tube and film cassette, which are interconnected by a metal bar moving about a fulcrum.

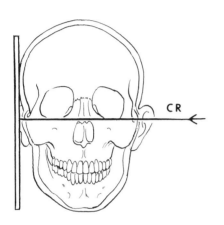
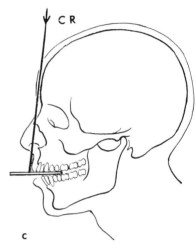

Diagram 6.   *A* and *B*, Lateral projection for nasal bones; *C*, Superoinferior axial projection for nasal bones. CR = central ray.

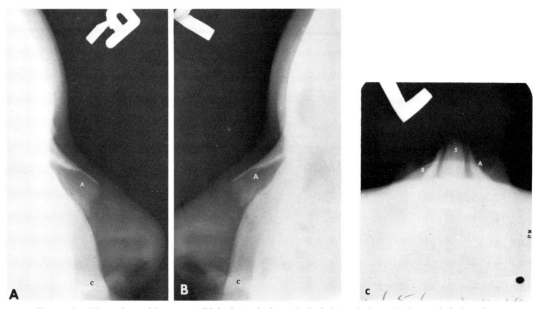

Figure 6.   Normal nasal bones, *A*, Right lateral view; *B*, Left lateral view; *C*, Superoinferior view.

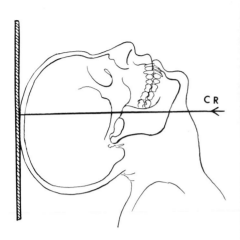

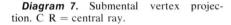

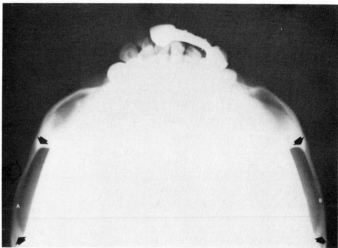

Diagram 7. Submental vertex projection. C R = central ray.

Figure 7. Underexposed submental vertex view for zygomatic arches. A, Right zygomatic arch (arrows); B, left zygomatic arch (arrows).

Alteration of the height of the fulcrum changes the layer of tissues brought into clear focus, since this is the only level not affected by motion of the x-ray tube and film cassette.

Tomography of the paranasal sinuses, nasal structures, orbits and base of skull and sella can be of great value in determining the presence of fracture (Fig. 8) or bone destruction due to tumor, particularly in the planning of surgical or radiotherapeutic procedures. This is the major application of tomography of the paransal sinuses and nose.

Contrast Radiography

On occasion aqueous or oily radiopaque contrast media may be utilized to outline ana-tomic or pathological abnormalities within the nasal cavities, paranasal sinuses, and nasopharynx, such as thickened membrane (Fig. 9), polyps or cysts, oroantral fistula (Fig. 10), congenital choanal atresia (Fig. 11), and neoplasms. The contrast medium may be injected by trocar through the bony nasoantral wall, or through its natural opening (Forestier and Sicard, 1922), or instilled by gravity (Proetz, 1930).

Angiography

Angiography may include both arterial and venous techniques (Krayenbuhl, 1952, 1962; Rosen et al., 1966). Carotid arteriography

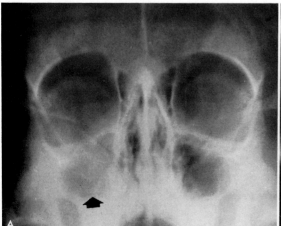

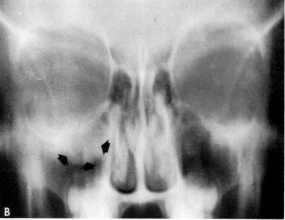

Figure 8. Blow out fracture of the right orbit. Trauma to right orbit 24 hours before examination was followed by diplopia. *A,* Waters view reveals an opaque right antrum (arrow). *B,* Anteroposterior tomography reveals a large orbital soft tissue herniation into the upper half of right antrum, typical of a blowout fracture (arrows).

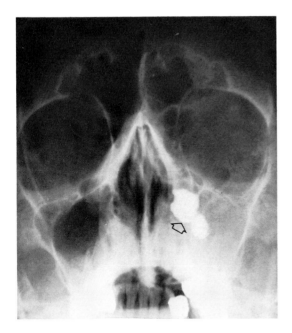

Figure 9. Contrast study with lipiodol reveals greatly diminished left antral lumen due to marked thickening of membrane (arrow).

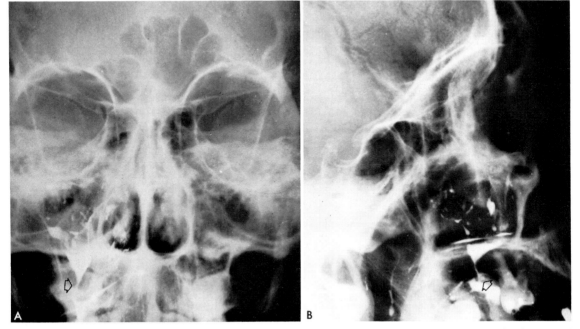

Figure 10. *A* and *B*, Man aged 56. Following extraction of a right upper molar tooth six months previously, pus and blood have drained intermittently from the extraction socket. Lipiodol outlines a nasoantral fistula (arrow).

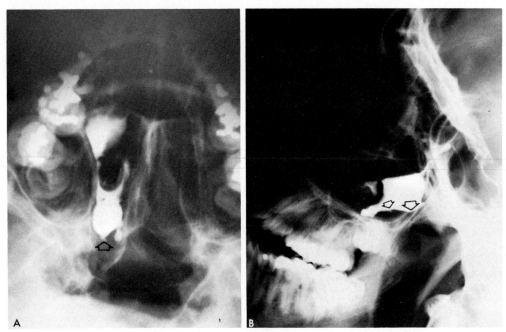

Figure 11. *A,* Base view reveals a right posterior choanal atresia (arrow) outlined with lipiodol in a woman aged 38. *B,* Lateral view reveals a posterior choanal atresia and blockage (arrows).

Figure 12. Right external carotid arteriography with subtraction technique reveals a mass (neurinoma) of right infraorbital nerve (arrows). A 54 year old man developed exophthalmos with upward displacement of the right eye over a four year period. Routine radiography revealed destruction of the right orbital floor. Right external carotid arteriogram revealed in the capillary phase a huge tumor in the plane of the right antrum and lower orbit profiled by capsular vessels of the internal maxillary artery in a pattern suggesting a benign tumor. This was surgically removed. Pathologic report revealed "neurinoma of infraorbital nerve." (Courtesy of Dr. H. Krayenbuhl, Zurich, Switzerland.)

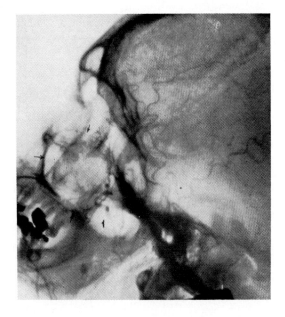

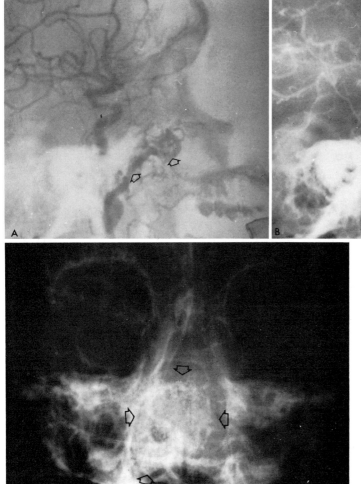

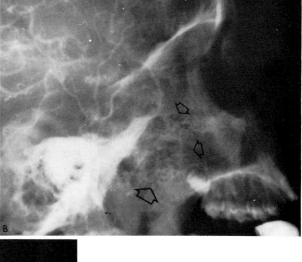

Figure 13. Angiofibroma of the naso-pharynx and nasal cavities in a 14 year old boy. *A, B,* and *C,* Left and right carotid arteriography reveals a network of fine vessels throughout a nasopharyngeal tumor (arrows), supplied mainly from the hypertrophied right internal maxillary branch of the external carotid artery (arrows) with (*C*) localized extensions of tumor vessels into the right midethmoidal region (arrows). The appearance is typical for a highly vascular tumor like angiofibroma. (Courtesy of Dr. D. F. Rideout, Toronto, Canada.)

may, in specific instances, indicate the benign nature of a mass in a paranasal sinus by the appearance of a circumscribing opacified ring of vessels (Fig. 12). In malignant lesions of the sinuses, the vasculature is of abnormal pattern and tumor stain may be noted. By the use of subtraction techniques in carotid arteriography, excellent visualization may be obtained of occult extensions of juvenile angiofibroma of the nasopharynx with its vascular connections (Fig. 13).

GENERAL STATEMENT ON RADIOGRAPHIC TECHNIQUE

1. Details of radiographic exposure, kilovoltage, milliampere-seconds, and tube film distance will not be reviewed since these vary with each radiographic machine and with each radiologist's preference.

2. Satisfactory films of the sinuses can be obtained with or without the use of the Potter-Bucky diaphragm by using par-speed screen cassettes.

3. The nasal bones are examined with nonscreen films.

4. Stereoscopic films can be made when desired for more detailed examination of the sinuses.

5. Tomography may be required to reveal evidence of fracture or neoplastic bone destruction when routine radiography of the paranasal sinuses, nasal cavities, and orbits is equivocal or negative.

6. Immobilization of the head during radiography is mandatory.

7. Radiography of the paranasal sinuses is

preferred in the erect sitting position, not only because of the increased ease of examination, but to demonstrate fluid levels in the paranasal sinuses and adjacent structures resulting from disease and fractures.

8. Extension cones of 3-inch width make for better film quality, with diminished secondary scatter radiation, while eliminating unnecessary roentgen exposure for the patient.

COMPARATIVE GROWTH AND DEVELOPMENT OF THE PARANASAL SINUSES AND NOSE (Fig. 14)

Frontal Sinuses

The frontal sinus is the only sinus that cannot be recognized radiologically in the neonate (Young, 1948; Pendergrass et al., 1956). The frontal diverticulum is present, but the frontal bone is not pneumatized until between the first and second years of life. The frontal sinus may assume its definitive shape as early as the third year of life, but continued growth and development are carried well into puberty. The frontal sinus is capable of extremes in under- and overdevelopment. Agenesis and massive pneumatization are both seen with regularity. The frontal sinus may extend widely laterally, posteriorly, and superiorly into the frontal bone, and cellular development into the orbital plate of the frontal bone may extend as far as the optic foramen on each side. The intersinus septum may or may not be in the midline and is occasionally deficient. The nasofrontal duct in the floor of the frontal sinus drains directly into the middle meatus in 50 per cent of instances, and in the remainder into the ethmoid infundibulum.

Ethmoid Sinuses

The anterior ethmoidal labyrinth is also present at birth, having derived its cellular development from the middle meatus as did the other two members of the anterior group of paranasal sinuses, the frontal and maxillary sinuses. The posterior cells of the ethmoid labyrinth are derived from the superior meatus and are associated with sphenoid sinus development. The ethmoid labyrinth is the only multicompartmentalized or honeycomb-type of sinus; it is opacified during the earliest days of life. The ethmoid labyrinth may demonstrate excessive development, and cells may be noted

in the ethmoid bulla, the middle turbinate itself, the crista galli, and the supraorbital area. Posterior ethmoid cells may envelop the optic foramina or bulge into the posterior aspect of the antra as so-called maxillo-ethmoid cells. Adequate roentgen diagnostic detail of the ethmoidal cells is rarely possible until the latter part of the first year of life.

Maxillary Sinuses

The maxillary antrum is evident radiologically at birth, though its lateral limit does not reach the level of the infraorbital foramen until sometime during the second year of life. The maxillary sinuses may appear cloudy during the initial days of life until their lumina become adequately aerated. The maxillary sinus typically has three processes: a prelacrimal, a zygomatic, and an alveolar process. The floor of the maxillary antrum descends below the level of the floor of the nose about the eighth year of life with development of the alveolar recess in the alveolar process and with the eruption of the secondary or adult dentition. The floor of the maxillary sinus in the alveolar recess is usually related to the second premolar and molar dental roots. In dental development the roots may project considerably into the antrum, and the sinus lumen may extend to the level of the canine tooth.

The maxillary antrum nearly always develops, and this stability in development is reflected in the usual absence of excessive pneumatization and the infrequency of compartmentalization and multiple septa. The usual adult maxillary antrum has a capacity of about 30 cc. Occasionally the lumen of the maxillary sinus may be small and its bony walls thick as a result of incomplete pneumatization and development. Complete failure of development of the antral lumen and total absence of the maxillary sinus are rare.

Sphenoid Sinuses

The rudimentary sphenoid sinus may be identified at birth and is quite well developed by the eighth year of life. It is in the posterior group of paranasal sinuses along with the posterior ethmoid cells. Sphenoid radiography shows evidence of abnormality less often than the other paranasal sinuses since primary and secondary infectious and neoplastic diseases are less common in this location. With the advent of transsphenoidal hypophysectomy, ra-

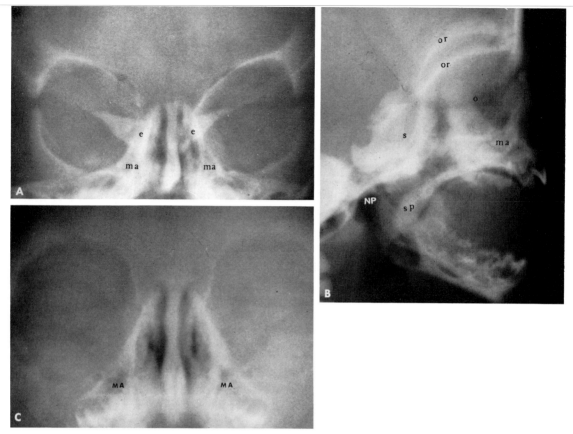

Figure 14. Development of sinuses in growing child.

A, Waters view, and *B,* lateral view of newborn show sinuses have not yet begun to develop. e = Plane of ethmoid cells; ma = maxillary antrum; or = orbital roof; o = orbit; s = unpneumatized body of sphenoid; NP = nasopharynx; SP = soft palate. (Courtesy of Dr. Herman Grossman, New York.)

C, Waters views, and *D* (opposite page), lateral view of sinuses of three month old child. MA = maxillary antrum; NP = nasopharynx; SE = sella; S = unpneumatized body of sphenoid. (Courtesy of Dr. B. J. Reilly, Toronto, Canada.)

(Illustration continued on opposite page.)

diographic study of the sphenoid sinuses and sella prior to surgical intervention has assumed greater importance, particularly with reference to the size of the sphenoid, the presence or absence of sphenoidal sinus disease, and the precise localization of the sella and pituitary. With failure of sphenoidal pneumatization which occurs in 1 per cent of instances, a mass of bone exists between the rostrum of the sphenoid and the pituitary fossa. Approximately two fifths of sphenoid bones exhibit presphenoid pneumatization in which cellular development is carried up to, but not beyond, the anterior aspect of the pituitary fossa. In the remainder, posterior sphenoid development may extend to the dorsum sellae and beyond, with extension reaching occasionally into the occipital bone. The sphenoid sinus may exhibit extremes of pneumatization, with cellular de-velopment being carried into the anterior and posterior clinoid processes and perisphenoidal cells in the greater and lesser wings of the sphenoid and the pterygoid plates.

The Nose

The external nose develops closely with the remainder of the middle third of the facial skeleton. The nasal bridge develops from the primitive frontal prominence, and the nasal ala and upper lateral cartilage develop from the lateral nasal process; the columella, anterior portion of the nasal septum, and upper lip are derived from the fusion of the median nasal process (of His) with its fellow across the midline and with the first arch maxillary process laterally. Imperfect fusion of these various pro-

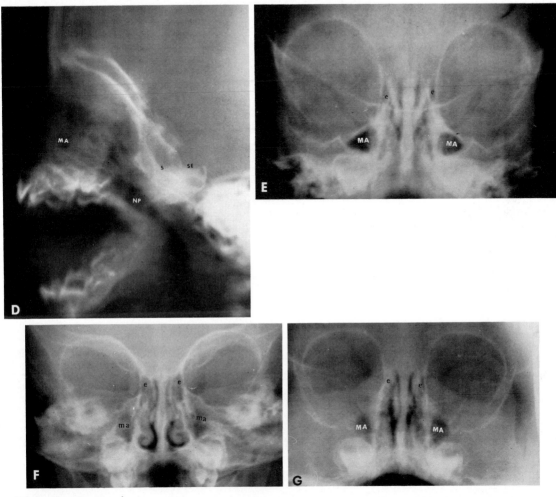

Figure 14. *Continued.*

E, Waters view of sinuses of seven month old child shows frontal sinuses are still undeveloped. e = Evidence of ethmoid pneumatization; MA = maxillary antrum development medial to infraorbital foramen and high above floor of nose and alveolus. (Courtesy of Dr. B. J. Reilly, Toronto, Canada.)

F, Caldwell view and *G*, Waters view of sinuses of one year old child show that frontal sinuses are still not developed. e = Some ethmoid pneumatization; ma (MA) = maxillary antra are small and still medial to infraorbital foramina. (Courtesy of Dr. B. J. Reilly, Toronto, Canada.)

Illustration continued on following page.

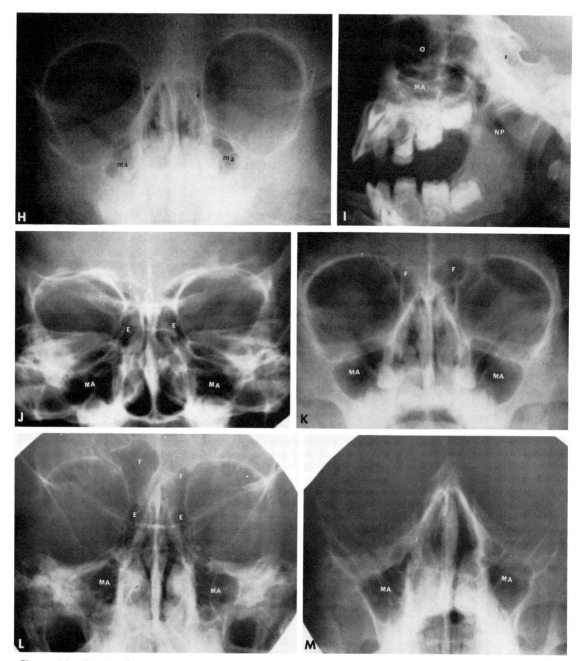

Figure 14. *Continued.*

H, Waters view, and *I*, lateral view of sinuses of two year old child. e = Ethmoid pneumatization; ma (MA), maxillary antrum; NP = nasopharynx; s = unpneumatized body of sphenoid. (Courtesy of Dr. Herman Grossman, New York.)

J, Caldwell view, and *K*, Waters view showing small frontal sinuses in six year old child. E = well pneumatized ethmoids; MA = well advanced but still incomplete development of the maxillary antrum. Note thick lateral bony wall. (Courtesy of Dr. B. J. Reilly, Toronto, Canada.)

L, Caldwell view, and *M*, Waters view showing small frontal sinuses in 12 year old child. F = sinuses; E = well pneumatized ethmoid cells; MA = well developed maxillary antra.

cesses results in a variety of congenital anomalies, such as cleft lip.

The primitive nasal pit on each side is surrounded by the medial and lateral nasal processes and, ultimately, becomes the nostril (anterior choana) anteriorly and extends to the posterior choana behind. The posterior choana is closed at the primitive bucconasal membrane initially, the site of fusion of nasal ectoderm and pharyngeal endoderm; should this membrane fail to disappear, a membranous or bony choanal atresia results. The septum is completed posteriorly by the tectoseptal expansion from the roof of the nose; this structure then fuses with the palatine processes of the maxilla which are developing laterally, and this completes the floor of the nose.

RADIOGRAPHIC SIGNS IN DISEASES OF THE NOSE AND PARANASAL SINUSES

The radiographic interpretation of diseases of the nose and paranasal sinuses depends on the recognition of the following abnormal signs:

1. Decreased aeration and luminal opacification
2. Mucosal thickening
3. Cyst formation
4. Soft tissue mass
5. Fluid level
6. Emphysema
7. Calcification
8. Ossification
9. One or more embryonic or fully developed teeth
10. Foreign bodies
11. Alterations in bony walls
    a. Decalcification
    b. Osteolysis
    c. Dehiscence
    d. Fractures
    e. Osteoblastosis and hyperostosis
    f. Expansion or displacement of bony walls
    g. Decreased luminal volume

Decreased Aeration and Luminal Opacification

Some evidence of decreased or absent aeration of the paranasal sinuses is usually present at birth (Samuel, 1952, 1968). Fluid may be present in the infantile antra and ethmoid cells in the absence of disease.

Developmental hypoplasia or agenesis, or other pathologic conditions later in life, may be associated with abnormally thick bony sinus walls and small lumina and may create the illusion of pathological nonaeration and opacification.

The commonest cause of decreased aeration is acute or chronic sinus infection (Fig. 15) which has extended either from the nose or, in 10 per cent of patients, from the dentition. Similar opacification is often found in allergic sinusitis (Fig. 16). When maxillofacial trauma and fractures extend into the sinuses, the edematous mucous membranes and intrasinus hemorrhage may diminish aeration and opacify the sinus. Neoplastic disease, either benign or

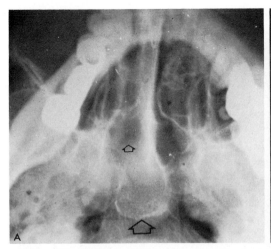
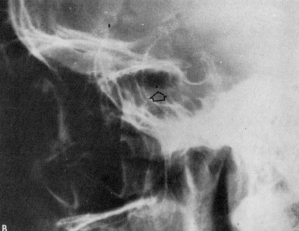

Figure 15. *A,* Base view reveals a very cloudy right sphenoid sinus (large arrow) with fluid level (small arrow). *B,* Lateral view reveals partial opacification of sphenoid sinus by fluid. Arrow points to fluid level. This 46 year old woman had a right optic neuritis. Treatment by drainage of pus and antibiotic medication resulted in clearing of the right sphenoid sinus and subsidence of the right optic neuritis.

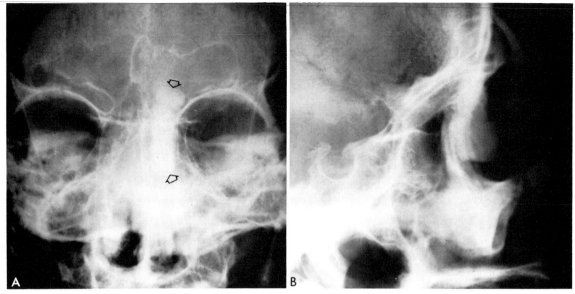

Figure 16. *A,* Caldwell view reveals chronic hypertrophic polypoid pansinusitis. This is a 69 year old man with a long history of chronic hypertrophic polypoid sinusitis. Note cloudy frontal and ethmoid sinuses, nasal obstruction by soft tissue masses (polyps), widened interorbital distance, and decalcification of ethmoid cell walls. An incidental finding is a large lobulated ethmoidal osteoma (between arrows). *B,* Lateral view. Note generalized opacification of ethmoid, antral, and nasal cavities by generalized hypertrophic polypoid sinusitis.

malignant (Fig. 17), diminishes aeration in proportion to the size of the tumor and by obstruction of drainage. Diminished aeration of the sinus lumen, whether due to inflammatory or allergic mucosal edema, purulent or nonpurulent fluid, traumatic hemorrhage, or benign or malignant soft tissue masses, may be described as slight, moderate, or marked clouding or opacification. A slight degree of opacification of a sinus is often an equivocal finding and difficult to evaluate because of variability of thickness and slight anatomic asymmetry of the right and left sides of the head. Bone dysplasias also produce opacification by increased density and thickness of the diseased bony sinus walls and encroachment on the lumina of the sinuses. Autoimmune disease such as Wegener's granulomatosis is a rare cause of opacification of the nasal cavities and sinuses; it may also cause bone destruction.

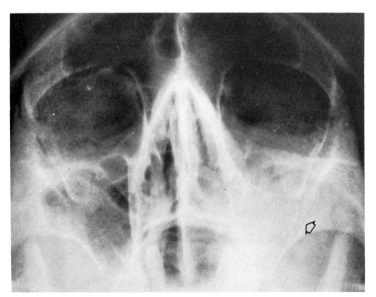

Figure 17. Waters view reveals very opaque left antrum with loss of mucoperiosteal cortical bony definition (arrow), laterally and medially, and increase of soft tissue in left nasal cavity. Diagnosis: squamous cell carcinoma.

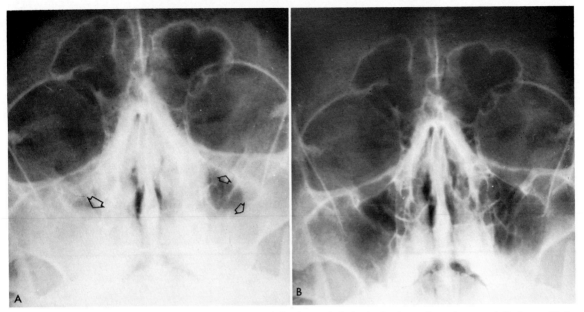

Figure 18. *A,* Man aged 31 with upper respiratory infection, pain in both cheeks, and purulent nasal discharge. Note cloudy antra with markedly thickened membrane and polyp formation in right antrum (arrows). *B,* Examination one year later reveals clear antra with no evidence of thickened membrane.

Mucosal Thickening

Mucous membrane thickening is one of the common signs of abnormality found in routine radiography of the sinuses. Mucosal thickening may be uniform or discretely polypoid. A thin white line of mucoperiosteum delimits the point of junction between mucosa and bony wall unless the mucoperiosteum is demineralized by local or systemic disease. Mucosal thickening of the sinuses is usually secondary to infection (Fig. 18), or allergy; it is rarely seen with malignant tumors (Fig. 19). Mucosal thickening may vary from a slight to a thick polypoid membrane which completely fills the sinus lumen. This is a frequent and easily de-

Figure 19. Waters view reveals squamous cell carcinoma of right antrum simulating marked thickening of membrane. The diagnosis of malignancy is suggested by the loss of bone in the inferolateral sinus wall (arrow).

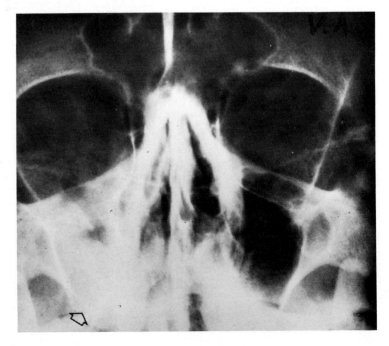

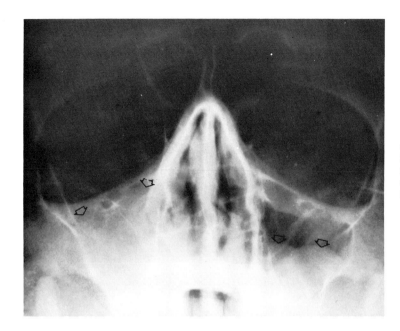

Figure 20. Waters view of man aged 44. The right antrum is filled by a large mucous cyst (arrows at superior margin of cyst). Mucoid fluid was drained through a trocar. Two smaller cysts are in the left antrum (arrow).

Figure 21. Waters view of a woman aged 47 with frontal headaches. Rhinological examination was negative. Note cysts in both antra. Puncture of right antrum elicited serous fluid. Diagnosis: serous cyst.

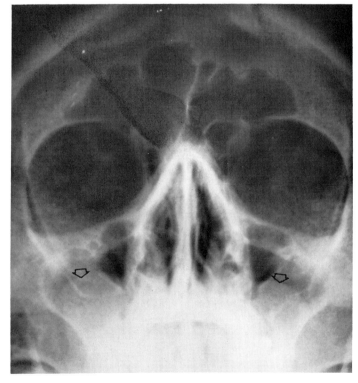

tectable radiographic finding in the maxillary antrum, and a common cause of opacification of the ethmoid sinuses. Thick membrane in the frontal sinuses is less common and usually not marked. In the sphenoid sinuses, membranous thickening is relatively rare and usually only slight.

Cyst Formation

Intrinsic Cysts. Cysts within the paranasal sinuses may be either intrinsic (that is, arising per primum within the paranasal sinuses) or extrinsic (that is, arising from extrasinus structures and secondarily involving the paranasal sinuses) (Paparella, 1963; Rosen et al., 1966; Samuel, 1968; Zizmor and Noyek, 1968). The intrinsic group of cysts may be further divided into those without evidence of associated bone destruction and those with bone destruction. Those with bone destruction will be dealt with in the section, "Alterations in Bony Walls."

There are two major intrinsic nonbone-destructive cysts. The mucous cyst (secretory retention cyst) (Fig. 20) is usually found in the maxillary antrum, although it is occasionally seen in the frontal and sphenoid sinuses. It is due to obstruction and dilatation of a duct of a minor seromucinous gland which results radiologically in a uniformly dense, homogeneous, dome-shaped mass.

The serous cyst (Fig. 21), which is a loculated collection of serous, amber fluid in the loose submucosal connective tissue of a sinus, usually occupies the antral floor. For this reason it is thought that gravity plays a role in its production. Interestingly the remainder of the paranasal sinus mucous membrane is rarely thickened in the presence of a serous cyst.

A differential diagnosis of these cystic lesions encompasses myxomatous polyps, loculated pus, various granulomatous lesions, dental cysts, tumor masses, and blowout fracture of the orbit.

Extrinsic Cysts. Various extrinsic cysts may involve the maxillary antrum and will produce a varying radiographic picture, depending on the site of origin, the type, and the size of the cyst (Stuart, 1944; Blumenfeld and Skolnik, 1965; Beekhuis and Watson, 1967; Zizmor and Noyek, 1968).

The radiologic appearance of dental cysts may be better appreciated in relationship to embryogenesis and development of dental structures. A follicular or primordial cyst develops in the tooth bud before enamel and dentin are produced (Fig. 22); hence, a follicular or primordial cyst will be visualized as a cystic lesion raising the antral floor. A dentigerous cyst (Fig. 23) arises following tooth bud maturation but prior to eruption; therefore, a dentigerous cyst always has a tooth present within the cyst with its crown pointing centrally. There are two types of dentigerous cysts, a central one in which the entire tooth is included, and a lateral type in which only a part of a tooth is included. The radiographic

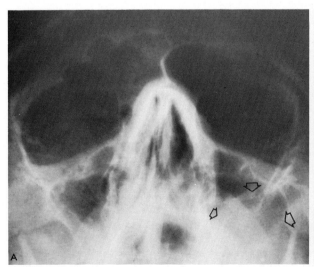
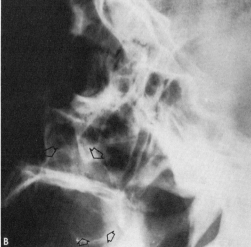

Figure 22. *A,* Waters view of man aged 59 with swelling of the left upper alveolus for two years. View shows a smooth dehiscence of the lateral wall of the left antrum in relation to a round soft tissue mass (arrows). *B,* Lateral view reveals dehiscence of upper alveolus and cyst expanding into the left antrum (arrows). Diagnosis: primordial cyst.

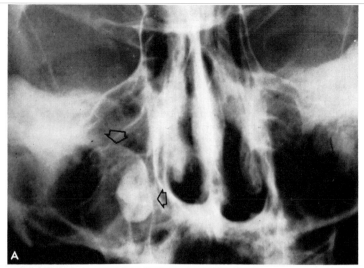

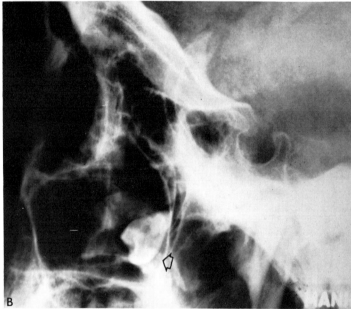

Figure 23. Dentigerous cyst in a 58 year old man. The radiographs reveal a large cyst (arrow), containing an adult tooth, extending into the right antrum from the right upper alveolus. Proved surgically. *A*, Caldwell view; *B*, lateral view.

appearance is similar to that of the follicular cyst except for the presence of a tooth, which is usually situated toward the periphery of the cyst.

A radicular or periodontal cyst arises after eruption of the tooth because of continued inflammatory stimulation of the epithelial cells within Hertwig's sheath of the periodontal membrane. In this instance a radicular cyst appears as a small radiolucent area of bone absorption at the root of the tooth. In some instances the cyst may enlarge and extend into the maxillary sinus. Extraction of the tooth connected with a radicular cyst is a common cause of oroantral fistula. Secondary infection

of a dental cyst may produce a pyocele (Fig. 24).

Neurogenic cysts involving the paranasal sinuses are of two types, the encephalocele (Fig. 25) and the meningocele (Fig. 26). Both are the result of congenital herniation of intracranial meningeal and neural tissue. These cystic lesions may present as extranasal, intranasal, or intrasinus masses, or as combinations of the three. In the usual instance a bony dehiscence in the base of the skull is recognized and a prolapsing cystic lesion is visualized between a widened nasal root and widened interorbital space.

Fissural cystic lesions, that is, those which

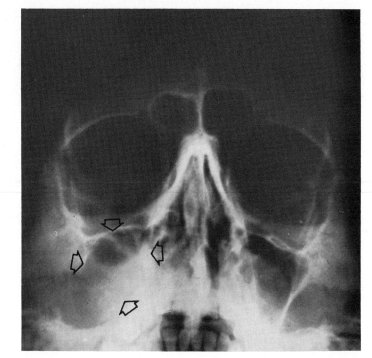

Figure 24. Waters view of infected radicular (periodontal) cyst. A 44 year old man had had a presumably abscessed right upper molar extracted six months previously. An oroantral fistula developed, with intermittent drainage of bloody pus. Radiography reveals a cyst filling the right antrum and eroding its lateral wall and floor. There is a fluid meniscus within the cyst. (arrows). A radicular cyst containing pus was found at surgery.

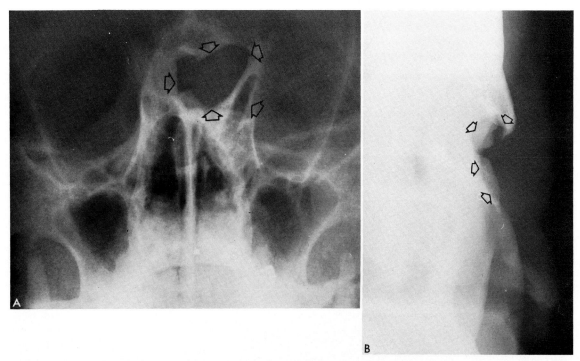

Figure 25. Typical dehiscence of bone through the cribriform plate and nasal bones in a 16 year old girl with widened interorbital distance, saddle nose, and compressible soft tissue mass over the nasal dorsum due to encephalocele (arrows). *A,* Waters view; *B,* lateral view.

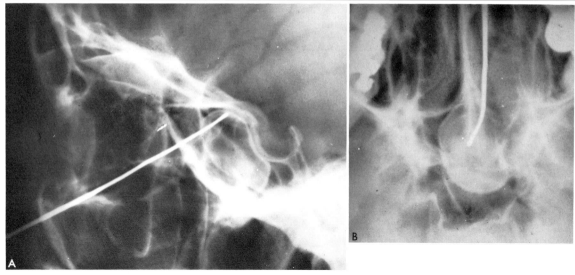

Figure 26. This 38 year old woman had headaches and rhinitis for several years. There is a 3-cm., cloudy, oval compartment in the left sphenoid which leaked cerebrospinal fluid after probing. *A*, Lateral view; *B*, base view. (Courtesy of Dr. M. H. Markham, New York.)

arise within lines of embryonal fusion in maxillofacial development, may also present radiologically. The medial cysts may be identified radiologically, e.g., cyst of incisive foramen (Fig. 27). The lateral cysts may cause an expanding erosion of bone, the globulomaxillary cyst, or merely a soft tissue mass, the naso-alveolar cyst. The globulomaxillary cyst classically separates the roots of the upper lateral incisor and canine teeth.

Other extrinsic cysts such as orbital cysts and dermoids have also been described.

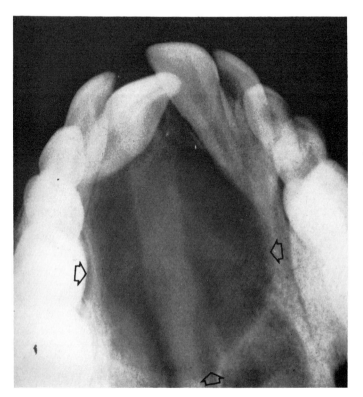

Figure 27. Occlusal film of hard palate, superoinferior view, reveals a large oval dehiscence of the hard palate and alveolus with separation of the incisor teeth. The bony nasal septum is exposed in the midline. A large infected cyst of the foramen incisivum was removed surgically.

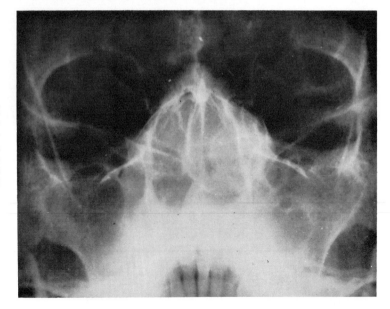

Figure 28. Waters view of nasal cavities packed with polyps; bony structures are thinned and expanded by continuous pressure of developing polyps. Both antra are opacified and filled with polyps. Diagnosis: Chronic hypertrophic polypoid disease of the nose and sinuses.

Soft Tissue Mass

Soft tissue masses in the lumina of sinuses, the nasal cavities and nasopharynx may be recognized in various non-neoplastic and neoplastic conditions (Larsson and Martensson, 1954; Pendergrass et al., 1956; Berdal and Myrhe, 1964; Lewin-Epstein et al., 1965; Cody, 1967; Zizmor and Noyek, 1968). The commonest soft tissue mass is that of the chron-ic, hypertrophic, allergic polyp (Fig. 28). This may be associated with chronic infections as well as being a mixed allergic infectious disorder. Polyps are noted within the sinus and may be profiled by air. Other polyps occur in the nasal cavity. The choanal polyp is usually associated with extrusion of mucosa from an opaque maxillary antrum (Fig. 29). A myxomatous choanal polyp (Fig. 30) may also arise from the nasal mucosa and extend into the

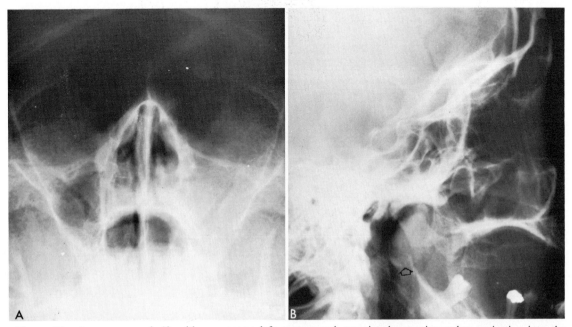

Figure 29. A woman aged 43 with an opaque left antrum and associated extrusion polyp projecting into the nasopharynx through the posterior nasal choana. *A*, Waters view; *B*, lateral view.

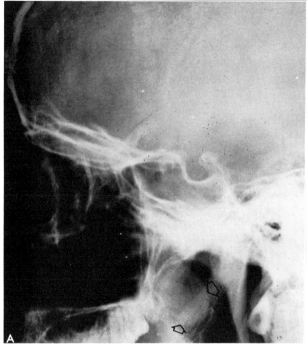
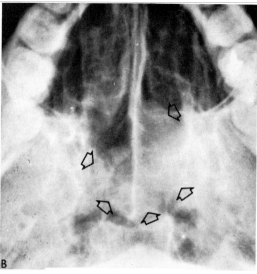

Figure 30. *A* and *B*, Lateral and base views reveal a fibromyxomatous polyp of posterior tip of left inferior turbinate protruding into the nasopharynx (arrows). Antra are normal.

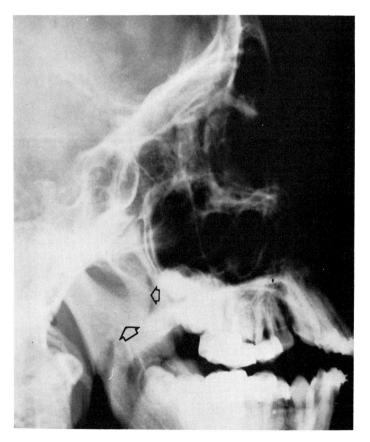

Figure 31. Lateral view reveals a large soft tissue mass arising from the posterior wall and vault of the nasopharynx, almost completely filling the airway. Diagnosis: adenoidal hypertrophy.

nasopharynx, where it is well outlined with air. A choanal polyp must be differentiated from the hypertrophied posterior tip of the inferior turbinate.

Adenoidal lymphoid tissue hypertrophy is the very common nasopharyngeal mass of early childhood (Fig. 31).

The neoplastic soft tissue masses include a variety of benign and malignant lesions. Benign tumors are rare and may be both epithelial and mesenchymal in origin. The epithelial tumor most frequently encountered, though relatively rare, is the inverting papilloma (Fig. 32). This may give rise to a lobulated soft tissue mass within the paranasal sinuses, usually the maxillary antrum; or it may arise in the ethmoid labyrinth or sphenoid or the nasal cavity. Of the mesenchymal soft tissue tumors, angio-

fibroma (Fig. 33), hemangioma, and neurofibroma (Fig. 34) are occasionally encountered. Intranasal glioma is very rare (Fig. 35).

Malignant soft tissue masses of the sinuses and nasal cavities may be of primary or secondary origin. The primary tumors include a variety of carcinomas, of which the squamous cell is the most common (Figs. 36 and 37). Of the adenocarcinomas, the cylindroma, though not common, is encountered most frequently. Melanoma is rare. All early primary epithelial malignancies may produce soft tissue masses without bone destruction, but by the time most of these lesions are apparent clinically, radiologic evidence of bone destruction is usually present, indicating an advanced stage of malignant disease. Sarcomata and lymphomata are also noted. Plasmacytoma (Fig. 38) has been de-

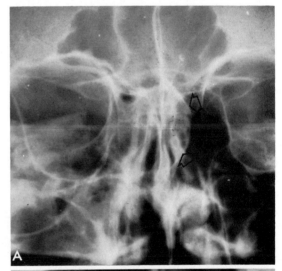

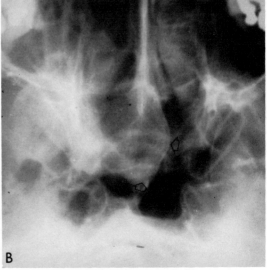

Figure 32. Epithelial papilloma in a 41 year old man with recurrent right serous otitis media due to eustachian tube obstruction. The frontal Caldwell (*A*) and basal (*B*) views reveal a mass in the right sphenoid that causes its medial wall to bulge to the left (arrows).

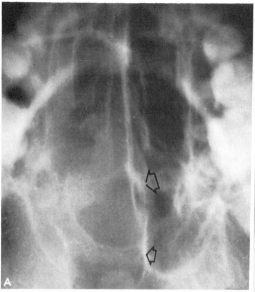

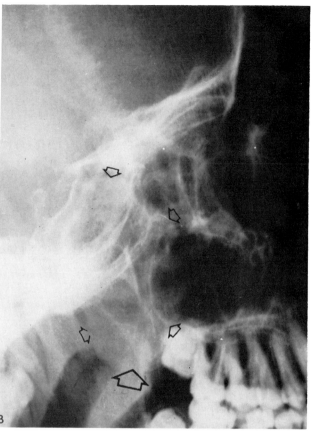

Figure 33. *A* and *B*, Base and lateral views of angiofibroma of the nasopharynx and sphenoid of a 16 year old boy who had a six months history of epistaxis. A soft tissue mass occupies the right side of the nasopharynx and right sphenoid sinus, and extends into the right posterior nasal cavity and posterior ethmoids (arrows). Surgically proved angiofibroma.

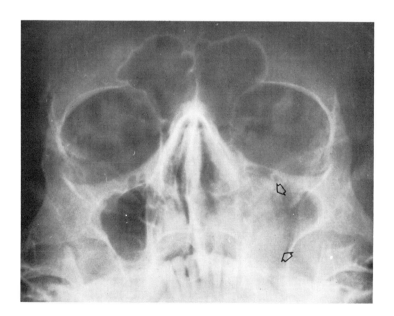

Figure 34. Waters view of a neurofibroma of the left antrum eroding into left nasal cavity of a woman aged 38.

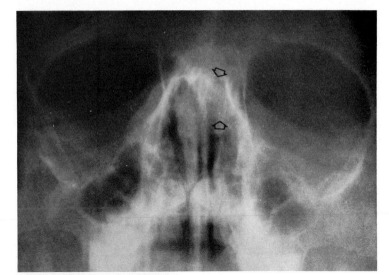

Figure 35. Waters view of intranasal glioma in a 14 year old boy with erosion of left nasal bone medially by soft tissue mass (arrows). Surgical specimen revealed intranasal glioma.

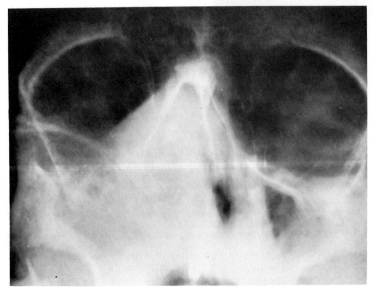

Figure 36. Waters view of primary squamous cell carcinoma of the right antrum. This 73 year old man had a painful swelling of the right cheek, right exophthalmos, and right nasal obstruction for six months. Radiography reveals a mass in the right antrum invading the right nasal cavity and orbit with extensive osteolysis. Pathologic report showed primary squamous cell carcinoma.

Figure 37. A 60 year old man had left exophthalmos for eight months and nasal obstruction for six months with epistaxis. Caldwell view shows the nasal cavities filled with soft tissue. The orbital plate of left ethmoids and the bony nasal septum are extensively destroyed. Intranasal biopsy revealed squamous cell carcinoma, presumably arising in the left ethmoidal labyrinth. (Arrows indicate destroyed orbital plate of ethmoids.)

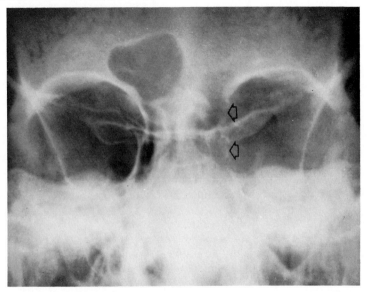

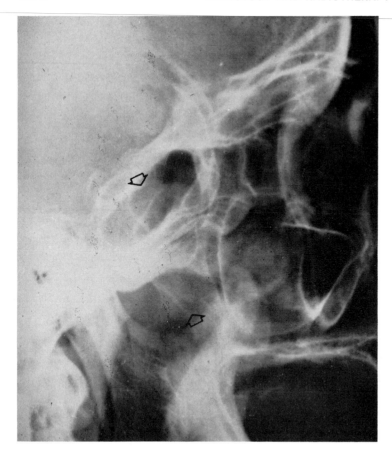

Figure 38. Lateral view of a woman aged 70 with epistaxis and nasal congestion. A large, round, soft tissue mass extends from the sphenoid sinus into the nasopharynx. Surgical specimen revealed plasma cell myeloma.

scribed within the paranasal sinuses, the nasal cavity, and the nasopharynx. Osteolysis associated with a soft tissue mass in a paranasal sinus in the pediatric and young adult group often indicates a sarcoma or, less commonly, a neuroblastoma.

Fluid Level

Intrasinus Fluid Level. Intrasinus fluid may be pus, blood, serous or mucoid secretion, or cerebrospinal fluid (Zizmor and Noyek, 1968). In acute infections an air-fluid level due to pus within a sinus may be recognized in the upright position. Intrasinus hemorrhage is usually secondary to fracture, rarely to a blood dyscrasia or malignant disease. In aerosinusitis the effusion may be serous or bloody, depending upon the extent and duration of negative pressure within the sinus. Not uncommonly a fluid level may be the result of a recent antral lavage. Cerebrospinal fluid may be found, though rarely, within the sphenoid sinus following a middle fossa fracture. In this instance there

may be other signs of middle fossa fracture, such as bubbles in the subarachnoid space, and a so-called "spontaneous ventriculogram." Demonstration of intra- and extrasinus fluid levels, as well as the increased ease of examination, are the important reasons for performing radiography of the skull and sinuses in the erect position (Fig. 39).

Extrasinus Fluid Level. Extrasinus fluid levels, secondary to suppurative disease of the sinuses with osteomyelitis and fistula formation, may result in orbital abscess (Fig. 40), in subcutaneous forehead abscess, or in brain abscess (Fig. 41) (Zizmor et al., 1964). Anaerobic or other gas-producing bacteria are rarely a cause of fluid levels in abscesses secondary to infectious disease of the sinuses.

Emphysema

Emphysema refers to the presence of gas outside the lumen of a sinus in adjacent soft tissues (Zizmor et al., 1962). Orbital emphysema is presumptive evidence of the fracture

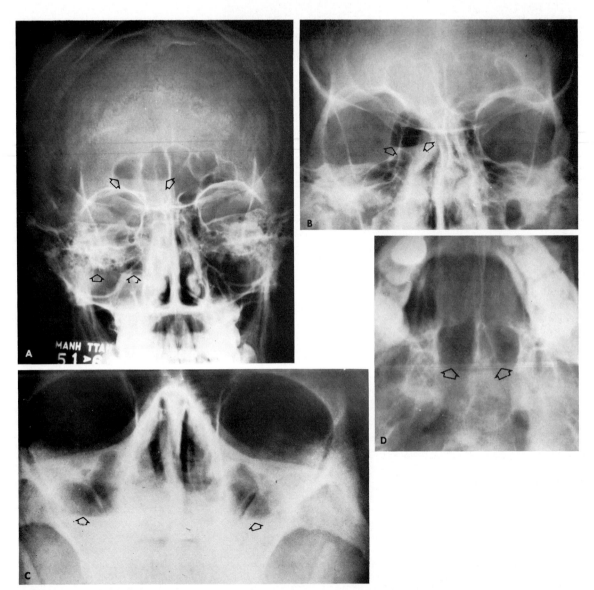

Figure 39. *A,* Caldwell view of boy aged 13 with acute sinusitis and right orbital cellulitis. Note fluid levels (arrows) in right frontal and maxillary sinuses and clouding of the right frontal, ethmoidal and maxillary sinuses. *B,* Caldwell view of a right ethmoidal pyocele with an air-fluid level in an 11 year old boy. An acute upper respiratory infection with right orbital cellulitis had been present for 11 days. There is an oval bone dehiscence with a gas-fluid level in the region of the right superior ethmoid cells. The right frontal and ethmoidal sinuses are cloudy. Diagnosis confirmed surgically. *C,* Waters view of man aged 23 with history of one week of upper respiratory infection. Note fluid levels in both antra, due to purulent fluid. *D,* Base view of man aged 43 with chronic hypertrophic polypoid sinusitis for many years. Patient now has sphenoid fluid level following an acute upper respiratory infection.

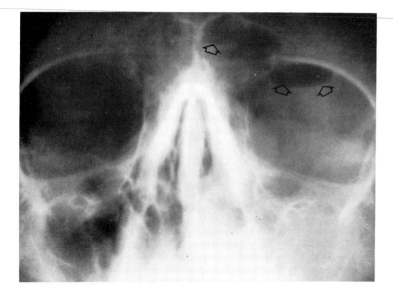

Figure 40. Waters view of left orbital fluid level secondary to frontal sinusitis. A 48 year old man with a long history of sinusitis developed left orbital cellulitis following an acute febrile upper respiratory infection. The left frontal, ethmoid, and antral sinuses are very cloudy. Fluid levels are present in the left frontal sinus and left orbit (arrows).

of a common bony wall between the orbit and a paranasal sinus, even if the exact site of fracture is not evident on routine radiography, as is so often the case in fractures of the orbital plate of the ethmoids. Blowout fracture of the orbital floor and antral roof is also a common cause of orbital emphysema (Fig. 42).

Malignant disease of the antrum extending into the orbit may produce a wide enough gap in the antral roof and orbital floor to permit the escape of air into orbital soft tissues.

Emphysema due to gas-producing bacteria in soft tissues in or adjacent to the sinuses is extremely rare.

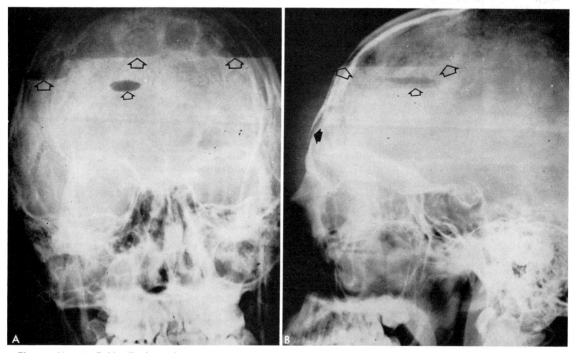

Figure 41. *A,* Caldwell view of a young man aged 19 who, two weeks following an upper respiratory infection, developed high fever, headaches, drowsiness, and massive swelling of his forehead. Note small fluid level in a frontal lobe abscess (small arrow), and large fluid levels in a huge forehead abscess (large arrows), both secondary to empyema of the frontal sinuses with osteomyelitis and fistula formation. Proved surgically. *B,* Lateral view. Black arrow points to osteolytic destruction of anterior wall of the frontal sinus by osteomyelitis.

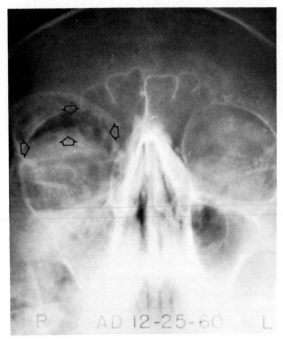

Figure 42. Waters view of emphysema of the right orbit, (indicated by mottled dark areas contrasting with the gray density of soft tissue [arrows]), following trauma which caused a blowout fracture of the floor of the right orbit. The right antrum is opacified by hemorrhage.

Calcification

Calcification in the paranasal sinuses is seen most frequently with mucocele (Fig. 43) (Samuel, 1952, 1968; Zizmor and Noyek, 1968). In 5 per cent of mucoceles there is macroscopic evidence of mural calcification. On occasion the mucocele may calcify heavily enough to mimic the radiographic appearance of an osteoma. Hemangioma produces discrete, round, dense phleboliths which are pathognomonic but occur rarely in the sinuses. Fibrous dysplasia may show tiny focal calcifications within its more radiolucent fibrous lesions (Fig. 44). The walls of mucous and serous cysts rarely calcify. Foreign bodies within the nose and paranasal sinuses, when they are of particularly long sojourn, may become encrusted and calcified and are called rhinoliths (Fig. 45). Homogeneous calcification, in moulage form, may develop at the site of osteoplastic frontal sinusectomy (Fig. 46).

Ossification

Osteoma is the commonest type of intrasinus ossification and most commonly arises from the periosteum in the region of the fronto-ethmoidal suture (Samuel, 1952; Pendegrass et al., 1956; Zizmor and Noyek, 1968). The frontal sinuses are most commonly involved (Fig. 47); the ethmoids less frequently (Fig. 48); antral and sphenoidal osteomata are rare. There are two histological types of osteoma — the hard cortical, and the soft cancellous. The cortical osteoma has an ivory-like, dense, homogenous, rounded or lobulated appearance. The soft osteoma has a lesser radiographic density, approaching that of soft tissue (Fig. 49).

Intrasinus ossification may also be a sequel of calcification secondary to inflammatory processes, organized traumatic hemorrhage, fractures, phleboliths, odontomata, chondroma and

Figure 43. Caldwell view of calcifying left frontal mucocele. A 72 year old woman with a history of sinusitis developed a left exophthalmos with swelling of the inner canthal region and left upper lid. Radiography reveals bone erosion of the left frontal sinus with peripheral calcific deposits on a mucocele that invades the superior medial quadrant of the left orbit (arrows).

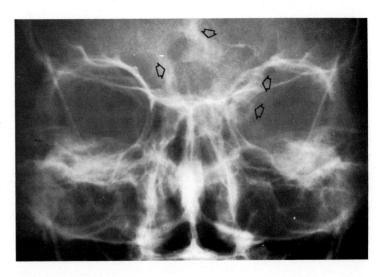

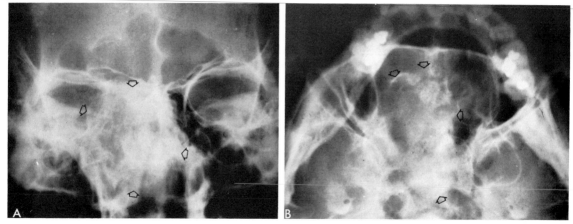

Figure 44.   Fibrous dysplasia in a 50 year old man with a 35 year history of right nasal obstruction and right exoph-thalmos. A soft tissue mass with calcific foci fills and expands the right nasal cavity and displaces the orbital plate of the right ethmoids laterally. *A*, Caldwell view; *B*, base view.

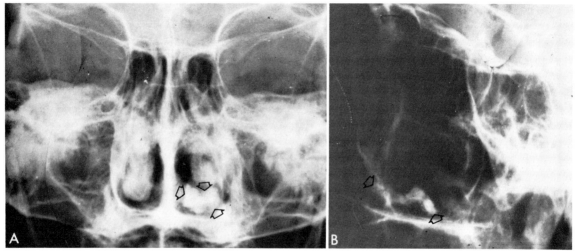

Figure 45.   *A*, Caldwell view reveals calcified rhinoliths along the floor of the left nasal passage (arrows). *B*, Lateral view. This 60 year old woman admitted that she had often inserted foreign bodies into her nose, i.e., bits of paper and wood.

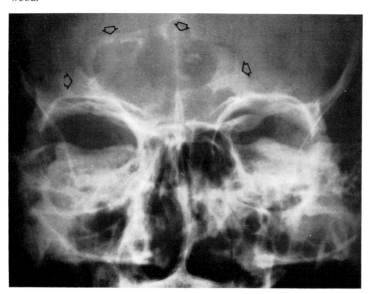

Figure 46.   This 31 year old man had an osteoplastic frontal sinusectomy for mucocele three years previously. He developed forehead tenderness and edema of the skin overlying the frontal sinuses two and one half years later. A calcifying cyst or mucocele was suggested radiologically. An infected calcified cyst was removed surgically. (Caldwell view.) (Courtesy of **Dr. D. G.** Voorhees, New York.)

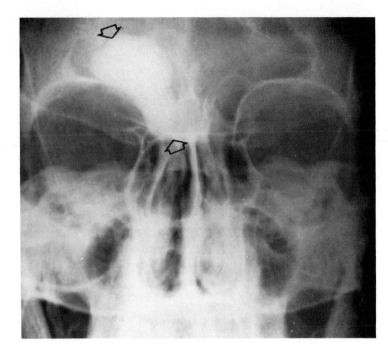

Figure 47. Caldwell view of a 43 year old man with frontal headaches. Note large cortical osteoma in the right frontal sinus and clouding of remaining sinus lumen as a result of blocking of the nasofrontal duct.

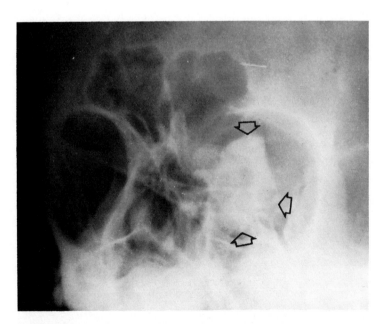

Figure 48. Oblique orbital view of cortical (hard) osteoma of the left posterior ethmoids in a 58 year old man with left exophthalmos for 10 years. Confirmed surgically.

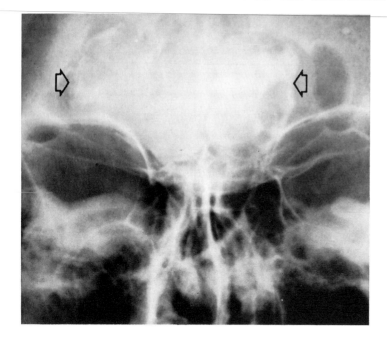

Figure 49. Caldwell view of a cancellous or soft osteoma, of lesser density than a cortical osteoma, which almost fills both frontal sinuses of a 58 year old man. Surgically proved.

osseous dysplasias like Paget's disease, fibrous dysplasia, and hypercalcemic ossification resulting from primary or secondary hyperparathyroidism.

Dentition Within the Maxillary Sinus

The presence of part or all of a fully developed tooth is a characteristic finding when a dentigerous cyst grows into the maxillary sinus from the upper alveolus. (See Figure 23.) Should an ameloblastoma develop in a dentigerous cyst and extend into a maxillary sinus, a tooth or part of a tooth, usually the crown, will be present (Fig. 50). A mass within the maxillary sinus containing myriads of embryonic teeth, with or without an adult tooth, is diagnostic of a compound odontoma that has invaded from the upper alveolus (Fig. 51) (Gorlin et al., 1963; Pantazopoulos and Nomikos, 1966; Zizmor and Noyek, 1968).

Figure 50. Waters view of ameloblastoma of the left maxillary sinus in a 29 year old woman with painless swelling of the left upper jaw and cheek for two years. The left antrum is almost filled with a soft tissue mass which has destroyed the lateral antral wall. A molar tooth within the ameloblastoma indicates its origin from a dentigerous cyst. (Courtesy of Dr. R. S. Sherman, New York.)

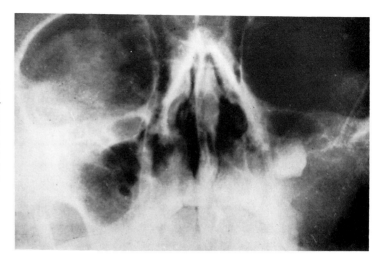

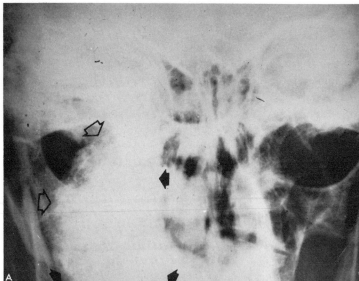

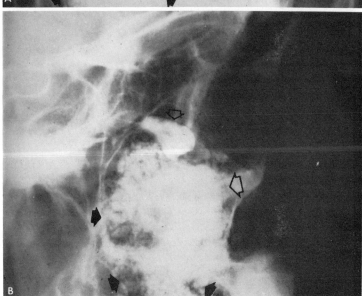

Figure 51. *A,* Caldwell view reveals a compound odontoma of the right maxilla and antrum. This is a 48 year old man with progressive swelling of the right upper alveolus for 10 years, and right exophthalmos for four years. *B,* An extensive opaque calcareous mass involves the right upper alveolus, fills the antrum and extends into the orbit. The mass consists of myriads of denticles, and a large adult tooth at its upper border. The roof of the antrum is displaced into the orbit (lateral view). Confirmed surgically.

Aberrant unerupted teeth along the floor of the nose or maxillary sinus are not uncommon, but are not usually of clinical significance.

Foreign Bodies

A variety of foreign bodies both within and adjacent to the paranasal sinuses and nasal cavities are encountered (Samuel, 1952; Pendergrass et al., 1956). These vary from radiographic contrast media to dental root canal fillings, bullets, shrapnel, buckshot, buttons, marbles, paper, and so forth. Intranasal foreign bodies may calcify and form rhinoliths (Fig. 45), or pseudotumors (Fig. 52). A residuum of Lipiodol within a sinus lumen, or Lipiodol injected submucosally, may cause chronic granuloma. Radioactive Thorotrast, (Buda et al., 1963) now abandoned although formerly used in contrast radiography of the paranasal sinuses, may cause granuloma and, ultimately, malignant disease if retained for many years within the lumen of a sinus (Fig. 53).

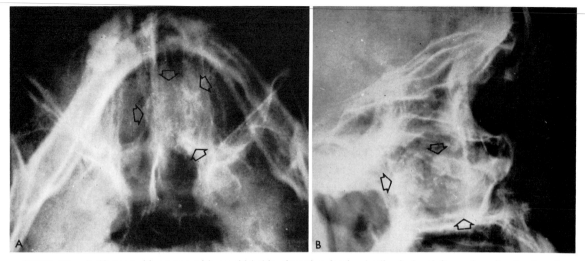

Figure 52. A 60 year old woman with an old habit of putting foreign bodies in her left nasal cavity developed an increasingly foul nasal discharge and left nasal obstruction. Radiographs reveal a large, round, soft tissue mass with calcific foci in the left nasal cavity. The mass erodes through the nasal septum. At surgery a pseudotumor, formed by the accretion of debris about multiple rhinoliths, was removed. The mass had eroded through the bony nasal septum. *A,* Base view; *B,* lateral view.

Alterations in Bony Walls

Decalcification. Decalcification of the bony wall of the sinus begins by demineralization of the mucoperiosteum and is indicated by disappearance of the mucoperiosteal white line (Samuel, 1952, 1968; Zizmor and Noyek, 1968). Resorption may be due to local or systemic diseases. The most common cause of decalcification is inflammatory mucosal hyperemia, either acute or chronic (Fig. 54). Systemic causes usually reflect abnormalities in calcium and phosphorus metabolism associated with parathyroid or renal diseases and bone dysplasias (Fig. 55). Pressure by benign and malignant tumors, polyps (Fig. 56), and cysts may also induce decalcification of the mucoperiosteum and thinning, displacement, and erosion of bone.

Interestingly, decalcification of the maxillary sinus mucoperiosteum, as well as of the nasal bones and anterior nasal spine of the maxilla, is a common finding in nasal leprosy. Loss of the anterior nasal spine of the maxilla is pathognomonic of leprosy (Fig. 57) in the absence of previous nasal surgery (Møller-Christensen and Inkster, 1965), trauma or congenital maxillonasal dysplasia (Gorlin and Sedano, 1968).

Osteolysis. Osteolysis describes a focal or diffuse dissolution of bone (Samuel, 1952; Larsson and Martensson, 1954; Pendergrass et al.,

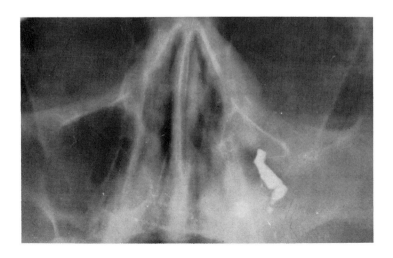

Figure 53. Thorotrast has remained in the left antrum for 20 years. Chronic granuloma and squamous cell carcinoma developed in the antral mucosa. There is a general loss of mucoperiosteal cortical white line and bone destruction in the antral roof. Note thinning of the left inferior orbital rim revealed in this Waters view. (Courtesy of Dr. H. P. Davis, New York.)

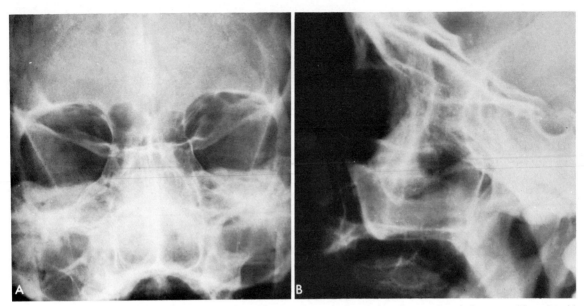

Figure 54. A 61 year old woman had a long history of nasal obstruction due to chronic hypertrophic polypoid sinusitis. Note diffuse decalcification of ethmoidal cell walls, nasal septum and orbital plates of ethmoids in association with blockage of nasal cavities by soft tissues (polyps). The interorbital distance has widened due to the chronic pressure of intransasal polyps. *A*, Caldwell view; *B*, lateral view.

Figure 55. Caldwell view of a 22 year old woman with osteoporosis circumscripta (phase I Paget's disease) of the frontoparietal area of the cranial vault with demineralization of the mucoperiosteal margins of the right frontal sinus (lower arrows).

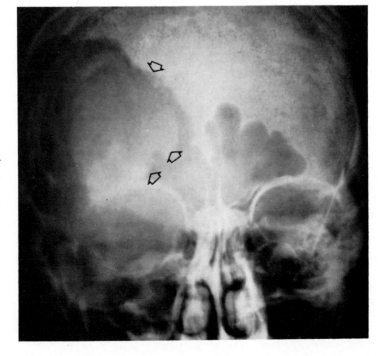

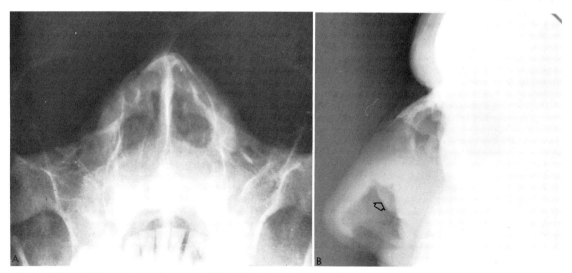

Figure 56. *A,* Waters view of man aged 53 with chronic hypertrophic polypoid pansinusitis of many years' duration and nasal obstruction. Note nasal cavities filled with soft tissue (polyps), decalcification, expansion, thinning and erosion of nasal bones and septum, and opaque antra. *B,* Lateral view of nasal bones. Lower border of polypoid tissue is profiled with air (arrow). Nasal bones decalcified, thinned, and eroded.

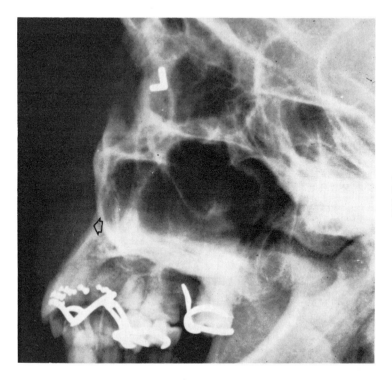

Figure 57. Lateral view of leprosy of the nose. Note the absence of the anterior nasal spine of the maxilla (arrow), a pathognomonic sign. Nasal bones are decalcified and atrophic.

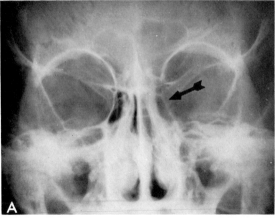
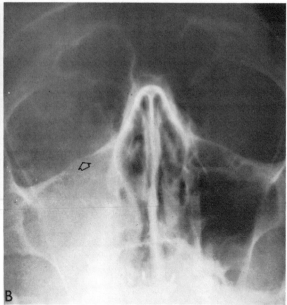

Figure 58. *A*, Caldwell view reveals cloudy left ethmoidal cells with decalcification and osteolysis of ethmoidal cell walls and orbital plate of ethmoids due to osteomyelitis (arrow) with associated left orbital cellulitis and exophthalmos for one month in a 38 year old woman. *B*, Waters view of man aged 52 who developed a painful, swollen right cheek and orbital cellulitis after an upper respiratory infection. Note opaque right antrum and osteolysis of right infraorbital rim (arrow) due to osteomyelitis associated with antral empyema.

1956; Berdal and Myrhe, 1964; Zizmor and Noyek, 1968). It is seen in acute osteomyelitis (Fig. 58) resulting from severe suppurative intrasinus infections caused by a variety of microorganisms. (See Figure 41 *B*.) Osteomyelitis of the sinuses secondary to dental infections, or as a complication of surgery, is not uncommon. Only rarely is septicemia a cause of os-

teomyelitis of the bony walls of the sinuses. Among the granulomatous proliferative lesions, tuberculosis, yaws, syphilis, and the mycoses may produce osteolysis.

Osteolysis is a common sign of primary, secondary, and metastatic malignant disease (Figs. 59 and 60), as well as histologically benign tumors such as hemangioma (Fig. 61),

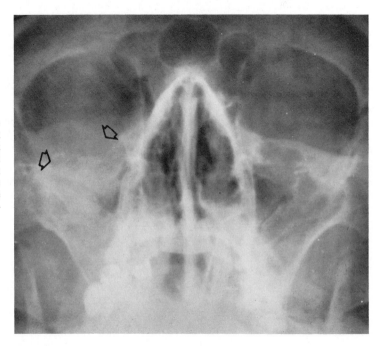

Figure 59. Waters view of a neglected basal cell carcinoma of the right lower lid that has invaded the right orbit and antrum, destroying the inferior orbital rim and floor (arrows). The opacification of the right antrum is due to neoplastic invasion of the mucosa, which mimics the radiographic appearance of thick membrane.

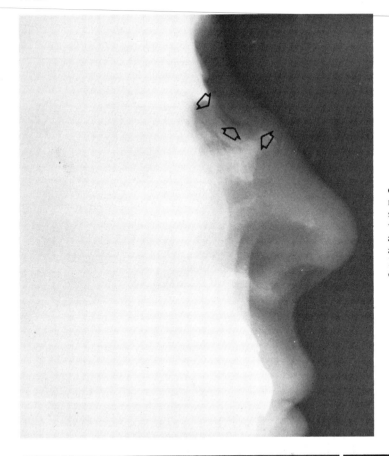

Figure 60. Lateral view of a 53 year old woman who had bumped her nose six months before. Pain and swelling persisted over the bridge of the nose. Lateral view of the nasal bones reveals osteolysis at the anterior aspect of the nasal bones associated with soft tissue swelling. Biopsy of the lesion revealed squamous cell carcinoma.

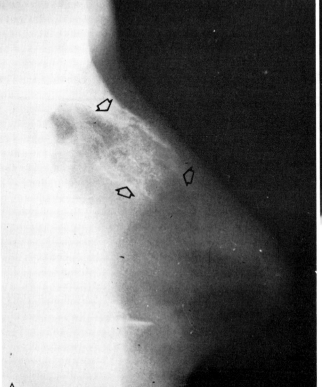

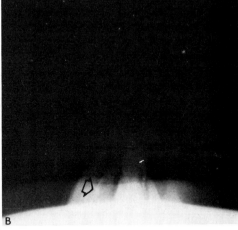

Figure 61. Hemangioma of the right nasal bone. Note the honeycombed osteolytic effect of the hemangiomatous involvement of the right nasal bone (arrows). *A*, Lateral view; *B*, axial view.

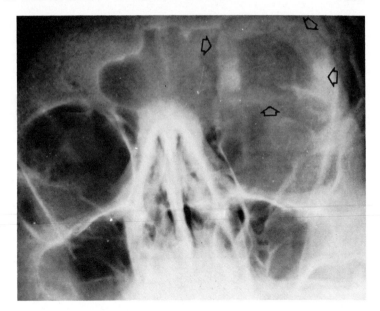

Figure 62. This 38 year old man had a two months' history of left exophthalmos. Osteolysis of the roof of the left orbit, lateral wall, and floor of the left frontal sinus is revealed on this Waters view (arrows). Pathologic report: Xanthoma.

angiofibroma, and chordoma. The reticuloendothelioses (Fig. 62), Wegener's granulomatosis (Fig. 63), and fibrous dysplasia with rhinologic and paranasal sinus involvement may also cause osteolysis.

Dehiscence. Dehiscence in a bony wall usually refers to a smooth, discrete, well defined bony defect. This is seen in several different conditions, the commonest being mucocele (Fig. 64) (Gorlin et al., 1963; Baxter,

1966; Zizmor and Noyek, 1968). The mucocele, as an intrinsic, expanding, destructive, cystic lesion, resulting from the continued accumulation of secretions within a blocked sinus cavity, commonly produces an expanding erosion of bone, with a loss of mucoperiosteum and scalloping. This results in a smooth bony dehiscence. Mucoceles occur in the frontal and ethmoid sinuses (Fig. 65) in a ratio of two to one; they are rare in the maxillary (Fig. 66),

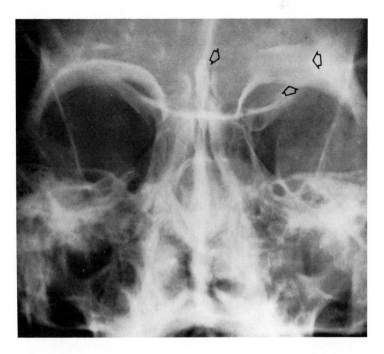

Figure 63. A 35 year old man had a two weeks' history of left exophthalmos, one month of malaise, anorexia, weight loss, and nasal obstruction. Note cloudy frontal and ethmoid sinuses and nasal cavities, smooth erosion of the roof of the left orbit and expansion of the left supraorbital ethmoid (Waters view). Surgical specimens from nasal cavities and left frontal sinus showed Wegener's granulomatosis.

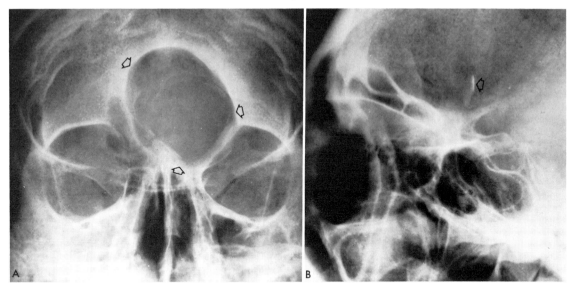

Figure 64. Waters view of a 55 year old woman with a long history of sinusitis, a three year history of left exophthalmos, and a compressible bulge of soft tissues over the left frontal sinus. Note the classic smooth dehiscence and expansion of the walls of the left frontal sinus, erosion into the left orbit, and marginal bone sclerosis. *B*, lateral view reveals a fragment of frontal bone displaced by deep intracranial extension of the mucocele. This radiographic finding may be associated with increased intracranial pressure due to displacement of the brain stem and interference with circulation of cerebrospinal fluid at the foramen magnum.

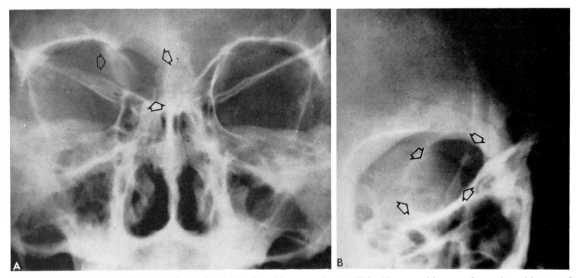

Figure 65. *A*, Caldwell view of classic right ethmoid mucocele. *B*, This 48 year old man after a long history of sinusitis developed a right exophthalmos. There is a large oval bony dehiscence in the medial wall of the right orbit in the plane of the right superior ethmoid cells. It is seen best in the oblique orbital view (*B*) (arrows).

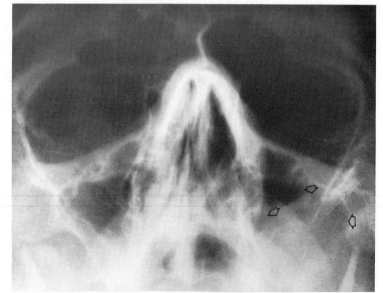

Figure 66. Waters view of left antral mucocele. This 61 year old man had a left maxillary antrotomy six years previously. He now presents with swelling in the left cheek and buccogingival fold. A mucocele was found at operation.

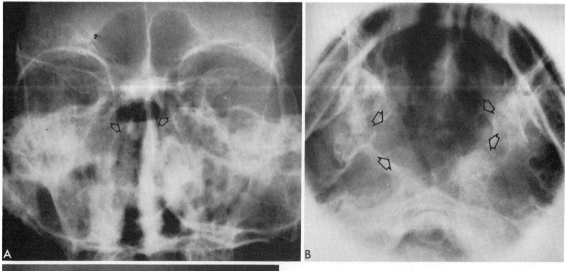

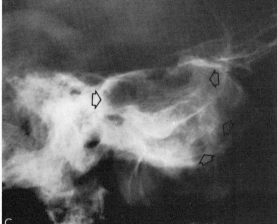

Figure 67. *A,* This is a 73 year old man with a long history of sinusitis, and frontal and occipital headaches. During instrumentation of the nasopharynx, a large cyst was punctured, and brown mucoid fluid was discharged. Caldwell view of sphenoid mucocele. There is a fluid level in the sphenoids (arrows). The basal (*B*) and lateral (*C*) views show erosion of the bony walls of the sphenoid sinuses associated with reactive sclerosing osteitis (arrows).

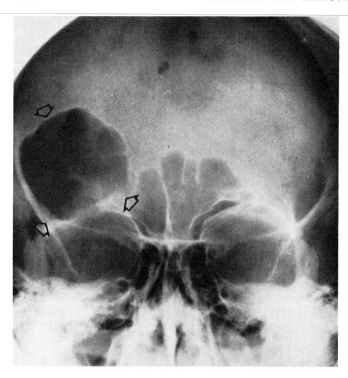

Figure 68. Caldwell view of primary cholesteatoma or epidermoidoma of the cranial vault invading the right orbit and frontal sinus. A woman aged 50 had a right forehead swelling and right proptosis for three years. Note the dehiscence of bone which has a well maintained mucoperiosteal border with short septal extensions and scalloping, in contrast to their usual absence with mucocele.

and extremely rare in the sphenoid (Fig. 67) sinuses. The high incidence of frontoethmoidal mucoceles suggests that blockage of drainage through their dependent ostia, most often by inflammation and rarely by fracture or osteoma, must be the important etiologic factor.

Cholesteatoma, a much rarer condition, may simulate mucocele as an expansile, benign, cystic, bone-eroding lesion (Figs. 68 and 69). Primary cholesteatoma or epidermoidoma may arise from congenital epithelial cell rests in the meninges, or in the diploe of the cranial vault or base of the skull. A second possible origin of cholesteatoma is by metaplasia of respira-

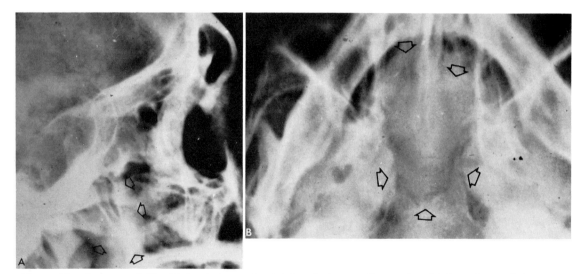

Figure 69. A man aged 68 with headaches and ophthalmoplegia was diagnosed as having primary cholesteatoma involving the sella and sphenoid sinuses with extension into the nasopharynx and posterior nasal cavities. *A,* Note opacification of sphenoids, disappearance of mucoperiosteal borders, erosion of sella, and nasopharyngeal mass (arrows) in lateral view. These radiographic findings could also be caused by sphenoidal mucocele. *B,* Arrows in basal view point to eroded margins of sphenoid sinuses and anterior extension of cholesteatoma into nasal cavities. Proved surgically.

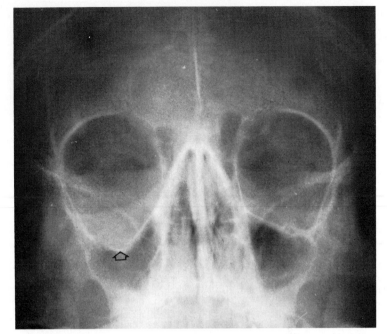

Figure 70. Waters view of blowout fracture of the right orbit with sagging of the orbital floor into the upper third of the right antrum (arrow).

tory epithelium to stratified squamous keratinizing epithelium within the sinus. Other lesions producing bony dehiscence are meningocele, encephalocele (Fig. 25), dental cysts (Figs. 22, 23, and 24), and surgical resections.

Fractures. Fractures are often obvious, but sometimes must be inferred from secondary signs such as emphysema of soft tissue of the orbit or cheek due to escape of air through a fractured sinus wall, or opacification of the sinus lumen with or without the appearance of

a fluid level as a result of hemorrhage (Pendergrass et al., 1956; Zizmor et al., 1962; Vinik and Gargano, 1966; Valvassori and Hord, 1968). Tomography is often of value for a precise diagnosis of fracture when routine radiographic studies are negative or equivocal. Most fractures are the result of trauma; occasionally pathologic fracture with fragmentation is due to underlying tumor or bone dysplasia (Figs. 70, 71, 72, and 73).

Osteoblastosis and Hyperostosis with Thicken-

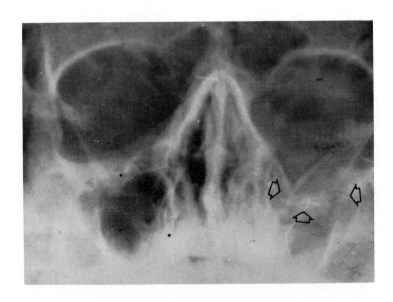

Figure 71. Waters view reveals comminuted fracture of the floor and rim of the left orbit from direct trauma. Note the displacement of bone fragments into the upper half of the left antrum (arrows), and clouding of the left antrum as a result of edema and hemorrhage.

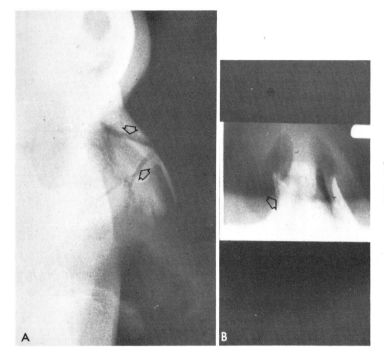

Figure 72. A, Lateral view reveals comminuted fracture of the right nasal bone (arrows). B, Superoinferior axial view reveals lateral displacement of fragment of right nasal bone (arrow).

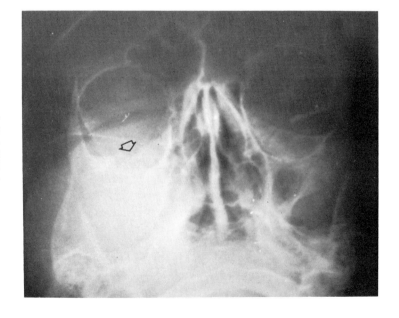

Figure 73. Waters view reveals advanced squamous cell carcinoma of the right antrum with extensive bone destruction, opaque antrum, and invasion of orbit, cheek, zygoma, nose, and hard palate. Note fracture of right inferior orbital rim and floor (arrow).

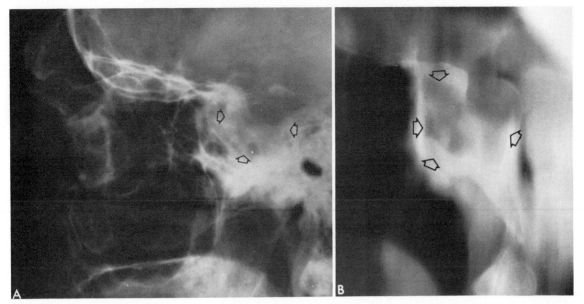

Figure 74. *A*, Lateral view of sinuses in a man aged 60 who had headaches and papilledema. Surgery had been performed for melanoma of lower extremity 10 years before. *B*, Lateral tomogram reveals a sphenoidal mucocele which has caused sclerosing osteitis with bony thickening of walls of the sphenoid sinus (arrows), sellar erosion, and intracranial extension. (Courtesy of Dr. E. Strong, New York.)

ing of Bony Walls. Chronic osteomyelitis (Fig. 74), meningioma, osteoblastic metastases, fibrous dysplasia (Fig. 75), Paget's disease (Fig. 76), infantile cortical hyperostosis, and Albers-Schönberg disease cause bony thickening with osteoblastosis and hyperostosis (Zizmor and Noyek, 1968). Healed fractures of nasal bones and sinus walls often show residual bony thickening. Thickening of the walls of the paranasal sinuses will diminish their lumina proportionately.

Expansion and Displacement of Bony Walls. Expansion and displacement of the bony walls of the paranasal sinuses can involve, in varying

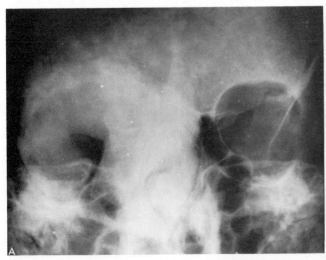

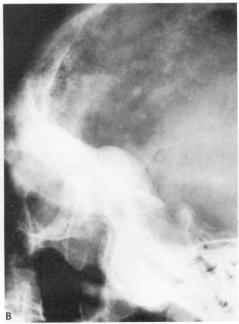

Figure 75. Hyperostotic bone of fibrous dysplasia blocks and expands the right nasal cavity and encroaches on the right orbit, causing unilateral exophthalmos. The right ethmoid and the sphenoid sinuses are obliterated by hyperostotic bone. *A*, Caldwell view; *B*, lateral view.

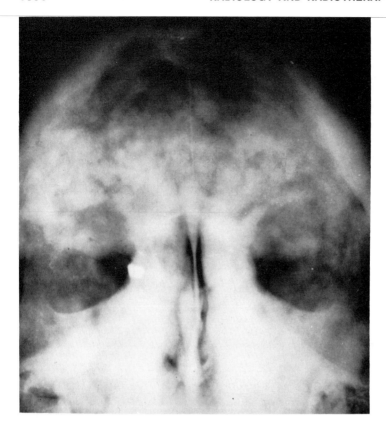

Figure 76. Caldwell view of dense bony thickening of Paget's disease, which largely obliterates frontals, ethmoids, antra, and nasal cavities, and blocks lipiodol in the right nasolacrimal sac. The interorbital distance has widened; the orbits are diminished in volume.

degrees, adjacent structures such as the dentition, the orbits, and various foramina in and about the paranasal sinuses (Gorlin et al., 1963; Lewin-Epstein et al., 1965; Zizmor and Noyek, 1968).

Chronic hypertrophic polypoid sinusitis (Figs. 54 and 56), usually indicated by mucosal thickening and polypoid change, may produce the picture of expansion of the sinuses and nasal cavities with decalcification, thinning, and displacement of adjacent bony walls. Granulomata associated with rhinoscleroma (Fig.

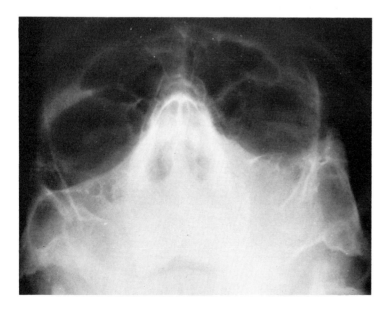

Figure 77. Waters view of expansion of both antra by rhinoscleroma. A 48 year old man from Central America had chronic nasal obstruction for years. Biopsy of granulomatous tissue from the nasal cavities and antra revealed rhinoscleroma. Radiography reveals very cloudy antra whose walls have expanded and thinned. Both antra have expanded into the zygomatic bodies. The floor of the left orbit is elevated. The nasal cavities are filled with soft tissue. The nasal bones are thinned.

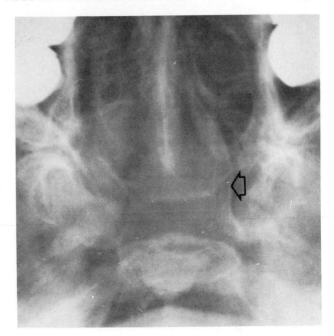

Figure 78. Base view of a woman aged 49 with occipital and frontal headaches. Note the cloudy expanded right sphenoid with bulge of the intersinus septum to the left (arrow). A sphenoid sinusectomy was performed and polypoid soft tissue was removed. Histological diagnosis: epithelial papilloma.

77) may expand the antra and nasal cavities. Among the tumors of the paranasal sinuses which may produce expansion, displacement, and thinning of bony walls are inverting papilloma (Fig. 78), the odontomas, both compound and complex, and ameloblastoma.

The compound odontoma (Fig. 51), contains masses of small malformed teeth which are referred to as denticles; the complex odontoma appears as a radiopaque irregular mass.

The ameloblastoma, a destructive epithelial tumor arising from the dental anlage of the enamel organ, arises in about one fifth of patients in the maxilla, usually in the canine region (Pantazopoulos and Nomikos, 1966). It may also arise in a dentigerous cyst. In either

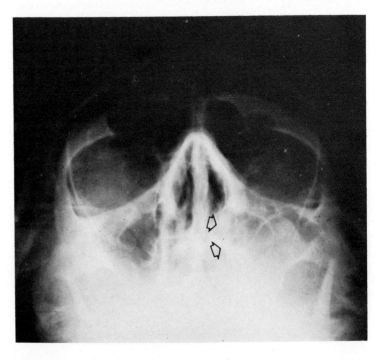

Figure 79. Waters view of a 43 year old man with a rounded mass in the left antrum displacing the nasoantral wall medially. Biopsy of the mass revealed adenocarcinoma.

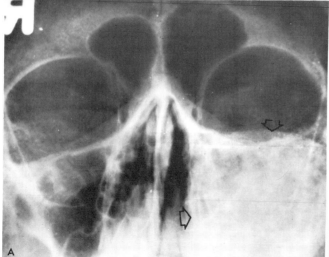

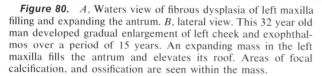

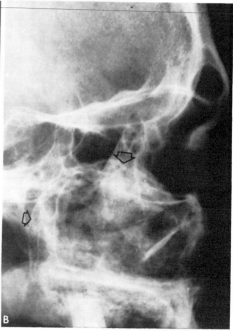

Figure 80. *A*, Waters view of fibrous dysplasia of left maxilla filling and expanding the antrum. *B*, lateral view. This 32 year old man developed gradual enlargement of left cheek and exophthalmos over a period of 15 years. An expanding mass in the left maxilla fills the antrum and elevates its roof. Areas of focal calcification, and ossification are seen within the mass.

event it tends to invade the maxillary antrum and to produce expansion, thinning, decalcification, and dehiscence of its bony walls.

A malignant tumor, in the course of its development, may cause a bony sinus wall to bulge outward (Fig. 79). Fibrous dysplasia may cause a similar expansion of the bony walls of the nasal and sinus cavities (Fig. 80).

Decreased Luminal Volume. Partial or complete failure to develop a lumen may be seen with agenesis (Fig. 81), or hypoplasia (Fig. 82), of any of the paranasal sinuses, or in choanal

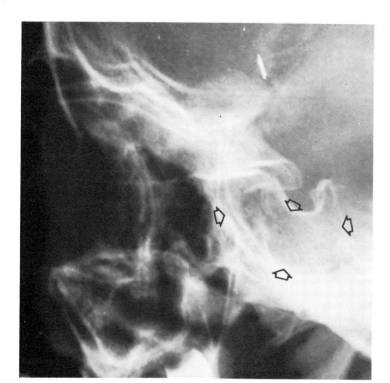

Figure 81. Note solid diploic bone in plane of the body of the sphenoid due to complete failure of pneumatization with resulting agenesis of sphenoid sinuses. Lateral view.

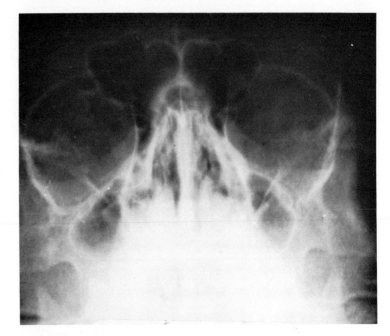

Figure 82. Waters view reveals clear antra with thick bony walls due to incomplete pneumatization in a 10 year old boy.

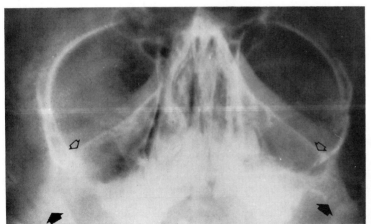

Figure 83. Waters view of a six year old boy with mandibulofacial dysostosis. Note downward slope of antral roofs laterally (hollow arrows) and hypoplastic zygomatic development (black arrows).

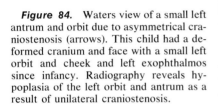

Figure 84. Waters view of a small left antrum and orbit due to asymmetrical craniostenosis (arrows). This child had a deformed cranium and face with a small left orbit and cheek and left exophthalmos since infancy. Radiography reveals hypoplasia of the left orbit and antrum as a result of unilateral craniostenosis.

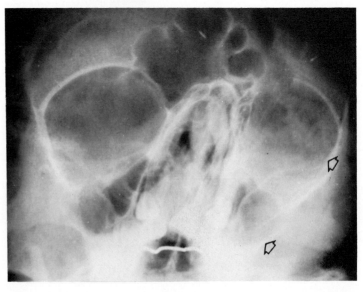

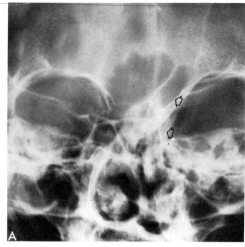 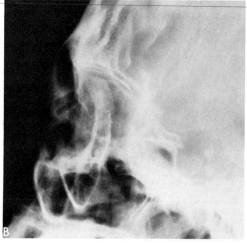

Figure 85. This is a 42 year old man with turricephaly, prominent eyes, and failing vision. *A,* Caldwell view. Note distortion of left frontal and ethmoidal sinuses (arrows) and widened interorbital distance. *B,* Lateral view. Note foreshortened anterior fossa, nasal passages, orbits, antra, sphenoids, and ethmoids. Diagnosis: craniostenosis with turricephaly.

atresia (Pendergrass et al., 1956). (See Figure 11.) Various congenital syndromes such as cleidocranial dysostosis, maxillonasal dysplasia, progeria, mandibulofacial dysostosis, and craniostenosis (Figs. 83, 84, and 85) may be associated with small or malformed lumina and bony walls of the paranasal sinuses (Gorlin and Sedano, 1968). In chronic infection with sclerosing osteitis (Fig. 74), thickening of bone may result in a diminution of sinus volume. Similarly, hyperostosis due to Paget's disease (Fig. 76), fibrous dysplasia (Fig. 75), and certain osteoblastic metastases may produce a decrease of sinus lumen by thickening of the bony walls. Radiation injury to bone in childhood will arrest normal sinus development. Surgical procedures may produce luminal obliteration, either partial or complete.

REFERENCES

Baxter, J. S. R.: Cholesteatoma of the maxillary antrum. J. Laryng. *80:*1059, 1966.

Beekhuis, G. J., and Watson, T. H.: Mid-facial cysts. Arch Otolaryng. *85:*62, 1967.

Berdal, P., and Myrhe, E.: Cranial chordomas involving the paranasal sinuses. J. Laryng. *78:*906, 1964.

Blumenfeld, R. L., and Skolnik, E. M.: Intranasal encephaloceles. Arch. Otolaryng. *82:*527, 1965.

Buda, J. A., Conley, J. J., and Rankow, R.: Carcinoma of the maxillary sinus following Thorotrast instillation. Amer. J. Surg. *106:*868, 1963.

Caldwell, W. E.: Further observations on the roentgen ray examination of the accessory nasal sinuses. Laryngoscope *18:*855, 1908.

Cody, C. C.: Inverting papilloma of the nose and sinuses. Laryngoscope *77:*584, 1967.

Forestier, J., and Sicard, J.: Méthode génerale d'exploration radiologique par l'huile iode (Lipiodol). Bull. Mém. Soc. Méd. d' Hôp Paris *46:*463–469, 1922.

Fuchs, A. W.: Optic foramina, ethmoidal sinuses and orbits (Rhese). Radiography *8:*6, 1932.

Gorlin, R. J., and Sedano, H. O.: Syndromes involving the sinuses—congenital and acquired. Seminars Roentgen. *3*(2):133–147, 1968.

Gorlin, R. J., Meskin, L. H., and Brodey, R.: Odontogenic tumors in man and animals. Pathologic classification and clinical behaviour — A review. Ann. N. Y. Acad. Sci. *108:*722, 1963.

Krayenbuhl, H.: Diagnostic value of orbital angiography. Brit. J. Ophthal. *42:*180–190, 1952.

Krayenbuhl, H.: The value of orbital angiography for diagnosis of unilateral exophthalmos. J. Neurosurg. *19:*281–301, April, 1962.

Larsson, L. G., and Martensson, G.: Carcinoma of the paranasal sinuses and the nasal cavities: A clinical study of 379 cases treated at Radiumhemmet and the otolaryngologic department of Karolinska Sjukhuset, 1940-1950. Acta Radiol. *42:*149–172, 1954.

Lewin-Epstein, J., Ulmansky, M., Oberman, M., and Gay, I.: Ameloblastic fibroma of the maxilla. J. Laryng. *79:*976, 1965.

Merrell, R. A., Jr., and Yanagisawa, E.: (1, Water's View): Yanagisawa, E., Smith, H. W., and Thaler, S. (2, Lateral View): Radiographic anatomy of the paranasal sinuses. Arch. Otolaryng. (Chicago) *87:*184–209, 1968.

Merrill, V.: Atlas of Roentgenographic Positions. St. Louis, The C. V. Mosby Co., 1967.

Møller-Christensen, V. L., and Inkster, R. G.: Cases of leprosy and syphilis in the Osteological Collection of the Department of Anatomy, University of Edinburgh. Danish Med. Bull. *12:*11, 1965.

Moore, S.: Body section roentgenography with laminography. Amer. J. Roentgen. *39:*514–522, 1938.

Pantazopoulos, P. E., and Nomikos, N.: Adamantinoma of the maxillary sinus. Ann. Otolaryng. *75:*1160, 1966.

Paparella, M. M.: Mucosal cyst of the maxillary sinus. Arch. Otolaryng. *77:*650, 1963.

Pendergrass, E. P., Schaeffer, J. P., and Hodes, P. J.: The

Head and Neck in Roentgen Diagnosis. Vol. 1. Springfield, Ill., Charles C Thomas, 1956.

Proetz, A. W.: Displacement method in sinus diagnosis and treatment; its advantages and limitations. Trans. Amer. Laryng. Ass. *52*:121–140, 1930.

Rosen, L., Hanafee, W., and Nahum, A.: Nasopharyngeal angiofibroma, an angiographic evaluation. Radiology *86*:103–107, 1966.

Samuel, E.: Clinical Radiology of the Ear, Nose and Throat. New York, Paul B. Hoeber, 1952.

Samuel, E.: Inflammatory diseases of the nose and paranasal sinuses. Seminars Roentgen. *3*(2):148–159, 1968.

Schuknecht, H. F., and Lindsay, J. R.: Benign cysts of the paranasal sinuses. Arch. Otolaryng. *49*:609, 1949.

Stuart, E. A.: An otolaryngic aspect of frontal meningocele. Arch. Otolaryng. *40*:171, 1944.

Valvassori, G. E., and Hord, G. E.: Traumatic sinus disease. Seminars Roentgen. *3*:160, 1968.

Vinik, M., and Gargano, F. P.: Orbital fractures. Amer. J. Roentgen. *97*:607, 1966.

Waters, C. A., and Waldron, C. W.: Roentgenology of the accessory nasal sinuses describing a modification of the occipito-frontal position. Amer. J. Roentgen. *2*:633, 1915.

Young, B. R.: The Skull, Sinuses and Mastoids. Chicago, Year Book Medical Publishers, Inc., 1948.

Zizmor, J., and Noyek, A. M.: Cysts and benign tumors of the paranasal sinuses. Seminars Roentgen. *3*:172, 1968.

Zizmor, J., Noyek, A. M., Bellucci, R. J., Gutkin, M. L., and Vermes, E.: The pre-operative diagnosis of brain abscess by the roentgenologic demonstration of an air-fluid level. Amer. J. Roentgen. *92*:844, 1964.

Zizmor, J., Smith, B., Fasano, C., and Converse, J. M.: Roentgen diagnosis of blow-out fractures of the orbit. Amer. J. Roentgen. *87*:1009, 1962.

Chapter 47

DIAGNOSTIC RADIOLOGY

DIAGNOSTIC RADIOLOGY OF THE SALIVARY GLANDS

by

George A. Gates, M.D.

Radiographic evaluation of patients with salivary gland disorders is a helpful and often indispensable method for differentiating between the many causes of salivary tumefactions and enlargements. This is particularly true when calculi and chronic inflammation are present. The two radiographic techniques for examination of the salivary glands are plain films and contrast studies. Plain films are used to detect radiopaque abnormalities in or around the salivary glands such as foreign bodies, calculi, or calcifying disorders, and to determine if abnormalities of the adjacent osseous structures exist. Contrast studies (sialograms) demonstrate abnormalities of the ductal system such as stricture, fistula, ectasia and neoplasm, and abnormalities within the ductal system such as radiolucent calculi. For sialography the contrast material is instilled in a retrograde manner. Intravenous excretory sialography must await future technical advances. Salivary gland scanning (radiosialography) is a newer diagnostic technique which has been of value in evaluating patients with salivary gland neoplasms. In some cases, especially those of recent onset, the radiographic findings may be subtle, equivocal, and subject to interpretation based upon other clinical findings. In most cases, however, the radiographic findings are sufficiently definitive to delineate the extent of the disease process and to substantiate the proper diagnosis.

INDICATIONS AND TECHNIQUE

Plain films are indicated when calculi are suspected; they should be made in every case of suppurative submandibular sialadenitis because of the high incidence of calculi. Calculi are rarely associated with acute suppurative parotitis but should be suspected in recurrent cases. The occasional case in which a calculus clinically simulates a parotid neoplasm warrants consideration of plain films in patients with solitary masses. Dystrophic calcification in or about the salivary glands is uncommon and usually results from tuberculous lymphadenitis. Anomalies and disease of the mandible (such as winged mandible or neoplasm, which may simulate a parotid mass) may be identified in the plain films. Involvement of adjacent bony structures by malignant salivary neoplasms may require plain film examination for documentation and assessment. Plain films are made routinely prior to sialography to determine the adequacy of exposure and to exclude the presence of radiopaque material before injection of the contrast agent.

A variety of head positions and film types are available and it may be necessary to employ all to detect calculi. The lateral and posteroanterior (PA) views are obtained routinely. In addition, the submentovertical view of the skull should be obtained because it displays the floor of the mouth without the overlying mandibular shadow. Intra–oral dental films provide good definition of the parotid and submandibular ductal areas. Superimposition of the stone and the facial skeleton is a common cause of non-visualization of calculi; multiple views from differing angles may be necessary (Fig. 1). Submandibular calculi may be nicely displayed if the patient depresses the floor of his mouth with his finger. This displaces the calculus below the mandibular shadow, and the finger becomes a built–in radiographic pointer (Fig. 2). The use of high definition industrial film and low voltage exposure overcomes problems in locating tiny calculi that may be encountered when coarse grained film is used.

Sialography

The principal indication for retrograde contrast sialography is for evaluation of patients with recurrent inflammatory swellings of the salivary glands. This clinical situation occurs in a number of heterogeneous pathological entities whose accurate diagnosis is often based upon the sialographic findings.

Sialography is indicated in the evaluation of patients with calculi: (1) when the calculus is radiopaque (20 per cent of patients); (2) when clinically suspected and the plain films are negative because of the small size of the stone or technical errors in taking the films; (3) to determine the location of the calculus in relationship to the gland parenchyma in order to plan for surgical removal; and (4) when the presence or absence of secondary ductal strictures or dilatation is important for therapeutic reasons.

Sialographic evaluation of patients with suspected neoplastic disease is considered when the clinician desires to know if the mass is intraglandular or extraglandular, when the mass is

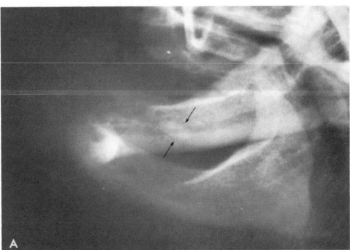

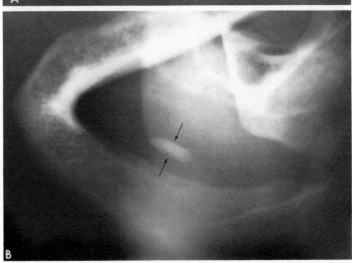

Figure 1. Calculus of the left submandibular duct. In *A* the calculus is obscured by the overlying shadow of the mandible. With rotation of the head as in *B* the calculus is seen to better advantage.

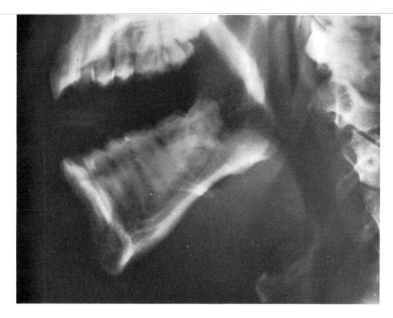

Figure 2. Submandibular duct calculus. The patient places his index finger over the calculus and depresses the floor of the mouth. Radiographically the calculus may be seen just ahead of the fingertip and well away from the body of the mandible.

poorly delineated by physical examination, or when routine studies cannot exclude a diagnosis of inflammatory disease. The frequent occurrence of inflammatory or allergic sialadenitis following contrast sialography limits its usefulness for routine preoperative assessment of clinically evident neoplasms.

Sialography is contraindicated in the presence of acute inflammatory disorders and when a history of sensitivity to iodides exists.

To perform sialography, the ductal orifices of the parotid and or submandibular glands must first be dilated to permit catheter placement. Following the use of a lacrimal dilator, the duct is probed with increasing sizes of probes to rule out the presence of stricture or stone. A number 60 polyethylene catheter is gently introduced into the duct and threaded proximally. Introduction of the catheter is facilitated by tapering of the end of the catheter and by the use of a stylet. The parotid duct is readily located and dilated, but the catheter can be advanced usually for only a short distance because of the bend where the duct curves around the anterior border of the masseter muscle. Undue pressure at this point leads to perforation and extravasation of the dye into the soft tissues. The submandibular duct orifice is smaller and more difficult to dilate, but once introduced the catheter advances easily and is less likely to become dislodged. After scout films are obtained, Pantopaque is slowly injected into the catheter until the patient notes fullness and discomfort in the gland. To avoid overinjection, it is important to fill the duct to the patient's tolerance, rather than to a predetermined volume. Overinjection produces a cloud effect which obscures ductal detail. Usually 0.6 to 0.8 ml. will produce satisfactory filling. Glands with large sialectatic spaces will accept a larger volume before discomfort results. Once filled, the catheter is occluded and radiographs are exposed. The developed films are examined and, if satisfactory, the catheter is withdrawn and the patient is instructed to chew on a fresh lemon for one minute. Normal glands will expel the contrast material within five minutes in response to this potent salivary stimulus. The term "secretory sialography," therefore, is used to indicate the physiological measurement obtained by this study (Blatt and Maxwell, 1957). If dye is retained in the five-minute postevacuation film, repeat films are obtained at 30 minutes, 60 minutes, and 24 hours. Pantopaque, (ethyl iodophenyl undecylate), is an oily iodized fatty acid which has proven to be ideal for sialography (Rubin et al., 1955). Its low viscosity permits excellent mixing with salivary secretions and little tendency toward droplet formation.

The radiographs are best taken in a room equipped for skull examination and may be made with the patient seated or recumbent. Scout films are obtained with the catheter(s) in place in the PA, Grainger, and lateral projections and are repeated following injection of contrast and again following emptying of the glands. Stereoscopic views of the filled glands are preferred.

Radiosialography

The indications for radiosialography (salivary gland scanning) depend upon the experience and surgical philosophy of the institution employing this diagnostic technique. Radiosialography is a relatively new procedure and has not yet been widely adopted. This procedure has been used routinely for patients with masses in the salivary gland areas since 1967 at the University of Michigan Medical Center. Based upon this experience, radiosialography has been helpful in the following situations: (1) in diagnosing the Warthin's tumor; (2) in searching for occult primaries in cases of cervical metastasis; (3) in confirming the presence and the extent of a neoplasm; and (4) occasionally, in distinguishing between benign and malignant disease.

Salivary gland scans utilize the same instrumentation and basic scintiscan techniques employed for thyroid scanning with 99m technetium pertechnetate. Atropine, 0.8 to 1.0 mg., is given 30 minutes prior to the intravenous injection of 4 mC. of pertechnetate, and scanning is begun 15 to 20 minutes later. Using the mandible, tragus, and outer canthi for landmarks, two lateral views are obtained on each side with the three inch, fine focus, low-energy collimator, positioned first at one inch and then at two and one half inches from the skin surface. This method, which produces scintiscan sections of both the deep and superficial parts of the gland, allows the lesion to be localized and produces more positive scans than with the single lateral view alone. Radiation exposure is minimal, and there have been no untoward reactions with this technique.

INTERPRETATION

Plain Films

In the normal person the salivary gland outlines are not evident on plain films nor is radiopaque material present (Fig. 3). It is generally accepted that approximately 80 per cent of salivary calculi are radiopaque, and it is commonly recognized that, because of technical problems, only about 50 per cent are seen on plain film x-ray. A negative x-ray, therefore, does not exclude a diagnosis of calculus disease, and further examination should be carried out.

Sialography

The normal ductal sialogram has an arboreal configuration; each distal branch is smaller than its predecessor and leaves it at an acute angle. The single, large, main collecting or excretory duct is from 40 to 60 mm. in length and 2 to 3

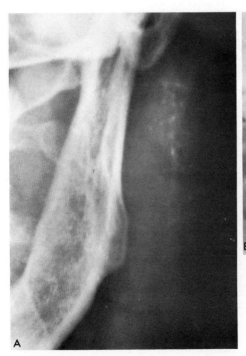
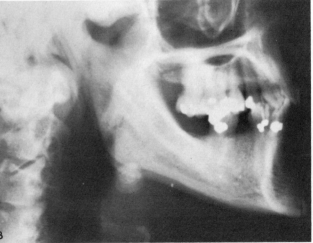

Figure 3. Multiple sialolithiases. *A*, Multiple calcifications are seen in the parotid gland in an adult patient with longstanding, recurrent, suppurative parotitis. The sialogram was normal; this represents a dystrophic calcification within the salivary gland. *B*, A large, spherical, laminated, submandibular calculus within the hilum of the gland is displayed in this lateral plain film.

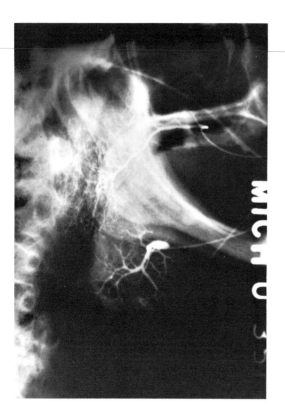

Figure 4. Simultaneous parotid and submandibular sialogram reveals normal architecture in both glands. The branching pattern of the ductal system is clearly visible in both glands. In this, the filling phase, the catheters through which the contrast was injected are also visible.

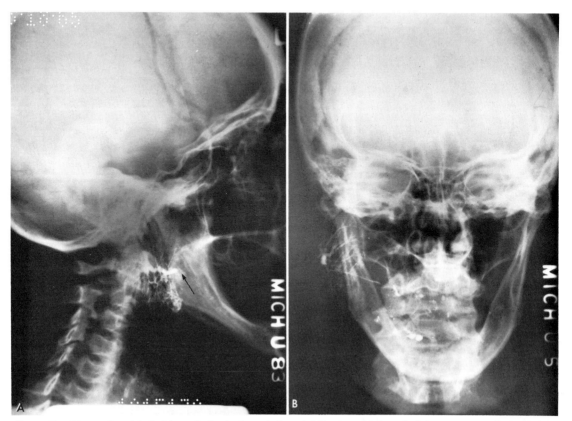

Figure 5. Obstructive sialodochiectasis. In the lateral view *A* following withdrawal of the catheter and stimulation of the gland (by chewing on a lemon), the contrast material is retained because of a radiolucent calculus (arrow) which is preventing expulsion of the Pantopaque. In the anterior view (*B*) the dilated main duct is also seen. In addition, the small amount of contrast material is seen in the floor of the mouth.

mm. in diameter, but its entire length is seldom seen because of the presence of the catheter within the distal lumen. The main duct receives the interlobar ducts, which are variable in number, the most distal one being from the accessory lobe. The interlobar ducts are formed by the interlobular ducts which, in turn, arise from the intralobular ducts. The latter drain secretions from the acini via the intercalated ducts. Normally the main duct and the first three orders of branches can be visualized sialographically (Fig. 4). The acini and intercalated ducts are too small and too numerous to be seen as discrete structures; when filled, as in the overinjected sialogram, they impart a hazy cloud effect to the sialogram.

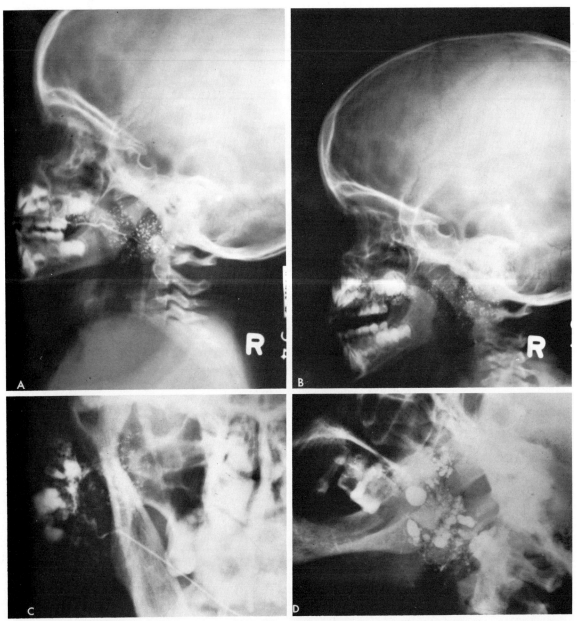

Figure 6. Nonobstructive sialodochiectasis. In the filling phase (*A*) the ductal system and sialectatic intralobular ducts are seen. In the secretory phase (*B*) the gland has incompletely emptied, and retained contrast material in the sialectatic spaces may be seen. This is congenital sialectasis seen in an eight year old child with recurrent episodes of suppurative parotitis. All degrees of sialectasis are seen in the PA filling film (*C*) and lateral emptying film (*D*) of a 45 year old female with Sjögren's syndrome. Nonemptying sialectatic spaces varying from punctate to cavitary in size are located throughout the gland.

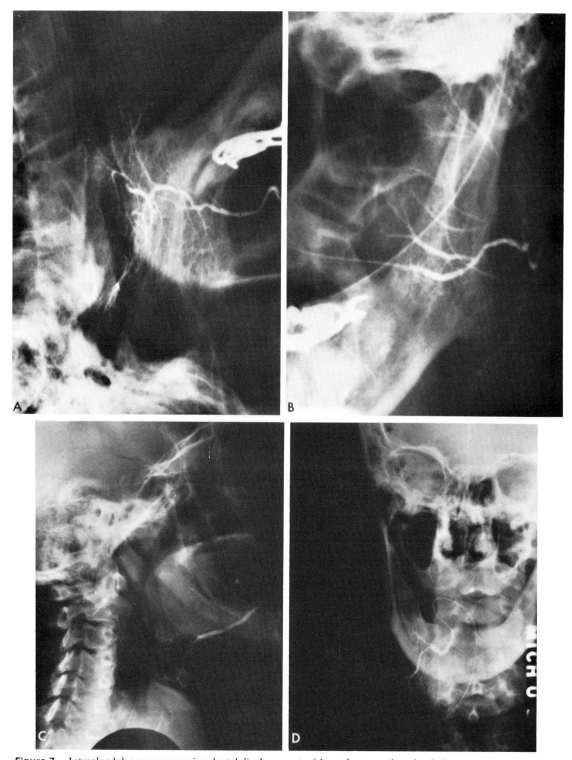

Figure 7. Intraglandular masses causing ductal displacement without dye retention simulating extraglandular masses. In the lateral (A) and PA (B) views stretching, straightening, and displacement of the ductal system is seen secondary to a benign mixed tumor of the parotid gland. A similar alteration of the submandibular ductal system is seen in the lateral (C) and PA (D) views of a patient with a benign mixed tumor.

(Illustration continued on opposite page.)

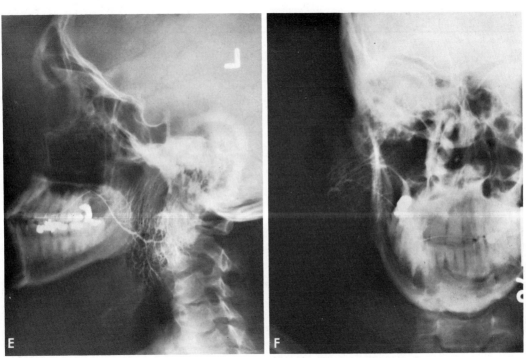

Figure 7 (*Continued*).   In a patient with fatty atrophy of the parotid gland the lateral (*E*) and PA (*F*) views disclose marked straightening and stretching of the ductal system, simulating an intraglandular neoplasm.

Sialographic examination will demonstrate the normal ductal architecture as well as any abnormalities causing obstruction, dilation, distortion, or destruction of the ductal system; and it provides, therefore, both positive and negative diagnostic information. Obstructive sialodochiectasis denotes the dilation and tortuosity of the main salivary duct, which occurs secondarily to the obstruction caused by calculi or by stricture (Fig. 5). Pneumococcal parotitis may result in multiple strictures, giving the main duct the appearance of a string of sausages. Nonobstructive sialodochiectasis describes the picture of dilated quaternary or intralobular ducts, which is commonly known as sialectasis (Fig. 6). The degree of ectasia is variable and progresses from the barely perceptible punctate stage to the globular, the cavitary, and, finally, in advanced conditions, the destructive stage. Many different pathological conditions produce sialectasis. It may be congenital, in which case all the glands are involved and infection is a secondary pheonomenon. It may be secondary to a suppurative sialadenitis and will be seen only in the affected gland. It is seen in all major salivary glands in established cases of benign lymphoepithelial lesion (Sjögren–Mikulicz disease). Retention of contrast material following gustatory stimulation is a prominent finding in sialectasis, but it is less commonly seen in obstructive sialodochiectasis except when ball-valving with calculi occurs.

Masses which displace the ductal system without causing significant dye retention in the emptying phase are probably benign in character and extrinsic to the gland proper (Fig. 7). When retention of the dye occurs without destruction of the ductal architecture, a benign intraglandular mass may be said to be present. Invasive masses not only displace the ductal system but invade the ductal walls and allow the contrast to pool within the destroyed segments of the gland (Fig. 8). Histologic identification of the tumor type cannot be inferred from the sialographic appearance (Blatt et al., 1956). It would be injudicious, therefore (on the basis of a normal sialogram or a sialogram that is interpreted as benign), to fail to obtain a tissue diagnosis when neoplasm is clinically suspected.

Radiolucent calculi appear as filling defects, but care must be taken to avoid injection of air bubbles which produce a similar appearance. The position of the calculus in relation to the hilum and duct orifice may be determined by sialography. With longstanding calculi and secondary inflammation, the sialographic presence of ductal strictures and poor gland emptying may signify the need for removal of the gland as well as of the calculus.

Radiosialography

The normal distribution of radioactivity within the salivary glands is shown in Figure 9*A*. The prior administration of atropine decreases or eliminates secretion of radioactive saliva into the oral cavity (Fig. 9 *B*). Excessive oral radioactivity interferes with visualization of the salivary glands because of overlapping areas of activity. The normal parotid gland outline is a smooth oval, being slightly wider above. The gland assumes a triangular shape in the superficial section because of the thin anterior part, which overlaps the masseter muscle. The submandibular gland may be round or multilobulated. The glands are symmetrical in the same patient but may vary considerably from patient to patient. The scan density of the gland is not uniform; it is greatest where the gland is thickest and least at the margins. When the uptake is low, the gland outline may appear irregular.

Abnormalities in the pictorial display of the salivary gland radioactivity provided by scintiscans fall into two general classes: radionegative (cold) lesions and radiopositive (hot) lesions. Radionegative lesions in salivary gland scans have been of two types, those with smooth margins and those with irregular margins. Smooth margined cold nodules appear in approximately 50 per cent of patients with benign, mixed tumors (Fig. 10). This scan finding occurs with other benign tumors as well as in patients with lymphoma, parotid cysts and, uncommonly, in cases of preinvasive malignant neoplasm (Fig. 11). Irregularly margined cold lesions involving 25 per cent or more of the scan outline of the gland have been principally associated with malignant primary salivary gland neoplasms, although patients with lymphoma, Sjögren's disease, and severe inflammatory disorders have occasionally exhibited the same scan abnormality (Fig. 12). Discrete radiopositive lesions have occurred only in cases of Warthin's tumor (Fig. 13).

A normal scan does not exclude disease; false negative scans occur in approximately 20 per cent of patients. This may be due to the size of the lesion, to a lack of radioactive contrast between the gland and the lesion, or to technical errors. Lesions less that 1 cm. in diameter cannot be accurately detected by radiosialography.

(*Text continued on page 1112*)

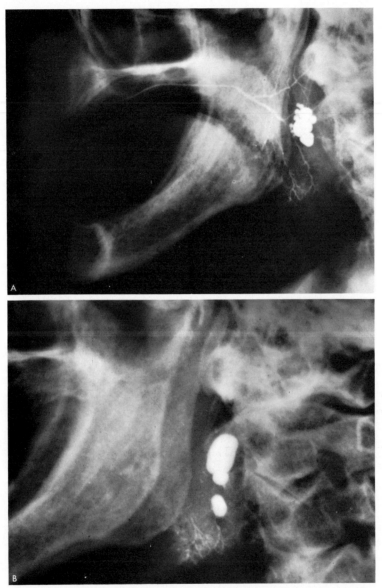

Figure 8. Malignant neoplasm. In the lateral view of the filling phase (*A*), displacement of the ductal system is seen as well as extravasation of dye into the glandular substance. In the secretory phase (*B*), retention of contrast material in the extravasated space as well as in the ductal lumina is noted.

Normal Radiosialogram
(no atropine)

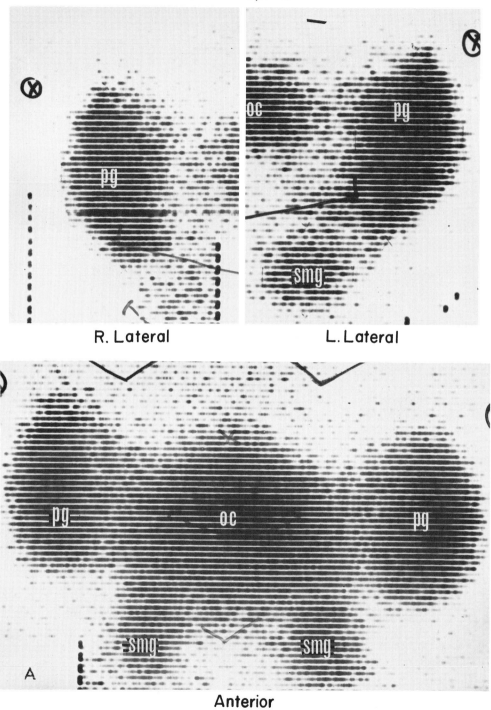

R. Lateral   **L. Lateral**

Anterior

Figure 9. *A,* A normal radiosialogram made with 4mC 99mTc without atropine is shown. Note the symmetrical distribution of radioactivity within the parotids (p.g.) and submandibular glands (smg) and the heavy radioactivity in the oral cavity (oc). (X = tragus; heavy line = mandible; broad V = orbital rim and chin.)

(Illustration continued on opposite page.)

Normal Radiosialogram
(with atropine)

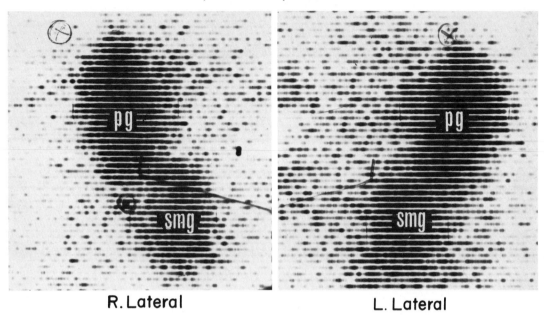

R. Lateral   L. Lateral

Anterior

Figure 9 (*Continued*). *B*, A normal radiosialogram made with 4mC 99mTc and 0.6 mg. atropine. Little radioactivity is present in the oral cavity (oc) which allows better visualization of the anterior border of the parotids (pg) and superior border of submandibular (smg).

Mixed Tumor R. Parotid Gland

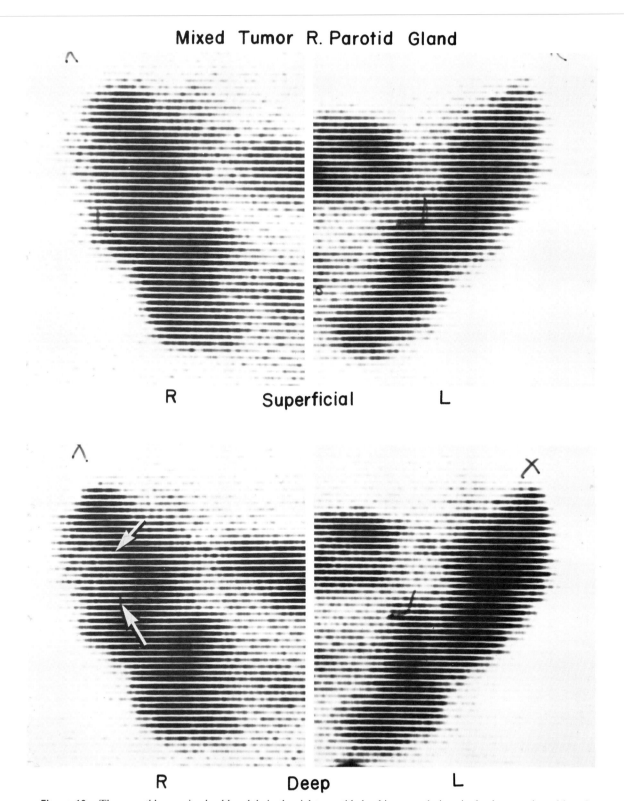

Figure 10. The smoothly margined cold nodule in the right parotid gland is more obvious in the deep section, although it can be seen in the superficial cut as well. Scan made with 4mC 99mTc and 0.8 mg. atropine. The tumor was deeply located in the gland immediately lateral to the facial nerve.

Acinic Cell Adenocarcinoma
L. Parotid Gland

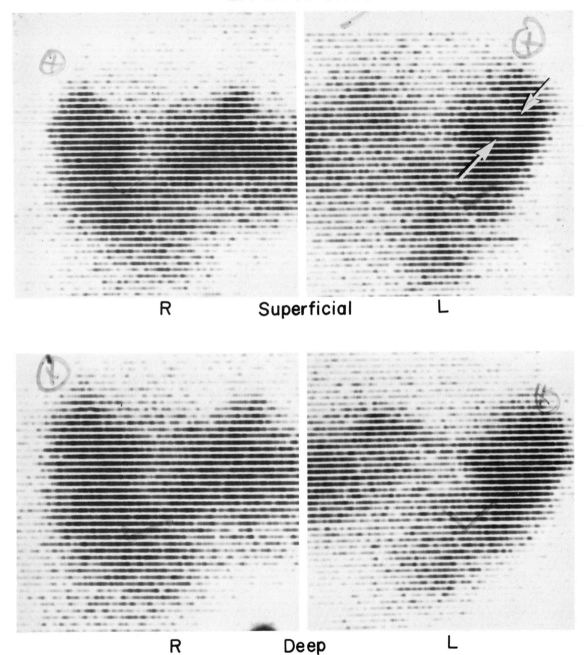

Figure 11. A smoothly margined cold nodule is seen in the superficial scan in the superior part of the gland (arrows). The tumor is not obvious in the deep section. This is an encapsulated acinic cell adenocarcinoma located lateral to the facial nerve.

Adenocarcinoma R. Parotid Gland

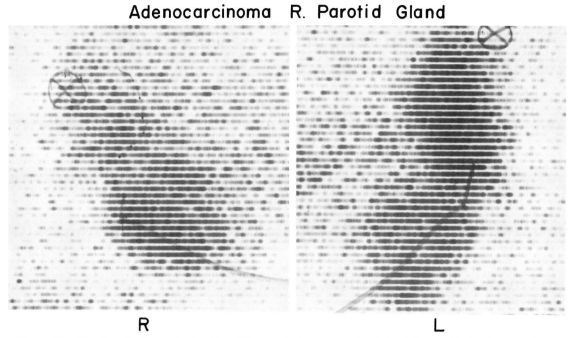

R   L

Figure 12. The irregularly margined cold nodule seen in the upper pole of the right parotid gland scan is due to a primary adenocarcinoma which had surrounded the facial nerve.

Warthins Tumor L. Parotid Gland

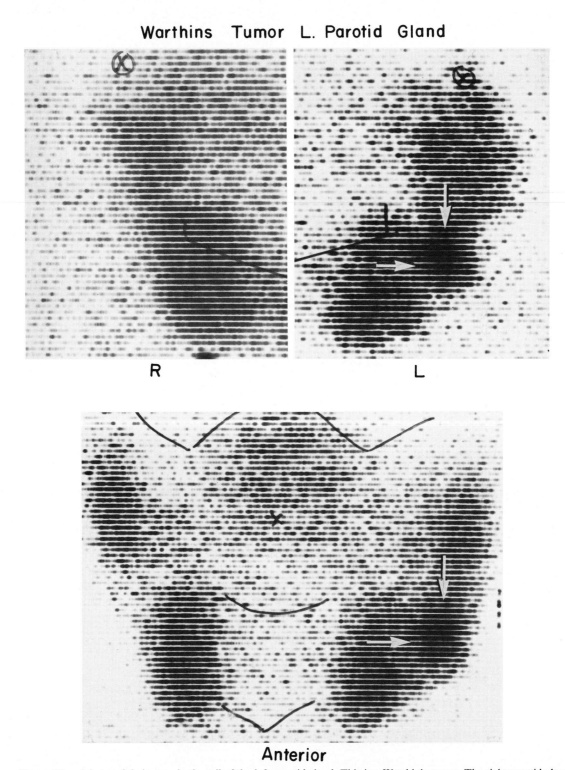

Figure 13.   A hot nodule is seen in the tail of the left parotid gland. This is a Warthin's tumor. The right parotid gland outline is smaller than the left. This patient had had a subtotal parotidectomy two years previously for a Warthin's tumor.

When the uptake in the tumor and in the gland is nearly equal, the scan will be normal. The larger the difference in uptake, the more marked will be the scan contrast between the abnormal and normal areas. The commonest technical difficulty relates to the focal length of the collimator; lesions superficial or deep to the plane of maximum response may not be detected and, hence, the need for two planes or more scanning. Section scanning is helpful for localization; lesions seen only in the deep section have been deep to the facial nerve, and vice versa.

In chronic inflammatory conditions the radiosialograms may be difficult to interpret because of the marked variations in gland uptake that are seen, particularly in cases of benign lymphoepithelial lesion. Here the scan may be normal, may show a unilateral or bilateral decrease in uptake, or may even show an irregularly margined cold nodule suggestive of neoplasm. Variations in salivary gland uptake between normal patients precludes making a judgment about the salivary gland function except when a marked difference exists between glands on opposite sides of the same patient.

REFERENCES

Blatt, I. M., and Maxwell, J. H.: Secretory sialography. Trans. Amer. Acad. Ophth. Otol., *61*:492–498, 1957.

Blatt, I. M., Rubin, P., French, A. J., Maxwell, J. H., and Holt, J. F.: Secretory sialography in diseases of the major salivary glands. Ann. Otol. *65*:295–318, 1956.

Rubin, P., Blatt, I. M., Holt, J. F., and Maxwell, J. H.: Physiological or secretory sialography. Ann. Otol. *64*:667–689, 1955.

RADIOLOGY OF THE
TRACHEOBRONCHIAL TREE AND LUNGS

by

Kenneth N. Hehman, M.D., Jack Brucher, M.D., and Jerome F. Wiot, M.D.

In the short space allotted it is impossible to discuss radiology of the tracheobronchial tree and the lungs in its entirety. The reader is therefore referred to the excellent texts on pulmonary diseases and encouraged to devote special attention to those writings dealing with fundamentals of interpreting radiographs. Because the tracheobronchial tree is of special interest to the otolaryngologist we will confine our remarks to this area.

The anatomy of the bronchial tree is quite variable but generally conforms to a basic pattern which, once learned, permits easy evaluation of bronchograms and the anatomic location of most lesions. The anatomic chart by Drs. J. Stanfer Lehman and J. A. Cullen, which can be obtained from the Medical Illustration Division of Eastman Kodak Company, is excellent for demonstrating the basic pattern and has been of great value both in evaluating and in teaching the anatomy of the bronchi. It should be available to anyone performing or interpreting bronchograms.

Although conventional films and tomograms may give considerable information concerning the tracheobronchial tree, bronchography is far more fruitful, when properly performed. This is true not only for congenital, inflammatory, and neoplastic lesions of the bronchi, but also for certain parenchymal diseases. Often, valuable information concerning alveolar lymphoma, alveolar cell carcinoma, and organized or unresolved pneumonia may be obtained because of the characteristic bronchographic pattern which these diseases may produce.

METHODS

No longer can the "blind" method of bronchography be accepted. This procedure, in which the entire study is done by positioning the patient and Bucky filming without fluoroscopic control, is subject to far too many diagnostic errors. Today fluoroscopic control of *all* bronchograms is essential.

We currently use two methods of broncho-

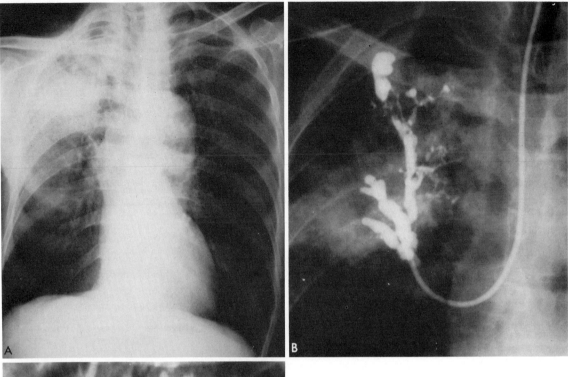

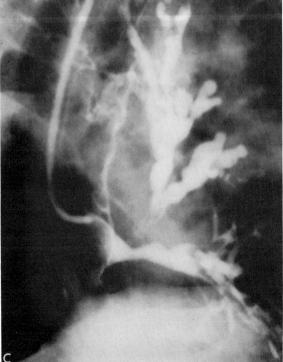

Figure 14. *A*, Routine chest film of 60 year old man with chronic cough shows extensive right upper lobe disease. *B*, Selective transcricoid bronchography of right upper lobe demonstrates bronchiectasis involving the apical and posterior segments of right upper lobe. *C*, Spot film of right upper lobe bronchogram demonstrating narrowed deformed bronchus to apical and posterior segment of right upper lobe, due to carcinoma, with distal bronchiectasis. The anterior segment shows invasion by tumor. Bronchoscopy showed a normal upper lobe orifice but failed to demonstrate the abnormality. Brush biopsy prior to bronchography revealed malignant cells.

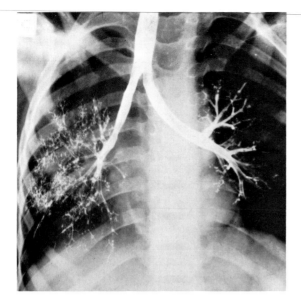

Figure 15. Agenesis of the right upper and right middle lobes. Note how the lower lobe bronchi rearrange themselves to approach a normal appearance.

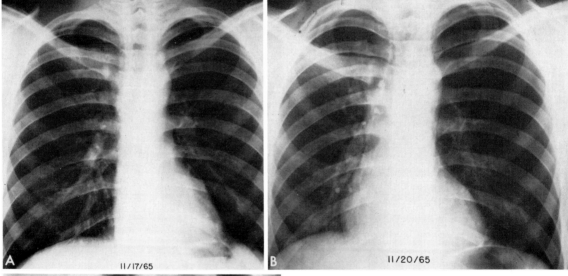

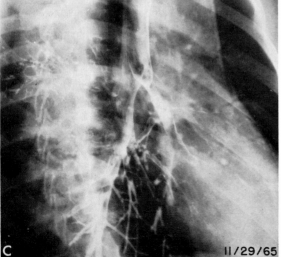

Figure 16. *A*, PA inspiration film of a patient with prior history of mild chest trauma. The chest appears normal. *B*, Expiration. Air trapping is noted on the left. *C*, Bronchogram reveals fracture of left main stem bronchus.

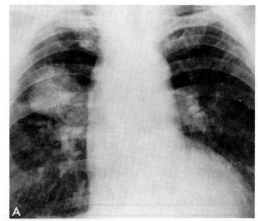

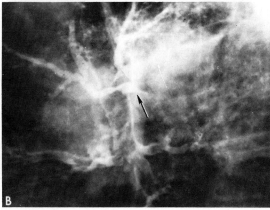

Figure 17. *A*, Chest film demonstrates diffuse fine nodularity with right upper lobe mass. The patient has a long history of silica dust exposure. *B*, Bronchogram demonstrates a rat-tail cut off of posterior segment, right upper lobe bronchus consistent with carcinoma. Surgical exploration proved this to be a silicotic conglomerate mass. Brush biopsy may have excluded this as being carcinoma.

graphy. In those patients in whom lung mapping is desired (i.e., study of all bronchial segments), after suitable topical anesthesia, a soft rubber catheter is passed from the nose or mouth through the larynx and placed in the trachea. When selective bronchography or brush biopsy of a lesion is desired, we use a transcricoid approach similar to the technique described by Seldinger for arteriography. The method may also be used for lung mapping studies if desired.

About 90 per cent of our studies are now performed via the transcricoid approach as described by Steckel and Grillo (1964). We find this method to be quick, safe, and less annoying to the patient; it requires a smaller amount of topical anesthetic and has the advantage of permitting selective studies of individual bronchi and allowing for brush biopsy.

Transcricoid Bronchography

The patient is placed supine on the fluoroscopy table and, after surgical preparation of the neck, about 0.5 ml. of lidocaine (Xylocaine) is infiltrated into the skin and subcutaneous tissues over the cricothyroid membrane. The membrane is then punctured and 1 ml. Xylocaine is injected rapidly into the trachea. The needle is then quickly removed and the patient is encouraged to cough to facilitate spread of the topical anesthetic. A small skin incision is made with a No. 12 Bard Parker blade and the tissues gently spread with a mosquito hemostate. A thin-walled, 18-gauge needle is then inserted and angled caudad with gentle suction. Once the needle is properly placed, a free flow of air occurs. A flexible guide wire is then inserted through the needle and the needle rapidly withdrawn. A red Odman catheter with side hole, which has been preformed with a gentle curve near its end, is then placed over the wire and into the trachea. After removal of the guide wire, the catheter is gently pushed into the bronchus of interest or, if a lung mapping is desired, into the right or left main stem bronchi. If coughing occurs, an additional small amount of topical anesthetic may be injected through the catheter to the area under study. If during the process of mapping, an individual bronchus fails to fill, the catheter can be passed into the area for additional study.

Brush Biopsy

When brush biopsy is desired, brushing is done prior to bronchography to prevent contrast medium from being within the specimen. Brush biopsy has proved to be of diagnostic value in appraising both central and peripheral pulmonary lesions. With the use of selective bronchus catheterization, it is possible to pass a brush into desired areas of the bronchial tree to obtain cultures and cells for study. The method is safe and effective and has permitted diagnosis to be made without resorting to thoracotomy or transthoracic needle biopsy.

Contrast Media

Currently, Dionosil (oily or aqueous) is the contrast medium of choice. Aqueous media appear to be slightly more irritating to the bronchial mucosa and, therefore, generally require a greater volume of topical anesthetic.

Recently considerable interest has been sti-

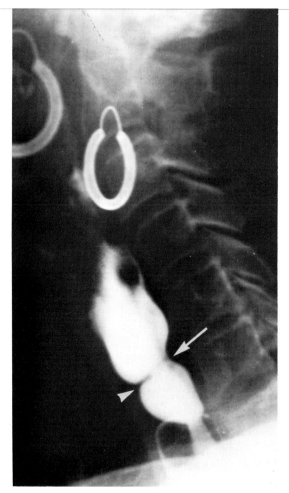

Figure 18. Note the web arising from the anterior wall of the hypopharynx (arrowhead). These may be multiple and originate in the upper esophagus, presenting as thin (less than 2 mm thick), filling defects projecting from the anterior wall at right angles (Seaman, 1967). The posterior aspect of the cricoid cartilage may occasionally produce a longer indentation of the esophagus in the same area. A distinct cricopharyngeal impression is seen posteriorly (arrow). This impression may be prominent after laryngectomy (Dey and Kirchner, 1961).

mulated in the use of barium sulfate and powdered tantalum for bronchography. Both have the advantage of being chemically inert. As yet both are experimental and not commercially available.

Filming

As mentioned previously, all bronchography must be done under fluoroscopic control to obtain optimal studies. When lung mapping is desired, we study the side of prime interest first; if there is no preference, the right side is investigated first. Spot films should be obtained during the filling stages in anteroposterior, oblique, and lateral projections and then Bucky films in the AP, lateral, and both oblique projections. The other side is similarly studied, except the lateral films are not obtained because of the problem of interpretation as a result of overlap of bronchi. With selective studies, similar films are obtained.

The use of fluoroscopy and spot filming facilitates complete filling of all bronchial segments and, in addition, permits careful study of individual bronchial segments for small lesions as they fill without superimposition. In addition, if certain bronchi fail to fill, this is evident at fluoroscopy, and additional effort can be directed toward that segment.

Cine bronchography is also of considerable
(*Text continued on page 1121*)

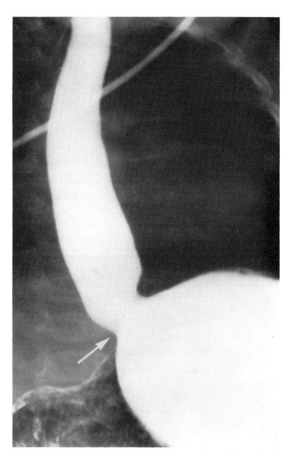

Figure 19. Chalasia. The cardioesophageal junction is patulous (arrow). Reflux into the esophagus is easily produced by manual pressure on the abdomen, or during crying or deep inspiration, or by placing the patient in the Trendelenburg position. Chalasia is best appreciated during fluoroscopy or on cine studies and is primarily seen in newborns (Silverman, 1955).

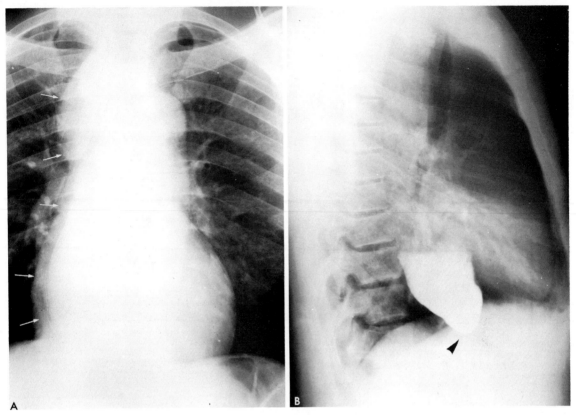

Figure 20. Achalasia. *A,* Note the large fluid-filled esophagus behind the heart shadow on the posteroanterior chest film (arrow). Frequently an air-fluid level is seen in the upper esophagus. *B,* Barium shows the smooth, tapering, distal esophagus (arrow). The esophagus may be tortuous and elongated, peristalsis weak and ineffective, and barium pass into the stomach in small intermittent amounts (Zboralske and Dodds, 1969). Drinking a carbonated beverage may cause prompt emptying of the esophagus, with the tapered segment opening momentarily but still maintaining a beaked appearance. Similar changes may occur in presbyesophagus (Zboralske, 1965). In contrast to carcinoma, there is no intraluminal mass in achalasia and the tapering is smooth.

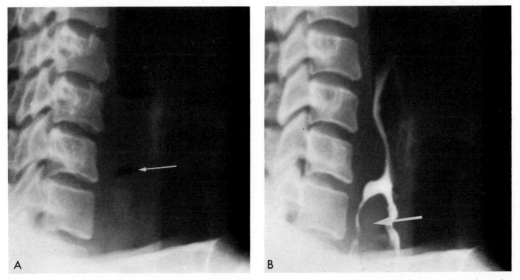

Figure 21. Foreign body (sparerib) stuck in upper portion of esophagus. *A,* Air in esophagus (arrow) just above the sparerib. *B,* Barium swallow demonstrates a filling defect (arrow) in the contrast column. Air may normally appear in the esophagus during eructation or swallowing but does not persist. Foreign bodies are usually arrested at the level of the cricoid cartilage, aortic arch, left bronchus crossing, or at the diaphragm. Air in the soft tissues or mediastinum and widening of the prevertebral soft tissues suggest perforation.

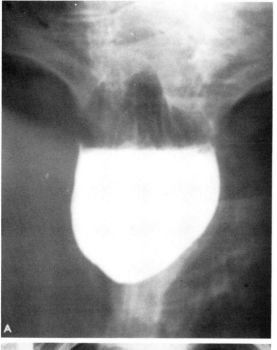

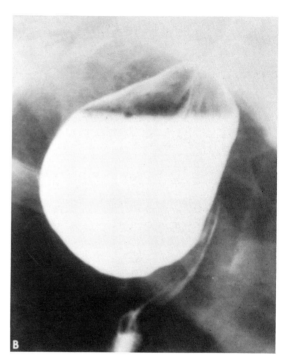

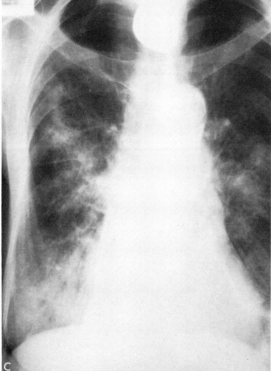

Figure 22. Zenker's diverticulum. *A* and *B* show a Zenker's diverticulum arising at the pharyngoesophageal junction and projecting posteriorly. As the diverticulum increases in size, it descends into the superior mediastinum behind the esophagus. The esophagus is pushed forward with larger lesions. Food or other foreign material may be seen within the diverticulum and aspiration pneumonia may develop (*C*).

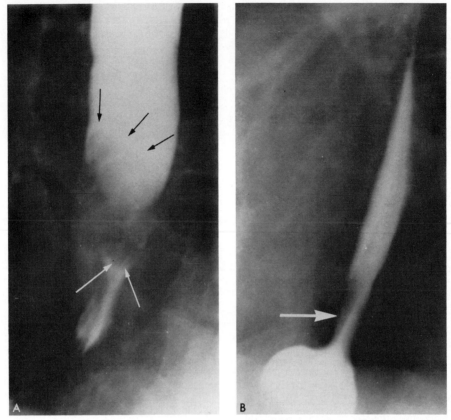

Figure 23. *A,* Food stuck in the distal esophagus (arrows) simulating carcinoma. *B,* After removal, barium swallow shows some narrowing and mucosal thickening (arrows) secondary to esophagitis, but no evidence of mass or mucosal destruction.

Figure 24. *A,* A small hiatus hernia (arrow) and some prominence of folds in the distal esophagus seen in film made in 1961. *B,* In 1966 a huge barium-filled ulcer (arrows) in the same area.

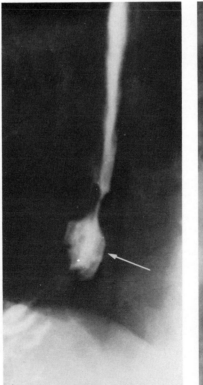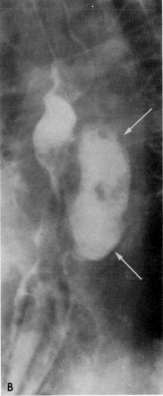

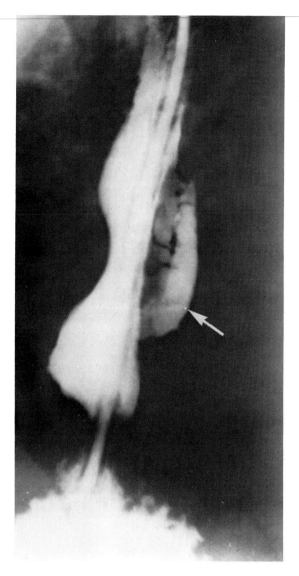

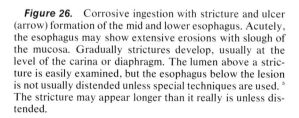

Figure 25. Huge esophageal ulcer (arrows) in a bedfast patient. Note the nasogastric tube in the esophagus. Most esophageal ulcers occur in the lower third and may be associated with columnar lined esophageal epithelium.[4,8] Esophagitis with ulceration and stricture also may follow esophageal intubation.

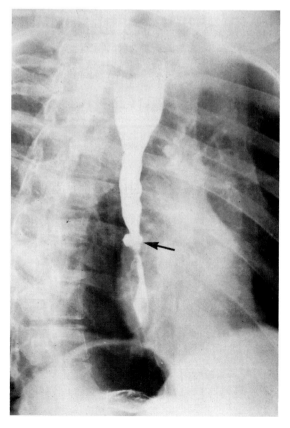

Figure 26. Corrosive ingestion with stricture and ulcer (arrow) formation of the mid and lower esophagus. Acutely, the esophagus may show extensive erosions with slough of the mucosa. Gradually strictures develop, usually at the level of the carina or diaphragm. The lumen above a stricture is easily examined, but the esophagus below the lesion is not usually distended unless special techniques are used.[5] The stricture may appear longer than it really is unless distended.

value in individual cases. Its advantage is primarily the study of bronchial physiology. Intrinsic bronchial motion can be studied by this method but cannot be appreciated with static filming. The motion or lack of motion has

proved to be helpful in the evaluation of chronic bronchitis, bronchiectasis, and in the length of involvement by intrinsic bronchial carcinoma.

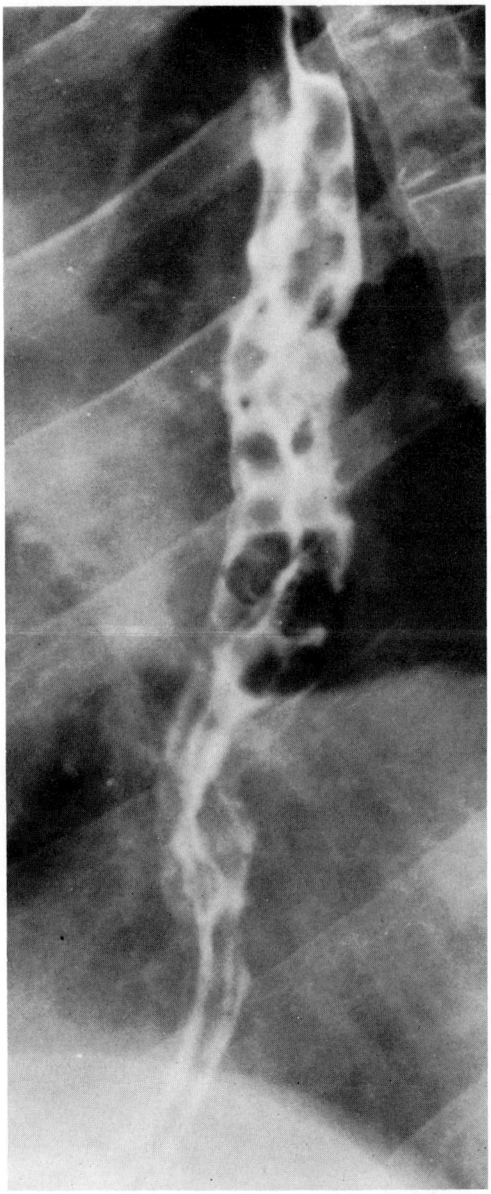

ESOPHAGUS

Radiographic examination of the esophagus is usually achieved by barium swallow, using both thick and thin barium mixtures. The thicker barium pastes give better coating of the mucosa and are used to show the transit of a barium bolus down the esophagus for better evaluation of esophageal motor function.

Fluoroscopy and spot films are often enough to fulfill the diagnostic needs, but cineradiography greatly improves the functional and anatomic evaluation, especially in the upper esophagus where physiologic events occur very rapidly. A small cotton pledget soaked in barium and swallowed may catch and hold on a foreign body for a short interval. Capsules of various sizes filled with barium may be used to demonstrate a stricture and its severity. Water-soluble contrast may be indicated when an esophageal perforation is suspected. When looking for aspiration, barium is probably better tolerated in the tracheobronchial tree than water-soluble contrast.

The roentgen examination is conducted in both upright and recumbent positions, using posterior, anterior, lateral, and oblique views. Inspiration, expiration, and the Valsalva maneuver are also used to modify the esophageal position and the intrathoracic dynamics.

The esophagus begins at the level of the cricoid cartilage and then passes to the left of the transverse aortic arch, resulting in a smooth indentation which becomes more prominent with advancing age. At the level of the left main stem bronchus, a slight indentation may also be noted. In elderly people the esophagus tends to follow the sweep of the aorta, which may be quite elongated and swings to the left and then back to midline. Enlargement of the left atrium or posterior displacement of the heart also displaces the adjacent esophagus.

The dynamics and anatomic detail of the distal esophagus are still disputed, and entire books have been written on this subject. Space does not permit an adequate radiographic discourse on this area, but the book by Zaino et al. (1963) provides an excellent discussion.

Figure 27. Large esophageal varices in a patient with cirrhosis of the liver. Varices appear earliest along the right anterolateral wall of the lower esophagus (Missakian et al., 1967). Varices appear as multiple serpiginous or oval filling defects in the lumen, best seen after the main bolus of barium has passed but while the mucosa is well coated. The esophageal wall remains distensible and peristalsis passes through the lesions. Felson and Lessure (1964) have demonstrated the occurrence of upper and mid esophagus varices in superior vena caval obstruction.

THE LARYNX AND HYPOPHARYNX

Radiographic examination of the larynx and

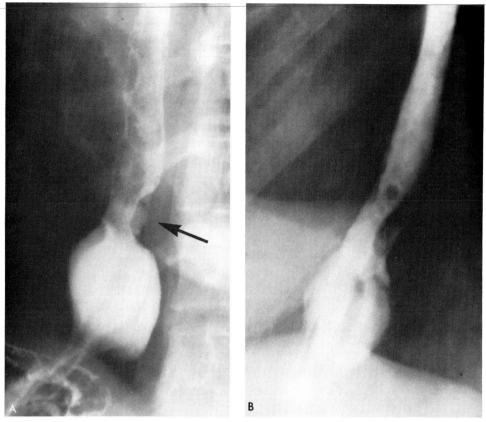

Figure 28. *A*, Carcinoma in the esophagogastric region (arrow). This mural lesion is located just above a small hiatus hernia. *B*, The defect remains even while the esophagus is distended. Cineradiography showed rigidity of this area.

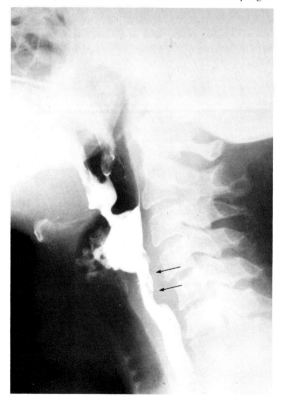

Figure 29. Note the flat esophageal carcinoma projecting inwardly from the posterior wall of the esophagus (arrows). The wall is irregular and the luminal narrowing minimal.

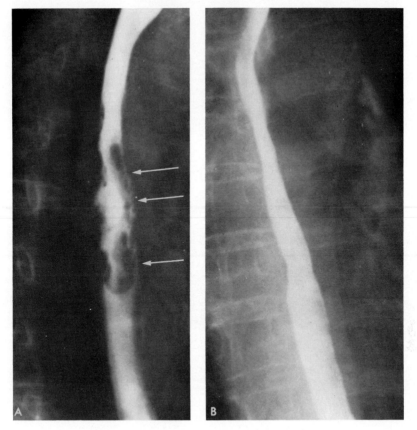

Figure 30. *A*, Mid esophageal carcinoma with prominent mucosal destruction (arrows). *B*, After radiation therapy some narrowing remains but there is no demonstrable mass.

hypopharynx is best accomplished with (1) soft-tissue, high KV, lateral radiographs taken at 6-foot distance with the patient erect; (2) frontal tomograms taken during phonation with the patient prone; and (3) positive contrast laryngography.

(*Text continued on page 1131*)

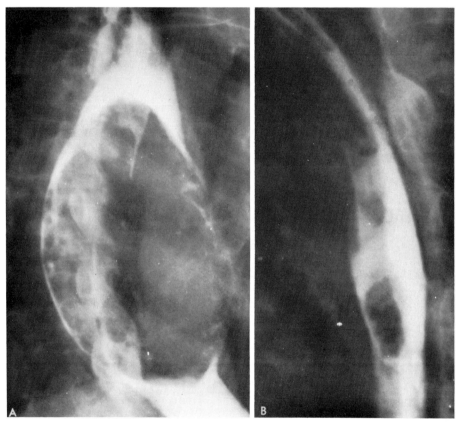

Figure 31. *A*, Huge intraluminal carcinoma of the esophagus. This mass resembles intramural extramucosal lesion (such as leiomyoma or other spindle cell tumors). *B*, Note the marked decrease in size after radiation therapy.

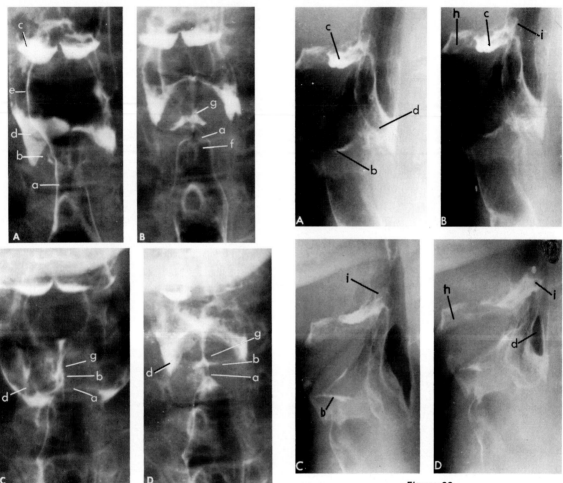

Figure 32

Figure 33

Figure 32 (AP) and Figure 33 (lateral). Quiet respiration. *AP*: The true cords (a) are in abduction and retracted superiorly obliterating the ventricles (b). The aryepiglottic folds (e) are outlined by a thin line of contrast medium. *Lateral*: The vallecula (c) and pyriform sinuses (d) fill passively. A thin line of contrast medium in the inferior portion of the vestibule outlines the collapsed ventricle (b). *B*, Phonation. *AP*: The true cords (a) approximate in the midline forming a sharp symmetrical subglottic concavity (f). The false cords (g) also become approximated, narrowing the inferior portion of the vestibule. *Lateral*: The hyoid bone (h) becomes elevated and the epiglottis (i) becomes more vertical, changing the configuration of the vallecula (c). *C*, Modified Valsalva. *AP*: The pyriform sinuses (d) distend and the true (a) and false (b) cords become approximated. The ventricles (b) are small. *Lateral*: The anterior larynx is elevated and the epiglottis (i) moves posteriorly. *D*, Valsalva, *AP*: There is close approximation of the true (a) and false (g) vocal cords, nearly obliterating the ventricles (b). The true cords appear thickened. The pyriform sinuses (d) and inferior portion of the vestibule become narrow. *Lateral*: The pyriform sinuses (d) are narrow in the AP dimension. The epiglottis (i) moves posteriorly tending to close the vestibule. The hyoid (H) descends to rest on the thyroid cartilage.

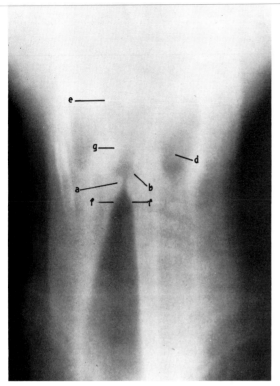

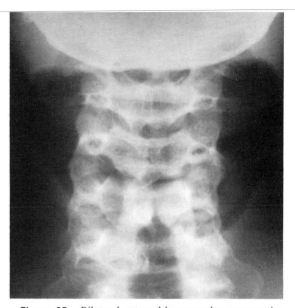

Figure 35. Bilateral external laryngoceles representing protrusions of the ventricular saccule through a weak point in the thyrohyoid membrane. The air-filled, or occasionally fluid-filled, pouch presents in the anterior triangle of the neck.

Figure 34. AP linear tomogram in phonation showing the true (a) and false (g) cords, ventricle (b), pyriform sinus (d), subglottic concavity (f) and aryepiglottic folds (e).

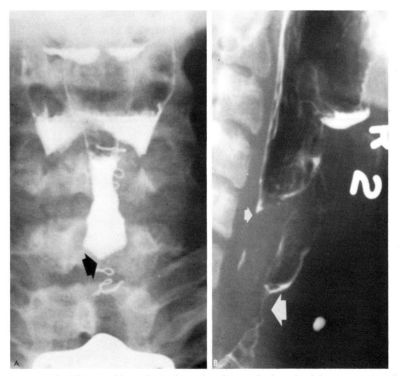

Figure 36. Laryngograms in AP (*A*) and lateral (*B*) views showing marked tracheal (large arrow) and esophageal (small arrow) stenosis at the site of a previous tracheostomy in which the tracheostomy tube had eroded through the trachea into the esophagus. The tracheostomy tube has been replaced at a lower level.

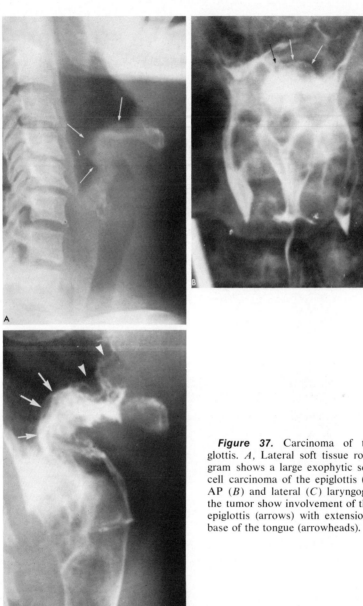

Figure 37. Carcinoma of the epiglottis. *A*, Lateral soft tissue roentgenogram shows a large exophytic squamous cell carcinoma of the epiglottis (arrows). AP (*B*) and lateral (*C*) laryngograms of the tumor show involvement of the entire epiglottis (arrows) with extension to the base of the tongue (arrowheads).

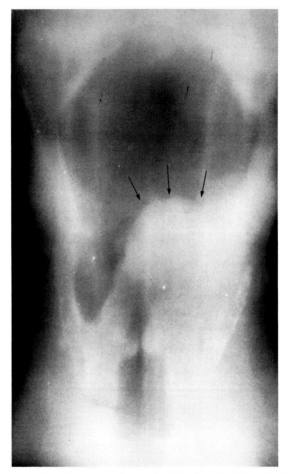

Figure 38. AP tomogram defines large mass (arrows) arising in and obliterating the left pyriform sinus.

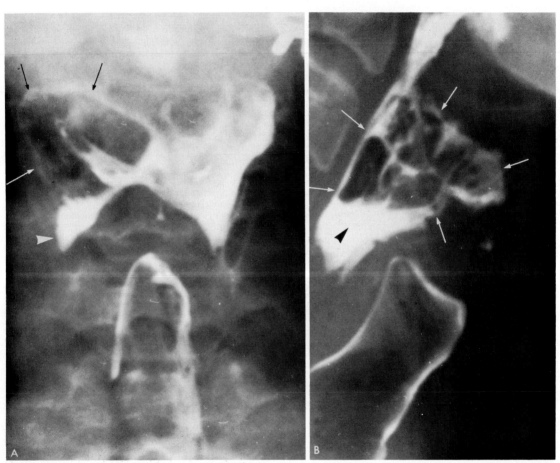

Figure 39. AP (*A*) and lateral (*B*) laryngograms demonstrate a polypoid squamous cell carcinoma (arrows) arising from the right aryepiglottic fold. Contrast medium in the bottom of the pyriform sinus (arrowhead) indicates the tumor arose high in the sinus. Tumors arising in the bottom of the sinus tend to be infiltrative, whereas those arising on the medial or lateral walls tend to be exophytic.

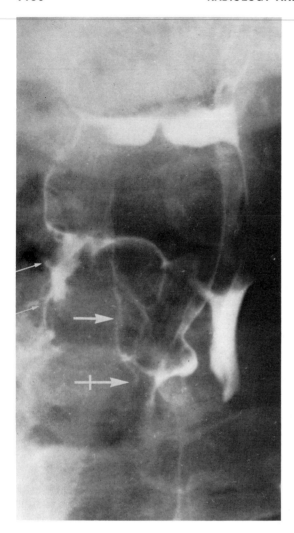

Figure 40. Infiltrative squamous cell carcinoma nearly obliterating the pyriform sinus (small arrows) and distorting the true (+→) and false (large arrow) cords.

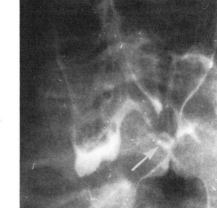

Figure 41. Small polypoid squamous cell carcinoma (arrow) arising from the superior aspect of the right true cord and obliterating the right ventricle.

Valsalva maneuver by forceful blowing against the cheeks with the mouth closed; and (4) regular Valsalva by straining down against a closed glottis), 5 to 10 ml. of oily Dionosil are dripped slowly over the back of the tongue intermittently during inspiration. Spot films are then taken in the AP and lateral positions during each of these maneuvers.

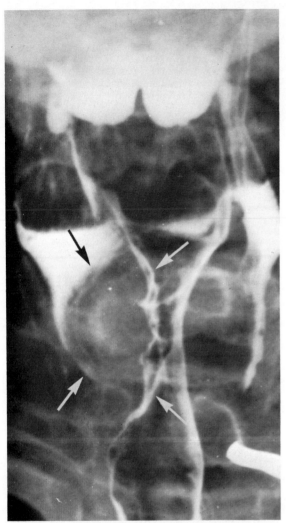

Figure 42. Transglottic extension of a squamous cell carcinoma (arrows) obliterating the right subglottic angle and ventricle, distorting the false cord and impinging on the medial aspect of the pyriform sinus.

Positive contrast laryngography has few disadvantages (most of which are related to iodine sensitivity), allows the most adequate evaluation of the anatomy and dynamics of the laryngopharyngeal apparatus, and is a relatively simple procedure. After allergy to iodine compounds and topical anesthetics has been excluded, the patient is premedicated with 100 mg. Nembutal and 0.4 mg. atropine. Lidocaine (Xylocaine) 4 per cent is sprayed on the posterior oro- and hypopharynx, and the pyriform sinuses are anesthetized with Xylocaine-soaked cotton pledgets. After the patient has been instructed in the various maneuvers (i.e., (1) quiet inspiration with the mouth closed; (2) phonation of the vowel *e* at high pitch; (3) modified

REFERENCES

The Tracheobronchial Tree and Lungs

Bronchography. Report of the Committee on Bronchoesophagology. American College of Chest Physicians. Dis. Chest *51*:663, 1967.

Felson, B.: Fundamentals of Chest Roentgenology. Philadelphia, W. B. Saunders Company, 1960.

Molnar, W., and Riebel, F. A.: Bronchography: An aid in the diagnosis of peripheral pulmonary carcinoma. Radiol. Clin. N. Amer., *1*(2):303, 1963.

Moskowitz, M., and Freihofer, A.: Seldinger brush biopsy. Chest *57*:426, 1970.

Nadel, J. A., Wolfe, W. G., and Graf, P. D.: Powdered tantalum as a medium for bronchography in canine and human lungs. Invest. Radiol. *3*:229, 1968.

Rinker, C. T., Garrotto, L. J., Lee, K. R., and Templeton, A. W.: Bronchography. Diagnostic signs and accuracy in pulmonary carcinoma. Amer. J. Roentgen. *104*:803, 1968.

Steckel, R. J., and Grillo, H. C.: Catheterization of the trachea and bronchi by modified Seldinger Technic: A new approach to bronchography. Radiology *83*:1035, 1964.

Trapnell, D. H., and Gregg, I.: Some principles of interpretation of bronchograms. Brit. J. Radiol. *42*:125, 1969.

Witt, R. L., and Wiot, J. F.: Cinebronchography. *In* Tice-Harvey Practice of Medicine *2*:223, 1965.

Dey, F. L., and Kirchner, J. A.: The upper esophageal sphincter after laryngectomy. Laryngoscope *71*:99, 1961.

Felson, B., and Lessure, A. P.: "Downhill" varices of the esophagus. Dis. Chest *46*:740, 1964.

Margulis, A. R., and Burhenne, H. J.: Alimentary Tract Roentgenology. Vol. I. St. Louis, The C. V. Mosby Co., 1967.

Missakian, M. M., Carlson, H. C., and Andersen, H. A.: The roentgenologic features of the columnar epithelial-lined lower esophagus. Amer. J. Roentgen. *99*:212, 1967.

Mortensson, W., and Sandmark, S.: Roentgen examination of stricture of the lower oesophagus. Acta Radiol. (Diagn.) *7*:355, 1968.

Seaman, W. B.: The significance of webs in the hypopharynx and upper esophagus. Radiology *89*:32, 1967.

Silverman, F. N.: Gastroesophageal incompetence, partial intrathoracic stomach, and vomiting in infancy. Radiology *64*:664, 1955.

Wright, J. T.: Allison and Johnstone's anomaly. Amer. J. Roentgen. *94*:308, 1965.

Zaino, C., Poppel, M. H., Jacobson, H. G., and Lepow, H.: The Lower Esophageal Vestibular Complex. Springfield, Ill., Charles C Thomas, 1963.

Zboralske, F. F.: The esophagus in the geriatric patient. Radiol. Clin. N. Amer. *3* (2):321, 1965.

Zboralske, F. F., and Dodds, W. J.: Roentgenographic diagnosis of primary disorders of esophageal motility. Radiol. Clin. N. Amer. 7(1):147, 1969.

The Larynx and Hypopharynx

Ardran, G. M., and Emrys-Roberts, E.: Tomography of the larynx. Clin. Radiol. *16*:369, 1965.

Brindle, M. J., and Stell, P. M.: Radiological assessment of laryngeal carcinoma. Clin. Radiol. *19*:257, 1968.

Burke, E. N., and Golden, J. L.: External ventricular laryngocele. Amer. J. Roentgen. *80*:49, 1968.

Lehmann, Q. H., and Fletcher, G. H.: Contribution of the laryngogram to the management of malignant laryngeal tumors. Radiology *83*:486, 1964.

Powers, W. E., McGee, H. H., Jr., and Seaman, W. B.: Contrast examination of the larynx and pharynx. Radiology *68*:169, 1957.

CERVICAL LYMPHANGIOGRAPHY
by
Melvin E. Sigel, M.D.

X-ray visualization of the human lymphatic system by utilization of radiopaque materials received its initial impetus in 1952 when Kinmonth injected water-soluble contrast agents directly into cannulated lymphatics of the lower extremities. This method provided a significantly superior lymphangiogram over that obtained by the indirect method of injecting contrast agents into perilymphatic tissue.

The application of direct lymphatic cannulization in radiographic demonstration of the cervical lymphatic system began in 1963 when Jackson was able to directly cannulate small cervical and supraclavicular lymph vessels. This technique was further refined by Fisch and delBuono in 1963 and by Fisch and Sigel in 1964.

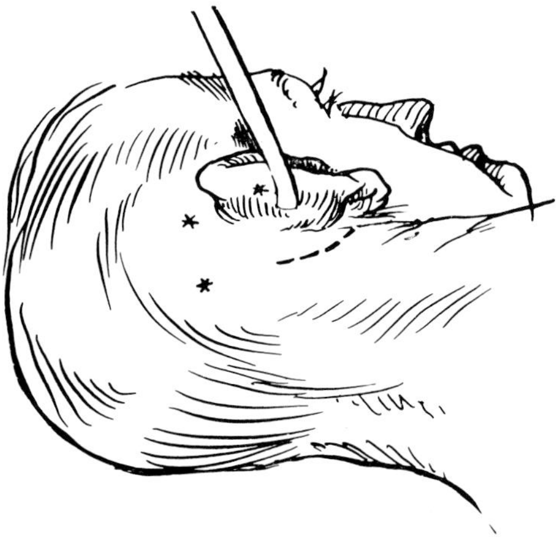

TECHNIQUE

The patient is placed in a supine position under sterile operating room conditions. The ear and retreauricular area are prepared with a

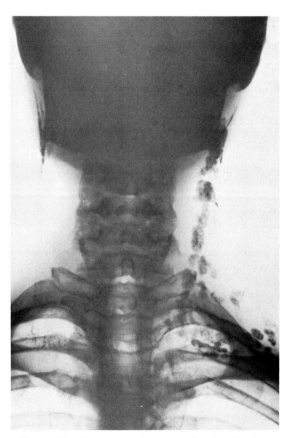

Figure 43. Sites of patent-blue dye injection. Broken line represents incision site (Fisch, U. P., and Sigel, M. E.: Ann. Otol. *73*:869, 1964.)

Figure 44. Anteroposterior x-ray of neck taken immediately after injection of contrast material, demonstrating normal cervical lymphogram.

surgical scrub. Anesthesia in the retroauricular region is obtained with procaine 2 per cent in three separate wheals. Patent blue dye is then injected, 0.3 to 0.4 cc. in each wheal. A skin incision is made (Fig. 43) and identification of the *deep* cervical retroauricular lymphatics is accomplished, using the magnification of the otomicroscope. These vessels, previously stained by the patent blue dye, are then fenestrated and cannulated with tapered PE 10 tubing. This cannulization has recently been accomplished more readily in experimental animals with a micromanipulator and No. 34 needle. Ethiodal is then injected, after which the cannula is removed and the incision closed. Anteroposterior (Fig. 44) and lateral (Fig. 45) x-rays of the neck are taken immediately and again after 24 hours. Complications such as fever and wound infection have rarely been observed.

FINDINGS OF CERVICAL LYMPHOGRAPHY

This method of roentgenographically studying the cervical lymphatic system has been of great value in following the physiologic action of cervical lymphatics in normal as well as in pathological situations.

Normal Cervical Lymphatic Physiology

A reclassification of the cervical lymphatic system into functional units rather than grouping by artificial anatomic boundries has been accomplished using lymphographic techniques.

Five specific lymph node groups have been classified lymphographically by filling sequence into junctional, jugular, supraclavicular, spinal, and retroauricular nodes (Figs. 46 and 47).

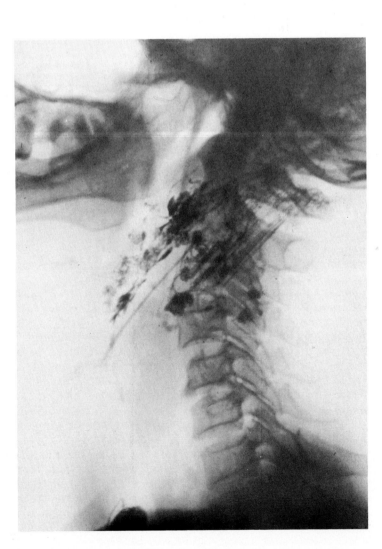

Figure 45. Lateral x-ray demonstrating filling of junctional and upper jugular lymph nodes.

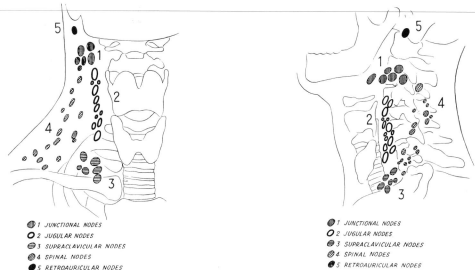

Figure 46. Schematic drawing of anteroposterior cervical lymphogram showing five functional lymph node units. (Fisch, U. P., and Sigel, M. E.: Ann Otol. *73*:869, 1964.

Figure 47. Schematic drawing of lateral cervical lymphogram, (Fisch, U. P., and Sigel, M. E.: Ann. Otol. *73*:869, 1964.)

Lymphatic flow patterns have also been demonstrated as to direction, with lymph observed seeking access into the main circulatory system in a caudal direction.

Lymphographic Studies of the Pathologic Neck

Although lymphographic demonstration of clinically inaccessible (nonpalpable) nodes has proved of value in studying such areas as abdominal and inguinal lymphatics, similar "filling-defect" patterns in cervical lymph nodes may be caused by reactive changes in the lymph nodes other than malignancy, such as reticular and follicular hyperplasia. Large groups of metastatic or hyperplastic nodes may also completely block the contrast agent from filling specific nodes or entire nodal groups so as to preclude satisfactory study of individual nodes. These findings make equivocal the diagnosis of cervical metastatic disease by lymphography alone.

The usual behavior of head and neck carcinoma in remaining localized for long periods of time in palpable lymphatics of the neck before more systemic involvement, the possible technical difficulty in the actual performance of the cervical lymphogram itself, as well as the large number of what could be considered false-positive results have all contributed to the spar-

ing use of lymphography in the search for occult cervical metastases.

However, this technique should not be dismissed too lightly, as it would appear that additional lymphographic work in this region may yield important findings in evaluating metastatic patterns of various head and neck malignancies as well as in diagnosing occult metastases.

EXPERIMENTAL CERVICAL LYMPHOGRAPHY

Cervical lymphography has proved of great value in studying alterations in lymphatic and lymph node patterns following surgical and radiation therapy of the cervical lymphatic chain in both the experimental animal and in humans.

Lymphographic studies of the radiated neck have demonstrated not only a diminution in numbers of nodes but also a decrease in the rate of lymph flow.

Following neck surgery, both in the experimental animal and in humans, a block in lymphatic flow has been seen at the site of radical neck resection, with eventual development of alternate or contralateral pathways observed lymphographically as healing progresses (Sigel and Fisch, 1964).

FUTURE OF CERVICAL LYMPHOGRAPHY

As cervical lymphography is used by more investigators concerned with malignant head and neck disease as well as by lymphologists, and when the interpretations of their findings become accepted, useful clinical information regarding radiographic study of the cervical lymphatic system and its relationship to various malignant diseases of the head and neck should be forthcoming.

Lymphographic techniques hold great promise not only for basic physiologic research but hopefully for significant clinical information.

REFERENCES

Fisch, U. P., and del Buono, M. S.: Zur Technik der cervicalen Lymphographie. Schweiz. Med. Wschr. 93:994, 1963.

Fisch, U. P., and Sigel, M. E.: Cervical lymphatic system as visualized by lymphography. Ann. Otol. 73:869, 1964.

Fisch, U. P.: Lymphography of the Cervical Lymphatic System. Philadelphia, W. B. Saunders Company, 1968.

Jackson, L., Wallace, S., Farb, S. N., and Parke, W. W.: Cervical lymphography. Laryngoscope 73:926, 1963.

Kinmonth, J. B.: Lymphangiography in man. Clin. Sci. 11:13, 1952.

Sigel, M. E., and Fisch, U. P.: The effect of surgery on the cervical lymphatic system. Laryngoscope 75:458, 1965.

Chapter 48

PRINCIPLES OF RADIATION THERAPY

by B. S. Aron, M.D.

RADIATION THERAPY AND THE RADIATION THERAPIST

Radiation therapy is a clinical specialty in which the treatment modality of ionizing radiation is used to treat patients with cancer and allied diseases. In the United States this specialty was developed by radiologists because of the initial use of a similar modality (x-rays) in diagnosis and treatment. However, radiation therapy is more closely allied to other specialties in oncology such as surgery and chemotherapy.

The radiation therapist is primarily a clinician whose background and interest lie in two areas—oncology and radiation therapy. The usual training period is three years; this includes experience in pathology, surgery, internal medicine, chemotherapy, and radiation physics. In the past this training was undertaken in conjunction with diagnostic radiology, but at present the fields are separating into two distinct disciplines.

Just as the radiation therapist who treats patients with cancer of the larynx must familiarize himself with the general outlines of otolaryngology, so must the otolaryngologist understand the basic principles of radiation therapy. This chapter presents an outline of these principles.

CLINICAL RADIATION BIOLOGY

Therapeutic Ratio—Radiation Sensitivity

The aim of a radiation therapy treatment is to destroy a malignant tumor and allow healing of the normal tissue within the treatment volume. The success or failure of this treatment depends on the therapeutic ratio of the radiation effect on the tumor and the normal tissue. A positive therapeutic ratio (greater effect on the tumor than normal tissue) is a necessity. This alone does not determine radiation curability; the biological behavior of a tumor is also significant.

Different normal tissues and different tumors vary in their sensitivities to radiation. Bergonie and Tribondeau, in 1906, formulated a general rule of radiation sensitivity: "X-rays are more effective on cells which have a greater reproductive activity, the effectiveness is greater on those cells which have a larger dividing future ahead, on those cells the morphology and function of which are least fixed."

The significant normal tissues and organs vary markedly in their sensitivity to radiation. In order of decreasing sensitivity they are: lens of the eye, bone marrow and lymph nodes, ovary and testes, gastrointestinal epithelium, kidney, lung, central nervous system, salivary glands, upper respiratory tract epithelium, mucous membrane of the oropharynx, skin, connective tissue, bone, and skeletal muscle.

The radiation effects on the normal tissues in the head and neck will be discussed in detail in a later section of this chapter.

In general, tumors have the same sensitivity to radiation as the normal tissue of origin. The significant primary tumors encountered in the field of otolaryngology are listed as radiation-sensitive tumors (Table 1) and radiation-resistant tumors (Table 2).

Clinically a markedly radiation-sensitive tumor is one which disappears quickly and

TABLE 1. *Radiation-Sensitive Tumors*

MARKEDLY SENSITIVE	MODERATELY SENSITIVE
1. Hodgkin's disease 2. Reticulum cell sarcoma 3. Lymphosarcoma 4. Multiple myeloma 5. Ewing's tumor	1. Epidermoid carcinoma (including differentiated and undifferentiated tumors and lympho-epithelioma)

TABLE 2. *Radiation-Resistant Tumors*

MODERATELY RESISTANT	MARKEDLY RESISTANT
1. Salivary and mucous gland tumors 2. Thyroid tumors 3. Rhabdomyosarcoma	1. Malignant melanoma 2. Connective tissue, bone and neurogenic sarcomas

permanently during treatment to a moderate dose of radiation (3000 to 4500 R in three to five weeks). Lymph nodes in Hodgkin's disease may shrink markedly after as low a dose as 2000 R in two weeks. A moderately sensitive squamous cell carcinoma of the tonsil starts to shrink after 3000 to 4000 R in three to four weeks—higher doses, up to 6000 to 6500 R in six to seven weeks, are necessary for cure (Perez et al., 1970). A moderately resistant salivary gland adenocarcinoma shrinks slowly after higher doses of radiation (6500 to 7500 R in seven to eight weeks) and rarely disappears completely. A markedly resistant osteogenic sarcoma of the mandible shrinks very little after even higher doses of radiation.

Four radiation biological factors determine the radiation effects on normal tissue and tumors: dose, time, volume, and quality of radiation.

Dose Factors

All radiation effects are proportional to dose—the greater the dose, the greater the effect. The units of dose commonly used indicate a measure of the ionization (roentgen) or of the absorbed energy (rad) of the radiation.

All dose effects follow a similar sigmoid-shaped dose response curve (Fig. 1). Below a certain dose (threshold dose) no effects are visible (see dose X on curve A in Figure 1). Larger doses produce proportionately greater effects (the straight portion of the curve). Once there has been complete destruction of the tissue or tumor (lethal dose Y on curve A), increasing the dose causes no further effect. This basic dose response curve describes radiation effects on normal tissue and tumors, both sensitive and resistant. Larger doses are needed to produce these effects on resistant tissues or tumors (see curve B in Figure 1).

A positive therapeutic ratio may be re-expressed as the ratio of effects on the dose response curves. If curve A represented a tumor and curve B represented the surrounding normal tissue (the clinical situation when Hodgkin's disease involving cervical nodes is treated with radiation therapy), the therapeutic ratio would be positive.

When a beam of x-rays or gamma radiation enters tissue, it ionizes the molecules into positive ions or molecules (very chemically reactive) and electrons. As the radiation is very energetic (thousands of electron volts—KV or orthovoltage—or millions of electron volts—MV or megavoltage), the electrons also are very energetic and cause further ionization. The roentgen is the unit of ionization and is that quantity of x-rays or gamma radiation such that the associated corpuscular emission (electrons and positive ions), per standard weight of air, produces in air ions carrying one electrostatic unit of electricity of either sign. This ionization is completed in about 10^{-21} seconds. The energy is transferred to the ions and molecules of tissue. The rad is the unit of energy transfer; this is defined as 100 ergs of energy absorbed per gram of tissue. The presence of oxygen facilitates this reaction. When megavoltage radiation is used in soft tissue, one roentgen equals approximately one rad.

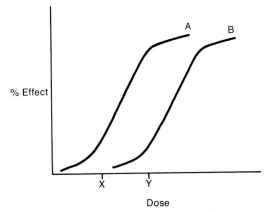

Figure 1. Dose response curve. *A* = sensitive tissue or tumor; *B* = resistant tissue or tumor.

This process of energy absorption is completed in 10^{-13} seconds.

Many biologically important reactions occur as a result of this radiation, and significant molecules are damaged both intra- and extracellularly. The most significant molecule for radiation effect is deoxyribonucleic acid (Andrews, 1962). When DNA molecules are irradiated in solution, chain scission occurs with resultant increased viscosity of the solution due to breaking of the twin coils into smaller fragments. This inactivation of DNA results ultimately in cell death, the main factor causing damage to normal tissues and destruction of tumors.

At the cellular level in the usual range of dose employed in radiation therapy three main effects are noted:

1. A small fraction of cells is killed immediately, in interphase or resting phase of their cycle. This occurs in small round cells with large nuclei and a thin rim of cytoplasm (lymphocytes, spermatogonia—the very radiosensitive cells).

2. A temporary arrest of mitosis and delay of growth occurs in all cells; the duration of this arrest depends on the dose of radiation. A dose of 500 R causes mitotic arrest of 24 hours in jejunal epithelium (normally mitosis occurs every 24 hours) and of several days in basal cell carcinoma. Single doses in the therapeutic range of 2000 R cause mitotic arrest of a few weeks in basal cell carcinoma.

3. A certain fraction of irradiated cells will suffer loss of reproductive integrity owing to DNA inactivation. These cells will survive as giant cells until the time for the next mitosis or even up to three or four mitoses, eventually to die in mitosis. Until cell death occurs, it is difficult to identify these cells histologically. A pathologist, examining a tumor which has received preoperative radiation, cannot distinguish these cells from other tumor cells which have the ability to continue to proliferate unless cell culture methods are used.

If, after a certain dose of radiation, 50 per cent of the cells survive and 50 per cent of the cells die in mitosis, we state that this dose of radiation causes a surviving fraction of $50/100 = 1/2$.

This loss of reproduction integrity, originally described by Puck and Marcus in 1956, is the specific effect on tumors with which radiation therapy is primarily concerned. It occurs in all tumors and normal tissues and may be expressed as the cell dose response curve (Fig. 2).

These cell dose response curves have a flat portion, or shoulder, suggesting that a certain dose must be accumulated before cell death occurs (threshold dose). The D_{37} value (37 per cent survival) is the mathematical slope of the straight portion of the curve and varies between 100 and 140 rads for mammalian cells and tumors. The slope of the curve varies with the radiosensitivity of the particular cell type and many other factors, such as environment during radiation, type and method of administration of radiation, and biological state of the cells. The extrapolation number varies between 2 and 12, suggesting that a multihit effect is necessary for cell death.

Time Factors

All radiation effects are modified by time—as the time (days) taken to deliver a certain dose is increased, the biological effect of that dose is decreased.

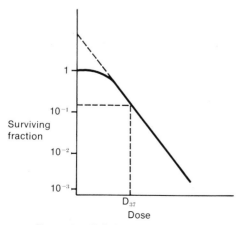

Figure 2.   Cell dose response curve.

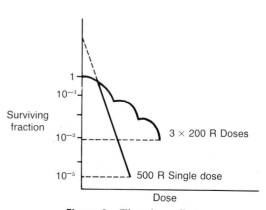

Figure 3.   Time dose effect.

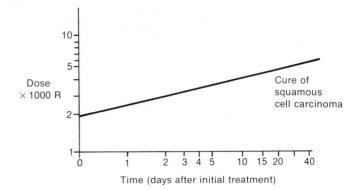

Figure 4. Dose time equivalence.

In terms of the basic cell dose response curve, Elkind and Sutton (1960) noted that there is less radiation effect (a greater surviving fraction) with three doses of 200 R delivered at six-hour intervals than with 500 R administered in a single dose (Fig. 3). Cell recovery (repair of sublethal injury) occurs during this time period between radiation doses. Thus, if radiation is given in daily fractions, the overall effect will be less than if the same total dose were given in a single dose. To achieve the same effect as a single dose, the total dose of a fractionated course of radiation therapy must be increased.

Strandquist (1944) documented this phenomenon in his clinical study of 280 skin cancers of skin and lip (Fig. 4). He plotted the results of treatment with various doses over different time intervals and noted that there was a zone in which the tumors were cured without necrosis of skin; thus, a single dose of 2000 R was equivalent to a dose of 600 R over 40 days, and so on. All dose-time treatments below this line resulted in recurrence of the tumor, and treatments above this line resulted in cure of the tumor with skin necrosis. Thus a 5000 R dose could cause skin necrosis if given in five days, recurrence of the tumor if given in 40 days, or cure of the tumor and healing of the skin (the desired effect of radiation therapy) if given in 21 days.

This phenomenon has been observed for small tumors. The units must be modified with larger tumors and large volumes of normal tissue; nevertheless, time-dose equivalence curve has been observed with other tumors and normal tissues. The slopes of the curves vary with the mitotic activity of the tumor or the normal tissue.

The overall dose and the overall time (protraction) are not the only factors of importance; the number of doses and the dose per fraction (fractionation) are also important. A dose of 6000 R given in 30 daily doses of 200 R five times a week (Monday through Friday) over a period of six weeks causes 10 to 20 per cent less biological effect than 6000 R given in 18 doses of 335 R three times a week (Monday, Wednesday, and Friday) over the same six-week period.

Ellis (1969) devised a general formula relating these variables based on normal connective tissue tolerance:

$$D = NSD \times N^{.24} \times T^{.11}$$

where D = total dose, N = number of fractions, NSD = nominal single dose, and T = overall times in days.

Volume Factors—Oxygen Effect

The volume of the tumor and the surrounding normal tissue modifies the radiation effect. The dose tolerated by normal tissue decreases as the volume of normal tissue increases, and the dose needed to cure tumors increases as the tumor becomes larger. As a result of these two factors, higher cure rates are obtained with small tumors than with larger tumors of the same pathological type at the same site.

The first factor is exemplified in the Skin Tolerance Table of Patterson (1963) (Table 3), which gives the tolerance dose in rads for skin reactions from orthovoltage radiation therapy. These doses must be adjusted for megavoltage by the appropriate R.B.E. (increase by 15

TABLE 3. *Skin Tolerance Dose (R)*

	FIELD SIZE (cm.)			
TIME	7 × 5	10 × 8	12 × 10	20 × 10
1 Day	2000	1700	1500	–
4 Days	3500	3000	2500	2000
10 Days	4500	4000	3500	3000
3 Weeks	5250	4500	4000	3500
5 Weeks	6000	5000	4500	4000

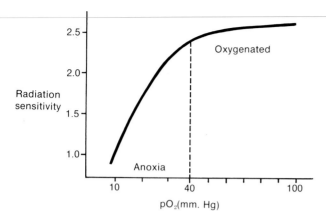

Figure 5. Oxygen effect.

per cent); they may then serve as a general outline for normal tissue tolerance (maximum tolerated dose). If these doses are compared to the Stranquist curve for squamous cell carcinoma, it can be seen that the tolerated doses are in the same range for the smaller field sizes (7 × 5 cm. and 10 × 8 cm.), but not for the larger field sizes.

Severe reactions caused by irradiation of large volumes of normal tissue to higher doses are not tolerated by patients. As an example, the posterior oropharynx will tolerate a tumoricidal dose of radiation (6000 R in five weeks); the patient will develop a severe mucositis and dysphagia. However, the patient will not tolerate the severe reaction when a larger volume is irradiated (oropharynx and oral cavity) to the same dose. Once the reaction occurs, he will stop eating and drinking or refuse radiation therapy.

The presence or absence of oxygen profoundly affects the basic cell response to radiation. Gray (1957) irradiated cell cultures in vitro under different concentrations of pO_2 (Fig. 5) and noted that "the radiation effect on living cells in anoxia rapidly increases with oxygenation until it reaches a near maximum at the pO_2 found in normal capillary and tissue fluids." The oxygen effect ratio was 2.5; similar results are obtained with cell dose response curves in vitro and in vivo.

Thomlinson and Gray (1955) studied oxygen diffusion in vitro and in vivo in intercapillary spaces and correlated this with the vascular microstructure of tumors and normal tissue. Microscopically squamous carcinoma consists of cord of tumor cells surrounding a normal capillary; the cells near the capillary were noted to be healthy, whereas the cells furthest away were frequently found to be necrotic. The measured distance from capillary to necrotic

area was reasonably constant at about 145 μ. The distance that oxygen can diffuse through tissue is about 150 μ. Normal tissues have a normal pO_2. Tumors vary considerably; many cells are hypoxic or anoxic, especially as the tumor grows larger. The blood supply of tumors is usually the normal capillary structure of the tissue of origin; but as the tumor enlarges, it outgrows this supply and becomes necrotic (this is especially prominent in ulcerated oropharynx cancers or large cervical nodes).

Thus as a tumor enlarges, hypoxic or anoxic cells, which are relatively more resistant to radiation by a factor of about 2.5, become a larger proportion of the tumor cell population. Also, as a tumor enlarges, the total number of tumor cells which have the capacity for unlimited proliferation increases. These two factors make larger radiation doses necessary to cure these tumors.

Attempts to favorably influence the radiation sensitivity of tumors through the oxygen effect have been made using the following methods:

1. Increased tumor oxygenation
2. Normal tissue anoxia
3. Avoidance of oxygen effect

The basic concepts of these methods are as follows:

Increased Tumor Oxygenation. If the local pO_2 in the tumor and the surrounding normal tissue is increased, there will be a marked increase in radiation sensitivity of the tumor with minimal increase in sensitivity of normal tissue (Fig. 5). Increasing the capillary pO_2 will increase the local tumor pO_2; this may be accomplished by having the patient breathe pure oxygen under three atmospheres of pressure in a hyperbaric tank (resulting in an increased capillary pO_2 from a normal of 100 to 2000 mm.Hg), having the patient breathe pure oxygen from a mask (less increase of capillary

pO_2), or by infusing hydrogen peroxide during radiation therapy. There will be a modest increase in capillary pO_2 if the patient's hemoglobin is raised above 11 gm. per cent before radiation therapy; this increase has been measured directly in cervical (uterine) squamous carcinoma.

A supervascularization effect is produced during a course of fractionated radiation therapy. As the bulk of tumor cells is destroyed, there is a relative increase in the capillary density. Thus the remaining tumor cells are better oxygenated. This has been verified experimentally by Badib and Webster (1959), who measured pO_2 in tumors before and during a course of fractionated radiation and showed a positive correlation between tumor control and increase in pO_2.

Normal Tissue Anoxia. If the local pO_2 in the tumor and the surrounding normal tissue is decreased, there will be a marked decrease in the sensitivity of the normal tissue with minimal decrease in sensitivity of the tumor. Normal tissue anoxia may be produced in the extremities by tourniquet occlusion of the blood vessels. This has been used in the treatment of connective tissue and bone sarcomas in the leg and arm. However, this is not applicable to the head and neck region because of the possibility of cerebral anoxia.

Avoidance of Oxygen Effect. Particle radiation (i.e., neutrons) does not show an oxygen effect. Thus anoxic tumor has an oxygen effect ratio of about 1.3 compared to oxygenated tumor. This represents a major advantage over x-radiation and accounts for the current interest in developing this modality.

Quality Factors

Quality of radiation refers to the type of radiation (i.e., x-rays, gamma rays, electrons, protons, etc.) or energy of the beam of radiation. A full discussion of these factors lies in the field of radiation physics; in this section only those parameters will be discussed insofar as they affect the patient.

When a beam of radiation enters a patient, there is relatively more absorption of energy near the surface than deeper in tissue. The peak absorption of energy (100 per cent dose) may be at the surface or a few centimeters below the surface, depending on the energy of the radiation. The energy absorbed at a certain depth is defined as the percentage depth dose relative to the 100 per cent depth dose.

Superficial Radiation Therapy (90–140 KV)

The peak dose is at the skin surface, and there is relatively little penetration into tissue—the 80 per cent depth dose is at 1.0 cm. and the 50 per cent depth dose is at 3.0 cm. below the skin surface. Therefore, if a dose of 6000 rads is delivered to the skin surface, the dose at 1.0 cm. is 4800 rads and the dose at 3.0 cm. is 3000 rads. This quality of radiation is useful only in treating superficial tumors such as skin tumors (Fig. 6).

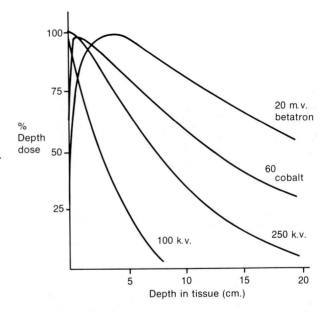

Figure 6. Central axis per cent depth dose curves.

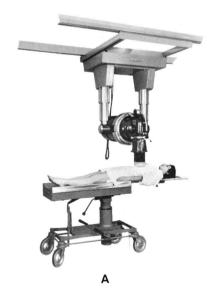

A

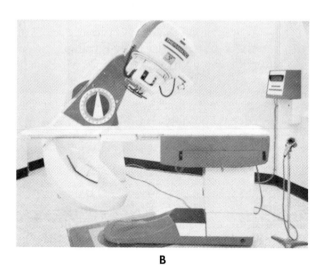

B

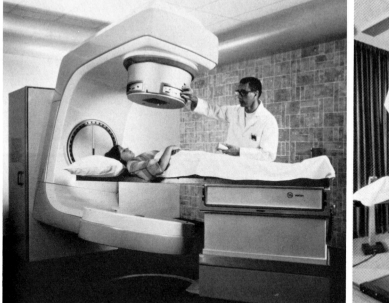

C

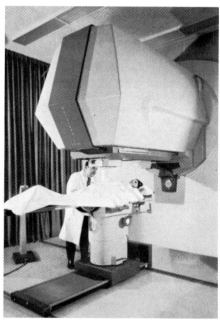

D

Figure 7.   Radiation therapy units. *A*, Orthovoltage therapy unit (100 kv. to 300 kv.). (Photo courtesy Picker X-Ray Corp.). *B*, ^{60}Cobalt teletherapy unit. (Photo courtesy Atomic Energy of Canada, Ltd.). *C*, 4 m.e.v. linear accelerator. (Photo courtesy Varian Radiation Division). *D*, 42 m.e.v. Betatron. (Photo courtesy Siemens Corp.)

Orthovoltage Radiation Therapy
(200–300 KV) (Fig. 7.)

This quality of radiation was the basis of clinical radiation therapy from 1925 to 1950; many orthovoltage units are still used in treating patients. The peak dose (100 per cent) is at the skin surface and there is moderate penetration into tissue. Percentage depth dose curves for different qualities of radiation are shown in Figure 6. The absorbed dose varies with the atomic number of the absorbing material. As bone contains a large amount of calcium (atomic number 20), it will absorb 40 per cent more of the dose (rads) than soft tissue, which is mostly carbon (atomic number 6), hydrogen (atomic number 1), and oxygen (atomic number 8).

Radiation skin reactions frequently limit the dose that can be delivered to a tumor. In treating carcinoma of the larynx the tumor is about 2 cm. below the skin surface (per cent D.D. = 95 per cent). Therefore, 6300 rads must be delivered to the skin surface to deliver 6000 rads to the tumor. This skin dose will be tolerated (see Table 3), and consequently this is a practical treatment. However, in treatment of carcinoma of the tonsil, where the tumor is about 6 cm. below the skin surface (per cent D.D. = 60 per cent), a single lateral field of radiation will require a 10,000 rad skin dose to deliver 6000 rads to the tumor. This excessive skin dose will cause necrosis of the skin, therefore, the required dose cannot be delivered to the tumor by this method. The tumor dose will be improved if two opposing lateral fields (right and left lateral) are used to crossfire the tonsil tumor; the tumor will receive 3000 rads from each field if the skin dose on each field is 5000 rads (tolerated by the skin). However, the mandible will actually absorb more radiation (40 per cent more) and receive a dose of 8400 rads (6000 rads plus 40 per cent). This high bone dose is one of the factors which lead to osteoradionecrosis.

There are many sites in the head and neck area where the dose that can de delivered to the tumor with orthovoltage radiation is limited by the tolerance of the skin. Some of these sites are nasopharynx, posterior oropharynx, maxillary antrum, and middle ear.

Megavoltage Radiation Therapy
(1–42 MV) (Fig. 7).

The era of megavoltage radiation therapy began in the 1950's. Currently most curative radiation therapy is performed on ^{60}Cobalt units (2 MV), linear accelerators (4–12 MV), or betatrons (22–42 MV). These therapy units are expensive, costing from \$75,000 to \$250,000, respectively, as compared to \$25,000 for an orthovoltage unit.

The peak dose (100 per cent) is below the skin surface, ranging from 0.5 to 5.0 cm. Therefore, there is skin sparing. Radiation skin reactions are no longer the bête noire of the radiotherapist. The peak dose is in the subcutaneous tissue where larger doses are better tolerated by normal connective tissue. If the tumor involves the skin, necessitating 100 per cent dose in the skin, appropriate thicknesses of soft tissue equivalent material (bolus) must be placed on the skin to bring the dose to 100 per cent. The increased energy of the radiation leads to greater penetration into tissue with resultant greater precentage depth dose (Fig. 6). The absorbed dose (rads) does not vary with the atomic number of the absorbing material so that the bone dose and the soft tissue dose are practically identical.

The same carcinoma of the tonsil described in the section on orthovoltage radiation is better treated with megavoltage radiation. The per cent D.D. at 6 cm. below the skin surface is 75 per cent for ^{60}Cobalt gamma rays; therefore, a subcutaneous peak dose of 8000 rads will deliver 6000 rads to the tumor and the mandible. This skin dose is still excessive, and a crossfire arrangement is preferred with 3000 rads delivered from each of two (right and left) lateral fields. The peak dose is 4000 rads. When megavoltage therapy units are used, any tumor dose desired can be easily delivered. The only limitations are those of normal tissue tolerance (i.e., cervical spinal cord, lens, etc.).

Electron Beam Therapy

Electron beam therapy came into clinical use in the 1960's. Megavoltage electron beams are produced by Van der Graaf generators, linear accelerators, and betatrons in the range of 2 to 42 MV.

The peak dose (100 per cent) is at the skin surface, as in orthovoltage radiation. However, the depth of penetration is determined by the energy and is approximately one third the energy in MV per centimeter. The dose falls off very rapidly at greater depths in tissue. This quality of radiation is advantageous only for superficial tumors; for deep-seated tumors (depth greater than 5 cm.) megavoltage x- or gamma radiation is as useful as electron beam therapy.

Brachytherapy refers to short-distance radiation therapy and involves placing radioactive materials in the form of seeds, needles, tubes, or other applicators into tumors (interstitial implants), into body cavities (intracavitary implants), or on the surface of tumors (molds). The radioactive sources used include ^{226}radium, ^{226}radon, ^{60}cobalt, ^{137}cesium, ^{182}tantalum, ^{192}iridium, and ^{198}gold.

All of these sources may emit alpha particles (helium nuclei), beta (electrons) and gamma rays. Their filtration (usually 0.5 mm. platinum) filters out all the rays except the gamma rays; these gamma rays, usually in the megavoltage range, deliver the dose to the tumor.

The dose distribution achieved by this method is characterized by a high local dose in the volume of the implant with rapid decrease of dose in the next few centimeters. The dose given to an interstitial tongue implant by means of radium needles for a small squamous cell carcinoma is 6000 rads—this dose ±10 per cent is delivered to the tumor. The dose 1 cm. away is about 2400 rads, and 2 cm. away is about 1500 rads. This rapid fall-off in dose is achieved by confining the radioactive sources to the tumor volume and because of the inverse square law (all radiation decreases inversely in intensity as the square of the distance from the source). Thus, a dose rate of 8.25 R per hour at 1 cm. from a 1 mg. radium source would decrease to .0825 R per hour at 10 cm. (8.25/10^2). No form of external radiation therapy can achieve the high local dose and rapid fall-off in dose that can be achieved with interstitial or intracavitary implants. When technically possible, these methods are to be preferred in treating small lesions.

Particle Radiation Therapy

Thus far our discussion of quality factors has included only x-rays or gamma rays and electrons. Qualitatively their radiobiological effects are similar, although there are quantitative differences. When particles are used in radiation therapy (i.e., neutrons, protons, pi mesons, etc.), there are different quantitative effects. At the present time cyclotron-produced fast neutrons (6MV) have been the only particles used clinically. Other particles are available only for experimental work.

The theoretical advantage of fast neutrons is an oxygen effect ratio of about 1.0 to 1.3 (Morgan, 1967). An anoxic or hypoxic tumor treated with neutrons would be affected in almost the same way as an oxygenated tumor. Thus, the central hypoxic nidus of tumor would be destroyed by fast neutrons just as the peripheral well oxygenated portion would be destroyed.

There is little recovery between fractionated doses of fast neutrons; the dose-time biological equivalence described for x- or gamma rays does not occur, because the local molecular energy transfer with neutrons is greater. Thus, ten doses (500 rads) of fast neutrons would have almost ten times the biological effect as a single dose of 500 rads.

Radiation Curability

Radiation curability implies two factors—a positive therapeutic ratio of the radiation effect on the tumor as compared to the surrounding normal tissue, and favorable tumor biology. The factors involved in radiation sensitivity (dose, time, volume, and quality) have been discussed previously. One other factor, favorable tumor biology, remains to be discussed in this section.

Clinical radiotherapists have noted that there is a greater chance of curing a large tumor when it is treated by a fractionated course of radiation rather than by a single dose. When a tumor is treated by fractionated radiation therapy, a supervascularization effect is produced as initial peripheral tumor cell destruction decreases the bulk of tumor, and the remaining tumor cells are better vascularized. The capillary and connective tissue stroma represents the normal tissue framework in which the tumor grows; as the tumor decreases in size, there is a relative increase in the capillary stroma—a supervascularization effect. As the remaining central tumor cells are better vascularized, oxygenation is improved and their radiation sensitivity is increased. The increase in local oxygen pO_2 during a course of fractionated radiation therapy has been measured in vivo by Badib (1959) and others. Thus, fractionation increases the therapeutic ratio and is used in all curative treatments.

Tumor biology profoundly affects radiation curability. Tumor biology encompasses the natural history of the tumor, stage at diagnosis, frequency of lymph node spread, and hematogenous dissemination. A squamous cell carcinoma of the lip usually presents in an early stage, at which the tumor size is 1 or 2 cm.

TABLE 4.   Radiation-Curable Tumors

MARKEDLY CURABLE (90% 5-year Survival)	MODERATELY CURABLE (50% 5-year Survival)
1. Early epidermoid carcinoma of skin, lip, oral cavity	1. Early epidermoid carcinoma of nasopharynx
2. Rhabdomyosarcoma of orbit	2. Moderately advanced epidermoid carcinoma of lip, oral cavity, oropharynx and larynx
	3. Localized lymphomas

TABLE 5.   Radiation-Incurable Tumors

LOW CURE RATES—PALLIATION (10% 5-year Survival)	MINIMAL PALLIATION
1. Advanced epidermoid carcinoma	1. Malignant melanoma
2. Salivary gland tumors	2. Connective tissue, bone and neurogenic sarcomas
3. Rhabdomyosarcoma	
4. Thyroid tumors	

Lymph node spread is infrequent and hematogenous dissemination is very rare, all factors implying favorable tumor biology. The cure rate for this tumor is in the 90 per cent range with radiation therapy (MacComb and Fletcher, 1967). A squamous cell carcinoma of the base of the tongue, which has the same radiation sensitivity as the lip, presents late and usually with invasion of surrounding structures. Lymph node spread is frequent even at the time of diagnosis, and hematogenous dissemination is not rare—all factors implying unfavorable tumor biology. The cure rate for this tumor is in the 30 per cent range with radiation therapy (Fletcher and MacComb, 1962).

Both a positive therapeutic ratio and favorable tumor biology are necessary for radiation curability. The radiation curable tumors are listed in Table 4 and the incurable tumors in Table 5 (MacComb and Fletcher, 1967; Fletcher and MacComb, 1962). Significant palliation, in terms of pain relief, healing of ulceration, relief of pressure symptoms, and so on, may be achieved in treating some tumors even though their advanced stage or poor therapeutic ratios do not allow curative treatment. These tumors are listed in Table 5. Other tumors are so radioresistant that little symptomatic relief is obtained with radiation therapy.

CLINICAL RADIATION THERAPY

The clinical treatment of patients with malignant disease by radiation therapy is a full-time job. Poor results will be obtained when patients are hastily positioned under a beam of external radiation and not followed closely either during or after treatment.

The aim of clinical radiation therapy is to deliver a tumoricidal dose of radiation to the tumor with minimal dose to the surrounding normal tissue. Precise treatment planning is necessary; this may involve a few days' work and is as exact as any surgical procedure. Treatment planning consists of the following steps.

(A) Evaluation of the tumor volume must be made. The tumor volume to which the high dose of radiation is to be delivered is evaluated clinically by examination of the patient (inspection and palpation) and use of diagnostic x-ray procedures (lateral soft tissue x-rays, tomograms, contrast studies, etc.).

(B) The tumor must be localized. Diagnostic x-rays are taken in various positions (anterior, posterior, lateral, and oblique) with radiopaque markers in the skin surface or immobilization shell (which fits over the skin) or in the tumor (with surgical clips or inactive radon seeds). The tumor volume may then be outlined on the

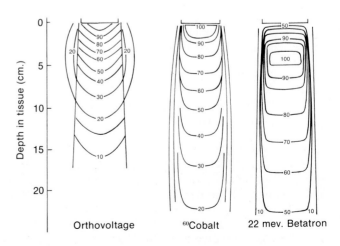

Figure 8.   Isodose curves.

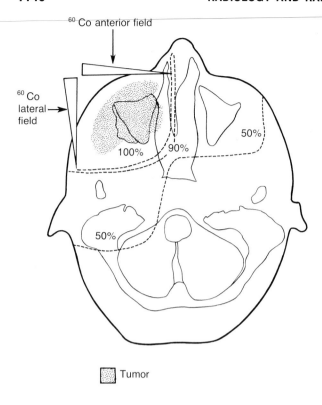

Tumor

Figure 9. Wedge pair treatment of maxillary sinus carcinoma.

x-rays. A contour is made of the cross-section of the patient at the level of the tumor by means of malleable wire or plaster of Paris. The surface marks are incorporated in this contour, which is transferred to paper. The tumor volume as well as the position of significant normal structures, such as the cervical spinal cord, mandible, and so forth, is drawn on this cross-section.

(C) The field arrangement to be used for a particular patient is then chosen. The area covered by individual radiation fields is outlined by isodose curves (two-dimensional "depth dose curves"; see Figure 8) for each field size and energy. The dose delivered to the tumor volume by individual fields (isodose curves) is then summated in an isodose distribution on the previously drawn cross-section map of the patient.

Specific field arrangements for individual sites are considered in a later discussion of individual tumors. Only a few examples will be included in this section.

Maxillary antral lesions are best treated by a pair of wedge fields directed at right angles to one another, as shown in Figure 9. Large tumors of the oropharynx with metastatic nodes are treated with parallel opposed right and left lateral fields, as shown in Figure 10.

(D) The dose to be delivered is mathematically determined and the treatment prescribed.

(E) Application of treatment is begun. The field arrangements are set up on the patient using beam direction and immobilization devices as necessary to ensure that the treatment may be successfully carried out over a three- to six-week period of daily treatments, five days a week.

During a course of external radiation therapy the patient is examined at least once a week, and more often if necessary, to evaluate the response to treatment and the reaction of the normal tissues. Minor adjustments in treatment technique may be made, and the patient is given the necessary medical care. Following the conclusion of the treatment, the patient is examined weekly to evaluate the complete response to therapy. This may not be manifest until four to six weeks later.

When interstitial implants are used, the implant is calculated according to the Patterson-Parker system based on the tumor volume (Meredith, 1958). The requisite number of radium needles is then brought to the operating room, and the tumor is implanted with a specific distribution (i.e., single-plane, two-plane, or volume) with the patient under general endotracheal anesthesia. Individual needles are

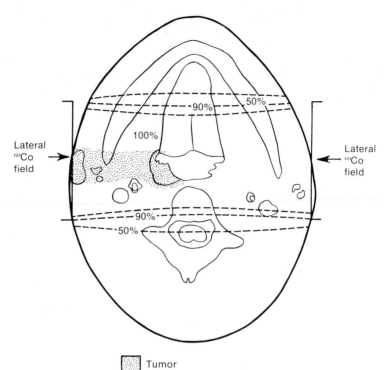

Figure 10. Lateral parallel opposed pair treatment of tonsil carcinoma.

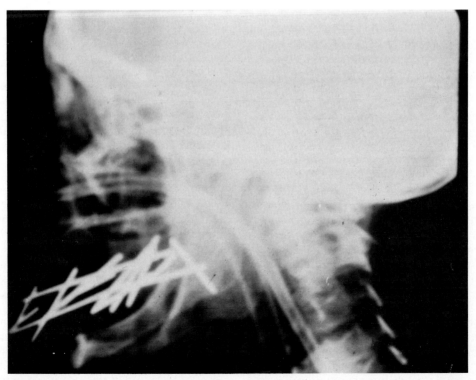

Figure 11. Interstitial implant. A single plane radium needle implant for epidermoid carcinoma of the dorsum of the tongue.

sewn into place. Needless to say, this procedure demands expertise on the part of the operator performing the implant as well as familiarity with operating room techniques. When the patient has left the recovery room after the implantation, diagnostic x-rays are taken so that the volume of the implant may be accurately calculated. The implant is left in place for four to seven days, delivering a dose to 4000 to 6500 rads, and then easily removed in the patient's room or the radiation therapy department. An example of a single-plane radium needle implant for a squamous carcinoma of the dorsum of the tongue is shown in Figure 11.

The lesions that are treated primarily by mold or interstitial therapy are early squamous cell carcinomas (T_1 and T_2) of the following sites:

1. Molds — skin, lip, and buccal mucosa
2. Interstitial implants — anterior floor of mouth, lateral border and surface of the tongue, and buccal mucosa.

Interstitial implants are also frequently used in the palliative treatment of metastatic cervical nodes.

COMBINATION OF RADIATION AND SURGERY

Radiation and surgery may be combined in a variety of ways in the treatment of malignant neoplasms of the head and neck area.

In some sites (nasopharynx, lip, anterior tongue) radiation may be used to treat the primary tumor, while surgery is used for the lymph node metastases. In other sites (early vocal cord carcinoma) radiation may be used primarily with surgery performed to control infrequent local recurrences. Conversely, radiation may be used to treat postoperative recurrences. These techniques will be discussed in a later section.

Planned combinations of radiation therapy and surgery may involve either preoperative or postoperative radiation and radical surgery in the treatment of the same lesion. Usually tumors with a moderate cure rate are treated in this fashion. If a high cure rate is obtained with a single treatment modality, then combination therapy is not needed; conversely, for very low cure rates combination therapy will probably not be effective. Tumors with high local recurrence rates, in which either radiation or surgery alone offers little chance of local control, are best treated by combination therapy. When both modalities are used, radiation is generally used preoperatively.

Preoperative Radiation Therapy

The aims of preoperative radiation therapy are as follows (Nickson and Glickman, 1966):

1. To render locally unresectable cancers resectable.
2. To render nonviable any tumor cells implanted in the wound or spread into the vascular system during surgery.
3. To increase the resistance of normal tissues to tumor cell implants.
4. To improve the cure rate in moderately advanced tumors when it is impractical or impossible to determine the extent of tumor preoperatively.

As tumors increase in size, the supporting normal connective tissue and blood vessels become incapable of supplying oxygen and nutritional requirements, with the result that the central portion of the tumor mass becomes hypoxic and eventually necrotic. The peripheral portion of the tumor invading normal tissue is well vascularized and tends to be well oxygenated. As we have noted previously, the oxygenated peripheral portion of the tumor is more radiosensitive than the hypoxic central portion by a factor of approximately three. The surgeon is usually able to resect the central portion of the tumor with a margin of apparently normal tissue; however, the peripheral extensions of tumor that are submucosal or in perineural lymphatics are frequently cut through at the time of resection. Therefore, radiation and surgery may be complimentary in their attack on tumors — radiation controlling the peripheral, well oxygenated extensions of tumor followed by surgical removal of the hypoxic central core of tumor.

The dose of radiation necessary to sterilize a tumor varies directly with the number of viable tumor cells. This has been formulated previously as the cell dose response curve. If a tumor consists of 10^{10} viable cells and the D_{10} (dose for 10 per cent survival or 90 per cent loss of reproductive integrity) single dose is 200 rads, then ten D_{10} doses (2000 rads) would be necessary to sterilize this tumor. A smaller dose of radiation — 1600 rads (eight D_{10} single doses biologically equivalent to 4000 rads in three weeks) — would result in a depopulation of 10^{-8}, leaving 10^2 viable tumor cells. Thus, doses of radiation that are less than tumoricidal would still sterilize the majority of tumor cells. These doses of radiation, commonly used in preoperative radiation therapy, may well sterilize the peripheral portion of the tumor (fewer tumor cells), leaving a remnant of viable tumor cells in the central core of tumor.

At the time of surgery there is spread of tumor cells into the vascular system; these cells may be recovered in 34 per cent of head and neck cancer operations (Delarue et al., 1964). Powers and Palmer (1968) have shown that in animal experiments there is a decrease in the frequency of tumor growths after implantation of tumor cells which have been exposed to subtumoricidal doses of radiation. Others have shown that there is a decrease in frequency of deaths from distant metastases after subtumoricidal doses of preoperative radiation and surgery as compared to surgery alone. It has also been noted that radiation of the recipient site in animals decreases the frequency of tumor growths after implantation of tumor cells in these sites, if radiation was given before implantation of tumor cells. All these experiments suggest that preoperative radiation may decrease the number of local recurrences and distant metastases after surgery.

The disadvantages of preoperative radiation therapy are as follows:

1. Impaired wound healing with increased postoperative morbidity. This is a real problem which can be minimized by proper surgical techniques; it cannot be avoided completely.

2. Delay in curative surgery. This should not affect the cure of the tumor for the reasons mentioned above.

3. Increased costs to patient. This is not significant if an increased cure rate is obtained.

The principles of preoperative radiation therapy are as follows (Moss and Brand, 1969):

1. The tumor volume irradiated should be more extensive than the anticipated surgical excision. Even if the tumor has not decreased markedly in size and the surgical excision extends through microscopic tumor, the tumor cells will be nonviable.

2. Megavoltage radiation therapy should be used, as the absence of severe skin reaction will allow adequate wound healing.

3. The dose of radiation therapy should usually be less than curative, so as to minimize surgical morbidity. Three dose levels are currently used:

(A) Rapid low dose schedules—1000 rads as a single dose the day before surgery or 2000 rads in one week with surgery performed a few days later. This should be effective in reducing recurrences in the operative site, but will allow little time for gross change in the tumor mass.

(B) Moderate dose schedules—4000 rads in three weeks to 5000 rads in five weeks with surgery performed three to six weeks later. This will allow time for maximum shrinkage of the tumor and maximum radiation effect. However, the extent of the surgical excision should be planned before radiation therapy and not changed later as subtumoricidal doses have been delivered.

(C) High dose schedules—6000 to 7000 rads in six to eight weeks with surgery performed six to eight weeks later. This treatment should be reserved for tumors of uncertain extent for which neither curative radiation nor curative surgery is possible. Surgery should be delayed as long as possible to obtain full regression from this tumoricidal dose of radiation. The limits of surgical excision are then planned on the basis of the existing tumor residue, not the initial tumor extent. Complications (i.e., postoperative morbidity) are anticipated with this method of treatment. Its use should be carefully evaluated in individual patients and not applied to hopelessly untreatable patients.

4. There should be a waiting period of approximately three to six weeks from the completion of moderate-dose radiation therapy to surgery. The acute radiation reaction, which includes mucositis, increased vascularity, dysphagia, and so on, will usually subside within this time period. If surgery is undertaken before the acute reaction subsides, there will be a marked increase in morbidity. The chronic radiation reaction, which includes endarteritis and fibrosis, usually begins at about two months after radiation; tissues already damaged by radiation poorly tolerate the added insult of surgery at this time. Thus, there is a "golden period" when surgery should be undertaken with minimal morbidity.

5. The pathological report of the excised tumor should be evaluated carefully. The presence of "viable" tumor cells does not imply that these cells have the capacity for unlimited growth—they might have died in the next mitosis. Conversely the absence of tumor cells in a cursory examination of one or two sections of the tumor should not imply complete destruction of the tumor by radiation.

The complication rate of postirradiation radical surgery is not prohibitive. Ditchik and

Lampe (1963) have reported that "the postoperative complication rates were low and interference with surgical technique was negligible." The complications mentioned include orocutaneous fistulas, slough of the skin (requiring skin graft), rupture of the carotid artery, and others. These occurred in five out of 50 patients treated by moderate- to high-dose preoperative radiation and radical surgery.

Although there is much theoretical and experimental basis for enthusiasm for preoperative radiation, Batley (1968) has noted that "the correct place for this regimen has yet to be proved by controlled studies, and there is a danger that overenthusiasm may produce disillusionment." Results in individual tumor sites are discussed in another chapter.

Postoperative Radiation Therapy

The aim of postoperative radiation therapy is to sterilize tumor which is residual within the volume of surgical excision or at the margins of the resection.

The residual tumor may consist of microscopic nests of tumor cells or gross tumor; in either case it is growing in a volume of normal tissue which has sustained maximum disturbance in vascularity. Therefore, this tumor is usually hypoxic and relatively radioresistant. Also, the normal tissues are less able to tolerate tumoricidal doses of radiation because of the reduction in vascularity and disturbance in connective tissue stroma secondary to the surgery.

The principles of postoperative radiation therapy are as follows:

1. The volume of tissue irradiated ideally consists of the entire surgical excision plus a margin of normal tissue.

2. Megavoltage radiation therapy should be employed, as this is best tolerated by the normal tissue that has been injured by surgery.

3. The dose of radiation therapy should be tumoricidal in the range of 6000 to 7000 rads in six to eight weeks.

4. There should be a waiting period of approximately three to six weeks to allow the surgical incisions to heal and normal tissues to recover as much as possible. Longer time periods are not advisable, since tumor regrowth may be rapid, rendering treatment impossible.

The disadvantages of postoperative radiation therapy are as follows:

1. The treatment volume is frequently too extensive in view of the impaired tissue tolerance to allow tumoricidal doses of radiation without prohibitive postradiation morbidity (i.e., necrosis, ulcerations, fistulas, fibrosis). Therefore, the radiation therapist is frequently faced with the choice of giving either tumoricidal doses of radiation to less than the optimal volume or subtumoricidal doses to the whole volume.

2. The patients referred for postoperative radiation usually have advanced cancer which has spread beyond anticipated limits. Cure rates for these patients will be poor even with surgery and radiation.

In summary, if postoperative radiation is necessary because of residual tumor, preoperative radiation should have been given. Successful postoperative radiation treatments can only be given as high dose-small volume treatments. If the entire resected volume is involved with tumor, radiation therapy usually fails to cure the patient.

NORMAL TISSUE REACTIONS TO RADIATION

Significant normal tissue reactions are frequently unavoidable in radical or curative radiation therapy; just as there is a surgical mortality and morbidity, there is also postradiation morbidity. Radiation treatments must be designed so as to minimize normal tissue reactions, but never at the price of decrease in cure rates.

Two general types of reactions by normal tissue are encountered. All patients suffer acute reactions of varying severity during and shortly after the treatment. These are practically unavoidable, but can be treated so that fatal complications are usually avoided. Some patients suffer chronic reactions (usually necrosis) for some time after radiation therapy has been completed. This time interval may be a few months to many years. These severe reactions should be avoided, if possible, because fatal complications may ensue despite proper management. Palliative treatments should be designed so that early reactions are minimized and late reactions avoided completely. For a detailed discussion of normal tissue reaction to radiation, the reader is referred to *Clinical Radiation Pathology* by Rubin and Casarett (1968).

The significant normal tissue reactions encountered in the head and neck area and the treatment of these reactions will be outlined for individual sites.

Eye

Many of the normal structures of the eye may be injured by radiation — cornea, ciliary apparatus, lens, and retina. Injury to periocular structures, such as eyelashes, eyelids, lacrimal glands, and nasolacrimal duct, contributes to injuries to the eye.

The eyelashes may be epilated following radiation in a manner similar to epilation elsewhere on the body (3000 rads in two weeks). This epilation abolishes the protective blink reflex. The eyelids will produce mucosal reactions and skin reactions similar to those of the oral cavity mucosa and skin. Chronic fibrosis and scarring will lead to contracture and deformity of the lid margin and secondary severe corneal reactions. The lacrimal gland has a radiation sensitivity similar to salivary glands; secretion of tears will be decreased at doses above 4000 rads in four weeks. Moreover, a "dry" eye deteriorates rapidly. The nasolacrimal duct is rarely injured by cancericidal doses of radiation. The cornea is injured by doses in the range of 5000 rads, with a resultant punctate keratitis and ulceration.

Changes in all these tissues result in a painful eye with decrease in vision, which is to be avoided if possible. With the surface-sparing properties of megavoltage radiation (100 per cent dose below the surface), the eye may be treated by a direct field of radiation. As long as the eye is open and looking directly at the beam of radiation, these reactions will be avoided. This represents a distinct advantage over orthovoltage therapy (100 per cent on the surface).

The significant radiation effect on the lens is cataract formation, which may occur with a dose as low as 200 rads in a single dose. There is increasing frequency of cataract formation with increasing dose up to 1200 rads (Merriman and Focht, 1957). Above this dose cataracts will occur in 100 per cent of irradiated eyes from several months to many years after radiation. These cataracts may not adversely affect vision, although they are visualized by the ophthalmologist. Significant visual loss occurs after higher doses, about 4000 rads; direct megavoltage irradiation of the globe does not usually spare the lens. The radiation-induced cataract may be treated surgically with results similar to those attained in treating normally occurring cataracts.

Irradiation to cancericidal doses may produce an iridocyclitis resulting in glaucoma; the severe pain ensuing may necessitate enucleation. Surgical procedures may relieve the tension and save the vision. Following doses in the range of 5000 to 7000 rads, the retina shows late changes which are characterized by narrowing of vessels, choroidal atrophy, and retinal degeneration. Retinal and vitrous hemorrhages may result from rupture of telangiectatic vessels, and retinal detachment is a possibility. These changes are infrequent even at cancericidal dose levels.

In summary, the significant changes in the anterior structures of the eye and orbit can be avoided. Cataract is an unavoidable sequela of high dose radiation. Uveal and retinal changes are infrequent even at these dose levels.

Ear

Radiation effects on the normal middle ear and inner ear may be acute or chronic. Approximately 50 per cent of patients treated to doses of 4000 to 6000 rads in four to six weeks will develop an acute radiation otitis media during the radiation or shortly thereafter (Borsanyi and Blanchard, 1962). Symptoms are a sensation of fullness in the ear, moderate loss of hearing, tinnitus, and earache. The pathophysiological mechanism is similar to serous otitis media with radiation-induced hyperemia and swelling of the eustachian tube. On examination the eardrums are bulging and show a mild to moderate hyperemia; there is a moderate conductive hearing loss. Radiation otitis media resolves spontaneously in a few weeks and treatment is symptomatic. Aspiration of fluid from the middle ear is rarely necessary. If a purulent infection develops, drainage and antibiotics become mandatory. Permanent hearing loss is very rare.

The late effects of high dose radiation (6000 to 7000 rads in five to eight weeks) are difficult to evaluate, as patients who are treated to this dose usually have middle ear tumors which cause similar changes. Late obliterative endarteritis may lead to damage to the cochlea, labyrinth, and auditory ossicles, resulting in a perceptive type of hearing loss. Surgical treatment may result in improvement in hearing. This late reaction is quite rare.

In summary, acute radiation otitis media is a frequent complication of radiation, but usually it is transient. Other late radiation reactions are infrequent.

Nose

There are no radiation effects specific to the nose or nasal cavity. The nasal mucous membrane and cartilage react to radiation in a fashion similar to the mucous membrane and bone of the oral cavity. Radiation damage to the olfactory nerve endings in the nasal cavity has not been reported.

Skin

All radiation therapy techniques involve irradiation of the skin. Skin reactions frequently were the limiting factor in treating deep-seated tumors with orthovoltage therapy. Megavoltage therapy may cause severe subcutaneous or dermal reactions with minimal epidermal reactions.

Reactions may be divided into early, or acute, reactions and delayed, or chronic, reactions. The severity of both early and late reactions depends on dose, time, and volume factors — more severe reactions will be caused by greater doses in shorter times to larger volumes of skin.

The cells composing the epidermis consist of a rapidly multiplying germinal or basal cell layer that serves as a source for the overlaying nondividing squamous cells. The squamous cells, in turn, become the overlying cornified layer of cells. These cells are shed, so a normal epithelium depends on the mitotically active basal cell layer to replace the loss. The time interval from origin of new cells in the basal cell layer to desquamation of cornified layer is about four weeks in normal skin.

Hair follicles, sweat glands, and sebaceous glands are interspersed in the epidermis. The dermis consists of capillaries within a connective tissue stroma. Pigment cells (chromatophores) are found in the dermis and in the basal cell layer of the epidermis.

Early or Acute Reactions

When a large single dose of superficial or orthovoltage radiation is given (1000 to 2000 rads skin dose), or occasionally during a course of fractionated treatment (300 to 400 rads daily skin dose), a treatment erythema may be noted within 24 hours. This is due to capillary dilation mediated by radiation-induced histamine release. This initial erythema fades within two to three days, and a second erythema appears during the second and third week of treatment. It reaches its peak about the fourth week of treatment, and there may be increased warmth in the skin owing to capillary dilation and congestion. In the early days of radiotherapy the minimal dose necessary to produce this reaction (erythema dose) was used as a unit of dose.

As the orthovoltage radiation therapy is continued in the dose-time-volume range noted in Table 3, there will be injury to the basal cell layer — mitotic arrest and loss of reproduction integrity. Clinically, at about three to four weeks after radiation is started, there will be dry desquamation or peeling of the skin. The dead cornified cells become dark before they flake off. If radiation injury to the basal cell layer has not been too severe, repopulation can occur with no further reaction. This occurs at doses of approximately one half to two thirds of those described in the Skin Tolerance Table (Table 3).

At higher doses radiation injury to the basal cell layer is more severe, and these cells are unable to replace the shed cornified cells. The dermis is exposed and serum oozes from its surface (moist desquamation). This usually occurs after a latent period (three to four weeks) after start of irradiation. Repopulation occurs from the basal cell layer (now dividing rapidly at 24-hour intervals as a response to radiation injury) of the epidermis within the irradiated area and from the periphery and from epithelial cells of the hair follicles. These islands of new epithelium enlarge and coalesce, covering the denuded area in the following three to four weeks. The new epidermis is thin and pink initially; eventually it thickens, but never attains normal thickness. It is atrophic, smoother than normal, is unable to form pigment (achromic), has little or no hair, and contains few sweat or sebaceous glands. This heavily irradiated skin is fragile and heals poorly after subsequent injury, which may be induced by further irradiation, surgery, heat, cold, or chemicals.

If the radiation dose has been above skin tolerance level, there is no recovery of the basal cell layer, and the moist desquamation never heals. Thus, a primary radiation necrosis is produced. Treatment of this necrosis will be discussed in a later section.

Radiation causes changes in pigmentation of the skin. There is an increase in pigmentation with dry desquamation and loss of pigment with moist desquamation. The hair follicle responds similarly to radiation — temporary epilation follows dry desquamation, and permanent epilation follows moist desquamation. The sweat and sebaceous glands also react in a similar manner — the dry smooth skin following moist desquamation is caused by absence of these glands. In the acute phase the dermis shows capillary congestion, edema, and leukocytic infiltration; these changes are clinically overshadowed by the changes in the epidermis.

There are regional differences in skin sensitivity to radiation. Skin in moist areas (axilla) or around body curvatures (supraclavicular areas) tends to show more severe reactions than flat areas (forehead and cheek).

The treatment of these reactions is supportive. Moist dressings are usually not necessary unless there are large areas of desquamation. Pain is usually not significant. Local antibiotics may be necessary if infection occurs. Combinations of steroids and antibiotics may be useful in minimizing severe reactions (Halnan, 1962). Large occlusive dressings are to be avoided.

These are the early changes following superficial or orthovoltage radiation therapy. They are rarely seen with megavoltage therapy owing to the skin-sparing effect. Following a tumoricidal dose, minimal dry desquamation usually occurs as long as no covering material (i.e., sheets, blankets, surgical dressings) is placed on the patient's skin while he is being irradiated.

Delayed or Chronic Reactions

The thin atrophic skin, which has healed after a moist desquamation, heals poorly after further injury. Healing may be slow, taking many weeks to a few months, and is frequently incomplete, resulting in a secondary necrosis. Medical treatment of this necrosis is difficult. It includes hydrogen peroxide dressings, medication to relieve pain, and antibiotics. Surgical treatment may be necessary and should involve skin grafting to the entire irradiated area, not just to the area of necrosis (Bennett and Carter, 1963).

Chronic reactions in the epidermis are rare with megavoltage radiation since moist desquamation is usually not produced. However, changes in the dermis may be more significant as this area receives the peak dose (100 per cent dose). The late dermal reactions consist of fibrosis, which gives the skin a woody texture, and subendothelial fibrosis of blood vessels. The overlying skin may show minimal reaction, while the subcutaneous tissues show a board-like rigidity. Necrosis is not common. Severe reactions occur after tumoricidal doses in about 5 per cent of patients.

Skin grafting is a common necessity after cancer surgery, and this may present problems in management to both the surgeon and radiotherapist. Irradiation of fresh grafts, up to several months postoperatively, with orthovoltage radiation is hazardous because the graft may slough. With megavoltage irradiation this is rare. Healed grafts (one or more years after surgery) tolerate radiation almost as well as normal skin. Irradiated skin should never be used for skin grafting. Although irradiation of the recipient site, as in preoperative radiation, will produce a decreased incidence of take, successful grafting can still be accomplished.

Oropharynx

The oropharynx is routinely irradiated in the treatment of malignancies arising in this area. Radiation reactions are frequent and may be severe. They are among the most important reactions encountered in clinical radiation therapy. The significant tissues involved are the mucous membrane, submucosal connective tissue, salivary glands, teeth, and mandible. Early acute reactions are frequent; chronic late reactions are infrequent.

Early or Acute Reactions

The stratified squamous epithelium lining the oropharynx is moderately radiosensitive. Reactions similar to skin reactions are produced by cancericidal doses of radiation, but as the mucous membrane is more sensitive than skin, the reactions appear earlier than skin reactions.

The mucous membrane varies in radiation sensitivity in different sites of the oropharynx. The most sensitive site is the soft palate, followed in order of decreasing sensitivity by the buccal mucosa, hypopharynx, vallecula, floor of mouth, gingiva, base of tongue, and dorsum of the tongue. When reactions occur after irradiation, they will occur first in the tumor and then in the most sensitive area of normal mucous membrane.

The earliest reaction noted during a course of fractionated radiation will be erythema, followed soon after by punctate or spotty mucositis, beginning in the second week. These yellow-white areas of ulceration (moist "epithelitis") will coalesce during the third and fourth weeks of radiation, and the mucous membrane will be covered by a confluent yellow diptheroid membrane (radiation mucositis). This membrane sticks to the underlying submucosa and cannot be easily lifted away with a tongue blade. Cure of epidermal carcinoma will not usually occur unless this radiation mucositis is produced. Healing starts earlier than with skin reactions and has frequently begun during the fifth and sixth week of radiation therapy. The mucositis has usually completely healed by the third or fourth week after radiation has been completed. The patient experiences pain on swallowing in the second or third week of therapy. This dysphagia increases in severity by the fourth and fifth week, and the patient may be limited to a liquid diet at this time. Local anesthetic gargles (e.g., Xylocaine Viscus), employed before swallowing, may reduce this discomfort. It is important that sufficient caloric and fluid intake be maintained; with severe reactions nasogastric feeding may be necessary.

When the posterior oropharynx and hypopharynx are irradiated with large fields of radiation, which extend from the palate to pyriform sinus, the reactions are so severe that tumoricidal doses of radiation are not tolerated. In these cases split course radiation therapy is planned (Scanlon, 1965), with 3000 to 3500 rads delivered in three to four weeks. This is followed by a two- to three-week rest period to allow healing of the severe mucositis, after which an additional dose of 3000 to 3500 rads is given. The overall dose of 6000 to 7000 rads in six to nine weeks is the maximum dose that this large volume of normal tissue can tolerate.

The healed mucous membrane is thin and fragile and its vessels are telangiectatic. The submucosal connective tissue shows progressive postradiation fibrosis, which with time contracts to produce shrinkage of the irradiated volume.

The major and minor salivary glands, as well as the small mucous glands, are affected by radiation. Occasionally an acute radiation-induced swelling of the submandibular salivary glands is noted after the first few treatments; this may be quite painful. There is an increase in salivary serum amylase, which subsides without treatment in a few days. As treatment progresses, the saliva becomes scanty and thick as radiation causes a progressive decrease in secretion of saliva, first affecting the serous acini and later the mucous acini. By the time treatment is complete, saliva and solid food will be difficult to swallow, and the patient will use liquids to wash down his food. This reaction is produced by doses of about 4000 rads in four weeks. The thick sticky saliva will persist for many months to years after radiation. Frequently the patient will permanently have a "dry" mouth and will constantly suck on hard candies to increase his saliva. This reaction, though it causes discomfort, is not significant in itself; its role in the pathogenesis of postradiation caries is significant.

Irradiation of the oropharynx invariably modifies the patient's sense of taste, both indirectly through modification of saliva and directly through damage to the taste buds. This is particularly bothersome at the time of acute mucositis when all foods have lost their flavor. During healing there is much recovery in taste sensation but it is rarely complete.

Late or Chronic Reactions

Severe late reactions include postradiation dental caries, osteoradionecrosis of the mandible and, rarely, soft tissue necrosis.

The postradiation scanty, thick, sticky saliva is very ineffective in preventing dental caries. Dental caries occurs rapidly after radiation, affecting teeth that were in good condition before radiation just as frequently as it affects teeth in poor condition (Frank et al., 1965). Characteristically the caries occurs at the gum line, but rampant caries occasionally effects the teeth in all areas. Factors which increase caries formation include:

1. Normally high susceptibility to caries.
2. Gingival recession with exposure of root surface (cementum).
3. Poor oral hygiene, which promotes formation of heavy plaques on all surfaces.
4. Dietary alterations during irradiation, especially to one high in carbohydrates.
5. Painful mucositis, which prevents proper brushing and cleansing of teeth.

As a general rule, all teeth that are in poor condition should be removed before beginning radiation therapy (Fletcher and MacComb, 1962). Removal should be done under antibiotic coverage, with careful smoothing of the mandibular surface with a rongeur and suturing of the mucous membrane. Healing should be allowed to occur before beginning radiation therapy; this is usually complete after a seven- to ten-day period. Opinion is divided as to whether all teeth in good condition should be removed prior to radiation. Perhaps a useful compromise is to remove only those good teeth within the treatment volume. Remaining teeth in good condition outside the treatment volume need not be removed, if the patient is one who will cooperate in caring for his teeth.

Daily fluoride treatments both during and after radiation therapy will reduce the incidence of dental caries. Meticulous oral hygiene is needed to properly care for the remaining teeth. Dental care should be performed on a regular basis, but teeth extraction after radiation therapy should not be performed for at least 18 months to two years. When teeth are extracted, great care must be taken to prevent infection, as this may incite an osteoradionecrosis of the mandible.

A significant proportion of patients irradiated with cancericidal doses will sooner or later develop osteoradionecrosis. This is caused by direct radiation damage to bone in conjunction with xerostomia and infection.

Orthovoltage radiation delivers a higher absorbed dose (rads) to bone than surrounding soft tissue by a factor of about 40 per cent. Megavoltage effectively delivers the same dose to bone and soft tissue; thus, less bone damage is produced by megavoltage radiation. Radiation damage to bone is due to periosteal damage and damage to the bone itself. There is damage to osteoblasts, osteoclasts, and endarteritis of vessels, leading to osteoporosis and eventual osteoradionecrosis. Typical changes include elevation of the periosteum, empty lacunae, and absence of marrow. This damaged bone is poorly able to withstand further injury, and trauma or infection rapidly leads to symptomatic osteoradionecrosis.

Patients who are alcoholics or heavy smokers, or who have poor oral hygiene and poor nutrition have a higher incidence of osteoradionecrosis. Also, irradiation of a mandible that is invaded by tumor (lesions visible on x-ray, not just tumor attached to the surface of the bone) or of a mandible with coexistent infection will almost invariably lead to osteoradionecrosis. This may occur from a few months to a few years after radiation. Local pain and swelling are the initial symptoms, and soon thereafter an area of bone is exposed. X-rays initially may show subperiosteal resorption of bone, but eventually there are areas of dense sclerotic bone with sequestrum formation. Pain is a most constant and distressing symptom. Differential diagnosis of necrosis versus recurrence of tumor may be difficult; severe pain is more frequent with necrosis. Biopsy is indicated, but may transform an incipient necrosis into a frank necrosis. Medical treatment consists of sufficient analgesics, appropriate antibiotics, oral hygiene, peroxide mouthwashes or soaks, and maintenance of adequate nutrition. Healing is a very slow process and may take months or years, with constant extrusion of sequestra of dead bone. Surgical treatment consists of removal of the necrotic portion of bone with wide margins of apparently normal bone (i.e., hemimandibulectomy) (Borsanyi and Blanchard, 1962). The surgical wound should be packed open, and no attempt to repair the resultant defect with a

TABLE 6. *Osteoradionecrosis*

SITE	INCIDENCE	PER CENT
Alveolar ridge	56/184	30
Floor of mouth	102/265	38
Buccal mucosa	56/234	24
Tongue	87/722	12
Tonsil	13/237	5
Lip	22/622	4
Palate	0/15	0
Nasopharynx	4/53	8
TOTAL	340/2332	15

bone graft or prosthetic device should be made, as this frequently results in further breakdown in these irradiated tissues.

The incidence of osteoradionecrosis reported by MacComb (1962), Watson and Scarborough (1938), and Wildermuth and Cantril (1953) is summated in Table 6. Surgical treatment (mandibulectomy) is required in about one third of patients; two thirds heal satisfactorily with medical treatment. Lesions of the floor of the mouth and alveolar ridge have the highest incidence of osteoradionecrosis, as the tumor is more likely to involve bone in these sites; also, radiation therapy (usually radium implants) produces a high dose in the adjacent mandible. With megavoltage external radiation therapy and avoidance of radiation therapy for tumors that involve bone, the overall incidence of necrosis will be 5 to 10 per cent.

Soft tissue necrosis is less frequent than bone necrosis (Fletcher and MacComb, 1962). Characteristically the patient complains of severe pain and dysphagia. On examination an ulceration with a yellowish slough at the base of a crater surrounded by hard edges is found. Treatment is similar to that outlined earlier for bone necrosis except that surgery is not possible for necrosis involving the posterior pharyngeal walls.

In summary, acute reactions are practically universal after irradiation of oropharyngeal neoplasms to cancericidal doses. Late reactions, in particular osteoradionecrosis, occur with significant incidence in the treatment of lesions of the floor of the mouth or alveolar ridge. Smaller doses of radiation should not be given to avoid these reactions as recurrence of the cancer is a more devastating complication.

Larynx

The larynx is irradiated in the treatment of laryngeal and hypopharyngeal malignancies.

The type of radiation reaction seen is quite similar to skin and oropharyngeal reactions. Both the soft tissues of the larynx (epithelium and subepithelial connective tissue) and the cartilage show significant acute and late reactions.

Early or Acute Reactions

The condition of the larynx prior to irradiation significantly determines the acute reaction to irradiation. Irradiation should not begin until the edema following direct laryngoscopy and biopsy or after vocal cord stripping has decreased—a one- to two-week period usually suffices. Gross infection should be treated with appropriate antibiotics before starting radiation therapy, especially in the presence of deeply infiltrating or ulcerating necrotic tumors. If the airway is compromised and significant laryngeal stridor is present, tracheostomy should be performed before radiation is begun. A scheduled tracheostomy performed in the operating room is much to be preferred to an emergency tracheostomy performed at the patient's bedside in the middle of the night. The stoma is included in the field of irradiation.

During the usual course of fractionated radiation therapy to the larynx few changes are noted in the first two weeks. Speckled fibrin deposits (reddish flecks) appear on the true vocal cords in the third week. These occasionally become confluent in the fourth and fifth weeks, forming a false membrane. At the same time erythema appears on the mucosa of the supraglottic portion of the larynx, particularly over the arytenoid cartilage. A mucositis forms, which is at first spotty and then confluent with a false membrane, at about the fourth to fifth week. This is most marked on the mucosa of the piriform sinuses, the aryepiglottic folds, and the interarytenoid region. Submucosal edema becomes a prominent feature at this time.

The patient experiences increasing hoarseness beginning in the third week and peaking in the fifth and sixth weeks of irradiation. If the hypopharynx is also in the volume of irradiation, dysphagia occurs. The patient is instructed to avoid irritation of his larynx by cessation of smoking and talking; oral local anesthetics (e.g., Xylocaine Viscus) may be given for dysphagia. This acute reaction usually begins to subside during the week after radiation is completed and takes an additional three to four weeks to subside completely. The voice may take longer to recover, and some hoarseness is present for one to three months postirradiation.

Occasionally there is a sudden increase in dyspnea. On examination marked edema is noted. Treatment with high doses of steroids (e.g., 40 to 60 mg. prednisone) for a few days will decrease this edema. These acute soft tissue reactions are more severe with orthovoltage than with megavoltage radiation.

Late or Chronic Reactions

There are two types of significant late reactions—laryngeal ulceration and edema and cartilage necrosis. These reactions are more severe in patients who develop severe acute reactions and in patients treated to a high dose of radiation in a large volume. Cartilage necrosis is almost certain to follow radiation with cancericidal doses if the cartilages are invaded by tumor or are infected before radiation therapy. If partial laryngectomy has proved inadequate for carcinoma, further treatment by total laryngectomy is preferred, since radiation therapy will frequently be followed by cartilage necrosis. Postradiation recurrences should be treated surgically, not by radiation for similar reasons.

Late reactions occur from a few months to a few years following radiation, the majority occurring within six months. The more severe reactions occur earlier. The patient notices increased hoarseness and pain. There is tenderness to palpation of the laryngeal cartilages. On examination the endolaryngeal structures are edematous, particularly the arytenoid areas. Ulceration may be present, and the differential diagnosis of necrosis versus recurrent carcinoma may be difficult to make. Local pain is more frequently present with necrosis than recurrent tumor. An immediate biopsy of the ulceration should be made, but that is frequently nonrepresentative of recurrence of cancer deep in the tissues. If no cancer is found on initial biopsy, then the patient is treated with antibiotics, a high protein-high caloric diet, and observed for one month. If there is no significant improvement, total laryngectomy is performed (Moss and Brand, 1969). With persistent edema and cartilage necrosis the voice is poor and the incidence of aspiration pneumonia is high; there is also significant local pain so that laryngectomy is the preferred treatment even in the absence of recurrent tumor. Frequently there is both recurrent tumor and necrosis.

The incidence of these severe complications is high after orthovoltage therapy of advanced lesions (stages III and IV); about 60 per cent of patients develop some form of cartilage necrosis. Fletcher and Klein (1964) reported an incidence with early lesions (stages I and II) of 12 per cent (5 out of 41 patients) with orthovoltage and an incidence of 6 per cent (11 out of 174 patients) treated with ^{60}Cobalt irradiation.

Central Nervous System

The central nervous system is infrequently involved by tumors of the head and neck area. Exceptions are primary malignancies of the nasopharynx, paranasal sinuses, and middle ear. Irradiation is usually incidental to treatment of large posterior cervical nodes or hypopharyngeal neoplasms when the cervical spinal cord is included in the treatment volume. Radiation tolerance of the central nervous system frequently limits the tumor dose that can be given to the adjacent neoplasm.

The adult brain, brain stem, and spinal cord are relatively radioresistant; damage to nerve tissue is slow in making its appearance, but once damage has occurred, patients recover slowly and incompletely. We recognize three phases of reaction—an acute phase of meningoencephalitis, a period of apparent normalcy, and a late reaction of vascular necrosis and nerve cell damage.

The acute reaction is caused by radiation doses far in excess of those used clinically (above 3000 rads in a single dose). There are no acute reactions within the normal clinical range of dose.

Chronic or late reactions occur for variable lengths of time after radiation therapy. Two syndromes are recognized:

Early Transient Myelopathy

Within two to four months after completion of radiation therapy the patient develops sensory defects, frequently complaining of "electric shocks" radiating down the back and into the extremities after neck flexion (Lhermitte's sign). This may reflect radiation-induced demyelinization due to damage to oligodendroglia. Recovery of these cells leads to increased myelin synthesis and repair of the damage. This syndrome is usually transient and spontaneous recovery occurs within the next one to two months without treatment. Rarely, late progressive irreversible injury follows.

Late Irreversible Injury

This syndrome occurs later than the transient myelopathy, beginning about 11 to 20 months after radiation. Initial symptoms depend on the area of central nervous system treated. If it is due to a cervical cord lesion, there may be sensory disturbances, such as paresthesia, and a high sensory level along with hyperactive reflexes, ankle clonus, and a positive Babinski reflex. Spinal tap, x-rays of the vertebral bodies, and myelograms are normal, thus ruling out metastatic carcinoma. High doses of steroids (e.g., prednisone, 40 mg. four times a day) may produce transient improvement, but usually there is slow steady progression to a Brown-Séquard syndrome or transverse myelopathy (with paraplegia or quadraplegia) over the next six to 12 months. The pathogenesis is a combination of vascular injury (endarteritis leading to necrosis) and irreversible nerve cell damage.

There is no treatment for the progressive irreversible injury. This is catastrophic, since it usually occurs in patients who have been cured of their neoplasm. Every effort must be made to avoid this reaction. Tolerance of the central nervous system varies with dose, time, and volume. Doses of 4000 rads in four weeks to a 20 cm. length of spinal cord, 4500 rads to a 10 cm. length, and 5000 rads to a 5 cm. length are tolerated and rarely lead to progressive irreversible injury. However, early transient myelopathy may be seen at this dose level. It is our practice to limit the dose to the cervical spinal cord to 4000 rads in four weeks (Maier et al., 1969). At this level we have encountered no progressive irreversible injuries. Portions of the brain may be treated to higher doses, as in the treatment of neoplasms of the nasopharynx, paranasal sinuses, or middle ear.

REFERENCES

Andrews, J. R.: A concept of radiosensitivity. Amer. J. Roentgenol., 87:601–605, 1962.

Badib, A. O., and Webster, J. H.: Changes in tumor oxygen tension during radiation therapy. Acta Radiol. Ther., 8:247–257, 1959.

Batley, F.: Fallacies of preoperative radiation. Arch. Otolaryngol., 87:30–34, 1968.

Bennett, J., and Carter, D.: Extensive necrosis after radiation for cancer. Arch. Surg., 86:203–210, 1963.

Bergonie, J. and Tribondeau, L.: Interprétation de quelques résultats de la radiothérapie et assai de fixation d'une technique rationale. C. R. Acad. Sci., 143:983–985, 1906.

Borsanyi, S. J., and Blanchard, C. L.: Ionizing radiation and the ear. J.A.M.A., 181:958–961, 1962.

Delarue, N., et al: Circulating "cancer cells." Arch. Surg., 89:392, 1964.

Ditchek, T., and Lampe, I.: Radical surgery after intensive high-energy irradiation. Arch. Surg., 86:534–539, 1963.

Elkind, M. M., and Sutton, H.: Radiation response of

mammalian cells grown in culture. Radiat. Res., 13:556–563, 1960.

Ellis, F. T.: Dose, time and fractionation: A clinical hypothesis. Clin. Radiol., 20:1–7, 1969.

Fletcher, G., and Klein, R.: Dose-time-volume relationships in squamous cell carcinoma of the larynx. Radiology, 82:1032–1042, 1964.

Fletcher, G., and MacComb, W.: Radiation Therapy in the Management of Cancer of the Oral Cavity and Oropharynx. Springfield, Ill., Charles C Thomas, 1962.

Frank, R. M., Herdley, J., and Phillips, E.: Acquired dental defects and salivary gland lesions after irradiation for carcinoma. J. Amer. Dent. Ass., 70:868–883, 1965.

Gray, L. H.: Oxygenation in radiotherapy: Radiological considerations. Brit. J. Radiol., 30:403, 1957.

Halnan, K. E.: The effect of corticosteroids on the radiation skin reaction. Brit. J. Radiol., 35:403–408, 1962.

MacComb, W.: Necrosis in treatment of intraoral cancer by radiation therapy. Amer. J. Roentgenol., 87:431, 1962.

MacComb, W., and Fletcher, G.: Cancer of the Head and Neck. Baltimore, The Williams & Wilkins Co., 1967.

Maier, J., Perry, R., Saylor, W., and Salak, M.: Radiation myelitis of the dorsolumbar spinal cord. Radiology, 93:153–160, 1969.

Meredith, W. J.: Radium Dosage. London, E. and S. Livingstone, Ltd., 1958.

Merriman, G. R., Jr., and Focht, E. F.: A clinical study of radiation cataracts and the relationship to dose. Amer. J. Roentgenol., 77:759, 1957.

Morgan, R. L.: Fast Neutron Therapy—Clinical Application. In Modern Trends in Radiotherapy, I (Deeley, T. and Wood, C., eds.). New York, Appleton-Century-Crofts, 1967.

Moss, W. T., and Brand, W. N.: Therapeutic Radiology. St. Louis, Mo., The C. V. Mosby Co., 1969.

Nickson, J., and Glicksman, A.: Preoperative radiotherapy in cancer. J.A.M.A., 195:138–142, 1966.

Patterson, R.: On the treatment of malignant disease by radiotherapy. London, Edward Arnold, Ltd., 1963.

Perez, C., Mill, W., Ogura, S., and Powers, W.: Carcinoma of the tonsil: Sequential comparison of four treatment modalities. Radiol., 94:649, 1970.

Powers, W., and Palmer, L. A.: Biological basis of preoperative radiation treatment. Amer. J. Roentgenol., 102:176–192, 1968.

Puck, T. T., and Marcus, P. I.: Action of x-rays on mammalian cells. J. Exp. Med., 103:653–666, 1956.

Rubin, P., and Casarett, G.: Clinical Radiation Pathology. Philadelphia, W. B. Saunders Company, 1968.

Scanlon, P.: Radiotherapeutic problems best handled with split-dose therapy. Amer. J. Roentgenol., 93:639–650, 1965.

Strandquist, M.: Studien unter die Kumulative Wirkung der Röntgenstrahlen der Fraktionierung. Acta Radiol. (suppl.), 55:1–300, 1944.

Thomlinson, R. H., and Gray, L. H.: Histological structure of some human lung cancers and possible implication for radiotherapy. Brit. J. Cancer, 9:539, 1955.

Watson, W. L., and Scarborough, J. E.: Osteoradionecrosis in intraoral cancer. Amer. J. Roentgenol., 40:524, 1938.

Wildermuth, O., and Cantril, S. T.: Radiation necrosis of the mandible. Radiology, 61:771–784, 1953.

INDEX

Numbers in *italics* indicate illustrations.

1159